Donglu Shi

NanoScience in Biomedicine

Donglu Shi

NanoScience in Biomedicine

With 292 figures

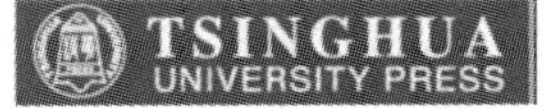

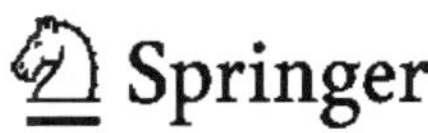

EDITOR:

Donglu Shi

Department of Chemical and Materials Engineering,
College of Engineering, University of Cincinnati,
Cincinnati, OH 45221, USA

The Institute for Advanced Materials and Nano Biomedicine,
Tongji University, Shanghai 200092, China

Research Institute of Micro/Nano Science and Technology,
Shanghai Jiao Tong University, Shanghai 200240, China

ISBN 978-7-302-17905-4 **Tsinghua University Press, Beijing**
ISBN 978-3-540-49660-1 **Springer Berlin Heidelberg New York**
e ISBN 978-3-540-49661-8 **Springer Berlin Heidelberg New York**

Library of Congress Control Number: pending

Co-published by Tsinghua University Press, Beijing and Springer-Verlag GmbH Berlin Heidelberg

Springer is a part of Springer Science+Business Media
springer.com

Cover design: Frido Steinen-Broo, EStudio Calamar, Spain
Printed on acid-free paper

Preface

The research on nanomaterials and nano biomedicine has been advancing rapidly in recent years, particularly in the development of unique nanostructures for specific biomedical applications. The research addresses the critical issues in medical applications including in vivo imaging, cell targeting, local drug delivery and treatment, bioactivity, compatibility, and toxicity. In the biomedical applications, traditional materials science and engineering have to deal with new challenges in the areas of synthesis, structure development, and biological, chemical, and physical behaviors, since medical needs place new demands in these respects.

The novel nanotechnologies included in this book are of great importance for biomedical applications. Based on these new developments, it is possible to alter the intrinsic properties of nanomaterials that cannot be achieved by conventional methods and materials. A key aspect of being able to manipulate the properties of the nanomaterials is the nanoscale architecture and engineering by various processing techniques. Some of the novel approaches introduced in this book can provide multi-functionality for a variety of substrates, be it biological, physical, or chemical, which can then be engineered for particular biomedical applications. For instance, novel surface functionalization methods have been developed for bio assays and cell targeting. In these approaches, a thin coating of polymer can be applied to the nano species and to provide various functional groups for passive or covalent coupling to biological molecules, such as antigens, antibodies, and DNA/RNA hybridization. However, the conventional synthesis of materials has only resulted in a single functionality which is generally not suitable for the complex procedures required for medical applications. The novel concept introduced in this book can be used to develop multiple functionalities, particularly suitable for medical diagnosis and treatment. The enhancement of properties is based on the study of the new nano structures and interfacial mechanisms.

This book summarizes the most recent research and development in nano biomedicine and addresses the critical issues in nanomaterials synthesis, structure, and properties. In particular, the major topics in nano biomedicine are covered in this book. The book devotes three parts of 25 chapters to various aspects of nanomaterials and their medical applications. Detailed experimental procedures are presented at a level suitable for readers with no previous training in these areas.

The first part of the book concentrates on the research works of design, synthesis, properties, and applications of nano scale biomaterials. Chapter 1 is on the topics of stem cells and related nanotechnology. In Chapter 2, an overview is documented on the recent progress of polymer nanofibers, mostly electrospun in biomedical applications, along with a brief description of history, principle, and operating parameters of electrospinning process. Chapter 3 introduces new concepts in assembly of biomaterials. In view of the emerging importance of bio-inspired materials in medical applications, this chapter is focused on describing the fundamentals of intermolecular interactions and their applications in biomaterials science. The particular focus will be on processes and structures that mimic the natural ECM. Chapter 4 is on the fabrication and assembly of nanomaterials for biological detections. In Chapter 5, the authors first introduce the peptide design strategies for the construction of nanostructured materials. It then gives a brief tutorial of amino acid structure and function. It further describes higher-order assemblies of peptides and peptidomimetics. Chapter 6 introduces an important category of nanomaterials: quantum dots. Chapter 7 focuses on the phosphate ceramics for applications in bio-related fields. In this chapter, the authors briefly review the progress made in the last decade on the microwave-assisted synthesis and processing of biomaterials both in nanometer- and micrometer-size range. Chapter 8 introduces the characterization of biointerfaces and biosurfaces in biomaterials design. In Chapter 9, the authors bring the focus of the discussion to one of the important nanomaterials: carbon nanotubes and their applications in biosensing. Chpater 10 discusses the issues on heparin-conjugated nanointerfaces for biomedical applications.

The second part of the book is on the new nanotechnologies in biomedicine. In Chapter 11, the authors introduce some of the novel technologies in drug delivery. Chapter 12 reports unique experimental results on nano metal particles for biomedical applications. Chapter 13 is on the micro- and nanoscale technologies in high-throughput biomedical experimentation. Chapter 14 introduces delivery system of bioactive molecules for regenerative medicine. Chapter 15 gives an overview on modification of nano-sized materials for drug delivery. Chapter 16 is another chapter on drug delivery, however via a different approach. Chapter 17 is about most recent developments in DNA nanotechnology. A major objective in this chapter deals with the creation of ordered nanostructures for executing complex operations. Chapter 18 provides an overview on the nanoscale bioactive surfaces and endosseous implantology. Chapter 19 gives an overview of potential applications of carbon nanotube smart materials in biology and medicine.

The last part of the book concentrates on some of the most recent experimental results on the nanomaterials synthesis and structure developments. These include the synthesis, properties, and application of intrinsically electroconducting nanoparticles of polypyrrole and pyrrole/sulfonic diphenylamine (20/80) Copolymers. Some studies focuse on the fracture processes in advanced nanocrystalline and nanocomposite materials. Unique nano properties such as field emission of carbon nanotubes are also introduced. Finally, the book concludes by introducing some theoretical aspects of the nanomaterials. In this chapter, the authors develop microscopic modeling of phonon modes in semiconductor nanocrystals.

Chapter 20 is on the physical origins of phonon behaviors in nanocrystals. Chapter 21 gives an overview on computer simulations and theoretical modeling of fracture processes in nanocrystalline metals and ceramic nanocomposites. Chapter 22 describes a detailed experimental study on the fabrication, structures, unique properties, and wide application potential of novel conducting polypyrrole (PPY) nanoparticles and nanocomposites. Chapter 23 introduces some of the most recent developments in the fascinating carbon nanotubes. Chapter 24 reviews the progress in the flexible dye-sensitized nanostructured thin film solar cells (DSSCs). Chapter 25 presents recent results on the synthesis of magnetic nanoparticles (MNP) and various types of magnetic nanofluids (MNF) or ferrofluids, their structural properties and behaviors in an external magnetic field.

We hope that these chapters will provide timely and useful information for the progress of nanomaterials and their applications in biomedicine.

Contents

1 Stem Cells and Nanostructured Materials

Vince Beachley[1] and Xuejun Wen[1,2,3]

[1] Department of Bioengineering, Clemson University, Charleston, SC 29425, USA
[2] Department of Cell Biology and Anatomy, Medical University of South Carolina, Charleston, SC 29425, USA
[3] Department of Orthopedic Surgery, Medical University of South Carolina, Charleston, SC 29425, USA

Abstract Stem cells and nanomaterials are currently two of the most promising technologies for tissue regeneration and the treatment of degenerative disease. Because of their ability to self-renew and differentiate into any cell type, stem cells offer the potential to regrow all types of damaged or degenerated tissues that are unrepairable by currently available treatment methods. Nanomaterials may prove to be ideal growth substrates for tissue regeneration as well as an ideal delivery vehicle for the diagnostic markers, growth factors, and drugs that are required to promote tissue regeneration and treat degenerative disease. Despite their great potential, stem cell behaviors such as proliferation and differentiation must be tightly regulated in order for this technology to be practical in a clinical setting. Experimental evidence has shown that the interactions of nanomaterials with stem cells can have a significant effect on many types of stem cell behaviors. In addition, nanomaterials can be used to provide targeted delivery of various agents in a controlled manner that allows for regulation of the chemical environment. Regulation of the chemical environment is critical for controlled guidance of stem cell behavior and for the treatment of degenerative disease. A precise understanding of the interactions between stem cells and nanomaterials is an important step toward unlocking the great potential of these two technologies.

Keywords nano, stem cell

1.1 Introduction

Stem cells and nanotechnology, two exciting and rapidly growing fields, have received extensive attention during the last decades. Stem cells and precursors

(1) Corresponding e-mail: xjwen@clemson.edu

bring new hope to regenerate functional tissue with native histological structures and properties, as opposed to simple replacement with artificial structures alone. The two main advantages of stem cells are the ability to self-renew, which means they can reproduce themselves, and the ability to potentially differentiate into all the possible cell types (Pedersen, 1999; Solter and Gearhart, 1999). Stem cells may be harvested from two different sources. Embryonic stem (ES) cells may be harvested from embryos and can be derived from germ cells as well. If problems such as immune rejection and the high possibility of tumorgenicity can be solved, ES cells may serve as a good source of cells for tissue regeneration. Their potential for the study of human developmental biology is always promising (Good, 1998). Stem cells can also be harvested from adult tissue, such as from muscle, cartilage, bone, nervous system, liver, pancreas, tooth, adipose tissue, etc. (Good, 1998). Like stem cells, precursor cells can differentiate into more than one cell type, but these cells have undergone some degree of differentiation (Weissman, 2000). For example, glial-restricted precursors (GRP) can differentiate into type Ⅰ and type Ⅱ astrocytes and oligodendrocytes, but not neurons (Foster and Stringer, 1999). Precursor cells can be harvested from adult tissue as well (Rizzoli and Carlo-Stella, 1997). Knowledge of stem cells can also bring profound insight to cancer research due to the fact that many cancer cells possess the characteristics of stem/progenitor cells and many cancer cells originated from stem cells. It is known that two key chemical signals, Hedgehog and Wnt, are active in the stem cells that repair damaged tissue. These signals also have been found in certain hard to treat cancers, supporting an old idea that some cancers may start from normal stem cells that have somehow gone bad. Therefore, a section about cancer treatment using nanostructured biomaterials is included in this chapter as well.

Nanostructured materials refer to certain materials with delicate structures of 'small' sizes, falling in the 1 – 100 nm range, and specific properties and functions related to the 'size effect' (Niemeyer, 2001; Safarik and Safarikova, 2002; Whitesides, 2003). Dramatic development of nanotechnology in material science and engineering has taken place in the last decade (Gao et al., 2004; Niemeyer, 2001; Whitesides, 2003). This does not come as a surprise considering that nanostructured materials have the capability to be adapted and integrated into biomedical devices, since most biological systems, including viruses and membrane and protein complex, are natural nanostructures (Laval et al., 1999). Currently, medicine and biomedical engineering are among the most promising and challenging fields involved in the application of nanostructured materials (Desai, 2000; Ziener et al., 2005). Rapid advancements of nanostructured materials have been made in a wide variety of biomedical applications, including novel tissue engineered scaffolds and devices, site-specific drug delivery systems, non-viral gene carriers, biosensor and screening systems, and clinical bio-analytical diagnostics and therapeutics (Mazzola, 2003; Ziener et al., 2005). For example, nanocomposites have been used to stabilize and regenerate bone matrices (Bradt et al., 1999; Du et al., 1998; Kikuchi et al., 2004; Kikuchi et al., 2004); biosensing with nanotubes and nanowires has demonstrated unprecedented sensitivity for biomolecule detection (Alivisatos, 2004; Drummond et al., 2003; Penn et al., 2003); and nanoscale assemblies and particles have been used to deliver high concentrations of therapeutic drugs and/or biomolecules, possessing high bioaffinity to specific host sites for precise drug administration (Moghimi and Szebeni, 2003; Muller et al., 2001; Takeuchi et al., 2001).

The combinational use of stem cells and nanostructured materials may help us to understand many scientific questions and also may bring many practical applications that promote the use of either or both components in biomedical research and clinical applications. In this chapter, the interactions between stem cells and nanostructured materials are discussed. In order to better present the contents, nanostructured materials are classified into two categories, one is nanotopographic substrate, which includes nanofibers and surface nano-textures, and the other is nanoparticles.

1.2 Interaction of Stem Cells with Nanotopographic Substrates

Cells in their natural in vivo surroundings are exposed to a complex chemical and structural environment. The natural extracellular matrix (ECM) is made up of structural components that are of nanoscale dimensions. Major fibrous extracellular molecules are in the nano-scale range, fibers such as collagen fibers, elastin fibers, keratin fibers, etc. are nanofibers. Mimicking the natural environment when culturing cells in vitro is highly important because cell behavior is determined by both genetic make up and the surrounding environmental cues. Cellular behaviors such as proliferation, differentiation, morphology, and migration are commonly controlled in culture by modulation of the chemical environment, cells also respond to different morphological cues that can be determined by the growth substrate in vitro and in vivo. Four components may be involved in the growth, differentiation, and morphology of cells on biomaterial surfaces: (1) adsorption of serum components, (2) extracellular matrix components secreted by the cell, (3) cell adhesion molecules, and (4) cytoskeleton mechanics (Matsuzaka et al., 1999). It has been shown that the structural substrate property of surface roughness can cause selective protein absorption, and that higher surface roughness increases total protein absorption (Deligianni et al., 2001). Increased protein adsorption could be attributed to an increase in surface area for rough surfaces and thus could be important in relation to nanotopographical materials because these exhibit extremely high surface areas. In relation to nanostructure and stem cell interactions, the cytoskeleton mechanics component is of importance because cells cultured on substrates with nanoscale features can take on different shapes in response to the specific features that are encountered. It is very apparent that nanotopography effects cellular behavior through the regulation of morphology, but it is likely that there are unknown effects associated with nanotopographies as well. Cells can react to objects as small as 5 nm (Curtis, 2001) and it is possible that nanostructures, especially those of similar dimensions to the natural ECM, can influence cell behavior through mechanisms other than determination of cell morphology, cytoskeletal mechanics, and protein absorption. It has been shown that stem cell behavior can be highly dependent on the substrate that they are cultured on and the understanding of stem cell interactions with nanosurfaces could provide valuable information about stem cells that could be utilized for desirable in vivo applications.

1.2.1 Cell Shape and the Cytoskeleton

While much is known about how various growth factors can regulate differentiation, the significance of cell density on cell differentiation is not well understood. It has been hypothesized that the differences in cell density cause differences in cell shape that in turn may act as differentiation cues (McBeath et al., 2004). The effect of cell shape on the differentiation of stem cells has been investigated. Spegelman and Ginty (1983) found that differentiation of an adipogenic cell line could be inhibited when it was allowed to attach and spread on fibronectin coated surfaces. The inhibitory effect on cell differentiation was reversed by keeping the cells rounded and by disrupting the actin cytoskeleton. On the contrary, cell spreading has been shown to cause an increase in osteoblast differentiation by osteoblastic progenitor cells as measured by increased osteocalcin expression (Thomas et al., 2002). It has been shown that regulation of cell shape can influence the differentiation of multipotent human mesenchymal stem cells (hMSCs) into adiogenic or osteoblastic fate (McBeath et al., 2004). hMSCs allowed to flatten and spread expressed osteoblastic markers, such as alkaline phosphatase, while constrained cells that remained unspread and rounded expressed adiogenic lipid production. In addition, more alkaline phosphatase activity was found at low hMSC plating density and more lipid staining was observed at high cell plating density. One proposed mechanism for the transduction of cell shape information into gene expression is by the transmission of mechanic forces directly from the myosin actin cytoskeleton to the nucleus (Maniotis et al., 1997). While cytoskeletal organization is related to cell shape, the cytoskeleton can influence gene expression independently of cell shape. In the study above, the inhibition of myosin-generated cytoskeletal tension in hMSCs caused decreased alkaline phosphatase activity and increased lipid production without changing cell shape (McBeath et al., 2004).

Stem cells have been cultured on a variety of nanotopographies including nanofibers, nanoparticle films, and etched nanosurfaces. Stem cells are highly responsive to nanotopagraphies for morphology, attachment, proliferation, and differentiation. Stem cells cultured on nanofibrous scaffolds can introduce two mechanical cues to cultured cells when compared to traditional culture methods. Nanofiber scaffolds present cells with a nanoscaled fibular microstructure and in many cases a three-dimensional 3-D growth environment. It is important to take both of these variables into consideration when analyzing the results from these studies. Because of differences in dimensionality, nanosurface interactions and nanofiber interactions will be described in separate sections.

1.2.2 Morphology, Attachment and Proliferation

1.2.2.1 Nanosurfaces

Several investigations have observed the effects that surface nanotopography can have on the attachment, spreading, and orientation of cultured stem cells. Nanoparticle films made by layer-by-layer assembly can be used to create nanotopographies of increasing surface roughness. Mouse mesenchymal stem cells (mMSCs) seeded on TiO_2 films of increasing particle desposition and surface roughness attached and spread better on the rough surfaces (Kommireddy et al., 2006).

Photolithographic techniques have been used to create nanotopographies of pits, bumps and grooves on polymer surfaces. Rat bone marrow mesenchymal stem cells (rBMCs) cultured on grooved surfaces with an applied groove depth of 0.5, 1.0 or 1.5 μm and a groove width of 1, 2, 5 or 10 μm induced alignment of the cells, matrix, actin filaments, and focal adhesion points to the surface grooves (Matsuzaka et al., 2000, et al., 1999). hMSCs were also cultured on wide grooves of 50 μm width and 327 nm depth and narrow grooves of 5 μm width and 510 nm depth (Dalby et al., 2006). In this case, cells cultured on narrow grooves developed stress fibers that were highly aligned in the direction of the grooves, while cells cultured on wider grooves only approximately aligned to the axis of the grooves. This would be expected, as grooves of 50 μm width are larger than the diameter of a cell. Bone marrow stem cell derived osteoblast-like cells cultured on 150 nm wide 60 nm deep grooves also directed cell orientation and actin fiber alignment with features of a much smaller scale(Zhu et al., 2005). hMSCs have also been cultured on pits of 30 μm and 40 μm widths and 310 nm and 362 nm depths respectfully and on bumps 10 – 45 nm in height(Dalby et al., 2006a, 2006b). For all sizes of pits and bumps significant increases in cell area and defined cytoskeletal fibers were observed.

Conflicting results on nanosurface effect on proliferation have been observed. Proliferation was enhanced for TiO_2 nanoparticle surface and 150 nm wide 60 nm deep grooved surfaces versus smooth surfaces (Kommireddy et al., 2006; Zhu et al., 2005). In contrast, in another study using 1 – 10 μm wide, 0.5 – 1.5 μm deep grooves, the differences in cell proliferation were not significant (Matsuzaka et al., 2000).

1.2.2.2 Nanofibers

Nanofiber meshes seeded with different types of stem cells have demonstrated the ability to promote cell adhesion, directional guidance and morphological changes. Osteoprogenitor cells cultured on electrospun polymer fiber meshes with diameters ranging from 140 nm to 2100 nm responded to fibrous nanotopography and osteogenic growth factors (Badami et al., 2006). Cells on fibers had a smaller projected area than cells on smooth surfaces, but cells on 2100 nm fibers had a higher aspect ratio. Proliferation was also effected by the fibrous nanotopography. Cells cultured on fibers exhibited a lower cell density than those on smooth surfaces in the absence of osteogenic factors, but when osteogenic factors were added the cell density of fiber surfaces was equal to or greater than that on smooth surfaces. In both cases cell density increased with fiber diameter. In contrast, osteoblast cells grown on carbon nanotubes of various diameters proliferated at much higher rates on smaller fibers with three times as many cells on 60 nm fibers than 125 nm fibers after 7 days in culture (Elias et al., 2002). Mouse (ES) cells cultured in a nanofibrullar network also greatly enhanced proliferation in comparison with the growth of tissue on culture surfaces without nanofibers (Nur et al., 2006). Another investigation observed hematopoietic stem cell proliferation to increase at a similar rate for both polymer films and nanofiber polymer meshes (Chua et al., 2006). Cell adhesion properties of nanofibers were also tested on hematopoietic stem cells grown on polymer nanofiber meshes and polymer films. After ten days of expansion culture, cells were gently washed three times and approximately 40% of total cells on nanofiber meshes were adherent as opposed to 25% of total cells on film substrates.

Similar to linear oriented etched surfaces, aligned nanofibers are able to promote directional guidance in stem cell culture. Neuronal stem cells seeded on random and aligned 300 nm and 1.5 μm nanofibers attached well and changed their shape from rounded to elongated and spindle-like for all fiber scaffolds. In addition, cells turned through large angles in order to grow parallel to the fiber alignment independent of fiber diameter (Yang et al., 2005).

1.2.3 Differentiation

1.2.3.1 Nanosurfaces

Nanotopography has been shown to have an effect on differentiation as measured by increased osteogenic gene expression in bone marrow cells. Rat bone marrow cells cultured on grooved polymer surfaces 500 – 1500 nm deep had greater alkaline phosphatase activity than cells cultured on smooth surfaces (Matsuzaka et al., 1999). The osteoblastic markers osteocalcin and osteopontin were expressed by human bone marrow stem cells (hBMCs) that were cultured on bumps 10 – 45 nm in height, while the same cells cultured on smooth surfaces displayed negligible positive staining (Dalby et al., 2006a). Increases in osteocalcin and osteopontin versus negligible staining in controls were also observed for hBMCs cultured on nanoscale pits 40 μm in width and 310 nm in depth (Dalby et al., 2006b).

1.2.3.2 Nanofibers

Different types of stem cells have been observed to differentiate in a variety of nanofiber scaffolds. hMSCs were induced to differentiate into adipogenic, chondrogenic, and osteogenic lineages in electrospun nanofibrous polymer scaffolds when cultured in specific differentiation media (Li et al., 2005). Neuronal stem cells were able to differentiate into neurons with sprouting neurites in a nanofibrous polymer scaffold made by liquid-liquid phase separation (Yang et al., 2004). Mouse embryonic fibroblasts cultured in 3-D peptide scaffolds were observed to undergo strong osteogenic differentiation after osteogenic induction while cells cultured in 2-D conditions did not differentiate (Garreta et al., 2006). Furthermore, mouse embryonic fibroblasts cultured in 3-D systems without osteogenic induction still maintained an adult stem cell-like phenotype and expressed the early stage markers of osteoblast differentiation.

Beyond having the capability to support stem cell differentiation, nanofibrous topography has been shown to selectively influence differentiation based on fiber diameter. Differentiation of neural stem cells cultured on aligned and random nanofiber meshes with fiber diameters of 300 nm and 1500 nm were observed to be highly dependent on fiber diameter (Yang et al., 2005). When the neural differentiation was evaluated on the basis of shape change it was found that the quantitative differentiation rates were ~80% and ~40% for 300 nm and 1500 nm, respectively. Fiber size dependent differentiation results were consistent for both randomly oriented and aligned nanofibers.

The ability of nanofibrous scaffolds in preventing differentiation has also been explored. Hematopoietic stem cells cultured in polymer nanofiber meshes for 10 days showed a slightly higher percentage of $CD34^+$ $CD45^+$ cells when compared to polymer film (Chua et al., 2006). Nanofiber meshes also mediated a lower monoblastic phenotype and greater number on primitive progenitor cells compared to films. Mouse ES cells also proliferated in 3-D polymer nanofiber meshes while maintaining their pluri-potency (Nur et al., 2006). While proliferation with self-renewal was allowed to continue in nanofiber topography, cells were observed to maintain their ability to differentiate when exposed to differentiation factors. In a separate study, a small fraction of mouse ES cells isolated during embryoid body development or after osteogenic induction appeared to develop into small ES cell-like colonies (Garreta et al., 2006). It was also found that the frequency of these colonies was remarkably higher in 3-D peptide nanofiber cultures than in 2-D culture, suggesting that 3-D microenvironment promoted the generation of a stem cell-like niche that allows undifferentiated stem cell maintenance.

1.2.4 Self-Assembling Peptide Nanofibers

The self-assembling peptide method used to create nanofibrous scaffolds for in vitro culture can be utilized for in vivo tissue engineering as well. When these peptides are injected into the body, the interaction with the physiological environment induces peptide nanofiber assembly. Peptide solution injected into the myocardium was able to assemble a 3-D nanofiber mesh and did not induce a major inflammatory response (Davis et al., 2005). This 3-D microenvironment recruited endothelial progenitor cells, smooth muscle cells, and myocyte progentitor cells and promoted vascularization. Implantation of matrigel as control resulted in few numbers of endothelial cells and no myocyte progenitors. In addition, the injection of neonatal myocytes with the peptide solution into the microenvironment increased the density of endogenous cardiac progenitors recruited and injected ES cells were able to differentiate into cardiac myocytes in the nanofiber microenvironment. Self-assembling nanofiber peptide networks have also been used as drug delivery vehicles. Improved differentiation of neural progenitor cells was observed when they were cultured in peptide nanofibers incorporated with isolucine-lysine-valine-alanine-valine (IKVAV) epitope found in laminin (Silva et al., 2004).. Nanofiber scaffolds incorporating the IKVAV epitope promoted rapid and selective differentiation of NSCs into neurons, with about 35% of cells differentiating after only 1 day. Neural stem cells cultured on 2-D laminin coated surfaces differentiated at a much lower percentage that did not exceed 15% even after 7 days. It was shown that the increase in differentiation was not due to 3-dimensionality when NSCs cultured in non-bioactive nanofiber meshes with soluble IKVAV did not promote differentiation, and was further shown when a 2-D substrate coated with IKVAV incorporated fibers promoted differentiation at the same level as 3-D IKVAV nanofiber meshes. The hypothesis for the success of this approach was that IKVAV nanofiber meshes could amplify the density of epitope presentation to the cells by a factor of 10^3 when compared to a laminin monolayer.

1.2.5 Summary

The results of nanofiber cell culture in relation to oriented cell guidance and improved attachment agree well with results from nanosurface culture; however, cell area was increased versus control for nanosurfaces and decreased on nanofibers. This could result from differences in the structure or dimensions, but it could also be a result of the three dimensionality of the nanofiber structure. Results for cell proliferation vary between similar studies for nanofiber scaffolds and for nanosurfaces. This discrepancy could be due to the differences in cell types and structures used in the individual studies, but it is certainly an indication that there may not be a direct relationship between topography and proliferation or that this relationship can be outweighed by other factors.

Nanofibrous topography has been shown to have a very strong effect on the differentiation of stem cells. Stem cells have been able to readily differentiate in nanofiber meshes and in some case the nanofiber mesh itself has been a requirement for differentiation. The influence of nanofibrous structures on stem cells differentiation lies in both its structural properties, such as fiber diameter, and its three dimensionality. It is important to note that there is evidence that dimensionality plays a role in maintaining stemness in proliferating ES cells and that nanofibrous structures could be the bioengineering tool used to exploit this role. It has been demonstrated that cells cultured on nanofiberous 3-D meshes experienced a loss of actin containing stress fibers and the absence of classic focal adhesions (Schindler et al., 2005). Stem cells cultured on nanosurfaces experience increased adhesion and formation of stress fibers that usually coincide with increased differentiation; therefore, it could be hypothesized that the loss of actin and focal adhesions could in fact be the reason for the ability of 3-D nanofiber networks to maintain stemness. The ability of nanostructures to affect stem cell behaviors such as attachment, proliferation, and differentiation shows the value of understanding and utilizing these special structures in advancing the applications of stem cells.

1.3 Stem Cell Interactions with Nanoparticles

Nanoparticles can be used for a variety of applications with stem cells and cancer cells. Magnetic or fluorescent nanoparticles are attached to the surface of stem cells in order to separate them from larger groups of cells by flow cytometry. Nanoparticles can also be internalized in stem cells and cancer cells after which the internalized nanoparticles can be exploited for a variety of functional purposes, such as gene delivery or transfection. For example, nanoparticles are used to deliver substances that need to be protected from the outside environment such as DNA to stem cells or drugs to cancer cells. Nanoparticles can also be used in vivo as markers to track transplanted stem cells or to locate tumor cells with selectively properties in vivo. In relation to stem cell applications, nanoparticles can be used as contrast agents or vehicles. Contrast agents such as magnetic nanoparticles are the target substance for delivery to the cell and are usually encapsulated by another substance before applied to the cell. These nanoparticles can be used as vehicles for delivery of target substance to the cell.

1.3.1 Nanoparticles as Contrast Agents

1.3.1.1 Super Paramagnetic Nanoparticles

Paramagnetic materials are materials that do not normally have magnetic properties, but become magnetic when exposed to an external magnetic field. Superparmagnetic nanoparticles are small particles that can act as imaging probes in magnetic resonance (MR) images. The most commonly used superparmagnetic nanoparticle is iron oxide (FeO_2), which is biocompatible and inert. Gadolinium (Gd) is another paramagnetic nanoparticle that can be visualized by MR imaging. Gd is strongly toxic as a free ion so it is nessecary that it be combined with ligands to form very stable chelates when used for biological purposes. Iron oxide nanoparticles usually consist of a FeO_2 core and an outer polymer shell and acts primaraly as a negative T_2 constrast agent producing dark spots in MR images. Gd acts to enhance T_1 MR images.

1.3.1.2 Quantum Dots

Quantum dots are inorganic semi-conductor nanoparticles that have been explored as fluorescent labeling agents for cells for biological imaging. Quantum dots are typically less than 10 nm in size. Quantum dots are advantageous over conventional organic probes because they can be excited by a wider range of wavelengths and they exhibit narrower emission bandwidths (Dubertret et al., 2002). Quantum dots (QDs) are coated with ligand shells for incorporation into cells. (Dubertret et al., 2002) CdSe/ZnS-core/shell quantum dots are of special interest because of their uniquely strong luminance and high photostability (Hoshino et al., 2004).

1.3.1.3 Nanoshells

Nanoshells are composed of a dielectric core and surrounded by a thin metal shell. Nanoshells cores and shells are typically silica and gold respectfully. Nanoshells can be designed with specific optical emission absorption properties. Nanoshells tunable optical resonance has also been exploited to generate heat (Cuenca et al., 2006).

1.3.2 Nanoparticles as Vehicles

1.3.2.1 Silica Nanoparticles

Organically modified silica nanoparticles surface functionalized with amino groups have been shown to bind and protect plasmid DNA from enzymatic digestion during the tranfection process. Silica nanoparticles are used as an immobilization matrix rather than in tracking. Silica nanopartilces have been used to deliver DNA to stem cells in vivo (Bharali et al., 2005). Mesoporous silica nanoparticles could be internalized by cells without modification (Huang et al., 2005).

1.3.2.2 Polymer Nanoparticles

Polymer nanoparticles can encapsulate substances to provide protection from the outside environment and add specificity for targeted cell delivery. Through controlled biodegradation, polymers can assure a controlled rate for sustained drug release. An important use of polymer nanoparticles is as a carrier for gene therapy. Catatonic polymers bind and condense plasmid DNA to protect it during intracellular transport. Polymer surfaces are also easy to modify which raises the prospect of targeting specific cellular receptors to avoid side effects resulting from expression of the genes in sites other than those intended (Corsi et al., 2003). Some polymers used as gene carriers are poly-*L*-lysine (PLL), polyethyleimine (PEI), chitosan, and poly (lactide-*co*-glycolide) (PLGA). Polymer nanoparticles show evidence of varying levels of cytotoxicity and transfection efficiency and can be modified to optimize these characteristics (Corsi et al., 2003).

1.3.3 Effect of Internalized Nanoparticles

1.3.3.1 Toxicity

The toxicity of commonly used nanoparticles is manner of debate. There is significant evidence for the toxicity of commonly used non-nanoparticle cationic liposome transfection agents (van den Bos et al., 2003). The limitation of cationic liposome is one of the reasons that the use nanoparticles as carriers for genes, and tracking agents is of such interest. Quantum dot tracking agents exhibit concentration dependent toxicity, but have not appeared to cause cytotoxicity at lower, but still functional levels and encapsulation can alleviate this effect (Dubertret et al., 2002; Hoshino et al., 2004). Polymer nanoparticles have also contributed to increased cytotoxicity at varying levels depending on conditions such as the type of polymer or the molecular weight (Corsi et al., 2003). FeO_2 particles can be toxic to cells at high concentration as well, but can be internalized at applicable concentration without apparent toxicity. The toxicity of nanoparticles is a however a subject of debate and there are conflicting reports on the toxicity of nanoparticles, but the overwhelming majority of published experiments reported negligible or minimal effects on cell viability for the specific type and concentration of nanoparticles that were transfected (Aime et al., 2004; Bulte et al., 2001; Corsi et al., 2003; Huang et al., 2005; Jendelova et al., 2004; Lewin et al., 2000; Miyoshi et al., 2005; Vuu et al., 2005; Zhao et al., 2002). Unfortunately, most viability tests conducted on nanoparticles are done over relatively short periods of time and with little detail. It has been stated that there is a serious lack of information concerning the impact of nanostructured materials on human health and the environment (Braydich-Stolle et al., 2005). An important issue in the assessment of the safety of nanoparticles may be the in vivo effects at the level of the organism and the long-term effects. Because of its sensitivity to environmental changes, a mouse spermatogonial stem cell line was used as a model to test the effect of different nanoparticles in vitro (Braydich-Stolle et al., 2005). Silver, aluminum, and molybdenum nanoparticles added into the spermatogonial cell line culture all demonstrated a concentration-dependent toxicity whereas the corresponding soluble salts had no effect. The effect of nanoparticle internalization was dependent of the material, as silver nanoparticles were very toxic and molybdenum did not affect metabolic activity at low concentrations.

1.3.3.2 Differentiation

The effect of internalized nanoparticles on differentiation is also a phenomena that is not well understood. Stem cells have been reported to differentiate normally with internalized iron oxide, quantum dots, and silica nanoparticles, but there are relatively few cases in which were this effect has been investigated (Bulte et al., 2001; Huang et al., 2005; Jing et al., 2004). In addition, many of the conclusions made about the normal differentiation of cells with internalized nanoparticles have been made based on morphological observations and gross analysis on the growth properties of cells without detailed characterization of molecular activities such as gene expression (Hsieh et al., 2006). Investigation of the differentiation properties of bone marrow stem cells (BMSCs) cultured with internalized CdSe/ZnS quantum dots showed that cells with quantum dots exhibited impaired linage specific gene expression for chondrogenesis and osteogenesis (Hsieh et al., 2006; Hsieh et al., 2006). The presence of quantum dots did not affect the proliferation of BMSCs or the size of chondrospheres after chondrogenesis induction, but mRNA, protein of type Ⅱ collagen and aggrecan was significantly inhibited. In a separate experiment, BMSCs induced to differentiate to an osteogenic lineage displayed lower alkaline phosphatase activity and significant inhibition of osteopontin and osteocalcin expression when compared to control cells. These results raise concerns about the effect of using quantum dots to label stem cells as well the possibility that internalization of other types of nanoparticles could have similar effects on stem cell differentiation.

1.3.3.3 Cell Internalization of Nanoparticles and Cell Tracking

In order to utilize nanoparticles to track stem cells or deliver agents to them, the nanoparticles must first be internalized in vitro or in vivo. Methods of labeling cells by surface attachment that are commonly used in cell sorting are not suitable for in vivo conditions because of the rapid reticuloendothelial recognition and clearance of cells thus labeled (Lewin et al., 2000). The most common modes of internalization are pinocytosis, which deals with the ingestion of fluid by means of small vesicles and endocytosis, which is a process where substances bound to the cell membrane and molecules present in the extracellular fluid are entrapped in endosomic vesicles. The high incubation concentration for absorption of straight iron oxide nanoparticles is toxic to cells so the particles must be modified in order to efficiently label stem cells. The use of DNA transfection agents such as cationic lipofectamins allow the internalization of enough iron oxide particles for visualization of in vivo tracking, but the use of these agents may cause toxic effects (Dokka et al., 2000; Lewin et al., 2000). A viral vector was able to transfer iron oxide nanoparticles into neural progenitor cells at 12 times the level of lipofectamine; however, viral vectors are accompanied by limitations such as their rapid clearance from the circulation and associated risks of toxicity and immunogenicity (Corsi et al., 2003; Miyoshi et al., 2005). An efficient method of internalization of FeO_2 particles by stem cells was developed that involved coating iron oxide particles with a dextran core and attaching tat peptides to the nano-FeO_2 surface (Lewin et al., 2000). The efficiency of cellular uptake of iron oxide nanoparticle conjugated with tat peptide has been measured for 1 – 15 tat peptide chains attached to the nanoparticle surface (Lewin et al., 2000). An exponential peptide number versus cellular uptake relationship was discovered and it was found that uptake efficiency was 100 times greater when tat peptide number per particle was above 10 as compared to 1.2 peptides per particle. Another method of cell internalization investigated is the encapsulation of nanoparticles by polymer dendrimers that can be internalized by stem cells through a nonspecific membrane absorption process facilitated by their high affinity for cellular membranes (Bulte et al., 2001).

1. Ex Vivo Stem Cell Tracking

While ex vivo tracking techniques have no clinical practicality, they are certainly useful for gaining an understanding of the behavior of transplanted stem cell in vivo in animal models. Labeled stem cells can be located by a number of different methods ex vivo. When fluorescently labeled cells are released in vivo they can be located ex vivo on histological sections using fluorescent microscopy. Histological sections can also be stained to label nanoparticles. Paramagnetic iron oxide particles can be visualized by Prussian blue staining. By tagging internalized nanoparticles with radioactive ligands it is possible to do gross analysis of stem cell distribution throughout the body on an organ-by-organ basis.

2. In Vivo Stem Cell Tracking

Fluorescent quantum dots can be visualized in vivo by whole body laser-based macroillumination systems (Bonde et al., 2004). Quantum dot accumulations in a prostate tumor site in a live mice were visualized as fluorescence signals and confirmed by subsequent histological analysis (Gao et al., 2004). This type of imaging is however limited by the penetration depth of visible light and it was noted that quantum dots in deep organs such as the liver and spleen were not detectable. One of the most exciting applications of combining nanotechnology and stem cell research is the possibility of in vivo magnetic resonance tracking of stem cells transplanted in the body for therapeutic purposes. It is theorized that the introduction of stem cells into damaged tissues could help to repair the damaged or diseased tissues through trophic support, proliferation, differentiation, and remodeling. Stem cell therapy is of particular interest in tissues that do not naturally regenerate, such as the central nervous system, heart, etc. Magnetic resonance imaging (MRI) can visualize superparamagnetic nanoparticles in vivo and therefore when magnetic nanoparticles are internalized by stem cells then they in turn can be visualized. Commonly, used superparamagnetic iron oxide (SPIO) nanoparticles act primarily as negative contrast agents producing dark spots in magnetic vesonance (MR) images and they are therefore particularly effective when dealing with anatomical regions of intense MR signaling intensity such as the brain (Aime et al., 2004). In the presence of an external magnetic field, internalized magnetic nanoparticles induce a local inhomogeneous magnetic field within and around the cells (Ziener et al., 2005). The induced local magnetic field caused by magnetic nanoparticles leads to the shorting of relaxation times by an order of magnitude greater than standard paramagnetic contrast agents (Jendelova et al., 2004). Analytical predictions can be made for the transverse relaxation rate as a function of the number and distribution of nanoparticles, the magnetic difference, and the diffusion coefficient of the tissue (Ziener et al., 2005). Reversing analysis can provide information about imaged tissue containing nanoparticles using the MR measured relaxation time (Ziener et al., 2005). The intensity of the MR signal disturbance is greater for greater numbers of nanoparticles and therefore a greater uptake of particles per cell allows for lower detection thresholds in vivo (Zhao et al., 2002). It has been reported that the MR visualization threshold for internalized Gd (III) chelates is of the order of $10^7 - 10^8$/cell (Aime et al., 2004). Single cells with internalized nanoparticles have been readily detected by MR imaging even when the spatial resolution per voxel is larger than that of individual cells (Lewin et al., 2000). This is possible because magnetic nanoparticles exert a magnetic susceptibility extending far beyond the cell margin.

Tracking of stem cells with internalized superparmagnetic nanoparticles by MR imaging has investigated extensively. Hemopoetic Stem cells containing SPIO particles were visualized in vitro in agar gels and ex vivo on tissue samples of bone marrow at the single cell level. It was also possible to separate single labeled stem cells from bone marrow tissue samples ex vivo using flow cytometry (Lewin et al., 2000). In vivo detection of stem cells labeled with paramagnetic nanoparticles has been confirmed by ex vivo staining. Prussian blue staining confirmed MR detection of nanoparticle labeled bone marrow and ES cells in the lesioned brain and spinal cord and in the intact and lesioned myocardium with good agreement (Jendelova et al., 2004; Kustermann et al., 2005). In another study an excellent correlation was noted between MR contrast images and sections stained for β-galactosidase for magnetically labeled oligodendroglial progenitors (Bulte et al., 2001).

3. Removal and Digestion of Nanoparticle in In Vivo Tracking

In MR stem cell tracking it is very important to consider the removal and digestion of nanoparticles from cells due to normal cell processes and cell division. It has been hypothesized that reduction of contrast agent over time can be attributed to dilution and or removal during cell division, exocytosis through the ATP binding cassette transportor, and lysosomal digestion (Miyoshi et al., 2005). When stem cells with internalized nanoparticles SPIO have been tracked by MR imaging the signal intensity gradually decreases until it is no longer detectable at around 6 or 7 weeks (Bulte et al., 2001; Jendelova et al., 2004; Jing et al., 2004). Theoretically, analysis of initial signal strength and signal strength decline as labeled cells divide could indicate whether the cells were merely residing in the tissue or actively dividing and integrating with host tissue (Bonde et al., 2004). After neural progenitor cells labeled with SPIO particles internalized by retrovirus or lipofectimine were cultured in high and low serum media the amounts of remaining nanoparticles versus initial concentration led to two hypothesis (Miyoshi et al., 2005). Because nanoparticles were cleared from retrovirus assisted internalized cells at a faster rate than lipofectamine mediated internalized cells, it was hypothesized that clearance rate could be internalization method dependent. Because nanoparticles were cleared at a faster rate in high serum media as compared to low serum media, it was hypothesized that labeling loss was related to cell division. It is also possible that a greater initial concentration of nanoparticles in retrovirus transfected cells caused an increased clearance rate in these cells because clearance rate is concentration dependent.

4. Possible Problems facing In Vivo MR Tracking

Despite the promise of MR imaging to track stem cell there are many potential problems that can be encountered when making conclusions about transplanted stem cell population based on data collected from MR images. One major obstacle is the complexity involved in nanoparticle clearance described in the previous section. Another is the assumptions made in analytical predictions of relaxation data such as the assumption that all cells contain the same number of internalized nanoparticles and the assumption the all internalized particles aggregate in an impermeable sphere (Ziener et al., 2005). In addition, uncleared nanoparticles released because of cell death could result in overestimation of calculated cell number (Freyman et al., 2006). Another potential problem was observed when nanoparticles internalized by neural progenitor cells were found to reside in growing axons and dendrites (Miyoshi et al., 2005). The spreading of these nanoparticles could be mistaken for cell proliferation. Yet another potential problem is interference with the MR signal of the nanoparticles. It was observed that ischemic myocardium tissue was characterized by signal attenuation similar to that of internalized paramagnetic particles, which could lead to false conclusions about stem cell number in vivo.

1.3.3.4 Gene Therepy

Advances in our ability to identify specific genes whose defect or absence is responsible for a particular pathological condition allow for the potential to treat these conditions by delivery of specific genes to the pathological cells. For gene therapy to be effective the genetic payload must enter the targeted cells and be transported to the nucleus where it either inhibits undesirable gene expression or synthesizes therapeutic proteins. An optimum gene delivery system should have good loading properties for DNA into the particles and for the particles into the target cells. Viral vectors have shown high tranfection efficiency, but accompanied significant drawbacks create the need for efficient non-viral vectors such as nanoparticles (Corsi et al., 2003). Biodegradable nanoparticles are of particular interest because of their ability to assure a controlled sustained gene release. It has been shown the gene delivery to stem cells using nanoparticles is feasible both in vitro and in vivo. DNA containing chitosan nanoparticles were synthesized from the complexation of the cationic polymer with a DNA plasmid (Corsi et al., 2003). These nanoparticles were successfully internalized into human stem cells. Ultrafine silica nanoparticles, functionalized with amino groups were successfully complexed with plasmid DNA and injected into the mouse brain where the in vivo transfection of fibroblast growth factor receptor type 1 resulted in significant inhibition of the in vivo incorporation of Bromodeoxyuridine (BrdU) into the DNA of the cells (Bharali et al., 2005). These results demonstrated that nanoparticle mediated gene therapy could be used to manipulate the biology of stem/progenitor cells in vivo.

1.3.3.5 Cancer Therepy

Nanoparticle technologies also have great promise in the diagnosis and treatment of cancer. Various types of nanoparticles have been utilized as a tool to locate cancer cells and to destroy them by means of chemical, thermal, and irradiation therapies (Cuenca et al., 2006). Nanoparticles can be used as vehicles to deliver drugs to cancer cells or the particles themselves can be utilized to locate or assault cancer cells. Nanoparticles can selectively target cancer cells passively, by taking advantage of the unique vasculature of tumor tissue or actively, by conjugation with tumor specific ligands or magnetic guidance. Tumor blood vessels are distinct from regular vessels by the existence wide fenestrations in the endothelial cell layer ranging from 200 nm to 1.2 μm. These large pores allow the preferential passage of nanoparticles into tumor containing extracellular spaces (Maeda et al., 2003). In addition, nanoparticles entering the tumor containing extracellular spaces tend to accumulate due to the lack of an effective lymphatic drainage system (Gao et al., 2004). Exploitation of these tumor specific features allowed unlabeled quantum dots to be successfully localized and visualized at a tumor site in a murine prostate cancer model (Gao et al., 2004). Active targeting of breast cancer with paramagnetic nanoparticles conjugated to the breast cancer expressing receptors, HER-2/neu and LHRH, have selectively internalized by breast cancer cells in vivo as confirmed by MRI and transmission electon microscopy (Artemov et al., 2003; Zhou et al., 2006). Cancerous neovasculature has also been targeted in vivo using receptor conjugated paramagnetic nanoparticles and imaged with MRI (Winter et al., 2003). A non-receptor method of actively targeting tumor cells is to direct a systemically injected magnetic nanoparticle-drug complex to a known region of cancer using external magnetic fields. Application of this method has resulted in tumor remission at 50% of the normally administered, systemic, chemotherapeutic dose (Alexiou et al., 2000). In addition to drug delivery and imaging, tumors that selectively uptake nanoparticles can be treated with external irradiation or thermal excitation. Systemically administered gold nanoparticles accumulated in a subcutaneous tumor model and greatly enhanced local radiation therapy compared to mice receiving radiation therapy without nanoparticles (Hainfeld et al., 2004). Cells containing nanoshells can be excited by moderately low exposures of near infared light to induce irreversible thermal tissue damage (Hirsch et al., 2003). Nanoshells have a tunable optical resonance that can be matched to external excitation to specifically induce thermal damage on nanoshell containing cells. In both in vitro and in vivo experiments cells containing nanoshells could be killed without damaging the non-nanoshell containing surrounding tissue (Hirsch et al., 2003).

1.3.4 Summary

Nanoparticles have a vast potential to revolutionize the field of biotechnology. The ability of nanoparticles to track stem cells could be a key factor in understanding the interaction of stem cells in the body and facilitate the future therapeutic use of stem cells in the repair of unregenerate damaged tissues such as the CNS tissue and heart. Nanoparticles also have the potential to allow fast and noninvasive diagnosis and treatment for cancer. Successful clinical progress in this complex field will require understanding and technological advances in all facets of nanoparticle technology. This will include the development of new and better nanoparticles and transfection methods, advances in the manipulation of internalized nanoparticles by in vivo non invasive imaging and excitation, and a greater understanding of the mechanics of nanoparticles in the cell and in response to external excitation.

1.4 Conclusions

Stem cells and nanostructures are two technologies that share both enormous potential and lack of understanding. Nanoparticles, nanofibers, and nanosufaces can currently be fabricated, and a vast amount of research is being conducted to continually find new ways to improve these nanostructures and expand their applications. Stem cells have demonstrated the potential to replace damaged tissues and provide new methods to treat currently untreatable diseases. As our understanding and ability to manipulate stem cells grows, nanostructures could be used as the tool to provide the required substrates for growth and the delivery of the appropriate cues required for controlled manipulation of stem cell biology. The integration of stem cells and nanotechnology may offer some of the most promising methods for the treatment of societies most difficult medical maladies, such as heart disease, nervous system degeneration, cancer, and organ failure.

Acknowledgements

This publication was supported by AO Research Fund (04-W55), Switzerland and The Wallace H. Coulter Foundation, USA.

References

Aime, S., A. Barge, et al. *Curr. Pharm. Biotechnol.* **5**: 509 – 518 (2004).
Alexiou, C., W. Arnold, et al. *Cancer. Res.* **60**: 6641 – 6648 (2000).
Alivisatos, P. *Nature Biotechnology* **22**: 47 – 52 (2004).
Artemov, D., N. Mori, et al. *Magn. Reson. Med.* **49**: 403 – 408 (2003).
Badami, A. S., M. R. Kreke, et al. *Biomaterials* **27**: 596 – 606 (2006).
Bharali, D. J., I. Klejbor, et al. *Proc. Natl. Acad. Sci. USA* **102**: 11,539 – 11,544 (2005).
Bonde, J., D. A. Hess, et al. *Curr. Opin. Hematol.* **11**: 392 – 398 (2004).
Bradt, J. H., M. Mertig, et al. *Chemistry of Materials* **11**: 2694 – 2701 (1999).
Braydich-Stolle, L., S. Hussain, et al. *Toxicol. Sci.* **88**: 412 – 419 (2005).
Bulte, J. W., T. Douglas, et al. *Nat. Biotechnol.* **19**: 1141 – 1147 (2001).
Chua, K. N., C. Chai, et al. *Biomaterials* **27**(36): 6043 – 6051 (2006).
Corsi, K., F. Chellat, et al. *Biomaterials* **24**: 1255 – 1264 (2003).
Cuenca, A. G., H. Jiang, et al. *Cancer* **107**: 459 – 459 (2006).
Curtis. *Trends in Biotechnology* **19**: 97 – 101 (2001).
Dalby, M. J., D. McCloy, et al. *Biomaterials* **27**: 2980 – 2987 (2006a).
Dalby, M. J., D. McCloy, et al. *Biomaterials* **27**: 1306 – 1315 (2006b).
Davis, M. E., J. P. Motion, et al. *Circulation* **111**: 442 – 450 (2005).
Deligianni, D. D., N. Katsala, et al. *Biomaterials* **22**: 1241 – 1251 (2001).
Desai, T. A. *Medical Engineering & Physics* **22**: 595 – 606 (2000).
Dokka, S., D. Toledo, et al. *Pharm. Res.* **17**: 521 – 525 (2000).
Drummond, T. G., M. G. Hill, et al. *Nature Biotechnology* **21**: 1192 – 1199 (2003).
Du, C., F. Z. Cui, et al. *Journal of Biomedical Materials Research* **42**: 540 – 548 (1998).

Dubertret, B., P. Skourides, et al. *Science* **298**: 1759 – 1762 (2002).
Elias, K. L., R. L. Price, et al. *Biomaterials* **23**: 3279 – 3287 (2002).
Foster, G. A. and B. M. Stringer. *Brain. Pathol.* **9**: 547 – 567 (1999).
Freyman, T., G. Polin, et al. *Eur. Heart J.* **27**: 1114 – 1122 (2006).
Gao, X., Y. Cui, et al. *Nat. Biotechnol.* **22**: 969 – 976 (2004).
Garreta, E., E. Genove, et al. *Tissue Eng.* **12**(8): 2215 – 2227 (2006).
Good, T. *IEEE Eng. Med. Biol. Mag.* **17**: 16, 18 (1998).
Hainfeld, J. F., D. N. Slatkin, et al. *Phys. Med. Biol.* **49**: N309 – 315 (2004).
Hirsch, L. R., R. J. Stafford, et al. *Proc. Natl. Acad. Sci. USA* **100**: 13,549 – 13,554 (2003).
Hoshino, A., K. Hanaki, et al. *Biochem. Biophys. Res. Commun.* **314**: 46 – 53 (2004).
Hsieh, S. C., F. F. Wang, et al. *J. Biomed. Mater. Res. B Appl Biomater* (2006).
Hsieh, S. C., F. F. Wang, et al. *Biomaterials* **27**: 1656 – 1664 (2006).
Huang, D. M., Y. Hung, et al. *Faseb. J.* **19**: 2014 – 2016 (2005).
Jendelova, P., V. Herynek, et al. *J Neurosci Res* **76**: 232 – 243 (2004).
Jing, M., X. Q. Liu, et al. *Zhonghua Yi Xue Za Zhi* **84**: 1386 – 1389 (2004).
Kikuchi, M., T. Ikoma, et al. *Composites Science and Technology* **64**: 819 – 825 (2004).
Kikuchi, M., T. Ikoma, et al. *Bioceramics* **16**: 561 – 564 (2004).
Kommireddy, D. S., S. M. Sriram, et al. *Biomaterials* **27**: 4296 – 4303 (2006).
Kustermann, E., W. Roell, et al. *NMR Biomed* **18**: 362 – 370 (2005).
Laval, J. M., P. E. Mazeran, et al. *Analyst* **125**: 29 – 33 (1999).
Lewin, M., N. Carlesso, et al. *Nat. Biotechnol.* **18**: 410 – 414 (2000).
Li, W. J., R. Tuli, et al. *Biomaterials* **26**: 5158 – 5166 (2005).
Maeda, H., J. Fang, et al. *Int. Immunopharmacol.* **3**: 319 – 328 (2003).
Maniotis, A. J., C. S. Chen, et al. *Proc. Natl. Acad. Sci. USA* **94**: 849 – 854 (1997).
Matsuzaka, K., F. Walboomers, et al. *Clin. Oral. Implants. Res.* **11**: 325 – 333 (2000).
Matsuzaka, K., X. F. Walboomers, et al. *Biomaterials* **20**: 1293 – 1301 (1999).
Mazzola, L. *Nature Biotechnology* **21**: 1137 – 1143 (2003).
McBeath, R., D. M. Pirone, et al. *Dev. Cell.* **6**: 483 – 495 (2004).
Miyoshi, S., J. A. Flexman, et al. *Mol. Imaging. Biol.* **7**: 286 – 7295 (2005).
Moghimi, S. M. and J. Szebeni. *Progress in Lipid Research* **42**: 463 – 478 (2003).
Muller, R. H., C. Jacobs, et al. *Advanced Drug Delivery Reviews* **47**: 3 – 19 (2001).
Niemeyer, C. M. *Angewandte Chemie-International Edition* **40**: 4128 – 4158 (2001).
Nur, E. K. A., I. Ahmed, et al. *Stem Cells* **24**: 426 – 433 (2006).
Pedersen, R. A. *Sci. Am.* **280**: 68 – 73 (1999).
Penn, S. G., L. He, et al. *Current Opinion in Chemical Biology* **7**: 609 – 615 (2003).
Rizzoli, V. and C. Carlo-Stella. *Crit. Rev. Oncol. Hematol.* **26**: 101-115 (1997).
Safarik, I. and M. Safarikova. *Monatshefte Fur Chemie* **133**: 737 – 759 (2002).
Schindler, M., I. Ahmed, et al. *Biomaterials* **26**: 5624 – 5631 (2005).
Silva, G. A., C. Czeisler, et al. *Science* **303**: 1352 – 1355 (2004).
Solter, D. and J. Gearhart. *Science* **283**: 1468 – 1470 (1999).
Spiegelman, B. M. and C. A. Ginty. *Cell* **35**: 657 – 666 (1983).
Takeuchi, H., H. Yamamoto, et al. *Advanced Drug Delivery Reviews* **47**: 39 – 54 (2001).
Thomas, C. H., J. H. Collier, et al. *Proc. Natl. Acad. Sci. USA* **99**: 1972 – 1977 (2002).

van den Bos, E. J., A. Wagner, et al. *Cell Transplant.* **12**: 743 – 756 (2003).
Vuu, K., J. Xie, et al. *Bioconjug. Chem.* **16**: 995 – 999 (2005).
Weissman, I. L. *Science* **287**: 1442 – 1446 (2000).
Whitesides, G. M. *Nature Biotechnology* **21**: 1161 – 1165 (2003).
Winter, P. M., S. D. Caruthers, et al. *Cancer. Res.* **63**: 5838 – 5843 (2003).
Yang, F., R. Murugan, et al. *Biomaterials* **25**: 1891 – 1900 (2004).
Yang, F., R. Murugan, et al. *Biomaterials* **26**: 2603 – 2610 (2005).
Zhao, M., M. F. Kircher, et al. *Bioconjug. Chem.* **13**: 840 – 844 (2002).
Zhou, J., C. Leuschner, et al. *Biomaterials* **27**: 2001 – 2008 (2006).
Zhu, B., Q. Lu, et al. *Tissue. Eng.* **11**: 825 – 834 (2005).
Ziener, C. H., W. R. Bauer, et al. *Magn. Reson. Med.* **54**: 702 – 706 (2005).

2 Biomedical Polymer Nanofibers for Emerging Technology

Kwideok Park[1], Won Ho Park[2], Jun Sik Son[1] and Dong Keun Han[1]

[1] Biomaterials Research Center, Korea Institute of Science and Technology, P. O. Box 131, Cheongryang, Seoul 130-650, Korea

[2] Department of Textile Engineering, College of Engineering, Chungnam National University, Daejeon 305-764, Korea

Abstract Nanofibers have been of great interest in the recent years, because of its huge potential to diverse fields, especially in biomedical applications. The most favorable feature is the dimension of nanofibers that resembles that of the natural collagen fibrils in nano scale. They thus provide extremely large surface area to volume ratio as compared to microfibers. Electrospinning is the most preferred method in producing nanofibers from polymers. In this chapter, an overview of polymer nanofibers is stated, specifically focusing on the electrospun nanofibers used in biomedical applications. Along with a brief description of history, principle, and operating parameters of electrospinning process, examples of specific functionalities are introduced through bulk and surface modifications of nanofibers. In addition, a broad range of biomedical application includes tissue-engineered scaffolds, wound dressings, medical device and implants, controlled drug release, and other applications in biosensor, biocatalyst, and bioenzyme. With the rapidly growing demand nanofibers should find its enormous potential for the future development of nanoscience and biomedicine.

Keywords electrospinning, nanofiber, surface/bulk modification, medical polymer, nanobioscience

2.1 Introduction

Polymer nanofibers have attracted much attention in the last decade, because of their unique nano-sized features. Nanofiber is generally referred to as a fiber which has a diameter less than 100 nm. However, one also calls it nanofiber with

(1) Corresponding e-mail: dkh@kist.re.kr

diameters less than 1000 nm (submicron) produced by ultra-thin fiber manufacturing techniques (Grafe and Graham, 2003). The size of nanofiber is clearly contrasted with a human hair in scanning electron microscopy (SEM) images (Fig. 2.1). Methods for the production of polymeric nanofibers include drawing (Ondarcuchu and Joachim, 1998), template synthesis (Feng et al., 2002; Martin, 1996), phase separation (Ma and Zhang, 1999), self-assembly (Liu et al., 1999; Whitesides and Grzybowski), and electrospinning (Reneker and Chun, 1996). Electrospinning is the most popular and preferred technique, which is simple, cost-effective and able to produce continuous nanofibers from polymers to ceramics. It is an efficient fabrication process that can be utilized to assemble nanofibrous polymer mats (Dietzel et al., 2001; Huang et al., 2004). A variety of polymers have been successfully electrospun into nanofibers, mostly in polymer solution and some in polymer melt. While the conventional fiber spinning techniques, such as wet spinning, dry spinning, and melt spinning, produce polymer fibers with diameters in micrometer scale, electrospinning can generate polymer fibers in nanometer range. When the diameters of polymer fibers are reduced from micrometer to submicron or nanometer scale, some fundamental changes in physical and mechanical characteristics occur: extremely large surface area to volume ratio, flexibility in surface functionality, and improvement of mechanical property (e.g. stiffness and tensile strength), as compared to other traditional forms of materials. These advanced properties make polymer nanofibers an optimal candidate for many biomedical and industrial applications (Huang et al., 2003).

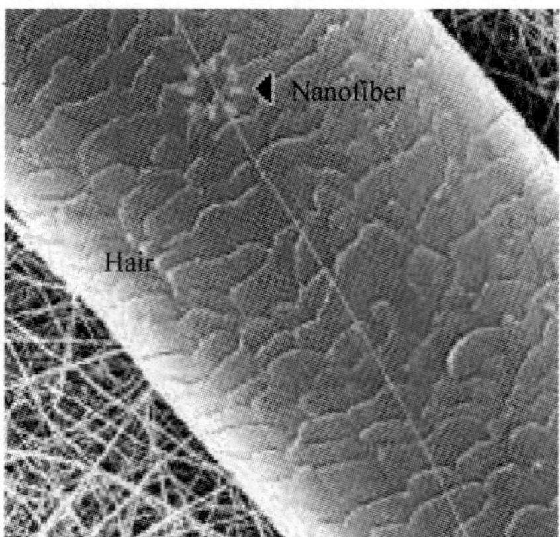

Figure 2.1 SEM images of the size of nanofiber and human hair

The use of polymer nanofibers for biomedical applications has some intrinsic benefits (Zhang et al., 2005). The most notable one is that they share a morphological proximity with natural extracellular matrix (ECM) components, for instance, collagen, which is composed of nanometer-scale (50 – 500 nm) multi-fibrils. The use of synthetic nanofibrillar matrix is thus expected to mimic the natural 3-D environment of ECM, in which tissue cells would attach, proliferate, and differentiate. It is believed that cells would organize a structural unit for normal cellular activity around fibers with diameter smaller than that of cells (Laurencin et al., 1999). Many studies have shown that apart from surface chemistry, nano-scale surface features have a significant impact on regulating cell behaviors in terms of cell adhesion, activation, proliferation, differentiation, alignment, and orientation (Flemming et al., 1999; Desai, 2000; Curtis, 2001; Craighead et al., 2001).

In this chapter, an overview is documented on the recent progress of polymer nanofibers, mostly electrospun in biomedical applications, along with a brief description of history, principle, and operating parameters of electrospinning process. Introduction of specific functionalities to nanofibers is mentioned through bulk and surface modifications. A broad range of biomedical applications of nanofibers deals with tissue-engineered scaffolds, wound dressings, medical device and implants, controlled drug release, and other applications for biosensor, biocatalyst, and bioenzyme (Fig. 2.2).

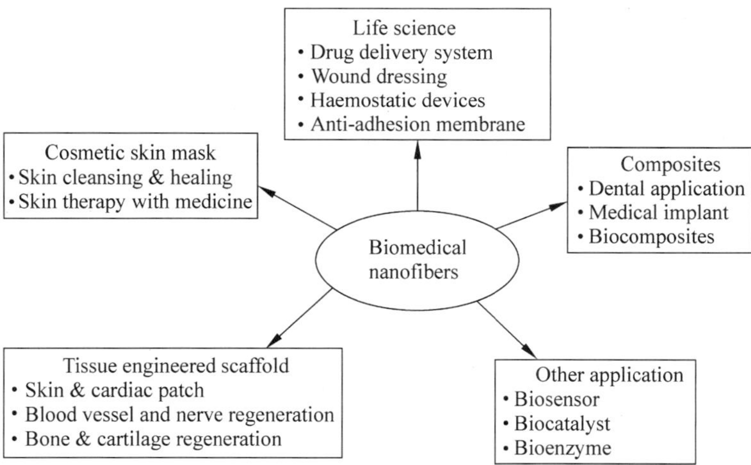

Figure 2.2 Biomedical applications of polymer nanofibers

2.2 Electrospinning Technology-History, Principle, Parameter

The history of electrospinning is dated back to the early 1930s. In 1934, Formhals (1934) patented electrospinning method, associated with the process and the apparatus for producing artificial filaments using electric charges. In fact, Lord Rayleigh already established theoretical and experimental background of electrospinning in the late 1800s. He determined the maximum charge that a liquid drop can withstand before electrostatic force overcomes surface tension of the drop and ejects a jet. In the early 1910s, Zeleny (1917) reported an electrospraying phenomenon. In the 1960s, Taylor (1964) investigated the deformation and disintegration of water drops in an electrical field and analyzed the conditions at the moment. During the past decade, Reneker and others (Doshi and Reneker, 1995; Reneker et al., 2000; Yarin et al., 2001; Spivak et al., 2000; Hohman et al., 2001; Tsai et al., 2002; Shin et al., 2001) studied the electrospinning process and contributed to intensifying in-depth knowledge and extending its applications.

The formation of nanofibers is based on the uniaxial stretching of a viscoelastic solution during electrospinning. Unlike the conventional fiber spinning methods, i.e. dry spinning and melt spinning, electrospinning takes advantage of electrostatic forces to stretch the solution as it solidifies. It involves using a high voltage electrostatic field to charge the surface of a polymer solution droplet and thus to induce the ejection of a liquid jet through a spinneret. In a typical process, an electrical potential is applied between a droplet of polymer solution, or melt, held at the end of capillary tube and ground target (collector). When the applied electric field overcomes the surface tension of droplet, a charged polymer jet is ejected. The jet experiences a bending instability caused by repulsive forces between the charges carried with the jet. The jet extends through spiraling loops, called as whipping. The jet grows longer and thinner until it is solidified or collected on the target (Frenot et al., 2003; Li and Xia, 2004; Deitzel et al., 2001). Schematic illustration of electrospinning is shown in Fig. 2.3.

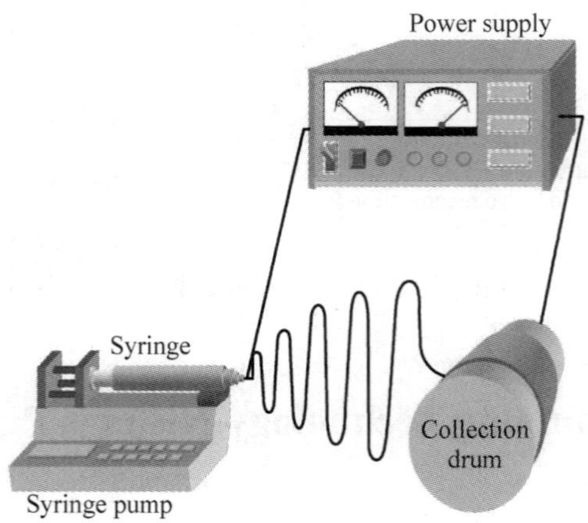

Figure 2.3 Schematic illustration of electrospinning process

There are some parameters and processing variables that affect electrospinning processes. Material parameters include molecular weight of polymer, molecular weight distribution, chemical composition, and polymer solution variables:

viscosity, surface tension, dielectric constant, conductivity, and charge density of spinning jet. Processing parameters encompass electric potential, flow rate, distance between capillary and collector, motion of the collector, and ambient parameters: humidity, temperature, and air flow in the chamber. Polymer solution needs to be concentrated high enough to cause polymer entanglements yet not so high that the viscosity interferes with polymer motion induced by an electric field. The solution should also have a surface tension low enough, a charge density high enough, and a viscosity high enough to prevent polymer jet from collapsing into droplets before the solvent evaporation. Increasing the distance between syringe needle and collector or decreasing the electric field can be a cause of reduced bead density, regardless of the concentration of polymer solution. In addition to producing round nanofibers, polymer solution can be electrospun into thin fibers with a variety of cross-sectional shapes, such as branched fibers, flat ribbons, and ribbons with other shapes (Koombhonge et al., 2001; Xinhua et al., 2002).

2.3 Functionalization of Nanofibers

2.3.1 Bulk Modification

Modification of electrospun nanofibers is primarily intended to introduce a new function on the pre-existing characteristics of base materials. Although two types of modifications exist: surface and bulk modifications, majority of functionalization of nanofibers occur through a bulk modification, due to relatively easy processing and diverse applicable options. Combination of different kinds of polymers, either synthetic or natural ones, is a common practice in achieving a bulk modification of electrospun nanofibers. To alter the hydrophobic nature of poly(L-lactide) (PLLA) itself, two synthetic polymers, PLLA and poly(ethylene glycol) (PEG) were blended and electrospun to produce a hydrophilic nanofibrous PLLA non-woven mat (Bhattarai et al., 2006). The PLLA/PEG (80/20, wt/wt) nanofibers could improve the hydrophilicity with a slow hydrolytic degradation. The effect was obvious with fibroblast attachment and proliferation better than the PLLA control. To take advantage of the benefits of natural polymers, some ECM components have been co-electrospun with synthetic polymers. Collagen-blended PLLA-*co*-poly(ε-caprolactone) (PLLA:PCL) (70:30, wt:wt) were electrospun into nanofiber (He et al., 2005). Its surface was smooth and distribution of fiber diameter was rather uniform, ranging from 100 to 200 nm. In vitro examination with human coronary artery endothelial cells (HCAECs) revealed that blended nanofibers could have a positive influence on the viability, attachment, and spreading of HCAECs. Gelatin, a natural protein was mixed with polyaniline (PANi), a conductive polymer, and electrospun into nanofibers (Li et al., 2006). When cardiac myoblast cells were cultured on the PANi-gelatin nanofibrous matrix, the cell attachment and proliferation were as similar as the control tissue culture plate. In addition, two different ECMs were blended to mimic a natural tissue composition for tissue engineering applications. Zhong et al. (2005) developed collagen-glycosaminoglycan (GAG) nanofibrous scaffold by electrospinning collagen and chondroitin sulfate in a mixed solvent of trifluoroethanol and water. Once crosslinked with glutaraldehyde vapor, the collagen-GAG scaffold was stable and resistant to collagenase degradation. In another study, nanofibrous collagen-elastin blend (1/1, wt/wt) was also successfully prepared by electrospinning in the addition of poly(ethylene oxide) (PEO) and NaCl, which was essential to spin continuous and homogeneous fibers (Buttafoco et al., 2006). Collagen/elastin nanofibrous mesh was then stabilized using *N*-(3-dimethylaminopropyl)-*N*'-ethylcarbodiimide hydrochloride (EDC) and *N*-hydroxysuccinimide (NHS).

Recent efforts made possible that conventional sol-gel precursor solution could be employed for electrospun bioceramic nanofibers. It is necessary to form a solution with viscoelastic behavior similar to that of a conventional polymer solution. A number of bioceramics including SiO_2, TiO_2, Al_2O_3, and ZnO were successfully fabricated into fibrous structures via sol-gel methods (Guan et al., 2003; Choi et al., 2003; Son et al., 2006). Several water-soluble polymers, i.e., poly(vinyl alcohol) (PVA), poly(vinyl pyrrolidine) (PVP), and PEO, are used as the polymer matrices to host inorganic precursors. Polymer nanofibers can also be functionalized blending functional molecules, for instance, growth factors, bioactive drugs, DNA, and enzymes with polymer solution. If these additives were insoluble in the solutions, they could be introduced in the form of emulsions. These components incorporated into nanofibrous matrix were rather stable in their activities and released in a controlled manner. Details are described in the section of 'Biomedical Applications'. Besides the blending technologies, various bulk modifications have been tested. As a new architecture for tissue-engineered bone, micro- and nanofibers were combined in a single structure (Tuzlakoglu et al., 2005). Starch/PCL nanofibers were randomly electrospun and distributed uniformly crossing and interconnecting the base microfibers. A leaching method was used to make a porous gelatin/PCL nanofiber by selectively removing the water-soluble component of gelatin (Zhang et al., 2006). The treatment led to a unique surface morphology of nanofibers containing elliptical pores, grooves, and ridges (Fig. 2.4). New electrospinning technology enabled a multilayering of fibers to build a structure, which has different polymers and fibers. Kidoaki et al. (2005) fabricated a bilayered tubular construct using collagen and segmented polyurethane (SPU). A thick SPU microfiber and thin type Ⅰ collagen nanofiber mesh consisted of an outer and inner layer, respectively.

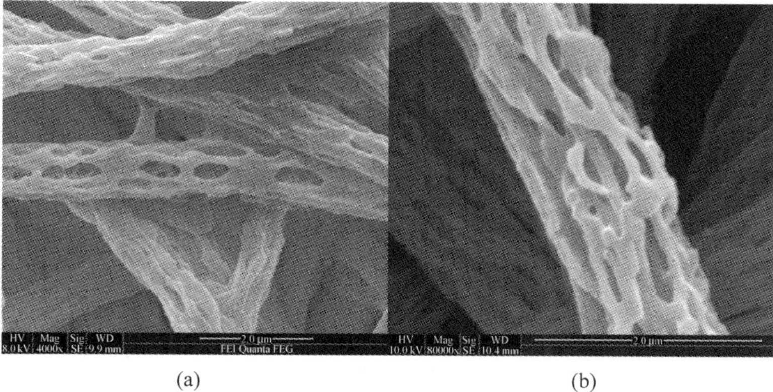

(a) (b)

Figure 2.4 High-resolution Field Emisson Scaning Electron Microscope (FESEM) images of the porous nanofibres at × 40,000(a) and × 80,000(b). Permission for reproduction from the publisher

2.3.2 Surface Modification

Surface modification of nanofibers has its significance in that cell-biomaterial interactions occur at the surface. Those interactions are very sensitive and easily affected by substrate chemistry, surface charges, and surface topography. Therefore, the goal of surface modification lies in the specific control of cellular reactions, i.e. cell attachment, migration, proliferation, and differentiation. Through surface modifications of nanofibers, their chemical, thermal, mechanical properties, wettability, protein adsorption, and biocompatibility can be significantly altered, yet barely changing the original fiber morphology and mechanical properties. Compared to the biodegradable microfiber scaffolds, selection of proper surface modification method requires a special attention to take advantage of nanofibrous 3-D architecture. Because of higher surface area and fiber thickness in nanoscale, the degradation of nanofibers would be uncontrollable after rather a harsh surface treatment.

Addition of functional groups on the surface is a simple modification technique. Polyethersulfone (PES) in dimethylsulfoxide was electrospun into nanofibers and surface-modified using acrylic acid (AA) in aqueous solution and following UV irradiation (Chua et al., 2006). The altered surfaces were further conjugated with ethylene diamine or ethanolamine to be animinated or hydroxylated, respectively. Interactions with hematopoietic stem/progenitor cells (HSPCs) showed that the aminated nanofiber mesh was more efficient in the selective expansion of $CD34^{+}/CD45^{+}$, as compared to the culture on tissue culture polystyrene. Chua et al. (2005) reported a galactosylated nanofiber poly(CL-*co*-ethy1 ethylene phosphate) (PCLEEP) scaffold. Once the electrospun PCLEEP was surface- modified to have AA grafts, galactose ligands were covalently conjugated to the nanofiber surface. Cultured hepatocytes on the galactosylaed PCLEEP nanofiber could form smaller aggregates of spheroids. Park et al. (2006, 2007) have performed plasma treatment to modify biodegradable poly(glycolide) (PGA), poly (lactide-*co*-glycolide) (PLGA), and PLLA nanofibrous meshes. These meshes were treated with nitrogen gas plasma and then subjected to in situ direct AA grafting in the plasma chamber. As compared to the unmodified control, fibroblasts adhesion and proliferation were significantly upregulated on the AA-grafted hydrophilic nanofibrous scaffolds (Fig. 2.5). Sanders et al. (2005) also introduced negatively or positively charged group on electrospun PU nanofiber surfaces through plasma-induced modification. The use of chemicals is also an effective method for surface modification. Electrospun PLLA nanofibrous scaffold was treated using NaOH aqueous solution (Chen et al., 2006). The hydrolysis of PLLA generated carboxylic acid group on the surface without compromising the structural integrity. In a simulated body fluid, the nanofibrous PLLA surface was mineralized with HA crystals, due to the calcium ions binding to the carboxylate groups.

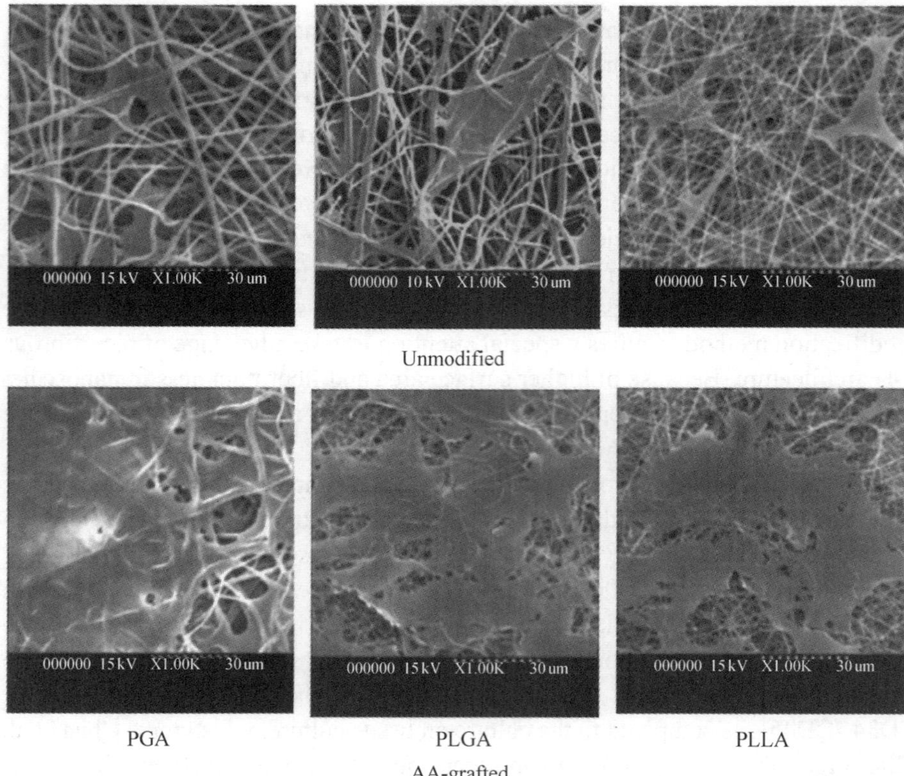

Figure 2.5 SEM micrographs: Fibroblast adhesion after 24 h in vitro culture on either unmodified or AA-grafted PGA, PLGA, and PLLA nanofibrous scaffolds

Some peptides that would elicit specific cellular behaviors can be incorporated in the nanofiber. Nanofibers were formed by self-assembly of isolucine-lysine-valine-alanine-valine (IKVAV) containing peptide amphiphile (Silva et al., 2004). It was found that when neural progenitor cells were encapsulated, relative to laminin or soluble peptide, the IKVAV-loaded nanofiber scaffold induced rapid differentiation of cells into neurons. This phenomenon may be linked to the bioactive epitope presentation to cells by nanofibers. In addition, ECM proteins, for instance, laminin, collagen, and fibronectin were coated on silk fibroin nanofiber surface to promote cell adhesion (Min et al., 2004). On the other hand, surface functionalization of polymer nanofibers can also find other applications in biosensors, biocatalyst, and enzyme immobilization. As a highly sensitive optical biosensor, cellulose acetate nanofibers were electrospun and a fluorescent probe was then assembled by electrostatic layer-by-layer adsorption (Wang et al., 2004). The fluorescent sensitivity was greatly enhanced, due to higher surface area of the nanofibers and efficient interaction between fluorescent conjugated polymer and analytes.

2.4 Biomedical Applications

2.4.1 Tissue-Engineered Scaffolds

2.4.1.1 Skin

Development of skin graft presents a significant implication for patients suffering from chronic nonhealing wounds, i.e., diabetic ulcer and venous ulcer. To utilize nanofibrous matrix for skin tissue regeneration, various electrospun polymers have been studied. Rho et al. (2006) fabricated biomimetic collagen nanofibers and chemically cross-linked them using a glutaraldehyde vapor. Once their efficacies were tested with normal human keratinocytes in vitro and wound healing effects in rats, they found that while cell adhesion rate was relatively lower in uncoated collagen nanofibers, the nanofibers treated with type I collagen or laminin were functionally active in response to human keratinocytes. These nanofibrous matrices were also very effective in early stage wound healing on rat model (Fig. 2.6). Two different types of polymers, mostly a combination of synthetic and natural ones, are widely used in the fabrication of electrospun polymer blends. Min et al. (2004) produced a nanostructured composite matrix from PLGA/chitin at the ratio of 80/20 (wt/wt). PLGA nanofibers in the average diameter of 310 nm was obtained by electrospinning 15 wt% PLGA solution in polar 1,1,1,3,3,3-hexafluoro-2-propanol (HFIP). Chitin was simultaneously electrospun in the form of nanosized particles, because chitin itself was unable to produce continuous fibers even at high concentration. When human keratinocytes were seeded on the nanofibrous matrix, the results suggested that the composite might be better than PLGA matrix in associated with cell adhesion and spreading. Pan et al. (2006) also combined dextran with PLGA for electrospun composite nanofibers. The cell-scaffold interactions were evaluated in attachment, proliferation, migration, ECM deposition, and gene expression. The overall results demonstrated that the nanofibrous composite was favorable to dermal fibroblasts and that cells could migrate into the highly porous matrix, building a multi-layered dermal-like structure.

2.4.1.2 Cartilage

Articular cartilage is critical for proper knee joint function. As a load-bearing tissue, it provides the articulating surface with a low friction and lubrication for repetitive gliding motions during daily activities. Unfortunately, cartilage has little capability of self-repair once damaged by traumatic injuries or osteoarthritic diseases. Since the concept of tissue engineering emerged in the late 1980s, many researchers have sought a way of making a hyaline-like articular cartilage tissue using both appropriate scaffolds and in vitro cultured chondrocytes or adult stem

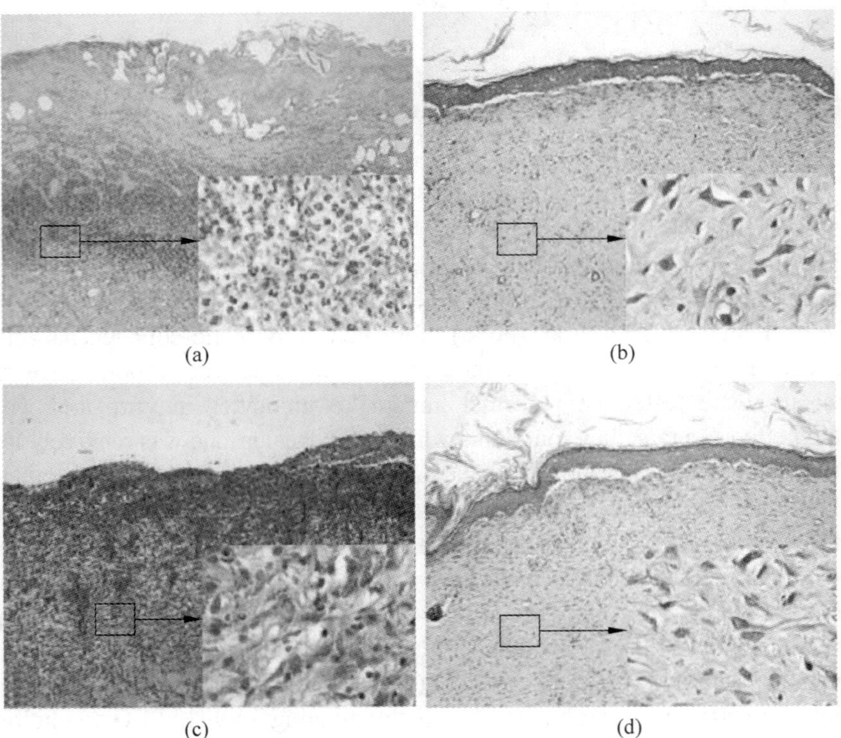

Figure 2.6 Representative photographs of wound healing of rat skin: control group at 1 week (a) and at 4 weeks (b), collagen nanofiber group at 1 week (c), and at 4 weeks (d) (H&E, × 100). Insets: × 400 magnification

cells (Langer and Vacanti, 1993; Gao et al., 2001; Solchaga et al., 2001). The primary function of scaffold is to deliver target cells into cartilage defect sites and to give a mechanical support from the physiological load. Once implanted, the ideal scaffold should encourage production of the ECM by the transplanted cells. Upon the recent applications of electrospinning technology, nanofibrous polymer scaffolds have been given much attention in tissue engineering. Various electrospun nanofibrous polymeric scaffolds have been fabricated and applied for tissue-engineered cartilage formation. Li et al. (2003) prepared an electrospun PCL nanofiber scaffold and then evaluated the biological activity of fetal bovine chondrocytes in vitro passaged between 2 – 6. Gene expression analysis for up to 3 weeks showed that the cells in the nanofibrous scaffold continuously maintained their chondrocytic phenotype by expressing cartilage-specific ECM genes, such as collagen type II and type IX, aggrecan, and cartilage oligomeric matrix protein (COMP). Phenotypic morphology of chondrocytes maintained well in the nanofibrous matrx (Fig. 2.7). In a series of study using human mesenchymal stem cells (MSCs), they used the same PCL nanofibrous scaffold, composed of randomly oriented nanofibers with a diameter of 700 nm, to examine its potential to encourage in vitro chondrogenesis of MSCs (Li et al., 2005). MSCs cultivated for 21 days in the addition of TGF-β1 could differentiate into a chondrocytic phenotype, as supported by chondrocyte-specific gene expression and cartilage-associated ECM proteins. The extent of chondrogenic differentiation in the nanofibrous environment was comparable to that of MSC pellets, a widely accepted model of chondrogenesis of MSCs. In a study of Bhattarai et al. (2005), chitosan-based nanofibers were fabricated by electrospinning the solutions of chitosan, PEO, and Triton X-100. The fibrous matrix with the ratio (wt%) of chitosan/PEO at 90:10 retained an excellent structural integrity in water and promoted the attachment of chondrocytes with characteristic cell morphology as confirmed by SEM analysis. PLGA nanofibrous scaffold was also evaluated for the purpose of cartilage reconstruction (Shin et al., 2006). When porcine articular

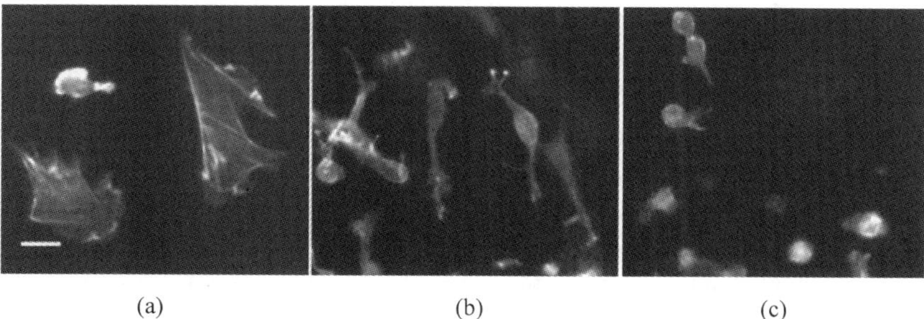

(a) (b) (c)

Figure 2.7 Organization of actin cytoskeleton and cell morphology of FBCs: (a) cells cultured on TCPs in ECM; (b) cells seeded onto PCL nanofibrous scaffolds and maintained in ECM; and (c) cells seeded onto PCL nanofibrous scaffolds and maintained in SEM. Bar, 20 μm. Permission for reproduction from the publisher

chondrocytes were seeded onto the nanofiber PLGA scaffolds, cell proliferation and ECM secretion was found to be superior to those in sponge-type PLGA scaffold. Intermittent hydrostatic pressure was helpful to chondrocyte-seeded nanofibrous scaffold in terms of cell proliferation and ECM production.

2.4.1.3 Bone

Over the past decades, autografts or allografts have been used for the treatment of bone defects, caused by bone diseases or trauma. Due to the limited sources of bone grafts, bioactive materials, such as HA, tricalcium phosphate (TCP), and glasses/glass ceramics have widely utilized in dentistry and orthopedics as a bone substitute. Some specific requirements include bioactivity (osteoconductivity and osteoinductivity), tissue compatibility, and mechanical strength. The biocompatibility of bioactive glasses is believed to be closely associated with the induction of a bone-like mineral phase on the surface, which can be directly integrated with the surrounding host tissues. In addition to the conventional macro/micro scaffolds, various nanofiber scaffolds are being developed for bone tissue engineering. Kim et al. (2006) recently introduced a bioactive glass nanofiber (BGNF) using an electrospinning method, with the diameter in 10s to 100s of nanometers. They reported that the glass nanofiber sustained excellent bioactivity in vitro and that showed favorable cellular responses. The bioactivity of BGNF was identified with the rapid deposition of bone-like minerals on the surface in a simulated body fluid (SBF). Bone marrow-derived stromal cells were attached and proliferated actively in the BGNF mesh and could differentiate into osteoblastic cells with great osteogenic potential. They also developed a nanocomposite, while combining inorganic BGNF with organic collagen as a novel bone regeneration matrix (Kim et al., 2006). Both electrospun BGNF and self-assembled collagen sol were hybridized in the aqueous solution and then crosslinked to make a BGNF-collagen nanocomposite. The composite matrix was excellent in forming bone-like apatite minerals. The osteoblastic cell growth was also great on the matrix and in particular, the alkaline phosphatase activity of the cells was significantly better than that on the collagen. Another bone scaffold was fabricated by electrospinning PCL solution containing nanoparticles of calcium carbonate ($CaCO_3$) or HA (Wutticharoenmongkol et al., 2006). The diameter of as-spun fibers increased with the increasing amount of nanoparticles. As the concentration of PCL solution rose from 8% to 12%, the mechanical strength and fiber diameter increased as well. Indirect cytotoxicity evaluation of PCL/$CaCO_3$ and PCL/HA composite fibers with human osteoblasts revealed their safety to the cells, suggesting their feasibility as a bone scaffold matrix. In another study, bone marrow-derived MSCs (BM-MSCs) were seeded on the PCL matrix and cultured in an osteogenic medium under a dynamic condition for up to 4 weeks (Yoshimoto et al., 2003). Penetration of cells and abundant ECM were noticed after 1 week and additionally, mineralization and type Ⅰ collagen were identified at 4 weeks.

The data supported that electrospun PCL scaffold might be a potential candidate for bone tissue engineering. Proliferation and osteogenic differentiation of MSC was investigated in a nanofiber formed by self-assembly of peptide-amphiphile (PA) (Hosseinkhani et al., 2006). A 3-D network was built by mixing cell suspension with dilute aqueous PA solution (1 wt%) at 1:1 volume ratio. The results showed that self-assembled arginine-glycine-aspartic acid (RGD) containing PA nanofibers had a great potential, showing much higher alkaline phosphatase (ALP) activity and osteocalcin content than the PA nanofibers without RGD during 3-week culture.

2.4.1.4 Blood Vessel

In the last two decades, many attempts have been made to develop small-diameter vascular grafts. Compared to large-diameter blood vessel like aorta, small-diameter blood vessels are much likely to be occluded and the sources of arterial substitutes are very limited. Design of vascular graft should satisfy some specific requirements, because of its unique role in the body, i.e., mechanical resilience and durability from repeated expansion and contraction. Electrospinning may offer great potential in mimicking composition, structure, and mechanical aspects of blood vessel. In an attempt to produce scaffold architecture similar to blood vessel in morphological and mechanical characteristics, Vaz et al. (2005) introduced a sequential multi-layering electrospinning method. It features a bi-layered tubular scaffold, which is composed of stiff, oriented PLLA outer layer and a pliable, randomly oriented PCL inner layer (Fig. 2.8). The flexibility of fiber orientation in the different layers was possible through control of the rotation speed of mandrel-type collector. The electrospun PLLA/PCL scaffolds retained acceptable level of mechanical properties: ultimate tensile stress of 4.3 MPa $\pm$ 0.2 MPa, failure strain of 47.0% $\pm$ 6.3%, and Young's modulus of 30.9 MPa $\pm$ 6.6 MPa. When 3T3 fibroblasts were cultured for 4 weeks on the scaffolds, cell-polymer constructs were proved to be capable of promoting cell growth and proliferation. The bi-layered PLLA/PCL tube scaffold thus presents suitable characteristics as a candidate for tissue-engineered blood vessel. Meanwhile, Stitzel et al. (2006) fabricated a vascular graft scaffold using electrospun polymer blends of type Ⅰ collagen (45%), elastin (15%), and PLGA (40%, 50:50 wt/wt, MW: 110,000) by weight. Three components were mixed in HFIP at a final concentration of 15% (wt/vol). They showed that the nanofibrous scaffolds were cell-compatible with an average of 83% and 72% viability of smooth muscle cells and endothelial cells, respectively during 1 week-culture. In another study, Kwon and Matsuda (2005) designed elastomeric nanofibers made from the combination of equimolar poly (L-lactide-*co*-caprolactone) (PLCL) with type Ⅰ collagen or heparin. Diameter of co-electrospun nanofibers was ranged from 120 to 520 nm. Both diameter and mechanical strength decreased with increasing collagen content in the solution. Transmission electron microscopy (TEM) uncovered that the added type Ⅰ collagen or heparin remained in a dispersed phase, which was localized within a continuous matrix

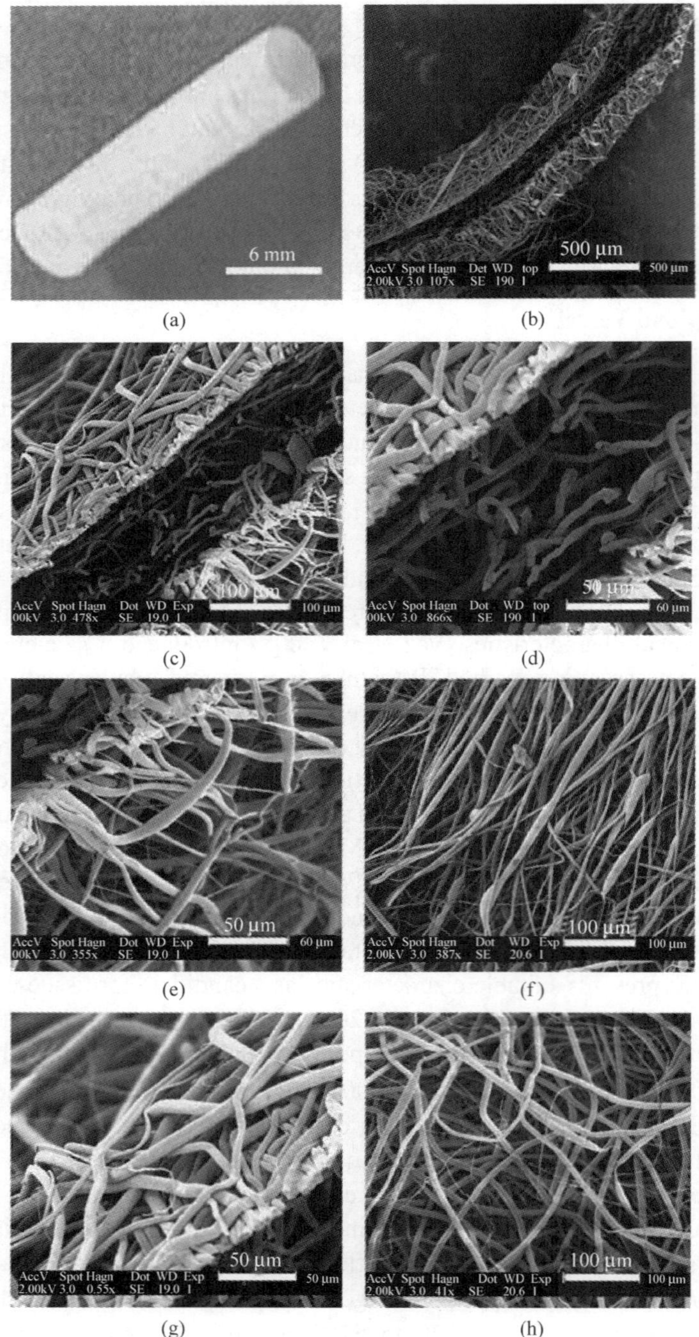

Figure 2.8 SEM micrographs of the bilayered tubular construct: (a) bilayered tube (entire view); (b) bilayered tube wall; (c), (d) details of the interface (mixing zone) between inner and outer layers; (e), (f) details of the outer layer (PLLA); and (g), (h) details of the inner layer (PCL). Permission for reproduction from the publisher

phase of PLCL fibers. Human umbilical vein endothelial cells (HUVECs) on the PLCL scaffold with 5 wt% or 10 wt% collagen exhibited higher elongation and better spreading. In addition, tubular PLCL electrospun nanofabrics, which have inner diameter of 2.3 – 2.5 mm with different wall thickness of 50 – 340 μm, were examined for their mechanical compliances as a small-diameter vascular graft (Inoguchi et al., 2006). Under static condition, based on the compliance-related parameters, i.e., stiffness and diameter compliance, it was found that the narrower the wall thickness, the more compliant the tubular scaffold. In a dynamic pulsatile condition (1 Hz, 90 mmHg/45 mmHg), relative inflation in diameter per pulse increased with the reduction of wall thickness. The results suggested that the preparation of a mechano-sensitive scaffold, responding to pulsatile flow could be possible using PLCL as a base material (Table 2.1).

Table 2.1 Applications of electrospun nanofibers in tissue-engineered scaffolds

Application	Nanofiber	Cell	Reference
Skin	Collagen	Human keratinocytes	(Rho et al., 2006)
	PLGA/chitin	Human keratinocytes	(Min et al., 2004)
	PLGA/dextran	Dermal fibroblasts	(Pan et al., 2006)
Cartilage	PCL	Chondrocytes	(Li et al., 2003)
	PCL	Human mesenchymal stem cells	(Li et al., 2005)
	Chitosan/PEO	Chondrocytes	(Bhattarai et al., 2005)
	PLGA	Chondrocytes	(Shin et al., 2006)
Bone	Bioactive glass	Mesenchymal stem cells	(Kim et al., 2006)
	Bioactive glass-collagen	Osteoblasts	(Kim et al., 2006)
	PCL/$CaCO_3$ and PCL/HA	Human osteoblasts	(Wuttícharoenmongkol et al., 2006)
	PCL	Mesenchymal stem cells	(Yoshimoto et al., 2003)
	Peptide-amphiphile (PA)	Mesenchymal stem cells	(Hosseinkhani et al., 2006)
Blood vessel	PLLA/PCL	Fibroblasts	(Vaz et al., 2005)
	Type I collagen/elastin/ PLGA	Smooth muscle/ endothelial cells	(Stitzel et al., 2006)
	PLCL	Human umbilical vein endothelial cells (HUVECs)	(Kwon and Matsuda, 2005)

2.4.2 Wound Dressing

The goal of wound dressing is to provide an ideal environment for wound healing, such as protection from infection, removal of exudates, and high gas permeation. In this sense, electrospun nanofibrous membrane is considered a good candidate of wound dressing. For wound healing test of nanofibrous PU, a wound (1 cm× 1 cm) was created on the back of guinea pig and then covered with an equal size of electrospun PU nanofibers (Khil et al, 2003). The dressing was changed every 3 days and healing of the wounds was monitored at 3, 6, and 15 days, postoperatively. They reported that from histological examination, the epithelialization rate increased and dermis was well organized in the use of electrospun PU membrane. On the other hand, PCL and PCL-collagen nanofibrous membranes were tested with human dermal fibroblast (HDF) adhesion and proliferation in vitro (Venugopal et al., 2006). The results indicated that cell proliferation significantly increased with PCL-blended collagen nanofibrous membrane up to 25% after 6 days, which was much better than PCL membrane itself. To take advantage of antimicrobial activity of silver, Hong et al. (2006) developed PVA nanofibers containing Ag nanoparticles for wound dressing application by electrospinning PVA/silver nitrate ($AgNO_3$) solution. After a brief heat treatment at 155℃, the PVA/Ag nanofibers became insoluble, while Ag^+ ions were reduced with the production of a large amount of Ag nanoparticles deposited on the surface. It was confirmed that the antibacterial activity of PVA/Ag nanofibers was effective in significantly reducing the number of bacteria colonies after 18 h incubation. In addition, silk fibroin nanofibers were also electrospun and further processed to examine the cell adhesion of human keratinocytes and fibroblasts (Wang et al., 2004). After a couple of pretreatment of raw silk fibers, the degummed silk (SF) sponge was dissolved in 98% formic acid and the concentrations of SF solution were ranged from 3% to 15%. Cell adhesion was assayed using methanol-treated SF nanofibers, in which they were coated with ECM proteins, i.e., type I collagen, fibronectin, and laminin in phosphate-buffered saline (PBS) solution by overnight adsorption at room temperature. Type I collagen-coated SF nanofibers were found to promote better adhesion and spreading of both keratinocyte and fibroblast than those in other groups.

2.4.3 Biomedical Devices and Implants

Recently, nanofibrous polymers have been utilized in medical devices or prostheses. Electrospun protein fibers were deposited onto a neural prosthetic device as a thin film coating. This coated film was supposed to play as an interface between neural tissue and prosthesis. This system is designed to minimize the stiffness difference between them at the interphase and thus improve the chance of successful performance of prosthetic device after implantation. Meanwhile, as abdominal surgery is routinely practiced, adhesion is a common cause of complications, including chronic debilitating pain, bowel obstruction, and female infertility. To prevent this, nanofiberous membrane has been utilized for the prevention of postoperation-induced abdominal adhesion. Zong et al. (2004) investigated the effect of electrospun PLGA impregnated with antibiotics as an anti-adhesion membrane. Rat model was used to evaluate the extent of abdominal adhesion after 4 weeks. They concluded that PLGA nanofibrous membrane was effective in reducing adhesion at the site of injury, in which the membrane acted as a physical barrier with delivery of the incorporated drug.

Nanofibers also find its application as reinforcement filler in the area of biomedical composites. Kim et al. (1999) produced electrospun polybenzimidazole nanofibers, mixed with epoxy matrix. The result showed that fracture toughness significantly increased as a function of the fiber content. Fracture toughness is an important factor in developing polymer composite dental device, i.e., orthodontic bracket. As a dental restorative composite, Fong et al. (2003) incorporated electrospun Nylon 6 nanfibers into 2,2'-bis-[4-(2'-hydroxy-3'-methacryloxypropoxy) phenyl]propane (Bis-GMA) and triethylene glycol dimethacrylate (TEGDMA) resins. A variety of mechanical tests revealed that the composite resin containing the nanofibers possessed considerably improved elastic modulus, flexural strength, and fracture toughness. Another study with electrospun Nylon-4,6 fibers also demonstrated that the mechanical properties of nanofiber/epoxy composite film were significantly advanced as compared to the epoxy resin alone (Bergshoef and Vancso, 1999).

2.4.4 Drug Delivery System

Drug delivery system (DDS) has been sought to boost therapeutic efficacy and minimize the side effects of overdoses. To do this, DDS, which can guarantee a controlled release profile of drug at the needed sites is definitely warranted. Recently, electrospun nanofibrous matrices have been documented as a novel DDS. The main function of biodegradable polymeric nanofiber-based DDS appears that it can act as not only a physical barrier in the target site but an efficient drug delivery vehicle, due mainly to their high surface area. Kim et al. (2004) demonstrated that a hydrophilic antibiotic drug could be successfully incorporated into electrospun PLGA-based nanofibrous scaffolds. Both morphology and density of the scaffold were highly dependent on the drug concentration. Sustained drug release and its antimicrobial effects were identified, inhibiting bacterial growth more than 90%. In another study, tetracycline hydrochloride-loaded electrospun poly(ethylene-*co*-vinylacetate) (PEVA), PLLA, and a 50:50 (wt/wt) blend nanofibers were fabricated, respectively (Kenawy et al., 2002). The drug (5%) was solubilized in methanol and mixed with polymer solution (14% wt/vol) in chloroform. Release of the drug was monitored by placing the samples in Tris buffer and by measuring the absorbance at 360 nm for up to 5 days. Assessment of the release profile indicated that PEVA and blend nanofibers could be better candidate than PLLA ones in the viewpoint of sustained release of the drug over time. When the release pattern was compared between film and electrospun mat, the benefit of nanofiber as a DDS was clear over film, which barely showed sustained release of the drug after initial burst. Verreck et al. (2003) also used the electrospinning technology to prepare drug-loaded nonbiodegradable PU nanofiber for topical drug administration and wound healing. Poorly water-soluble, amorphous drugs, itraconazole and ketanserin, were chosen and the drug/polymer solution in dimethylformamide (DMF) or dimethylacetamide, respectively were electrospun. Release rates and profiles of the incorporated drugs were monitored for up to 60 days and found highly dependent on the nanofiber morphology and drug concentration (10% or 40%). While the diameter of 10% drug-loaded fibers was about 2 μm, that of 40% loaded fibers was ranged from 300 – 700 nm. It was interesting that at lower drug content, itraconazole was released as a linear function of the square root of time, whereas a biphasic release pattern was observed for ketanserin in which two sequential linear components were noticed. Besides the vehicle of drug delivery, electrospun scaffold is utilized in the delivery of DNA for therapeutic applications. Luu et al. (2003) developed a nanofibrous DNA delivery scaffold via electrospinning of PLGA, PLLA-PEG block copolymers, and pCMVβ plasmid (5 mg/mL in Tris- EDTA buffer) together. Release of plasmid DNA from the scaffold was monitored for over 20 days, with the maximum release at ~2 h. Upon the successful incorporation of plasmid DNA, the results presented that DNA released from the nanofibrous scaffold was intact and thus it could hold capability of cellular transfections and encoding of protein β-galactosidase.

2.4.5 Other Applications

Immobilization of enzyme on inert, insoluble substrates represents a significant impact in order to lift the functionality and performance of enzymes for bioprocessing applications. In many cases, the major barriers are low catalytic efficiency and stability of enzymes. Reduction of the size of carrier materials would effectively improve the efficiency of immobilized enzyme. In addition, porous structure can reduce diffusional resistance. With high specific surface area and porous structure, electrospun membrane is considered a good candidate for immobilization of enzymes. Wu et al. (2005) immobilized cellulase in nanofibrous PVA membrane. Both PVA and cellulase were dissolved together in an acetic buffer solution (pH = 4.6) and then electrospun in the diameter of 200 nm. Once crosslinked, the catalytic activity of cellulase in PVA nanofibers was more than 65% the activity of free enzyme. In another study, PS nanofibers were prepared by electrospinning, followed by the chemical attachment of α-chymotrypsin (Jia et al., 2002). The hydrolytic activity of the enzyme-carrying PS nanofibers in aqueous carboxymethyl cellulose (CMC) solution (2%, wt/vol) was over 65% that of the native enzyme, suggesting a high catalytic efficiency as compared to other immobilized ones. Since the covalent binding appeared to have improved the enzyme's functional stability against structural denaturation, the half-life of the nanofibrous enzyme in methanol was 18-fold longer than that of the native one. On the other hand, electrospun nanofibers are also applied in the area of high sensitive sensors. The sensitivity of sensor that detects analytes by interacting with molecules on the surface would increase in parallel with surface area per unit mass. Wang et al. (2002) synthesized poly (AA)-poly (pyrene methanol) (PAA-PM), a fluorescent polymer and mix it with cross-linkable polyurethane latex in DMF. They were electrospun into nanofibrous membrane and tested as a highly responsive fluorescence quenching-based optical sensor for metal ions (Fe^{3+} and Hg^{2+}) and 2, 4-dinitrotoluene (DNT). The resultant sensors exhibited high sensitivity due to the high surface area-to-volume ratio of nanofibrous membrane.

2.5 Concluding Remark

For the past decade, electrospun nanofibers have found the great potential in the area of biomedical applications. They encompass tissue-engineered scaffolds for diverse target tissues, wound dressing, biomedical devices/implants, drug delivery system, and other applications, i.e., biosensor, bioenzyme, and biocatalyst. The most notable benefit of 3-D nanofibrous structure is that its unique architecture can be suitable in providing a biomimetic environment, similar to natural fibrillar network. Technical progress is rapidly underway, including core/shell nanofibers, hollow nanofibers, porous nanofibers, and peptide nanofibers. Along with the promise, some challenges are still pending. Infilteration of seeded cells into nanofibrous structure and even distribution of them are essential for successful performance as a tissue-engineered scaffold. Construction of nanofibrous scaffold with a critical thickness is also necessary for application toward engineering of sizable tissue. For a wide variety of applications of polymer nanofibers, specific functionalization of nanofiber surface and development of novel functional nanofibers are truly justified. Bioengineering of nanofibers is certainly promising technology in the future...

Acknowledgement

This work was supported by KIST grant, 2E20340, from Ministry of Education, Science and Technology, Korea.

References

Bergshoef, M.M. and G.J. Vancso. *Adv. Mater.* 11: 1362 (1999).

Bhattarai, N., D. Edmondson, O. Veiseh, F.A. Matsen and M. Zhang. *Biomaterials* **26**: 6176 (2005).

Bhattarai, S.R., N. Bhattarai, P. Viswanathamurthi, H.K. Yi, P.H. Hwang and H.Y. Kim. *J. Biomed. Mater. Res.* **78A**: 247 (2006).

Buttafoco, L., N.G. Kolkman, P.E. Buijtenhuijs, A.A. Poot, P.J. Dijkstra, I. Vermes and J. Feijen. *Biomaterials* **27**: 724 (2006).

Chen, J., B. Chu, and B.S. Hsiao. *J. Biomed. Mater. Res.* **79A**: 307 (2006).

Choi, S.S., S.G. Lee, S.S. Im and S.H. Kim. *J. Mater. Sci. Lett.* **22**: 891 (2003).

Chua, K.N., C. Chai, P.C. Lee, Y.N. Tang, S. Ramakrishna, K. W. Leong and H.Q. Mao. *Biomaterials* **27**: 6043 (2006).

Chua, K.N., W.S. Lim, P. Zhang, H. Lu, J. Wen, S. Ramakrishna, K.W. Leong and H.Q. Mao. *Biomaterials* **26**: 2537 (2005).

Craighead, H.G., C.D. James and A.M.P. Turner. *Curr. Opin. Solid State Mater. Sci.* **5**: 177 (2001).

Curtis, A. and C. Wilkinson. *Trends Biotech.* **19**: 197 (2001).

Deitzel, J.M., J. Kleinmeyer, D. Harris and N.C.B. Tan. *Polymer* **42**: 261 (2001).

Desai, T.A. *Med. Eng. & Phys.* **22**: 595 (2000).

Deitzel, J.M., J. Kleinmeyer, J.K. Hivonen and T.N.C. Beck. *Polymer* **42**: 8163 (2001).

Doshi, J. and D.H. Reneker. *J. Electrost.* **35**: 151 (1995).

Feng, L., S. Li, H. Li, J. Zhai, Y. Song. and L. Jiang. *Angew. Chem. Int. Ed.* **41**: 1221 (2002).

Flemming, R.G., C.J. Murphy, G.A. Abrams, S.L. Goodman and P.F. Nealey. *Biomaterials* **20**: 573 (1999).

Fong, H. *Polym. Prepr.* **44**: 100 (2003).

Formhals, A. US Patent 1,975,504 (1934).

Frenot, A., and I.S. Chronakis. *Curr. Opin. Colloid Interf. Sci.* **8**: 64 (2003).

Gao, J., J.E. Dennis, L.A. Solchaga, A.S. Awadallah, V.M. Goldberg and A.I. Caplan. *Tissue Eng.* **7**: 363 (2001).

Grafe, T. and K. Graham. *Inter. Nowov. J.* **12**: 51 (2003).

Guan, H., C. Shao, B. Chen, J. Gong, and X. Yang. *Inorg. Chem. Commun.* **6**: 1409 (2003).

He, W., T. Yong, W.E. Teo, Z. Ma, and S. Ramakrishna. *Tissue Eng.* **11**: 1574 (2005).

Hohman, M.M., M. Shin, G. Rutledge and M.P. Brenner. *Phys. Fluids* **13**: 2201 (2001).

Hong, K.H., J.L. Park, I.H. Sul, J.H. Youk and T.J. Kang. *J. Polym. Sci. Part B: Polym. Phys.* **44**: 2468 (2006).

Hosseinkhani, H., M. Hosseinkhani, F. Tian, H. Kobayashi and Y. Tabata. *Biomaterials* **27**: 4079 (2006).

Huang, Z.-M., Y.-Z Zhang, M. Kotaki and S. Ramakrishna. *Comp. Sci. Tech.* **63**: 2223 (2003).

Huang, Z.-M., Y.-Z Zhang, S. Ramakrishna and C.T. Lim. *Polymer* **15**: 5361 (2004).

Inoguchi, H., I.K. Kwon, E. Inoue, K. Takamizawa, Y. Maehara and T. Matsuda. *Biomaterials* **27**: 1470 (2006).

Jia, H., G. Zhu, B. Vugrinovich, W. Kataphinan, D.H. Reneker and P. Wang. *Biotechnol. Prog.* **18**: 1027 (2002).

Kenawy, E.R., G.L. Bowlin, K. Mansfield, J. Layman, D.G. Simpson, E.H. Sanders, and G.E. Wnek. *J. Control. Rel.* **81**: 57 (2002).

Khil, M.S., D.I. Cha, H.Y. Kim I.S. Kim, and N. Bhattarai. *J. Biomed. Mater. Res. Appl. Biomater.* **67B**: 675 (2003).

Kidoaki, S., I.K. Kwon and T. Matsuda. *Biomaterials* **26**: 37 (2005).

Kim, H.W., H.E. Kim and J.C. Knowles. *Adv. Funct. Mater.* **16**: 1529 (2006).

Kim, H.W., J.H. Song and H.E. Kim. *J. Biomed. Mater.* Res. **79A**: 698 (2006).

Kim, J.S. and D.H. Reneker. *Polym. Comp.* **20**: 124 (1999).

Kim, K., Y.K. Luu, C. Chang, D. Fang, B.S. Hsiao, B. Chu and M. Hadjiargyrou. *J. Control. Rel.* **98**: 47 (2004).

Koombhonge, S., W. Liu and D.H. Reneker. *J. Polym. Sci. Polym. Phys. Ed.* **39**: 2598 (2001).

Kwon, I.K. and T. Matsuda. *Biomacromol.* **6**: 2096 (2005).

Langer, R. and J.P. Vacanti. *Science* **260**: 920 (1993).

Laurencin, C.T., A.M. Ambrosio, M.D. Borden and J.A. Cooper Jr. *Ann. Rev. Biomed. Eng.* **1**: 19 (1999).

Li, D. and Y. Xia. *Adv. Mater.* **16**: 1151 (2004).

Li, M., Y. Guo, Y. Wei, A.G. MacDiarmid and P.I. Lelkes. *Biomaterials* **27**: 2705 (2006).

Li, W.J., K.G. Danielson, P.G. Alexander, and R.S. Tuan. *J. Biomed. Mater. Res.* **67A**: 1105 (2003).

Li, W.J., R. Tuli, C. Okafor, A. Derfoul, K.G. Danielson, D.J. Hall and R.S. Tuan. *Biomaterials* **26**: 599 (2005).

Liu, G.J., J.F. Ding, L.J. Guo, B.P. Dymov and J.T. Gleeson. *Chem. A Eur. J.* **5**: 2740 (1999).

Luu, Y.K., K. Kim, B.S. Hsiao, B. Chu and M. Hadjiargyrou. *J. Control. Rel.* **89**: 341 (2003).

Ma, P.X. and R. Zhang. *J. Biomed. Mater. Res.* **46**: 60 (1999).

Martin, C.R. *Chem. Mater.* **8**: 1739 (1996).

Min, B.M., G. Lee, S.H. Kim, Y.S. Nam, T.S. Lee and W.H. Park. *Biomaterials* **25**: 1289 (2004).

Min, B.M., Y. You, J.M. Kim, S.J. Lee and W.H. Park. *Carbohyd. Polym.* **57**: 285 (2004).

Ondarcuchu, T. and C. Joachim. *Europhys. Lett.* **42**: 215 (1998).

Pan, H., H. Jiang and W. Chen. *Biomaterials* **27**: 3209 (2006).

Park, K., Y.M. Ju, H.J. Jung, J.-J. Kim, K.-D. Ahn, and D.K. Han. *Macromol. Res.* **14**: 552 (2006).

Park, K., Y.M. Ju, J.S. Son, K.-D. Ahn, and D.K. Han. *J. Biomater. Sci. Polym. Edn.* **18**: 369 (2007).

Reneker, D.H. and I. Chun. *Nanotech.* **7**: 216 (1996).

Reneker, D.H., A.L. Yarin, H. Fong and S.J. Koombhongse. *Appl. Phys.* **87**: 4531 (2000).

Rho, K.S., L. Jeong, G. Lee, B.M. Seo, Y.J. Park, S.D. Hong, S. Roh, W.H. Park and B.M. Min. *Biomaterials* **27**: 1452 (2006).

Sanders J.E., S.E. Lamont, A. Karchin, S.L. Golledge and B.D. Ratner. *Biomaterials* **26**: 813 (2005).

Shin, H.J., C.H. Lee, I.H. Cho, Y.J. Kim, Y.J. Lee, I.A. Lee, K.D. Park, N. Yui and J.W. Shin.

J. Biomater. Sci. Polym. Edn. **17**: 103 (2006).
Shin, Y.M., M.M. Hohman, M.P. Brenner and G.C. Rutledge. *Polymer* **42**: 9955 (2001).
Silva, G.A., C. Czeisler, K.L. Niece, E. Beniash, D.A. Harrington, J.A. Kessler and S.I. Stupp. *Science* **303**: 1352 (2004).
Solchaga, L.A., V.M. Goldberg, and A.I. Caplan. *Clin. Orthop. Res.* **391S**: S161 (2001).
Son, W.K., D. Cho, and W.H. Park. *Nanotech.* **17**: 439 (2006).
Spivak, A.F., Y.A. Dzenis and D.H. Reneker. *Mech. Res. Commun.* **27**: 37 (2000).
Stitzel, J., J. Liu, S.J. Lee, M. Komura, J. Berry, S. Soker, G. Lim, M.V. Dyke, R. Czerw, J.J. Yoo and A. Atala. *Biomaterials* **27**: 1088 (2006).
Taylor, G.. *Proc. R. Soc.* **A 280**: 383 (1964).
Tsai, P., H. Schreuder-Gibson and P. Gibson, *J. Electrost.* **54**: 333 (2002).
Tuzlakoglu, K., N. Bolgen, A.J. Salgado, M.E. Gomes, E. Piskin and R.L. Reis. *J. Mater. Sci. Mater. Med.* **16**: 1099 (2005).
Vaz, C.M., S. van Tuijl, C.V.C. Bouten and F.P.T. Baaijens. *Acta Biomater.* **1**: 575 (2005).
Venugopal, J.R., Y. Zhang and S. Ramakrishna. *Artif. Organs* **30**: 440 (2006).
Verreck, G., I. Chun, J. Rosenblatt, J. Peeters, A.V. Dijck, J. Mensch, M. Noppe and M.E. Brewster. *J. Control. Rel.* **92**: 349 (2003).
Wang, X., C. Drew, S.H. Lee, K.J. Senecal, J. Kumar and L.A. Samuelson. *Nano lett.* **2**: 1273 (2002).
Wang, X.Y., Y.G. Kim, C. Drew, B.C. Ku, J. Kumar and L.A. Samuelson. *Nano Lett.* **4**: 331 (2004).
Whitesides, G.M. and B. Grzybowski. *Science* **295**: 2418 (2002).
Wu, L., X. Yuan and J. Sheng. *J, Membr. Sci.* **250**: 167 (2005).
Wutticharoenmongkol, P., N. Sanchavanakit, P. Pavasant and P. Supaphol. *Macromol. Biosci.* **6**: 70 (2006).
Xinhua, Z., K. Kim, R. Shaofeng, B.S. Hsiao and B. Chu. *Polymer* **43**: 4403 (2002).
Yarin, A.L., S.J. Koombhongse and D.H. Reneker. *J. Appl. Phys.* **90**: 4836 (2001).
Yoshimoto, H., Y.M. Shin, H. Terai, and J.P. Vacanti. *Biomaterials* **24**: 2077 (2003).
Zeleny, J. *Phys. Rev.* **10**: 1(1917).
Zhang, Y., C.T. Lim, S. Ramakrishna and Z.M. Huang. *J. Mater. Sci. Mater. Med.* **16**: 933 (2005).
Zhang, Y.Z., Y. Feng, Z.M. Huang, S. Ramakrishna and C.T. Lim. *Nanotech.* **17**: 910 (2006).
Zhong, S., W.E. Teo, X. Zhu, R. Beuerman, S. Ramakrishna and L.Y.L. Yung. *Biomacromol.* **6**: 2998 (2005).
Zong, X., S. Li, E. Chen, B. Garlick, K.S. Kim, D. Fang, J. Chiu, T. Zimmerman, C. Brathwaite, B.S. Hsiao and B. Chu. *Annals Surg.* **240**: 910 (2004).

3 Nanoscale Mechanisms for Assembly of Biomaterials

Zhijie Sui[1] and William L. Murphy[1,2,3]

[1] Department of Biomedical Engineering, University of Wisconsin-Madison, Madison, WI 53706, USA

[2] Department of Pharmacology, University of Wisconsin-Madison, Madison, WI 53706, USA

[3] Department of Materials Science and Engineering, University of Wisconsin-Madison, Madison, WI 53706, USA

Abstract Non-covalent interactions are a ubiquitous mechanism directing assembly of natural materials. Similarly, these types of interactions have become an important component of emerging approaches in biomaterials science. In view of the emerging importance of bio-inspired materials in medical applications, this chapter will be focused on describing the fundamentals of intermolecular interactions and their applications in biomaterials science. The particular focus will be on processes and structures that mimic the natural ECM.

Keywords tissue engineering, bioinspired, biomimetic, self-assembly, and scaffold.

3.1 Introduction

Biomaterials have been broadly defined as synthetic or naturally derived materials used in therapeutic or diagnostic systems (Langer and Tirrell, 2004). They are typically chosen based on their favorable interaction with natural tissues, and are commonly used as implants, prostheses, or surgical instruments. Many biomaterials, such as polyurethane, hydroxyapatite and metal alloys, have been developed and successfully applied in clinical practice, such as artificial hips, vascular stents, artificial pacemakers, and catheters. However, these traditional biomaterials are typically assembled at the macroscopic scale by processing inorganic crystals or organic macromolecules, and this limits one's ability to control molecular level interactions. In contrast, the structure and function of natural biological materials

(1) Corresponding e-mail: wlmurphy@wisc.edu

are often tailored via molecular self-assembly. It is becoming evident that novel biomaterials that can interact with cells and tissues or carry out biologically specific functions at a molecular level with a high degree of specificity could expand the capabilities of biomaterials in a variety of medical applications.

One way of designing materials at the molecular level is to mimic natural materials, since nature has been evolving such materials for billions of years. A particularly relevant example is the structurally well-defined and functionally interactive scaffold in which cells reside—the extracellular matrix (ECM) (Alberts et al., 2004). The ECM is an intricate network composed of mainly proteins and polysaccharides, and it provides a physical support for cells to survive and perform their biological functions such as proliferation during tissue growth and motility during muscle contraction. The ECM interactively influences cell behavior by providing biological signals, including binding sites to facilitate cell attachment, enzyme-labile sequences to enable cell-mediated remodeling, and sequestered signaling molecules (e.g. growth factors) to regulate cell function. The ECM also provides physicochemical signals, including porosity, mechanical stability, elasticity, and mass transport conduits. A fundamental premise guiding recent biomaterials design is that by understanding how the ECM interacts with cells on the molecular level, one can develop novel biologically-derived or 'bio-inspired' materials that interact with cells and respond to their biological environment. The general premise guiding recent research in this area is that direct mimicry of biological systems or processes with well-designed modifications may yield novel biomaterials with enhanced properties.

If one is to create bio-inspired materials, then a first logical question is 'how are natural materials assembled'? Mother Nature generates biomaterials largely through directed molecular self-assembly, which is a spontaneous process that results in stable, structurally well-defined supramolecular architectures (Whitesides et al., 1991). Indeed, self-assembly is a key mechanism that underlies formation of macroscopic biological entities (e.g. cells, ECMs) from biological precursor molecules like proteins. For example, in the natural ECM, biopolymers such as proteins and polysaccharides self-assemble into nanometer-scale fibrous three-dimensional structures, then intertwine to form macroscopic, porous, and stable network architectures. Recent research in fields ranging from materials chemistry to tissue engineering has attempted to determine how biological materials are formed and, in turn, how their assembly mechanisms might be exploited.

In view of the emerging importance of bio-inspired materials in medical applications, this chapter will be focused on describing the fundamentals of intermolecular interactions and their applications in biomaterials science. The particular focus will be on the processes and structures that mimic the natural ECM. The next section will introduce the fundamental physics of intermolecular interactions and their relevance in the ECM. We will use protein folding throughout this section as a specific example to highlight the importance of each type of interaction. The third section of the chapter will describe self-assembly approaches that have been used to generate biomimetic materials. The fourth section will briefly review some recently developed biomaterials that are constructed based on molecular-level self-assembly or possess the ability to interact with biologically active macromolecules through non-covalent interactions. Particular emphasis will be placed on the potential application of these biomaterials in medical applications (e.g. drug delivery, tissue engineering).

3.2 Non-Covalent Intermolecular Interaction

Molecular self-assembly directs supramolecular assemblies mainly through non-covalent interactions. Non-covalent interactions are different from covalent bonding, in that they are reversible, relatively weak, and in many cases specific. As a result of these properties, non-covalent interactions are a ubiquitous mechanism in nature and the basis for directing assembly of many supramolecular biological systems. For example, although covalent bonds form the backbone of a polypeptide chain, it is the 3-D structure that largely dictates a protein's functionality and bioactivity, and this complex, properly folded 3-D structure is almost exclusively manipulated through various non-covalent interactions. Many cell signaling pathways also use reversible non-covalent interactions as a mechanism to efficiently transduce signals. Therefore, understanding the principles of these interactions is essential to understand natural systems and may be beneficial in modern biomaterials design and synthesis.

A non-covalent interaction is defined as (Kollman, 1977) an interaction between molecules in which there is no change in either chemical bondings or electron pairings. In contrast to the strong (typically >100 kJ/mol), stoichiometric (i.e. one-to-one interaction between atoms) and directional nature of covalent bonds, non-covalent interactions are generally weaker, non-stoichiometric, less directional, and more sensitive to the environment. Several specific contrasts can be drawn between these types of interactions. While covalent bonds are generally shorter than 2 Å, non-covalent interactions usually function within a range of several angstroms. The formation of a covalent bond requires overlap of partially occupied electron orbitals of interacting atoms, which share a pair of electrons, whereas no orbital overlapping or electron sharing takes place in non-covalent interactions. Furthermore, although the entropy change during formation of an irreversible covalent bond contributes to the overall free energy change less than enthalpy change, it often plays a more important role in non-covalent self-assembly processes, especially when the enthalpies of the interactions holding the molecules together are relatively weak. For example, non-covalent complexation between oppositely charged polyelectrolytes was theoretically predicted (Michaels, 1965) and recently experimentally observed to be an entropy-driven, athermal process (Bucur et al., 2006).

Although in general weaker than covalent bonds, non-covalent interactions are the primary mechanism dictating the conformations of biomacromolecules (e.g.

proteins, DNA). They are also the prominent mechanism directing assembly of hierarchical structures in supramolecular biological assemblies, such as the coiled coil structure of some protein fibrils. It is cooperativity that allows these weak non-covalent interactions to build into strong, stable molecular interactions and hierarchical structures. If the simultaneous presence of multiple interactions in a single molecule or a supramolecular assembly produces positive cooperativity, then the overall interaction can be much stronger than might be expected from the sum of their individual strengths. For example, individual ions such as sodium and chloride ions are dissociated and solvated in aqueous solution due to (1) the entropy increase upon ion dissociation and (2) the strong interactions of ions with water molecules. In contrast, oppositely charged polyelectrolytes bind strongly to one another in aqueous solution to form insoluble complexes. These systems behave quite differently despite the fact that each is driven by electrostatic interactions between oppositely charged ions. Chemical complementarity and structural compatibility is essential in creating the kind of positive cooperative interaction observed in polyelectrolyte complexes.

Compared to strong and irreversible covalent bonds, the non-covalent interactions seem to be a poor choice of interaction to hold macromolecules and supramolecular assemblies together. However, since biological processes are dynamic and need constant remodeling and reorganizing, relatively weak and reversible non-covalent interactions are indeed advantageous energetically. For example, in order to produce large quantity of hierarchically structured proteins and keep the structural fidelity, it is more efficient to synthesize simple linear polypeptides first, and then allow them to self-assemble into 'correct' structures based on the built-in structural information in their sequences.

In the following sections the fundamental physics of non-covalent interactions will be briefly reviewed (readers are referred to (Israelachvili, 1991) for a comprehensive description of intermolecular interactions). Throughout this section we will highlight the importance of each type of non-covalent interaction during protein folding (Fig. 3.1), as this process is: (1) ubiquitous in biological systems; (2) driven almost exclusively by non-covalent interactions; (3) a key mechanism for the assembly of natural and synthetic ECMs.

3.2.1 Electrostatic Interaction

All intermolecular interactions are thought to be essentially electrostatic in origin [p11 in (Israelachvili, 1991)]. Electrostatic interactions are originated between ions, permanent dipoles and induced dipoles. They can be either attractive or repulsive and are non-directional. Specific types of electrostatic interactions will be introduced in the following subsections. The intention of this subsection is to classify the types of electrostatic interactions and briefly introduce the physics governing each interaction. Examples of the importance of the interactions in protein folding or assembly will be given in some cases to highlight the importance of the interactions.

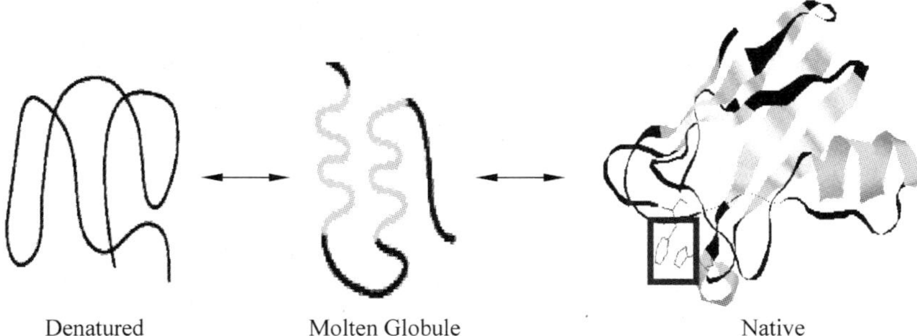

Figure 3.1 Schematic representation of the interactions that direct protein (plastocyanin) assembly during initial folding (Color Fig. 1). The structure is color-coded by the types of noncovalent interactions. Hydrogen bonding is represented by red (α-helix) or yellow (β-sheet), salt bridges are shown between lysine (blue) and glutamate (orange) residues, and π-π interaction is shown in purple (included in the blue box) between the side chains of histidine and phenylalanine residues. The protein crystal structure is from the Protein Data Bank (PDB ID: 1KDI)

3.2.1.1 Ion-Ion Interaction

The interaction between two ions is also known as the Coulomb force. The energy of such an interaction is given by

$$E \propto \frac{q_1 q_2}{4\pi\varepsilon_0\varepsilon_r r} \tag{3.1}$$

where q represents the charge the ions carry; ε_0 is the vacuum permittivity; ε_r is the relative permittivity or dielectric constant of the medium; and r is the distance between the two ions. The dependence on $1/r$ makes this a relatively strong and long-range force when compared to other types of non-covalent interactions (see below).

In the context of protein structure and folding, interactions between proximal, oppositely charged moieties are known as 'salt bridges'. These charged entities include cationic residues (Lys, Arg, His, and the *N*-terminus) and anionic residues (Glu, Asp, and the C-terminus) in the protein. During protein folding the ion-ion interaction plays a critical role in allowing a protein to fold into its native state (Fig. 3.1). Ionic interactions are an important component of several biomimetic assembly processes, in which cooperative binding takes place (see Section 3.3.1 below).

3.2.1.2 Ion-Dipole Interaction

An ion-dipole interaction is the force between a charged group and a polar group. The energy of this type of interaction is given by

$$E \propto \frac{qu}{4\pi\varepsilon_0\varepsilon_r r^2} \tag{3.2}$$

where u refers to the dipole moment of the polar group, and other variables are as defined above for ion-ion interactions. Interactions between charged amino acid residues (listed above) and polar residues (e.g. Ser, Thr, Tyr, Asn, and Gln) in a protein fall under this category. A common ion-dipole interaction in a protein structure is the interaction between the negative charge on a carboxylate group and the dipole of a hydroxyl or amine group. This kind of interactions is commonly considered hydrogen bonding, and will be introduced in Section 3.2.2.

A cation-π interaction is a special kind of non-covalent ion-dipole interaction between the electron-rich π orbitals of an aromatic ring and an adjacent cation. These interactions are relatively strong (5 – 80 kJ/mol), approximately equivalent in energy to a hydrogen bond (Ma and Dougherty, 1997). Cation-π interactions are remarkably common in protein structures, as over 25% of all tryptophan residues are involved in energetically favorable cation-π interactions (Dougherty, 1996; Gallivan and Dougherty, 1999).

3.2.1.3 Ion-Induced Dipole Interaction

An ion-induced dipole interaction is the force between a charged group and a nonpolar group. The energy of this type of interaction is given by

$$E \propto \frac{q^2 \alpha}{(4\pi\varepsilon_0\varepsilon_r)^2 r^4} \tag{3.3}$$

where α refers to the polarizability of the nonpolar group and other variables are as defined above for ion-ion interactions. When nonpolar molecules or groups interact with adjacent charged or polar molecules, transient dipole moments can be induced through polarization. Interactions between charged amino acid residues and nonpolar residues such as Leu and Ile in a protein fall under this category.

3.2.1.4 Dipole-Dipole Interaction

A dipole-dipole interaction is defined as an interaction between molecules or groups having a permanent electric dipole moment (IUPAC Compendium of Chemical Terminology). When the dipole moments are in fixed orientation (e.g. when they are close to each other), energy is given by

$$E \propto \frac{u_1 u_2}{4\pi\varepsilon_0\varepsilon_r r^3} \tag{3.4}$$

When the two dipole moments are free to rotate, generally at large separations or in a high ε media, the net strength of the dipole-dipole interaction is angle-averaged. The energy of such an interaction, also termed Keesom force, is given by

$$E \propto \frac{u_1^2 u_2^2}{(4\pi\varepsilon_0\varepsilon_r)^2 r^6} \tag{3.5}$$

where u_1 and u_2 are the dipole moments of the interacting species. Interactions between polar residues (e.g. Ser, Tyr, and Thr) in a protein fall under this category.

A special kind of dipole-dipole interaction between aromatic rings is called a π-π interaction (2 – 10 kJ/mol). The π electrons present in aromatic rings are localized above and below the face of the ring. This excess of electrons gives the face of the ring a partial negative charge whereas the hydrogen atoms on its edge have a corresponding net positive charge. The electrostatic interactions between these partial charges result in the so-called π-π interaction. It dominates the interactions between aromatic side chains during protein folding, thus play an important role in the tertiary and even quaternary structure of proteins that contain Phe, Tyr or Trp residues (Fig. 3.1) (McGaughey et al., 1998). According to Burley and Petsko's analysis of 4 biphenyl peptides and 34 proteins (Burley et al., 1985), on average 60% of aromatic side chains are involved in π-π interactions, and 80% form networks of three or more interacting aromatic side chains. 80% of these energetically favorable interactions stabilized tertiary structure, and 20% stabilized quaternary structure.

3.2.1.5 Dipole-Induced Dipole Interaction

A dipole-induced dipole interaction takes place between one polar molecule and one nonpolar molecule. It is often termed an induction force or Debye force. The energy of this type of interaction is given by

$$E \propto \frac{u^2 \alpha}{(4\pi \varepsilon_0 \varepsilon_r)^2 r^6} \tag{3.6}$$

This interaction is usually categorized as one subset of the van der Waals forces (see the next subsection for the definition of the van der Waals force).

3.2.1.6 Induced Dipole-Induced Dipole Interaction

An induced dipole-induced dipole interaction is also known as a dispersion force or a London force (p83 in (Israelachvili, 1991)). It acts between all atoms and molecules. The energy of this type of interaction is given by the same equation described above for dipole-induced dipole interactions.

Keesom, Debye (induction) and London (dispersion) forces together make up what are generally called van der Waals forces (<5 kJ/mol). These ubiquitous interactions are relatively weak and short-range ($1/r^6$ distance dependence). They essentially contribute to all types of self-assembly in biology and biomaterials science. Van der Waals forces may act as an important stabilizing factor in the closely packed interiors of a native protein, because these forces act over only short distances and hence are lost when the protein is unfolded. Although weak individually, careful design of chemical complementarity and structural compatibility can result in positive cooperativity, which enables van der Waals interactions to serve as an essential component of the structural integrity of certain biological materials. For example, neighboring β-sheets in silk fibroin are held together through van der Waals forces, resulting in the mechanically stable yet flexible property of silk (Voet et al., 2001).

Although non-covalent intermolecular interactions are considered primarily electrostatic in this chapter, a couple of special interactions, hydrogen bonding and hydrophobic interactions, are worth describing more specifically and in more detail due to their prevalence in biological systems. These interactions are often a combination of different types of electrostatic interactions.

3.2.2 Hydrogen Bonding

A hydrogen bond, D—H···A, is formed between a hydrogen atom, which is formally bonded to an electronegative donor atom (D), and a neighboring acceptor atom (A). The main component of the hydrogen bond is an electrostatic interaction between the dipole of the donor-hydrogen bond, in which the hydrogen atom has a partial positive charge, and a partial negative charge on the acceptor atom. The hydrogen atom is special in being able to interact strongly with one electronegative atom while being covalently attached to another. The length of hydrogen bonds depends on bond strength, temperature, and pressure and the bond strength itself is dependent on temperature, pressure, bond angle, and the environment, usually characterized by local dielectric constant. The typical length of a hydrogen bond in water is 1.97 Å and the strength of most hydrogen bonds lies between 10 – 40 kJ/mol. The strength of O—H···N, O—H···O, N—H···N, and N—H···O interactions is approximately 29 kJ/mol, 21 kJ/mol, 13 kJ/mol, and 8 kJ/mol, respectively (Jeffrey, 1997; Scheiner, 1997).

Hydrogen bonding plays an important role in determining a protein's secondary structures. For example, α-helix and β-sheet secondary structures are formed through numerous hydrogen bonds on the polypeptide backbone. In an α-helix, the hydrogen bonds are between the backbone C═O groups and N—H groups that are four residues farther along the same polypeptide chain, whereas in a β sheet, hydrogen bonding occurs between neighboring polypeptide chains (Fig. 3.1).

3.2.3 Hydrophobic Interactions

Ion-ion interactions and hydrogen bonding between two polar or charged molecules in an aqueous environment are not particularly favorable energetically because there are competing interactions between the molecules and the water surrounding them. However, the interactions between nonpolar molecules and water molecules are less favorable because these molecules lack the ability to form hydrogen bonds. This relative absence of interactions among the nonpolar molecules and water molecules results in interactions among the nonpolar groups themselves, and this preference is known as hydrophobic interaction.

Hydrophobic interactions, which cause nonpolar substances to minimize their contacts with water, are an important determinant of native protein structure (Kellis et al., 1988; Spolar et al., 1989). Most folded proteins have a hydrophobic core in which side chain packing stabilizes the folded state, and charged or polar side chains are largely partitioned to the solvent-exposed surface where they interact with surrounding water molecules. An illustrative example is the coiled coil structure of the extracellular matrix (ECM) protein α-keratin, in which two α-helical polypeptide chains are twisted to form a left-handed coil, and this structure is formed through a hydrophobic interaction between the two hydrophobic strips on each α-helical chain (Voet et al., 2001).

3.2.4 Non-Covalent Interactions in Biological Systems

Each of the interactions described in this section plays a role not only in the aforementioned protein folding and stabilization processes, but also intermolecular interactions between proteins and various ligands. The ligands may be small molecules (e.g. metabolites, peptides, oligonucleotides) or macromolecules (e.g. DNA, RNA, other proteins), and the binding between a protein and a ligand is often very strong and specific. These binding events, often termed 'molecular recognition' (Fig. 3.2(c)), are a key element of virtually all biological processes, from enzyme-mediated metabolism to tissue and organ development. Molecular recognition plays a prominent role in cell-ECM interactions, as cell adhesion and migration are regulated by integrin binding to adhesion ligands in the ECM, and cell proliferation and differentiation are regulated by binding of cell surface receptors to specific signaling cues (e.g. protein growth factors) in the ECM. Instead of taking advantage of any individual non-covalent force, molecular recognition interactions are usually dictated by a collection of non-covalent interactions working cooperatively, and 'affinity'—meaning the strength of the binding—is largely determined by the efficiency of this cooperativity. We will often refer to these types of interactions as 'affinity-based' interactions in this chapter, to distinguish these interactions from those in which one dominant type of non-covalent force is operative.

The equilibrium dissociation constant (K_d) is commonly used to quantitatively represent the binding affinity. When a ligand (L) and a protein (P) are associated to form a complex (PL) in a solution, the corresponding equilibrium dissociation constant is defined as:

$$K_d = \frac{[P][L]}{[PL]} \tag{3.7}$$

where [P], [L] and [PL] represent the concentrations of the protein, ligand and bound complex, respectively. The dissociation constant has units of molarity (M), and corresponds to the concentration of ligand [L] at which the binding site on the protein is half occupied, i.e. when the concentration of protein with ligand bound [PL] equals the concentration of protein with no ligand bound [P]. The smaller the dissociation constant, the more tightly bound the ligand is; for example, a ligand with a nanomolar (nM) dissociation constant binds more tightly than a ligand with a micromolar (μM) dissociation constant. Molecular recognition events in natural systems often have dissociation constants lower than nM, and therefore show significant binding even at very low protein and ligand concentrations. When these interactions are used for self-assembly, they can have a wide range of affinities, and the affinity of the interaction impacts the stability and dynamics of a molecular assembly (see (Whitesides et al., 1991; Whitesides, and Grzy bowski, 2002) for a more comprehensive review of molecular self-assembly interactions).

3.2.5 Summary

The interactions between biological molecules are often complex, but can ultimately be understood as a composite of the several types of non-covalent interactions described in this section. Thus, non-covalent interactions represent the driving force behind natural processes ranging from protein dimerization to organogenesis. The same fundamental interactions may also be used as driving forces to assemble novel synthetic biomaterials, which will be discussed in the following section. Non-covalent interactions are also the driving force behind molecular recognition events in biological systems, and these interactions can be mimicked to create materials that act as synthetic mimics of the extracellular matrix. We will discuss this concept in Section 3.4.

3.3 Approaches for Bioinspired Nanoscale Assembly of Biomaterials

Recent research has begun to unveil nature's delicate design of hierarchical structures, and yet most biological assembly processes remain incompletely understood and unpredictable. Furthermore, it has proven difficult to duplicate the sophisticated structure and function of biological assemblies with synthetic molecules. In order to establish supramolecular structure through self-assembly one must build sufficient information into the molecular building blocks so that the desired structure forms spontaneously, and this is a daunting task. Moreover, nature is capable of designing interactive assemblies that change their properties in response to specific biochemical or physical stimuli, such as pH, temperature, ligand binding, ionic strength, or electric field, and it is uniquely challenging to mimic these functions.

However, the emergence of molecular biology and genetic engineering coupled with recent advances in peptide and nucleic acid synthesis has enabled many functional and biologically active supramolecular structures to be built. Micelles, vesicles, lamella, bicontinuous structures, and fibrils are some common types of structures assembled via the non-covalent interactions introduced in the previous section. Many biologically derived molecules, such as peptides, nucleotides and lipids, have been successfully used as the building blocks of these biomimetic assemblies. Some specific examples will be given below, and they are categorized based on their dominant assembly mechanism (Fig. 3.2). Although we do not explicitly focus on biomedical applications in this section, each of the assemblies described may ultimately have relevance to the biomaterials-related applications described in Section 3.4, including tissue engineering and drug delivery.

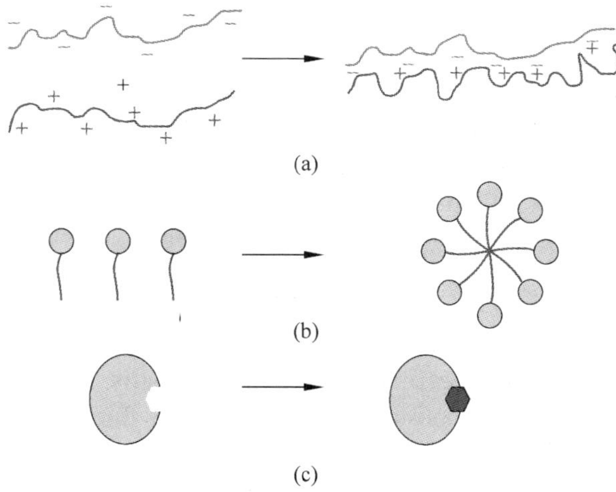

Figure 3.2 Schematic representations of molecules self-assembling into hierarchical structures; (a) cooperative assembly of polyelectrolytes into a complex based via ion-ion interactions; (b) assembly of micellar structure via hydrophobic interactions; (c) Binding of complementary molecules via molecular recognition or 'affinity-based interactions'

3.3.1 Supramolecular Assembly Based Primarily on Ion-Ion Interactions

Thanks in part to the emergence of solid-phase peptide synthesis (Fields and Noble, 1990), which established a routine synthetic protocol to create short peptides (typically <100 amino acids), bio-molecules are becoming important building blocks for supramolecular assembly. They provide versatility of monomeric units (e.g. natural and unnatural amino acids, modified or unmodified nucleotides) and control over molecular architecture. Furthermore, peptides allow one to borrow well-defined structural motifs from nature, and these motifs have been evolved over millions of years (Tu and Tirrell, 2004). Therefore, investigators have developed many peptide-based self-assembling systems with a variety of supramolecular structures and biologically active functions.

Ion-ion interactions between peptides have been used to build a variety of nanometer-scale structures. For example, Zhang and coworkers have developed a class of ionic self-complementary peptides (Zhang, 2003; Zhao and Zhang, 2006), and used these molecules to form nanofiber-like structure spontaneously. These peptides fold into β-sheet structures in aqueous solution with one hydrophilic and one hydrophobic surface. The unique structural feature of these peptides is that they have regular spacing between ionic groups on the hydrophilic surface, and thus form complementary ionic bonds between molecules. Upon the addition of monovalent alkaline cations or the introduction of the peptide solutions into physiological media, these oligopeptides spontaneously assemble to form matrices. The matrices are made of interwoven nanofibers, which typically have 10 – 20 nm in diameter and a few hundred nanometers to a few microns in length (Yokoi, 2005).

In an alternative approach, Pandya et al. used ion-ion interactions to assembly two 28-residue peptides into an extended coiled-coil fiber (Pandya, 2000). Inspired from nature's leucine zipper-like motif and α-helical coiled-coil structure, the peptides were designed to form staggered heterodimers. These heterodimers had 'sticky-ends' to promote the formation of fibers of at least several hundred micrometers long and 20 times thicker than expected for the dimeric coiled-coil design. The 'sticky-ends' were generated by staggering the ends of the peptides so that residue 1 – 14 of the first peptide preferentially interacts with residue 15 – 28 of the second via ion-ion interactions. The thickness of these fibers implied lateral association of the designed structures. Pandya et al. proposed that complementary features present in repeating structures promoted lateral assembly, and that a similar mechanism may underlie fibrillogenesis in certain natural systems. This example illustrates another theme in biomimetic self-assembly—the use of synthetic systems to gain insight into natural assembly processes. It is noteworthy that these extended fibers can be supplemented with special 'fiber shaping' peptides, which are subunits of the original peptides designed to introduce morphological variations and produce kinked, waved and branched fibers (Ryadnov and woolfson, 2003).

In another approach, Zhang and coworkers have extended peptide-based self-assembly to include structurally dynamic peptides based in part on ion-ion interactions. For example, one 16-residue peptide has a β-sheet structure at ambient temperature with 5 nm in length but undergoes an abrupt structural transition at high temperatures to form a stable α-helical structure with 2.5 nm in length (Zhang and Rich, 1997; Altman et al., 2000). These peptides have a cluster of negatively charged aspartate or glutamate residues close to the N-terminus and a cluster of positively charged lysine or arginine residues near the C-terminus. Because of the unique sequence, the side chain charges favor helical structure formation, while the alternating hydrophilic and hydrophobic residues as well as the ionic self-complementarity favor stable beta-sheet formation. Thus these peptides are able to transform their secondary structures under the appropriate conditions.

3.3.2 Assembly of Amphiphilic Biomaterials

Amphiphilic molecules have hydrophobic regions, which usually comprise hydrocarbon chains, and hydrophilic regions, which usually contain either ionic or uncharged polar functional groups. The hydrophobic regions of these molecules aggregate due to the aforementioned hydrophobic interactions, resulting in assembly of various structures such as micelles (Fig. 3.2(b)). Many biological macromolecules are amphiphilic, including phospholipids, cholesterol, glycolipids and fatty acids, and these molecules have been shown to form supramolecular structures, such as vesicles, micelles and tubules, in vivo and in vitro. A comprehensive discussion of amphiphilic assembly is beyond the scope of this chapter. We will instead focus on illustrative demonstrations of amphiphilic assembly in the synthesis of peptide-based biomaterials.

The sequence of an amphiphilic peptide typically contains a hydrophilic region composed of one or more charged or polar amino acid residues on one terminus and a hydrophobic region composed of nonpolar amino acid residues or a hydrocarbon chain on the other terminus. For example, Stupp and coworkers (Stupp and Braun, 1997a; Stupp et al., 1997b) have developed a class of molecules termed 'peptide amphiphiles' by attaching a long hydrophobic alkyl tail to a hydrophilic oligopeptide head (Fig. 3.3). These peptide amphiphiles self-assemble into cylindrical micelles in an aqueous environment, with the alkyl tails packed in the center of the micelle and the peptide headgroups exposed to the aqueous environment.

Applications of these 'peptide amphiphiles' have been exploited in tissue engineering. In one particular example, Hartgerink et al. (Hartgerink et al., 2001) described an attempt to mimic the biomineralization process by using self-assembled amphiphilic peptide nanofibers to guide the nucleation and growth of bone-like mineral crystals. On the surface of the fibrils, a flexible trio of glycine residues efficiently presents both a phosphoserine residue, which induces mineral nucleation and growth, and a peptide sequence, which promotes cell adhesion. The resultant mineralized matrix bears some similarity to the mature bone matrix, as the mineral is aligned with the direction of the self-assembled fibrils. In another example, Silva et al., (Silva et al., 2004) incorporated the Ile-Lys-Val-Ala-Val

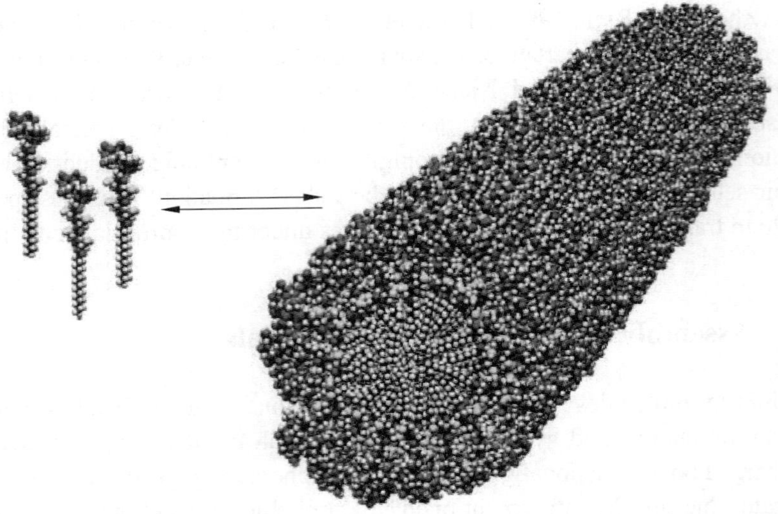

Figure 3.3 Schematic representation of the self-assembly of amphiphilic peptide molecules into a cylindrical micelle (reproduced from (Hartgerink, 2001) with permission)

(IKVAV) pentapeptide into a peptide amphiphile. IKVAV is an amino acid sequence found in laminin, an extracellular matrix protein that promotes neurite adhesion, sprouting, and growth. These IKVAV-containing peptide amphiphiles self-assemble in aqueous media to form nanofibers 5 – 8 nm in diameters and hundreds of nanometers to a few micrometers in length. These intermeshed fibers form 3-D hydrogels, which contain a remarkably high concentration of IKVAV sequences throughout the network. Due in part to the high desity of IKVAV these self-assembled hydrogels are able to promote specific differentiation of encapsulated neural progenitor cells into neurons while discouraging the production of astrocytes. This study represents an example of the importance of biomaterial properties in directing cell activity during formation of a new tissue, and it particularly emphasizes the potential of molecular self-assembly as a mechanism for biomaterials design.

In an alternative approach, Zhang and coworkers synthesized a series of peptide-based amphiphiles, which have tails composed of six repeated hydrophobic residues (Val, Ala or Leu) and head groups consisting of one or two hydrophilic amino acids (Asp) (Santoso et al., 2002; Vauthey et al., 2002). Although individually they have different compositions and sequences, these surfactant-like peptides each have a hydrophilic head and a hydrophobic tail that allow for self-assembly into a network of open-ended, helical nanotubes with an average diameter of 30 – 50 nm. Nanovesicles can 'fuse' with these nanotubes or 'bud' out of them to increase or decrease the length of the tubes, and this phenomenon makes these structures dynamic.

3.3.3 Biomimetic Supramolecular Assembly Based on Hydrogen Bonding

Amino acid side chains in polypeptides and heterocyclic bases in polynucleotides each have a well-defined tendency to form intramolecular and intermolecular hydrogen bonds. Investigators have developed a variety of peptide- or nucleotide-based biomaterials by exploiting the capacity of these molecules to interact and undergo supramolecular assembly. For example, Ghadiri and coworkers (Ghadiri et al., 1993; Ghadiri et al., 1994; Hartgerink et al., 1996; Fernandez-Lopez et al., 2001) designed a series of cyclic peptides (Fig. 3.4), which exhibit an anti-parallel β-sheet structure and self-assemble into nanochannel-like structures. These nanostructures are held together by intermolecular hydrogen bonds, and they remain stable during solvent, temperature or pH variation. The diameter of the cyclic peptides, and therefore the cylindrical diameter of the assembled nanochannels, can be defined by varying the number of amino acids in the peptides. The exterior functionality of the cylinder can also be controlled by varying the amino acid side chains (Bong et al., 2001), which makes this a particularly flexible

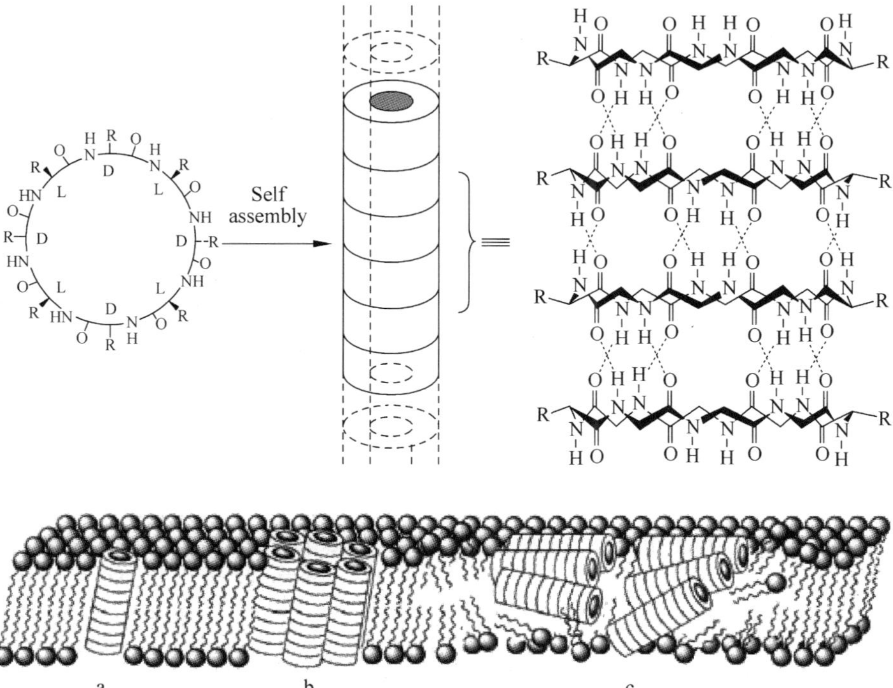

Figure 3.4 Schematic representation of a β-sheet-like, hydrogen-bonded tubular architecture created via self-assembly of eight-residue cyclic peptides. Also shown is a schematic of membrane permeation by peptide nanotubes (reproduced from (Fernandez-Lopez, 2001) with permission)

design methodology. Ghadiri and coworkers have demonstrated that these biomimetic assemblies can function as transmembrane channels to selectively transport hydrophilic molecules (e.g. glucose) across a lipid bilayer (Ghadiri et al., 1994) or as antibiotic agents that destabilize bacterial cell membranes in vitro and in vivo. (Fernandez-Carneado et al., 2004).

Other investigators have instead used complementary DNA molecules as building blocks for assembly. These molecules are capable of assembling into a double helical structure, in which two polynucleotide backbones are held together by hydrogen bonds between complementary nucleotide bases. Due to advances in modern molecular biology and solid phase oligonucleotide synthesis, it is possible to create sequences that are programmed at the level of their sequence to assemble into functional 3-D structures with predefined topologies (Yan, 2004; Tirrell, 2005). Pioneering studies by Seeman and coworkers originally showed that branched DNA building blocks could be used to construct ordered arrays (Seeman, 1982; Seeman, 2003), and more recently Mirkin (Mirkin, 2000) and Alivisatos (Alivisatos et al., 1996) have assembled nanoparticle arrays via cDNA interactions. DNA was also used to make nano-scale materials with moving parts (e.g. nanotweezers (Yurke et al., 2000)), and used as linker to direct assembly of metal nanoparticles (Mucic et al., 1998; Loweth et al., 1999; Maeda et al., 2001), metal nanowires (Braun et al., 1998; Martin et al., 1999), semiconductor particle arrays (Coffer et al., 1996; Torimoto et al., 1999), carbon nanotubes (Shim et al., 2002) and field effect transistors (Keren et al., 2003). Taken together, these studies demonstrate that hydrogen bonds between complementary DNA strands are a robust and adaptable mechanism for assembly of a variety of nanostructured materials.

3.3.4 Biomimetic Assembly Based on Affinity-Based Interactions

The molecular assemblies described in the last few sections can be generally characterized by: (1) one dominating type of non-covalent force directing assembly; (2) the use of relatively small synthetic molecules as building blocks. This is largely in contrast to natural systems, in which relatively large molecules interact via a composite of many different non-covalent interactions. The large number of distinct interactions leads to molecular recognition (Fig. 3.2(c)) (described in Section 3.2.4), which enhances specificity and, in some cases, increases the affinity of an interaction. These affinity-based interactions are prevalent in all biological systems, and investigators have also used these interactions to develop biomimetic self-assembly approaches ex vivo. For example, hydrogel networks have been assembled via specific recognition events such as reversible antibody-antigen interactions (Miyata et al., 1999), streptavidin-biotin interactions (Stayton et al., 1995; Kim et al., 2005; Kulkarni et al., 2006) and coiled-coil interactions (Petka et al. 1998; Wang et al., 1999). In one illustrative example, Miyata et al. assembled a hydrogel network by immobilizing both an antigen and the corresponding antibody in an interpenetrating polymer network (Miyata et al., 1999). These hydrogels changed their volume upon exposure to antigen-containing or antigen-free solutions, and this change was a result of changes in antibody-antigen binding within the network. In another example (Kim and Lyon, 2005), Kim and coworkers fabricated a class of bioresponsive hydrogel microlenses using biotinylated polymers and developed a new protein detection technology based on the well-studied avidin-biotin interaction. Using poly (*N*-isopropylacrylamide-*co*-acrylic acid) as the basic building block, biotinylated hydrogels were synthesized and then assembled onto a silane-modified glass substrate via ion-ion interactions. The binding of avidin was visualized by monitoring optical properties and modulation of gel swelling using a brightfield optical microscopy technique. These examples demonstrate the utility of affinity-based interactions in design of materials, and there are a wide variety of other materials design approaches in this general category. Readers are referred to Yeates et al. for a more comprehensive description of self-assembled, protein-based materials (Yeates et al., 2002).

3.3.5 Summary

Due to the pragmatic issues associated with biomaterials development, including biocompatibility, toxicity, production cost, and FDA approval, many of the specific self-assembled biomaterials described in this section have not yet been optimized for widespread clinical use. Therefore, molecular self-assembly largely represents a 'next generation' approach to assembling biomaterials, and there is not a well-established history of using most types of assembled materials in vivo. However, investigators have begun to apply some of the more general assembly mechanisms and schemes described thus far in this chapter to biomedical applications, most notably drug delivery and tissue engineering. In many cases the utility of self-assembly mechanisms stems from their ability to mimic the manner in which cells and proteins interact with the natural matrix that surrounds them in vivo.

3.4 Development of Biomaterials That Mimic The Natural ECM

3.4.1 Introduction

Animal tissues are made up of not only cells, but also an extracellular space, which is typically filled with an extensive and intricate network of macromolecules.

This network, called the extracellular matrix (ECM), serves as: (1) a structural support for cells; (2) an adhesive substrate for anchorage and migration of cells; (3) a storage depot for soluble signaling molecules; and (4) a conduit for mass transport. The ECM is capable of assembling and dissembling in response to cell activities and environmental conditions, which makes it a particularly dynamic, stimulus-responsive material. This wide variety of functional ECM properties makes it an inherently difficult structure to mimic. Furthermore, the diversity of ECM properties adds an extra layer of complexity, as ECM properties are dependent on the anatomical location, the tissue type, the health status, age, and genetic make-up of an organism, among other variables. Despite this daunting complexity, investigators have made substantial progress in recreating specific properties of the ECM to create biomaterials for medical applications ranging from biosensors to tissue engineering scaffolds. This section will describe some basic non-covalent interactions present in the natural ECM and discuss methods that have been used to mimic these interactions in biomaterials design. We specifically focus on ECM functions related to non-covalent assembly, as a more comprehensive description of all ECM-mimetic materials is beyond the scope of this chapter.

3.4.2 Non-Covalent Interactions in Natural Extracellular Matrices

The ECM of most tissue types is mainly composed of polysaccharides, proteins and their conjugates (Alberts et al., 2004). The polysaccharides are highly negatively charged, and hence attract osmotically active sodium ions via ionic interactions. This specific property of polysaccharides enables the ECM to draw in large amount of water molecules and behave as a natural hydrogel. Structural ECM proteins such as collagen and elastin are interwoven in the ECM largely via non-covalent interactions (Fig. 3.5) and assembled into fiber ropes and mesh 10 – 300 nm in diameter. These enmeshed fibers provide tensile strength and elasticity and form the structural backbone many ECMs.

A particularly important ECM property is the ability to interact non-covalently with resident cells. The ECM facilitates cell attachment and migration via specific non-covalent interactions between ECM proteins (e.g. laminin, fibronectin) and a class of specific receptors on the cell surface called integrins (Fig. 3.5). The ECM also acts as a local depot for a wide range of soluble proteins called growth factors (Fig. 3.5), which regulate myriad cell activities by interacting specifically with receptors on the cell surface. These soluble proteins are often sequestered via non-covalent interactions with molecules linked to the ECM (e.g. heparin).

The intriguing dynamic properties of many ECMs can also be tied to non-covalent interactions. There is a dynamic, reciprocal relationship between cells and the matrix in which they reside. The ECM actively regulates cell behavior by providing structural support, promoting cell attachment and regulating signaling molecules. Meanwhile, cells detect and respond to numerous features of the ECM,

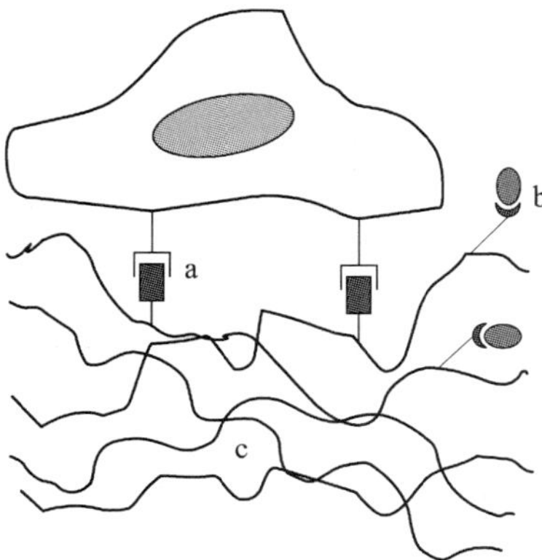

Figure 3.5 Schematic representation of a cell interacting with a natural ECM via non-covalent interactions. Specific interactions shown include: (a) integrin receptor binding to an adhesion ligand (FILLED SQUARE). (b) soluble protein (FILLED OVAL) binding to an ECM-linked ligand; and (c) interactions between protein fibers in the ECM

such as the composition and availability of adhesive ligands, soluble factors, mechanical stiffness, and spatial and topological organization of the matrix. Therefore, on one hand the structure of the ECM affects cell activity, and on the other hand cell activity often leads to structural remodeling of the ECM via synthesis of new ECM proteins and realignment of ECM fibrils.

It is clear that several unique functions of the ECM are a result of designed non-covalent interactions, and the importance of natural ECM functions in medical applications (e.g. tissue engineering) has led several investigators to mimic these interactions directly or indirectly. The following sections will describe a number of examples in which interactions in the ECM are mimicked to build functional biomaterials.

3.4.3 Biomaterials That Mimic ECM Structures and Properties

ECM-mimetic biomaterials can be designed based on the same structural features and cell-interactive mechanisms the natural ECM possesses. There are several natural ECM characteristics that are desirable for these synthetic biomaterials (Pratt et al., 2004). Structurally, these materials should be porous and highly hydrated. They should present specific adhesion sites to actively accommodate cell attachment and facilitate cell migration. They should be susceptible to enzymatic matrix remodeling, which allows for cell invasion and ECM re-organization. In many cases it may also be desirable to incorporate binding sites for cell signaling molecules (e.g. growth factors) to allow more active control of cell behavior,(e.g. proliferation, differentiation). Although natural ECMs typically possess all of the above merits, it remains a great challenge to design synthetic biomaterials that simultaneously perform the broad range of ECM functions. Instead, many of the biomimetic matrices explored to date focus on achieving one or two features of the natural ECM. The following sections will describe some of these approaches, highlighting key non-covalent assembly mechanisms.

3.4.3.1 Non-Covalent Assembly of Structural 3-D Hydrogel Matrices for Cell Culture

As described above, natural ECMs are highly hydrated, porous matrices. In designing biomimetic materials for tissue engineering and cell development, synthetic hydrogels have drawn great attention because their structural properties resemble many fundamental structural features of natural ECMs (Graham 1998). For example, hydrogels are networks of water-interactive or water-soluble molecules, which have water-absorbing capacity and thus high porosity, similar to natural ECMs. Hydrogels are viscoelastic, which also mimics the mechanical properties of some natural ECMs. These structural properties make synthetic hydrogels a suitable base material for design of novel biomaterials for tissue engineering (Hutmacher, 2001; Langer and Tirrell, 2004; Almany and Selikar, 2005; Dankers et al. 2005; Hollister, 2005; Lutolf and Hubbell, 2005; Salvay and Shea, 2006; Zhao and Zhang, 2006), as they offer 3-D matrices to support cell growth and have some degree of structural flexibility and biochemical adaptability, similar to natural tissue. Investigators have developed a number of approaches for generating biocompatible hydrogels based on molecular self-assembly through several intermolecular pathways as described in section 3.3 (Stupp et al., 1997b; Schneider et al., 2002; Pochan et al., 2003; Mahler et al., 2006).

Many synthetic hydrogel networks require gelation conditions that may compromise cell viability, such as ultraviolet radiation or reactive chemical cross-linkers. Hydrogels that assemble via non-covalent interactions can circumvent this issue by assembling in environments that are cell-friendly and similar to physiological conditions. In addition, self-assembly may potentially provide a minimally invasive surgical technique if matrices can be formed in vivo. In view of these potential advantages, investigators have begun to use the assembly methods described in Section 3.3 to generate hydrogels in physiological environments. Zhang and colleagues (Holmes et al., 2000) have developed a class of peptide nanofibril-based hydrogel networks that undergo gelation at physiological pH and temperature. These scaffolds have 5 – 200 nm pores and greater than 99.5% water content, which closely mimics the porosity and structure of the native ECM. These peptide-based matrices have demonstrated the ability to support 3-D culture of cells (e.g. neurons, endothelial cells) and maintain their functional behavior, including migration, proliferation and differentiation. Remarkably, these matrices promote proper cell function in the absence of any specific biologically functional ligands, which suggests that cells or cell-secreted proteins may have a mechanism for directly interacting with the materials. For example, Holmes et al. constructed self-assembling peptides and applied them as matrices for culture of neurons. The matrices supported neuronal cell attachment and differentiation as well as extensive neurite outgrowth and synapse formation between the attached neurons (Holmes et al., 2000). Peptide-based scaffolds also provide an angiogenic environment (Narmoneva et al., 2005) by inhibiting endothelial cell apoptosis in the absence of added pro-angiogenic factors. As a result, the scaffolds promote long-term cell survival and capillary-like network formation in 3-D cultures of human microvascular endothelial cells. Other peptide- and nucleotide-based hydrogels formed via non-covalent assembly (described in Section 3.3) may be similarly useful as structural matrices for 3-D cell culture.

3.4.3.2 Substrates and Scaffolds That Interact Specifically and Non-Covalently with Cells

Cells in connective tissues don't float around freely. Instead, they are immobilized by attaching to ECM proteins. These proteins, such as fibronectin, contain adhesion domains that facilitate specific binding to cell surface receptors. This binding is mediated by affinity-based, non-covalent interactions, as described in Section 3.2.4. In addition, the density and spatial distribution of such regions regulate cell behavior. In view of these important natural interactions, investigators have designed synthetic biomaterials that interact with cell surface receptors in a similar manner. Synthetic biomaterials can mimic the cell-adhesive property of the natural ECM through incorporation of adhesion-promoting ligands, such as ECM proteins or short peptides bearing cell-adhesion motifs. Incorporation of these biomimetic adhesion sites provides a means to promote cell adhesion and migration on materials, enabling scientists and engineers to study cell-substrate interactions in a well-controlled manner. Moreover, controlling receptor-mediated interactions between cells and their substrates is one of the central themes in many tissue engineering approaches (Hubbell, 1995; Sakiyama-Elbert et al., 2001).

Perhaps the most commonly used cell adhesion ligand in biomaterials-related applications is the Arg-Gly-Asp (RGD) sequence from the native ECM protein fibronectin. In 1984, Ruoslahti and coworkers discovered this motif (Pierschbacher et al., 1984), and their discovery has resulted in the development of numerous materials containing RGD attachment sites (Hersel et al., 2003). Similarly, many other adhesion-promoting peptides with short primary sequences have been developed based on the receptor-binding domains of adhesion proteins, such as the Arg-Glu-Asp-Val (REDV) and Leu-Asp-Val (LDV) (Mould et al., 1991) sequences from fibronectin, the Tyr-Ile-Gly-Ser-Arg (YIGSR) and Ile-Lys-Val-Ala-Val (IKVAV) sequences from laminin (Vukicevic et al., 1990) and the Asp-Gly-Glu-Ala (DGEA) sequence from type I collagen (Dalton et al., 1995). Short peptides are often advantageous in design of synthetic biomaterials when compared with full-length ECM proteins, as they are stable, relatively easy to synthesize and purify, and can be covalently linked to a wide range of hydrogel matrices. In contrast, full-length adhesion proteins are large, expensive, and often difficult to modify without influencing biological activity. Myriad studies have demonstrated that these adhesion-promoting biomaterials are able to promote integrin-mediated molecular interactions (Massia et al., 1991; Ruoslahti 1996), stimulate cell spreading, and enable differentiation (Schlaepfer et al., 1994; Humphries 1996; Palecek et al., 1997). It is noteworthy that the interaction between cell adhesion ligands and their receptors are governed by complex, and often poorly understood, non-covalent interactions. Therefore, these interactions can be described quantitatively by equilibrium dissociation constants (see Section 3.2.4), which provide information about the strength of the interaction. For example, binding between the surface of NRK cells and oligopeptides containing the RGD motif have equilibrium dissociation constants of 300 – 600 μM (Pierschbacher et al., 1984).

As in the native ECM, the density and spatial distribution of adhesion-promoting ligands actively affect cell adhesion and migration on biomaterials. For example, Massia et al. reported approximately 10^5 copies of RGD per cell were required to induce cell adhesion, spreading, focal contact formation, and cytoskeletal organization on 2-D cell culture substrates (Massia et al., 1991). Palecek et al. demonstrated that cell migration speed was dependent on substrate ligand density, integrin expression level, and integrin-ligand binding affinity (Palecek et al., 1997). Maheshwari et al. showed that as the degree of ligand clustering was increased, the average ligand density required to support cell migration decreased, suggesting that the spatial distribution of ligand is important for cell motility (Maheshwari et al., 2000). Taken together, these studies indicate that the affinity and number of non-covalent interactions have important consequences for cell function on synthetic substrates that mimic the natural ECM.

Mimicry of cell-ECM adhesion can also be used as a mechanism to enhance biocompatibility of traditional biomaterials. In vivo, cell recognition of traditional biomaterials, such as polytetrafluoroethylene, silicone rubber, or polyethylene, occurs indirectly. Proteins from body fluids adsorb nonspecifically onto the surfaces of these materials, and some of the adsorbed proteins, such as fibronectin, vitronectin, and fibrinogen, promote cell adhesion. This nonspecific, uncontrolled cell adhesion often times can cause negative effects, including poorly controlled inflammatory reactions that can lead to a poor implant-tissue interface. Incorporation of cell type-specific adhesion ligands into traditional biomaterials may allow one to define the interactions between synthetic implants and natural tissues, leading to more predictable biological responses. For example, Hubbell et al. (Hubbell et al., 1991) found that the integrin receptor $\alpha_4\beta_1$ is present on human endothelial cells but not on platelets. When immobilized on otherwise bio-inert substrates, the REDV peptide sequence selectively promoted the adhesion and spread of endothelial cells by interacting specifically with the $\alpha_4\beta_1$ integrin, while fibroblasts, vascular smooth muscle cells, and platelets did not attach. Furthermore, the endothelial cell monolayers on REDV were non-thrombogenic. One can imagine this ligand could be useful for biomaterials designed to support the adhesion and migration of endothelial cells but prevent the adhesion of blood platelets (e.g. vascular grafts).

3.4.3.3 Dynamic Matrices That Dissemble in Response to Cell Activity

The ECM is anything but a static pool simply holding cells together. As described above, the ECM is dynamic and interactive with the cells it hosts. It is responsive to many stimuli, both physical (e.g. temperature, mechanical stress) and chemical (e.g. pH, ionic strength), and undergoes constant remodeling and reorganization via local proteolytic enzyme activity. Although numerous scaffolding systems have been developed that are biodegradable, degradation often occurs via a cell independent mechanism, such as hydrolysis in aqueous solution. In many cases it would be preferable to allow cells to degrade their surrounding matrix via proteolysis, as this would mimic the cell-mediated remodeling that occurs in the natural ECM. Furthermore, when cells are encapsulated in non-biodegradable synthetic matrices, they are often not able to synthesize and assemble their own matrix. Cell-mediated degradation in dynamic matrices would allow the cells to assemble a more natural matrix, and this not only mimics natural ECM reorganization, but could also be advantageous in tissue engineering.

To that end, recent work has used clever chemistries to enable cell-mediated remodeling in synthetic matrices (Hubbell, 1999; Hubbell, 2003; Lutolf and Hubbell, 2005). Hubbell and coworkers developed a matrix synthesis strategy, in which poly(ethylene glycol) (PEG) is copolymerized with short peptides bearing a sequence that can be recognized by specific proteases (West and Hubbell, 1999). One matrix contained the Ala-Pro-Gly-Leu (APGL) sequence derived from the ECM protein collagen, and this matrix was specifically degraded by collagenase. Another matrix contained the Val-Arg-Asn (VRN) sequence derived from fibrinogen and this matrix was specifically degraded by plasmin. Both matrices remained stable in the presence of the other protease, indicating that protease-mediated degradation was specific. In another study (Lutolf et al., 2003a; Lutolf et al., 2003b), when matrix metalloproteases (MMPs) cleavable peptides were incorporated into a PEG hydrogel network, exposure to MMPs resulted in hydrogel swelling as a result of peptide cleavage, ultimately leading to complete erosion of the network. When these networks were exposed to human fibroblasts, cell-secreted MMPs were found to locally degrade the incorporated peptides, and allow for cell migration through the hydrogel matrix.

It is worth mentioning that the hydrogel systems described in the subsection are covalently cross-linked materials, in contrast to the self-assembled matrices that are more common in natural ECMs. However, enzyme-mediated remodeling to the matrix enables the encapsulated cells to assemble a natural matrix around them in place of the synthetic matrix that has been degraded, and such processes involve many molecular recognition events via a number of non-covalent interactions.

3.4.3.4 Matrices That Interact with Growth Factors via Non-Covalent Interactions

Besides providing structural support and acting as a dynamic substrate for cell adhesion and remodeling, the native ECM also plays a significant role in regulation of cell development and tissue development by influencing growth factor signaling pathways. One way in which the ECM influences cell activity is by sequestering growth factors, thereby regulating their availability to cells. Natural ECMs can 'store' these growth factors through non-covalent interactions, and due to the reversibility of the interactions, the sequestered growth factors can be released and allowed to interact with cell surface receptors. In some cases, growth factors can also be released actively through enzyme-mediated degradation of the matrix. Therefore, developing matrices able to interact with growth factors and maintain their bioactivity is desirable for tissue engineering applications, where cell-secreted growth factors could be sequestered, concentrated and regulated in the matrix. These types of matrices could also be important in localized drug delivery applications, as the matrix could potentially release growth factors on site in a spatially and temporally controlled manner. Previously developed polymer-based matrices that immobilize growth factors using physical entrapment (Richardson et al., 2001) or covalent immobilization (Zisch et al., 2003) can delivery growth factors in a sustained manner. However, strong and reversible interactions between a matrix and a growth factor may offer unique capabilities in tissue engineering approaches, including spatial and temporal control over growth factor signaling during new tissue growth. Furthermore, it is possible that matrices designed to interact with growth factors with controlled affinity can either sequester these signals from cells or present them to cells, thereby actively agonizing or inhibiting specific cell signaling pathways. Some recent progress from our group in this area will be introduced in the last part of this chapter.

1. Heparin-based sequestering

Several growth factors contain heparin-binding motifs, and therefore bind to the highly sulfated glycosaminoglycan heparin. For example, basic fibroblast growth factor (bFGF) is bound to heparin in the ECM (K_d ~10 nM (Nugent and Edelman, 1992)) and can be released in an active form when the ECM-heparin linkage is degraded by heparanase (Vlodavsky et al., 1991). Thus, incorporation of heparin into hydrogel networks may provide affinity sites to sequester heparin-binding growth factors, thus allowing the release of these growth factors in a controlled manner.

One successful strategy of heparin incorporation is to covalently immobilize it in a matrix. For example, Edelman and coworkers (Edelman et al., 1991) encapsulated heparin-conjugated Sepharose beads in alginate hydrogel matrices to sequester bFGF, therefore protecting bFGF from degradation and enabling sustained release. Wissink and coworkers (Wissink et al., 2000a; Wissink et al., 2000b) covalently immobilized heparin in collagen matrices by cross-linking collagen with EDC/NHS and then immobilizing heparin with a similar scheme. These matrices were then used to sequester bFGF, which enhanced endothelial cell proliferation. Tanihara and coworkers (Tanihara et al., 2001) cross-linked alginate and heparin with diamine using carbodiimide chemistry to construct a hydrogel, which released loaded bFGF in a sustained manner. Heparin-linked matrices have also been used to bind and release vascular endothelial growth factor (VEGF). For example, Tae and coworkers (Tae et al., 2006) crosslinked hydrazide-functionalized heparin with the N-hydroxysuccinimidyl ester of poly(ethylene glycol)-bis-butanoic acid to form a heparin-containing gel, and VEGF was directly injected into the hydrogel. The loaded VEGF displayed a sustained release over 3 weeks with little initial burst phase. The biological activity of the released VEGF was confirmed with a proliferation assay utilizing human umbilical vein endothelial cells. This VEGF-loaded gel was then implanted subcutaneously in the dorsal region of mice, resulting in an increased density of the endothelial cell marker platelet endothelial adhesion molecule in the tissues surrounding the implanted gel. These data suggest that heparin-based controlled release systems could be an important component of emerging pro-angiogenic therapies.

An alternative strategy involves restraining heparin non-covalently with the help of heparin-binding peptides (HBPs). For example, Seal and Panitch (Seal and Panitch, 2003) covalently attached HBPs to multi-arm poly(ethylene glycol)s (PEGs), which were then incubated with heparin to form a self-assembled matrix. The K_d of the HBP-heparin interaction ranges from 30 – 600 nM. These gels were able to sequester heparin-binding peptides and release these peptides over several days at rates dependent on heparin-HBP affinity. Sakiyama and Hubbell (Sakiyama-Elbert and Hubbell, 2000) developed a fibrin-based heparin-containing delivery system, in which heparin is sequestered via non-covalent interactions (mainly ion-ion interactions) through a covalently linked heparin-binding peptide derived from the heparin-binding domain of antithrombin III. As a model system, neurite extension from dorsal root ganglia was tested to determine the ability of the delivery system to release bioactive growth factor in response to cell-mediated processes. The results demonstrated that the immobilized bFGFs within fibrin enhanced neurite extension by up to about 100% relative to unmodified fibrin. The results suggest that these matrices could serve as therapeutic materials to enhance peripheral nerve regeneration through nerve guide tubes and may have more general usefulness in tissue engineering. Recently, a nerve growth factor neurotrophin-3 was also successfully sequestered in these heparin-based fibrin scaffolds and the effect of the controlled delivery on tissue regeneration following spinal cord injury was assessed (Taylor et al., 2004; Taylor et al., 2006a; Taylor and Sakiyama-Elbert, 2006b).

Recently, Kiick's group developed another route of fabricating heparin-contained hydrogel systems, which possesses the characteristics of both strategies described above. These hydrogels were assembled non-covalently on the basis of the interaction between a heparin-modified PEG star copolymer and an HBP-bearing PEG star copolymer, whose sequence was derived from the heparin-binding regions of antithrombin III (Yamaguchi et al., 2005a; Yamaguchi and Kiick, 2005b). In a later study, a heparin-binding, coiled-coil peptide, $PF4_{ZIP}$, was employed to mediate the assembly of heparinized matrix (Zhang et al., 2006). The $PF4_{ZIP}$ sequence is based on a GCN4 coiled-coil and mimics the heparin-binding domain of human platelet factor 4. $PF4_{ZIP}$ demonstrates a higher heparin-binding affinity and heparin association rate when compared to the heparin-binding domains of antithrombin III. Viscoelastic hydrogels were formed upon the association of $PF4_{ZIP}$-functionalized PEG star copolymer with the heparin-modified PEG star copolymer. Both systems demonstrated the feature of sustained release of basic fibroblast growth factor (bFGF) as a function of matrix erosion.

2. Gelatin-based sequestering

Gelatin is a denatured, biodegradable material obtained by acidic or basic processing of collagen, and it has been extensively utilized for pharmaceutical and medical applications. The processing yields gelatin with different acidity. When mixed with acidic (positively charged) or basic (negatively charged) gelatin, an oppositely charged protein will interact to form a polyelectrolyte complex via ion-ion interactions (Tabata 2003). Tabata and coworkers developed gelatin-based hydrogels by chemical crosslinking of acidic or basic gelatin. Based on this non-covalent interaction, these hydrogels demonstrated controlled release of various protein growth factors, including bFGF (Tabata and Ikada, 1999), transforming growth factor- β1 (TGF-β1) (Holland et al., 2003), TGF-β2 (Kojima et al., 2004), platelet-derived growth factor (PDGF) (Hokugo et al., 2005), hepatocyte growth factor (HGF) (Ozeki and Tabata, 2006b; Ozeki and Tabata, 2006a) and bone morphogentic protein 2 (BMP-2) (Okamoto et al., 2004) while maintaining their biological activities.

3. Specific sequestering interactions for growth factor delivery

Both heparin and gelatin based hydrogels are capable of binding to many different growth factors non-specifically, which is beneficial when one desires to sequester or deliver multiple growth factors. However, if one wishes to sequester a specific growth factor or a specific combination of growth factors, the specificity of the interaction becomes important. Furthermore, control over the affinity between growth factors and the matrix is an important factor determining one's ability to regulate the release profile of immobilized growth factors.

An approach that has begun to emerge in the area of growth factor-material interactions involves using molecules, typically peptides or oligonucleotides, which bind strongly and selectively to a molecule of interest. In this approach, a sequestering molecule is linked covalently to a synthetic matrix, and a particular growth factor then interacts non-covalently with the matrix. A class of molecules termed 'aptamers' (from the latin *aptus*, meaning 'to fit') may be particularly useful in this general approach. Aptamers are oligonucleotide or peptide molecules that bind to target molecules (e.g. proteins, small molecules) specifically and with variable affinity, and these molecules have been commonly used as protein antagonists. The interactions between aptamers and their target proteins are based on affinity, as described in Section 3.2.4, and the specific mechanisms of interaction are often poorly understood. Due to their ability to interact non-covalently with specified target molecules it is possible that aptamer-linked biomaterials may be used to both agonize and antagonize growth factor activity, which may be useful in tissue engineering applications. To that end, aptamers have recently been used to localize growth factors in materials and to modulate growth factor release from biomaterial matrices.

Based on their unique properties, we (Hudalla and Murphy, 2007) and others (Willerth et al., 2007) have begun to use aptamers as building blocks for assembly of smart biomaterials. Our laboratory has recently used aptamers as building blocks to develop PEG-based hydrogel systems for growth factor sequestering (Hudalla and Murphy, 2007). Briefly, our approach covalently immobilizes two peptide aptamers (CVEPNCDIHVMWEWECFERL and CEELWCFDGPRAWVCGYVK), which bind specifically to vascular endothelial growth factor (VEGF) with differing affinities (~200 nM, and ~10,000 nmol/L, respectively) into a PEG hydrogel. When the hydrogels are exposed to a solution containing VEGF, fluorescent microscopy showed these gels are able to sequester VEGF, and the amount of protein non-covalently bound is dependent on the aptamer-VEGF affinity (Fig. 3.6). The sequestered VEGF undergoes sustained release over days to months, dependent on the amount of aptamer included into the hydrogel matrix. These aptamer-based sequestering interactions may become an enabling tool for growth factor delivery and tissue engineering applications. These non-covalent sequestering approaches exemplify a theme of emerging biomaterials design approaches, which involves using synthetic materials to actively regulate of cell activity.

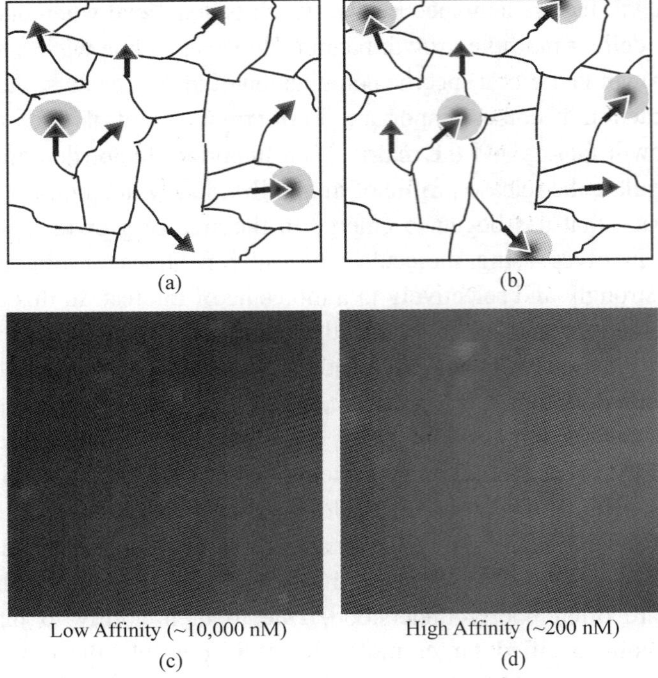

Figure 3.6 Schematic representation of sequestering Rhodamine-labeled VEGF (•) in PEG hydrogels containing (a) a low affinity peptide ligand (K_d ~10,000 nM); and (b) a high affinity ligand (K_d ~200 nM) (▲). Also shown are the fluorescence images of hydrogels containing low affinity (c) and high affinity (d) peptide ligands after incubation in 10 nM VEGF and rinsing with PBS. Results suggest that the amount of VEGF sequestered in a hydrogel is dependent on the affinity of the ligand-VEGF interaction (color Fig.2)

3.5 Concluding remarks

Non-covalent interactions have been a ubiquitous mechanism for assembly in various biological systems, from exquisitely folded proteins to structurally sophisticated and functionally adaptable ECMs. Recent progress in understanding the mechanistic underpinnings of biological assembly has led scientists and engineers to mimic natural systems, with the goal of designing next-generation biomaterials. Yet the complexity of natural processes creates inherent challenges in biomimetic assembly. However, the emergence of modern tools, from nanotechnology to molecular biology, presents new opportunities for biomimetic self-assembly.

The concepts and previous studies reviewed in this chapter demonstrate the tremendous promise and formidable challenges associated with biomimetic self-assembly. A variety of novel biomaterials have been developed using non-covalent assembly mechanisms, and these materials are now being applied to medical applications such as tissue engineering and drug delivery. The variety of non-covalent assembly mechanisms in existence (Section 3.2 herein) coupled with the advantages of non-covalent interactions in biomaterials design (Section 3.3 herein) and bio-medical applications (Section 3.4 herein) suggests that molecular self-assembly will continue to be an important theme in biomaterials science.

Acknowledgements

The authors acknowledge funding from the National Institutes of Health (R21EB005374) and the American Chemical Society Petroleum Research Fund (44235-G7).

References

Alberts, B., A. Johnson, J. Lewis, M. Raff, K. Roberts and P. Walter. *Molecular Biology of the Cell,* New York: Garland Science, (2004).

Alivisatos, A. P., K. P. Johnsson, X. Peng, T. E. Wilson, C. J. Loweth, M. P. Bruchez, Jr. and P. G. Schultz. *Nature* **382**: 609 – 611 (1996).

Almany, L. and D. Seliktar. *Biomaterials* **26**: 2467 – 2477 (2005).

Altman, M., P. Lee, A. Rich and S. Zhang. *Protein Science* **9**: 1095 – 1105 (2000).

Bong, D. T. and M. R. Ghadiri. Angew. *Chem. Int. Edit.* **40**: 2163 – 2166 (2001).

Braun, E., Y. Eichen, U. Sivan and G. Ben-Yoseph. *Nature* **391**: 775 – 778 (1998).

Bucur, C. B., Z. Sui and J. B. Schlenoff, J. Am. *Chem. Soc.* **128**: 13,690 – 13,691 (2006).

Burley, S. K. and G. A. Petsko. *Science* **229**: 23 – 28 (1985).

Coffer, J. L., S. R. Bigham, X. Li, R. F. Pinizzotto, Y. G. Rho, R. M. Pirtle and I. L. Pirtle. *Appl. Phys. Lett.* **69**: 3851 – 3853 (1996).

Dalton, B. A., C. D. Mcfarland, P. A. Underwood and J. G. Steele. *J. Cell. Sci.* **108**: 2083 – 2092 (1995).

Dankers, P. Y., M. C. Harmsen, L. A. Brouwer, M. J. van Luyn and E. W. Meijer. *Nat. Mater.* **4**: 568 – 574 (2005).

Dougherty, D. A. *Science* **271**: 163 – 168 (1996).

Edelman, E. R., E. Mathiowitz, R. Langer and M. Klagsbrun. *Biomaterials* **12**: 619 – 626 (1991).

Fernandez-Carneado, J., M. J. Kogan, S. Pujals and E. Giralt. *Biopolymers* **76**: 196 – 203 (2004).

Fernandez-Lopez, S., H. S. Kim, E. C. Choi, M. Delgado, J. R. Granja, A. Khasanov, K. Kraehenbuehl, G. Long, D. A. Weinberger, K. M. Wilcoxen and M. R. *Ghadiri. Nature* **414**: 329 – 329 (2001).

Fields, G. B. and R. L. Noble. *Int. J. Pept. Protein. Res.* **35**: 161 – 214 (1990).

Gallivan, J. P. and D. A. Dougherty. *Proc. Natl. Acad. Sci. USA* **96**: 9459 – 9464 (1999).

Ghadiri, M. R., J. R. Granja and L. K. Buehler. *Nature* **369**: 301 – 304 (1994).

Ghadiri, M. R., J. R. Granja, R. A. Milligan, D. E. McRee and N. Khazanovich. *Nature* **366**: 324 – 327 (1993).

Graham, N. B. *Med. Device. Technol.* **9**: 18 – 22 (1998).

Hartgerink, J. D., E. Beniash and S. I. Stupp. *Science* **294**: 1684 – 1688 (2001).

Hartgerink, J. D., J. R. Granja, R. A. Milligan and M. R. Ghadiri. *J. Am. Chem. Soc.* **118**: 43 – 50 (1996).

Hersel, U., C. Dahmen and H. Kessler. *Biomaterials* **24**: 4385 – 4415 (2003).

Hokugo, A., Y. Sawada, K. Mushimoto, S. Morita and Y. Tabata. *Journal of Hard Tissue Biology* **14**: 288 – 290 (2005).

Holland, T. A., Y. Tabata and A. G. Mikos. *J. Control. Release* **91**: 299 – 313 (2003).

Hollister, S. J. *Nat Mater* **4**: 518 – 524 (2005).

Holmes, T. C., S. de Lacalle, X. Su, G. S. Liu, A. Rich and S. G. Zhang. *P. Natl. Acad. Sci. USA* **97**: 6728 – 6733 (2000).

Hubbell, J. A. *Bio-Technol.* **13**: 565 – 576 (1995).

Hubbell, J. A. *Curr Opin Biotechnol.* **10**: 123 – 129 (1999).

Hubbell, J. A. *Curr Opin Biotechnol.* **14**: 551 – 558 (2003).

Hubbell, J. A., S. P. Massia, N. P. Desai and P. D. Drumheller. *Biotechnology (N Y)* **9**: 568 – 572 (1991).

Hudalla, G. A. and W. L. Murphy. *American Chemical Society PMSE* preprints (2007).

Humphries, M. J. *Curr. Opin. Cell. Biol.* **8**: 632 – 640 (1996).

Hutmacher, D. W. J. *Biomater. Sci. Polym. Ed.* **12**: 107 – 124 (2001).

Israelachvili, J. N. *Intermolecular and Surface Forces.* London: Academic Press (1991).

Jeffrey, G. A. *An Introduction to Hydrogen Bonding (Topics in Physical Chemistry).* New york: Oxford University Press (1997).

Kellis, J. T., Jr., K. Nyberg, D. Sali and A. R. Fersht. *Nature* **333**: 784 – 786 (1988).

Keren, K., R. S. Berman, E. Buchstab, U. Sivan and E. Braun. *Science* **302**: 1380 – 1382 (2003).

Kim, J., S. Nayak and L. A. Lyon. *J. Am. Chem. Soc.* **127**: 9588 – 9592 (2005).

Kojima, K., R. A. Ignotz, T. Kushibiki, K. W. Tinsley, Y. Tabata and C. A. Vacanti. *J. Thorac. Cardiovasc. Surg.* **128**: 147 – 153 (2004).

Kollman, P. A. *Accounts of Chemical Research* **10**: 365 – 371 (1977).

Kulkarni, S., C. Schilli, B. Grin, A. H. E. Muller, A. S. Hoffman and P. S. Stayton. *Biomacromolecules* **7**: 2736 – 2741 (2006).

Langer, R. and D. A. Tirrell. *Nature* **428**: 487 – 492 (2004).

Loweth, C. J., W. B. Caldwell, X. G. Peng, A. P. Alivisatos and P. G. Schultz. Angew. *Chem. Int. Edit.* **38**: 1808 – 1812 (1999).

Lutolf, M. P. and J. A. Hubbell. *Nat. Biotechnol.* **23**: 47 – 55 (2005).

Lutolf, M. P., G. P. Raeber, A. H. Zisch, N. Tirelli and J. A. Hubbell. *Adv. Mater.* **15**: 888 (2003a).

Lutolf, M. P., F. E. Weber, H. G. Schmoekel, J. C. Schense, T. Kohler, R. Muller and J. A. Hubbell. *Nat. Biotechnol.* **21**: 513 – 518 (2003b).

Ma, J. C. and D. A. Dougherty. *Chemical. Reviews* **97**: 1303 – 1324 (1997).

Maeda, Y., H. Tabata and T. Kawai. *Appl. Phys. Lett.* **79**: 1181 – 1183 (2001).

Maheshwari, G., G. Brown, D. A. Lauffenburger, A. Wells and L. G. Griffith. *J. Cell. Sci.* **113 (Pt 10)**: 1677 – 1686 (2000).

Mahler, A., M. Reches, M. Rechter, S. Cohen and E. Gazit. *Adv. Mater.* **18**: 1365 – 1370 (2006).

Martin, B. R., D. J. Dermody, B. D. Reiss, M. M. Fang, L. A. Lyon, M. J. Natan and T. E. Mallouk. *Adv. Mater.* **11**: 1021 – 1025 (1999).

Massia, S. P. and J. A. Hubbell. *J. Cell. Biol.* **114**: 1089 – 1100 (1991).

McGaughey, G. B., M. Gagne and A. K. Rappe. *J. Biol. Chem.* **273**: 15,458 – 15,463 (1998).

Michaels, A. S. *Journal of Industrial and Engineering Chemistry* **57**: 32 – 40 (1965).

Mirkin, C. A. *Inorg. Chem.* **39**: 2258 – 2272 (2000).

Miyata, T., N. Asami and T. Uragami. *Nature* **399**: 766 – 769 (1999).

Mould, A. P., A. Komoriya, K. M. Yamada and M. J. Humphries. *J. Biol. Chem.* **266**: 3579 – 3585 (1991).

Mucic, R. C., J. J. Storhoff, C. A. Mirkin and R. L. Letsinger. *J. Am. Chem. Soc.* **120**: 12,674 – 12,675 (1998).

Narmoneva, D. A., O. Oni, A. L. Sieminski, S. G. Zhang, J. P. Gertler, R. D. Kamm and R. T. Lee. *Biomaterials* **26**: 4837 – 4846 (2005).

Nugent, M. A. and E. R. Edelman. *Biochemistry-Us* **31**: 8876 – 8883 (1992).

Okamoto, T., Y. Yamamoto, M. Gotoh, C. L. Huang, T. Nakamura, Y. Shimizu, Y. Tabata and H. Yokomise. *J. Thorac. Cardiovasc. Surg.* **127**: 329 – 334 (2004).

Ozeki, M. and Y. Tabata. *J. Biomater. Sci. Polym. Ed.* **17**: 139 – 150 (2006a).

Ozeki, M. and Y. Tabata. *J. Biomater. Sci. Polym. Ed.* **17**: 163 – 175 (2006b).

Palecek, S. P., J. C. Loftus, M. H. Ginsberg, D. A. Lauffenburger and A. F. Horwitz. *Nature* **385**: 537 – 540 (1997).

Pandya, M. J., G. M. Spooner, M. Sunde, J. R. Thorpe, A. Rodger and D. N. Woolfson. *Biochemistry-Us* **39**: 8728 – 8734 (2000).

Petka, W. A., J. L. Harden, K. P. McGrath, D. Wirtz and D. A. Tirrell. *Science* **281**: 389 – 392 (1998).

Pierschbacher, M. D. and E. Ruoslahti. *Nature* **309**: 30 – 33 (1984).

Pochan, D. J., J. P. Schneider, J. Kretsinger, B. Ozbas, K. Rajagopal and L. Haines. *J. Am. Chem. Soc.* **125**: 11,802 – 11,803 (2003).

Pratt, A. B., F. E. Weber, H. G. Schmoekel, R. Muller and J. A. Hubbell. *Biotechnol. Bioeng.* **86**: 27 – 36 (2004).

Richardson, T. P., M. C. Peters, A. B. Ennett and D. J. Mooney. *Nat. Biotechnol.* **19**: 1029 – 1034 (2001).

Ruoslahti, E. *Annu. Rev. Cell. Dev. Bi.* **12**: 697 – 715 (1996).

Ryadnov, M. G. and D. N. Woolfson. *Nat. Mater.* **2**: 329 – 332 (2003).

Sakiyama-Elbert, S. E. and J. A. Hubbell. *J. Control. Release* **65**: 389 – 402 (2000).

Sakiyama-Elbert, S. E. and J. A. Hubbell. *Ann. Rev. Mater. Res.* **31**: 183 – 201 (2001).

Salvay, D. M. and L. D. Shea. *Mol. Biosyst.* **2**: 36 – 48 (2006).

Santoso, S., W. Hwang, H. Hartman and S. G. Zhang. *Nano. Lett.* **2**: 687 – 691 (2002).

Scheiner, S. *Hydrogen Bonding: A Theoretical Perspective.* New York: Oxford University Press. (1997).

Schlaepfer, D. D., S. K. Hanks, T. Hunter and P. van der Geer. *Nature* **372**: 786 – 791 (1994).

Schneider, J. P., D. J. Pochan, B. Ozbas, K. Rajagopal, L. Pakstis and J. Kretsinger. *J. Am. Chem. Soc.* **124**: 15,030 – 15,037 (2002).

Seal, B. L. and A. Panitch. *Biomacromolecules* **4**: 1572 – 1582 (2003).

Seeman, N. C. *J. Theor. Biol.* **99**: 237 – 247 (1982).

Seeman, N. C. *Nature* **421**: 427 – 431 (2003).

Shim, M., N. W. S. Kam, R. J. Chen, Y. M. Li and H. J. Dai. *Nano Lett.* **2**: 285 – 288 (2002).

Silva, G. A., C. Czeisler, K. L. Niece, E. Beniash, D. A. Harrington. J. A. Kessler and S. I. Stupp. *Science* **303**: 1352 – 1355 (2004).

Spolar, R. S., J. H. Ha and M. T. Record, Jr. *Proc. Natl. Acad. Sci. USA* **86**: 8382 – 8385 (1989).

Stayton, P. S., T. Shimoboji, C. Long, A. Chilkoti, G. H. Chen, J. M. Harris and A. S. Hoffman. *Nature* **378**: 472 – 474 (1995).

Stupp, S. I. and P. V. Braun. *Science* **277**: 1242 – 1248 (1997a).

Stupp, S. I., V. V. LeBonheur, K. Walker, L. S. Li, K. E. Huggins, M. Keser and A. Amstutz. *Science* **276**: 384 – 389 (1997b).

Tabata, Y. *Tissue Eng* **9 Suppl 1**: S5 – 15 (2003).

Tabata, Y. and Y. Ikada. *Biomaterials* **20**: 2169 – 2175 (1999).

Tae, G., M. Scatena, P. S. Stayton and A. S. Hoffman. *J. Biomat. Sci-Polym. E.* **17**: 187 – 197 (2006).

Tanihara, M., Y. Suzuki, E. Yamamoto, A. Noguchi and Y. Mizushima. *J. Biomed. Mater. Res.* **56**: 216 – 221 (2001).

Taylor, S. J., J. W. McDonald and S. E. Sakiyama-Elbert. *J. Control. Release.* **98**: 281 – 294 (2004).

Taylor, S. J., E. S. Rosenzweig, J. W. McDonald and S. E. Sakiyama-Elbert. *J. Control. Release* **113**: 226 – 235 (2006).

Taylor, S. J. and S. E. Sakiyama-Elbert. *J. Control. Release* **116**: 204 – 210 (2006).

Tirrell, M. Aiche. J. **51**: 2386 – 2390 (2005).

Torimoto, T., M. Yamashita, S. Kuwabata, T. Sakata, H. Mori and H. Yoneyama. *J. Phys. Chem.* B **103**: 8799 – 8803 (1999).

Tu, R. S. and M. Tirrell. *Adv. Drug. Deliv. Rev.* **56**: 1537 – 1563 (2004).

Vauthey, S., S. Santoso, H. Gong, N. Watson and S. Zhang. *Proc. Natl. Acad. Sci. USA* **99**: 5355 – 5360 (2002).

Vlodavsky, I., Z. Fuks, R. Ishaimichaeli, P. Bashkin, E. Levi, G. Korner, R. Barshavit and M. Klagsbrun. *J. Cell. Biochem.* **45**: 167 – 176 (1991).

Voet, D., J. G. Voet and C. W. Pratt *Fundamentals of Biochemistry*. Wiley (2001).

Vukicevic, S., F. P. Luyten, H. K. Kleinman and A. H. Reddi. *Cell* **63**: 437 – 445 (1990).

Wang, C., R. J. Stewart and J. Kopecek. *Nature* **397**: 417 – 420 (1999).

West, J. L. and J. A. Hubbell. *Macromolecules* **32**: 241 – 244 (1999).

Whitesides, G. M. and B. Grzybowski. *Science* **295**: 2418 – 2421 (2002).

Whitesides, G. M., J. P. Mathias and C. T. Seto. *Science* **254**: 1312 – 1319 (1991).

Willerth, S. M., P. J. Johnson, D. J. Maxwell, S. R. Parsons, M. E. Doukas and S. E. Sakiyama-Elbert. *J. Biomed. Mater. Res.* A **80**: 13 – 23 (2007).

Wissink, M. J. B., R. Beernink, A. A. Poot, G. H. M. Engbers, T. Beugeling, W. G. van Aken and J. Feijen. *J. Control. Release* **64**: 103 – 114 (2000a).

Wissink, M. J. B., R. Beernink, N. M. Scharenborg, A. A. Poot, G. H. M. Engbers, T. Beugeling, W. G. van Aken and J. Feijen. *J. Control. Release* **67**: 141 – 155 (2000b).

Yamaguchi, N., B. S. Chae, L. Zhang, K. L. Kiick and E. M. Furst. *Biomacromolecules* **6**: 1931 – 1940 (2005).

Yamaguchi, N. and K. L. Kiick. *Biomacromolecules* **6**: 1921 – 1930 (2005).

Yan, H. *Science* **306**: 2048 – 2049 (2004).

Yeates, T. O. and J. E. Padilla. *Curr. Opin. Struc. Biol.* **12**: 464 – 470 (2002).

Yokoi, H., T. Kinoshita and S. G. Zhang. *P. Natl. Acad. Sci.* USA **102**: 8414 – 8419 (2005).

Yurke, B., A. J. Turberfield, A. P. Mills, Jr., F. C. Simmel and J. L. Neumann. *Nature* **406**: 605 – 608 (2000).

Zhang, L., E. M. Furst and K. L. Kiick. *J. Control Release* **114**: 130 – 142 (2006).

Zhang, S. *Nat. Biotechnol* **21**: 1171 – 1178 (2003).

Zhang, S. and A. Rich. *Proc. Natl. Acad. Sci.* U S A **94**: 23 – 28 (1997).

Zhao, X. J. and S. G. Zhang. *Adv. Polym. Sci.* 145 – 170 (2006).

Zisch, A. H., M. P. Lutolf, M. Ehrbar, G. P. Raeber, S. C. Rizzi, N. Davies, H. Schmokel, D. Bezuidenhout, V. Djonov, P. Zilla and J. A. Hubbell. *Faseb. J.* **17**: 2260 – 2262 (2003).

4 Fabrication and Assembly of Nanomaterials and Nanostructures for Biological Detections

Qingkai Yu[1] and Jie Lian[2]

[1] Department of Electrical and Computer Engineering, University of Houston, Houston, TX 77204, USA

[2] Departments of Geological Sciences and Materials Sciences & Engineering, University of Michigan, Ann Arbor, MI 48109, USA

Abstract Due to the rapid development of nanotechnologies, the concept and design of biological and chemical sensors are changing correspondingly. In this chapter, the recent advances in the application of nanostructures for biological sensors are briefly reviewed. 0-D, 1-D, and 2-D nanomaterials and nanostructures for biological detection are discussed in three sections respectively. In every section, in order, principles of detection, biodiagnostic application, fabrication, and assemblies of nanomaterials and nanostructures are discussed.

Keywords biological detection, nano particles, nano dots, nanotube, nanowire, cantilever

4.1 Introduction

A biosensor can be defined as a device that can detect biological signals through a sensing element connected to a transducer. A biological sensing element is a selective element, which can attach itself to a specific target chemical or biological agent but not to others. The four main groups of biological sensing elements are enzymes, antibodies, nucleic acids, and receptors (Eggins, 1996). A transducer converts the variation of the biological sensing element into a measurable signal, such as an electronic or photonic signal. Based on the different ways of delivering signals, transducers can be categorized as electrochemical, field-effect-transistor (FET), optical, mechanical, piezoelectric, surface acoustic wave, and thermal types (Eggins, 1996; Jain, 2006). Due to the rapid development of nanotechnologies, the concept and design of biological and chemical sensors, mainly at transducer parts, are changing correspondingly, and significant progress has been achieved

---

(1) Corresponding e-mail: qyu2@uh.edu; jlian@umich.edu

for biological detection based on novel nanomaterials and nanostructures. Because the sizes of nanostructures are comparable to the sizes of biological and chemical species such as proteins, DNA and viruses, biological and chemical sensors based on novel nanostructures have significant advantages (e.g. high sensitivity, rapid response, and low toxicity) over their traditional counterparts.

In this chapter, the recent advances in the application of nanostructures for biological sensors are briefly reviewed. Specifically, we will discuss 0-D (semiconductor quantum dots (QDs) and metal nanoparticles), 1-D (semiconductor nanowires and carbon nanotubes (CNT)), and 2-D (micro-cantilevers) nanomaterials and nanostructures for biological detection. The approaches of detection based on the above 0-D, 1-D, and 2-D nanomaterials and nanostructures are mainly optical, microelectronic and mechanical measurements, respectively. For multiplex detection, a rational, addressable array of such sensors on one chip is necessary. Therefore, the architecture of arrays of nanostructures is an important issue in the fabrication of biological sensors. The following three successive sections are focused, respectively, on 0-D, 1-D, and 2-D nanomaterials and nanostructures for biological detections, and every section describes, in order, principles of detection, biodiagnostic application, fabrications, and assemblies of nanomaterials and nanostructures.

4.2 Semiconductor Quantum Dots and Metal Nanoparticles

Semiconductor quantum dots (QDs) and metal nanoparticles have been extensively explored for application for biological detection mainly because of their unique optical properties and small sizes (Alivisatos, 2004; Hutter and Fendler, 2004, Rosi and Mirkin, 2005). The wavelength of the photoluminescence or scattering from these nanostructures is tunable by controlling their sizes, shapes and compositions. The sizes of these nanostructures can be as small as a typical protein; therefore they can be used in such biodiagnostics applications as cell labeling, cell tracking, in vivo imaging, and DNA detection. Semiconductor QDs and metal nanoparticles possess great advantages as compared with conventional organic fluorophores, which have shortcomings such as photobleaching, sensitivity to environmental conditions, and inability to excite multiple fluorophores using a single wavelength (Stroscio and Dutta, 2004).

4.2.1 Principles of Semiconductor QDs and Metal Nanoparticle Biosensors

Although both the semiconductor QDs and metal nanoparticles are in nanometer scales and can be used for biosensor applications—typically through optical detection, the detection principles are different as a result of different natures of interaction between light and nanostructures. Semiconductor QDs emit light using the same mechanisms as their bulk counterparts, except that the bandgap of the semiconductor QDs can be tuned through variations in size. If the energy of a single incident photon is equal to or larger than the band-gap of a semiconductor, the energy of the incident photon can be absorbed by the semiconductor, and then a photon with energy equal to the band-gap is emitted. Because the band-gap varies with the size of QDs at the nanometer level, the color of light emitted by QDs can be tuned. Detection through metal nanoparticles is realized by localized surface plasmons (LSPs), which are charge density oscillations confined in metallic nanoparticles and nanostructures (Hutter and Fendler, 2004). LSPs strongly interact with incident light. In solution, metal nanoparticles can lead to brilliant colors, which can be attributed to both their absorption and scattering properties (Hutter and Fendler, 2004). Since the absorption and scattering are sensitive to sizes, shapes, and structures (e.g. hollow or solid) of metal nanoparticles, as shown in Fig. 4.1, they are ideal for multiplexed biological detection (Rosi and Mirkin, 2005).

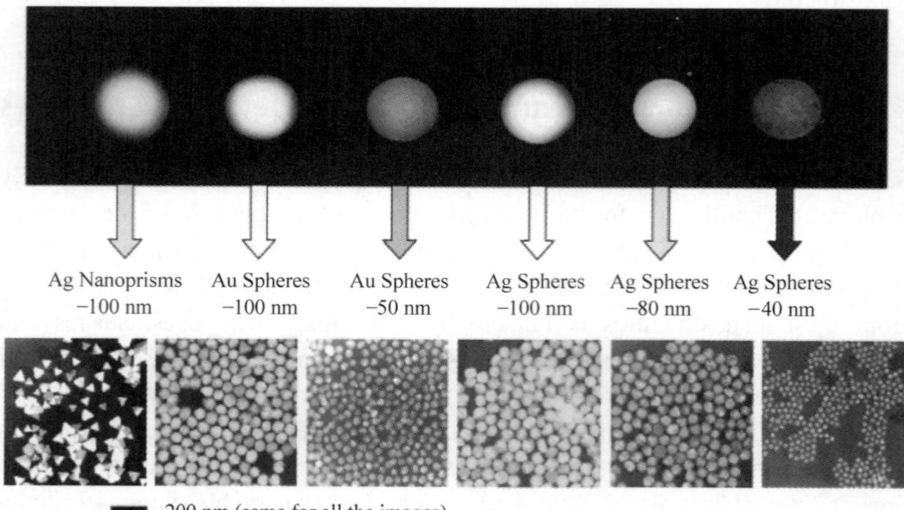

Figure 4.1 The sizes, shapes, and compositions of metal nanoparticles can be systematically varied to produce materials with distinct light-scattering properties (Rosi and Mirkin, 2005; Color Fig. 3)

Colloidal semiconductor QDs were first used for biological labeling by Alivisatos and Nie (see Bruches et al., 1998; Chan and Nie, 1998) who reported the advantages of their photochemical stability and tunable wavelength. Chan and Nie (1998) further demonstrated that by covalent coupling of ZnS-capped CdSe

QDs with biomolecules, the luminescence of the QDs can be used for ultrasensitive biological detection. In the case of coupling of ZnS-capped CdSe with transferrin, receptor-mediated endocytosis occurred, and the luminescent QDs were transported into the cell. In the absence of transferrin, no QDs were observed inside the cell, and only a weak cellular autofluorescence was obtained, as shown in Fig. 4.2(a). Moreover, such QDs, labeled with immunomolecules, can recognize specific antibodies or antigens (Chan and Nie, 1998). Recently, with the development of functionalization of QDs, more applications of semiconductor QDs were achieved, including in vivo molecular and cellular imaging (Dubertret et al., 2002; Gao et al., 2004; Gao et al., 2005), DNA detection (Taylor et al., 2000; Xu et al., 2003) and cell tracking (Parak et al., 2002).

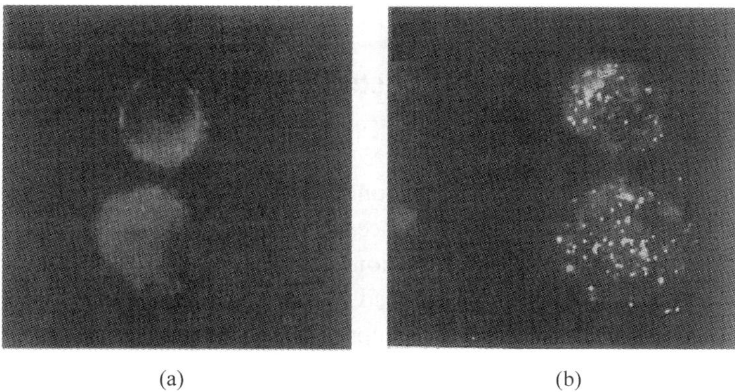

(a) (b)

Figure 4.2 Luminescence images of cultured HeLa cells incubated with (a) QDs without coupling with transferrin and (b) QD-transferrin conjugates (Chan and Nie, 1998)

The scattering and adsorption in the near field region around metal nanoparticles are greatly enhanced as the size of metal particles approaches the nanometer scale (Kreibig and Vollmer, 1995). Depending on the size of the nanoparticles and the space between them, the color of metal nanoparticle colloids varies. Mirkin and colleagues used gold nanoparticles for colorimetric polynucleotide detection (Mirkin et al., 1996). When two sets of 13-nm-diameter gold particles, conjugated with non-complementary strands of DNA (*a* and *b* in Fig. 4.3(a)), were mixed in the presence of a linking strand with ends complementary to both sets of particles, the color of the solution changed from red (dispersed particles) to blue (particle aggregates). The change of color is a consequence of interacting particle surface plasmons and aggregated scattering properties (Fig. 4.3(b)) (Mirkin et al., 1996). Metal nanoparticles also can be used to detect proteins and biologically relevant small molecules (Nam et al., 2003; Hirsch et al., 2003).

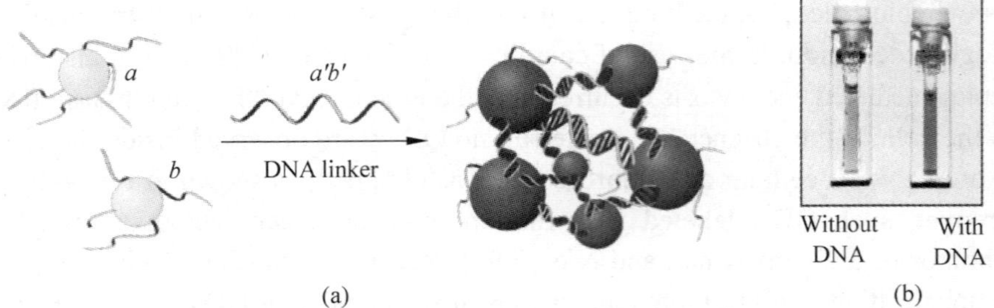

Figure 4.3 Scheme for (a) DNA-directed nanoparticle assembly (Elghanian et al., 1997) and (b) colorimetric detection. When target DNA (*a'b'*) is added to a solution of gold nanoparticles modified with DNA '*a*' and DNA '*b*,' the particles aggregate results in a change of color from red to blue that can be monitored visually (Rosi and Mirkin, 2005; Color Fig. 4)

4.2.2 Fabrication of semiconductor QDs and metal nanoparticles for biosensors

The methods for synthesizing semiconductor QDs and metal nanoparticles include sol process, micelles, sol-gel process, chemical precipitation, hydrothermal synthesis, pyrolysis, and vapor deposition (Burda et al., 2005). Except pyrolysis and vapor deposition, other methods need to employ solutions. The sol process is a common method for preparing semiconductor QDs and metal nanoparticles. Nucleation and growth should be controlled for preparing monodispersed nanostructures. A single, temporally short nucleation event followed by slower growth on the existing nuclei, which is helpful for monodispersed nanostructures, can be achieved through controlling temperature and speed of addition of reagents. The sol process is a low-cost method and can be used to synthesize nanostructures in many different material systems including Ⅱ – Ⅳ, Ⅲ – Ⅴ, Ⅳ – Ⅵ semiconductor, core/shell structures, metal, metal alloy and metal oxide (Murray et al., 1993; Hines and Guyot-Sionnest, 1998; Sun et al., 2000; Murray 1999; Murray et al., 2001; Peng and Peng, 2003; Steckel et al., 2003; Shevchenko et al., 2003; Wiley et al., 2005). Micelles and the sol-gel process can be used to synthesize metal oxides. Vapor deposition is generally used for depositing nanostructures on substrates directly.

The shape of the nanostructures can be sphere, rod, cube, triangle, and even branched structures. Peng (2003) systematically studied CdSe nanostructures and found that monomer concentration in the growth solution is a key factor for nanoparticle shape-controlling and shape-evolution. The classic model, the Gibbs-Curie-Wulff theorem based on pure thermodynamic argument, cannot explain the shape-evolution of an elongated structure, which occurs far away from the thermodynamic equilibrium. The formation of an elongated CdSe nanostructure was found to be a highly kinetics-driven reaction. In the nucleation stage, the magic-sized nanoclusters formed in a tetrahedral closed-shell configuration with a zinc blende core. If the remaining monomer concentration is extremely high, the tetrapoles form through the growth of four arms from the four (111) facets of the nanoclusters. A moderately-high monomer concentration can lead to rod-shaped nanostructures. A median monomer concentration generates rice-shaped structures. For a relatively-low monomer concentration, the growth of any of the elongated nanostructures cannot occur, and only nanodots form instead.

The structure of the nanoparticles can be solid or empty. Sun and Xia (2002) synthesized monodispersed Ag nanocubes by reducing $AgNO_3$ with ethylene glycol in the presence of poly(vinylpyrrolidone). These nanocubes had a mean edge length of 175 nm, with a standard deviation of 13 nm. Using these Ag nanocubes as sacrificial templates, Sun and Xia (2002) also synthesized gold nanoboxes with a well-defined shape and hollow structure, and the reaction can be described as $3Ag(s) + HAuCl_4(aq) \rightarrow Au(s) + 3AgCl(aq) + HCl(aq)$. Based on this stoichiometric relationship, the silver nanocubes can be converted into soluble species and leave behind a pure, solid product in the form of gold nanoboxes. Pinholes existed in the surfaces of boxes and allowed the transport of chemical species into and out of the gold boxes. From TEM study, an epitaxial relationship might exist between the surfaces of the Ag cubes and these of the gold boxes.

4.2.3 Assembly of QD and Metal Nanoparticle Arrays for Biosensor Applications

The QD and nanoparticle arrays on substrates are necessary for a chip-based biodiagnostic detection format, which allows for massive parallel screening of various analytes in a small area. Such arrays also have the benefits, such as repeated usage and controllable space between the nanoparticles. The fabrication of surface patterns in a controllable and repeatable manner has been extensively studied, and the controlled patterning of nanostructures has been achieved in predefined templates fabricated by top-down approaches. A variety of alternative methods have been developed for patterning nanostructures, such as advanced photolithographic techniques utilizing extreme ultraviolet or hard X-ray radiation as the light source (Ito and Okazaki, 2000), soft lithography (Yang et al., 2000) and replica molding (Xia et al., 1996), micro-contact (Xia et al., 1999) and nanoimprinting (Chou et al., 1996; Chou et al., 1997; Chou et al., 2002), direct-writing methods by e-beam (Huang et al., 2003) and ion beam (Albrecht et al., 2002) and dip-pen nanolithography (Piner et al., 1999; Demers et al., 2002; Zhang and Mirkin, 2004). In contrast to top-down methods, bottom-up methods assemble the atomic or molecular constituents into organized surface structures, and it is highly desirable to develop alternative approaches for the bottom-up fabrication of functional nanostructures and patterns by self-assembly processes at well-defined surfaces that have been created using top-down methods. Lian et al. (2006) have developed a simple method that allows one to pattern metallic surface nanostructures with precisely controlled size, spacing, and location using ion-beam-induced dewetting and Rayleigh instability, although at present most of such arrays are only metal nanoparticles. Predefined patterns created by focused ion beam direct-writing were used as the templates for the self-organization of ordered nanostructures. This approach represents a maskless process that combines the top-down and bottom-up patterning methods, and no chemical etching or pattern transfer steps are involved. Arrays of nanodots fabricated by dip-pen lithography and focused ion-beam lithography are shown in Fig. 4.4.

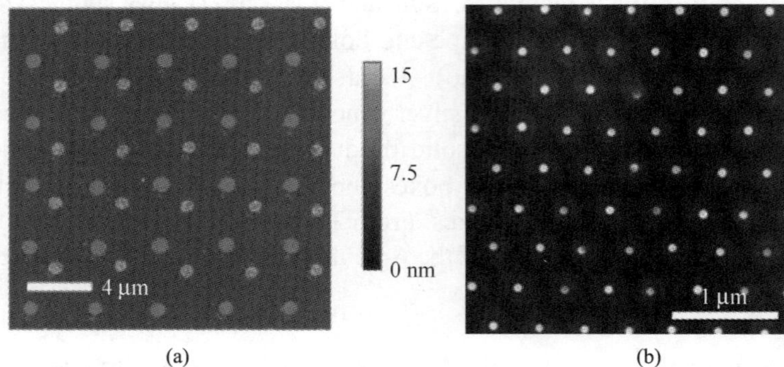

Figure 4.4 Arrays of metal nanoparticles: Au (a) by dip-pen lithography (Demers et al., 2002) and Co (b) by focused ion beam lithography (Lian et al., 2006)

4.3 Field Effect Sensors Based on Nanowires and Nanotubes

4.3.1 Detection Principles of 1-D Nanowire and Nanotube-Based Biosensors

1-D nanomaterials, such as semiconductor nanowires (NWs) and carbon nanotubes (CNTs) have been explored as signal transducers based on electrical field effects for biodiagnostics. Field effect sensors for chemicals and biological agents have been studied for more than 30 years (Bergveld, 1970; Bergveld, 1972). The principle of field effect sensors is based on the Field-effect-transistor (FET), which is used ubiquitously in electronic integrated circuits. Fig. 4.5 shows the principle of a *p*-Si planar FET device (Patolsky and Lieber, 2005), in which S, D, and G denote the source, drain, and gate electrodes, respectively. Electrical bias

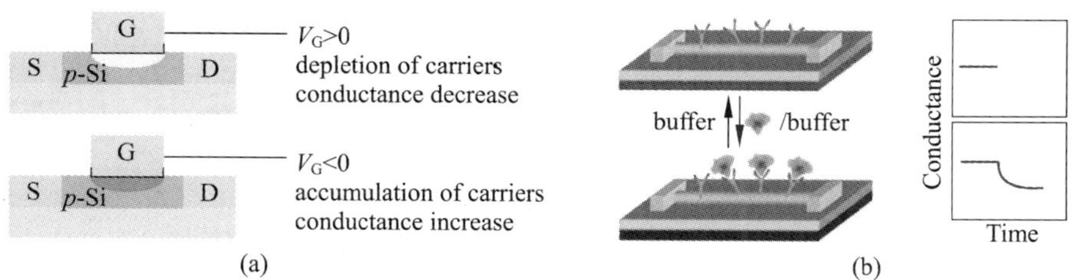

Figure 4.5 Principle of the FET NWs sensor (Color Fig. 5). (a) schematic of a regular planar FET. (b) schematic of an NWs FET sensor (Patolsky and Lieber, 2005)

is applied on S and D to drive current flowing through the *p*-Si channel. The voltage of the gate above the *p*-Si channel can adjust the carrier density in the conductive channel and thus the conductance of the Si channel of the FET (Sze, 1999). For a field effect sensor for biological agents, the gate in a FET is replaced by a biological sensing element. When a target biological agent binds with the biological sensing element, an electrical field is applied on the conductive channel because of the binding of charged biological agents. By monitoring the change in the conductance of the channel, the biological agent can be detected.

The poor sensitivity of field effect sensors based on planar FETs limits their application. However, in recent years, the progress in synthesis and assembly of semiconductor NWs has significantly enhanced the performance of field effect sensors, and the detection of a single virus was achieved (Patolsky et al., 2004; Patolsky and Lieber, 2005). The higher sensitivity of field effect sensors based on NWs can be attributed to the fact that the binding charges of biological agents only affect the conductivity of the semiconductor channel near the surface. In contrast to a bulk material, the entire volume of an NW is near its surface; therefore, the conductance of whole NWs is affected by the target biological agents. Fig. 4.5(b) shows the schematic of a biological sensor based on a Si NW-based FET (Patolsky and Lieber 2005) with antibody receptors (green) which can bind positive-charged proteins (red), leading to a decrease in conductance. At present, Si NWs and CNTs are used to build field effect sensors for chemical and biological detection (Zheng et al., 2005; Kojima et al., 2005; Byon and Choi 2006; Patolsky et al., 2006).

4.3.2 Fabrication of 1-D Nanowires and Nanotubes

Semiconductor NWs and CNTs can be synthesized through vapor-liquid-solid (VLS) growth mode by physical vapor deposition (PVD), chemical vapor deposition (CVD) and laser ablation (Morales and Lieber 1998; Kong et al., 1998; Gole et al., 2000; Hochbaum et al., 2005; Meister et al., 2006). Micelles are also used for the synthesis of NWs (Qi et al., 1997). The VLS growth mechanism is an important mode for the growth of 1-D nanomaterials by PVD and CVD. The VLS growth mechanism was first proposed in 1964 by Wagner and Ellis, who studied the growth of silicon whiskers (Wagner and Ellis, 1964). The thermodynamic and kinetic aspects were justified by Givargizov (1975) and its in situ TEM observation was done by Law et al. (2004). A typical VLS process for 1-D nanomaterials is described in Fig. 4.6 (Hu et al., 1999). A metal catalyst in nano-size is used as a template for the growth of 1-D nanomaterials, and it is liquid at growth temperature. The species of 1-D nanomaterials in the vapor phases are transported to the vapor-liquid interface. The species are dissolved into and diffused in liquid catalysts. With more dissolution of the species, the catalyst is supersaturated with the species, leading to the nucleation of solid 1-D nanomaterial. By continuing supplement of the species, the 1-D nanomaterials grow longer. The diameter of 1-D material is defined by the size of the catalyst, and in general, the size of the catalyst does not change during the VLS process. An appropriate catalyst is selected by analyzing the equilibrium phase diagrams. As a major requirement, a good solvent capable of forming a liquid alloy with the target material should exist, and ideally eutectic compounds should form.

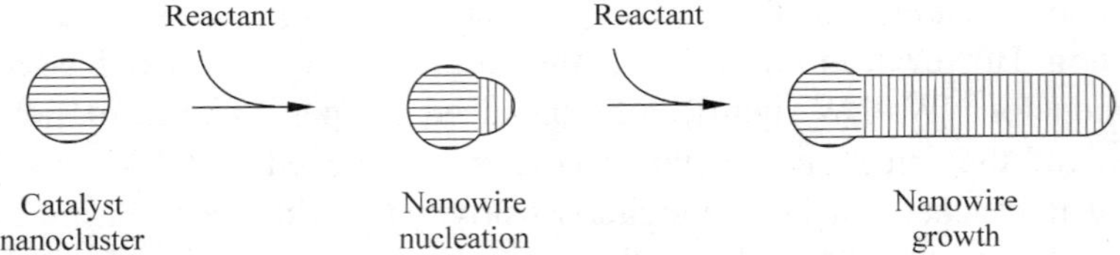

Figure 4.6 Schematic diagram illustrating the catalytic synthesis of nanowires. Reactant material, which is preferentially absorbed on the catalyst cluster, is added to the growing nanowire at the catalyst-nanowire interface (Hu et al., 1999)

Because 1-D nanomaterials with binary and more complex stoichiometries can be synthesized by the VLS mechanism, it is possible for one of these elements to serve as the VLS catalyst, which is termed self-catalytic VLS. Stach and coworkers used in situ TEM to observe directly self-catalytic growth of GaN nanowires by heating a GaN thin film in a vacuum of 10^{-7} torr (Stach et al., 2003). The major advantage of a self-catalytic process is that it avoids undesired contamination from foreign metal atoms typically used as VLS catalysts.

At present, the VLS process is extensively used to grow 1-D nanomaterials from a wide variety of pure and doped inorganic materials, including Ⅳ semiconductors (Si, Ge) (Westwater et al., 1997; Wu and Yang 2000; Zhang et al., 2001a), Ⅲ – Ⅴ semiconductors (GaN, GaAs, GaP, InP, InAs) (Gudiksen and Lieber 2000; Wu et al., 2002), Ⅱ – Ⅵ semiconductors (ZnS, ZnSe, CdS, CdSe) (Wang et al., 2002), oxides (indium-tin oxide, ZnO, MgO, SiO_2, CdO) (Yang and Lieber 1996; Peng et al., 2002; Ma and Bando 2002), carbides (SiC, B_4C) (Kim et al., 2003a), and nitrides (Si_3N_4) (Kim et al., 2003b). The 1-D nanomaterials grown by VLS are typically single crystals and are dislocation free.

4.3.3 Assembly of Ordered Nanowire and Nanotube Arrays

For practical and complex detection of biological agents, an addressable array of NWs or CNTs is necessary. Although vertically-aligned NW and CNT arrays are relatively easy to grow, horizontally-aligned 1-D nanomaterials are more useful for sensors employing field effects. In general, there are two approaches to achieving this goal: post-growth assembly and *in situ* horizontal alignment during the growth process.

Mainly, two methods are employed as post-growth assembly processes—fluidic flow-directed assembly and dip-pen nanolithography. Fluidic flow-directed assembly (Huang et al., 2001), explored by Lieber's group, is based on the Langmuir-Blodgett (LB) technique, in which the alignment of NWs was achieved through the flow of liquid in a channel. The LB technique is an effective method to assemble arrays of NWs or nanorods on a large scale (Kim et al., 2001; Kwan et al., 2001; Whang et al., 2003a, 2003b). As a common process, a drop of NW suspension in nonpolar solvent is spread on the surface of aqueous solutions, then a layer of NWs float on the air-liquid interface. During the compression, NWs become aligned along their long axes with the average spacing (center-to-center distance) controlled by the compression process, as shown in Fig. 4.7.

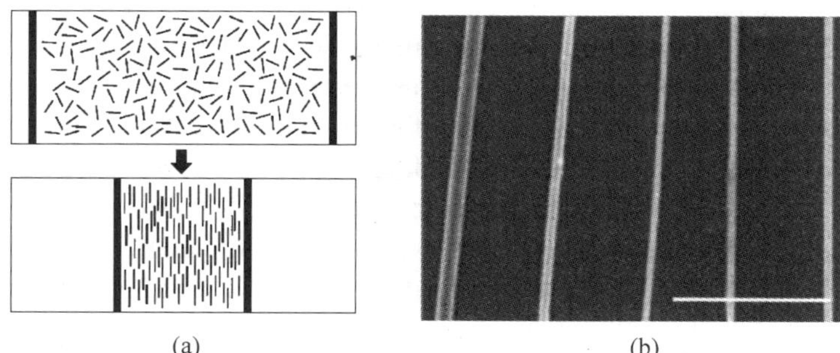

(a) (b)

Figure 4.7 (a) NWs (blue lines) in a monolayer of surfactant at the air-liquid interface are compressed on a LB trough to a specified pitch. (b) The aligned NWs are transferred to the surface of a substrate to make a uniform parallel array (Whang et al., 2003a)

Dip-pen nanolithography (DPN) has been used to assemble CNT arrays (Rao et al., 2003; Wang et al., 2006). This method is based on the phenomenon that functionalized CNTs can have strong attraction with polar chemical groups, such as COOH-terminated self-assembled monolayer (SAM), while no attraction exists between functionalized CNTs with the non-polar chemical groups, such as CH_3-terminated SAM. Fig. 4.8 shows the self-assembled CNT arrays based on DPN method (Rao et al., 2003). Wang et al., (2006) further enhanced this method such that a complex shape can be patterned.

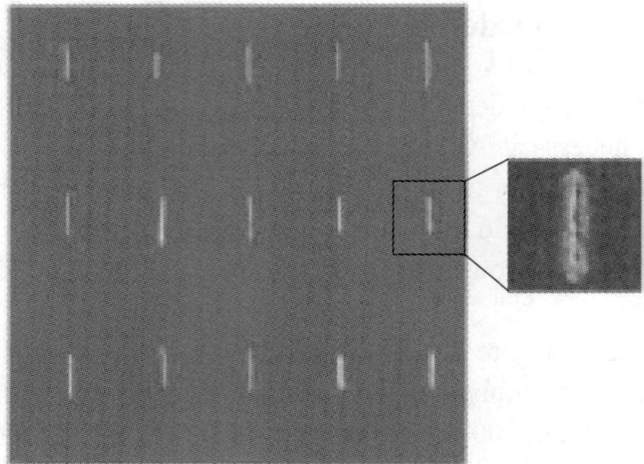

Figure 4.8 AFM images showing large-scale self-assembly of SWNTs. Topography (30 μm × 30 μm) of an array of individual SWNTs covering about 1 cm^2 of gold surface. The friction-force image (inset) shows an individual SWNT, and the regions containing 2-mercaptoimidazole (bright area) and 1-octadecanethiol (dark area)

4.3.4 Horizontally-Aligned Growth of Single-Walled Nanotubes (SWNTs) on Substrates

In situ horizontal alignment during the growth process is mainly used for aligning SWNTs. Horizontally-aligned growth can be achieved using outside forces to align the SWNTs in a certain direction. For example, electrical fields, magnetic fields and gas flows are used as external forces to drive SWNT growth in a given direction by CVD (Zhang et al., 2001b; Joselevich and Lieber, 2002; Ural et al., 2002; Huang et al., 2003). It was also discovered that SWNTs can grow in certain crystallographic directions on a single crystal wafer (Ago et al., 2005; Han et al., 2005) or in directions relative to atomic steps (Ismach et al., 2004; Ismach et al., 2005; Kocaba et al., 2005), which can be described as atomic- arrangement-programmed (AAP) mechanism. Gas-flow- and electrical-field-directed assembly are intuitive methods to align the CNTs, but currently, AAP growth shows more advantages, such as large area, high density and clean substrates. These methods for aligned growth are further discussed in detail below. The following discussion is limited to the growth by CVD because it is the only approach available to get aligned growth of SWNTs at present.

SWNTs can grow along the direction of a gas flow by CVD (Ural et al., 2002). However, in many cases growth is not aligned by gas flow; instead, the SWNTs grow in random directions on the substrate and form a network. An important factor for this aligned growth is that SWNTs must grow to a sufficient length. Because of the surface velocity profile, the velocity of the gas flow is much slower near the surface than its velocity far from the surface. Only long SWNTs can couple with the gas flow to obtain a force strong enough for the alignment.

Electrical fields have also been explored as an effective way to align SWNTs during the CVD growth. In general, the electrical field is locally created by a pair of micro-fabricated electrodes on the substrate, as schematically represented in Fig. 4.9(a). The dipole moment, P was induced by an applied field of E (Fig.4.9(b)) and can be described as: $\boldsymbol{P} = \boldsymbol{\alpha} \boldsymbol{E}$, for an SWNT with length of L. The static polarizability tensor, α, of a long SWNT is highly anisotropic. The polarizability along the tube axis, $\alpha_{//}$, is much higher than that perpendicular to the tube axis, $\alpha_{\perp}$. The coupling strength can be calculated by the electrical field and the dipole moment. According to Zhang's calculation and experiments (Zhang et al., 2001b), when $\boldsymbol{E}$ is larger than 1 V/μm, the coupling force is large enough to align the SWNTs.

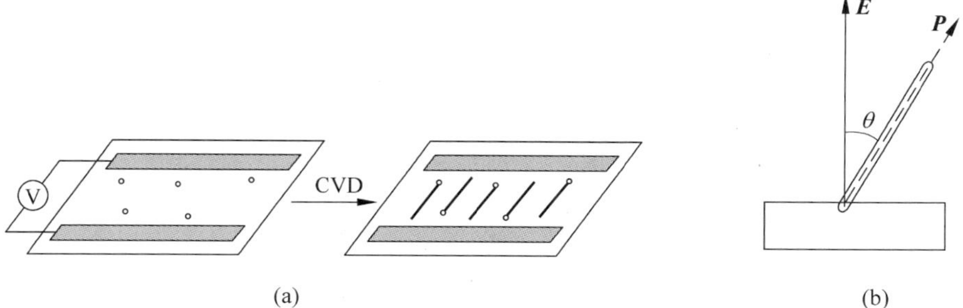

Figure 4.9 The scheme of SWNTs growth aligned by electrical field. (a) The electrical field is applied by a pair of micro-fabricated metal stripes (in grey). The dots between the metal stripes are catalysts (Joselevich and Lieber 2002). (b) An SWNT in an electrical field. E: intensity of electrical field. P: Dipole moment. θ: the angle between E and P (Zhang et al., 2001b)

Horizontally-aligned growth of SWNTs without outside forces was obtained by several groups recently (Ismach et al., 2004; Ismach et al., 2005; Han et al., 2005; Yu et al., 2006a). The growth directions of the SWNTs are related to certain lattice indexes on some crystalline planes or to the atomic steps due to the miscut of the wafer plane. The directional growth of SWNTs in certain lattice indexes can be described by AAP mode. For example, SWNTs can grow along the $[1\bar{1}0\bar{1}]$ and $[\bar{2}201]$ direction on R-plane and A-plane sapphire substrates, respectively, as shown in Fig. 4.10 However, on C-plane sapphire substrates, SWNTs grew in random directions. It is indicated that the SWNTs are strongly influenced by Al atoms on sapphire substrates. There are two possible interactions between SWNTs and Al atoms: (i) electrostatic charges transfer from Al to C atoms and (ii) the formation of a covalent bond between them. A similar phenomenon also occurred on quartz substrates [92]. However, $[1\bar{1}0\bar{1}]$ in R-plane is not the impact arrangement direction of Al atoms, which conflicts with the assumption of the strongest interaction between Al and C atoms in this direction. Recently, Yu et al. (2006a) suggested the surface of sapphire is depleted of O atoms in the growth environment due to the high temperature and hydrogen. The depletion of O atoms can make $[1\bar{1}0\bar{1}]$ the impact arrangement direction of Al atoms. Yu et al. (2006a) also synthesized horizontally-aligned SWNTs with two alignment modes on the same R-plane sapphire wafer by CVD with cationized ferritins as catalysts. In the middle part of the wafer, SWNTs were aligned on the R-plane sapphire in the direction $[1\bar{1}0\bar{1}]$. At the edge of the wafer, SWNTs were aligned in the tangential direction to the wafer edge. The comparison of these two groups of SWNTs suggests the competition between the two alignment modes and indicates that high-density atomic steps may strongly influence the SWNTs' alignment relative to the crystal structure on the sapphire substrate.

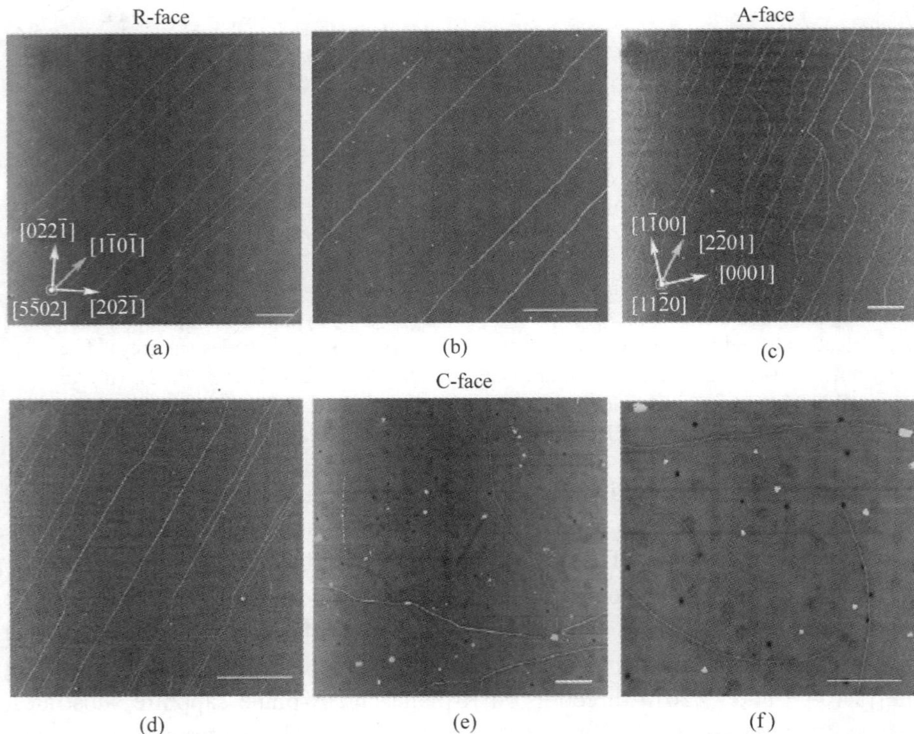

Figure 4.10 AFM images of SWNTs grown over Fe nanoparticles on three different crystalline surfaces of sapphire substrates: (a), (b) R-face $(1\bar{1}02)$, (c), (d) A-face $(11\bar{2}0)$, and (e), (f) C-face (0001). Scale bars are 1 μm. Crystalline directions were determined by an EBSD analysis (Ago et al., 2005)

Horizontally-aligned growth is very important for semiconductive NWs. However, the very limited research reported in this area reflects the difficulty of this goal. Horizontally-aligned ZnO nanowires on sapphire substrates were reported in 2004 without much discussion of the mechanisms involved (Nikoobakht et al.,

2004). The systematic investigation of the horizontal growth of semiconductor nanowires is required before such nanowires could be used for device applications.

4.4 Micro-cantilever sensors

4.4.1 Detection Principle of Micro-Cantilever Sensors

The principle of chemical and biological sensors based on micro-cantilevers is similar to that of the atomic force microscope (AFM), as shown in Fig. 4.11. An AFM consists of a micro-cantilever with a sharp tip (probe) at its end which is used to scan the specimen surface. When the tip is brought into proximity with a sample surface, forces between the tip and the sample lead to a deflection of the cantilever and a change of its resonance frequency, which can be monitored through a laser beam reflection from the cantilever's backside. A chemical and biological sensor based on micro-cantilevers requires neither a sharp tip nor a sample surface. A micro-cantilever sensor is an array of cantilever beams functionalized by deposition of a sensitive layer of biological detection elements. The micro-cantilevers are tens to hundreds of micrometers long, tens of micrometers wide and tens to hundreds of nanometers thick. The sensitive layer can be either highly-specific for molecular recognition or only partially-specific to produce response patterns for various analytes, provided that each cantilever is coated with a different partially-specific sensor layer. The binding of target agents with biological detection elements can change some characteristics of the cantilever, such as mass, stress and temperature, which lead to the deflection or change of the cantilever's resonance frequency. The changes can be monitored by laser-photodiode or piezoelectric system. The sensitivity of sensors based on

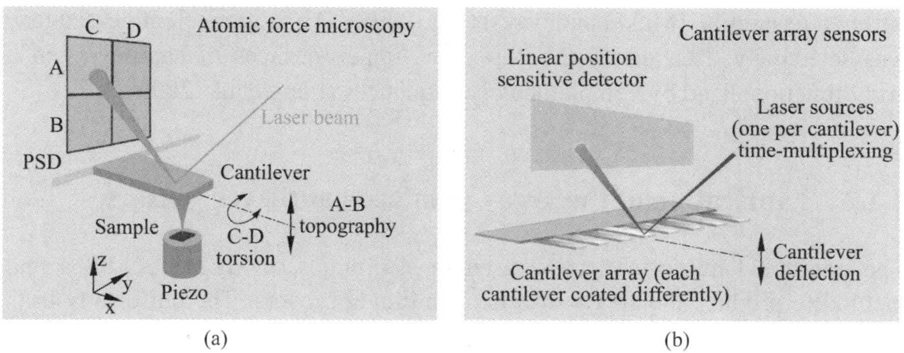

Figure 4.11 Schematic of the AFM technique (a) and the cantilever-array sensor readout (b). Different sensing layers are shown in different colors (Lang et al., 2005; Color Fig. 6)

micro-cantilevers is as high as a picogram. The miniaturization of cantilevers can improve their sensitivity to sub-picogram measurement (Viani et al., 1999; Yu et al., 2006b). However, the improvement of sensitivity by miniaturization is limited when the thickness of the cantilever is comparable with the thickness of coated receptors and the caught target species on the cantilever (Gupta et al., 2006). Specifically, when the mass of the attached biological agent is large and comparable with that of the cantilever, the change of the net stiffness constant of the cantilever is not negligible and may lead to the increase in the cantilever's resonant frequency.

Two-dimensional micro-cantilever arrays on one chip have been developed to simultaneously perform multiple biomolecular analyses and thereby rapidly provide a large database to study the underlying science (Yue et al., 2004).

The micro-cantilever is a sensitive tool for detecting biological agents and can be operated in static, dynamic and heat modes. In static mode, a sensitive layer is deposited onto one surface of the cantilever for molecule recognition and the surface stress induced by the adsorption process bends the cantilever. Surface stresses of several 10^{-3} N/m can result in deflections of about 10 nm for the cantilever sensors used (McKendry et al., 2002). In dynamic mode, the resonance frequency of the cantilever shifts to a lower value because of the adsorbed mass. A mass change of 1 pg can lead to a change of 1 Hz in resonance frequency for the cantilever sensors (Battiston et al., 2001). Using cantilevers with bilayer materials, a heat mode can detect temperature variations due to biological adsorption. Temperature changes of 10^{-5} K produce cantilever deflections of several nanometers, which can be measured easily (Gimzewski et al., 1994).

Microporous silica and mesoporous alumina film were used to selectively detect dimethyl methylphosphonate, a simulant of the nerve agent, sarin (Zhao et al., 2006). Some polymer films can be used to detect organic vapors, such as *n*-octane, 1-butanol, toluene and a mixture of them (Then et al., 2006). The conformation-specific peptides β/α I and β/α II were used to detect oestrogen receptor with or without oestradiol (Mukhopadhyay et al., 2005). An oligonucleotide sequence was selectively detected by the Au-coated upper surfaces of cantilevers in an array functionalized by complementary-sequences (Lang et al., 2005).

4.4.2 Fabrication of the array of micro-cantilever sensors

The traditional micro-fabrication used in electronics or MEMS is still a main method to produce the arrays of micro-cantilever sensors. The uniformity in the sizes of cantilevers in an array is critical for comparing the responses of different cantilevers. A silicon-on-insulator technique is used to obtain uniform thickness of the cantilever arrays. It is still a challenge to functionalize the cantilevers individually. Traditional photolithography fails to functionalize cantilevers because photoresist is difficult to apply to cantilevers and is not compatible with many solvents during the functionalization process (Bietsch et al., 2004). Bietsch et al. (2004) used ink jet and microcapillaries to functionalize micro-cantilevers with high efficiency, as shown in Fig.4. 12.

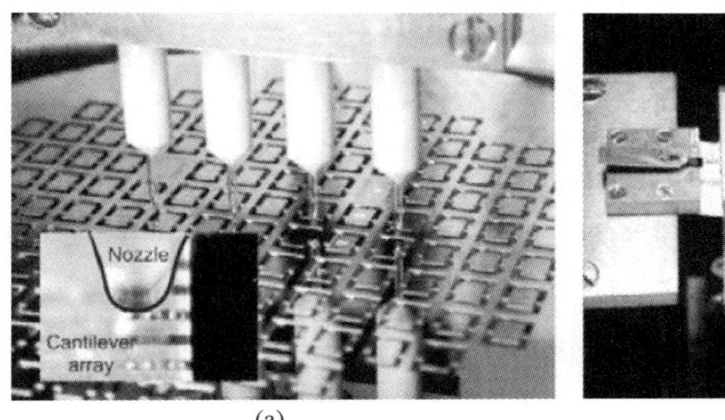

(a)

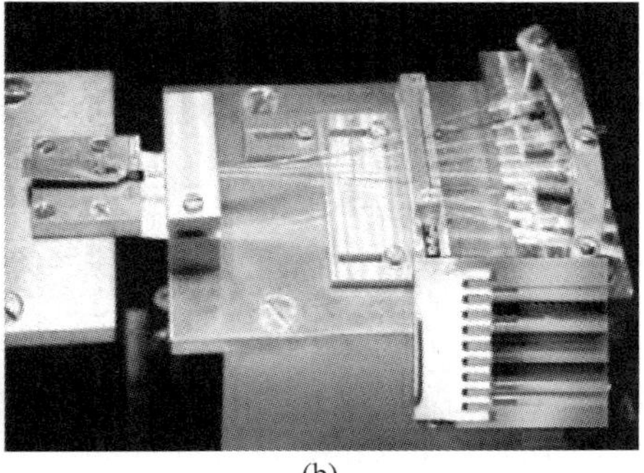

(b)

Figure 4.12 Cantilever array functionalization using (a) a four-nozzle ink-jet device (the inset shows spotted liquid droplets at the upper surface of the cantilever) and (b) an array of eight microcapillaries (the inset shows how the individual cantilevers of the array are inserted into the array of microcapillaries; the colored liquids are for visualization purposes only) (Lang et al., 2005; Color Fig.7)

4.5 Summary

The significant development of nanotechnology brings new approaches for biological detection. Semiconductor QDs, metal nanoparticles, semiconductor NWs, CNTs and micro-cantilevers have been broadly explored for biological detection by the surveillance of changes in optical, electrical and mechanical properties. Despite the significant advances in using novel nanostructures for biological detection, great challenges still exist before nano-biosensors can be fully utilized for practical clinical use. For example, the assembly of ordered semiconductor QDs and metal nanoparticle arrays on chips and the horizontal growth of desired nanowires and nanotubes on substrates should be realized. The fabrication of micro-cantilever arrays with well-controlled size uniformity and functionality is a critical issue for the application of micro-cantilever-based biosensors, and the effects of variations in the mass and stiffness constants and thus the resonance frequency of the cantilever arrays upon the attachment of the biological agents should be compensated in order to improve sensitivity. With the advantages over their conventional counterparts—such as rapid response, high sensitivity and multiplex detection on one chip—and with the rapid development of nanotechnology, we believe that biological sensors based on novel nanomaterials and nanostructures will move from the research arena to mainstream clinical use.

References

Ago, H., K. Nakamura, K. Ikeda, N. Uehara, N. Ishigami and M. Tsuji. *Chem. Phys. Lett.* **408**: 433 (2005).

Albrecht, M., C. T. Rettner, A. Moser, M. E. Best and B. D. Terris. *Appl. Phys. Lett.* **81**: 2875 (2002).

Alivisatos, P. *Nat. Biotechnol* 22: 47 (2004).

Battiston, F.M., J.P. Ramseyer, H.P. Lang, M.K. Baller, C. Gerber, J.K. Gimzewski, E. Meyer and H.J. Guntherodt. *Sens. Actuators* **B 77**: 122 (2001).

Bergveld, P. *IEEE Trans. Biomed. Eng.* **17**: 70 (1970).

Bergveld, P. *IEEE Trans. Biomed. Eng.* **19**: 342 (1972).

Bietsch, A., J. Zhang, M. Hegner, H. P. Lang and C. Gerber. *Nanotechnol* **15**: 873 (2004).

Bruches, M., M. Moronne, P. Gin, S. Weiss and A.P. Alivisatos. *Science* **281**: 2013 (1998).

Burda, C., X. Chen, R. Narayanan and M. A. El-Sayed. *Chem. Rev.* **105**: 1025 (2005).

Byon, H. R., and H. C. Choi. *J. Am. Chem. Soc.* **128**: 2188 (2006).

Chan, W.C.W. and S.M. Nie. *Science* **281**: 2016 (1998).

Chou, S. Y., P. R. Krauss and P. J. Renstrom. *Science* **272**: 85 (1996).

Chou, S. Y., P.R. Krauss, W. Zhang, L. Guo and L. Zhuang. *J.Vac. Sci. Technol.* B **15**: 2897 (1997).

Chou, S. Y., C. Keimel and J. Gu. *Nature* **417**: 835 (2002).

Demers, L.M., D. S. Ginger, S.J. Park, Z. Li, S.W. Chung and C.A. Mirkin. *Science* **296**: 1836 (2002).

Dubertret, B., P. Skourides, D. J. Norris, V. Noireaux, A. H. Brivanlou and A. Libchaber. *Science* **298**: 1759 (2002).

Eggins, B. *Biosensors: An Introduction,* Wiley and Teubner (1996).

Elghanian, R., J.J. Storhoff, R.C. Mucic, R.L. Letsinger and C.A. Mirkin. *Science* **277**: 1078 (1997).

Gao, X., Y. Cui, R. M. Levenson, L. W. K. Chung and S. Nie. *Nat. Biotechnol.* **22**: 969 (2004).

Gao, X., L. Yang, J. A Petros, F. F Marshall, J. W Simons and S. Nie. *Curr. Opin. Biotechnol.* **16**: 63 (2005).

Gimzewski, J.K., C. Gerber, E. Meyer and R.R. Schlittler. *Chem. Phys. Lett.* **217**: 589 (1994).

Givargizov, E. I. *J. Cryst. Growth* **31**: 20 (1975).

Gole, J.L., J.D. Scout, W.L. Rauch and Z.L. Wang. *Appl. Phys. Lett.* **76**: 2346 (2000).

Gudiksen, M. S., and C. M. Lieber. *J. Am. Chem. Soc.* **122**: 8801 (2000).

Gupta, A. K., P. R. Nair, D. Akin, M. R. Ladisch, S. Broyles, M. A. Alam and R. Bashir. *Proc. Natl. Acad. Sci.* **103**: 13,362 (2006).

Han, S., X. Liu and C. Zhou. *J. Am. Chem. Soc.* **127**: 5294 (2005).

Hines, M.A. and P. Guyot-Sionnest. *J. Phys. Chem. B* **102**: 3655 (1998).

Hirsch, L.R., J.B. Jackson, A. Lee, N.J. Halas and J. West. *Anal.Chem.* **75**: 2377 (2003).

Hochbaum, A.I., R. He, R. Fan and P. Yang. *Nano Lett.* **5**: 457 (2005).

Hu, J., T. W. Odom and C. M. Lieber. *Acc. Chem. Res.* **32**: 435 (1999).

Huang, S., X. Cai and J. Liu. *J. Am. Chem. Soc.* **125**: 5636 (2003).

Huang, Y., X. Duan, Q. Wei and C. M. Lieber. *Science* **291**: 630 (2001).
Huang, W.S., W. He, W. Li, W.M. Moreau, R. Lang, D.R. Medeiros, K.E. Petrillo, A.P. Law, M., J. Goldberger and P. Yang. *Annu. Rev. Mater. Res.* **34**: 83 (2004).
Hutter, E., and J. H. Fendler. *Adv. Mater.* **16**: 685 (2004).
Ismach, A., L. Segev, E. Wachtel and E. Joselevich. Angew. *Chem. Int. Ed.* **43**: 6140 (2004).
Ismach, A., D. Kantorovich and E. Joselevich. *J. Am. Chem. Soc.* **127**: 11,554 (2005).
Ito, T., and S. Okazaki. *Nature* **406**: 1027 (2000).
Jain, K.K. *Nanobiotechnology in Molecular Diagnostics: Current Techniaues and Application*, Horizon Bioscience (2006).
Joselevich, E. and C. Lieber. *Nano Lett.* **2**: 1137 (2002).
Kim, F., S. Kwan, J. Akana and P. Yang. *J. Am. Chem. Soc.* **123**: 4360 (2001).
Kim, H. Y., J. Park. and H. Yang. *Chem. Commun.* **21**: 256 (2003a).
Kim, H. Y., J. Park and H. Yang. *Chem. Phys. Lett.* **372**: 269 (2003b).
Kocabas, C., S. H. Hur, A. Gaur, M. A. Meitl, M. Shim and J. A. Rogers. *Small* **1**: 1110 (2005).
Kojima, A., C. K. Hyon, T. Kamimura, M. Maeda and K. Matsumoto. *Jap. J. Appl. Phys.* **44**: 1596 (2005).
Kong, J., A. Cassell and H. J. Dai. *Chem. Phys. Lett.* **292**: 567 (1998).
Kreibig, U. and M. Vollmer. *Optical Properties of Metal Clusters*. Berlin: Springer Verlag (1995).
Kwan, S., F. Kim, J. Arkana and P. Yang. *Chem. Commun.* **5**: 447 (2001).
Lang, H. P., M. Hegner and C. Gerber. *Mater. Today* **8**: 30 (2005).
Lian, J., L. M. Wang, X. C. Sun, Q. Yu, R. C. Ewing, *Nano Lett.* **6**: 1047 (2006).
Liu, J., M. J. Casavant, M. Cox, D. A. Walters, P. Boul, W. Lu, A. J. Rimberg, K. A. Smith, D. T. Colbert and R. E. Smalley. *Chem. Phys. Lett.* **303:** 125 (1999).
Ma, R. and Y. Bando. *Chem. Mater.* **14**: 4403 (2002).
Mahorowala, M. Angelopoulos, C. Deverich, C. Huang and P.A. Rabidoux. *Proc. SPIE-Int. Soc. Opt. Eng.* **5130**: 58 (2003).
McKendry, R., J. Zhang, Y. Arntz, T. Strunz, M. Hegner, H. P. Lang, M. K. Baller, U. Certa, E. Meyer, H.-J. Güntherodt and C. Gerber. *Proc. Natl. Acad. Sci. USA* **99**: 9783 (2002).
Meister, S., H. Peng, K. McIlwrath, K. Jarausch, X.F. Zhang and Y. Cui. *Nano Lett.* 6: 1514 (2006).
Mirkin, C.A., R.L. Letsinger, R.C. Mucic and J.J. Storhoff. *Nature* **382**: 607 (1996).
Morales, A.M., and C.M. Lieber. *Science* **279**: 208 (1998).
Mukhopadhyay, R., V. V. Sumbayev, M. Lorentzen, J. Kjems, P. A. Andreasen and F. Besenbacher. *Nano Lett.* **5**: 2385 (2005).
Murray, C.B., D.J. Norris and M.G. Bawendi. *J. Am. Chem. Soc.* **115**: 8706 (1993).
Murray, C. B., S. Sun, W. Gaschler, H. Doyle, T.A. Betley and C.R. Kagan. *IBM J. Res. Rev.* **45**: 47 (2001).
Nam, J.M., C.S. Thaxton and C.A. Mirkin. *Science* **301**: 1884 (2003).
Nikoobakht, B., C.A. Michaels, S. Stranick and M.D. Vaudin. *Appl. Phys. Lett.* **85**: 3244 (2004).
Parak, W.J., R. Boudreau, M. Le Gros, D. Gerion, D. Zanchet, C.M. Micheel, S.C. Williams, A.P. Alivisatos and C. Larabell. Adv. Mater. **14**: 882 (2002).

Patolsky, F., G. Zheng, O. Hayden, M. Lakadamyali, X. Zhuang and C. M. Lieber. *Proc. Natl. Acad. Sci. USA* **101**: 14,017 (2004).

Patolsky, F. and C. M. Lieber. *Mater. Today* **8**: 20 (2005).

Patolsky, F., G. Zheng, and C.M. Lieber. *Nanomedicine* **1**: 51 (2006).

Peng, X. S., G. W. Meng, X. F. Wang, Y. W. Wang, J. Zhang J, X. Liu, and L. D Zhang. *Chem. Mater*. **14**: 4490 (2002).

Peng, X. *Adv. Mater*. **15**: 459 (2003).

Peng, Z.A. and X. Peng. *J. Am. Chem. Soc*. **123**: 183 (2001).

Piner, R. D., J. Zhu, F. Xu, S. Hong and C. A. Mirkin. *Science* **283**: 661 (1999).

Qi, L.M., J. Ma, H. Chen and Z. Zhao. *J. Phys. Chem. B* **101**: 3460 (1997).

Rao, S.G., L. Huang, W. Setyawan and S. Hong. *Nature* **425**: 36 (2003).

Rosi, N. L. and C. A. Mirkin. *Chem. Rev*. **105**: 1547 (2005).

Shevchenko, E.V., D.V. Talapin, H. Schnablegger, A. Kornowski, O. Festin, P. Svedlindh, M. Haase and H. Weller. *J. Am. Chem. Soc*. **125**: 9090 (2003).

Stach, E. A., P. J. Pauzauskie, T. Kuykendall, J. Goldberger, R. He and P. Yang, *Nano Lett*. **3**: 867 (2003).

Steckel, J.S., S. Coe-sullivan, V. Bulovic and M.G. Bawendi. *Adv.Mater*. **15**: 1862 (2003).

Stroscio, M. and Mitra Dutta. *Biological Nanostructures and Applications of Nanostructures in Biology: Electrical, Mechanical, & Optical Properties*. New York: Kluwer Acaademic/ Plenum Publishers (2004).

Sun, S. and C.B. Murray. *J. Appl. Phys*. **85**: 4325 (1999).

Sun, S., C.B. Murray, D. Weller, L. Folks and A. Moser. *Science* **287**: 1989 (2000).

Sun, Y. and Y. Xia. *Science* **298**: 2176 (2002).

Sze, S.M. *Semiconductor Devices: Physics and Technology*, 2nd edn. Wiley (1999).

Taylor, J. R., M. M. Fang and S. Nie. *Anal Chem*. **72**: 1979 (2000).

Then, D., A. Vidic and Ch. Ziegler. *Sens Actuators* B **117**: 1 (2006).

Ural, A., Y. Li and H. Dai. *Appl. Phys. Lett*. **81**: 3464 (2002).

Viani, M. B., T. E. Schaffer, A. Chand, M. Rief, H. E. Gaub and P. K. Hansma. *J. Appl. Phys*. **86**: 2258 (1999).

Wagner, R. S. and W. C. Ellis. *Appl. Phys. Lett*. **4**: 89 (1964).

Wang, Y., L. Zhang, C. Liang, G. Wang and X. Peng. *Chem. Phys. Lett*. **357**: 314 (2002).

Wang, Y., D. Maspoch,S. Zou, G.C. Schatz, R.E. Smalley and C.A. Mirkin. *Proc. Natl. Acad. Sci* **103**: 2026 (2006).

Westwater, J., D. P. Gosain, S. Tomiya, S. Usui and H. Ruda. *J. Vac. Sci. Technol. B* **15**: 554 (1997).

Whang, D., Song Jin, Yue Wu and C. M. Lieber. *Nano Lett*. **3**: 1255 (2003a).

Whang, D., S. Jin and C.M. Lieber. *Nano Lett*. **3**: 951 (2003b).

Wiley, B., Y. Sun, J. Chen,H. Cang, Z. Y. Li, X. Li and Y. Xia. *MRS Bull*. **30**: 356 (2005).

Wu, Y., and P. Yang, *Chem. Mater*. **12**: 605 (2000).

Wu, Y., H. Yan, M. Huang, B. Messer, J. H. Song and P. Yang. *Chem. Eur. J*. **8**: 1260 (2002).

Xia, Y. N., E. Kim, X. M. Zhao, J. A. Rogers, M. Prentiss and G. M. Whitesides. *Science* **273**: 347 (1996).

Xia, Y. N., J. A. Rogers, K. E. Paul and G. M. Whitesides. *Chem. Rev.* **99**: 1823 (1999).

Xu, H., M. Y. Sha, E. Y. Wong, J. Uphoff, Y. Xu, J. A. Treadway, A. Truong, E. O'Brien, S. Asquith, M. Stubbins, N. K. Spurr, E. H. Lai and W. Mahoney. *Nucleic Acids Res.* **31**: E43 (2003).

Yang, P. and C. M. Lieber. *Science* **273**: 1836 (1996).

Yang, P. D., G. Wirnsberger, H. C. Huang, S. R. Cordero, M. D. McGehee, B. Scott, T. Deng, G. M.Whitesides, B. F. Chmelka, S. K. Buratto and G. D. Stucky. *Science* **287**: 465 (2000).

Yu, Q., G. Qin, H. Li, Z. Xia, Y.Nian, S. S. Pei. *J. Phys. Chem. B* **110**: 22676 (2006a).

Yu, Q., G. Qin, C. Darne, C. Cai,W. Wosik, S. S. Pei. *Sens. Actuators A* **126**: 369 (2006b).

Yue, M., H. Lin, D. E. Dedrick, S. Satyanarayana, A. Majumdar, A. S. Bedekar, J. W. Jenkins and S. Sundaram. *J. Microelectromech. Syst.* **13**: 290 (2004).

Zhang, H. and C.A. Mirkin. *Chem. Mater.* **16**: 1480 (2004).

Zhang, Y. J., Q. Zhang, N. L. Wang, Y. J. Yan, H. H. Zhou and J. Zhu. *J. Cryst. Growth* **226**: 185 (2001a).

Zhang, Y., A. Chang, J. Cao, Q. Wang, W. Kim, Y. Li, N. Morris, E. Yenilmez, J. Kong and H. Dai. *Appl. Phys. Lett.*, **79**: 3155 (2001b).

Zhao, Q., Q. Zhu, W. Y. Shih, W.-H. Shih. *Sens. Actuators B* **117**: 74 (2006).

Zheng, G., F. Patolsky, Y. Cui, W. U Wang and C. M Lieber. *Nat. Biotechnol.* **23**: 1294 (2005).

5 Nanostructured Materials Constructed from Polypeptides

Peng Jing, Jangwook P. Jung and Joel H. Collier[1]

Department of Biomedical Engineering,
University of Cincinnati, Cincinnati, OH 45221-0048,USA
[1] Department of Surgery and Committee on Molecular Medicine,
University of Chicago, Chicago, IL60637

Abstract This chapter describes peptide design strategies for the construction of nanostructured materials. It begins with a brief tutorial of amino acid structure and function and then describes higher-order assemblies of peptides and peptidomimetics. Primarily β-sheet fibril-forming peptides and α-helical coiled coil systems are discussed, as these systems have received particular attention in recent years for building nanostructured materials. Useful properties that arise from peptide construction are addressed, including stimulus-responsiveness, modularity, and multifunctionality, and a number of technological applications are described, including Tissue Engineering, antimicrobials, drug delivery, and nanoscale electronics. The chapter is meant to be an introduction for researchers or students in nanotechnology who may wish to extend their approaches into the biomolecular realm, and it also provides a compendium of recent advances for experts in the field of nanoscale peptide materials.

5.1 Introduction

Proteins and peptides are nanostructured biological materials. In their native roles in biology, they exhibit a staggering diversity, taking part in such wide-ranging functions as chemical catalysis, force generation, signaling, transport, optical responsiveness, and load bearing. Owing to these diverse and technologically relevant natural roles, proteins and peptides represent one of the most compelling inspirations for creating synthetic or semi-synthetic materials that can perform similarly wide-ranging functions in engineered systems.

This chapter aims to provide a synopsis of strategies that utilize peptides,

---

(1) Corresponding e-mail: collier@uchicago.edu

peptide derivatives, and peptidomimetics for building synthetic or semi-synthetic nanostructured materials. In the most successful recent examples of such strategies, these materials approach the functionality of native protein structures but also retain the engineerability inherent in synthetic materials. The chapter also aims to provide a general background in protein and peptide design necessary for a working understanding of these strategies in nanoscience. Although engineered peptide materials are useful in a variety of medical and non-medical applications, this chapter will emphasize strategies that are impacting or likely to impact biomedical science, with special emphasis on biomaterials. Current target applications in this regard include utilizing these materials as matrices for tissue engineering/ regenerative medicine and as controlled drug release materials.

The chapter is intended to be useful to those potentially interested in expanding their nanoscience approaches into the biological realm but who may not have had significant experience in protein and peptide design. It also provides a compendium of recent approaches for producing nanostructured peptide biomaterials that should be useful to readers of all levels. The chapter begins with a tutorial in the general underpinnings of protein and peptide science: amino acid structure, secondary structures, and the design rules necessary for producing nanostructured materials from these peptides and proteins. In particular, β-sheet fibrillar materials and α-helical filamentous materials will be discussed. Useful materials properties that arise from these engineered structures will be outlined, including stimulus-responsiveness, complex bioactivity, multi-functionality, and modularity, and recent advances in these regards will be discussed. The chapter will conclude with a discussion of several technological hurdles facing the advancement of such materials, particularly with respect to their use in biomedicine.

5.2 Amino Acids and Their Derivatives: Building Blocks for Nanostructured Materials

5.2.1 Canonical Amino Acids

The common structure of the 20 genetically encoded amino acids consists of a C_α atom to which an amino group, a carboxylic acid group, a hydrogen atom, and a side chain are attached (Fig. 5.1). Amino acids in naturally occurring proteins are almost always L-amino acids, with D-isomers occurring only infrequently, for example in bacterial cell walls. In biology, peptides and proteins are produced through the action of ribosomes, which catalyze the condensation polymerization of amino acids to produce polypeptides. To produce peptides synthetically, amino acids are polymerized using amino acids whose primary amines and side chains are chemically protected. Using sequential deprotection, activation, and condensation reactions, peptides are polymerized step-wise on solid phase resins using the procedures originally outlined by Nobel laureate Bruce Merrifield (Merrifield, 1963). For a given application in nanotechnology, the choice between chemical synthesis or biosynthesis of a target peptide or protein is frequently made based on the molecule's size, as peptides approaching 50 amino acids tend to be challenging to produce synthetically, though this limit is continually being extended.

Amino acids can be divided into a number of categories. Among the more useful subdivisions are: hydrophobic (non-polar), hydrophilic (polar), and charged (Fig. 5.1). The hydrophobic/hydrophilic character of the 20 naturally occurring

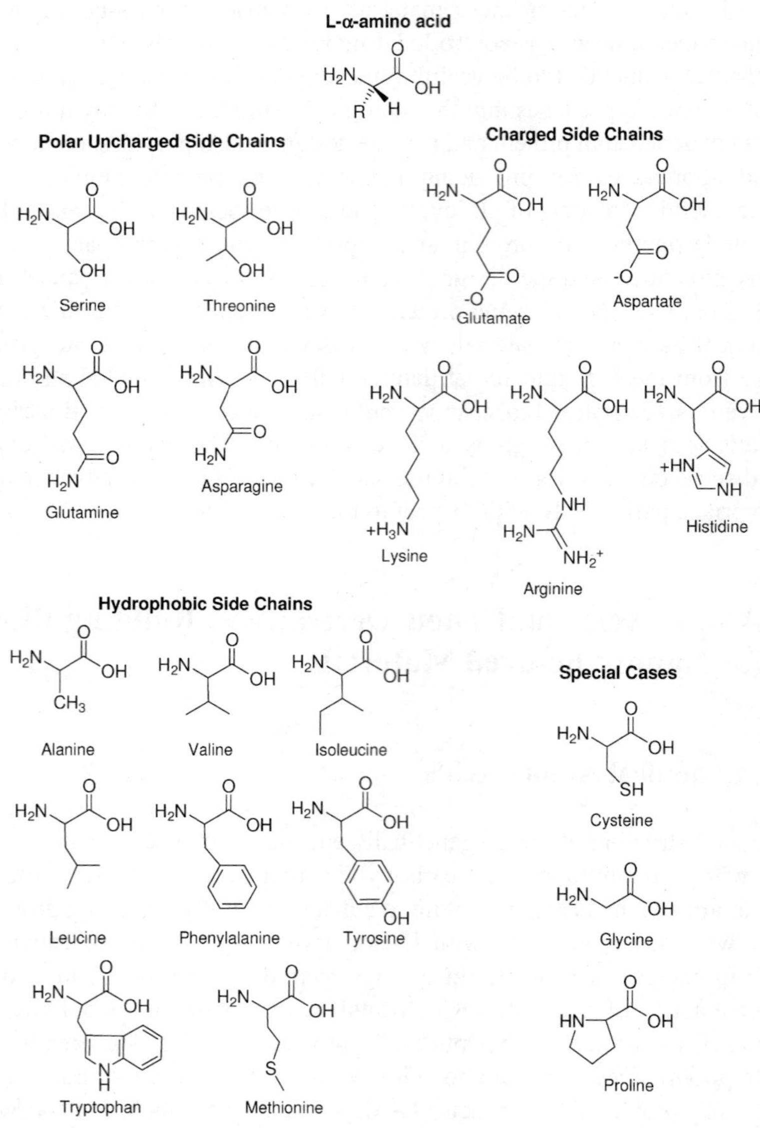

Figure 5.1 The twenty genetically encoded amino acids

amino acids varies widely, with phenylalanine, leucine, and isoleucine being the most hydrophobic. In proteins, these residues tend to be buried in solvent-hidden sites. Consideration of the positioning of these hydrophobic residues represents one of the most significant factors in designing nanostructured protein and peptide materials, as will be discussed later in the chapter. Polar residues tend to occupy solvent-exposed positions in proteins. Within this category, acidic and basic amino acids exhibit pH-dependent ionization of their side chains that enables electrostatic interactions between and within polypeptides. Two amino acids, proline and cysteine merit particular mention due to their uniqueness. Proline can act to constrain the positioning of the peptide backbone due to the rigidity of its cyclic side chain. It is thus infrequently found in the secondary structures discussed in this chapter, but it is often found at the ends of helices, at the edges of sheets, and in turns. Cysteine can act to stabilize protein folding through the generation of disulfide bonds, formed between the thiol side chains of two closely approximated cysteine residues.

5.2.2 Non-canonical Amino Acids

Although the 20 genetically coded amino acids represent a diverse collection of chemical functionality, non-natural or post-translationally modified amino acids can be utilized to confer additional features such as unique chemical reactivity or enhanced thermal or chemical stability (Fig. 5.2). Here we will illustrate a few notable examples; for more complete reviews of non-canonical amino acids in protein engineering, see (Dougherty, 2000; Hohsaka and Sisido, 2002; Link et al., 2003). One useful group of non-canonical amino acids are those with very hydrophobic fluorinated side chains such as trifluoroisoleucine, hexafluoroleucine, or trifluorovaline, which may be utilized for enhancing the thermal or chemical stability of engineered proteins without significantly altering their folding (Montclare and Tirrell, 2006; Son et al., 2006). To provide for covalent stabilization of nanostructures or other chemoselective conjugation chemistry, amino acids with unsaturated side chains such as allylglycine, homoallylglycine, or homopropargylglycine (Fig. 5.2) may be incorporated either synthetically (Clark and Ghadiri, 1995) or biosynthetically (Tang and Tirrell, 2002; van Hest et al., 2000). Incorporation of azide-containing amino acids such as azidohomoalanine (Kiick et al., 2002) further enables copper (I)-catalyzed triazole chemistry or Staudinger ligation for the 'covalent capture' of nanostructures. Beyond those residues useful for stabilization or functionalization, another interesting example of a useful non-canonical amino acid is 3,4-dihydroxyphenylalanine (DOPA), an amino acid produced biologically by the posttranslational hydroxylation of tyrosine (Waite and Tanzer, 1981). It is one of the key components of the adhesive plaques of marine animals, including mussels, so it has recently garnered attention for producing nanoscale adhesives and coatings (Lee et al., 2007a; Lee et al., 2007b). In one example, conjugates of DOPA-containing peptides and polyethylene glycol (PEG) have been designed such that the DOPA anchors the PEG chains to a variety of surfaces to produce non-fouling coatings (Dalsin et al., 2003; Lee et al., 2006).

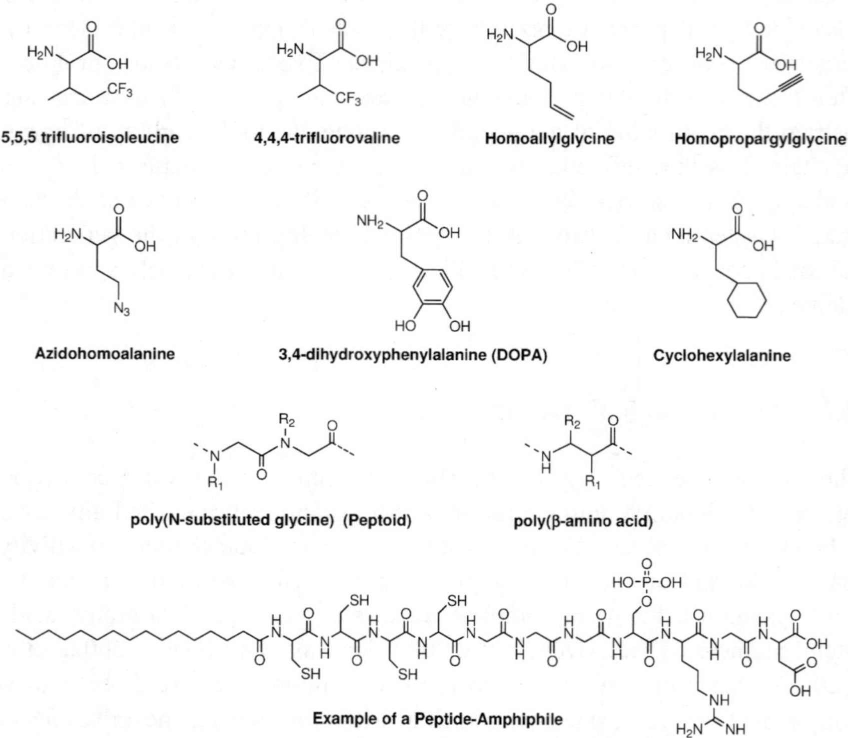

Figure 5.2 A selection of non-canonical amino acids and peptidomimetics useful for the construction of nanoscale peptide materials. The peptide amphiphile shown is described in Hartgerink et al., *Science*, **294**: 5547, 1684 – 1688 (2001)

5.2.3 Peptidomimetics and Peptide Derivatives

As an alternative to L-α-amino acid-based peptides and proteins, significant advances are continually being made in the engineering of peptidomimetics, protein-like oligomers designed to mimic the structure of peptides. This large class of molecules often provides advantageous properties over peptides for a variety of biomedical applications, including greater resistance to proteolysis, improved bioavailability, greater target specificity, enhanced stability of folding, or potentially reduced immunogenicity. In this section, we provide a few examples of peptidomimetic systems and peptide derivatives that have found application in nanostructured biomaterials. For a more complete recent review, see (Gentilucci et al., 2006).

Oligomers of *N*-substituted glycines, also known as peptoids, feature side chains attached to the amide nitrogen instead of the α-carbon (Fig. 5.2). A significant advantage of peptoids is their resistance to proteolytic cleavage, making them generally attractive drug candidates; however, peptoids do not have an amide proton or a chiral α-carbon, so their ability to fold into predictable structures or take part in self-assembly processes can be diminished in comparison to peptides. Approaches to overcome this diminished folding and assembly have included the introduction of chiral centers not in the peptoid backbone but in the side chains. Such an approach has been utilized to bias peptoid folding towards polyproline helix configurations (Wu et al., 2001a, 2001b, 2003a). This folding in peptoids mimics in some respects the helical conformation found in natural surfactant proteins, providing new routes for synthetic and proteolytically stable replacements for lung surfactant (Seurynck et al., 2005; Wu et al., 2003b).

Oligo (β-amino acids) or β-peptides also exhibit enhanced resistance to enzymatic degradation and additionally have more conformational freedom than α-peptides due to an additional methylene group in each monomer (Fig. 5.2). For example in contrast to α-peptide helices existing primarily in α-helical conformations, β-peptides can adopt several different helical conformations depending on the substitution of the α- and β-carbons. In this regard, 12-helix folding (Porter et al., 2000) and 14-helix folding (Arvidsson et al. 2001; Hamuro et al., 1999) have been successfully demonstrated for antibacterial β-peptide mimics. For a more complete review of β-peptides, see (Cheng et al., 2001).

Peptide amphiphiles contain a peptide domain and one or more alkyl tails. These peptide derivatives can self-assemble in aqueous environments to form nanostsructures such as cylindrical nanofibers (Hartgerink et al., 2001, 2002) or may also assemble in two dimensions to form Langmuir-Blodgett films (Mardilovich et al., 2006; Mardilovich and Kokkoli, 2004). Fibrillar self-assembly is in part due to the overall conical shape of the amphiphiles (Israelachvili, 1992), but it is becoming increasingly clear that secondary structure in the peptide domain is also an important contributor (Guler et al., 2006; Paramonov et al., 2006). One of the most significant advantages of peptide amphiphiles is that in two dimensions or three, the alkyl tails are packed on the interior of the fibers or films, presenting high densities of peptide on the surfaces of these structures. With specific regard to the design of cell-interactive biomaterials, this dense packing greatly enhances the interaction of receptors involved in cell adhesion, migration, and phenotypic expression (Silva et al., 2004; Stevens and George, 2005). Peptide amphiphiles will be discussed in greater detail later in the chapter in the section on applications of nanoscale biomaterials.

Rigid backbone frameworks are also useful for producing peptidomimetics useful as nanoscale biomaterials. For example, the dibenzofuran templates introduced by Kelly and coworkers (LaBrenz and Kelly, 1995; Lashuel et al., 2000) pre-organize two covalently attached peptides for the formation of supramolecular β-sheet fibrils. Depending on the pH, buffer concentration, and ionic strength, the nanostructures of these fibrillar physical gels could be controlled and in some cases specified.

5.3 Secondary, Tertiary, and Quaternary Structures in Nanomaterials

Building from the primary structures of amino acids, we now address the engineering of a peptide's sequence so as to predictably produce higher-order organization that leads to the formation of a nanostructured material. Predicting the folding of a polypeptide from its sequence is one of the most challenging scientific questions of our time, so it is not surprising that the secondary, tertiary, and quaternary structures that have found utility in nanomaterials to date are among the simpler and more clearly understood protein folds. Of particular interest in this chapter are those protein folds that form fibrils or networks, as these lead to the formation of 3-D materials. In this regard, β-sheet fibrils and α-helical coiled coils are particularly useful. While these are not remotely the only protein folds capable of forming nanostructured three-dimensional materials, they have seen particularly active investigation in recent years and so warrant special attention in this chapter.

5.3.1 β-Sheet Fibrils

β-sheets, the conformations of which were first accurately described by Linus Pauling and Robert Corey in the 1950 s (Pauling and Corey, 1950, 1951), are fundamental secondary structure elements in proteins and peptides. They are composed of two or more β-strands arranged in either a parallel or antiparallel configuration (Fig. 5.3). The amide N—H and C=O groups are hydrogen-bonded to the C=O and N—H groups (respectively) of adjacent peptide chains, generating a 'pleated' conformation, and the side chain residues project alternately above and below the plane of the sheet. Although the backbone hydrogen bonding patterns of β-sheets are their defining characteristics, the β-sheet structure is also significantly supported by hydrophobic effects, van der Waals forces, and electrostatic interactions between their side chains and the backbone. β-sheets also commonly possess a twist of $0-30^\circ$ between each consecutive strand. For a review of β-sheet structure, see (Nesloney and Kelly, 1996) and (Nelson and Eisenberg, 2006).

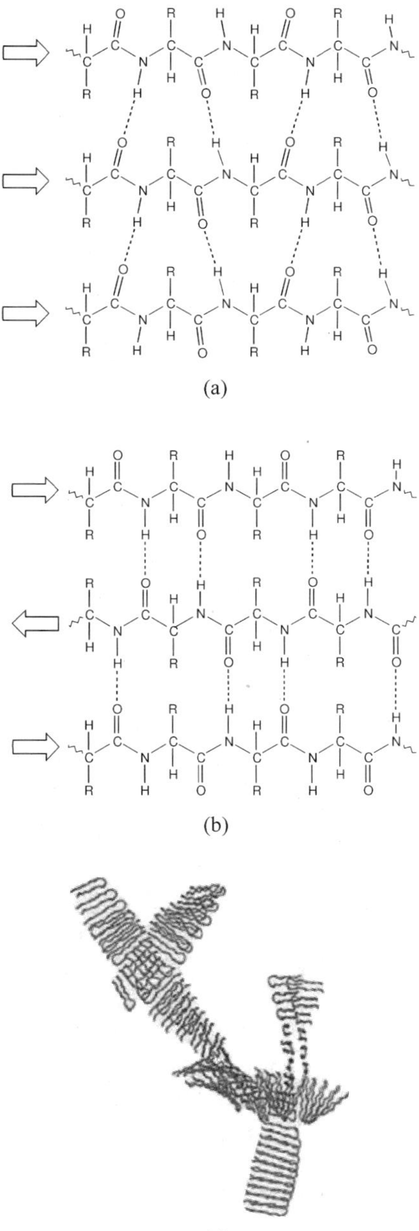

Figure 5.3 Parallel (a) and anti-parallel (b) β-sheet folding. β-sheet fibrils often possess 'cross- β' structure, in which the backbone of the peptide is perpendicular to the fibrillar axis (c) schematic of the self-assembly of a designed β-hairpin peptide, reprinted from *Biomaterials*, **26**, Kretsinger, et al., 'Cytocompatibility of self-assembled β-hairpin peptide hydrogel surfaces,' 5177 – 5186, © 2005, with permission from Elsevier

Although it is generally difficult to predict whether a given amino acid sequence will form β-sheets, it is known that certain patterns of hydrophobic and hydrophilic amino acids have a high propensity for forming β-sheet structures in water. Since 1975 it has been recognized that peptides exhibiting a strictly alternating hydrophobic-hydrophilic primary structure tend to form β-sheets (Brack and Orgel, 1975b). Many such peptides have been utilized to engineer nanostructured materials since these early findings, as described later in this chapter. In alternating hydrophobic-hydrophilic-hydrophobic-hydrophilic sequences, each subsequent residue is positioned above, then below the plane of the sheet, placing all hydrophobic residues on one side of the sheet and all hydrophilic residues on the other. This amphiphilicity then drives further assembly of the β-sheets into tertiary structures such as β-sandwiches or fibrils.

β-sheet fibrils are remarkably consistent in their geometries, even when they are composed of peptides or proteins with widely differing primary structures or lengths. The fibrils are typically about 10 nm in diameter, relatively unbranched, and tend to be laterally associated into bundles and tangles (Fig. 5.4). In these fibrillar structures, the β-sheets are believed to run across the width of the fibrils and perpendicular to the fibrillar axis in a conformation known as 'cross- β' (schematic shown for a β-hairpin peptide in Fig. 5.3(c)). It is curious that while there is a tendency for alternating peptides to form β-sheet fibrils, many proteins and peptides of significantly divergent sequences, lengths, and patterning of hydrophobicity/hydrophilicity are also able to form β-sheet fibrils. For example, transthyretin, the SH3 domain, and lysozyme are three distinctly different proteins, yet they are able to form similar β-sheet fibrillar structures, and none of them possess strictly alternating primary structures (Chamberlain et al., 2000). Also, proteins that generally do not form β-sheet fibrils in vivo may be coerced to do so in certain conditions in vitro, as has been shown for proteins like myoglobin (Fandrich et al., 2001) β-lactoglobulin (Gosal et al., 2002), and others. Also consider the fibrils shown in Fig. 5.4. Similar fibrils are produced from a 20-amino acid peptide (Fig .5.4(a)), a peptide-amphiphile (Fig. 5.4(b)), and a β-hairpin peptidomimetic (Fig. 5.4(c)). This suggests that β-sheet fibril formation is an intrinsic property potentially possessed by most peptides and proteins, as the structure is stabilized by hydrogen bonding between the amide chain backbone, not by the interactions of specific side chain residues (Dobson, 2002; MacPhee and Dobson, 2000). In terms of the utility of β-sheet fibrils for producing nanostructured materials, this provides a great deal of latitude for creating fibers on the 10 nm scale from a diversity of different proteins.

β-sheet fibril growth is believed to start in many instances with a 'seed' of aggregated protein or peptide. This seed then nucleates the further denaturation of nearby peptides or proteins, which then add to the growing fibril to form a 2 – 4 nm wide protofibril. This protofibril then laterally associates with up to four other protofibrils to produce a mature amyloid fibril with a width of about 10 nm (Sipe and Cohen, 2000). Often a helical twist is observed in these more mature

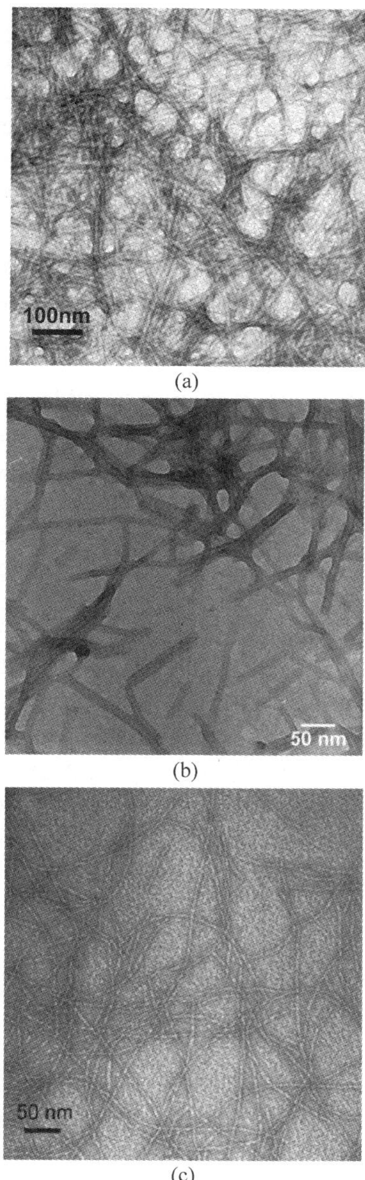

Figure 5.4 Negative-stained transmission electron micrographs of nanostructures created by β-sheet folding. (a) fibrils formed from the peptide GGRGDSGGGQQ-KFQFQFEQQ. (b) fibers formed by a peptide amphiphile terminated by a cyclic RGD sequence reported by Stupp and coworkers, reprinted with permission from Guler et al., *Biomacromolecules* **7** (6), 1855 – 1863 (2006). (c) fibrils formed by a β-hairpin peptide reported by Schneider, Pochan, and coworkers, reprinted with permission from Ozbas et al., *Macromolecules* **37** (19), 7331 – 7337 (2004). Note the similarity of the fibrils even when they are formed from relatively dissimilar peptides and peptide derivatives

fibrils. Aggregates then form from extended and insoluble tangles of fibrils to produce mature self-assemblies. This entire process of nucleation and fibrillization is affected by the local solution conditions (pH, salt content, temperature, the presence of other small molecules or proteins, and tissue-specific events). This idea of local condition specificity is supported by the observation that most amyloidoses are localized to a specific tissue or organ, e.g. Alzheimer's plaques in the brain (Kisilevsky, 2000).

In terms of building materials from β-sheet fibrils, the dependence of their assembly on solution conditions is an attractive aspect. In particular, the addition of salts can be utilized to trigger rapid fibrillization. This salt-sensitivity of self-assembly has been investigated in solutions of salts with varying valences by Caplan et al., who found that for a given peptide $(FKFE)_3$, the critical salt concentration for causing fibrillization was dependent on the valency of the salt, with higher valences requiring less salt to cause peptide self-assembly (Caplan et al., 2000). This is in general agreement with the Derjaguin-Landau-Verwey-Overbeek (DLVO) theory and the Schultz-Hardy rule. DLVO theory states that when electrostatic repulsive forces are decreased by charge-shielding and reduction of the Debye length in solutions, attractive van der Waals forces can become dominant and cause aggregation/self-assembly. The Schultz-Hardy rule is an empirical observation that the critical salt concentration for coagulation typically varies with the inverse sixth power of the valency of the electrolyte. Caplan and coworkers also found that increasing the hydrophobicity of the hydrophobic amino acids decreases the critical salt concentration for self-assembly, which further supports that DLVO theory is an appropriate method for understanding the self-assembly behavior of β-sheet peptides (Caplan, et al., 2000).

Salt-sensitivity is one of the more advantageous properties of β-sheet fibrillizing peptides with regards to their use as nanomaterials. It enables the in situ formation of materials at specific desirable moments, for example upon injection into the body for a tissue-engineered scaffold. Other technologically advantageous properties of β-sheet fibrillar peptides include their typically short length, which facilitates their synthesis, and the fact that β-sheet structure can accommodate a wide variety of primary structures. Peptides, proteins, peptidomimetics, and peptide-amphiphiles may all form β-sheet fibrillar structures. Also, in contrast to globular proteins, β-sheet fibrils are exceedingly stable, allowing them to perform in denaturing environments, in the presence of proteases, and in greater temperature ranges than materials built from globular proteins. This extreme stability has facilitated the use of β-sheet fibrils in applications ranging from nanoelectronics (Scheibel et al., 2003) to tissue engineering (Davis et al., 2005). However, as is the case with nearly all materials, with these useful properties come attendant challenges. For example, β-sheet fibrillar structures can be complex, heterogeneous, and difficult to control at the molecular level. Alternating hydrophobic and hydrophilic structures do not always give well-defined fibrous scaffolds (Schneider et al., 2002), and lateral aggregation can be difficult to control. A number of strategies have been applied to control lateral aggregation, including conjugation of hydrophilic polymers to the peptide so as to produce a hydrophilic exterior to the fibril (Burkoth et al., 1998; Collier and Messersmith, 2004). Other challenges in engineering β-sheet fibrillar materials include the fact that the final nanostructure can be very sensitive to processing history. For example, seemingly insignificant processing details can have major impacts on fibrillar structure, including how the peptide is freeze-dried or whether it was able to undergo any pre-aggregation in the work-up stage after synthesis. In this way, β-sheet fibrillar systems are useful engineering structures for nanomaterials, but care must be exercised in their handling so as to produce consistent structures. Lastly, one potentially significant issue with the use of β-sheet fibrillar materials in biomedical applications revolves around the fact that the β-sheet fibril is not representative of a well-folded and properly functioning protein. In this way, β-sheet fibrils are rather non-functional biologically. They must be decorated, modified, or conjugated to other bioactive components to render them biospecific or bioactive. Furthermore, β-sheet fibrils are prominent components of diseases including Alzheimers' disease, Parkinson's disease, and prion diseases. Whether engineered β-sheet fibrillar materials likewise could participate in these or similar protein aggregation disorders remains to be seen, but at the very least their similarity to natural amyloids warrants thorough and careful evaluation prior to their use within the body.

5.3.2 α-Helices and Coiled Coils

The α-helix is a rigid helical arrangement of the polypeptide chain. It is a common secondary structural element of both fibrous and globular proteins, and it represents one of the most highly investigated structures for producing nanoscale materials. This section will outline the major structural features of α-helices and one of their most useful structural motifs, the coiled coil. Alpha- helices are right-handed spirals. With each amino acid, the helix rotates 100° and translates 0.15 nm along its axis. In this way the helix makes one complete revolution every 3.6 residues, and the helical pitch is 0.54 nm. This structure is stabilized by hydrogen bonding between the backbone N—H group of an amino acid with the C=O group of the amino acid preceding it by four residues, and it is this hydrogen bonding pattern that defines the structure. Further, the core of the α-helix is tightly packed, maximizing van der Waals interactions, which further stabilize the structure. Other helical structures exist, including the 3_{10} helix, where hydrogen bonding occurs between an N-H group and the C=O group from the residue preceding it by three residues; and the π-helix, where hydrogen bonding occurs between an N—H group and the C=O group from the residue preceding it by five residues. Among these helical structures, however, the α-helix is by far the most prevalent.

Being one of the fundamental secondary structures in nature, α-helices represent attractive engineering templates for nanomaterials; however, α-helices are generally unstable as monomers in solution. This is due to the fact that water can readily interact with the backbone N—H and C=O groups, making the entropic costs for helix formation relatively high. This may be overcome by designing peptides where α-helix formation is stabilized by multiple non-covalent intermolecular interactions between more than one helix. The coiled coil has been the most pursued motif in this regard. Other strategies for stabilizing helical folding in water include the use of co-solvents such as trifluoroethanol, but these approaches are less relevant to the work described in this chapter because many nanomaterials are based on supramolecular network formation, and solvent-based strategies that render soluble monomeric helices are less useful toward this end.

The coiled coil is a common structural motif that packs two or more α-helices into a stable bundle. Coiled coils are found in a diversity of proteins (Lupas, 1996), including fibrous proteins (Cohen and Parry, 1986), DNA-binding proteins (Ellenberger, 1994), load-bearing proteins (Kammerer, 1997), and membrane-spanning, fusogenic proteins (Harbury, 1998; Skehel and Wiley, 1998). Their utility as construction elements for forming engineered nanostructured networks is suggested by their natural roles within network-forming proteins both inside the cell (e.g. intermediate filaments, tropomyosin) and in the extracellular matrix (e.g. laminin, fibrinogen). Coiled coils are formed by two or more right-handed α-helices that wrap around each other to form a left-handed superhelix (Fig. 5.5). When the N- and C-termini of individual helices are all oriented in the same direction, we designate them as parallel coiled coils. Opposing orientations are designated anti-parallel.

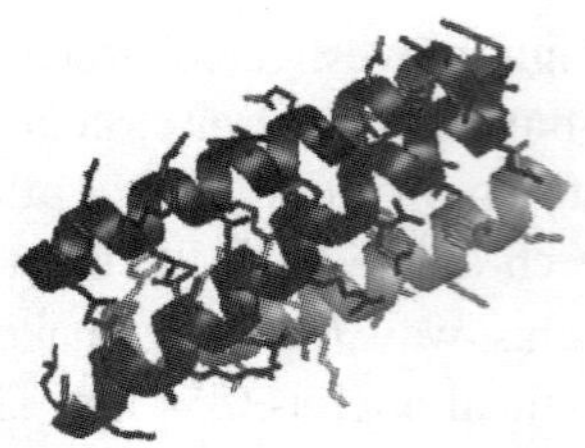

Figure 5.5 Ribbon diagram of a short parallel triple helical coiled coil from the central region of bovine fibrinogen. The N-termini of each chain is to the right. Side chains are displayed (Color Fig. 8)

The most distinguishing feature of the primary structure of coiled coils is the well-known heptad repeat (Fig. 5.1), denoted $(\boldsymbol{abcdefg})_n$. In general, the ***a*** and ***d*** positions are occupied by hydrophobic amino acids, and the 3.6 residue pitch of the helix results in the placement of these residues along a hydrophobic stripe. Burial of this hydrophobic stripe in the core of the coiled coils drives their formation (Fig. 5.6), and packing of the *a* and *d* residues within the core significantly impacts the coiled coil's stability and multimerization state. In 1953

Crick originally proposed a knobs-into-holes model for two-stranded α-helical homodimeric parallel coiled coils (Crick, 1953), in which α-helices mesh together when their axes are inclined at about 18° to one another. At the hydrophobic interface, there is a hole located between positions a_n, d_n, d_{n-1}, and g_{n-1} on the first helix, into which the side chain at the position a'_n from the neighboring helix fits (Fig. 5.6). In the same way, a side chain at the d'_n position on the neighboring helix acts as a knob to insert into the hole formed by the residues at positions a_n, d_n, a_{n+1}, and e_n (Note: *n* refers to n^{th} heptad on the helix). Although hydrophobic interactions between *a* and *d* residues are present in both parallel and anti-parallel coiled coils, the two geometries are distinguished from each other by the way in which *a* and *d* residues are paired between different helices. For example, in parallel coiled coils, residues at positions *a* and *a'* (and *d'* and *d*) are most closely paired. Conversely, in anti-parallel coiled coils, residues at positions *a* and *d'* (and *d* and *a'*) are paired (Note: The prime symbol means a residue at an analogous position on the opposite helix).

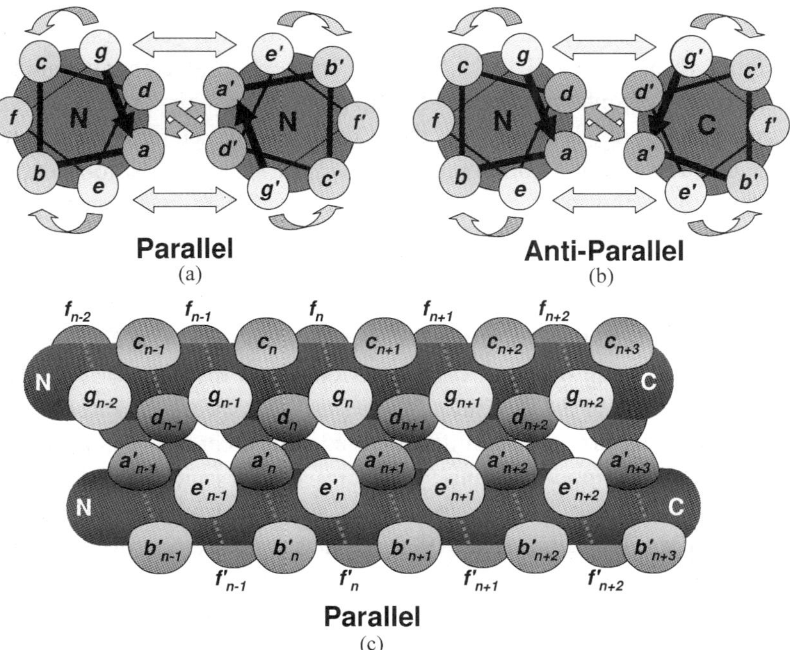

Figure 5.6 Intermolecular and intramolecular interactions in parallel and anti-parallel coiled coils. (a-b) helical wheel projections. (c) 3-D representation. Coiled coil folding is primarily driven by hydrophobic interactions (pink arrows) between ***a*** and ***d*** residues (pink residues). Hydrophobic interactions are stabilized by additional electrostatic interactions between ***e*** and ***g*** residues (yellow arrows and residues) and by tertiary interactions between ***g-c*** and ***e-b*** pairs (blue arrows and residues). (Color Fig. 9)

In addition to hydrophobic interactions between *a* and *d* residues, residues in the *e* and *g* positions are often charged, and those in the *b*, *c*, and *f* positions tend to be either polar or charged and solvent-exposed. Close approximation of *e* and *g* residues (Fig. 5.6) permits either stabilization or destabilization of the coiled coil through attractive or repulsive charge pairs, respectively. In parallel coiled coils, these electrostatic interactions can exist between $e-g'$ and $g-e'$ pairs, whereas in anti-parallel coiled coils, these interactions exist between $e-e'$ and $g-g'$ pairs.

The simplicity and regularity of the coiled coil structural motif has made it an attractive system for exploring fundamental questions concerning protein folding and protein-protein interactions. Owing to its extensive use as a model system, much is known regarding the major factors relevant to coiled coils' stability, specificity, and parallel versus antiparallel orientation. These insights directly facilitate the engineering of coiled coil-based nanomaterials and are briefly outlined here. To engineer the global stability of coiled coils, it is not surprising that hydrophobic residues in the *a* and *d* positions play the most dominant role. In particular, the packing of these residues is a major determinant of both stability and oligomerization state. In the *a* and *d* positions, aliphatic residues are generally preferred to aromatic residues owing to the steric constraints presented by the latter (Lupas et al., 1991). Although tryptophan and phenylalanine have been utilized as hydrophobic core residues to produce 'Trp-zipper' and 'Phe-zipper' structures, (Liu et al., 2004; 2006), these residues are relatively uncommon in naturally occurring coiled coil cores. For residues in the *d* position, leucine has been shown to be the most stabilizing residue for coiled coil dimer formation, and other amino acids have been ranked in the order Leu>Met>Ile>Val>Cys>Ala>Ser from most stabilizing to least stabilizing (Moitra et al., 1997) in bZIP leucine zipper models. Similar results were also obtained by evaluating the 20 natural amino acids in the *d* positions of a model peptide system in which coiled coil peptides were conjugated at their N-termini by a disulfide bridge (Tripet et al., 2000). In contrast to the *d* position, the *a* position appears to prefer β-branched amino acids to maximize the stability of coiled coil dimers (Zhu et al., 1993). By comparing leucine zipper mutants with any amino acid in the *a* position, Wagschal and coworkers concluded that Ile and Val produced the most stable coiled coil dimers (Wagschal et al., 1999). This is primarily owing to the fact that branched residues in the dimeric core (i.e. Leu in *d* positions and β-branched residues in *a* positions) fill the packing space between the two helices, pack well with adjacent residues between the helices, and make close contacts with adjacent layers. As discussed below, manipulation of this hydrophobic packing is also a primary means for engineering the oligomerization state of coiled coils. Chain length is another factor that significantly impacts coiled coil stability, as the number of stabilizing contacts increases with more heptads. It is generally challenging to produce stable coiled coil bundles with fewer than three heptads (Su et al., 1994), though shorter de novo peptides have been shown to produce stable coiled coils, including those designed recently by Hartgerink and coworkers (Dong and Hartgerink, 2006) and Lustig and coworkers (Burkhard et al., 2002), which contain only 14 and 15 amino acids, respectively. Also, although it is generally true that increasing chain length leads to more stable coiled coils, in certain contexts the added entropy of extending a coiled coil chain can negatively impact its stability, particularly for heptads that are only moderately stable to begin with (Kwok and Hodges, 2004). Stability of coiled coils can be enhanced to a lesser degree by capitalizing on charge pairing between *e* and *g* residues. A number of studies have indicated that $e-g$ interactions contribute significantly to coiled coil stability (Hu et al., 1993; Krylov et al., 1998; Zhou et al., 1994), but other experiments have shown that these residues may only provide a small contribution to the global stability of coiled coils (Lumb and Kim, 1995b; O'Shea et al., 1993). Importance of $e-g$ charge pairing is also significantly impacted by ionic strength (Lazo and Downing, 2001; Yu et al., 1996). Other means to improve coiled coil stability include using α-helix-favoring residues such as alanine or glutamic acid (Spek et al., 1998), avoiding helix-disfavoring residues such as proline and glycine, and adjusting helix dipoles such that negatively charged side chains are positioned more toward the N-terminus and positively charged side chains are positioned more toward the C-terminus (Kohn et al., 1998).

To engineer the oligomerization state of coiled coils, a number of strategies have been outlined. Coiled coils can exist as dimers, trimers, tetramers, and larger oligomeric assemblies of α-helices (Harbury et al. 1993; Kajava, 1996). Despite this diversity, the canonical heptad repeat sequence is maintained. As described above, packing of the *a* and *d* residues has major bearing on coiled coils' stability; it also directs their oligomerization. For example, in the GCN4 leucine-zipper, a dimeric coiled coil is formed when β-branched residues occupy the *a* positions and leucine occupies the *d* positions. If the *a* and *d* residues are all mutated to isoleucine, trimeric coiled coils are favored; conversely leucine in the *a* positions and isoleucine in the *d* positions favors tetramers (Harbury et al., 1994, 1993). These preferences arise from the distinct packing of the core residues; geometrical complementarity determines the oligomerization state. For crystal structures and details of these geometries, see (Harbury, et al., 1994). Other means for engineering the oligomerization state of coiled coils include incorporating polar or charged residues in the hydrophobic core (Akey et al., 2001; Harbury, et al., 1993). Alignments and oligomerization states that position two or more buried polar residues together are favored, as this is less destabilizing than two independently acting buried polar residues. This is one mechanism by which natural coiled coils specify oligomerization state, as about 20% of residues at the a an d positions of natural coiled coils are in fact polar or charged (Conway and Parry, 1990, 1991). Even when buried polar residues are paired, however, some degree of destabilization results, so a compromise between oligomerization state specification and stability must often be made when using this strategy to design coiled coil peptides de novo. As an example, Woolfson and coworkers have successfully utilized buried asparagine residues to specify the dimerization and registration of coiled coils for constructing long coiled coil fibers (Ryadnov and Woolfson, 2003a, 2003b). Electrostatic pairing between *e* and *g* residues can also influence the oligomerization state, especially when used in conjunction with appropriate packing of the hydrophobic core (Schnarr and Kennan, 2003).

Heterospecificity and orientation of coiled coil bundles can be tailored through a number of approaches, but most take advantage of the differential side chain packing that exists between parallel and anti-parallel orientations. For example, in parallel coiled coils, the hydrophobic core contains alternating layers of *a* and *d* side chains, and interhelical electrostatic interactions occur between *e* residues on one chain and *g* residues on another (Fig. 5.5). In antiparallel orientations, *a* residues contact *d* residues, and $e-g$ interactions are mixed depending on the oligomerzation state. In one strategy developed by Kennan and coworkers for producing a parallel heterotrimeric bundle, matched core layers were designed where one bulky cyclohexylalanine side chain was positioned against two smaller alanine side chains. Assembly geometries which did not result in this sterically matched core (for example those that positioned multiple cyclohexylalanines together or three alanines together) were disfavored in relation to the matched parallel trimer (Schnarr and Kennan, 2002). Switching of this bundle from a parallel orientation to an anti-parallel one could be achieved simply by moving the cyclohexylalanine residues from *a* positions to *d* positions (Schnarr and Kennan, 2004). In addition these models employed productive $e-g$ electrostatic interactions, which served as an additional level of control (Schnarr and Kennan, 2003). Lastly, in addition to engineering the packing of the hydrophobic core and making use of complementary $e-g$ electrostatic interactions, buried polar residues have also been successfully employed to form heterotypic coiled coils (Akey, et al., 2001; Lumb and Kim, 1995a) or anti-parallel coiled coils (Monera et al., 1996; Oakley and Kim, 1998).

To apply our understanding of coiled coil folding towards the construction of materials, several strategies have been demonstrated for producing fibers, fibrils, or networks (Fig. 5.7). These have included their use as controllable oligomerizing structures for joining together multiple proteins, nanoparticles, or surfaces (Pack and Pluckthun, 1992; Stevens et al., 2004; Willcox et al., 2005) (Fig.5.7(a)), for physically cross-linking stimulus-sensitive polymer-peptide bioconjugate hydrogels (Wang et al., 2001; 1999; Jing et al., 2008) (Fig. 5.7(b)), or for oligomerizing designed proteins (Petka et al., 1998; Stevens et al., 2005; Xu et al., 2005) into stimulus-responsive biomaterials. In other approaches, the peptide is the primary component of the material, as with coiled-coils polymerized via 'sticky-ended' assembly (Pandya et al., 2000; Ryadnov and Woolfson 2003a, 2003b, 2005) (Fig. 5.7(c)), or the assembly of α-helical peptide dendrimers into 3-D networks (Zhou et al., 2004; Zhou and Ghosh, 2004) (Fig. 5.7(d)). Each of these approaches affords complex, nanostructured, and bioactive matrices with significantly greater structural and compositional control than is possible with conventional synthetic polymers or biologically derived extracellular matrices and biopolymers.

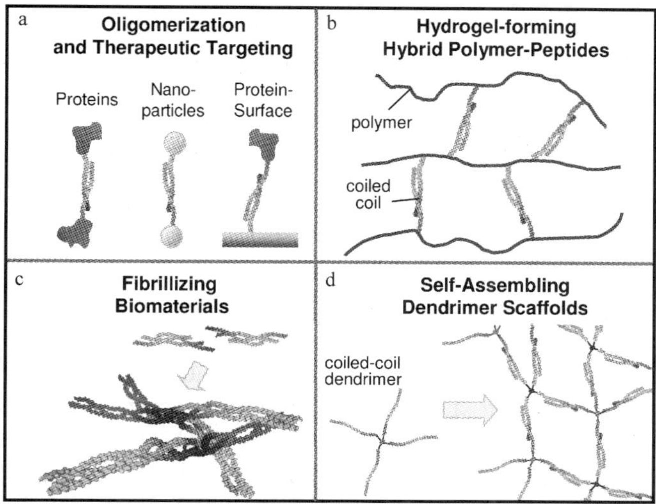

Figure 5.7 Applications of coiled-coils in Biomaterials. Coiled-coils are useful folding motifs for tethering proteins, nanoparticles, or surfaces together (a) and for nanostructured scaffold construction (b-d). For scaffolds, coiled-coils can be utilized to cross-link biocompatible polymers into stimulus-responsive hydrogels (b), to form fibrillar networks through sticky-ended assemby (c), or to form networks by the oligomerization of multi-arm molecules (d). See text for corresponding references. (Color Fig. 10)

As was the case for β-sheet fibrillar materials, there are a number of advantages and disadvantages associated with using coiled coils as building blocks for nanoscale materials. One significant advantage of coiled coils with particular relevance to biomedical applications is that unlike β-sheet fibrils, coiled coils' folding is highly predictable and representative of properly folded native proteins. Whereas β-sheet fibrillar materials are primarily found in association with disease states such as Alzheimers' disease, Parkinson's disease, and prion diseases and are somewhat non-functional biologically, coiled coils are major components of an incredibly wide range of important proteins. In the field of biomaterials, the prevalence of coiled coils in matrix-forming proteins such as fibrin, laminins, and matrilins indicates that use of these structures in engineered systems is likely to produce materials for which specific and controllable bioactivity is more achievable. This specific functionality is exemplified by coiled coil-based pharmaceuticals, for example viral fusion inhibitors such as enfuvirtide, a 36 amino acid peptide which acts by interfering with the coiled coil entry protein of HIV. For review, see (Matthews et al., 2004). Additional advantageous features of coiled coils include the precision of assembly that can be engineered using the design rules described in this section. Stability, oligomerization state, strand orientation, and specificity can be tailored by careful peptide design. Disadvantages concerning the use of coiled coils in the field of biomaterials arise from these properties, however. For example, coiled coils are much more dynamic than β-sheet fibrils, and in some cases the dynamic nature of coiled coils may compromise the mechanical properties of materials constructed from them. Also, coiled coil-forming peptides are generally longer than β-sheet forming peptides and so require more time and reagents for their synthesis and purification.

5.4 Materials Properties Arising from Peptide Construction

Peptides provide an attractive profile of materials properties that make them unique building blocks for nanoscale materials. Because aqueous self-assembly processes are employed in many materials applications of peptides, these materials tend to be sensitive to pH, ionic strength, temperature, and other factors from which stimulus-responsive strategies can be built. Moreover, peptide materials can be bioactive, particularly when their design mimics functional elements of native proteins. Additionally, being accessible synthetically, peptide materials are by nature easily tailored, and the materials from which they are built are likewise highly engineerable. This aspect arises from these materials' inherent modularity.

5.4.1 Stimulus-Responsiveness

Given that many peptide-based materials are constructed through peptide folding and aqueous self-assembly, the factors that govern these processes are convenient triggers for rapidly altering the properties of these materials. Self-assembly mechanisms are covered in depth in this book in the chapter by Sui and Murphy entitled 'Nanoscale Mechanisms for Assembly of Biomaterials'. In particular, self-assembly is sensitive to pH, ionic strength, temperature, and co-solvents. Stimulus-responsiveness is a useful property that enables such applications as triggered release of drug payloads, injectable gels for minimally invasive surgery, or biosensing, where changes in the sensing environment trigger large scale changes in the properties of the material. Here we will provide a few examples of peptide-based materials that employ such strategies. For a more complete review of stimulus-responsive peptide-based biomaterials, see (Mart et al., 2006).

In β-sheet fibrils, many strategies for producing stimulus-sensitive materials have capitalized on the sensitivity of β-sheet fibril assembly to the presence of salts. As described in Sec. 5.3.1, β-sheet fibrillization is dramatically accelerated when salts are present in solution. This primarily arises from the ionic shielding of electrostatic repulsive forces, allowing hydrophobic forces, hydrogen bonding, and van der Waals forces to dominate (Caplan, et al., 2000). Salt sensitivity in peptides with alternating polar/non-polar residues was first observed by Brack and Orgel (1975a) but more recently has been pioneered in materials applications by Zhang and colleagues (Davis, et al., 2005; Holmes et al., 2000; Zhang et al., 1993). In these studies, alternating peptides such as $(RADA)_4$, $(FEFEFKFK)_2$, or $(AEAEAKAK)_2$ are initially soluble and only partially oligomerized in aqueous solutions. However, when these solutions are added to salt-containing buffers such as phosphate buffered saline, transparent hydrogels form nearly instantaneously. These materials have been reviewed (Zhang 2003; Zhang et al., 2002) and have been explored in a variety of applications described in the following section. Other efforts to trigger the gelation of alternating polar/non-polar peptides include that of Collier and Messersmith, who sequestered calcium chloride within liposomes whose bilayers could be switched from calcium-impermeable to calcium-permeable when warmed from room temperature to body temperature or when exposed to near-infrared light (Collier et al., 2001). Light-induced or heat-induced calcium release from these liposomes caused alternating peptides in the extravesicular space to rapidly fibrillize and form gels.

Beta hairpin peptides developed by Schneider, Pochan, and coworkers have also proven to be usefully stimulus-sensitive, and they serve as useful examples for this chapter. In this work, a family of peptides containing a central Val-^{D}Pro-Pro-Thr turn and alternating polar/non-polar N- and C-termini was engineered so as to be sensitive to ionic strength (Ozbas et al., 2004), pH (Lamm et al., 2005; Schneider, et al., 2002), temperature (Pochan et al., 2003), or exposure to light (Haines et al., 2005). Ionic strength sensitivity and pH sensitivity arose from the placement of positively charged residues (primarily Lys) in hydrophilic positions of the alternating polar/non-polar portions of the peptides. Assembly was triggered by ionic screening or by raising pH so as to neutralize the charge repulsion between the multiple positively charged lysine residues. To achieve light-induced assembly, a caged cysteine residue with a negatively charged α-carboxy-2-nitrobenzyl photoactive group was placed in a hydrophobic amino acid position in the hairpin. This negative charge prevented assembly because its burial in the hydrophobic layer of the β-sheet was energetically unfavorable. However, exposure to UV light removed the α-carboxy-2-nitrobenzyl group to leave a much more hydrophobic cysteine residue, allowing the peptide to fold into the β-hairpin configuration and undergo intermolecular assembly. Significantly, a major difference between the β-hairpin approach and those utilizing linear peptides is that with β-hairpins, the triggered response involves intramolecular folding from an extended conformation to the hairpin conformation, and it is this folding event that allows self-assembly into fibrillar gels. This aspect leads to reversible assembly (Pochan, et al., 2003), which is a significant advantage given that most other β-sheet fibrils are difficult to disassemble.

The convenient property of reversible stimulus-responsiveness has also been demonstrated within systems of peptide amphiphiles (see Fig. 5.2 for example), notably by Stupp and co-workers (Beniash et al., 2005; Bull et al., 2005; Guler, et al., 2006; Hartgerink, et al., 2001; Niece et al., 2003). In the first of these studies, pH was utilized to switch from soluble peptide-amphiphiles at neutral pH to gels at pH = 4 (Hartgerink, et al., 2001). This switch was reversible, as gels could be disassembled by raising the pH (Hartgerink, et al., 2002). Peptide amphiphiles were later designed which form gels at neutral pH in salt-containing cell culture medium. By placing a glutamic acid residue in the peptide amphiphile, the peptide was negatively charged at neutral pH, but addition of cell culture medium with its relatively high ionic strength shielded this negative charge and allowed assembly and gelation (Silva, et al., 2004). These materials were additionally employed as 3-D culture matrices for the differentiation of neural progenitor cells into neurons, as described in the next section.

In α-helical coiled coil systems, stimulus-responsiveness has been achieved through routes similar to those employed for β-sheet fibrils and peptide-amphiphiles. In this regard, ionic strength adjustment and pH control have seen the most widespread use. Most stimulus-responsive coiled coil systems take advantage of the roles of the *e* and *g* residues in the $(abcdefg)_n$ heptad repeat (Fig. 5.6). These residues can participate in inter-helical electrostatic interactions that either stabilize or de-stabilize the coiled coil. Placement of amino acids whose protonation states are responsive to pH (e.g. Glu, Lys) in *e* and *g* positions affords systems for which attractive electrostatic pairings only occur in specified pH regimes. Also, in some cases repulsive $e-g$ electrostatic contacts can be overcome by shielding them through ionic strength increase, affording systems that are responsive to the addition of salts. In one example, pH sensitivity was engineered into peptide-nanoparticle conjugates through control of the acidic and basic amino acids in the *e* and *g* positions of leucine zipper peptides (Stevens, et al., 2004). At high pH, repulsive electrostatic interactions between these residues prevented coiled coil formation and gold particle aggregation, but at low pH these interactions were rendered favorable by protonation. This system represents a simple and compact pH sensor. Ionic strength and pH are also critical control points for the self-replicating coiled coil systems outlined by Chmielewski and coworkers, reviewed by (Li and Chmielewski, 2003). Another example is provided by the work of Woolfson and coworkers, who placed stabilizing $e-g$ contacts in their 'sticky-ended' fibril-forming coiled coil dimers (Pandya, et al., 2000). In these systems, raising the ionic strength screened these stabilizing interactions, leading to a stimulus-responsive unwinding of the helices. Collectively, these examples of β-sheet fibrillar systems and α-helical coiled coil systems highlight how control of solution conditions (particularly pH and ionic strength) and appropriate peptide design can afford a variety of stimulus-responsive systems.

5.4.2 Multifunctionality and Modularity

Interactions between biological systems and synthetic materials involve complex combinations of chemical, biological, and mechanical signaling. In this context, systematically engineering a synthetic biomaterial to predictably drive a specific biological response requires the concerted and precise adjustment of many distinct signaling pathways (Lutolf and Hubbell, 2005). Multifunctional materials that can engage more than one biological signaling pathway are therefore attractive, and in order to facilitate the experimental optimization of such multifunctional materials, it is highly advantageous that these materials be modular. In this way, multiple discrete functional elements can be independently swapped, combined, and adjusted (Dankers et al., 2005; Lutolf and Hubbell, 2005). Appreciation for the utility of modular biomaterials has been increasing, as evidenced by a number of recently described peptide strategies that feature modularity, including those based on ureido-pyrimidinone-containing polymers able to non-covalently incorporate various pendant peptides (Dankers, et al., 2005) and self-assembling peptide systems (Genove et al., 2005; Mi et al., 2006). As an example of modular biomaterials, Collier and coworkers have designed peptides which contain a β-sheet fibrillizing domain and one of five different cell binding domains from either fibronectin or laminin. The fibrillizing domain consists of the sequence QQKFQFQFEQQ (Q11) (Collier and Messersmith, 2003) and is used to incorporate a variety of short biofunctional sequences into multi-peptide gels (Fig. 5.7). These gels are then easily tuned by mixing the peptides in any specified formulation in solution and inducing gelation by overlaying the peptide solution with phosphate-buffered saline. Other similar approaches for multifunctional peptide-based materials include work by Semino and coworkers, who also used β-sheet fibril-forming peptides to incorporate pendant cell-binding sequences into fibrillar hydrogels (Genove, et al., 2005). In another example, Nomizu and coworkers utilized a β-sheet fibril-forming sequence from laminin with cell-binding activity of its own to incorporate amino acid sequences with additional orthogonal cell-binding activity (Kasai et al., 2004). In α-helical systems, structural modularity is exemplified by the family of coiled coil peptides developed by Woolfson and co-workers which polymerize into long helical fibers via 'sticky-ended' coiled coils (Fig. 5.8). These coiled coils feature complementary $e-g$ pairs and a buried Asn-Asn interaction which register the

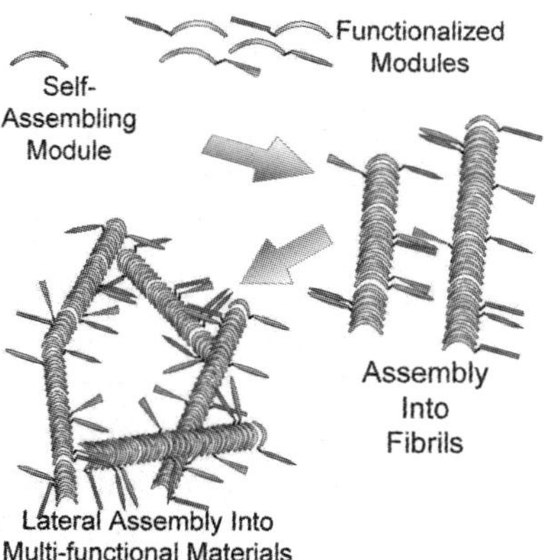

Figure 5.8 Modularity in β-sheet peptide systems. Functionalized co-assembling peptides form mixed fibrils, which laterally associate into gel materials. (Color Fig. 11)

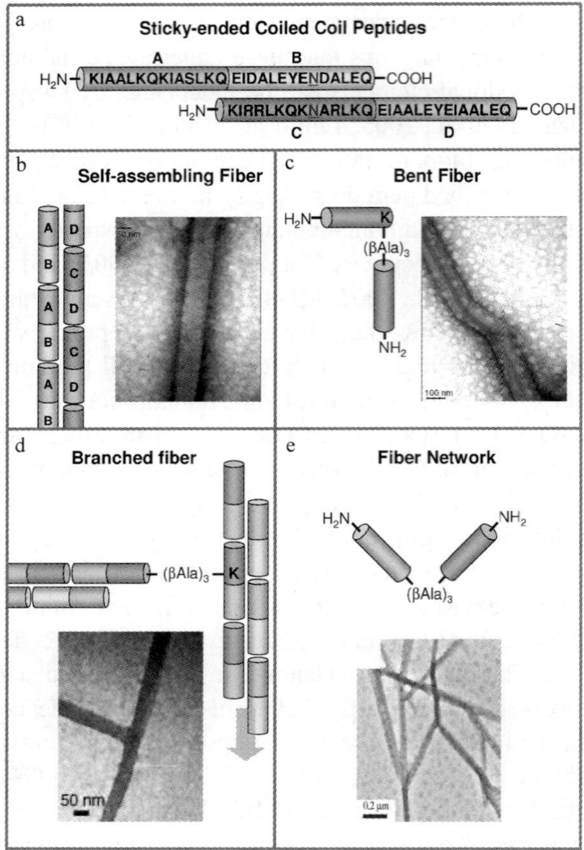

Figure 5.9 Modularity in coiled coil fibrils described by Woolfson and coworkers. Sticky ended coiled coil dimers (a) form straight fibers (b), the morophology and interconnectedness of which can be varied through the addition of one or more modifying peptide modules (c-e). See text for details. TEM images in (b-c) reprinted by permission from Macmillan Publishers Ltd: Ryadnov et al., *Nature Materials* **2**, 329-332 (2003). TEM image in (d) reprinted by permission from Wiley-VCH: Ryadnov et al., *Angewandte Chemie, Int'l Ed.* **42**, 3021-3023 (2003). TEM image in (e) reprinted with permission from Ryadnov et al., *J. Am. Chem. Soc.* **127** (35), 12407-12415 (2005). Copyright 2005 American Chemical Society. (Color Fig. 12)

coiled coil dimer such that self-complementary overhangs (sticky ends) are produced. Oligomerization of these two peptides produces long unbranched peptide fibers (Fig. 5.9(a)-(b)), (Pandya, et al., 2000). To modify the shape of these fibers in a modular fashion, several additional structure-directing peptides have since been designed. These include flexible peptides joined at their N-termini by a flexible $(\beta\text{-Ala})_3$ linker (Ryadnov and Woolfson, 2003a), which produces bent fibers (Fig. 5.9(c)); T-shaped peptides produced from a lysine branch point (Ryadnov and Woolfson, 2003b), which produce branched fibers (Fig. 5.9(d)); and several Y-shaped or bent peptides that are able to join two different fibrils together

(Fig. 5.9(e)), (Ryadnov and Woolfson, 2005). These modular peptides can be mixed in various combinations to tailor the fiber shape and connectivity in fine degrees. As biomaterials science matures, it is likely that multifunctional and modular approaches such as these will help provide finely tuned biomaterials.

5.5 Technological Applications of Nanoscale Peptide Materials

In this section we provide a brief discussion of notable examples of nanostructured peptide materials applied towards various technological ends. We emphasize biomedical applications, including regenerative medicine, antimicrobial strategies, and drug delivery, and we also include a brief section addressing nanoelectronics.

5.5.1 Tissue Engineering and Regenerative Medicine

Owing to peptide materials' inherent bioactivity, stimulus responsiveness, multifunctionality, and modularity, a number of peptide systems are currently being explored as scaffolds for use in the repair or regeneration of diseased or damaged tissues. The field of regenerative medicine has achieved notable but finite success in recent years, primarily in simpler tissues such as skin and cartilage. One challenge for the continued growth and development of the fields of Tissue Engineering and Regenerative Medicine is that available materials for use as synthetic extracellular matrices or scaffolds generally do not possess the complex bioactivity necessary for supporting specific regenerative processes. Those materials that do possess such complex bioactivity tend to be naturally derived and are thus not easily defined or tailored. Nanostructured materials constructed from peptides and proteins represent steps towards addressing these issues. Here we provide a few examples of recent successes in this regard.

The alternating β-sheet fibril-forming peptides originally described by Zhang and coworkers have shown some promise as a scaffold material (Zhang et al., 1993). Like most β-sheet fibrillar materials, these assemblies are remarkably stable with respect to temperature (up to 90℃), pH (between pH = 1.5 and 11), proteases (trypsin, chymotrypsin, papain, protease K, pronase), and denaturation agents (0.1% SDS, 7 mol/L guanidine HCl, 8 mol/L urea). Mechanically, these peptide assemblies were found to be soft, with tensile strengths between 50 and 200 Pa, elastic moduli on the order of 1 – 10 kPa, and maximum elongations between 1% and 6%. These properties appear to be appropriate for supporting cells in 3-D culture environments, and since their introduction many variations of the originally identified peptide have been investigated. Under certain culture conditions these matrices are able to maintain the functions of differentiated neural cells (Holmes et al., 2000), chondrocytes (Kisiday et al., 2002), and liver cells (Semino et al., 2003). They also have been explored for creating myocardial microenvironments conducive to regeneration (Davis et al., 2005). One of the main advantages of these peptide materials appears to be their relative biological neutrality. Although their primary structures do not contain any biological recognition sequences, they are able to biomechanically organize cells in a 3-D fashion. In vitro, this enables the creation of 3-D microenvironments in which cells are suspended in a gel-like matrix that is mechanically somewhat similar to the native extracellular matrix. Additional bioactivity has been recently added to these materials in the work of Semino and coworkers, who created fusion peptides with the self-assembling β-sheet sequence on the C-termini and a number of different cell-binding sequences on the N-termini. These materials were capable of modulating the attachment and behavior of endothelial cells depending on the incorporation of the bioactive sequences (Genove et al., 2005). As a family of materials for regenerative medicine, these alternating hydrophobic-hydrophilic β-sheet fibril-forming peptides appear to be very promising, though it will need to be resolved whether the materials are appropriately tolerated in vivo and that they do not induce any aggregation of endogenous proteins as some β-sheet fibrils can.

Another approach for producing scaffolds for regenerative medicine that shows promise and versatility is the peptide-amphiphile system developed by Stupp and coworkers. These molecules consist of a C16 alkyl tail conjugated to the *N*-terminus of a multifunctional peptide (Fig. 5.2, Fig. 5.4(b)). The alkyl tail drives clustering and fibrillization of the molecule, which additionally possesses significant β-sheet structure not unlike that of β-sheet fibrils. In the first of a series of reports, the peptide component contained multiple cysteines, a phosphoserine residue, and an RGD cell-binding sequence (Hartgerink et al., 2001). The cysteine residues enabled stabilization of the self-assembled fibers through disulfide bond formation, and the phosphoserine and aspartic acid residues facilitated mineralization to form aligned crystals of hydroxyapatite on the fibrils. Subsequent to this initial contribution, variations on the original peptide amphiphile design have been developed and applied towards various biotechnological ends. These variations have included the adjustment of the pH sensitivity of the original peptide amphiphiles so that they assemble at neutral pH (Niece, et al., 2003), entrapment of cells in these matrices (Beniash, et al., 2005), decoration of the fibers with high densities of cell-binding ligands to promote neural cell differentiation (Silva, et al., 2004), formation of cadmium sulfide nanoparticles on the original peptide amphiphile (Sone and Stupp, 2004), production of MRI-active peptide amphiphiles through gadolinium chelation (Bull et al., 2005), and production of branched and cyclic versions of the peptide amphiphiles to tailor the presentation of cell-binding sequences (Guler et al., 2006). These two technologies, peptide-amphiphiles and alternating hydrophobic-hydrophilic peptides, are examples of peptide-based nanostructured materials that are currently being applied towards tissue engineering and regenerative medicine.

For a more complete review of peptide-based nanostructured materials in tissue engineering, see Lutolf and Hubbell (Lutolf and Hubbell, 2005).

5.5.2 Antimicrobials

Many natural antimicrobials are derived from peptides, and so it is not surprising that engineered peptide systems can also be designed to have antimicrobial activity. For example, in an interesting example of β-sheet peptide self-assembly, Ghadiri and coworkers have engineered cyclic 8-amino acid peptides with alternating D- and L-amino acids. These form ring structures that are able to stack with a β-sheet hydrogen bonding pattern into 3-D nanotubules (Ghadiri et al., 1993). These self-assembled tubes were then engineered to span lipid bilayers and serve as artificial ion channels (Ghadiri et al., 1994) or bacteria-puncturing antimicrobials (Fernandez-Lopez et al., 2001). Also, stacked rings bearing homoallylglycine residues (Fig. 5.2) have been covalently crosslinked to each other via olefin metathesis to produce unimolecular nanotube structures (Clark and Ghadiri, 1995). This work by Ghadiri and coworkers shows the versatility in utilizing β-sheet self-assembly for producing interesting and useful nanostructures.

5.5.3 Controlled Drug Release

Peptide scaffolds may provide useful depots for the controlled release of pharmacological agents. In a simple example, several different dye molecules were entrapped within gels formed by alternating hydrophobic/hydrophilic peptides (Nagai et al., 2006). Depending on the size and charge of the dye, variable release from the matrices was observed. Also, because many self-assembled β-sheet fibrillar systems possess unresolved hydrophobicity, they have been explored as a means to entrap and slowly release hydrophobic cargos (Keyes-Baig et al., 2004). At the same time, because β-sheet fibrillar gels also have an extremely high water content, they are able to sequester hydrophilic species in their aqueous pores (Rarnachandran et al., 2005). Such approaches show promise for the controlled release of protein therapeutics, as the protein could be protected from proteolysis by the highly stable β-sheet fibrillar network until it is released. Peptide-based matrices that are specifically sensitive to a particular protease have also been produced, and these may prove to be the foundation for stimulus-responsive drug delivery materials. For example, Hartgerink and coworkers have developed a peptide-amphiphile which forms fibrils but is proteolytically degradable by the matrix metalloproteinase MMP-2 (Jun and Hartgerink, 2005). Materials such as this can be envisioned to release their drug cargoes only under the influence of degradative enzymes that may be associated with a particular disease state.

5.5.4 Nanoscale Electronics

β-sheet self-assemblies have recently been utilized as templates for the deposition of inorganic materials for nanoscale device and wire fabrication. Two examples include the use of dipeptides (Phe-Phe and Phe-Trp) (Reches and Gazit, 2003; Yemini et al., 2005a, 2005b) or a fragment of a yeast prion determinant protein, the N-terminal and middle region (NM) of Sup35p (Scheibel et al., 2003). Both of these polypeptides were found to self-assemble into β-sheet structures that could be subsequently metallized, yet they each have somewhat distinctive properties. For example, the dipeptides form stiff, hollow tubules with widths of about 100 – 150 nm, while NM fibrils have a solid core and form more traditional amyloid fibrils of about 9 – 11 nm in width. While FTIR spectra showed a predominance of β-sheet structure for the self-assembled dipeptide Phe-Phe, the large tubules are somewhat atypical of natural amyloid and may self-assemble in a different mechanism than amyloid. Also, the different structures of Phe-Phe tubules and NM fibrils provided different metallization templates: whereas silver was deposited within the lumens of Phe-Phe tubules, the NM fibrils were surface-functionalized with gold, resulting in a gold-coated amyloid fibril. These materials show promise as components of compact biosensors (Yemini, et al., 2005a). These two contrasting approaches give a good example of the range of possible β-sheet nanostructures for constructing nanoscale devices and wires, and they highlight the versatility of the β-sheet fibril in general.

5.6 Concluding Remarks

As our understanding of protein and peptide folding becomes deeper and more nuanced, the complexity, specificity, and functionality of peptide-based nanostructured materials will become more advanced. Clearly, the strategies outlined in this chapter are encouraging first steps towards providing materials where fine nanostructural control affords bioactive, complex, multifunctional, and finely tuned materials. Although this chapter has focused predominantly on β-sheet fibrils and α-helical coiled coil systems, increasingly complex assembly strategies more akin to the folding of full-length proteins are sure to lead this field into exciting new territories of material functionality. Additionally, advancements in our ability to vary the spatial and temporal positioning of bioactive features within these materials will also likely represent a fruitful area. However, realization of many of the technologies described will require a much deeper understanding of how these materials interact with biological systems. For example, although a number of the peptide-based nanostructured materials described have been preliminarily evaluated in vivo, it is not yet clear what general rules may be applied for preventing or at least minimizing their immunoreactivity. Although peptides in general are not highly immunoreactive owing to their small size, conformational flexibility, and consequent diminished ability to form epitopes, oligomerization and assembly into nanostructured protein-like materials may well present proteinaceous surfaces capable of binding antibodies or B-cell receptors. Ultimately, this may prove to be both a challenge to overcome for areas such as Tissue Engineering and an opportunity for producing immunomodulating nanostructures. As the field of peptide nanomaterials evolves and extends to more applications within biomedicine, such issues are likely to be raised.

References

Akey, D.L., V.N. Malashkevich and P.S. Kim. *Biochemistry* **40** (21): 6352 – 6352 (2001).

Arvidsson, P.I., J. Frackenpohl, N.S. Ryder, B. Liechty, F. Petersen, H. Zimmermann, G.P. Camenisch, R. Woessner and D. Seebach, *Chem. Bio. Chem.* **2** (10): 771 – 773 (2001).

Beniash, E., J.D. Hartgerink, H. Storrie, J.C. Stendahl and S.I. Stupp. *Acta Biomaterialia.* **1** (4): 387 – 397 (2005).

Brack, A. and L. Orgel. *Nature* **256** (5516): 383 – 387 (1975a).

Brack, A. and L.E. Orgel. *Nature* **256** (5516): 383-387 (1975b).

Bull, S.R., M.O. Guler, R.E. Bras, T.J. Meade and S.I. Stupp. *Nano Lett.* **5** (1): 1 – 4 (2005).

Burkhard, P., S. Ivaninskii and A. Lustig. *Journal of Molecular Biology.* **318** (3): 901 – 910 (2002).

Burkoth, T.S., T.L.S. Benzinger, D.N.M. Jones, K. Hallenga, S.C. Meredith and D.G. Lynn. *J. Am. Chem. Soc.* **120** (30): 7655 – 7656 (1998).

Caplan, M.R., P.N. Moore, S. Zhang, R.D. Kamm and D.A. Lauffenburger. *Biomacromolecules* **1** (4): 627 – 631 (2000).

Chamberlain, A.K., C.E. MacPhee, J. Zurdo, L.A. Morozova-Roche, H.A.O. Hill, C.M. Dobson and J.J. Davis. *Biophysical Journal* **79** (6): 3282 – 3293 (2000).

Cheng, R.P., S.H. Gellman and W.F. DeGrado. *Chem. Rev.* **101** (10): 3219 – 3232 (2001).

Clark, T.D. and M.R. Ghadiri. *J. Am. Chem. Soc.* **117** (49): 12,364 – 12,365 (1995).

Cohen, C. and D.A.D. Parry. *Trends in Biochemical Sciences* **11** (6): 245 – 248 (1986).

Collier, J.H., B.H. Hu, J.W. Ruberti, J. Zhang, P. Shum, D.H. Thompson and P.B. Messersmith, *J. Am. Chem. Soc.* **123** (38): 9463 – 9464 (2001).

Collier, J.H. and P.B. Messersmith. *Bioconjugate Chem.* **14** (4): 748 – 755 (2003).

Collier, J.H. and P.B. Messersmith. *Advanced Materials* **16** (11): 907 – 910 (2004).

Conway, J.F. and D.A. Parry. *Int. J. Biol. Macromol.* **12** (5): 328 – 334 (1990).

Conway, J.F. and D.A. Parry. *Int. J. Biol. Macromol.* **13** (1): 14 – 16 (1991).

Crick, F.H.C. *Acta crystallographica* **6**: 689 – 697 (1953).

Dalsin, J.L., B.H. Hu, B.P. Lee and P.B. Messersmith. *J. Am. Chem. Soc.* **125** (14): 4253 – 4258 (2003).

Dankers, P.Y.W., M.C. Harmsen, L.A. Brouwer, M.J.A. Van Luyn and E.W. Meijer. *Nat. Mater.,* **4**: 568 – 574 (2005).

Davis, M.E., J.P. Motion, D.A. Narmoneva, T. Takahashi, D. Hakuno, R.D. Kamm, S. Zhang and R.T. Lee. *Circulation* **111** (4): 442 – 450 (2005).

Dobson, C.M. *Nature* **418** (6899): 729 – 730 (2002).

Dong, H. and J.D. Hartgerink. *Biomacromolecules* **7** (3): 691 – 695 (2006).

Dougherty, D.A. *Curr. Op. Chem. Biol.* **4** (6): 645 – 652 (2000).

Ellenberger, T. *Curr. Op. Struct. Biol.* **4** (1): 12 – 21 (1994).

Fandrich, M., M.A. Fletcher and C.M. Dobson. *Nature* **410** (6825): 165 – 166 (2001).

Fernandez-Lopez, S., H.S. Kim, E.C. Choi, M. Delgado, J.R. Granja, A. Khasanov, K. Kraehenbuehl, G. Long, D.A. Weinberger, K.M. Wilcoxen and M.R. Ghadiri. *Nature* **412** (6845): 452 – 455 (2001).

Genove, E., C. Shen, S. Zhang and C.E. Semino. *Biomaterials* **26:** 3341 – 3351 (2005).

Gentilucci, L., A. Tolomelli and F. Squassabia. *Curr. Med. Chem.* **13** (20): 2449 – 2466 (2006).

Ghadiri, M.R., J.R. Granja and L.K. Buehler. *Nature* **369** (6478): 301 – 304 (1994).

Ghadiri, M.R., J.R. Granja, R.A. Milligan, D.E. McRee and N. Khazanovich. *Nature* **366** (6453): 324 – 327 (1993).

Gosal, W.S., A.H. Clark, P.D.A. Pudney and S.B. Ross-Murphy. *Langmuir* **18** (19): 7174 – 7181 (2002).

Guler, M.O., L. Hsu, S. Soukasene, D.A. Harrington, J.F. Hulvat and S.I. Stupp. *Biomacromolecules* **7** (6): 1855 – 1863 (2006).

Haines, L.A., K. Rajagopal, B. Ozbas, D.A. Salick, D.J. Pochan and J.P. Schneider. *J. Am. Chem. Soc.* **127** (48): 17,025 – 17,029 (2005).

Hamuro, Y., J.P. Schneider and W.F. DeGrado. *J. Am. Chem. Soc.* **121** (51): 12,200 – 12,201 (1999).

Harbury, P.A. *Structure* **6** (12): 1487 – 1491 (1998).

Harbury, P.B., P.S. Kim and T. Alber. *Nature* **371** (6492): 80 – 83 (1994).

Harbury, P.B., T. Zhang, P.S. Kim and T. Alber. *Science* **262** (5138): 1401 – 1407 (1993).

Hartgerink, J.D., E. Beniash and S.I. Stupp. *Science* **294** (5547): 1684 – 1688 (2001).

Hartgerink, J.D., E. Beniash and S.I. Stupp. *Proc. Nat. Acad. Sci. USA* **99** (8): 5133 – 5138 (2002).

Hohsaka, T. and M. Sisido. *Curr. Op. Chem. Biol.* **6** (6): 809 – 815 (2002).

Holmes, T.C., S. de Lacalle, X. Su, G. Liu, A. Rich and S. Zhang. *Proc. Nat. Acad. Sci. USA* **97** (12): 6728 – 6733 (2000).

Hu, J.C., N.E. Newell, B. Tidor and R.T. Sauer. *Protein. Sci.* **2** (7): 1072 – 1084 (1993).

Israelachvili, J.N. In: *Intermolecular and Surface Forces*. London: Academic Press (1992).

Jun, H.-W., V. Yuwono, S.E. Paramonov and J.D. Hartgerink. *Advanced Materials* **17** (21): 2612 – 2617 (2005).

Jing, P., Rudra, J.S., Herr, A.B., and Collier, J.H., Biomaro Molecules, in Press (2008). DOT: 10.1021/BM800459V.

Kajava, A.V. *Proteins* **24** (2): 218 – 226 (1996).

Kammerer, R.A. *Matrix. Biol.* **15** (8 – 9): 555 – 565; discussion 67 – 68 (1997).

Kasai, S., Y. Ohga, M. Mochizuki, N. Nishi, Y. Kadoya and M. Nomizu. *Peptide. Sci.* **76**: 27 – 33 (2004).

Keyes-Baig, C., J. Duhamel, S.Y. Fung, J. Bezaire and P. Chen. *J. Am. Chem. Soc.* **126** (24): 7522 – 7532 (2004).

Kiick, K.L., E. Saxon, D.A. Tirrell and C.R. Bertozzi. *Proc. Natl. Acad. Sci. USA* **99**(1): 19 – 24 (2002).

Kisiday, J., M. Jin, B. Kurz, H. Hung, C. Semino, S. Zhang and A.J. Grodzinsky. *Proc. Natl. Acad. Sci. USA* **99** (15): 9996 – 10,001 (2002).

Kisilevsky, R. *Journal of Structural Biology* **130** (2 – 3): 99 – 108 (2000).

Kohn, W.D., C.M. Kay and R.S. Hodges. *Journal of Molecular Biology* **283** (5): 993 – 1012 (1998).

Krylov, D., J. Barchi and C. Vinson. *J. Mol. Biol.* **279** (4): 959 – 972 (1998).

Kwok, S.C. and R.S. Hodges. *Biopolymers* **76** (5): 378 – 390 (2004).

LaBrenz, S.R. and J.W. Kelly. *J. Am. Chem. Soc.* **117** (5): 1655 – 1656 (1995).

Lamm, M.S., K. Rajagopal, J.P. Schneider and D.J. Pochan. *J. Am. Chem. Soc.* **127** (47): 16,692 – 16,700 (2005).

Lashuel, H.A., S.R. LaBrenz, L. Woo, L.C. Serpell and J.W. Kelly. *J. Am. Chem. Soc.* **122**: 5262 – 5277 (2000).

Lazo, N.D. and D.T. Downing. *Journal of Peptide Research* **58** (6): 457 – 463 (2001).

Lee, H., N.F. Scherer and P.B. Messersmith. *Proc. Natl. Acad. Sci. USA* **103** (35) 12,999 – 13,003 (2006).

Lee H., Dellatore, S.M., Miller, W.M., Messersmith, P.B., *Science* 318 (5849): 426 – 430 (2007a).

Lee H, Lee, B.P., Messersmith, P.B., *Nature* **448** (7151): 338 – 341 (2007b).

Li, X.Q. and J. Chmielewski. *Organic & Biomolecular Chemistry* **1** (6): 901 – 904 (2003).

Link, A.J., M.L. Mock and D.A. Tirrell. *Curr. Op. Biotechnology* **14** (6): 603 – 609 (2003).

Liu, J., W. Yong, Y.Q. Deng, N.R. Kallenbach and M. Lu. *Proc. Natl. Acad. Sci. USA* **101** (46): 16,156 – 16,161 (2004).

Liu, J., Q. Zheng, Y.Q. Deng, N.R. Kallenbach and M. Lu. *Journal of Molecular Biology* **361** (1): 168 – 179 (2006).

Lumb, K.J. and P.S. Kim. *Biochemistry* **34** (27): 8642 – 8648 (1995a).

Lumb, K.J. and P.S. Kim. *Science* **268** (5209): 436 – 439 (1995b).

Lupas, A. *Trends in Biochemical Sciences* **21** (10): 375 – 382 (1996).

Lupas, A., M. Van Dyke and J. Stock. *Science* **252** (5010): 1162 – 1164 (1991).

Lutolf, M.P. and J.A. Hubbell. *Nat. Biotechol.* **23:** 47 – 55 (2005).

MacPhee, C.E. and C.M. Dobson. *J. Am. Chem. Soc.* **122** (51): 12,707 – 12,713 (2000).

Mardilovich, A., J.A. Craig, M.Q. McCammon, A. Garg and E. Kokkoli. *Langmuir* **22** (7): 3259 – 3264 (2006).

Mardilovich, A. and E. Kokkoli. *Biomacromolecules* **5** (3): 950 – 957 (2004).

Mart, R.J., R.D. Osborne, M.M. Stevens and R.V. Ulijn. *Soft Matter* **2** (10): 822 – 835 (2006).

Matthews, T., M. Salgo, M. Greenberg, J. Chung, R. DeMasi and D. Bolognesi. *Nat. Rev. Drug Discovery* **3** (3): 215 – 225 (2004).

Merrifield, R.B. *J. Am. Chem. Soc.* **85**: 2149 (1963).

Mi, L.X., S. Fischer, B. Chung, S. Sundelacruz and J.L. Harden. *Biomacromolecules* **7** (1): 38 – 47 (2006).

Moitra, J., L. Szilak, D. Krylov and C. Vinson. *Biochemistry* **36** (41): 12,567-12,573 (1997).

Monera, O.D., N.E. Zhou, P. Lavigne, C.M. Kay and R.S. Hodges. *J. Biol. Chem.* **271** (8): 3995 – 4001 (1996).

Montclare, J.K. and D.A. Tirrell. *Angew. Chem. Int'l. Ed.* **45** (27): 4518 – 4521 (2006).

Nagai, Y., L.D. Unsworth, S. Koutsopoulos and S.G. Zhang. *J. Controlled Release* **115** (1): 18 – 25 (2006).

Nelson, R. and D. Eisenberg. *Curr. Op. Struct. Biol.* **16** (2): 260 – 265 (2006).

Nesloney, C.L. and J.W. Kelly. *Bioorg. Med. Chem.* **4** (6): 739 – 766 (1996).

Niece, K.L., J.D. Hartgerink, J.J.J.M. Donners and S.I. Stupp. *J. Am. Chem. Soc.* **125** (24): 7146 – 7147 (2003).

O'Shea, E.K., K.J. Lumb and P.S. Kim. *Curr. Biol.* **3** (10): 658 – 667 (1993).

Oakley, M.G. and P.S. Kim. *Biochemistry* **37** (36): 12,603 – 12,610 (1998).

Ozbas, B., J. Kretsinger, K. Rajagopal, J.P. Schneider and D.J. Pochan. *Macromolecules* **37** (19): 7331 – 7337 (2004).

Pack, P. and A. Pluckthun, *Biochemistry* **31** (6): 1579 – 1584 (1992).

Pandya, M.J., G.M. Spooner, M. Sunde, J.R. Thorpe, A. Rodger and D.N. Woolfson, *Biochemistry* **39** (30): 8728 – 8734 (2000).

Paramonov, S.E., H.W. Jun and J.D. Hartgerink. *J. Am. Chem. Soc.* **128** (22): 7291 – 7298 (2006).

Pauling, L. and R.B. Corey. *J. Am. Chem. Soc.* **72:** 5349 (1950).

Pauling, L. and R.B. Corey. *Proc. Natl. Acad. Sci. U S A* **37**: 729 – 740 (1951).

Petka, W.A., J.L. Harden, K.P. McGrath, D. Wirtz and D.A. Tirrell. *Science* **281** (5375): 389 – 392 (1998).

Pochan, D.J., J.P. Schneider, J. Kretsinger, B. Ozbas, K. Rajagopal and L. Haines. *J. Am. Chem. Soc.* **125** (39): 11,802 – 11,803 (2003).

Porter, E.A., X. Wang, H.S. Lee, B. Weisblum and S.H. Gellman. *Nature* **404** (6778): 565 (2000).

Rarnachandran, S., P. Flynn, Y. Tseng and Y.B. Yu. *Chem. Mater.* **17** (26): 6583 – 6588 (2005).

Reches, M. and E. Gazit. *Science* **300** (5619): 625 – 627 (2003).

Ryadnov, M.G. and D.N. Woolfson. *Nature Materials* **2** (5): 329 – 332 (2003a).

Ryadnov, M.G. and D.N. Woolfson. *Angew. Chem. Int'l. Ed.* **42** (26): 3021 – 3023 (2003b).

Ryadnov, M.G. and D.N. Woolfson. *J. Am. Chem. Soc.* **127** (35): 12,407 – 12,415 (2005).

Scheibel, T., R. Parthasarathy, G. Sawicki, X.-M. Lin, H. Jaeger and S.L. Lindquist. *Proc. Natl. Acad. Sci. U S A* **100** (8): 4527 – 4532 (2003).

Schnarr, N.A. and A.J. Kennan. *J. Am. Chem. Soc.* **124** (33): 9779 – 9783 (2002).

Schnarr, N.A. and A.J. Kennan. *J. Am. Chem. Soc.* **125** (3): 667 – 671 (2003).

Schnarr, N.A. and A.J. Kennan. *J. Am. Chem. Soc.* **126** (44): 14,447 – 14,451 (2004).

Schneider, J.P., D.J. Pochan, B. Ozbas, K. Rajagopal, L. Pakstis and J. Kretsinger. *J. Am. Chem. Soc.* **124** (50): 15,030 – 15,037 (2002).

Semino, C.E., J.R. Merok, G.G. Crane, G. Panagiotakos and S. Zhang. *Differentiation* **71** (4 – 5): 262 – 270 (2003).

Seurynck, S.L., J.A. Patch and A.E. Barron. *Chemistry & Biology* **12** (1): 77 – 88 (2005).

Silva, G.A., C. Czeisler, K.L. Niece, E. Beniash, D.A. Harrington, J.A. Kessler and S.I. Stupp. *Science* **303** (5662): 1352 – 1355 (2004).

Sipe, J.D. and A.S. Cohen. *J. Struct. Biol.* **130** (2 – 3): 88 – 98 (2000).

Skehel, J.J. and D.C. Wiley. *Cell* **95** (7): 871 – 874 (1998).

Son, S., I.C. Tanrikulu and D.A. Tirrell. *Chem.Bio.Chem.* **7** (8): 1251 – 1257 (2006).

Sone, E.D. and S.I. Stupp. *J. Am. Chem. Soc.* **126** (40): 12,756 – 12,757 (2004).

Spek, E.J., A.H. Bui, M. Lu and N.R. Kallenbach. *Protein Science* **7** (11): 2431 – 2437 (1998).

Stevens, M.M., S. Allen, M.C. Davies, C.J. Roberts, J.K. Sakata, S.J.B. Tendler, D.A. Tirrell, P.M. Williams. *Biomacromolecules* **6** (3): 1266 – 1271 (2005).

Stevens, M.M., N.T. Flynn, C. Wang, D.A. Tirrell and R. Langer. *Advanced Materials* **16** (11): 915 – 918 (2004).

Stevens, M.M. and J.H. George. *Science* **310** (5751): 1135 – 1138 (2005).

Su, J.Y., R.S. Hodges and C.M. Kay. *Biochemistry* **33** (51): 15,501 – 15,510 (1994).

Tang, Y. and D.A. Tirrell. *Biochemistry* **41** (34): 10,635 – 10,645 (2002).

Tripet, B., K. Wagschal, P. Lavigne, C.T. Mant and R.S. Hodges. *J. Mol. Biol.* **300** (2): 377 – 402 (2000).

van Hest, J.C., K.L. Kiick and D.A. Tirrell. *J. Am. Chem. Soc.* **122** (7): 1282 – 1288 (2000).

Wagschal, K., B. Tripet, P. Lavigne, C. Mant and R.S. Hodges, *Protein Sci.* **8** (11): 2312 – 2329 (1999).

Waite, J.H. and M.L. Tanzer. *Science* **212** (4498): 1038 – 1040 (1981).

Wang, C., J. Kopecek and R.J. Stewart. *Biomacromolecules* **2** (3): 912 – 920 (2001).

Wang, C., R.J. Stewart and J. Kopecek. *Nature* **397** (6718): 417 – 420 (1999).

Willcox, P.J., C.A. Reinhart-King, S.J. Lahr, W.F. DeGrado and D.A. Hammer. *Biomaterials* **26** (23): 4757 – 4766 (2005).

Wu, C.W., K. Kirshenbaum, T.J. Sanborn, J.A. Patch, K. Huang, K.A. Dill, R.N. Zuckermann and A.E. Barron. *J. Am. Chem. Soc.* **125** (44): 13,525 – 13,530 (2003a).

Wu, C.W., T.J. Sanborn, K. Huang, R.N. Zuckermann. A.E. Barron. *J. Am. Chem. Soc.* **123** (28): 6778 – 6784 (2001a).

Wu, C.W., T.J. Sanborn, R.N. Zuckermann and A.E. Barron. *J. Am. Chem. Soc.* **123** (13): 2958 – 2963 (2001b).

Wu, C.W., S.L. Seurynck, K.Y.C. Lee and A.E. Barron. *Chemistry & Biology* **10** (11): 1057 – 1063 (2003b).

Xu, C., V. Breedveld and J. Kopecek. *Biomacromolecules* **6** (3): 1739 – 1749 (2005).

Yemini, M., M. Reches, E. Gazit and J. Rishpon. *Anal. Chem* **77** (16): 5155 – 5159 (2005a).

Yemini, M., M. Reches, J. Rishpon and E. Gazit. *Nano Lett.* **5** (1): 183 – 186 (2005b).

Yu, Y., O.D. Monera, R.S. Hodges and P.L. Privalov. *Journal of Molecular Biology* **255** (3): 367 – 372 (1996).

Zhang, S. *Nat. Biotechnol.* **21** (10): 1171 – 1178 (2003).

Zhang, S., T. Holmes, C. Lockshin and A. Rich. *Proc. Natl. Acad. Sci. USA* **90** (8): 3334 – 3338 (1993).

Zhang, S., D.M. Marini, W. Hwang and S. Santoso. *Curr. Opin. Chem. Biol.* **6** (6): 865 – 871 (2002).

Zhou, M., D. Bentley and I. Ghosh. *J. Am. Chem. Soc.* **126** (3): 734 – 735 (2004).

Zhou, M. and I. Ghosh. *Organic Letters* **6** (20): 3561 – 3564 (2004).

Zhou, N.E., C.M. Kay and R.S. Hodges. *Protein Eng.* **7** (11): 1365 – 1372 (1994).

Zhu, B.Y., N.E. Zhou, C.M. Kay and R.S. Hodges. *Protein Science* **2** (3): 383 – 394 (1993).

6 Photoluminescent Carbon Nanomaterials: Properties and Potential Applications

Yaping Sun, Fushen Lu, Xin Wang, Li Cao, Yi Lin, Mohammed J. Meziani, Haifang Wang, Pengju G. Luo, Bing Zhou, Barbara A. Harruff, Wei Wang, L. Monica Veca, Puyu Zhang, Suyuan Xie, Hua Yang

Department of Chemistry and Laboratory for Emerging Materials and Technology, Clemson University, Clemson, SC 29634-0973, USA

Abstract Carbon nanoparticles and nanotubes upon surface passivation or modification via chemical functionalization exhibit strong photoluminescence in the visible and into the near-IR. In this Chapter, the general features and related optical characteristics of the photoluminescence are highlighted, mechanistic issues discussed, and their potential material and biomedical applications explored. For single-walled carbon nanotubes, the similarities and differences between the defect-derived emission and the band-gap fluorescence (emission from individualized single-walled carbon nanotubes) are also discussed.

6.1 Introduction

Carbon nanomaterials, especially fullerenes and carbon nanotubes, have attracted much interest for their novel properties and potential technological and biological applications (Baugh man et al., 2002). Much effort has been devoted to the study and understanding of their photoexcited states and related optical characteristics. As predicted theoretically, the electronic states in semiconducting single-walled carbon nanotubes (SWNTs) are characterized by sharp spikes in the density of states (DOS) (Dressel haus et al., 1996). Experimentally, electronic transitions in these nanotubes are featured as broad absorption bands in the near-infrared region, corresponding to the first (S_{11}) and second (S_{22}) van Hove singularity pairs (Kataura et al., 1999). The band-gap fluorescence mirroring the S_{11} absorption band was reported and studied first by O'Connell, et al. and then by a number of other research groups for SWNTs mostly produced from the high-pressure carbon monoxide disproportionation (HiPco) process (O'Connell et al., 2002;

---

(1) Corresponding e-mail: syaping@clemson.edu

Bachilo et al., 2002; Lebedkin et al., 2003a, 2003b; Jones et al., 2005; Graff et al., 2005; Lefebvre et al., 2004). An accurate quantum yield value for the fluorescence is still being determined or decided, with current numbers ranging from 0.001% to 0.1% presumably depending on the degree of nanotube bundling/aggregation, surface doping, etc. (O'Connell et al., 2002; Bachilo et al., 2002; Lebedkin et al., 2003a, 2003b; Jones et al., 2005; Graff et al., 2005). There is apparently a required condition for the observation of band-gap fluorescence in SWNTs, namely, that the nanotubes must be dispersed very well to minimize inter-nanotube quenching effects (O'Connell et al., 2002; Bachilo et al., 2002; Graff et al., 2005). Recently, there were reports on the detection of band-gap fluorescence for suspended SWNTs in ambient environment (Lefebvre et al., 2004) and also for nanotubes produced by the laser ablation method (Lebedkin et al., 2003a, 2003b; Hennrich et al., 2005; Arnold et al., 2004).

Even before the first report on band-gap fluorescence from semiconducting SWNTs, carbon nanotubes including both single-walled and multiple-walled ones (MWNTs) upon their surface modification or functionalization were found to be strongly emissive in visible and near-infrared regions (Riggs et al., 2000). In that report, Sun and coworkers referred the emission as luminescence because the nature of the emissive excited state was not well-defined or understood. The luminescence was bright, with quantum yields more than 10% under some conditions (Riggs et al., 2000). While there were questions on the assignment of the strong emission to carbon nanotube species (Zhao et al., 2001), several other research groups confirmed the observation and assignment in subsequent investigations (Guldi et al., 2002; Banerjee and Wong, 2002). For example, Guldi and coworkers reported that the luminescence was associated with carbon nanotube samples from different production methods, including laser ablation and arc discharge, and with heavily oxidized nanotubes (Guldi et al., 2002). Similarly, Wong and coworkers reported strong visible luminescence from carbon nanotubes that are functionalized with Wilkinson's catalyst (Banerjee and Wong, 2002). Mechanistically, Sun and coworkers suggested that the broad visible luminescence could be attributed to the presence of passivated surface defects on carbon nanotubes, which serve as trapping sites for the excitation energy. The passivation as a result of the surface modification and functionalization with oligomeric and polymeric species stabilizes the emissive sites in their competition with other excited state deactivation pathways (Riggs et al., 2000; Sun et al., 2002; Lin et al., 2005).

Recently, mechanistically similar photoluminescence was found and reported in surface-passivated small carbon particles (Sun et al., 2006). These photoluminescent carbon particles, which are being compared with fluorescent semiconductor quantum dots (QDs) (Chan and Nie, 1998; Klimov et al., 2000; Bruchez et al., 1998) are dubbed carbon dots (Sun et al., 2006). The carbon dots offer potentially benign (non-toxic or less toxic) alternatives to currently best performing but mostly heavy metal-based QDs (Esteves and Trindade, 2002; Green, 2002). On the other hand, the defect-derived luminescence of surface-modified or functionalized carbon nanotubes represents an interesting optical property of the nanotubes because surface defects should be considered as the norm rather than exception in typical SWNTs and MWNTs. These carbon nanomaterials of vastly different aspect ratios and other properties (such as optical polarization characteristics) may find many applications complementarily, such as luminescence imaging with visible and near-infrared colors, sensors based on luminescence quenching properties, and other uses in biological systems in vitro and in vivo. In this article, we will discuss the characteristics of the photoluminescence in carbon dots and surface-modified or functionalized carbon nanotubes, and some mechanistic and application relevant issues.

6.2 Photoluminescent Carbon Particles-Carbon Quantum Dots

The finding and development of carbon dots are against the backdrop of rapid advances in the synthesis, property control, and applications of traditional semiconductor QDs (Klimov et al., 2000; Bruchez et al., 1998; Alivisatos, 1996; Larson et al., 2003; Michalet et al., 2005; Parak et al., 2003; Medintz et al., 2005; Kim et al., 2004), and the continued search for alternative QDs based on non-toxic elements (Ding et al., 2002; Chen et al., 2006; Bharali et al., 2005; Seydack, 2005; Wilson et al., 1993; Burns et al., 2006). Traditional QDs are often composed of atoms from groups II – VI or III – V elements in the periodic table, and are defined as particles with physical dimensions smaller than the exciton Bohr radius (a few nanometers in general) (Chan and Nie, 1998). Several characteristics resulted from the quantum confinement distinguish QDs from traditional fluorophores, such as broad excitation spectra, size-tunable emission properties, longer emission lifetimes, photostability, etc., which are expected to offer substantial advantages in a wide variety of promising applications, especially those in biology and medicine (Michalet et al., 2005). For both in vitro and in vivo uses, however, the known toxicity and potential environmental hazard associated with many of these materials may represent serious limitations (Michalet et al., 2005; Derfus et al., 2004; Kirchner et al., 2005; Lovric et al., 2005). Therefore, the search for benign nanomaterials of similar optical properties continues (Bharali et al., 2005; Seydack, 2005; Wilson et al., 1993; Burns et al., 2006). For quantum-sized silicon, the discovery of Brus and coworkers (Wilson et al., 1993) on the strong luminescence in surface-oxidized nanocrystals has attracted extensive investigations of silicon nanoparticles and nanowires (Holmes et al., 2000; Belomoin et al., 2002; Hua et al., 2005; Li and Ruckenstein, 2004; Huisken et al., 2002). For example, silicon nanoparticles capped with water-soluble polymers, thus compatible with physiological media, have been studied for the luminescence labeling of cells (Li and Ruckenstein, 2004).

Sun and coworkers (Sun et al., 2006) found and reported carbon-based QDs or carbon dots, which are nanoscale carbon particles with simple surface passivation to exhibit strong photoluminescence in both solution and the solid-state. The emission spectral features and properties of the available carbon dots are comparable to those of surface-oxidized silicon nanocrystals. The starting pristine carbon nanoparticles can be produced from the laser ablation of a graphite target in inert atmosphere under reduced pressure (Lin et al., 2003). Raman spectra of the as-produced samples (Fig. 6.1) are characterized by the typical tangential mode peak (G-band) at 1590 cm^{-1} and the disorder band (D-band) centered at 1320 cm^{-1}. The former is related to the graphitic sp^2 carbons, while the latter is usually associated with the disorder or defect sp^3 carbons. The comparable intensities of the two peaks (the D-band slightly higher) and their broadness suggest that these carbon nanoparticles are largely amorphous. This is supported by results from transmission electron microscopy (TEM) and X-ray diffraction (XRD) analyses of the carbon particles.

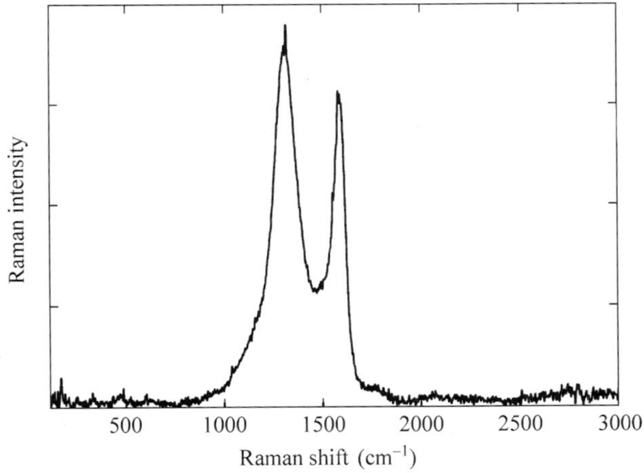

Figure 6.1 Raman spectrum of carbon nanoparticles (633 nm excitation) shows contributions of both sp^2 (G-band at 1590 cm^{-1}) and sp^3 carbons (D-band at 1320 cm^{-1}) (Reproduced from (Sun et al., 2006) with permission. Copyright ©2006 American Chemical Society)

The carbon nanoparticles as produced or after treatments such as refluxing with nitric acid are largely aggregated. They are non-emissive either in the solid state or in suspensions. However, upon simple surface passivation by attaching organic molecules, the particles become soluble in common organic solvents and/or water depending upon the attached functionalities. For example, the use of a diamine-terminated oligomeric polyethylene glycol (PEG_{1500N}, Fig. 6.2) or an aminopolymer poly(propionylethylenimine-*co*-ethylenimine) (PPEI-EI, Fig. 6.2) for the surface passivation imparts solubility in both water and chloroform. Microscopy results (Fig. 6.3) suggest that these soluble surface-modified carbon

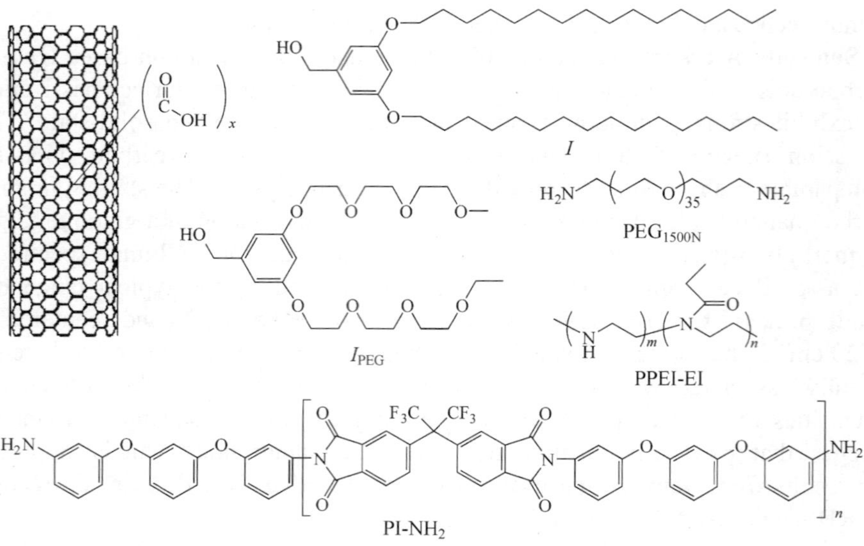

Figure 6.2 Defect-derived functionalization of carbon nanotubes

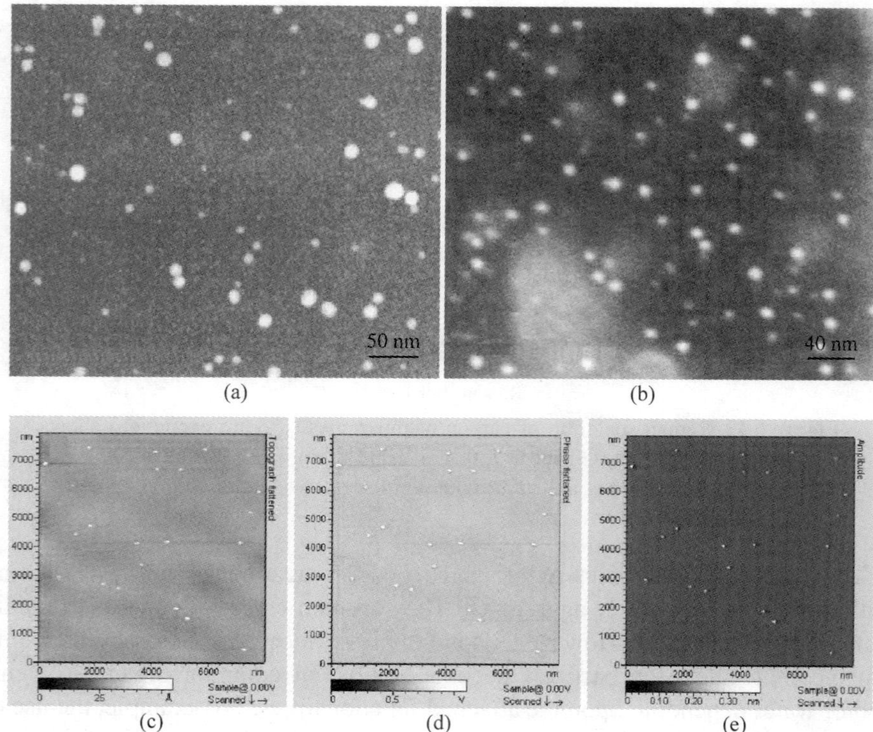

Figure 6.3 Representative S-TEM images (Color Fig. 13) of carbon dots surface-passivated with (a) PEG_{1500N} and (b) PPEI-EI, and AFM images of carbon dots surface-passivated with PPEI-EI (c) topography, (d) phase, and (e) amplitude. (Reproduced from (Sun et al., 2006) with permission. Copyright ©2006 American Chemical Society)

nanoparticles are well dispersed as individual particles with diameters of a few nanometers.

The surface passivation makes carbon nanoparticles into carbon dots, which exhibit bright and colorful photoluminescent in the visible to the near infrared (Sun et al., 2006) (Fig. 6.4). Since the organic functional groups are colorless and non-emissive in the wavelength ranges, the emission must be due to the passivated carbon nanoparticles (carbon dots). Mechanistically, the photoluminescence may be attributed to the presence of surface energy traps, likely related to the abundant surface defect sites that become emissive upon passivation. It should be noted that surface passivation is also required in the luminescent silicon nanocrystals, though the emissions there were widely attributed to band-gap transitions (radiative recombination of excitons).

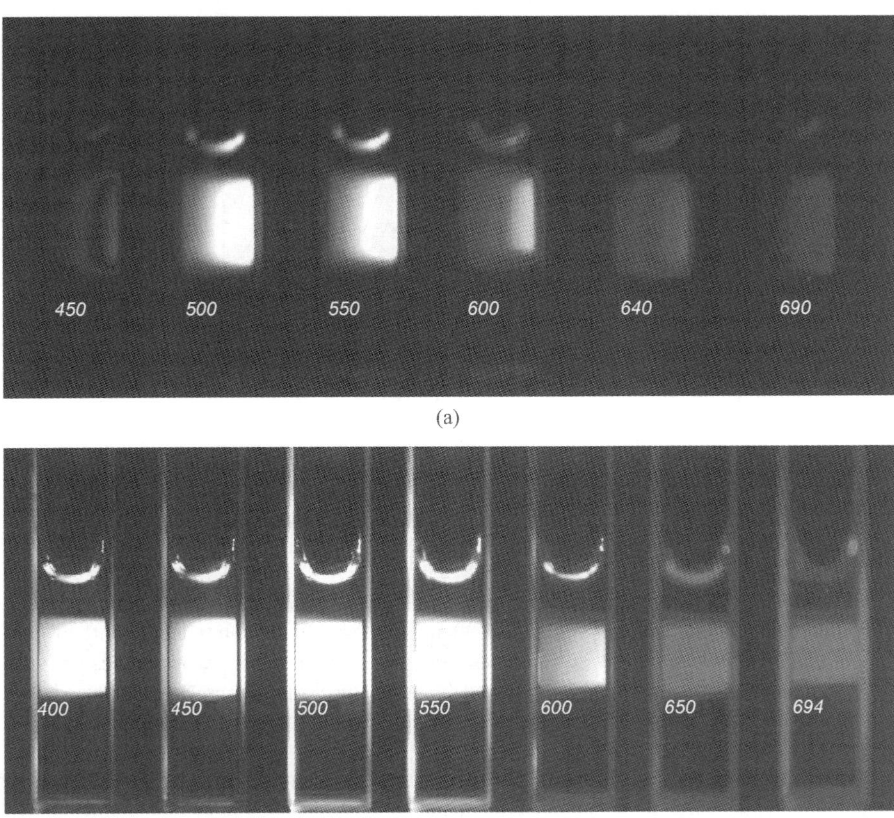

Figure 6.4 Aqueous solutions of the PEG_{1500N}-attached carbon dots (Color Fig. 14) (a) excited at 400 nm and photographed through band-pass filters of different wavelengths as indicated, and (b) excited at the indicated wavelengths and photographed directly (Reproduced from (Sun et al., 2006) with permission. Copyright ©2006 American Chemical Society)

Nevertheless, the surface emissive sites of the carbon dots are likely quantum confined in the sense that a large surface-to-volume ratio is required for the strong photoluminescence. In fact, larger carbon particles (30 – 50 nm in diameter) with the same surface passivation are much less luminescent (Sun et al., 2006).

Photoluminescence spectra of carbon dots are generally broad and dependent on excitation wavelengths, moving progressively to the red as the excitation wavelength becoming longer (Fig. 6.5). As in silicon nanocrystals (Wilson et al., 1993) and some other nanoscale optical materials (Riggs et al., 2000; Bruchez et al., 1998), such emission characteristics are indicative of the inhomogeneity in underlying emissive species. There are not only particles of different sizes in the sample but also a distribution of different emissive sites on each carbon dot (Sun et al., 2006).

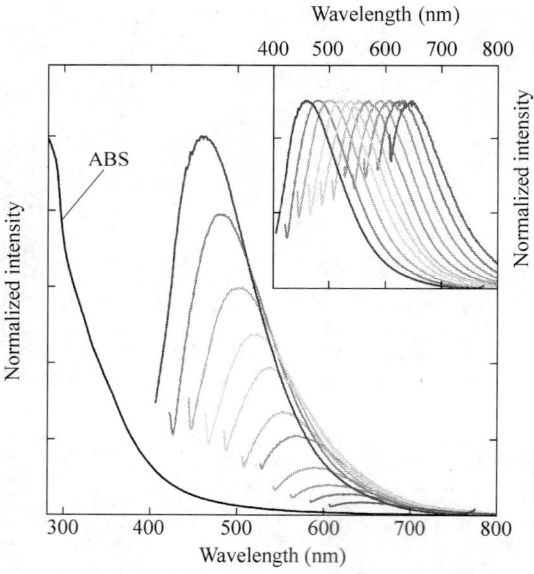

Figure 6.5 The absorption spectrum (ABS) and emission spectra (with progressively longer excitation wavelengths from 400 nm on the left in 20 nm increment) of PPEI-EI-carbon dots in an aqueous solution. The emission spectral intensities are normalized to quantum yield (normalized to spectral peaks in the inset) (Reproduced from (Sun et al., 2006) with permission. Copyright ©2006 American Chemical Society)

The reported carbon dots have photoluminescence quantum yields from about 4% to more than 10% at 400 nm excitation, and the yields decrease progressively with longer excitation wavelengths. The observed emission quantum yields are obviously dependent on how well is the surface passivation in the carbon dots. When the dots with relatively lower quantum yields are subject to a repeat of the same surface passivation reaction, they become more emissive with higher quantum yields.

The luminescence decays of carbon dots can be measured by using the time-correlated single photon counting (TCSPC) technique. The observed decays are generally not mono-exponential. When fitted with multi-exponential functions, the average lifetimes of the carbon dots are on the order of 4 – 5 ns.

The photoluminescence of carbon dots is stable against photobleaching in irradiation with a 450-W xenon lamp for hours. There is also no blinking in the photoluminescence (Fig. 6.6), in contrast to the commonly observed fluorescence blinking in many other QDs (such as CdSe (Kuno et al., 2001; Shimizu et al., 2001), InP (Kuno et al., 2001), Si (Sychugov et al., 2005) and Au (Geddes et al., 2003).

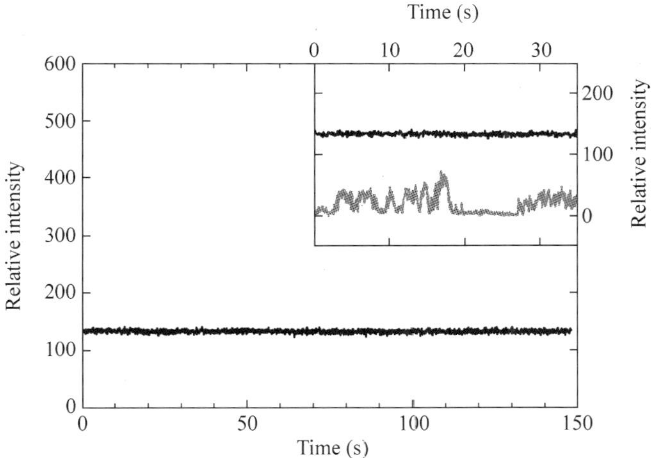

Figure 6.6 The time-dependence of luminescence intensity of PEG_{1500N}-carbon dots measured in confocal microscopy (Leica TCS SP2, the frame rate 37 ms/frame at 514 nm excitation). Shown in the inset is a comparison of the same data (black) with that (grey) of a commercially available blinking gold nanoparticle sample (Ted Pella, Inc, diameter ~50 nm). (Reproduced from (Sun et al., 2006) with permission. Copyright ©2006 American Chemical Society)

In summary, carbon dots are potentially competitive alternatives to traditional semiconductor QDs. Carbon as an element is obviously non-toxic and environmentally benign. With further improvement in performance, carbon dots will likely find many applications in biology and medicine, especially those that require photoluminescent labels in vivo.

6.3 Photoluminescent Carbon Nanotubes

Carbon nanotubes typically contain surface defects that structurally resemble the surface of a nanoscale carbon particle, and may thus be made brightly photoluminescent just like carbon dots (Riggs et al., 2000; Guldi et al., 2003; Banerjee and Wong, 2002; Sun et al., 2002; Lin et al., 2005; Sun et al., 2003;

Zhou et al., 2006; Kose et al., 2006). In fact, it took almost a decade since the discovery of carbon nanotubes to the realization that these nanotubes are in fact strongly luminescent under well-defined conditions (Riggs et al., 2000). The revealing of the luminescence was a direct result of the significant advance in the chemical modification and functionalization of carbon nanotubes for their solubilization and dispersion at the individual nanotube level (Lin et al., 2005; Sun et al., 2002).

6.3.1 A Consequence of Functionalization

As-produced carbon nanotubes are generally insoluble in common organic solvents and water (Bahr et al., 2001). The insolubility is due to the fact that these species are relatively large in sizes and also significantly bundled (strong van der Waals interactions between adjacent nanotube graphitic surfaces). The bundling of nanotubes has made it difficult to observe many of their intrinsic properties, including the band-gap fluorescence and the defect-derived luminescence due to their sensitivity to inter-nanotube quenching (O'Connell et al., 2002; Riggs et al., 2000).

The field of chemical functionalization of carbon nanotubes has become very active and diversified, driven primarily by application needs in the processing of nanotube-based materials. The functionalization leads to the homogeneous dispersion (the exfoliation of nanotube bundles, especially for SWNTs) and solubilization of the nanotubes. The chemical functionalization methods may be classified roughly into two categories, i.e. noncovalent and covalent modifications (Sun et al., 2002; Bahr and Tour, 2002; Hirsch, 2002; Tasis et al., 2003; Niyogi et al., 2002). The noncovalent functionalization methods usually take advantage of the hydrophobic or π-π interactions between functional molecules (such as surfactants and some polymers) and the nanotube surface. The reagents in covalent methods target either the nanotube graphitic sidewall (Bahr et al., 2002; Hirsch, 2002; Tasis et al., 2003) or surface defect sites (carboxylic acid moieties from oxidative acid treatment of the defect carbons on nanotubes, see below) (Sun et al., 2002; Niyogi et al., 2002). Compared to noncovalent functionalization, covalent methods have provided a higher degree of flexibility in functional groups selection and generally higher efficiency in the resulting nanotube dispersion and solubilization.

The nanotube sidewall chemistry is largely derived from the previously well-developed graphite and fullerene chemistry, since the reactivity of nanotube sp^2 carbons, as a result from π-orbital misalignment and curvature-induced pyramidalization, is in fact intermediate between those two carbon allotropes (Niyogi et al., 2002). A less attractive feature with the dispersion and solubilization via the sidewall chemistry in some applications is that it disrupts the nanotube graphitic surface and thus alters the nanotube electronic structures, again making it difficult to observe and study many intrinsic properties of the underlying carbon nanotubes. The functionalization targeting nanotube surface defects (including open ends) seems preserving the nanotube electronic structures much better (Niyogi et al., 2002; Chen et al., 1998).

Experimentally, a typical estimate on the population of defects on the nanotube surface suggests that the defects represent a few percent of the nanotube carbons (Kuznetsova et al., 2000; Hu et al., 2001). After oxidative treatments, these defect nanotube carbons are converted into oxygen-containing groups (especially carboxylic acid moieties). These functional groups on the nanotube surface may be derivatized with a variety of reagents in functionalization reactions. For example, Sun and coworkers have explored many oligomeric and polymeric molecules containing hydroxyl or amino groups for esterification or amidation reactions with the nanotube-bound carboxylic acids (Fig. 6.2) (Sun et al., 2002).

The functionalization of carbon nanotubes with the selected oligomeric or polymeric molecules typically improves dramatically their solubility in common organic solvents and/or water, depending upon the properties of the molecules. For example, solubilities of carbon nanotubes in both water and organic solvents were afforded by the functionalization with PEG_{1500N} (Huang et al., 2003) or PPEI-EI polymer (Fig. 6.2) (Lin et al., 2002). The nanotube-equivalent solubilities for the functionalized carbon nanotubes are usually on the order of a few mg/mL to as high as about 100 mg/mL with the right functional groups and functionalization reactions (Fernando et al., 2004). The soluble functionalized carbon nanotubes are generally in individual nanotubes or thin bundles, which can be probed and visualized by imaging with state-of-the-art electron microscopy techniques (Fig. 6.7) (Lin et al., 2003).

The solubility has allowed the characterization and investigations in the solution phase. For example, nanotube carbons in soluble functionalized sample of SWNTs were recently detected in solution by ^{13}C NMR (Kitaygorodskiy et al., 2005). It has also been shown that the solubilization by functionalization targeting defect sites largely preserves the electronic structures and optical transitions in SWNTs, especially the observation that the band-gap absorptions associated with the van Hove singularity pairs are little changed when measured in both solution-phase and the solid state (Fig. 6.8) (Lin et al., 2005; Zhou et al., 2003).

6.3.2 Photoluminescence Features and Properties

The solubilization of carbon nanotubes via chemical functionalization has provided great opportunities for studying optical properties of nanotubes in solution phase under the condition of homogeneous dispersion. The most relevant was the discovery by Sun and coworkers that polymer-functionalized carbon nanotubes are luminescent or strongly luminescent in homogeneous organic or aqueous solution, exhibiting broad luminescence emission bands in the visible and well extending into the near-IR region (Fig. 6.9) (Riggs et al., 2000). The luminescence

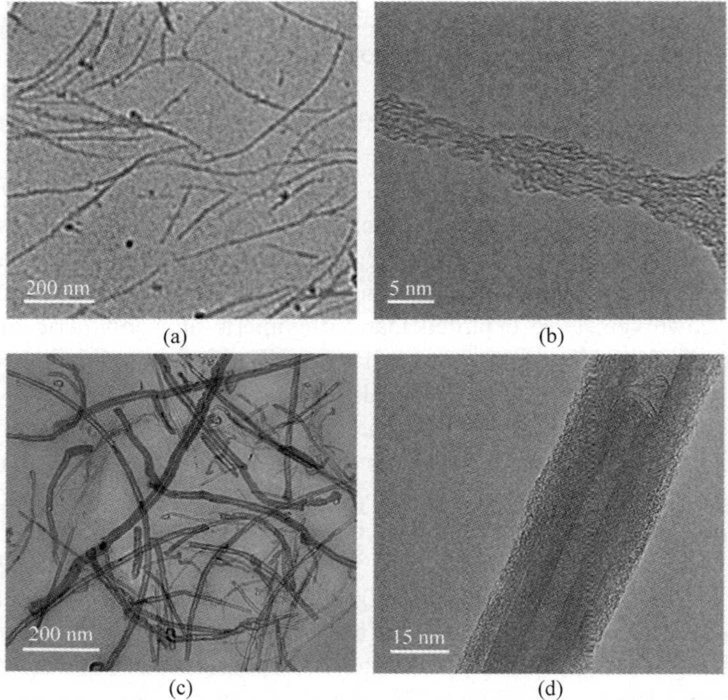

Figure 6.7 TEM images of (a), (b) a PPEI-EI-functionalized SWNT sample and (c) ,(d) a PI-NH_2-f unctionalized MWNT sample

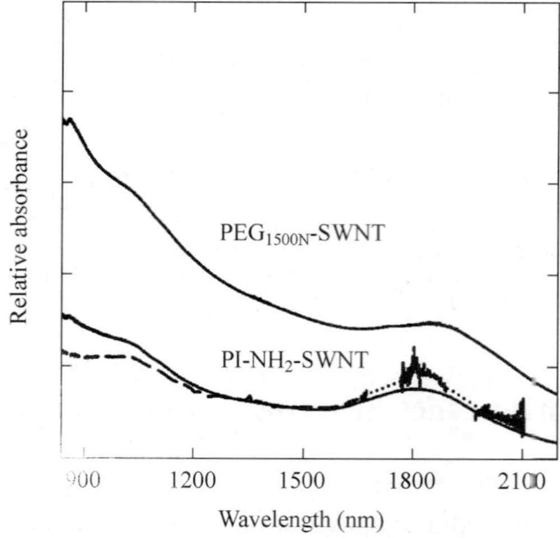

Figure 6.8 Absorption spectra of PEG_{1500N}-SWNT in the solid-state (solid line) and PI-NH_2-SWNT in DMF solution (dashed line, the dotted line region subject to overwhelming solvent background) and the solid-state (solid line) (Reproduced from (Lin et al., 2005) with permission. Copyright ©2005 American Chemical Society)

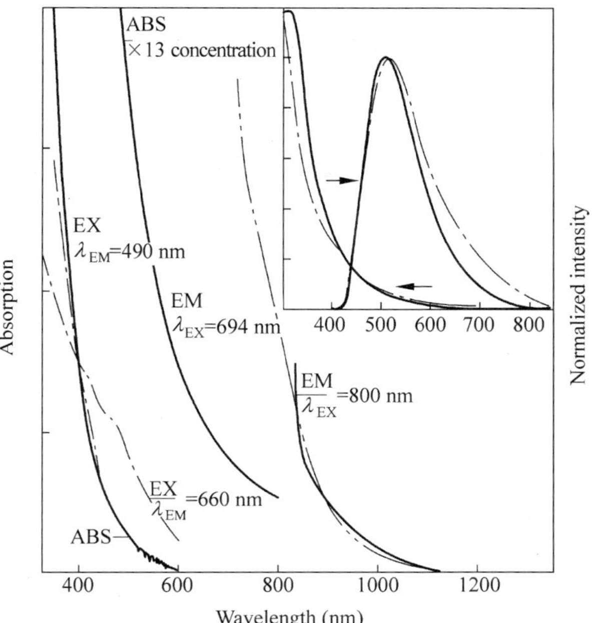

Figure 6.9 Absorption (ABS), luminescence (EM), and luminescence excitation (EX) spectra of the PPEI-EI-MWNT in room-temperature chloroform. Inset: A comparison of absorption and luminescence (440 nm excitation) spectra of PPEI-EI-MWNT (solid line) and PPEI-EI-SWNT (dashed line) in homogeneous chloroform solutions at room temperature (Reproduced from (Riggs et al., 2000) with permission. Copyright ©2000 American Chemical Society)

of functionalized carbon nanotubes is not specific to any particular polymeric or oligomeric functionality on the nanotube surface. In fact, the luminescence has been observed in all well-functionalized carbon nanotube samples of diverse functional groups (Riggs et al., 2000; Guldi et al., 2002; Banerjee and Wong, 2002; Lin et al., 2005; Sun et al., 2002). Much effort was made to eliminate other possible explanations on the observed strong luminescence emission. For example, fluorescence contribution from the polymers or oligomers used in the functionalization was ruled out because these molecules have no absorption at the excitation wavelength. The possibility of luminescent impurities and small aromatic species induced from the solubilization was also excluded in various control experiments.

The luminescence excitation spectra of functionalized carbon nanotubes monitored at different emission wavelengths are consistent with the broad UV-vis absorption spectra. However, the emission spectra are strongly dependent on excitation wavelengths in a progressive fashion. The excitation wavelength dependence indicates the presence of significant inhomegeneity or a distribution of emitters in the sample (nanotubes of different diameters, in particular) or emissive excited states (trapping sites of different energies) (Riggs et al., 2000; Banerjee and Wong, 2002; Sun et al., 2002; Lin et al., 2005).

The observed luminescence quantum yields are generally high. As shown in Fig. 6.10, for example, the luminescence quantum yields of PPEI-EI-functionalized SWNTs (PPEI-EI-SWNT) and PEG_{1500N}-functionalized SWNTs (PEG_{1500N}-SWNT) at 450 nm excitation are 4.5% and 3%, respectively (Lin et al., 2005). Generally speaking, the luminescence quantum yields of SWNTs and MWNTs are on the same order of magnitude. The luminescence decays of functionalized nanotubes are relatively fast and non-exponential, with average lifetimes on the order of a few nanoseconds. The non-exponential nature of the luminescence decays is consistent with the presence of multiple emissive entities in the sample and the observed excitation wavelength dependence of luminescence.

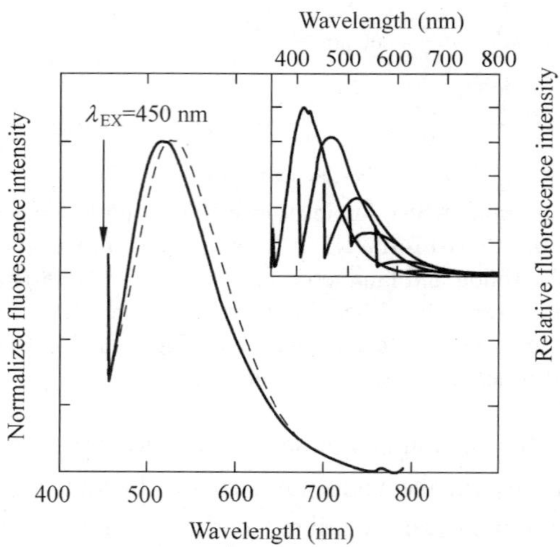

Figure 6.10 Luminescence emission spectra (normalized, 450 nm excitation) of PPEI-EI-SWNT (solid line) and PEG_{1500N}-SWNT (dashed) in aqueous solution. Inset: the spectra of PPEI-EI-functionalized SWNT excited at 350 nm, 400 nm, 450 nm, 500 nm, 550 nm, and 600 nm (intensities shown in relative quantum yields) (Reproduced from (Lin et al., 2005) with permission. Copyright ©2005 American Chemical Society)

6.3.2.1 Effect of Dispersion

There is ample experimental evidence suggesting that the defect-derived luminescence is sensitive to the degree of functionalization and dispersion of the carbon nanotubes. The higher observed luminescence quantum yields are generally associated with better functionalized carbon nanotubes, as supported by results from the experiments of repeated functionalization and the defunctionalization of functionalized carbon nanotubes (Lin et al., 2005; Sun et al., 2002). The repeated functionalization reactions of a carbon nanotube sample with the same polymer results in a substantial increase in the luminescence quantum yield of the final functionalized nanotube sample. Conversely, the luminescence can be quenched or eliminated upon partial or complete defunctionalization process through thermal evaporation or acid/base hydrolysis to remove the functional groups from the nanotube surface. The polymer-functionalized carbon nanotube samples obtained from different functionalization routes may have different luminescence quantum yields due to the nature of the functionalization reactions with respect to the nanotube dispersion. It is commonly observed that the amidation/esterification of carbon nanotubes through the acyl chloride route (Chen et al., 1998; Lin et al., 2002) is more effective than other reactions (such as the diimide-activated coupling (Huang et al., 2002) in the functionalization, corresponding to a higher degree of nanotube dispersion in the resulting sample.

The functionalization of carbon nanotubes for their solubilization is likely more than just dragging the nanotubes into aqueous or common organic solution through covalently wrapping the nanotube with the oligomeric or polymeric molecules. In the functionalization reaction, the functional groups exfoliate the nanotube bundles by either reducing the bundle size or completely disintegrating the bundle into individual nanotubes (thus, the degree of nanotube dispersion greatly enhanced) (Lin et al., 2003). Better functionalized carbon nanotubes and the associated better dispersion result in higher luminescence quantum yields. Conversely, stronger luminescence serves as an indication that the underlying nanotubes are better dispersed, which may be verified or supported by other complementary techniques such as high-resolution electron microscopy or atomic force microscopy. In fact, because of the sensitivity of fluorescence spectroscopy, the luminescence measurements may be used as an experimental tool for probing the dispersion of carbon nanotubes.

Lin, et al. have demonstrated the sensitivity of the defect-derived luminescence to the nanotube dispersion (Lin et al., 2005). In a comparison of non-functionalized and functionalized SWNTs, the former were dispersed in DMF with the assistance of polyimide under sonication. The latter (SWNTs functionalized with polyimide) were dissolved in DMF to afford another solution. At the same equivalent nanotube content, the two solutions had comparable optical density at the same excitation wavelength (450 nm). However, the luminescence measurements of the two solutions revealed that the latter was much more luminescent than the former (Fig. 6.11). This is a piece of evidence strongly in support of the conclusion that the dispersion of carbon nanotubes plays a critical role in their luminescence.

The effective exfoliation to obtain individually dispersed nanotubes is a necessary prerequisite to observe strong defect-derived luminescence. This requirement seems the same as that for the detection of band-gap fluorescence (O'Connell et al., 2002) because both emissions are subject to the inter-nanotube quenching effect. Again, the high quantum yield of defect-derived luminescence combined with the sensitivity to nanotube bundling may be exploited as a convenient, effective, and non-invasive technique to monitor the dispersion of carbon nanotubes in polymer and other matrices.

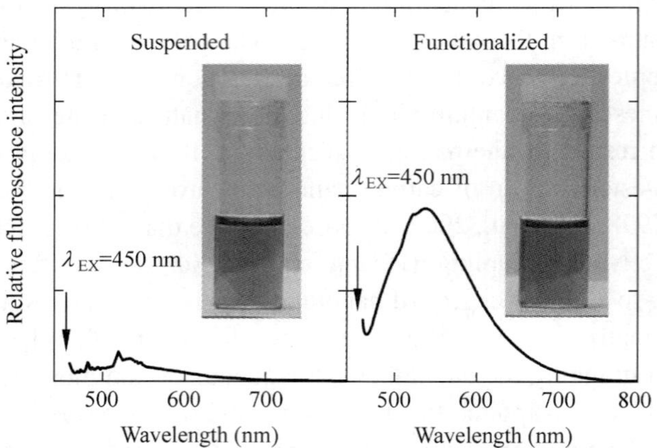

Figure 6.11 Luminescence emission spectra and pictures from SWNTs dispersed with the aid of polyimide in DMF (a) and the PI-NH_2- SWNT in DMF solution (b). The nanotube and polymer contents in the two samples were comparable (Reproduced from (Lin et al., 2005) with permission. Copyright ©2005 American Chemical Society)

6.3.2.2 Effect on Raman

The strong luminescence in functionalized carbon nanotubes often becomes overwhelmingly interfering in the Raman characterization of the nanotube samples. Resonant Raman spectroscopy has been identified as one of the most important experimental tools for probing and studying carbon nanotubes because of the sensitivity of Raman features to the nanotube diameter, chirality, environmental effect, etc. For example, a typical Raman spectrum of a pristine SWNT sample shows characteristic peaks including the radial breathing mode (100 – 300 cm^{-1}), D-band (~1300 cm^{-1}), G-band (~1600 cm^{-1}), and D*-band (~2600 cm^{-1}). However, for functionalized carbon nanotubes, these characteristic Raman bands are generally obscured or overwhelmed by the strong luminescence background, which essentially turns the Raman spectrum into a luminescence spectrum (Lin et al., 2005; Sun et al., 2002). The extent of luminescence interference in Raman measurements is consistent with the intensities in directly measured luminescence spectra. Better-functionalized nanotube samples with better solubility and dispersion are usually associated with more intensive luminescence interference, which often buries the Raman features completely. For example, the Raman spectrum of I-MWNT is simply a broad curve (Fig .6.12) (Sun et al., 2002).

The luminescence background in Raman spectra could be removed by reducing the degree of nanotube functionalization. Typically, a chemical or thermal defunctionalization process may be used to remove the functional groups from the nanotube surface. The characteristic Raman features of carbon nanotubes are restored upon the defunctionalization, as shown in Fig. 6.12 for I-MWNT.

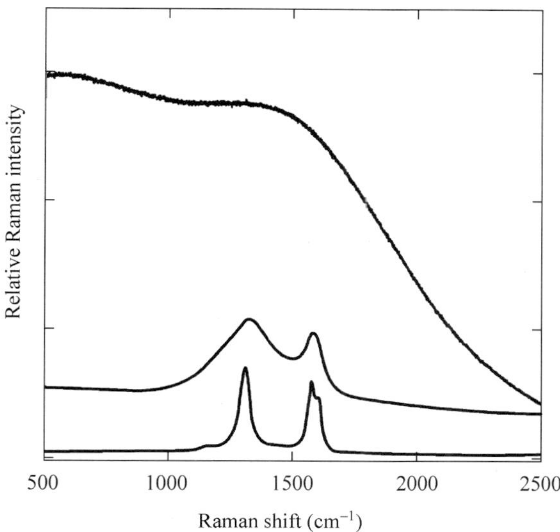

Figure 6.12 Raman spectra (785 nm excitation) of the I-MWNT sample (Fig. 6.2) before (top) and after (middle) thermal defunctionalization in a TGA scan to 650℃. The spectrum of the pristine MWNT sample (bottom) is also shown for comparison (Reproduced from (Sun et al., 2002) with permission. Copyright ©2002 American Chemical Society)

6.3.3 Defect-Derived vs Band-Gap Emissions

The two emissions of carbon nanotubes are obviously different in origin, but complementary in some properties. As observed by Kappes, et al. in the measurement of band-gap fluorescence, there was a significantly stronger and structureless luminescence background toward the visible region with the intensity increasing smoothly toward the excitation wavelength for stable dispersion of acid-treated SWNTs (Lebedkin et al., 2003a). It suggests the coexistence of the two kinds of emissions in the same carbon nanotube sample.

The band-gap emission is likely much weaker and very sensitive to any effects on the electronic structure of SWNTs (easily quenched or diminished by doping or chemical treatment). For example, the emission spectrum of dispersed SWNTs after the acid-treatment is weak and poorly structured (Lebedkin et al., 2003a). However, the defect-derived luminescence is much improved by the same procedure that induces or generates more defects sites. The excellent surface passivation is critical to the observation of strong defect-derived luminescence (Lin et al., 2005).

The band-gap emission is strongly dependent on the nanotubes diameter d and diameter distribution (O'Connell et al., 2002; Lebedkin et al., 2003a). It has been reported that the quantum efficiency of SWNTs from the arc-discharge production ($d \sim 1.5$ nm) are weaker in band-gap fluorescence because of their larger average diameter than that of SWNTs produced from the HiPco method ($d \sim 0.7 - 1.2$ nm) (Lebedkin et al., 2003a). The band-gap emission is more prominent in the small-diameter nanotubes with an upper diameter limit of 1.5 nm. For example, the observed quantum yield of SWNTs from the laser ablation production ($d \sim 1.4$ nm) is on the order of 1×10^{-5}, two orders of magnitude lower than that of the HiPco nanotubes. SWNTs from arc-discharge are predicted to have an even lower quantum yield, which may actually represent a technical challenge in the observation of their band-gap fluorescence.

A shared requirement between the two kinds of emissions is that the emission is highly sensitive to the nanotube dispersion. For the band-gap emission, the dispersion is often assisted by the use of surfactants with the carbon nanotubes and also ultra-high-speed centrifugation. The functionalization is effective in the exfoliation of nanotubes bundles to the level of individual nanotubes and very thin bundles, but it is hardly applicable to the investigation of band-gap fluorescence. Despite the extensive effort on the elucidation of the two kinds of emissions, there are still significant technical and mechanistic issues for both. For example, the accurate determination of quantum yield for the band-gap fluorescence remains difficult because of the wavelength region, while the nature and properties of the emissive excited states for the defect-derived luminescence require further investigations.

6.4 Dots vs Tubes—Luminescence Polarization

A significant difference in the photoluminescence properties of carbon dots vs carbon nanotubes is in their different polarization characteristics. The luminescence emissions of carbon dots with oligomeric passivation agents on the dot surface are hardly polarized in solution (Zhou and Sun, unpublished). However, the luminescence emissions of functionalized carbon nanotubes are highly polarized both in solution at ambient temperature and in polymer thin films. The anisotropy values r can be calculated for the nanotube luminescence in terms of the well-established equations (Lakowicz, 1999).

$$P = (I_{HH}I_{VV} - I_{HV}I_{VH})/(I_{HH}I_{VV} + I_{HV}I_{VH}) \quad (6.1)$$

$$r = 2P/(3-P) \quad (6.2)$$

At each excitation wavelength, the anisotropy values are essentially independent of emission wavelengths. Shown in Fig. 6.13 are typical luminescence anisotropy results for the functionalized SWNTs, where each value is averaged over all emission wavelengths (Sun et al., 2002).

The luminescence anisotropy values are strongly dependent on the excitation wavelengths, exhibiting obvious increases with progressively longer excitation wavelengths, approaching the limiting anisotropy value of 0.4 (Table 6.1). The excitation wavelength dependence of the anisotropy value is less significant in polymer films than in solution (Zhou et al., 2006).

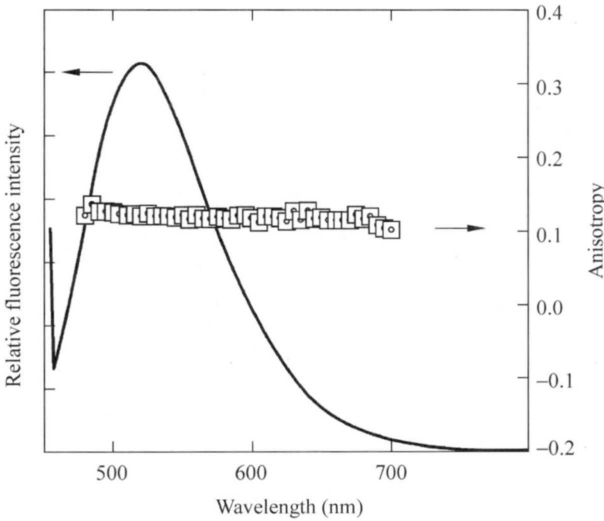

Figure 6.13 Luminescence anisotropy values at different emission wavelengths for I PEG-MWNT (Fig. 6.2) in room-temperature chloroform solution with 450 nm excitation. The luminescence spectrum at the same excitation wavelength is also shown for comparison (Reproduced from (Sun et al., 2002) with permission. Copyright ©2002 Elsevier Science B.V.)

Table 6.1 Luminescence anisotropy (r) values at different excitation wavelengths (Zhou et al., 2006)

Excitation Wavelength (nm)	$r_{solution}$ [(1)]	r_{film}	Excitation Wavelength (nm)	$r_{solution}$ [(1)]	r_{film}
400	0.052	0.32	525	0.15	0.38
425	0.069	0.34	550	0.16	0.39
450	0.10	0.35	575	0.18	0.39
475	0.12	0.35	600	0.19	0.39
500	0.14	0.37			

[(1)] From repeating the experiments reported in ref (Sun et al., 2006).

The luminescence emission is likely associated with excited state energy trapping sites (well-passivated nanotube surface defects). The luminescence polarization indicates that the absorption and emission dipole moments are correlated. The excitation wavelength dependence of luminescence polarization seems to suggest that the excitation is at least partially localized in a distribution of electronic states in the functionalized carbon nanotubes. For the functionalized carbon nanotubes embedded in the polymeric matrix, the anisotropy values are generally larger than those in solution. This may be attributed to the more restrictive environment in the films toward rotational diffusion, thus minimizing or completely eliminating the depolarization induced by molecular motion.

The absorption and emission dipole moments are close to being parallel for the functionalized carbon nanotubes dispersed in the polymeric matrix. However, the orientation of parallel dipoles with respect to the nanotube structure can not be revealed from only the luminescence anisotropy results. The alignment of the luminescent carbon nanotubes is required. The alignment has been achieved by uniaxial mechanic stretching of PVA thin films embedded with functionalized SWNTs. The large aspect ratio of carbon nanotubes makes them good candidates for the alignment by mechanical stretching, as already reported in the literature (see, for example, (Rozhin et al., 2005)). Experimentally, the nanotube-embedded PVA films (about 100 microns in thickness) can usually be stretched to 5 – 7 fold. The observed dichroic ratios are strongly in favor of the film stretching direction (Fig. 6.14), indicating that the electronic absorption responsible for the luminescence properties are along the nanotube long axis (Zhou et al., 2006). When combined with the luminescence anisotropy results, an obvious conclusion is that both the absorption and emission dipole moments are coaxial with the functionalized carbon nanotubes. It should be noted that the measurement of luminescence emissions from the stretched films is a more sensitive alternative to the direct determination of absorption polarization in reference to the film stretching direction.

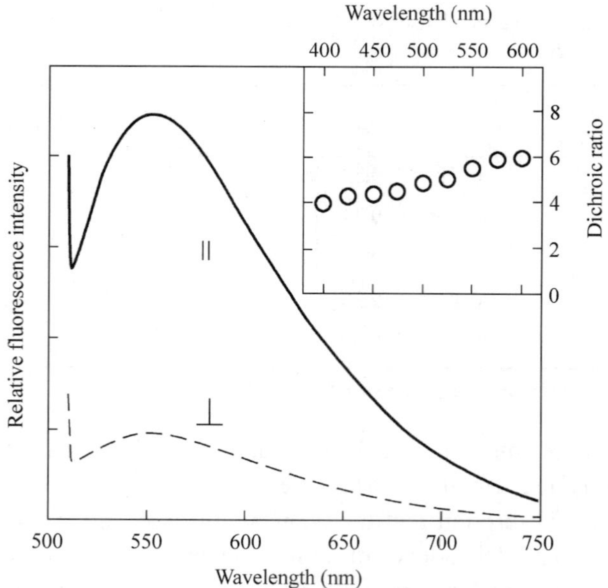

Figure 6.14 Luminescence emission spectra of PPEI-EI-SWNT in stretched PVA film (draw ratio ~ 5) excited with polarized light parallel (||, solid line) and perpendicular (⊥, dashed line) to the stretching direction. Shown in the inset is the excitation wavelength dependence of the observed dichroic ratio (Reproduced from (Zhou et al., 2006) with permission. Copyright ©2006 American Chemical Society)

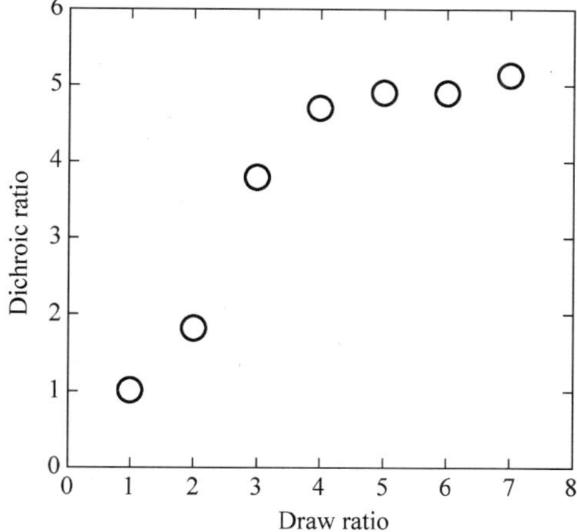

Figure 6.15 The observed dichroic ratio for PPEI-EI-SWNT in stretched PVA film as a function of the draw ratio (500 nm excitation) (Reproduced from (Zhou et al., 2006) with permission. Copyright ©2006 American Chemical Society)

The alignment of the functionalized SWNTs in the stretched PVA film has also been evaluated in terms of the dependence of the observed dichroic ratio on the draw ratio (Zhou et al., 2006). As shown in Fig. 6.15 for the stretching with the film draw ratio from 1 to 7, the dichroic ratio initially increases rapidly with the increasing draw ratio and then reaches almost a plateau.

Further investigations on the similarities and differences between photoluminescence properties of carbon dots and functionalized carbon nanotubes are in progress.

6.5 Potential Applications

Most excitements generated by fluorescent quantum dots (QDs) are for their potential applications in biological and medical sciences, such as bio-tagging and bio-imaging (Michalet et al., 2005; Park et al., 2003, 2005; Alivisatos et al., 2005; Alivisatos, 2004; Fu et al., 2005; Gao et al., 2004). However, there are many serious concerns on traditional QDs, especially those based on cadmium and lead, for their toxicity both in vitro and in vivo (Michalet et al., 2005; Derfus et al., 2004; Kirchner et al., 2005; Holmes et al., 2000). Recent results suggest that the photoluminescent carbon dots may serve as competitive alternatives to the traditional QDs in similar bio-applications. For example, Sun and coworkers used water-soluble PEG_{1500N}-passivated carbon dots to label Escherichia coli (E. coli) cells (Fig. 6.16) and Bacillus subtilis spores (commonly used simulant for anthrax spores, Fig. 6.17) (Sun et al., 2006).

The bright photoluminescence in functionalized carbon nanotubes may find similar bio-tagging and bio-imaging applications, as demonstrated by the existing

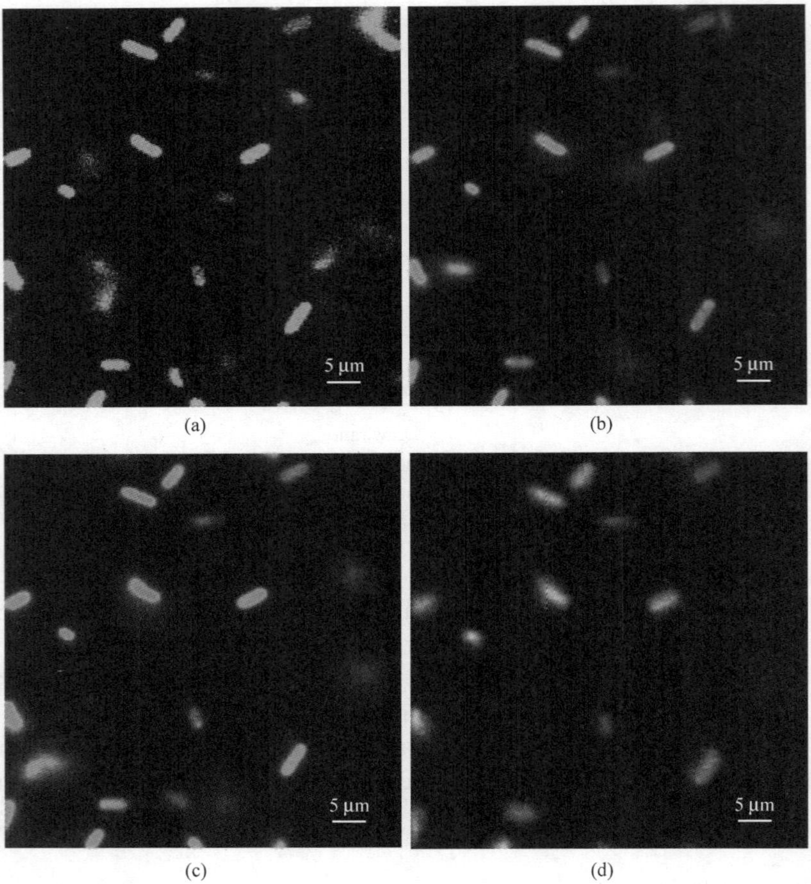

5 μm (a) 5 μm (b)

5 μm (c) 5 μm (d)

Figure 6.16 Confocal microscopy images of E. coli ATCC 25922 cells labeled with luminescent carbon dots (Color Fig.15): (a) λ_{EX} = 458 nm, detected with 475 nm long pass filter; (b) λ_{EX} = 477 nm, detected with 505 nm long pass filter; (c) λ_{EX} = 488 nm, detected with 530 long pass filter (d) λ_{EX} = 514 nm, detected with 560 nm long pass filter (Reproduced from (Sun et al., 2006) with permission. Copyright © 2006 American Chemical Society)

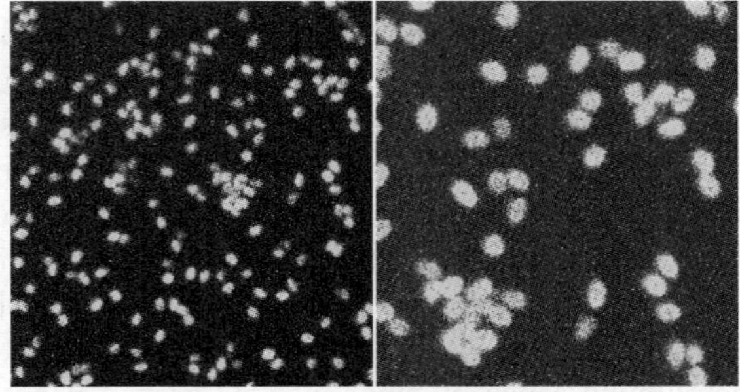

Figure 6.17 Confocal microscope images of Bacillus subtilis spores labeled with luminescent carbon dots (λ_{EX} = 488 nm, detected with 545 nm neutral density long pass filter)

confocal imaging results on the evaluation of polymeric nanocomposite materials (Zhou et al., 2006). Shown in Fig. 6.18 are confocal microscopy images of the PVA film dispersed with PPEI-EI-SWNT. The images at different depths beneath the film surface suggest that these are representative of the whole film matrix (not any surface effects). The compatibility of the functionalized nanotubes with and their well-dispersion in the PVA matrix are also reflected in the confocal images, with bright and homogeneous emissions (spatial resolution about 0.5 μm)

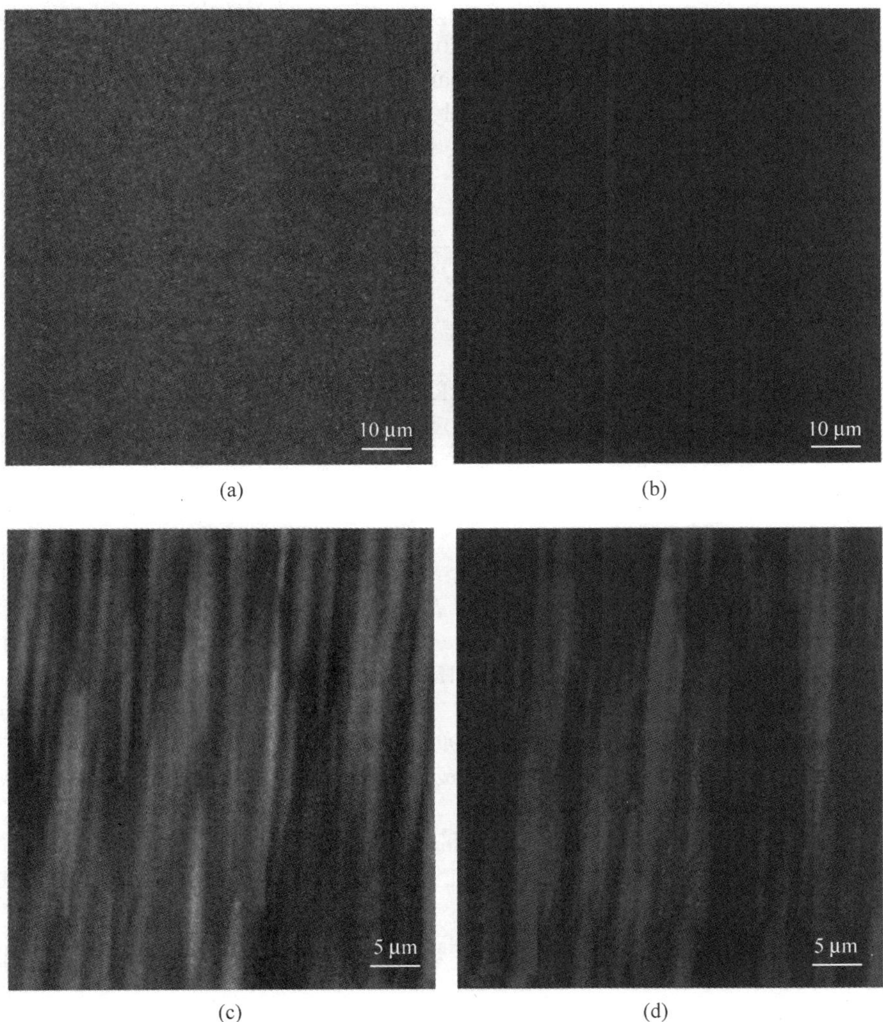

Figure 6.18 Confocal microscopy images of PPEI-EI-SWNT in PVA film (Color Fig. 16) (a), (b) before and (c), (d) after mechanical stretching to a draw ratio of about 5. (a), (c) 514 nm excitation, >530 nm detection; (b), (d) 633 nm excitation, >650 nm detection (Reproduced from (Zhou et al., 2006) with permission. Copyright © 2006 American Chemical Society)

across the whole film. The emission light intensity as expressed by the color intensity from across the film is uniform, without obvious deviation (such as bright or dark spots from local aggregation, locally enrichment or absence of functionalized nanotubes, etc.). Different excitation wavelengths can be used (such as 514 nm and 633 nm in Fig. 6.18). For the stretched films, while the nanotubes remain well-dispersed according to confocal microscopy images (Fig. 6.18), their preferential orientation along with the stretching direction is also well illustrated in the images.

The conceptually similar material configuration can obviously be applied to the fluorescence microscopy imaging of biological systems. In this regard, carbon dots and specifically functionalized carbon nanotubes serve as luminescence agents of somewhat different characteristics, mostly physical such as dramatically different aspect ratios and optical polarizations, but also potentially biological in their interactions with bio-systems.

Acknowledgement

Financial support from NSF, NASA, USDA, ONR, Center for Advanced Engineering Fibers and Films (NSF-ERC at Clemson University), and South Carolina Space Grant is gratefully acknowledged.

References

Special issue on carbon nanotubes. *Acc. Chem. Res.* **35** (2002).

Dresselhaus, M.S. and H.J. Dai. *Theme: Advances in Carbon Nanotubes, MRS Bull vol* **29** (2004)

Baughman, R.H., A.A. Zakhidov and D.H. de Heer. *Science* **297**: 787 (2002).

Dresselhaus. M.S., G. Dresselhaus and P.C. Eklund. *Science of Fullerenes and Carbon Nanotubes.* New York: Academic Press (1996).

Kataura, H., Y. Kumasawa, Y. Maniwa, I. Umezu, S. Suzuki, Y. Ohtsuka and Y. Achiba *Synth. Met.* **103**: 2555 (1999).

O'Connell, M.J., S.M. Bachilo, C.B. Huffman, V.C. Moore, M.S. Strano, E.H. Haroz, K.L. Rialon, P.J. Boul, W.H. Noon, C. Kittrell, J. Ma, R.H. Hauge, R.B. Weisman and R.E. Smalley. *Science* **297**: 593 (2002).

Bachilo, S.M., M.S. Strano, C. Kittrell, R.H. Hauge, R.E. Smalley and R.B. Weisman. *Science* **298**: 2361 (2002).

Lebedkin, S., F. Hennrich, T. Skipa and M.M. Kappes. *J. Phys. Chem. B* **107**: 1949 (2003a).

Lebedkin, S., K. Arnold, F. Hennrich, R. Krupke, B. Renker and M.M. Kappes. *New. J. Phys.* **5**: 140 (2003b).

Jones, M., C. Engtrakul, W.K. Metzger, R.J. Ellingson, A.J. Nozik, M.J. Heben and G.P. Rumbles. *Phys. Rev. B* **71**: 115,426 (2005).

Graff, R.A., J.P. Swanson, P.W. Barone, S. Baik, D.A. Heller and M.S. Strano. *Adv. Mater.* **17**: 980 (2005).

Lefebvre, J., J.M. Fraser, P. Finnie and Y. Homma . *Phys. Rev. B* **69**: 075,403 (2004).

Hennrich, F., R. Krupke, S. Lebedkin, K. Arnold, R. Fischer, D.E. Resasco and M.M. Kappes. *J. Phys. Chem. B* **109**: 10,567 (2005).

Arnold, K., S. Lebedkin, O. Kiowski, F. Hennrich and M.M. Kappes. *Nano. Lett.* **4**: 2349 (2004).

Riggs, J.E., Z. Guo, D.L. Carroll and Y.P. Sun. *J. Am. Chem. Soc.* **122**: 5879 (2000).

Zhao, B., H. Hu, S. Niyogi, M.E. Itkis, M.A. Hamon, P. Bhowmik, M.S. Meier and R.C. Haddon. *J. Am. Chem. Soc.* **123**: 11,673 (2001).

Guldi, D.M., M. Holzinger, A. Hirsch, V. Georgakilas and M. Prato. *Chem. Commun.* 1130 (2003).

Banerjee, S. and S.S.Wong. *J. Am. Chem. Soc.* **124**: 8940 (2002).

Sun, Y.P., B. Zhou, K. Henbest, K. Fu, W. Huang, Y. Lin, S. Taylor and D.L. Carroll. *Chem. Phys. Lett.* **351**: 349 (2002).

Lin, Y., B. Zhou, R.B. Martin, K.B. Henbest, B.A. Harruff, J.E. Riggs, Z.X. Guo, L.F. Allard and Y.P. Sun. *J. Phys. Chem. B* **109**: 14,779 (2005).

Sun, Y.P., B. Zhou, Y. Lin, W. Wang, K.A.S. Fernando, P. Pathak, M.J. Meziani, B.A. Harruff, X.Wang, H.F. Wang, P.J.G. Luo, H. Yang, M.E. Kose, B.L. Chen, L.M. Veca and S.Y. Xie. *J. Am. Chem. Soc.* **128**: 7756 (2006).

Chan, W.C.W and S. Nie. *Science* **281**: 2016 (1998).

Klimov, V.I., A.A. Mikhailovsky, S. Xu, A. Malko, J.A. Hollingsworth, C.A. Leatherdale, H.J. Eisler and M.G. Bawendi. *Science* **290**: 314 (2000).

Bruchez, M., M. Moronne, P. Gin, S. Weiss and A.P. Alivisatos. *Science* **281**: 2013 (1998).

Esteves, A.C.C. and T. Trindade. *Curr. Opin. Solid. State Mater. Sci.* **6**: 347 (2002).

Green, M. *Curr. Opin. Solid. State Mater. Sci.* **6**: 355 (2002).

Alivisatos, A.P. *Science* **271**: 933 (1996).

Larson, D.R., W.R. Zipfel, R.M. Williams, S.W. Clark, M.P. Bruchez, F.W. Wise and W.W. Webb. *Science* **300**: 1434 (2003).

Michalet, X., F.E. Pinaud, L.A. Bentolila, J.M. Tsay, S. Doose, J.J. Li, G. Sundaresan, A.M. Wu, S.S. Gambhir and S. Weiss. *Science* **307**: 538 (2005).

Parak, W.J., D. Gerion, T. Pellegrino, D. Zanchet, C. Micheel, S.C. Williams, R. Boudreau, M. A. Le Gros, C.A. Larabell and A.P. Alivisatos. *Nanotechnology* **14**: R15 (2003).

Medintz, I.L., H.T. Uyeda, E.R. Goldman and H. Mattoussi. *Nat. Mater.* **4**: 435 (2005).

Kim, S., Y.T. Lim, E.G. Soltesz, A.M. De Grand, J. Lee, A. Nakayama, J.A. Parker, T. Mihaljevic, R.G. Laurence, D.M. Dor, L.H. Cohn, M.G. Bawendi and J.V. Frangioni. *Nat. Biotechnol.* **22**: 93 (2003).

Ding, Z.F., B.M. Quinn, S.K. Haram, L.E. Pell, B.A. Korgel and A.J. Bard. *Science* **296**: 1293 (2002).

Chen, C.S., J. Yao and R.A. Durst. *J. Nanopart. Res.* **8**: 1033 (2006).

Bharali, D.J., D.W. Lucey, H. Jayakumar, H.E. Pudavar and P.N. Prasad. *J. Am. Chem. Soc.* **127**: 11,364 (2005).

Seydack, M. *Biosens. Bioelectron.* **20**: 2454 (2005).

Wilson, W.L., P.F. Szajowski and L.E. Brus. *Science* **262**: 1242 (1993).

Burns, A., H. Ow and U. Wiesner. *Chem. Soc. Rev.* **35**: 1028 (2006).

Derfus, A.M., W.C.W. Chan and S.N. Bhatia. *Nano Lett.* **4**: 11 (2004).

Kirchner, C., T. Liedl, S. Kudera, T. Pellegrino, A.M. Javier, H.E. Gaub, S. Stolzle, N. Fertig and W.J. Parak. *Nano Lett.* **5**: 331 (2005).

Lovric, J., S.J. Cho, F.M. Winnik and D. Maysinger. *Chem. Biol.* **12**: 1227 (2005).

Holmes, J.D., K.P. Johnston, C. Doty and B.A. Korgel. *Science* **287**: 1471 (2000).

Belomoin, G., J. Therrien, A. Smith, S. Rao, R. Twesten, S. Chaieb, M.H. Nayfeh, L. Wagner and L. Mitas. *Appl. Phys. Lett.* **80**: 841 (2002).

Hua, F., M.T. Swihart and E. Ruckenstein. *Langmuir*. **21**: 6054 (2005).

Li, Z.F. and E. Ruckenstein. *Nano Lett.* **4**: 1463 (2004).

Huisken, F., G. Ledoux, O. Guillos and C. Reynaud. *Adv. Mater*. **14**: 1861 (2002).

Lin, Y., D.E. Hill, J. Bentley, L.F. Allard and Y.P. Sun. *J. Phys. Chem. B* **107**: 10,453 (2003).

Kuno, M., D.P. Fromm, H.F. Hamann, A. Gallagher and D.J. Nesbitt. *J. Chem. Phys.* **115**: 1028 – 1040 (2001).

Shimizu, K.T., R.G. Neuhauser, C.A. Leatherdale, S.A. Empedocles, W.K. Woo and M. G. Bawendi. *Phys. Rev. B* **63**: 205,316 (2001).

Kuno, M., D.P. Fromm, A. Gallagher, D.J. Nesbitt, O.I. Micic, A.J. Nozik. *Nano Lett.* **1**: 557 (2001).

Sychugov, I., R. Juhasz, J. Linnros and J. Valenta. *Phys. Rev. B* **71**: 115,331 (2005).

Geddes, C.D., A. Parfenov, I. Gryczynski and J.R. Lakowicz *Chem. Phys. Lett.* **380**: 269 (2003).

Sun, Y.P., K. Fu, Y. Lin and W. Huang. *Acc. Chem. Res*. **35**: 1096 (2002).

Kose, M.E., B.A. Harruff, Y. Lin, L.M. Veca, F.S. Lu and Y.P. Sun. *J. Phys. Chem. B* **110**: 14,032 (2006).

Zhou, B., Y. Lin, L.M. Veca, K.A.S. Fernando, B.A. Harruff and Y.P. Sun. *J. Phys. Chem. B* **110**: 3001 (2006).

Bahr, J.L., E.T. Mickelson, M.J. Bronikowski, R.E. Smalley and J.M. Tour. *Chem. Commun* 193 (2001).

Bahr, J.L. and J.M. Tour. *J. Mater. Chem*. **12**: 1952 (2002).

Hirsch, A. *Angew. Chem. Int. Ed.* **41**: 1853 (2002).

Tasis, D., N. Tagmatarchis, V. Georgakilas and M. Prato. *Chem. A. Euro. J.* **9**: 4001 (2003).

Niyogi, S., M.A. Hamon, H. Hu, B. Zhao, P. Bhowmik, R. Sen, M.E. Itkis and R.C. Haddon. *Acc. Chem. Res*. **35**: 1105 (2002).

Chen, J., M.A. Hamon, H. Hu, Y. Chen, A.M. Rao, P.C. Eklund and R.C. Haddon. *Science* **282** :95 (1998).

Kuznetsova, A., D.B. Mawhinney, V. Naumenko, J.T. Yates, J. Liu and R.E. Smalley. *Chem. Phys. Lett*. **321**: 292 (2000).

Hu, H., P. Bhowmik, B. Zhao, M.A. Hamon , M.E. Itkis and R.C. Haddon. *Chem. Phys. Lett.* **345**: 25 (2001).

Huang, W.J., S. Fernando, L.F. Allard and Y.P. Sun. *Nano Lett*. **3**: 565 (2003).

Lin, Y., A.M. Rao, B. Sadanadan, E.A. Kenik and Y.P. Sun. *J. Phys. Chem. B* **106**: 1294 (2002).

Fernando, K.A.S., Y. Lin and Y.P. Sun. *Langmuir* **20**: 4777 (2004).

Kitaygorodskiy, A., W. Wang, S.Y. Xie, Y. Lin, K.A.S. Fernando, X. Wang, L.W. Qu, B. Chen and Y.P. Sun. *J. Am. Chem. Soc.* **127**: 7517 (2005).

Zhou, B., Y. Lin, H. Li, W. Huang, J.W. Connell, L.F. Allard and Y.P. Sun. *J. Phys. Chem. B* **107**: 13,588 (2003).

Huang, W., Y. Lin, S. Taylor, J. Gaillard, A.M. Rao and Y.P. Sun. *Nano Lett.* **2**: 231 (2002).

Zhou, B. and Y.P. Sun, et al. Unpublished.

Lakowicz, R.J. *Principles of Fluorescence Spectroscopy, 2nd edn.* New York: Kluwer Academic/Plenum Publisher (1999).

Rozhin, A.G., Y. Sakakibara, H. Kataura, S. Matsuzaki, K. Ishida, Y. Achiba and M. Tokumoto. *Chem. Phys. Lett.* **405**: 288 (2005).

Parak, W.J., T. Pellegrino and C. Plank. *Nanotechnology* **16**: R9 (2005).

Alivisatos, P. *Nature Biotechnol.* **22**:47 (2004).

Alivisatos, A.P., W.W. Gu, and C. Larabell. *Annu. Rev. Biomed. Eng.* **7**: 55 (2005).

Fu, A.H., W.W. Gu, C. Larabell and A.P. Alivisatos. *Curr. Opin. Neurobiol.* **15**: 568 (2005).

Gao, X., Y. Cui, R.M. Levenson, L.W.K. Chung and S. Nie. *Nat. Biotechnol.* **22**: 969 (2004).

7 Microwave-assisted Synthesis and Processing of Biomaterials

Yingjie Zhu[1] and Jiang Chang

Shanghai Institute of Ceramics, Chinese Academy of Sciences, Shanghai 200050, China

Abstract Microwave heating has received considerable attention as a new promising method for rapid volumetric heating, which results in higher reaction rates and selectivities, reduction in reaction times often by orders of magnitude, and increasing yields of products compared to conventional heating methods. As a result, this has opened up the possibility of realizing fast synthesis of materials in a very short time, leading to relatively low cost and high efficiency of materials production. The application of microwave heating in the synthesis of materials especially in solution is a fast-growing area of research. In this chapter, we will briefly review the progress made in the last decade on the microwave-assisted synthesis and processing of biomaterials both in nanometer- and micrometer-size range. The biomaterials reviewed in this chapter include hydroxyapatite (HA, $Ca_{10}(PO_4)_6(OH)_2$), β-tricalcium phosphate (β-TCP, β-$Ca_3(PO_4)_2$), calcium carbonate ($CaCO_3$), the composite biomaterials and functionally graded material (FGM).

7.1 Introduction

Microwave heating has received considerable attention as a new promising method for the fast synthesis of materials, especially in solution. The application of microwave heating in synthetic chemistry is a fast-growing area of research (Perreux and Loupy, 2001, Varma 2001, Zhu et al., 2004). Since the first reports of microwave-assisted synthesis in 1986 (Gedye et al., 1986, Giguere et al., 1986), microwave heating has been accepted as a promising method for rapid volumetric heating, which results in higher reaction rates and selectivities, reduction in reaction times often by orders of magnitude, and increasing yields of products compared to conventional heating methods. As a result, this has opened up the possibility of realizing fast synthesis of materials in a very short time, leading to relatively low cost and high efficiency of materials production.

---

(1) Corresponding e-mail: y.j.zhu@mail.sic.ac.cn

Microwaves are the electromagnetic waves with frequencies in the range of 300 MHz to 300 GHz. The commonly used frequency is 2.45 GHz. The principle of microwave heating is related to the polar characteristic of molecules. In the microwave frequency range, polar molecules such as H_2O try to orientate with the fast changing of electric field. When dipolar molecules try to re-orientate with an alternating electric field, they lose energy in the form of heat by molecular friction. The microwave power dissipation per unit volume in a material (*P*) is given by Eq. (7.1) (Tsuji et al., 2005):

$$P = cE^2 f \varepsilon_1 = cE^2 f \varepsilon_2 \tan\delta \tag{7.1}$$

where *c* is a constant, *E* is an electric field in the material, *f* is frequency of radiation, and ε_1 and ε_2 are the dielectric loss and dielectric constants, respectively. ε_2 represents the relative permittivity, which is a measure of the ability of a molecule to be polarized by an electric field and $\tan\delta = \varepsilon_1 / \varepsilon_2$ is the energy dissipation factor or loss tangent. Equation (7.1) indicates that ε_1 is the most important physical parameter that describes the ability of a material to heat in the microwave field.

The physical parameters of some typical solvents used in microwave heating are listed in Table 7.1. From Table 7.1 one can see that water, alcohols, *N*, *N*-dimethyl formamide, and ethylene glycol have high dielectric losses, they also have *a* high reduction ability. Therefore, they are ideal solvents for microwave rapid heating.

Table 7.1 Physical parameters of typical solvents used for microwave heating (Kingston and Haswell, 1997)

Substance	Boiling point (℃)	ε_1	ε_2	$\tan\delta$
Water	100	12.3	78.3	0.157
Methanol	65	20.9	32.7	0.639
Ethanol	78	6.08	24.3	0.200
N, *N*-dimethyl formamide	153		36.71	
Ethylene glycol	198	41.0	41.0	1.00
N-methyl pyrrolidone	202	8.855	32.0	0.277

Calcium-phosphate-based biomaterials have received considerable attention due to their bioactive and biocompatible property. Major phases of the calcium phosphate are hydroxyapatite (HA, $Ca_{10}(PO_4)_6(OH)_2$), octacalcium phosphate (OCP, $Ca_8H_2(PO_4)_6$), tricalcium phosphate (TCP, $Ca_3(PO_4)_2$), $CaHPO_4$ $2H_2O$ and $Ca_2P_2O_7$. HA and TCP are mainly used as bone-substituted biomaterials hydroxyapatite (HA) has a non-biodegradable property, whereas tricalcium phosphate (TCP) is used as biodegradable bone replacement material. Calcium carbonate ($CaCO_3$) is also an important biomineral which exists in both nature and biosystems. Although many methods such as hydrothermal, direct precipitation and solid state reaction have been reported for the synthesis of biomaterials, the reports on the microwave-assisted synthesis and processing of biomaterials has been relatively few despite of the advantages of microwave heating. However, this situation is changing. There are increasing interest and research effort in the area of synthesis of biomaterials by microwave heating nowadays.

In this chapter, we will briefly review the progress reported in the literature on the microwave-assisted synthesis and processing of inorganic biomaterials. The review is not confined in nanometer-size inorganic biomaterials, but submicrometer- and micrometer-size inorganic biomaterials are also included. The inorganic materials which are covered in this review include HA, TCP ($Ca_3(PO_4)_2$) and $CaCO_3$. Next, we will give a brief review on the progresses in microwave-assisted synthesis and processing of inorganic biomaterials.

7.2 Synthesis of Hydroxyapatite

Hydroxyapatite (HA, $Ca_{10}(PO_4)_6(OH)_2$) is one of the most important biomaterials for bone and dental applications because it is the main inorganic constituent of the natural bone and teeth (Hench, 1991) and it has excellent biocompatibility. The natural bone consists of nanostructured nonstoichiometric HA with 20 nm in diameter and 50 nm in length, together with substitution of ions like magnesium, fluoride and carbonate in minor concentrations. Nanocrystalline HA has proved to be of biological importance in terms of osteoblast adhesion, proliferation, osseointegration and formation of new bone on its surface (Webster et al., 2001). There is a great demand for HA in odontology and traumatology. The properties of HA depend on its stoichiometry, crystallinity, particle size and morphology. In this regard, to develop new methods for the control over these factors is of great importance for biomedical applications of HA. Many synthesis methods of HA powders are known, such as precipitation, solid state synthesis, hydrolysis, hydrothermal and sol-gel methods. The microwave heating method is very promising in the controlled synthesis and processing of biomaterials due to its advantages.

In general, the formation of HA involves the reaction between Ca^{2+}, PO_4^{3-} and OH^- ions, which can be simplified as a following reaction:

$$10Ca^{2+} + 6\,PO_4^{3-} + 2OH^- = Ca_{10}(PO_4)_6(OH)_2 \tag{7.2}$$

The usual starting reagents used for the synthesis of HA are soluble calcium salt such as $CaCl_2$, $Ca(NO_3)_2$, soluble compound containing PO_4^{3-} such as Na_3PO_4, Na_2HPO_4, NaH_2PO_4, $(NH_4)_2HPO_4$, $NH_4H_2PO_4$, and H_3PO_4. In some cases, a hydroxide is also used to create an alkaline environment for the synthesis.

There has been the progress achieved to synthesize HA by microwave heating method. HA with various morphologies such as spherical particles, nanorods and nanosheets has been synthesized using a microwave heating method. There are relatively more reports on the synthesis of 1-D HA nanostructures (nanorods, nanoneedles, nanofibers) than spherical particles or 2-D nanosheets. The hexagonal structure of HA may be a possible reason for the common formation of rod-like morphology.

7.2.1 Synthesis in Aqueous Solution

Microwave-assisted synthesis of HA through precipitation from the aqueous solution within less than one hour was reported in 1991 by Lerner et al. (Lerner et al., 1991). Murugan et al. (2003) reported microwave synthesis of bioresorbable carbonated HA using goniopora. Under microwave irradiation, the carbonated HA was prepared by using goniopora as calcium precursor and $CaHPO_4$ as phosphate precursor. The X-ray powder diffraction (XRD) pattern confirmed the formation of a single phase of HA without any other phases. The Fourier transform infrared (FTIR) spectrum of HA showed the presence of carbonate ions, indicating carbonate substitution into the apatite phase. The goniopora was found to decompose all the organic debris and carbonate phases at 900℃. The prepared carbonated HA did not show significant weight loss up to 1000℃ indicating its thermal stability. *In-vitro* solubility test showed an increase in the solubility of carbonated HA than that of pure HA. These findings imply the feasibility of carbonated HA production using goniopora by microwave irradiation.

Siddharthan et al. (2004) used microwave heating to accelerate the formation of nanometer-size needles of calcium deficient HA (Ca/P ratio = 1.5) with a shorter processing time as compared to other available methods reported. The aqueous solution containing $Ca(NO_3)_2 \cdot 4H_2O$, H_3PO_4 and NH_3H_2O was subjected to microwave irradiation in a domestic microwave oven for 15 min. The morphology of the calcium deficient HA powder was needle-shaped and mostly agglomerated. The needles were 16 – 39 nm in length and 7 – 16 nm in width. The thermal decomposition of calcium deficient HA was also studied. The HPO_4^{2-} ions in calcium deficient HA converted to $P_2O_7^{4-}$ at around 500℃. The calcium deficient HA transformed to β-$Ca_3(PO_4)_2$ (β-TCP) at about 650℃.

Mahabole et al. (2005) reported HA synthesized by three different routes via wet chemical process, microwave irradiation and hydrothermal technique. The XRD pattern of the product revealed HA with a hexagonal structure. The average crystallite size was found to be in the range 31 – 54 nm. Absorption bands corresponding to phosphate and hydroxyl functional groups, which are characteristic of HA, were confirmed by FTIR. HA could be used as CO gas sensor at an optimum temperature near 125℃. X-ray photoelectron spectroscopy (XPS) studies showed that the Ca/P ratio was 1.63 for the HA sample prepared by wet chemical process. The microwave irradiation technique yielded calcium rich

HA whereas calcium deficient HA was obtained by hydrothermal method. This study indicates that heating method has an influence on the composition of crystal phase of HA.

Yang et al. (2004) reported the microwave-assisted synthesis of thermally stable HA prepared using $Ca(NO_3)_2 \cdot 4H_2O$, H_3PO_4, and glucose. The experiments showed that various parameters such as aging time, microwave irradiation power and time had significant effects on thermal stability of HA. The thermal stability of HA increased with increasing aging time, microwave irradiation time and power, respectively. The morphology of HA is not known since no TEM or SEM micrographs were given in the paper.

The microwave-assisted molten salt method was also reported to synthesize HA whiskers using an aqueous solution containing $Ca(NO_3)_2 \cdot 4H_2O$, KH_2PO_4, $NaNO_3$ and HNO_3 (with or without urea) (Jalota et al., 2006). The reactants were irradiated in a household microwave oven at about 500 – 550℃ for 5 min. The as-prepared precursor was then simply stirred in water at room temperature for 1 h to obtain the whiskers of HA. HA whiskers were found to possess apatite-inducing ability when soaked in simulated body fluid (SBF). Osteoblast attachment and proliferation on the surfaces of whisker compacts was evaluated by scanning electron microscopy (SEM) (Fig. 7.1). Osteoblasts were attached to the surfaces of all the whisker compacts tested, however, the high-magnification micrographs showed slight differences in osteoblast proliferation. The osteoblast viability and protein concentrations were found to be the highest on HA whiskers compared with β-TCP and HA-TCP whiskers. Upon soaking in SBF solution at 37℃ for 1 week, all the whiskers were observed to form petal- or flake-like morphology on their surfaces, while still retaining their global whisker-like shapes. In vitro cell culture tests performed with the mouse osteoblasts (7F2) on the whisker compacts showed decreasing number of cells attached and protein concentration values in the following order: HA > biphasic HA-TCP >β-TCP (Fig. 7.1).

A novel microwave-assisted combustion synthesis (auto ignition)/molten salt synthesis hybrid route was developed by the same group for the synthesis of HA, TCP, and biphasic HA-TCP nanowhiskers (Jalota et al., 2004). Aqueous solutions containing $Ca(NO_3)_2 \cdot 4H_2O$, KH_2PO_4, and $NaNO_3$ (with or without urea) were irradiated in a household microwave oven for 5 min at 600 W of power. The as-synthesized precursors were then simply stirred in water at room temperature for 1 h to obtain the nanowhiskers of the calcium phosphate product.

Kundu et al. (1998) prepared HA by microwave irradiation of $Ca(NO_3)_2 \cdot 4H_2O$ and $(NH_4)_2HPO_4$ in aqueous solution. HA prepared was subjected to biocompatibility assay by a cell-culture method using the hybridoma cell line AE9D6 in both conventional Dulbecco's modification of Eagle's medium (DMEM) and SBF, both supplemented with 5% fetal calf serum. HA synthesized by the microwave method showed the presence of TCP. Biocompatibility assays showed reproducible growth and secretion patterns of cells both in DMEM as well as in SBF, thereby indicating the effectiveness of the microwave method for the production of biocompatible HA.

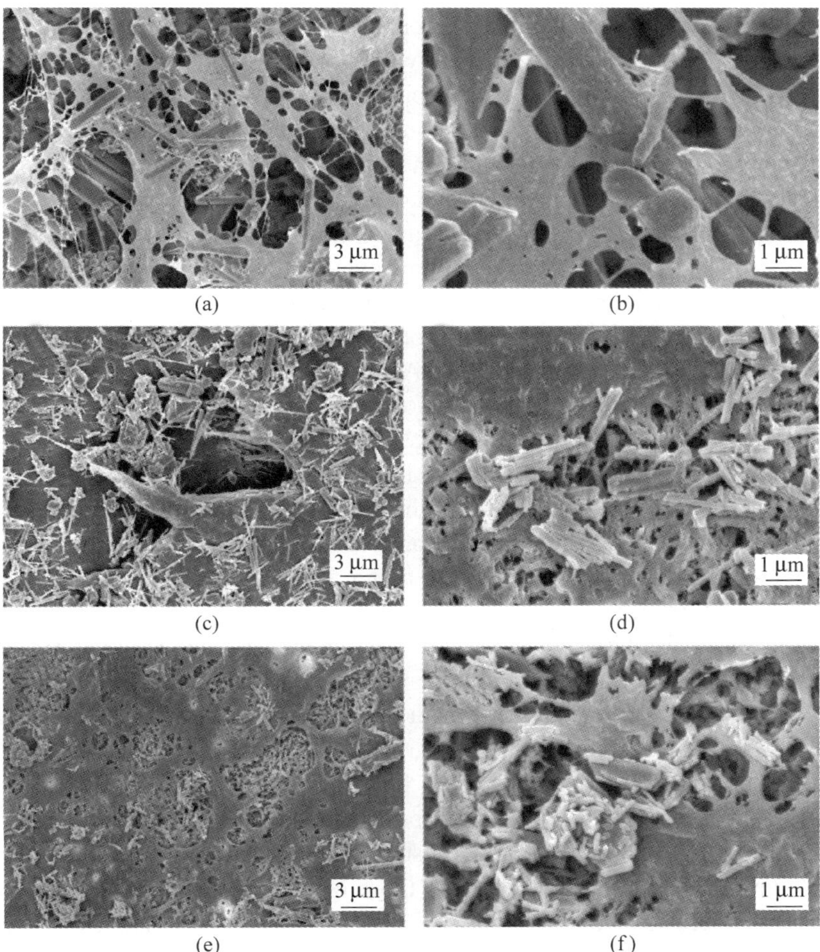

Figure 7.1 SEM micrographs of osteoblast proliferation on whiskers: (a), (b) β-TCP whiskers. (c), (d) biphasic HA-TCP whiskers. (e), (f) HA whiskers. (Reprinted from (Jalota et al., 2006))

$Ca(OH)_2$ and $(NH_4)_2HPO_4$ were used as the starting reagents to prepare HA by a microwave heating method (Vaidhyanathan and Rao, 1996, Meejoo et al., 2006). Meejoo et al. reported the preparation of calcium deficient HA needle-like nanocrystals using an aqueous solution containing $Ca(OH)_2$ and $(NH_4)_2HPO_4$ by a microwave-assisted method. The needle-shaped nanocrystals were about 50 nm in diameter and 200 nm in length. The as-prepared calcium deficient HA was B-type carbonated HA with PO_4^{3-} sites substituted by CO_3^{2-}. However, carbonate can be removed after annealing at 800℃, but the secondary phases β-TCP and α-TCP also formed after heating HA at 900℃ or above.

In order to control the concentration of free Ca^{2+} ions in solution and thus control the reaction rate, complexing ligand was used in the synthesis of HA.

López-Macipe et al. studied the precipitation of nanosized HA needles at atmospheric pressure by a rapid microwave heating of the solution containing $CaCl_2$, Na_2HPO_4, sodium citrate (Na_3(cit)) and compared this technique with a conventional heating method. Citrate ions could act as the Ca-complexing agent and also exhibit crystal-growth-inhibition activity. A comparison between products obtained by microwave irradiation and a conventional heating method using a similar heating rate (7.8℃/min) and heating time (2 – 120 min) was carried out. The experiments showed that the microwave heating did not seem to favor a decrease in HA crystal size compared with the conventional heating, this result is different from the results obtained on other system such as calcite (Rodríguez-Clemente and Gómez-Morales, 1996). A possible explanation was proposed by examining the rate-controlling factors for precipitation of the two solids. In the case of calcite, with an activation energy $E_a = 40$ kJ/mol for crystal growth, the rate-limiting step is the dehydration of ions at the surface, which is favored by microwave radiation. However, the higher Ea value (186 kJ/mol) calculated for HA indicates the appearance of additional surface processes that influence the rate of precipitation, such as diffusion along the crystal surface or into vacant sites in the crystal lattice.

Torrent-Burgués et al. (1999) also used citrate ions as a complexing reagent to prepare nanoneedles of calcium deficient HA (Ca/P ratio ~ 1.5) by a continuous microwave-assisted precipitation method. The starting solution containing $CaCl_2 \cdot 2H_2O$, $Na_3cit \cdot 2H_2O$ (where $cit^{3-} = C_6H_8O_7{}^{3-}$) and Na_2HPO_4 was used and the solution was microwave heated to boiling point, ensuring that the reactor worked as a mixed suspension-mixed product removal (MSMPR) reactor. The chemical and morphological characteristics of the product did not change with the residence time, and were similar to those of HA obtained in a batch process using also microwave heating and Ca/citrate/phosphate solution. On the other hand, the steady state in the precipitation of HA was reached faster than that in an MSMPR reactor using a noncomplexing solution and conventional heating. In the latter process submicrometer (< 1 μm) needle-like particles were obtained. Similarly, HA with a needle-like morphology (in submicrometer range) was prepared from highly concentrated $CaCl_2$ and K_2HPO_4 solution by a continuous method in a MSMPR reactor at 85℃ in N_2 atmosphere (pH = 9.0) (Gómez-Morales et al., 2001). Under these conditions HA with a Ca to P ratio equal or close to the stoichiometric composition (Ca/P = 1.667) was obtained at steady state with a high yield (up to 99%) and a high production rate (up to 1.17 g/min).

In addition to citrate ions, EDTA was also selected as the complexing ligand to Ca^{2+} ions. Liu et al. (2004) reported the formation of HA nanorods by microwave heating the solution containing $Ca(NO_3)_2$, Na_2HPO_4 and EDTA. The pH of solution was adjusted to 9 – 13 by adding NaOH solution. The aqueous solution was put into a household type microwave oven and the reaction was performed under ambient air for 30 min. The microwave oven followed a working cycle of

6 s on and 10 s off (37% power). The shape of HA crystals could be controlled by changing the stability of Ca-EDTA and the hindrance effect of OH^- on the crystallite facets. The pH value had a significant influence on the morphology of HA since the stability of Ca-EDTA complex was different in the solution with a different pH value. HA powder synthesized from the solution with pH = 9 consisted of single crystalline nanorods with an average diameter of ~ 40 nm and a length of up to ~400 nm. However, bowknot-like bundles of HA were obtained at pH = 11. The bundle consisted of HA nanorods with a typical width of 150 nm and lengths up to 2 μm. The bowknot-like HA nanostructures were stable after long-period ultrasonic treatment, indicating the nanostructures were not due to aggregation. The morphology of HA prepared at pH = 13 was flower-like structures consisting of leaf-like flakes of 150 – 200 nm in width and 1 – 2 μm in length. The corresponding SAED pattern taken from an individual leaf-like flake confirmed that the flakes were well-crystallized single crystals.

Yoon et al. (2005) reported the synthesis of HA whiskers by a microwave-assisted hydrolysis of α-$Ca_3(PO_4)_2$ (α-TCP) at 70 – 90℃ for 6 – 15 h (pH = 11) (Fig. 7.2). Microwave heating increased the hydrolysis rate and enhanced the development of HA whiskers. From Fig. 7.2 one can see that the diameter and length increase with increasing microwave heating time. The optimum hydrolysis reaction time at 90℃ was about 10 h and was significantly

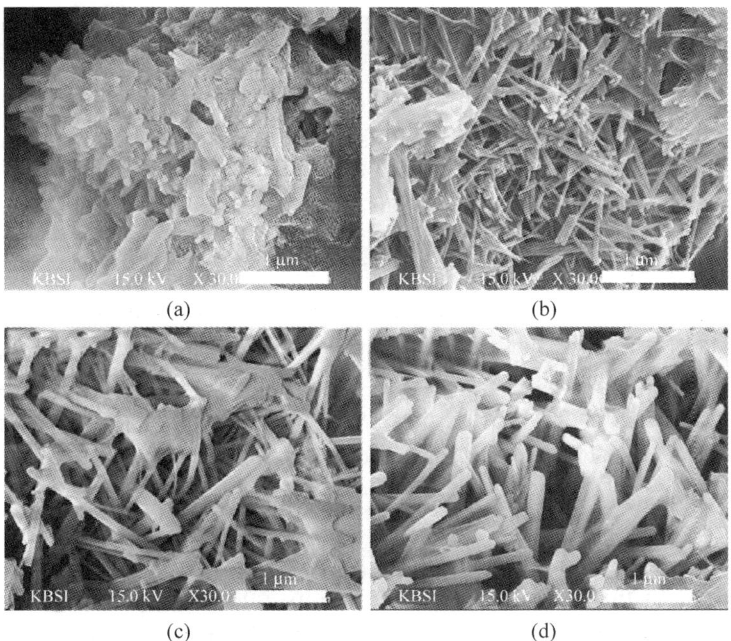

Figure 7.2 SEM micrographs of the products obtained by microwave heating at 70℃ for (a) 4 h, (b) 6 h, (c) 10 h and (d) 15 h. (Reprinted from (Yoon et al., 2005))

shorter compared with conventional heating (24 h). The morphology of the product was controlled by varying the hydrolysis temperature and time. The conversion rate at 70℃ for 15 h was 95%, and HA whiskers (Ca/P molar ratio = 1.66) had an aspect ratio >10 ($\leqslant$ 0.2 μm in diameter) and a specific surface area of 5.34 m^2/g.

In addition to rod-like morphology of HA, HA nanosheets have also been synthesized by microwave-assisted method. Rameshbabu et al. (2005) synthesized HA nanocrystals with a plate-like morphology by microwave heating a solution of $Ca(OH)_2$ and $(NH_4)_2HPO_4$ at Ca/P molar ratio of 1.67. The microwave heating reduced the HA crystallization time and improved crystallinity of the final product. The XRD pattern of HA formed by conventional heating showed a low crystallinity. The HA powder heat treated at 1000℃ did not show any secondary phase formation (e.g., TCP or CaO), indicating its high thermal stability. Sarig and Kahana (2002) reported the microwave-assisted synthesis of HA using an aqueous solution of $CaCl_2$ and NaH_2PO_4 with small amounts of additives L-aspartic acid and $NaHCO_3$. The powder was composed of spherulites with diameters of about 2 – 4 μm. Each spherulite consisted of nanoplatelets of about 300 nm on edge, loosely aggregated. Siddharthan et al. (2006) synthesized nanometer-size HA by a microwave-assisted co-precipitation process using $Ca(NO_3)_2$, H_3PO_4 and $NH_3 \cdot H_2O$. The precipitate in paste form was subjected to microwave irradiation in a domestic microwave oven at various powers until the precipitate was dry. The results showed the variation of particle size with the power of microwave irradiation. The shape of the particles also changed from needle-like to platelet-like form with the increase in microwave power. However, temperatures in the synthesis were not reported, which could significantly influence the particle size and morphology.

7.2.2 Microwave-Hydrothermal Synthesis

The microwave-hydrothermal method was also used to synthesize HA (Katsuki and Furuta, 1999). HA nanorods were prepared using gypsum ($CaSO_4 \cdot 2H_2O$) powder and $(NH_4)_2HPO_4$ at 100 ℃ for 0.5 – 120 min by microwave-hydrothermal treatment. Gypsum powder could be completely converted to HA nanorods for 5 min. The reaction for the formation of HA was proposed as follows:

$$
\begin{aligned}
&10CaSO_4 \cdot 2H_2O + 6(NH_4)_2HPO_4 \\
&= Ca_{10}(PO_4)_6(OH)_2 + 6(NH_4)_2SO_4 + 4H_2SO_4 + 18H_2O
\end{aligned}
\tag{7.3}
$$

Compared with the formation of HA by conventional-hydrothermal treatment, microwave-hydrothermal treatment led to increased HA formation rate by two orders of magnitude.

7.2.3 Synthesis of HA by the Conversion of Precursor Monetite Prepared in Mixed Solvents

Recently, we have developed a simple microwave-assisted method for synthesis of flowerlike and bundlelike monetite ($CaHPO_4$) consisting of nanosheets using $CaCl_2 \cdot 2.5\ H_2O$, NaH_2PO_4 and sodium dodecyl sulfate (SDS) in mixed solvents of water and ethylene glycol at 95℃ for 1 h. (Ma et al., 2006). Monetite is also bioactive, it is usually used as a precursor to synthesize HA. In this regard, the control over the morphology of the precursor monetite to obtain the specific morphology of HA is a useful route. The prepared sample consisted of a single phase of crystalline monetite with a triclinic structure. The chemical reaction for the formation of monetite can be simplified as follows:

$$Ca^{2+} + H_2PO_4^{-} = CaHPO_4 + H^{+} \tag{7.4}$$

SEM micrographs (Fig. 7.3) showed that of the prepared monetite had a flowerlike and bundlelike morphologies. Each flowerlike or bundlelike microstructure was formed by the assembly of nanosheets with thicknesses ranging from 80 nm to 100 nm and with sizes up to 3.5 μm.

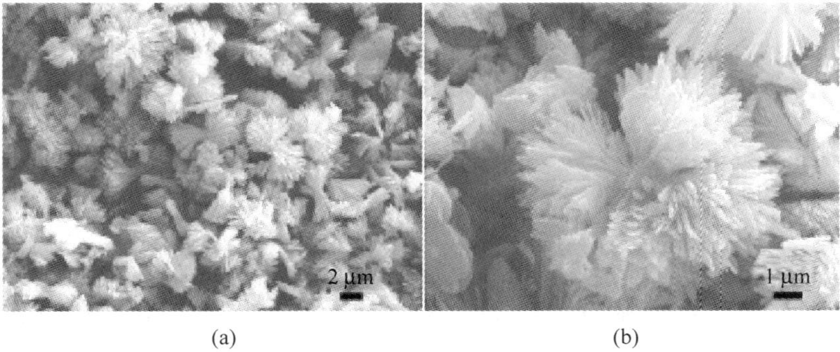

(a) (b)

Figure 7.3 SEM micrographs of monetite prepared by microwave heating at 95℃ for 1 h: (a) at a low magnification and (b) at a high magnification (Reprinted from reference by Ma et al., 2006)

In order to investigate the formation mechanism of flowerlike monetite, the monetite samples were prepared at 95℃ for different heating time, while other reaction conditions were the same. When the heating time was 1 min (Fig. 7.4(a)), many irregular polyhedra and spindlelike nanosheets were observed. Only a few low-symmetry bundlelike monetite was observed, and the degree of assembly was low. When the heating time was increased to 5 min, the congeries and bundles of nanosheets dominated (Fig. 7.4(b)). When the heating time was increased to 20 min, the highly oriented nanosheets were assembled to form the flowerlike morphology (Fig. 7.4(c)). The degree of assembly increased with increasing time, although the sizes of the monetite structures increased. From Figs. 7.4(a) – (c), one can clearly see the process of oriented-aggregation-based growth from nanosheets to a flowerlike morphology.

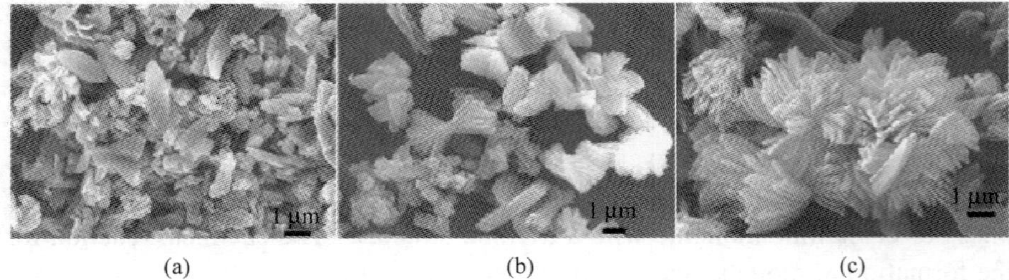

Figure 7.4 SEM micrographs of monetite prepared by microwave heating at 95℃ for different times: (a) 1 min, (b) 5 min, and (c) 20 min. (Reprinted from (Ma et al., 2006))

SDS was used as a surfactant to control the morphology of the monetite. SDS was favorable for the formation of a flowerlike morphology of monetite. In the absence of SDS, the morphologies of monetite were sheets and a small number of bundles. No flowerlike morphology was obtained. However, the flowerlike and bundlelike morphologies were formed in the presence of SDS. Because of the electrostatic interaction with Ca^{2+} ions, the negatively charged SDS polar groups acted as active sites for the nucleation of monetite. Ca^{2+} ions strongly adsorbed on the micellar surface of the opposite charge, leading to a much faster nucleation rate on the surface of the SDS micelles. Because of the high viscosity of ethylene glycol at room temperature, the diffusion of Ca^{2+} and HPO_4^{2-} ions and fast nucleation were restrained. With the elevation of temperature by microwave heating, the viscosity of ethylene glycol rapidly decreased, and the polarization of ethylene glycol and water molecules under the rapidly changing electric field of the microwave reactor may facilitate the anisotropic growth of monetite nanosheets. The flowerlike morphology was formed by the assembly of nanosheets with the help of SDS through the oriented attachment mechanism.

Monetite is an excellent precursor for the formation of HA. We used flowerlike monetite as a precursor to obtain HA by immersing flowerlike monetite powder in 0.1 mol/L NaOH solution at 60℃ for 15 min and 1, 4, 8, and 12 h, respectively. The XRD pattern of the monetite sample immersed in NaOH solution for 15 min indicates the presence of HA with a hexagonal structure as a major phase and a minor phase of the residual monetite. The monetite sample immersed in NaOH solution for 1 h consisted of a single phase of crystalline HA. The transformation from monetite to HA was complete within 1 h, which was much shorter than previously reported (4 h) (Da Silva et al., 2001).

Figure 7.5 shows SEM micrographs of HA samples after immersion of the monetite powder in a NaOH solution at 60℃ for 15 min and 1, 4, and 8 h, respectively. One can see that the flower-like morphology of monetite was sustained and flower-like agglomerated nanorods of HA were formed. The sizes of the HA nanorods increased with increasing the immersing time in the NaOH solution. This interesting result indicates that it is feasible to prepare the agglomerated nanorods of HA through the conversion of the monetite in NaOH solution, providing a simple route to the synthesis of HA.

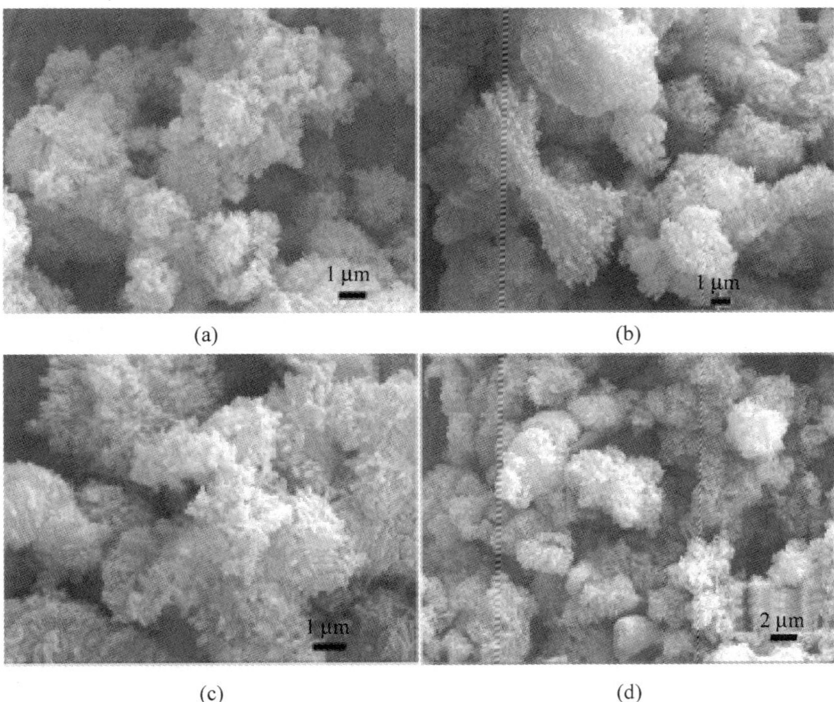

Figure 7.5 SEM micrographs of nanocrystalline HA prepared by immersing monetite powder in 0.1 mol/L NaOH solution at 60℃ for (a) 15 min, (b) 1 h, (c) 4 h, and (d) 8 h (Reprinted from (Ma et al., 2006))

7.2.4 Prepration of HA Thin Film

The progress on the microwave-assisted preparation of HA thin films has also been achieved. Adams et al. (2005) studied the influence of geometrically configured HA thin films prepared by microwave-assisted sol-gel method on osteoblast adhesive response. High-quality crystalline HA thin films with thickness about 350 nm on titanium substrates with underlying micro-channels were prepared by microwave annealing at 400℃ for 30 min. A comprehensive in vitro study was conducted to assess the osteoblast adhesive response to the well-defined micro-scale topographical features on HA coated and uncoated surfaces. The study confirmed the osteoblast's response to the HA coated micro-channels with an elongated morphology. The results suggest that osteoblast adhesion can be improved through optimal micro-channel design and may provide a possible route for improving the long-term performance of prosthetic orthopedic and dental implants.

7.2.5 Synthesis by Solid State Reaction

Microwave-assisted solid state reaction process was also used to synthesize nanocrystalline HA (Parhia et al., 2004; Feng et al., 2005). Parhia et al. synthesized nanocrystalline spherical particles (~100 nm) of HA by microwave treatment of $CaCl_2$ and Na_3PO_4 at a stoichiometric ratio by solid-state reaction. Use of sodium carbonate or sodium fluoride in addition to calcium chloride resulted in the formation of carbonate- or fluoride-substituted HA.

HA nanorods with diameters from 60 nm to 80 nm and lengths of about 400 nm were prepared using $Ca(NO_3)_2 \cdot 4H_2O$ and $Na_3PO_4 \cdot 12H_2O$ at a stoichiometric ratio by a microwave-assisted solid-state reaction (Cao et al., 2005). The product obtained under conventional heating for 6 h at 80℃ was poorly crystallized, while well-crystallized HA was obtained by a domestic microwave oven heating for only 1 min. Unfortunately, no temperature was reported for microwave synthesis in the paper, making the comparison between the two heating method difficult. The microwave heating time had a significant influence on the morphology of HA. Spherical HA nanoparticles were produced by microwave interval heating for 0.5 min; while HA nanorods were obtained by microwave interval heating for 1 min. In this case, temperature was not known and it may also have an influence on the morphology of HA.

7.3 Synthesis of β-Tricalcium Phosphate (β-$Ca_3(PO_4)_2$)

β-$Ca_3(PO_4)_2$ (β-TCP) is another important biomaterial which has many biomedical applications. Microwave-assisted synthesis of β-TCP was rarely reported. Jalota et al. (2006) synthesized single-phase β-TCP rods using $Ca(NO_3)_2 \cdot 4H_2O$, KH_2PO_4, $NaNO_3$ and HNO_3 (with or without urea) by a microwave-assisted molten salt process. The reactants were irradiated in a household microwave oven for 5 min at about 500℃ to 550℃. As-prepared precursor was stirred in water at room temperature for 1 h to obtain β-TCP rods. The morphology of β-TCP rods is shown in Fig. 7.6.

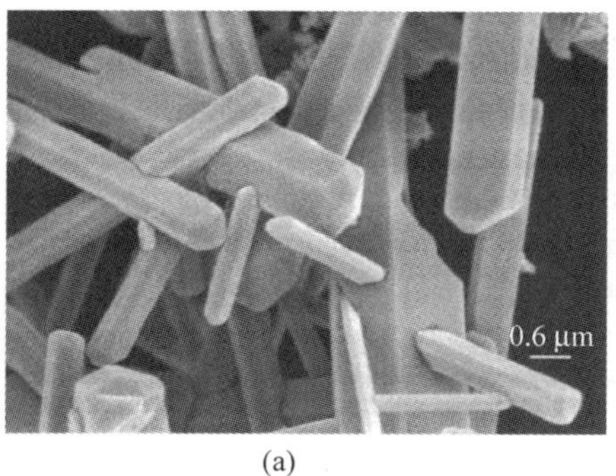

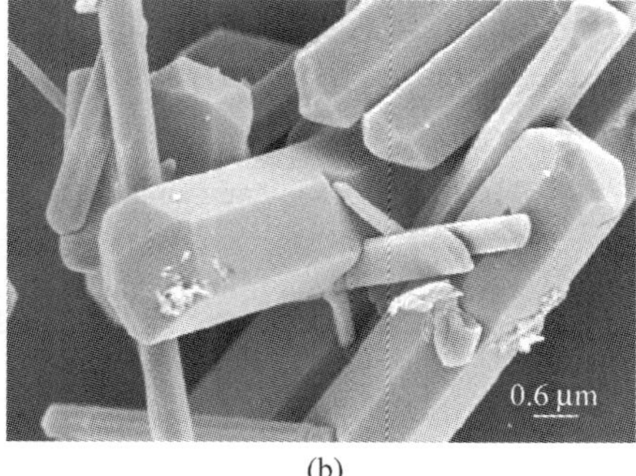

(a) (b)

Figure 7.6 SEM micrographs of β-TCP whiskers (reprinted from (Jalota et al., 2006))

7.4 Synthesis of Calcium Carbonate ($CaCO_3$)

Calcium carbonate ($CaCO_3$) is an attractive model mineral for studies because the morphology control of $CaCO_3$ has been an important subject in biomineralization processes. $CaCO_3$ can crystallize as calcite, aragonite, and vaterite. Calcite and aragonite are the most common biologically formed $CaCO_3$ polymorphs. Vaterite, a less stable polymorph, will transform into calcite via a solvent-mediated process. However, vaterite is expected to have potential applications for various purposes. Unlike calcite, vaterite is rarely found in either biological or nonbiological systems. Vaterite transforms easily and irreversibly into thermodynamically stable form when in contact with water, so it can only be fabricated in the presence of specific additives in a controlled environment.

So far, most of the preparations of $CaCO_3$ were carried out at room temperature; very few reports investigated the influence of temperature on the morphology and crystalline phase of $CaCO_3$. Rodríguez-Clemente and Gómez-Morales (1996) reported microwave-assisted precipitation of $CaCO_3$ (calcite) from a Ca-citrate and HCO_3^- / CO_3^{2-} solution both in batch and MSMPR reactor. In the batch experiments, monodisperse calcite crystals with ellipsoidal or peanut-like shapes were obtained, while in the continuous precipitation experiments the calcite crystals showed ellipsoidal shape. These morphologies are unusual for the calcite phase. In the continuous precipitation experiments, the rate of nucleation was higher than that in a conventional MSMPR reactor under the same conditions.

Recently, we have found that microwave heating has a great effect on the morphology of $CaCO_3$. The unique morphologies of $CaCO_3$ which cannot form at room temperature can be obtained by microwave heating. We have reported microwave-assisted synthesis of $CaCO_3$ (vaterite) in a water/ethylene glycol (EG) system with surfactants (Qi and Zhu, 2006). Vaterite with various morphologies has been obtained by controlling the experimental parameters. The self-assembly played an important role in the formation of these vaterite crystals with various morphologies. The experimental conditions for typical samples and their morphologies are listed in Table 7.2.

Table 7.2 Experimental conditions for typical samples and their morphologies[(1)]. SDS stands for sodium dodecyl sulfate and CTAB for cetyltrimethylammonium bromide. (Reprinted from (Qi and Zhu, 2006))

Sample	Solution	Time(min)	Morphology
1	SDS(1.5 mmol)/EG (10 mL)/0.75 mol/L $Ca(CH_3COO)_2$ aqueous solution (2 mL) +SDS(1.5 mmol)/EG (10 mL)/0.75 mol/L Na_2CO_3 aqueous solution (2 mL)	8	dagger-like
2	same as sample 1	5	bicone-like
3	same as sample 1	6	dagger-like
4	same as sample 1	7	dagger-like
5	same as sample 1	10	dagger-like
6	same as sample 1	30	irregular
7	EG (10 mL)/0.75 mol/L $Ca(CH_3COO)_2$ aqueous solution (2 mL) +EG (10 mL)/0.75 mol/L Na_2CO_3 aqueous solution (2 mL)	10	irregular
8	SDS(3 mmol)/EG (10 mL)/0.75 mol/L $Ca(CH_3COO)_2$ aqueous solution (2 mL) +SDS(3 mmol)/EG (10 mL)/0.75 mol/L Na_2CO_3 aqueous solution (2 mL)	10	irregular
9	Same as sample 8	20	shuttle-like
10	CTAB(1.5 mmol)/EG (10 mL)/0.75 mol/L $Ca(CH_3COO)_2$ aqueous solution (2 mL) +CTAB(1.5 mmol)/EG (10 mL)/0.75 mol/L Na_2CO_3 aqueous solution (2 mL)	10	regular microspheres

(1) All samples were prepared by microwave heating at 100℃.

XRD patterns of the products prepared by the microwave-assisted method in the water/EG/SDS system at 100℃ showed a well-crystalline vaterite with a hexagonal structure. It was reported that calcite was formed in the water/SDS system (Wei et al., 2005). This indicates that the presence of EG affected the precipitation rate of vaterite and limited its phase transformation into calcite and therefore was favorable for the formation of vaterite. Samples 1 – 5 have similar XRD patterns, which can be indexed to a hexagonal vaterite. However, in addition to the main phase of vaterite, samples 3, 4, and 5 had a small quantity of calcite. The main phase of sample 6 was calcite in coexistence with a minor phase of vaterite. This indicates that when the reaction time is prolonged, vaterite, as a less stable polymorph which is stabilized kinetically, will transform into calcite.

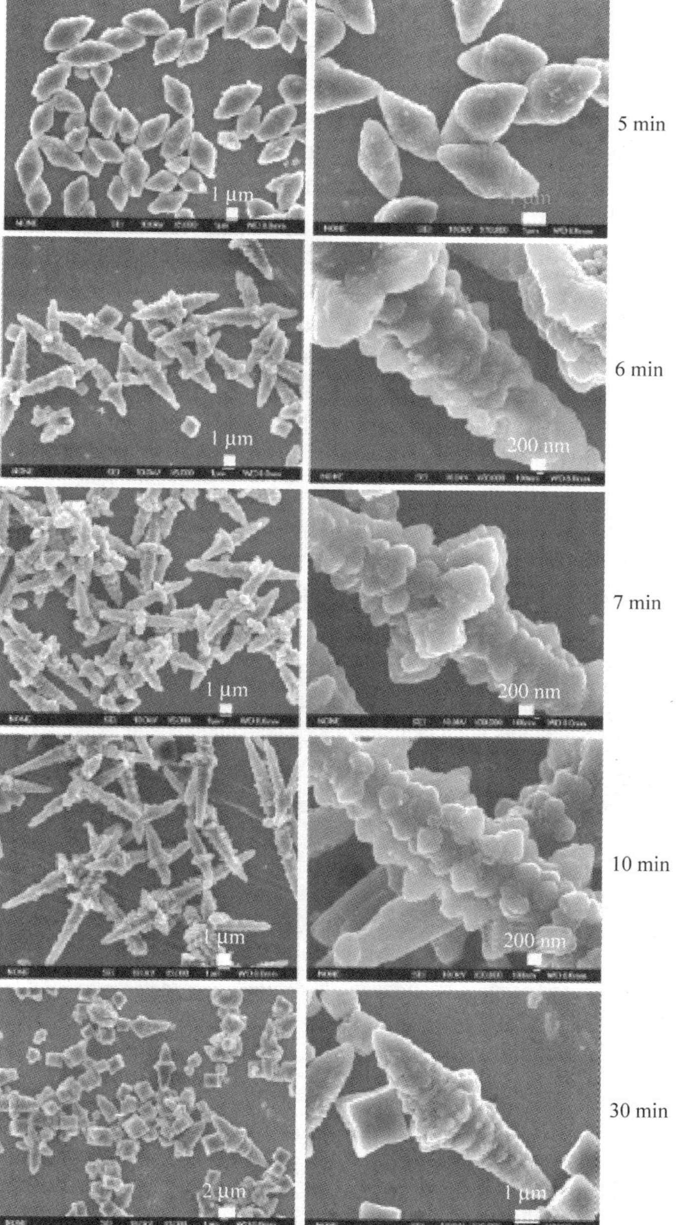

Figure 7.7 SEM micrographs of samples 2 – 6. Samples 2, 3, 4, 5, and 6 correspond to the microwave heating time of 5, 6, 7, 10, and 30 min, respectively. (Reprinted from (Qi and Zhu, 2006))

The microwave heating time played an important role in the morphology of vaterite. Figure 7.7 shows SEM micrographs of samples prepared in the water/EG/SDS system by microwave heating at 100℃ for different heating time. Bicone-like vaterite structures were obtained when the heating time was 5 min (sample 2). It is interesting that dagger-like vaterite structures could be obtained when the heating time was increased to 6 min (sample 3). Each daggerlike structure consisted of ellipsoid-like vaterite nanoparticles. Similar dagger-like vaterite structures formed for samples prepared for 7 min (sample 4), 8 min (sample 1), or 10 min (sample 5). In contrast, daggerlike vaterite structures were not observed by using an oil bath at 100℃ for 10 min instead of microwave heating. A large number of rhombohedral calcite crystals were formed, although some dagger-like vaterite structures were still present when the heating time was prolonged to 30 min, which was consistent with the main phase of calcite in the XRD pattern. This implies that phase transformation of vaterite to calcite occurs with increasing the heating time. These results indicate that the morphology and size of vaterite structures were sensitive to the microwave heating time.

When CTAB instead of SDS (sample 10) was used, the product consisted mainly of hexagonal vaterite and a small quantity of calcite. SEM (Fig. 7.8(a), (b) and TEM (Fig. 7.8(c), (d)) micrographs of sample 10 show monodisperse vaterite microspheres with an average size of 1 μm. One can see that each vaterite microsphere consists of self-assembled vaterite nanoparticles with diameters of

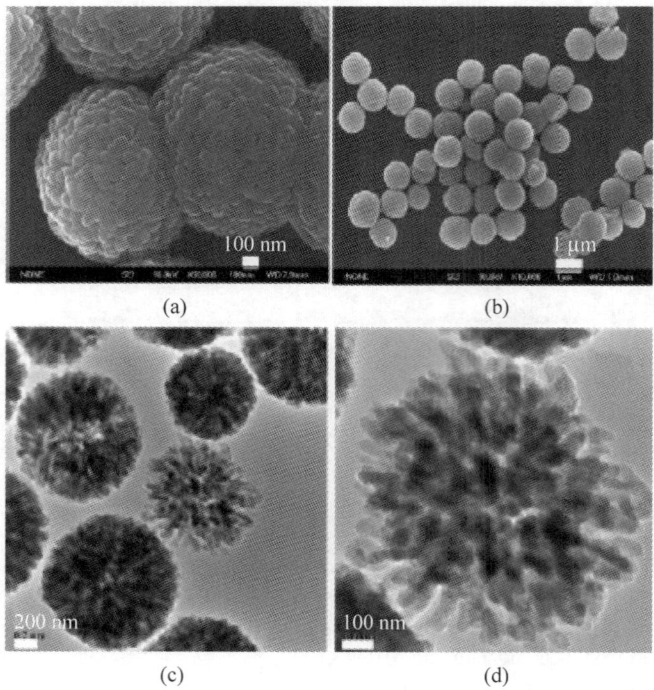

(a) (b) (c) (d)

Figure 7.8 (a), (b) SEM and (c), (d) TEM micrographs of sample 10 prepared by using CTAB by microwave heating in a mixed solvents of water and EG. (Reprinted from (Qi and Zhu, 2006))

about 50 nm. This implied a multistep growth mechanism where small nanoparticles were first formed, and then microspheres were formed by self-assembly of smaller nanoparticles.

7.5 Synthesis of Composite Biomaterials

Although HA is well recognized for its use as a bone substitute for filling bone defects and as a coating on orthopaedic and dental implants due to its biocompatibility, osteoconductiity, non-toxicity and structural similarity to natural bone, unfortunately, it cannot be used as heavy-loaded implant due to the lack of fracture toughness compared to the human bone. The non-bioresorbability of HA in body fluid (BF) is unfavorable to the host tissue surrounding the implant. β-TCP was used as a bioresorbable bone-replacing material. However, the rate of bioresorption of β-TCP is too rapid in an uncontrolled way. A material with ideal biodegradability will be replaced by newly formed bone as it degrades in the biological medium. In this regard, the use of composite biomaterials is a good choice for improvement of the mechanical and other biological properties of HA (Ji and Marquis, 1992). Biphasic calcium phosphate (BCP) biomaterials containing HA and TCP phases have recently attracted attention as an bone graft substitute due to their controlled resorption in the BF. They exhibit high fracture toughness and good biocompatibility and high bioactivity to the surrounding tissue upon implantation, which are more efficient than HA alone for biomedical applications. The bioactivity and biodegradation of BCP can be controlled by varying HA/TCP ratio because β-TCP is more soluble component and HA allows significant biological apatite precipitation. This unique composite biomaterial provides new bone formation as it releases calcium and phosphate ions into the BF upon implantation (Daculsi, 1998). As the BCP is prepared conventionally by mixing the HA and TCP phases at required ratio, the one-step in situ method under microwave heating provides homogeneous phase and hence provides better conditions for new bone formation compared to conventional methods.

Jalota et al. (2006) synthesized biphasic HA-TCP whiskers using $Ca(NO_3)_2 \cdot 4H_2O$, KH_2PO_4, $NaNO_3$ and HNO_3 (with or without urea) by a microwave-assisted molten salt mediated process. Manjubala et al. (Manjubala and Sivakumar, 2001) reported the in situ formation of BCP consisting of a mixture of HA and β-TCP at various ratios using $Ca(OH)_2$ and $(NH_4)_2HPO_4$ by microwave irradiation. The content of β-TCP phase increased as the Ca/P ratio decreased from 1.67 to 1.52. The in vitro solubility study of BCP powders in phosphate buffer (pH = 7.2) showed the resorbable nature of BCP. This study demonstrates the feasibility of in situ formation of BCP using a microwave heating method. BCP samples which contain TCP phase showed continuous dissolution, leading to a decrease in the pH value. The variation in the pH depended on the amount of TCP present in the samples.

Recent studies by Ferranis et al. (2000) and Piconi and Maccauro (1999) proved the suitability of zirconia as a good implant material for hard tissue repair due to its higher bending strength and fracture toughness. Murugan et al. (Murugan and Ramakrishna, 2003) reported the preparation of zirconia-reinforced HA by a microwave-assisted method. HA was prepared using an aqueous solution of goniopora, $CaHPO_4$ under microwave irradiation. The zirconia-reinforced HA was prepared by adding 5 mol% or 10 mol% of zirconia, while retaining the stoichiometric HA under microwave irradiation. The precipitate without zirconia showed a single phase of HA. The XRD patterns of zirconia- reinforced HA samples showed a mixture of HA and β-TCP. To improve the crystallinity, the zirconia-reinforced HA samples were calcined at 900℃ for 2 h. The heat treatment substantially improved the crystallinity. The occurrence of β-TCP may be due to the partial decomposition of HA in the presence of zirconia. The rate of decomposition of HA could be controlled by the amount of zirconia in the reaction medium. In general, the decomposition of HA occurs at 1150℃ (Wu and Yeh, 1988) according to

$$Ca_{10}(PO_4)_6(OH)_2 = 3\beta\text{-}Ca_3(PO_4)_2 + CaO + H_2O \tag{7.5}$$

However, the decomposition of HA depends on the reaction temperature. If the reaction occurs at 1150℃, HA decomposes into the β-TCP phase, whereas α-TCP forms at above 1200℃. The reinforcement of zirconia changed the actual decomposition temperature of HA, resulting in the formation of bi-phasic HA and β-TCP. The addition of zirconia improved the resorbable property of HA by producing a β-TCP phase. The prepared BCP ceramics had a better bioresobability than HA, and it is anticipated that it may have an excellent mechanical strength due to zirconia reinforcement. The in vitro physiological stability of prepared samples was performed in phosphate-buffered saline (pH = 7.4) at 37℃ in a thermostatic water bath, and the results indicated that the resorbable nature of BCP was in between the resorption levels of HA and β-TCP.

Sampath Kumar et al. (2000) synthesized carbonated HA by the substitution of $CaCO_3$ (10 mol%, 20 mol%, 30 mol%, and 40 mol%) for $Ca(OH)_2$ while maintaining the stoichiometry of HA during the reaction with $(NH_4)_2HPO_4$ under microwave irradiation. The magnesium-substituted carbonated apatite was also prepared using $MgCO_3$ (5 mol% and 10 mol%) instead of calcium carbonate in the above process. The XRD analysis indicated the decrease of *a*-axis up to 20 mol% of carbonate substitution confirming the formation of the B-type carbonated HA. Further increase of carbonate content showed the presence of TCP in addition to carbonated HA. Reaction of substituted magnesium carbonate instead of calcium carbonate in the above process resulted in the formation of BCP consisting of both carbonated HA and TCP phases. The in vitro solubility study in phosphate buffer (pH = 7.2) at 37℃ showed the resorbable nature of the BCP samples. This study indicates the feasibility of in situ formation of BCP ceramics using microwave irradiation.

$CaCO_3$/Ca-P biphasic materials prepared by microwave processing of natural aragonite and calcite was also reported (Pena et al., 2000). Particles of coral (natural aragonite) and a porous limestone (natural calcite) were suspended in phosphate solutions of different pH and concentrations and heated for different time (up to 5 h) using a domestic microwave oven. Parallel experiments were carried out using hydrolysis method. Higher extent of transformation was observed with microwave processing. Partial transformation of aragonite (coral) or calcite (limestone) to acidic calcium (monetite) or basic (carbonated hydroxyapatite) calcium phosphates was achieved by adjusting the pH and reaction time.

Mandubalal et al. (2005) reported the bone in-growth induced by biphasic calcium phosphate ceramic in the experimentally created circular defects in the femur of dogs. This BCP ceramic consisted of 55% HA and 45% β-TCP prepared in situ by the microwave method. The defective sites were radiographed at a period of 4, 8, and 12 weeks postoperatively. The radiographical results showed that the process of ossification started after 4 weeks and the defect was completely filled with new woven bone after 12 weeks. Histological examination of the tissue showed the formation of osteoblast inducing the osteogenesis in the defect. The collageneous fibrous matrix and the complete Haversian system were observed after 12 weeks. The blood serum was collected postoperatively and biochemical assays for alkaline phosphatase activity were carried out. The measurement of alkaline phosphatase activity levels also correlated with the formation of osteoblast-like cells. This BCP ceramic prepared by microwave method is a good biocompatible implant as well as osteoconductive and osteoinductive materials to fill bone defects.

7.6 Synthesis of Functionally Graded Bioactive Materials

Biomaterials must simultaneously satisfy a number of requirements and posses properties such as biocompatibility, bioactivity, strength, corrosion resistance and sometimes aesthetics. A single composition material with a uniform structure cannot satisfy all these requirements. A functionally graded material (FGM) is characterized by a gradual change of properties with position. The property gradient in the FGM is realized by a position-dependent chemical composition and microstructure. Recently, the potential importance and applications of FGM have attracted the biomedical community (Watari et al., 1997; Iwasaki 1997).

BCP is based on an optimum balance of HA and TCP phases. The functional gradient of BCP with the surface covered with TCP and the composition gradually changing to HA with increasing depth from the surface may provide better conditions for the bone formation. The TCP surface of the FGM will face BF and will dissolve to supply calcium and phosphate ions for new bone growth. Katakam et al. (2003) reported microwave processing of FGM by gradually changing the composition of calcium phosphates from the surface to the interior.

Silver oxide (5 mol% and 10 mol%) was spread on the surface of compact HA powder and exposed to microwave irradiation in a domestic microwave oven for 3 h. The sintered samples consisted of a mixture of β-TCP, metallic silver (Ag) and HA. The content of TCP and Ag gradually decreased with increasing depth from the surface. They also investigated the influence of microwave processing and conventional heat treatment at 900℃ for 12 h with 5% Ag_2O. For comparison, a pellet with 5% Ag_2O was heated in a furnace at 900℃ for 12 h in air. The experiments showed that more amounts of TCP and Ag were formed on the surface by the microwave heating compared with those by a conventional heating, suggesting the possibility of better compositional control in FGM fabrication by microwave processing. The microwave heating was rapid and throughout the volume, the silver oxide in the top region converted nearly all HA to TCP in that region. These results suggest that microwave processing is advantageous to prepare the FGM structures with desired gradient.

7.7 Microwave Sintering of Biomaterials

The production of porous BCP ceramics is generally based on a conventional heat sintering process with a relatively long sintering time at a high temperature, during which the bioactivity of the final products is reduced. Microwave heating is a faster sintering process compared with the conventional heating. Energy can be deposited volumetrically throughout the material during the microwave heating rather than thermal conduction in a conventional heating. Due to these advantages, microwave sintering shows a promising potential in ceramics processing. Readers are referred to a review article by Sutton for early work done on microwave sintering (Sutton, 1989).

For microwave sintering of calcium phosphate bioceramics, the investigation was focused on the fabrication of porous or dense HA or biphasic ceramics (Fang et al., 1992, 1994; Yang et al., 2002; Sun et al., 2003, Goren et al., 2004). Porous HA ceramics with porosity up to 73% were obtained by microwave sintering at 1150 – 1200℃ for 1 to 5 min (Fang et al., 1992). Two kinds of HA precursor powders, whiskers of HA (200 nm in diameter) synthesized by the hydrolysis of α-TCP at 60℃ (pH = 7.5 – 8.5) and aggregates of fine HA crystals with typical size of 50 – 300 nm prepared by the hydrolysis of brushite ($CaHPO_4 \cdot 2H_2O$) followed by ripening treatment with $CaCl_2 \cdot 2H_2O$, were used. For the sample with 50% porosity, 82% – 100% of the pores were connected. The porosity and pore size of the ceramics could be controlled by adjusting the starting material, green density, sintering time and temperature. The microstructure of the microwave sintered porous ceramics was homogeneous and the tensile strengths were reasonably good (up to about 45 MPa). Vijayan and Varma (2002) reported that nanocrystalline HA powder with crystallite size of 35 nm was sintered to high densities (above 95%) by short-time microwave processing for 5 min. The sintered sample had grain sizes of 200 – 300 nm and microhardness of 5.25 GPa.

Microwave sintering of both porous HA and porous HA/β-TCP ceramics (BCP) in a dual frequency microwave sintering furnace was reported (Wang et al., 2005, 2006). Through the optimization of sintering conditions, such as the sintering temperature, the heating rate and the holding time, porous bioceramics with average crystal size of 300 nm, porosity of 65%, and compressive strength of 6.40 MPa were obtained. Microwave sintered samples had a much smaller and more uniform grain size compare with the conventional sintering. The variation of the grain size was from 200 – 400 nm by microwave radiation with only 5 min holding time at 1100℃, however the variation of the grain size ranged from 1.0 to 1.5 μm by conventional sintering with 2 h holding time at the same temperature. The results showed that the microwave sintering could obtain a sintered ceramic more rapidly at lower sintering temperature for much shorter sintering time compared with the conventional sintering, leading to smaller grain size and more uniform microstructure and higher compressive strength than those obtained by conventional sintering. The smaller grain size and higher compressive strength of the samples sintered by microwave heating were probably due to lower sintering temperature and shorter sintering time. Another reason for the higher mechanical strength of the sample by microwave sintering was the uniform microstructure where large pores and defects as cracking origin were reduced. Therefore, the microwave processing is a promising method for sintering porous bioceramics.

Fang et al. (1995) reported the fabrication of transparent HA ceramics by microwave sintering at ambient pressure. The starting material used was crystalline HA powder synthesized by hydrothermally treating an aqueous solution of $Ca(NO_3)_2$ and $(NH_4)_2HPO_4$ (pH = 10.2) at 200℃, 1.5 MPa for 24 h. The as-synthesized HA powder was composed of crystalline nanometer-size hexagonal prisms. The microwave sintering was carried out at 1150℃ for 5 min in a 500 W domestic microwave oven. The microwave-sintered HA was a single phase of HA and the average grain size was around 200 nm.

Ji et al. (2005) reported microwave plasma sintering and in vitro study of porous HA/β-TCP biphasic bioceramics. The microwave plasma-sintered samples exhibited a higher densification rate, smaller grain size and higher compressive strength compared with those of conventional sintered samples. The Ca^{2+} concentration and the dissolution rate were also higher than those of conventional sintered samples in physiological saline. After immersed in SBF and simulated inflammation BF, the amount of bone-like apatite formed on microwave plasma-sintered samples was more than that formed on conventionally sintered samples. The experiments indicated that microwave plasma sintered porous BCP bioceramics had better mechanical and biological properties. On the other hand, the surface of samples that underwent a simulated inflammation procedure was smoother and the amount of bone-like apatite formed on them was less than that formed on the samples immersed in normal SBF all the time, indicating that the acid in an inflammation response would affect the bone reconstruction when Ca-P biocerarnics implanted in living body.

References

Adams D, R.D. Smith, G.F. Malgas, S.P. Massia, T.L. Alford and J.W. Mayer. *Bioceramics 17 Key Eng. Mater.* **284 – 286**: 569 (2005).

Cao, J.M., J. Feng, S.G. Deng, X. Chang, J. Wang, J.S. Liu, P. Lu, H.X. Lu, M.B. Zheng and G. Daculsi. *Biomaterials* **19**: 1473 (1998).

Da Silva, M.H.P., J.H.C. Lima, G.A. Soares, C.N. Elias, M.C. de Andrade, S.M. Best and I.R. Gibson. *Surf. Coat. Technol.* **137**: 270 (2001).

Fang, Y., D.K. Agrawal, D.M. Roy and R. Roy. *J. Mater. Res.* **7**: 490 (1992).

Fang, Y., D.K. Agrawal, D.M. Roy and R. Roy. *J. Mater. Res.* **9**: 180 (1994).

Fang, Y., D.K. Agrawal, D.M. Roy and R. Roy. *Mater. Lett.* **23**: 147 (1995).

Feng J., J.M. Cao and S.G. Deng. *Chin. J. Inorg. Chem.* **21**: 801 (2005).

Ferraris, M., E. Verné, P. Appendino, C. Moisescu, A. Krajewski, A. Ravaglioli and A. Piancastelli. *Biomaterials* **21**: 765 (2000).

Gedye, R., F. Smith, K. Westaway, A. Humera, L. Baldisera, L. Laberge and L. Rousell. *Tetrahedron Lett.* **27**: 279 (1986).

Goren S., H. Gokbayrak and S. Altintas. *Euro ceram. Key Eng. Mater.* **264 – 268**: 1949 (2004).

Giguere, R., T.L. Bray, S.M. Duncan and G. Majetich. *Tetrahedron Lett.* **27**: 4945 (1986).

Gómez-Morales, J., J. Torrent-Burgués, T. Boix, J. Fraile and R. Rodríguez-Clemente. *Cryst. Res. Technol.* **36**: 15 (2001).

Ji, H. and P.M. Marquis. *Biomaterials* **13**: 744 (1992).

Katakam, S., D. Siva Rama Krishna and T.S. Sampath Kumar. *Mater. Lett.* **57**: 2716 (2003).

Kingston, H.M. and S.J. Haswell. *Microwave-Enhanced Chemistry: Fundamentals, Sample Preparation, Applications*. Washington DC: American Chemical Society (1997).

Siddharthan, A., S.K. Seshadri and T.S. Sampath Kumar. *Scripta Materialia* **55**: 175 (2006).

Hench, L.L. *J. Am. Ceram. Soc.* **74**: 1487 (1991).

Iwasaki, K. *Mater. Res. Innov.* **1**: 180 (1997).

Jalota, S., S.B. Bhaduri and A.C. Tas. *J. Biomed. Mater. Res.* A **78A**: 481 (2006).

Jalota, S., A.C. Tas and S.B. Bhaduri. *J. Mater. Res.* **19**: 1876 (2004).

Ji, J.G., J.G. Ran, L. Gou, F.H. Wang and L.W. Sun. High-performance ceram. *Key Eng. Mater.* **280 – 283**: 1519 (2005).

Katsuki, H. and S. Furuta. *J. Am. Ceram. Soc.* **82**: 2257 (1999).

Kundu, P.K., T.S. Waghode, D. Bahadur and D. Datta. *Med. Biolog. Eng. Comput.* **36**: 654 (1998).

Lerner E., S. Sarig and R. Azoury. *J. Mater. Sci.-Mater. Med.* **2**: 138 (1991).

Liu, J. B., K.W. Li, H. Wang, M.K. Zhu and H. Yan. *Chem. Phys. Lett.* **396**: 429 (2004).

López-Macipe, A., J. Gómez-Morales and R. Rodríguez-Clemente. *Adv. Mater.* **10**: 49 (1998).

Ma, M.G., Y.J. Zhu and J. Chang. *J. Phys. Chem. B* **110**: 14,226 (2006).

Mahabole M.P., R.C. Aiyer, C.V. Ramakrishna, B. Sreedhar and R.S. Khairnar. *Bull. Mater. Sci.* **28**: 535 (2005).

Mandubalal I., T.P. Sastry and R.V.S. Kumar. *J. Biomater. Appl.* **19**: 341 (2005).

Manjubala, I. and M. Sivakumar. *Mater. Chem.Phys.* **71**: 272 (2001).

Meejoo, S., W. Maneeprakorn and P. Winotai. *Thermochimica Acta* **447**: 115 (2006).

Murugan, R., K.P.Rao and T.S.S. Kumar. *Bioceram. Key Eng. Mater.* **240 – 242**: 51 (2003).

Murugan, R. and S. Ramakrishna. *Mater. Lett.* **58**: 230 (2003).

Parhia, P., A. Ramananb and A.R. Raya. *Mater. Lett.* **58**: 3610 (2004).

Pena, J., R.Z. LeGeros, R. Rohanizadeh and J.P. LeGeros. *Bioceram. Key Eng. Mater.* **192 – 1**: 267 (2000).

Perreux, L. and A. Loupy. *Tetrahedron* **57**: 9199 (2001).

Piconi, C. and G. Maccauro. *Biomaterials* **20**: 1 (1999).

Qi, R.J. and Y.J. Zhu. *J. Phys. Chem. B* **110**: 8302 (2006).

Rameshbabu, N., K. Prasad Rao and T.S. Sampath Kumar. *J. Mater. Sci.* **40**: 6319 (2005).

Rodríguez-Clemente, R. and J. Gómez-Morales. *J. Cryst. Growth* **169**: 339 (1996).

Sampath Kumar, T.S., I. Manjubala and J. Gunasekaran. *Biomaterials* **21**: 1623 (2000).

Sarig, S. and F. Kahana. J. Cryst. Growth **237 – 239**: 55 (2002).

Siddharthan, A., S.K. Seshadri and T.S. Sampath Kumar. *J. Mater. Sci.: Mater. Med.* **15:** 1279 (2004).

Sun, L.W., J.G. Ran, L. Gou, F.H. Wang and J.G. Ji, K.J. Xie. *Rare Metal Mater. Eng.* **32** (Suppl. 1): 106 (2003).

Sutton, W.H. *Am. Ceram. Soc. Bull.* **68**: 376 (1989).

Torrent-Burgués, J., J. Gómez-Morales, A. López-Macipe and R. Rodríguez-Clemente. *Cryst. Res. Technol.* **34**: 757 (1999).

Tsuji, M., M. Hashimoto, Y. Nishizawa, M. Kubokawa and Takeshi Tsuji. *Chem. Eur. J.* **11**: 440 (2005).

Varma, R.S. *Green Chem.* **3**: 98 (2001).

Vaidhyanathan, B. and K.J. Rao. *Bull. Mater. Sci.***19**: 1163 (1996).

Vijayan, S.and H. Varma. *Mater. Lett.* **56**: 827 (2002).

Wang, X.L., Z. Wang, H.S. Fan, Y.M. Xiao and X.D. Zhang. *Adv. Biomater. VI Key Eng. Mater.* **288 – 289**: 529 (2005).

Wang, X.L., H.S. Fan, Y.M. Xiao and X.D. Zhang. *Mater. Lett.* **60**: 455 (2006).

Watari, F., A. Yokoyama, F. Saso, M. Uo and T. Kawasaki. *Composites B* **28B**: 5 (1997).

Webster, T.J., C. Ergun, R.H. Doremus, R.W. Siegel and R. Bizios. *Biomaterials* **22**: 1327 (2001).

Wei, H., Q. Shen, Y. Zhao, Y. Zhou, D.J. Wang and J.F. Xu. *J. Cryst. Growth* **279**: 439 (2005).

Wu, J.M. and T.S. Yeh. *J. Mater. Sci.* **23**: 3771 (1988).

Yang, Z.W., Y.S. Jiang, Y.J. Wang, L.Y. Ma and F.F. Li. *Mater. Lett.* **58**: 3586 (2004).

Yang, Y.Z., J.L. Ong and J. M. Tian. *J. Mater. Sci. Lett.* **21**: 67 (2002).

Yoon, S.Y., Y.M. Park, S.S. Park, R. Stevens and H.C. Park. *Mater. Chem. Phys.* **91**: 48 (2005).

Zhang, F. and J. Tao. *J. Mater. Sci.* **40**: 6311 (2005).

Zhu Y.J., W.W. Wang, R.J. Qi and X.L. Hu. *Angew. Chem. Int. Ed.* **43**: 1410 (2004).

8 Characterizing Biointerfaces and Biosurfaces in Biomaterials Design

Kalpana S. Katti, Devendra Verma and Dinesh R. Katti

Department of Civil Engineering, North Dakota State University, Fargo ND 58105, USA

Abstract Often in composite biomaterials, molecular interactions at various interfaces are known to have significant role on mechanical response of the composite system as well as biocompatibility of the biomaterials. The biomaterial surface elicits a response from tissue that is specific to the nature of the surface and several surface modification techniques are used to analyze the response. Currently, many physical and spectroscopic methods are available to characterize the nature of the biomaterial surface. This Chapter introduces various characterization techniques for characterizing biointerfaces and biosurfaces in biomaterials Design. The important characterization tools used by biomaterials researchers are outlined in the chapter and the fundamental principles governing these tools are elaborated.

8.1 Introduction

Biomaterial is a material that is defined as 'a nonviable material used in a medical device, intended to interact with biological systems' (Williams, 1987). In another definition by Black, a biomaterial is defined as 'materials of natural or manmade origin that are used to direct, supplement, or replace the functions of living tissues' (Black, 1992). For biomaterials to function appropriately, it is paramount that these materials maintain integrity, do not exhibit toxicity, and lead to appropriate signal transduction. In addition, for the case of biomaterials used for tissue engineering, they must exhibit controlled degradation. Many of these properties are influenced by the response of tissue to the biomaterial surface. Thus surface characterization remains an important step for biomaterials design. The characterization of the surface involves characterizing its:

(1) Microstructure,
(2) Roughness,
(3) Wettability,
(4) Molecular structure, bonding,
(5) Chemical composition.

(1) Corresponding e-mail: Kalpana.Katti@ndsu.edu

Table 8.1 Surface characterization techniques in biomaterials surface analysis

Technique	Primary detection principle	Information obtained	Spatial resolution	Analysis depth	Destructive/ nondestructive
Contact angle measurement	Liquid is allowed to wet the biomaterial surface and the angle of wetting-contact angle is precisely measured	Surface energies of surfaces	~1 mm	~10 Å	Nondestructive
X-ray photoelectron spectroscopy (XPS)	X-rays are bombarded on biomaterial surface and electrons of characteristic energy are emitted from the biomaterial surface. Energy of the emitted electrons are measured	Binding energy of core electrons from atoms of biomaterial. The nature and the environment of the atoms in biomaterial surface are measured	10 – 150 μm	10 – 250 Å	Somewhat destructive on long exposure to X-rays
Fourier transform infrared spectroscopy (FTIR)-ATR, PAS	Infrared light impinges on the sample and causes vibrations of bonds in the biomaterial. Reflected infrared light or generated photoacoustic waves are detected	Nature of bonding in molecules of the biomaterial	~1 μm for micro-spectroscopic reflection investigation. And 1 μm for photoacoustic investigation	~ 1 μm for ATR and ~30 μm for PAS	Nondestructive
ToF secondary ion mass spectroscopy (SIMS)	Biomaterial surface is bombarded with a beam of accelerated ions. As a result, ions from the surface of the biomaterial sputter from the surface and mass to charge ratio of the emitted ions is measured using a time-of-flight analyzer	Exact elemental nature of the surface of biomaterial surface is ascertained	100 Å	10 Å – 1 μm	Destructive

Continued

Technique	Primary detection principle	Information obtained	Spatial resolution	Analysis depth	Destructive/ nondestructive
Atomic force microscopy (AFM)	Deflection of a tip terminating in a single atom in close proximity of the biomaterial surface due to weak non bonded interactions (van der Waals, electrostatic) between tip atoms and biomaterial surface atoms. The extent of this deflection is accurately measured using a laser bouncing off from the top of the cantilever arm that has the tip attached	Surface topography and structure are detected	1 Å	1 Å – 100 s of μm	Nondestructive
Auger electron spectroscopy (AES)	The Auger process is initiated by creation of a hole in the core level with an impinging focused electron beam on the biomaterial surface. The resulting ionized atom is in a highly excited state and rapidly relaxes to original state by X-ray fluorescence or Auger emission. The kinetic energy of the emitted electrons is measured	Oxidation states and nature of atoms on biomaterial surface are detected	50 – 100 Å	100 Å	Destructive
Scanning electron microscopy (SEM)	High energy focused electron beam impinges on sample and secondary electrons are emitted from the surface	The biomaterial surface is imaged at high spatial resolution.	~5 Å	~10 Å	Destructive

Many physical and spectroscopic methods are available to characterize the nature of the biomaterial surface. The biomaterial surface elicits a response from tissue that is specific to the nature of the surface and several surface modification techniques are available to analyze the response. A summary of these techniques and their primary principles of detection is shown in Table 8.1. The reader should refer to one of the several comprehensive texts in surface science that are available (Vickerman, 1997; Feldman and Mayer, 1986; Briggs and Seah, 1996; Vanselow and Howe, 1982; Watts and Wolstenholme, 2003). An exhaustive overview of these techniques is also covered in the text by Ratner et al. (2004). The following is detailed description of the more commonly used surface characterization techniques used for biomaterials design.

8.2 Characterization of Biointerfaces

8.2.1 Surface and Interface Analysis Using Fourier Transform Infrared Spectroscopy

Vibrational spectroscopy is a useful tool to experimentally characterize the bonding of proteins to biomaterial surfaces. Fourier transform infrared spectroscopy is a widely used technique for analysis of surfaces and interfaces (Urban, 1993; Hirschmugl, 2002; Mueller, 2001; Nakamoto, 1997; Koenig, 1997). Recent advancements in interferometer design and control electronics have led to significant improvement in data quality and analysis techniques. The (FTIR) spectrum can be acquired using various methods of measurement such as transmission, reflection, attenuated total reflection (ATR) and photoacoustic modes. Usually, transmission methods provide spectra with the best signal-to-noise ratio (SNR) but require samples with a relatively short path length through their thickness. Reflection methods require the surface to be measured to be well polished. Reflection absorption infrared (RAIR) spectroscopy has been used to analyze molecular orientations of organic monolayer on metallic substrates. The ATR method does not require polishing of the sample and it is well-suited for samples that are not easy to polish. In the ATR method, however, a good contact between the ATR crystal and the surface of the sample must be achieved.

ATR is the most commonly used and preferred technique for study of biomaterials surfaces and interfaces (Chittur, 1998; Ratner et al., 2004). Figure 8.1 shows schematic of the ATR setup. Here, IR radiation is focused onto the end of the ATR crystal. Light enters the ATR crystal and due to total internal reflection, light is reflected back at the ATR crystal-sample interface. However, at each internal reflection, the IR radiation actually penetrates a short distance (~1 μm) from the surface of the crystal into the polymer membrane, also known as the evanescent wave. The interaction of evanescent wave with the sample surface enables one to obtain infrared spectra of samples placed in contact with the ATR crystal.

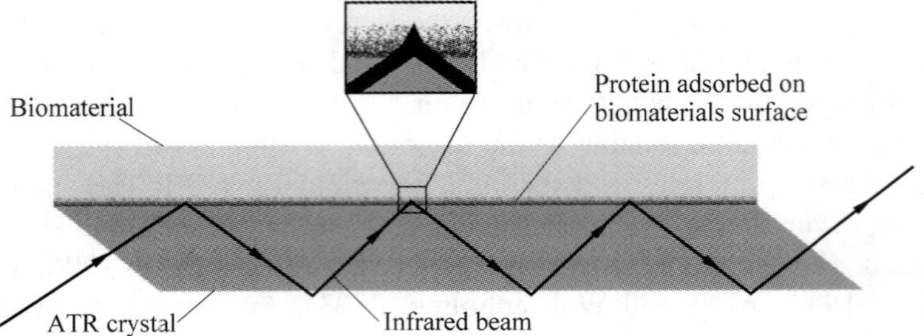

Figure 8.1 Schematic for use of ATR for study of adsorbed protein of biomaterials surface

Although vibrational spectroscopy has been extensively used in biology and medicine, here specifically the role of protein adsorbtion, on surfaces is described in detail. The adsorption of proteins at the surfaces of biomaterials is the first initial response of the tissue to biomaterial. Protein adsorption precedes cellular interactions with biomaterials. The adsorbed proteins mediate interactions between biomaterial and surrounding cells and tissues. The adsorption of proteins may be specific or non-specific and that depends upon surface characteristics of biomaterials (Recum, 1999). The non-specific adsorption of proteins may lead to failure of the implant. For this reason, several studies have focused on adsorption of proteins on biomaterials surfaces (Andrade, 1973; Blomberg et al., 1998; Ishihara et al., 2003; Ratner and Brant, 2004). Roach et al. have studied effect of topography and surface chemistry on adsorption behavior of bovine serum albumin (BSA) and bovine fibrinogen (Fg) on silica sphere (Roach et al., 2006). The conformation and intermolecular interactions of BSA and Fg have been investigated using ATR-FTIR. The ATR study revealed that BSA exhibits a disordered structure on larger silica sphere (< 10 – 40 nm), whereas Fg exhibits a more disordered structure on smaller silica sphere (> 30 nm). The disorder is more pronounced on hydrophilic surfaces.

FTIR has also been used to determine the secondary structure of proteins over biomaterials surfaces (Frushour and Koenig, 1975; Jackson, 1991; Lenk et al., 1991). For conformation analysis of proteins, amide Ⅰ regions (~1640 cm^{-1}) bands are used. The frequency of vibrations of C=O bonds in the amide region depends on the strength of hydrogen bonds formed. The stronger the hydrogen bond, the lower the frequency in the amide Ⅰ absorption. Intermolecular β-sheets form the strongest hydrogen bonds and show band in the interval 1620 – 1640 cm^{-1}. Antiparallel β-sheets and parallel β-sheets show band around 1620 cm^{-1} and 1640 cm^{-1}, respectively. Unordered structures (hydrogen bonded water or side groups) appear around 1640 – 1650 cm^{-1}. α-Helices with weak hydrogen bonds absorb at 1652 – 1660 cm^{-1}. Hole et al. have analyzed grafting and conformation changes of polypeptide on a graft using diffusion spectroscopy (Hole et al., 2005). The changes in conformation of polypeptide were determined from deconvolution of bands in the regions of amide Ⅰ. The attachment was shown to cause a decrease in β-sheets and increase in disordered structure of the polypeptide. Recently, studies on adsorption of Fg on polystyrene have shown that there is almost no difference in conformation of adsorbed Fg and Fg present in solution (Wang et al., 2006).

It has been realized that surface properties are the key parameter, which dictate implant's fate in body environment (Ratner et al., 2004). In order to tailor the surface behavior of the implants and grafts, usually surfaces are modified by adsorbing or surface grafting the necessary chemical species. ATR-FTIR has been proved to be a valuable tool in studying surface modification of biomaterials (Kannan et al., 2006; Mansur et al., 2002).

Polyethylene, polyurethane and Teflon are the three most commonly used polymers for biliary stent. It is postulated that failure of stents starts with adsorption of proteins and bacteria which further cause occlusion of stent by buildup of biofilm and other materials (Tsang et al., 1997; Speer et al., 1988). To decrease the rate of occlusion in polyethylene stents, Peng et al. used sulfonation of the surface of stent by exposing them to fuming sulfuric acid (Peng et al., 2004). The sulfonation of surface was confirmed by ATR-FTIR. Klee et al. have modified poly(vinylidenefluoride) (PVDF) with fibronectin using different method (Klee et al., 2003). The attachment of fibronectin was investigated by ATR-FTIR.

Although ATR remains one of the most commonly used vibrational spectroscopic techniques its use is limited to surface analysis of biomaterials. For biomaterials design, the interfacial behavior in the composite biomaterials bulk is also important. Phatoacoustic FTIR spectroscopy (PAS-FTIR) is a useful technique to study molecular interfacial behavior in composites (Urban, 1993; Rosencwaig and Gersho, 1975). PAS-FTIR has been used to study interfacial interactions in polycaprolactone-polyacrylic acid-hydroxyapatite composites (Verma et al., 2006a). The mechanism of nucleation and growth of apatite on these composites has also been investigated using reflectance microspectroscopy (Verma et al., 2006b). Kazarian et al. applied FTIR imaging using ATR acquisition mode to materials of interest in tissue engineering (Kazarian et al., 2004). They demonstrate the distribution of the growing hydroxyapatite (HA) layers on the surface of porous PDLLA/Bioglasss composites, which occurs upon immersion of the materials in simulated body fluid (BF).

8.2.2 Surface and Interface Analysis Using Atomic Force Microscopy

Atomic force microscopy (AFM) is a high resolution microscopy technique that provides unique opportunity to investigate biointerfaces and interfaces in terms of structure, composition and molecular interactions in natural environment (Morra and Cassinelli 2006; Chrstopher et al., 1998). A schematic of AFM is shown in Fig. 8.2. In this technique, the deflection of a tip terminating in a single atom in close proximity of the biomaterial surface due to weak non bonded interactions (van der Waals, electrostatic) between tip atoms and biomaterial surface atoms is measured. The extent of this deflection is accurately measured using a laser bouncing off from the top of the cantilever arm that has the tip attached. AFM has several operating modes and they differ from each other in the manner in which the tip moves over the surface. In the contact mode, the AFM tip rasters over the sample, while the applied force to the tip is kept constant using a feedback control. In the tapping mode, the AFM tip oscillates at a frequency close to its resonance and the tip is allowed to make contact with the sample only for a short duration in each oscillation cycle. Because lateral forces during imaging are greatly reduced, this mode may be advantageous for imaging soft biological samples. Further information on the different imaging modes can be found in literature (Jena and Hörber, 1999; Morris et al., 1999). Several examples illustrating the extensive use of AFMs are described below.

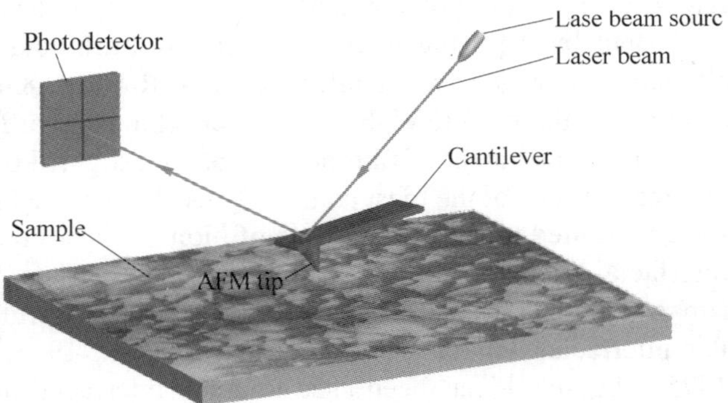

Figure 8.2 Schematic of AFM tip rastering over surface

8.2.2.1 Atomic Force Microscopy for Surface Imaging

Silk from the silkworm, Bombyx mori, has been used as biomedical suture material for centuries (Mori and Tsukada, 2000). The unique mechanical properties of the silk fibers and ability to genetically tailor the protein provide additional rationale for the silk as a biomaterial. Silk Ⅰ is a water soluble form, whereas Silk Ⅱ is water insoluble form. One approach is to transform Silk Ⅰ to Silk Ⅱ by treatment of Silk Ⅰ with methanol solution. Servoli et. al. have investigated the topography and phase distribution using phase imaging and lateral force imaging (Servoli et al., 2005). AFM phase images showed presence β-sheet crystals of Silk Ⅱ.

Morra et al. have surface modified the Titanium bone implant by first grafting acrylic them coupling collagen to it (Morra et al., 2003). The morphology of all the samples was characterized by AFM in contact mode in both wet and dry conditions. Significant differences in morphology were observed in case of acrylic acid grafted and collagen coupled samples in wet conditions.

It has been known that surface roughness has significant influence on the cellular response (Cacciafesta et al., 2001). Cacciafesta et al. have created surface features using a variety of methods. The effect of surface features on adsorption of human plasma Fg has been studied by AFM in phase imaging mode. A direct visualization of protein has been achieved. Polyurethane block co-polymers are some of the most important polymeric biomaterials. They are widely used in a variety of blood contacting applications, because of their excellent mechanical properties and hemo-compatibility. Agnihotri et al. have investigated surface morphology of poly(urethane urea) block co-polymer under wet and dry conditions using AFM in phase imaging mode (Agnihotri et al., 2006). AFM height images showed occurrence of 50 – 70 nm sized raised features under wet conditions. AFM phase images revealed that due to wetting redistributions of soft and hard phases occur at the surface and this distribution is retained even after dehydration.

8.2.2.2 Atomic Force Microscopy in Study of Cellular Adhesion

Adhesion of cells to substrate is preceded by other cellular activities such as proliferation, growth and differentiation. Cellular adhesion is an important step for the cell to perform its natural biological activities. Cell morphology is a direct indication of cellular adhesion. Well adhered cells have spreading morphology whereas spheroid morphology is an indication of non-adhering cells. Quantitative measurement of adhesive forces between cells and substrate can also be performed by applying external forces on the cells. The cells can be visualized by optical and electron microscopy. Optical microscopy is a simplest way to distinguish non-adhered cell morphology from well adhered cell morphology. Electron microscopy methods such as scanning electron microscopy require fixing of cells. AFM is an emerging tool for studying cellular adhesion. It allows observation of cells in their culture media without causing any irreversible changes caused by fixing.

Domke et al. have utilized AFM in contact mode to investigate adhesion of osteoblasts cells on metals, glass and polystyrene substrates (Domke et al., 2000). The cellular adhesion was determined qualitatively from cross section area and height information colleted from AFM data. Because, large cell deformation occurs even under very low load, the actual height of cells was determined from the force-curve plots. Elastic modulus was calculated following Hertz model.

Various cytoskeletal structures have different role in mechanical stiffness of the cell, where microtubules provides compressive strength, and actin fibers and intermediate filaments provide tensile strength. Takai et al. have shown that the elastic modulus of cytoskeleton depends upon the substrate to which cell is attached (Takai et al., 2005). It was observed from the AFM force plots of osteoblasts attached on fibronectin and vitronectin, which bind cells via integrins showed higher elastic modulus than cells attached on glass, where adhesion is non-integrin mediated.

Sagvolden et al. modified AFM to measure force required to laterally dislodge the cell from the surface (Sagvolden et al., 1999). This modified AFM consists of canted tip which was aligned with the cells using Inverted microscope. It was reported that the force required to detach the cell depends on substrate and varies between 100 – 200 nN. Doneva et al. used a novel technique to study cell-biomaterials interactions (Doneva et al., 2004). They immobilized single osteoblasts cell on AFM cantilever, which was used as a probe to measure interaction forces between cell and surface. Both short term (5 min and 10 min.) and long term (60 min and 120 min.) adhesion studies were performed. Results were compared with force required for detachment from glass substrate. It was observed that cellulose acetate samples showed significant increase in adhesion compared to poly(lactin-*co*-glycolic acid) samples.

8.2.2.3 Evaluating Molecular Mechanics Using AFM

The cellular response depends on ligand-receptor interactions at biointerfaces. For the development of biomaterials surfaces giving desirable cellular response, it is important to have a detailed understating of molecular interactions between biomaterial surfaces and cells. AFM is a valuable tool for exploration of these molecular interactions and due to the high sensitivity of the instrument, even single molecules can be investigated. For this purpose, AFM force spectroscopy is used. A schematic diagram of pulling of single molecules is shown in Fig. 8.3. In force spectroscopy, the sample is pushed towards the tip and then retracted. The cantilever deflection is recorded as a function of the vertical displacement of the piezoelectric scanner, which can be transformed into a force-distance curve by converting the cantilever deflection into a force by multiplying deflection with cantilever spring constant. A schematic of protein pulling is shown in Fig. 8.4.

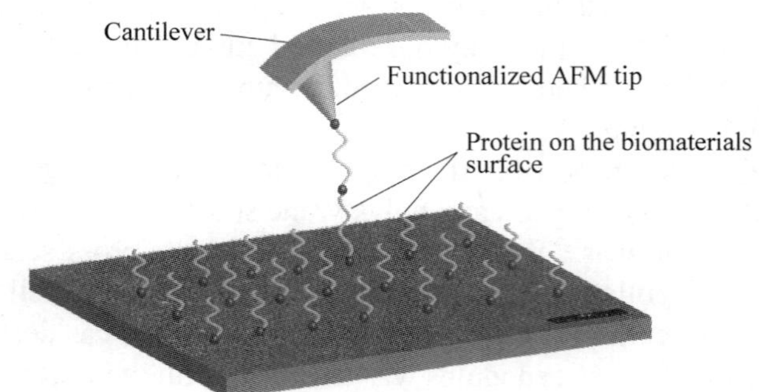

Figure 8.3 Schematic of protein pulling by functionalized AFM tip

The AFM tips can be functionalized for protein-specific adherence. Wang et al. functionalized the AFM tips with BSA and gold wafers with BSA, anti-BSA and dextran over $—CH_3$, —OH, —COOH and $—NH_2$ terminated monolayers (Wang et al., 2004). Highest pull-off force was registered between BSA and —OH terminated monolayers. Dextran being hydrophilic, did not adhere to BSA functionalized tip. Recently, AFM force spectroscopy was used to determine force of adhesion between Fg and two different dental implant materials (Titanium and hydroxyapatite coated Titanium) (Boukai et al., 2006). The average adhesion force was significantly higher for Titanium implant after interaction time of 1000 ms. The difference in adhesion forces between two implants is attributed to difference in mechanism of adsorption of Fg.

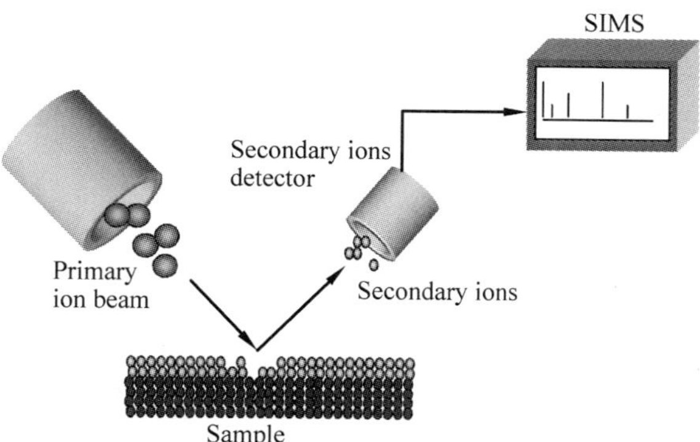

Figure 8.4 Schematic diagram of the operation of Time of flight secondary ion mass spectrometer (ToF-SIMS)

Cell-matrix adhesion is mediated by integrin, which in turn affect other cellular processes like growth, differentiation and adhesion. It is known that integrins bind to specific domains (Arg-Ghy-Asp (RGD) and PHSRN) of the extracellular matrix. Thus, several studies have focused on modifying biomaterials surfaces with RGD and PHSRN sequence to enhance cellular adhesion. Mardilovich and Kokkoli have investigated interaction between integrin and these peptides by functionalizing AFM tip with integrin and surface with novel peptide, PHSRN$(SG)_3$-SGRGDSP (Mardilovich and Kokkoli, 2004).

8.2.3 X-ray Photoelectron Spectroscopy

X-ray photoelectron spectroscopy (XPS) technique was developed by Siegbahn in the 1960s for which he received a Nobel prize in physics in 1981. The XPS technique is based on the photoelectric effect as described by Einstein in 1905. The photoelectric effect consists of photons impinging on surfaces of materials resulting in the ejection of electrons (Fig. 8.5). The total energy of the photon ($h\nu$) equals the sum of the work function (ϕ) of material impinged on and the maximum kinetic energy (KE_p) of the photons as given by:

$$h\nu = \phi + KE_p \tag{8.1}$$

For XPS, often the photon energies used are the Al K_α (1486.6 eV) or Mg K_α (1253.6 eV). The XPS technique is highly surface specific due to the short range of the photoelectrons that are excited from the solid. In this technique, the energy of the photoelectrons ejected from the sample is measured resulting in a spectrum consisting of several peaks. The specific energy of the peaks is characteristic of each element in the sample. The shape and position of the peaks can be altered by the surrounding state of the element and hence this technique gives information on chemical bonding. The XPS experiments need to be conducted under ultra high vacuum. This technique is often used for biomaterials (McArthur,

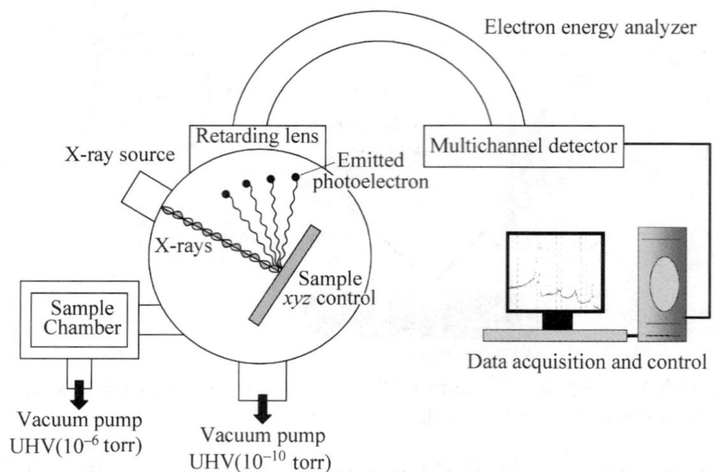

Figure 8.5 Schematic diagram of the operation of an X-ray photoelectron spectrometer

2006). Protein adsorption is the very first event that occurs on the surface of biomaterial in the biological environment. Often structure of the protein molecules is altered on adsorption to biomaterial. The structure of the adsorbed protein determines the nature of tissue-biomaterial interactions. XPS is often used to study the structure of adsorbed proteins. Recently, adsorption of fibronectin on Fe-Cr alloys was studied using XPS (Galtayries et al., 2006). Immobilization of proteins on biomaterials surface is a very promising method to improve the biocompatibility of the implant. Bonding of gelatin over Ti surface by covalently immobilized gelatin was confirmed by XPS (Dubruel et al., 2006). Also, coating of collagen on nanofiber mesh of poly(L-lactic acid)-*co*-poly(ε-caprolactone) (70:30) has been studied using XPS (Wei et al., 2005).

8.2.4 Contact Angle

Contact angle is defined as the geometric angle formed by liquid on solid substrate at the three phase interface of solid-liquid-vapor. A schematic of the contact angle is illustrated in Fig. 8.6. Contact angle gives the quantitative measurement of wetting of solid by liquid. A contact angle value lower than 90° indicates wetting of substrate whereas contact angle greater than 90° indicates non-wetting of substrate. For complete understanding of wetting of substrate, it's necessary to measure the contact angle over time. If there is drop in contact angle in a given time, that is called receded contact angle and if contact angle rises over given time then it's called advanced contact angle. Receding contact angle and advanced contact angles are called dynamic contact angles. The contact angle depends on interfacial energies between solid/liquid/gas and is defined as:

$$\gamma_{lv}\cos\theta = \gamma_{sv} + \gamma_{sl} \tag{8.2}$$

where γ_{lv} is interfacial energy at liquid/vapor interface, γ_{sv} is interfacial energy at solid/vapor interface, γ_{sl} is interfacial energy at solid liquid interface and θ is the contact angle.

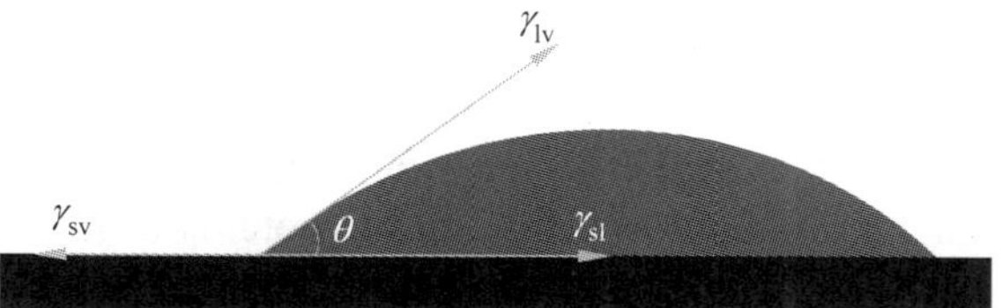

Figure 8.6 Schematic diagram for spreading of liquid on substrate and contact angle measurement

8.2.5 Time-of-Flight Secondary Ions Mass Spectrometry (ToF-SIMS)

Time-of-Flight Secondary Ion Mass Spectrometry (ToF-SIMS) uses a pulsed primary ion beam source (with short pulses ~1 nm) to desorb and ionize molecular species from the surface of a sample. Secondary ions are ejected from the sample and are accelerated into a mass spectrometer, where they are mass analyzed by measuring their time-of-flight from the sample surface to the detector (Belu et al., 2003) (Fig. 8.4). There are three types of methods used in ToF-SIMS. These methods are:

(1) Mass spectra are acquired to determine the molecular and elemental species on a surface.

(2) Images are acquired to ascertain the distribution of individual molecular species on the surface (Winograd, 2003).

(3) Depth profiles are used to determine the distribution of different chemical species as a function of depth from the surface of the sample.

The mass spectrum and the secondary ion images are used to determine the composition and distribution of the different constituents on the sample surface. ToF-SIMS provides characterization of chemical composition, and images showing distribution of chemical species, and depth profiling at small depths are obtained. The secondary ions are extracted into a ToF analyzer by applying a high voltage potential between the sample surface and the mass analyzer. The secondary ions travel through the ToF analyzer at different velocities, depending on their mass to charge ratio. For each primary ion pulse, a full mass spectrum is obtained by measuring the arrival times of the secondary ions at the detector and performing a simple time to mass conversion.

ToF-SIMS is commonly used to study the proteins adsorbed on biomaterial surfaces. The very high surface sensitivity of ToF-SIMS allows probing very low levels of protein adsorption. In addition to specific identification of adsorbed proteins, static ToF-SIMS can be used to study the conformation, the orientation and the degree of denaturation of an adsorbed protein. This information is obtained in ToF-SIMS by examining the changes in the nature and/or in the intensity of the amino acid SI fragments detected at the upper most surface of the adsorbed protein.

Quantification of adsorbed proteins on biomaterials surface is important for understanding the interfacial interaction between biomaterials and tissues. ToF-SIMS can be used for the identification of the proteins adsorbed on biomaterials. Wagner et al. has used ToF-SIMS for identification of proteins present in serum and plasma (Wagner et al., 2003). In this study, proteins from serum and plasma was allowed to get adsorbed on mica sheet and then the ToF-SIMS spectra was compared with pure albumin, Fg and immunoglobulin G films. The attachment of RGD (Arginine-Glycine-Aspartic acid) peptides on Ti-6Al-4V alloy has also been investigated.(Poulin et al., 2006). Aoyagi et al. investigated metallic surfaces after culturing cell on them. They used for information theory and principal components analysis to characterize proteins specifically produced by cells (Aoyagi et al., 2004). ToF-SIMS has also been utilized to investigate the mechanism of bonding of Sr substituted hydroxyapatite (Sr-HAP) to cancellous and cortical bone (Ni et al., 2006). SIMS images provided spatial distribution of ions at the interface of biomaterial and bone. They observed that the concentration of Ca, Na, P, PO_2 and O was higher in cortical bone/Sr-HAP interface than cancellous bone/Sr-HAP interface.

Researchers have also used ToF-SIMS to evaluate the bacterial infection on implants. Bacterial infection is often a major reason for failure of implant. Speranza et al. studied adhesion of Escherichia coli bacteria on polyvinyl chloride (PVC), polymethylmethaacrylate (PMMA) and low density polyethylene (LDPE) thin films (Speranza et al., 2004). Thin films were made by spin coating to ensure flat surface. For the enhancement of secondary ions Murayama et al. treated peptides with aqueous droller containing trifluoroacetic acid (TFA) (Murayam et al., 2006).

8.3 Nano-Structuring Surfaces

The currently used biomaterials are often prone to inflammatory responses by the body, which subsequently lead to their failure. Therefore, there is a thrust for developing biomaterials with tailored surfaces, which can induce biocompatibility, haemocompatibility and osseointegration. In the last few years it has been realized that phenotypic modification of cell can be achieved by chemical signaling and topography of the implant surface. A significant number of studies have shown that both micro and nanotopographies such as grooves, pits, pillars and pyramids affect adhesion, motility, cytokine release, gene expression and differentiation. Efforts have also been made to control the cellular response by patterning proteins and peptides on the surfaces.

8.3.1 Nanotopology

Initial studies on the effect of topology on cellular behavior were performed on features in micron range. The advancement in semiconductor industry has benefited the development of new approaches for creation of nanoscaled topography on biomaterials. Random nanostructured surfaces can be created by chemical treatment of polymer membranes. Miller et al. treated poly(lactide-co-glycolic acid) (PLGA) with NaOH, which is a biodegradable polymer used for biomedical implants. The etching of PLGA created pits of different height, width, and spacing, and also altered the surface chemistry of the polymer. A negative cast of PLGA membrane was made using PDMS and this negative cast was used as a mold for development of PLGA membrane having original nano features without altered surface chemistry. It was observed that smooth muscle cells seeded onto the nanostructured PLGA achieved greater adhesion than on the flat PLGA substrates, which demonstrated that the effect of topology can be independent of surface chemistry.

Teixeira et al. investigated responses of human keratocytes on nanopatterns created using electron beam lithography (Teixeira et al., 2004). Electron lithography uses electron beam to scan over surfaces and is capable of producing feature size as small as 5 – 10 nm. They coated silicon wafers with UV3 photoresist and baked on a vacuum hotplate at 130℃ for 60 s. Then resist films were exposed to electron beam to create patterns. The dissolution of patterned area to developing solution created topographic patterns. The resist patterns were transferred to silicon by etching and then the remaining resist was also removed. About 70% of keratocytes showed alignment along the patterns with pitches of 800 nm compared to 35% for epithelial cells. On 70 nm wide ridges on a 400 nm pitch, keratocytes aligned dropped to 45%, whereas epithelial cell alignment remained constant.

Nanoimprinting techniques have been used to create various patterns (Yim et al., 2005). Yim et al. have developed a nanoimprinting technique and investigated the effect of nanopattern on morphology and motility of smooth muscle cells. In nanoimprinting technique a prepatterned SiO_2 grating mold was pressed against PMMA film at 180℃, which is well above glass transition temperature of PMMA. This allowed viscous flow of PMMA and creation of negative gratings on the PMMA surface. Nanopattern was also reproduced on poly(dimethylsiloxane) (PDMS) using soft lithography. In this technique, nanoimprinted PMMA was used as a master sample. The PMMA master was fluorinated and cleaned by blowing nitrogen gas. The PDMS and cross-linking agent were poured over mold and baked at 50℃. More than 90% of smooth muscle cells aligned along grating on nanopatterned surface than non-patterned surfaces.

Colloidal lithography has been utilized to create nanotopographies. In this technique nano colloidal particles are monolayer dispersed over the substrate. Further, the pattern formed by the colloidal particles can be transferred to substrate by ion etching. The size and distribution of nanotopography can be controlled by size of colloidal particles and its concentration. Wood et al., used colloidal nanolithography technique to fabricate irregular nanotopographies with features of either 20 or 50 nm in diameter (Wood et al., 2006). Before deposition of nano colloidal particles silica base substrate was treated with an aminosilane. They observed that colloidal topographies altered fibroblast adhesion and morphology with respect to planar substrates. Both 20 and 50 nm diameter colloidal topographies resulted in increased fibroblast adhesion at 20 min and 1 h, however, by 3 h, adhesion was similar to planar surfaces.

8.3.2 Nanopatterning Surfaces with Biomolecules

Cell-matrix adhesion is mediated by integrin, which in turn affects other cellular processes like growth, differentiation and adhesion. Integrin binding site on extracellular material is the Arg-Gly-Asp (RGD) sequence that is present in fibronectin, Fg, vitronectin, and other adhesive proteins. Previous studies have shown that specific recognition of integrin receptor is significantly increased for a surface that also contains PHSRN. The distance between RGD and PHSRN is very critical and found to around 50 nm for optimum recognition. These findings emphasized that the control over positioning of proteins over biomaterials is necessary for proper cell response.

Further, various techniques have been developed for patterning surfaces with biomolecules in nanoscale. Nanografting is an AFM-based fabrication method (Fig. 8.7). First, self assemble monolayer (SAM) is formed on gold substrate and then this monolayer is immersed in solution containing the desired replacement thiol molecules. At the site where desired molecules are to be deposited, the load on the AFM tip is increased to scrap away the adsorbed molecules and molecules from the solution gets deposited at that site. This method was first demonstrated by Liu's group at UC Davis (Xu and Liu, 1997). They nanografted patterns of $HS(CH_2)_2COOH$ into a $CH_3(CH_2)_9S/Au(111)$ SAM. The grafting of $HS(CH_2)_2COOH$ was confirmed by incubating the surface with lysozyme, which specifically adsorbed to the COOH terminated pattern and then imaging with AFM. The increase in height due to adsorbed lysozyme confirmed the grafting of $HS(CH_2)_2COOH$ protein patterns as small as 10 nm × 150 nm and 40 nm × 40 nm were created. Several other studies have used similar approach to create nanopatterns (Xu et al., 1999; Yu et al., 2006).

Dip-pen nanolithography (DPN) (Piner et al., 1999; Lee et al., 2002; Lim et al., 2003) is another AFM based technique in which AFM tip is first dip in solution

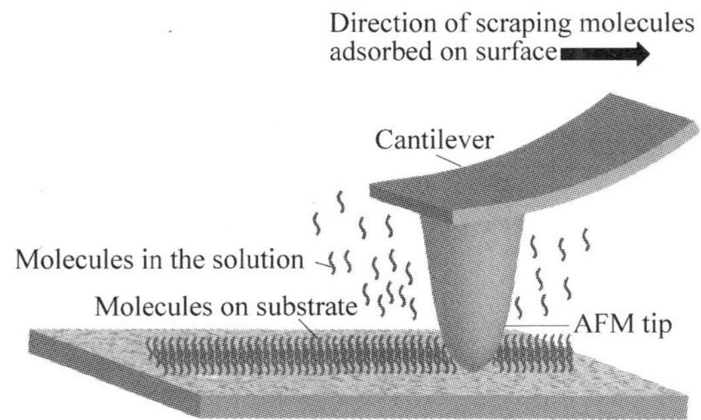

Figure 8.7 Schematic of nanografting performed by AFM tip

containing desired molecules (Fig. 8.8). This tip is moved to the surface, where molecules diffuse to the surface via water meniscus that forms between tip and the surface. There are two variations of DPN, one is indirect DPN and second is direct DPN. In indirect DPN methodology, first protein adsorbing molecules are patterned over the surface and then this nanopatterned surface is exposed to protein solution to form protein nanopatterns. In case of direct DPN, proteins are directly patterned over surface. Nanopattern as small as 10 nm can be created using DPN. Salazar et al. have demonstrated application of DPN methodology for fabrication of nanopatterned high-molar-mass polyamidoamine (PAMAM) dendrimers onto reactive *N*-hydroxysuccinimide (NHS) terminated SAMs on gold and NHS-activated polystyrene-block-poly(tert-butyl acrylate) (PS_{690}-b-$PtBA_{1210}$) block copolymer (Salazar et al., 2006). They fabricated nanopatterns of dendrimers down to 30-nm length scales. Kwak et al. and Lee et al. deposited 16-mercaptohexadecanoic acid (MHA) onto gold substrate. Lysozyme and IgG were shown to specifically adsorb on MHA. Before attachment of proteins, the non-patterned area was made protein resistant.

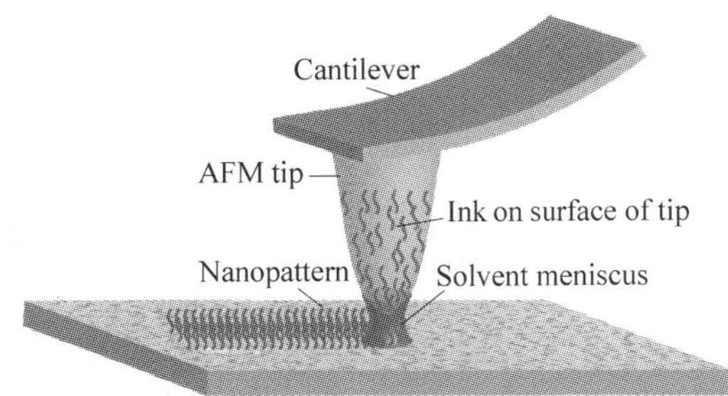

Figure 8.8 Schematic of dip-pen lithography performed by AFM tip

Nanopen is another AFM based technique in which nanopippet is used as a protein (Fig. 8.9). Bruckbauer et al. have used nanopipett of 90 – 130 nm inner diameter and 240 – 280 nm outer diameter biomolecules, including antibodies and DNA, onto a surface to create multicomponent and functional submicron features

Table 8.2 Surface modification of biomaterials for applications pertaining to different tissues

Tissue	Materials	Surface modification
Bone	Titanium metal and alloys	Oxidation (Sul et al., 2006), sandblasting (Goransson et al., 2006; Gorrieri et al., 2006), anodization (Goransson et al., 2006; Yao et al., 2006), coating with collagen (Wolf-Brandstetter et al., 2006; Morra et al., 2006), coating with apatite (Yao et al., 2006; Harle et al., 2006; Hosaka et al., 2006; Wu et al., 2006; Zreiqat et al., 2005), immobilization of biomolecules (Morra, 2006; Yoshinari et al., 2006; Zurlinden et al., 2005), Titanium aluminium nitride coating (Freeman and Brook, 2006), sandblasting and acid-etched surface modification by alkali and heat treatments (Feng et al., 2006).
	Polymers	Apatite coating (Ngiam et al., 2007; Oyane et al., 2005), functionalization by peptides (Santiago et al., 2006; Smith et al., 2005; Fan et al., 2005), Glow discharge surface modifications (Mwale et al., 2006 ; Alves et al., 2004), Surface treatment with alkaline solution (Park et al., 2005; Kokubo, 2005; Zhao et al., 2005; Pashkulewa et al., 2005).
Heart		Sulfonated PEO-grafted polyurathene (Han et al., 2006), immobilization of gene vectors on prosthetic heart valve (Fishbein et al., 2005), grafting of polydimethylsiloxane on polyurethane (Dabagh et al., 2005), surface modification of bovine pericardium by hyaluronic acid (Hahn et al., 2005; Ohri et al., 2004), surface modification by plasma immersion ion implantation (Huang et al., 2004).
Vascular	Poly-tetra-fluoro-ethylene (PTFE)	Exposure to RF plasma in argon, oxygen or ammonia (Jardine and Wilson, 2005), Binding of chitosan/heparin complex (Zhu et al., 2005), immobilization of vascular endothelial growth factor (Crombez et al., 2005).
	Polyurethane	Sulfonated poly(ethylene oxide) (PEO) grafting (Han et al., 2006), Ozonization method to graft N,N-dimethyl-Nmethacryloxyethyl-N-(sulfopropl) ammonium (Yuan et al., 2004).
	Polyethylene terephthalate (PET)	Covalent attachment of gentamicin (Ginalska et al., 2005), gelatin grafting (Ma et al., 2005), applying coating of cyclodextrin (Blanchemain et al., 2005).
	Poly methyl methacrylate (PMMA)	Peptide bonding (Kaladhar and Sharma, 2006).
	Polyester	gelatin grafting (Ma et al., 2005), coating of bacterial cellulose with the help of UV/ozone and plasma treatment (Charpentier et al., 2006).
	Polycarbonate	Surface immobilization of PGI2, synthetic PGI2, heparin and antitheombin III(Sharma, 2004).
Coronary	Metallic, polymeric and biopolymeric stents	(Mani et al., 2007).
Dental		Plasma discharge treatment (Pier et al., 2006; Silva et al., 2006), sandblasting and acid etching (Ferguson et al., 2006; Giordano et al., 2006; Vanzillotta et al., 2006), Peptide grafting or coating (Schuler et al., 2006; Ku et al., 2005), surface modification by Zn, Mg or apatite (Petrini et al., 2006; Zreiqat et al., 2005; Zhao et al., 2005), Micro-arc oxidation (Elias et al., 2005), anodization (Yao et al., 2005).

(Bruckbauer et al., 2004). The number of molecules exiting the tip depends on a combination of electroosmotic flow, electrophoresis, and dielectrophoresis, depending on the size, charge, and polarizability of the molecules (Bruckbauer et al., 2003). Rodolfa et al. used double-barreled pipette as nanopens (Rudolfa et al., 2005). Use of two pipettes allowed them to deposit two species independently from each of the pipette barrels of a single tip. Taha et al. delivered proteins though cantilevered nanopipette using a near field scanning optical microscopy (NSOM)/SPM confocal system (Taha et al., 2003). In this technique patterns of protein G and green fluorescent protein were deposited with resolution of 250 nm.

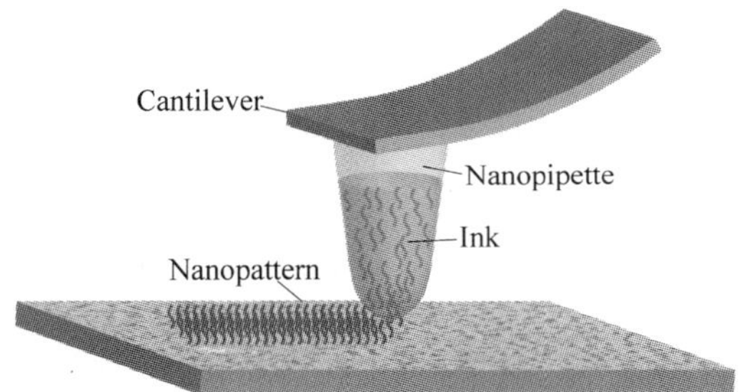

Figure 8.9 Schematic of Nanopen. In this technique nanopen nano pipette is used as a pen

In addition several surface modification studies have been conducted as shown in Table 8.2.

8.4 Conclusions

As a field at the intersection of medicine and engineering and science, biomaterials research is a major thrust area worldwide. The ability to design bio-replacements for tissue, organs and devices is of high importance to the human race. Both for the evaluation and testing of new biomaterials and biomedical devices, as well as design of new nanomaterials systems in biomedical engineering applications, the analysis of surface and interfaces is becoming increasingly significant. With the availability of advanced instrumentation and recent advancements in technology, very detailed molecular, structural, chemical and biochemical interactions between biomaterials and tissue can be probed. As biomaterials research remains at the cutting edge of science and technology, the ability to understand and characterize surface and interfaces associated with biomaterials remains an important research and industry thrust. This chapter gives an overview of the current techniques and applications of surface characterization methods used in biomaterials design.

References

Alves, C.M., Y. Yang, D.L. Carnes, J.L. Ong, V.L. Sylvia, D.D. Dean, R.L. Reis and C.M. Agrawal. Gas plasma treatment of poly(DL-lactic acid) films and its influence on the adhesion and proliferation of osteoblast-like cells. Transactions—7th World Biomaterials Congress, 2004. pp. 768.

Agnihotri, A., J.T. Garrett, J. Runt and C.A. Siedlecki. Atomic force microscopy visualization of poly(urethane urea) microphase rearrangements under aqueous environment. *Journal of Biomaterials Science Polymer Edition* **17**(1): 227 – 238 (2006).

Andrade, J.D. Interfacial phenomena and biomaterials. *Medical Instrumentation* 7(2): 110 – 120 (1973).

Aoyagi, S., S. Hiromoto, T. Hanawa and M. Kudo. TOF-SIMS investigation of metallic material surface after culturing cells. *Applied Surface Science* **231** – **232**: 470 – 474 (2004).

Belu, A.M., D.J. Graham and D.G. Castner. Time-of-flight secondary ion mass spectrometry: Techniques and applications for the characterization of biomaterial surfaces. *Biomaterials* **24**: 3635 – 3653 (2003).

Black, J. *Biological Performance of Materials*: *Fundamentals of Biocompatability*. New York: Marcel Deckker Inc. (1992).

Blanchemain, N., S. Haulon, B. Martel, M. Traisnel, M. Morcellet and H.F. Hildebrand. Vascular PET prostheses surface modification with cyclodextrin coating: Development of a new drug delivery system. *European Journal of Vascular and Endovascular Surgery* **29**(6): 628 – 632 (2005).

Blomberg, E., P.M. Claesson and J.C. Frö berg. Surfaces coated with protein layers: A surface force and ESCA study. *Biomaterials* **19**(4 – 5): 371 – 386 (1998).

Boukari, A., G. Francius and J. Hemmerlé. AFM force spectroscopy of the fibrinogen adsorption process onto dental implants. *Journal of Biomedical Materials Research-Part A* **78**(3): 466 – 472 (2006).

Briggs, D. and M.P. Seah. *Practical Surface Analysis*: *Auger and X-Ray Photoelectron Spectroscopy* (*Practical Surface Analysis*), 2nd edn. John Wiley & Sons (1996).

Bruckbauer, A., D.J. Zhou, D.J. Kang, Y.E. Korchev, C. Abell and D. Klenerman. An addressable antibody nanoarray produced on a nanostructured surface. *J. Am. Chem. Soc.* **126**: 6508 – 6509 (2004).

Bruckbauer, A., D.J. Zhou, L.M. Ying, Y.E. Korchev, C. Abell and D. Klenerman. Multicomponent submicron features of biomolecules created by voltage controlled deposition from a nanopipet. *J. Am. Chem. Soc.* **125**: 9834 – 9839 (2003).

Cacciafesta, P., K.R. Hallam, A.C. Watkinson, G.C. Allen, M.J. Miles and K.D. Jandt. Visualization of human plasma fibrinogen adsorbed on titanium implant surfaces with different roughness. *Surface Science* **491**(3): 405 – 420 (2001).

Charpentier, P.A., A. Maguire and W.K. Wan. Surface modification of polyester to produce a bacterial cellulose-based vascular prosthetic device. *Applied Surface Science* **252**(18): 6360 – 6367 (2006).

Chittur, K.K. FTIR/ATR for protein adsorption to biomaterial surfaces. *Biomaterials* **19**(4 – 5): 357 – 369 (1998).

Christopher, A., C.A. Siedlecki and R.E. Marchant. Atomic force microscopy for characterization of the biomaterial interface. *Biomaterials* **19**(4 – 5): 441 – 454 (1998).

Crombez, M., P. Chevallier, R.C. Gaudreault, E. Petitclerc, D. Mantovani and G. Laroche. Improving arterial prosthesis neo-endothelialization: Application of a proactive VEGF construct onto PTFE surfaces. *Biomaterials* **26**(35): 7402 – 7409 (2005).

Domke, J., S. Dannöhl, W.J. Parak, O. Müller, W.K. Aicher and M. Radmacher. Substrate dependent differences in morphology and elasticity of living osteoblasts investigated by atomic force microscopy. *Colloids and Surfaces B: Biointerfaces* **19**(4): 367 – 379 (2000).

Dabagh, M., M.J. Abdekhodaie and M.T. Khorasani Effects of polydimethylsiloxane grafting on the calcification physical properties and biocompatibility of polyurethane in a heart valve. *Journal of Applied Polymer Science* **98**(2): 758 – 766 (2005).

Doneva, T.A., H.B. Yin, P. Stephens, W.R. Bowen and D.W. Thomas. Development and AFM study of porous scaffolds for wound healing applications. *Spectroscopy* **18**(4): 587 – 596 (2004).

Dubruel, P., E. Vanderleyden, M. Bergadà, P.I. De, H. Chen, S. Kuypers, J. Luyten, J. Schrooten, H.L. Van and E. Schacht. Comparative study of silanisation reactions for the biofunctionalisation of Ti-surfaces. *Surface Science* **600**(12): 2562 – 2571 (2006).

Elias, C.N., J.H.C. Lima, E. Costa F. Silva, C. Muller and D.C. Figueira. Surface modification of titanium dental implants by micro-arc oxidation Surface. In: Engineering in Materials Science III-Proceedings of a Symposium sponsored by the Surface Engineering Committee of the(MPMD) of the Minerals Metals and Materials Society TMS, 2005. pp.177 – 183.

Feng, Y., W. Yan, D. Yang, J. Feng, X. Wang and S. Zhang. Biological and biomechanical properties of chemically modified SLA titanium implants in vitro and in vivo. *Key Engineering Materials* **309 – 311** I: 399 – 402 (2006).

Ferguson, S.J., N. Broggini, M. Wieland, M. De Wild, F. Rupp, J. Geis-Gerstorfer, D.L. Cochran and D. Buser. Biomechanical evaluation of the interfacial strength of a chemically modified sandblasted and acid-etched titanium surface. *Journal of Biomedical Materials Research - Part A* **78**(2): 291 – 297 (2006).

Fan, V.H., J.W. Wright, A.H. Wells and L.G. Griffith. Tethered epidermal growth factor as a substrate for bone regeneration. Transactions—7th World Biomaterials Congress, 2004. pp. 926.

Feldman, L.C. and J.W. Mayer. *Fundamentals of surface and thin film analysis*. New York: North Holland (1986).

Fishbein, I., S.J. Stachelek, J.M. Connolly, R.L. Wilensky, I. Alferiev and R.J. Levy. Site specific gene delivery in the cardiovascular system. *Journal of Controlled Release* **109**(1 – 3): 37 – 48 (2005).

Freeman, C.O. and I.M. Brook. Bone response to a titanium aluminium nitride coating on metallic implants. *Journal of Materials Science: Materials in Medicine* **17**(5): 465 – 470 (2006).

Frushour, B.J. and J.L. Koenig Raman spectroscopy of proteins. *Advances in Infrared and Raman Spectroscopy* **1**: 35 – 97 (1975).

Galtayries, A., R. Warocquier-Clérout, M.D. Nagel and P. Marcus. Fibronectin adsorption on Fe-Cr alloy studied by XPS. *Surface and Interface Analysis* **38**(4): 186 – 190 (2006).

Ginalska, G., D. Kowalczuk and M. Osińska. A chemical method of gentamicin bonding to gelatine-sealed prosthetic vascular grafts international. *Journal of Pharmaceutics* **288**(1): 131 – 140 (2005).

Giordano, C., E. Sandrini, V. Busini, R. Chiesa, G. Fumagalli, G. Giavaresi, M. Fini, R. Giardino and A. Cigada. A new chemical etching process to improve endosseous implant osseointegration: In vitro evaluation on human osteoblast-like cells International. *Journal of Artificial Organs* **29**(8): 772 – 780 (2006).

Göransson, A., C. Gretzer, A. Johansson, Y.T. Sul and A. Wennerberg. Inflammatory response to a titanium surface with potential bioactive properties: An in vitro study Clinical Implant. *Dentistry and Related Research* **8**(4): 210 – 217 (2006).

Gorrieri, O., M. Fini, K. Kyriakidou, A. Zizzi, M. Mattioli-Belmonte, P. Castaldo, A. De Cristofaro, D. Natali, A. Pugnaloni and G. Biagini. In vitro evaluation of biofunctional performances of Ghimas titanium implants. *International Journal of Artificial Organs* **29**(10): 1012 – 1020 (2006).

Hahn, S.K., R. Ohri and C.M. Giachelli. Anti-calcification of bovine pericardium for bioprosthetic heart valves after surface modification with hyaluronic acid derivatives. *Biotechnology and Bioprocess Engineering* **10**(3): 218 – 224 (2005).

Han, D.K., K. Park, K.D. Park, K.D. Ahn and Y.H. Kim. In vivo biocompatibility of sulfonated PEO-grafted polyurethanes for polymer heart valve and vascular graft. *Artificial Organs* **30**(12): 955 – 959 (2006).

He, W., Z. Ma, T. Yong, W.E. Teo and S. Ramakrishna. Fabrication of collagen-coated biodegradable polymer nanofiber mesh and its potential for endothelial cells growth. *Biomaterials* **26**(36): 7606 – 7615 (2005).

Huang, N., P. Yang, Y.X. Leng, J. Wang, H. Sun, J.Y. Chen and G.J. Wan. Surface modification of biomaterials by plasma immersion ion implantation. *Surface and Coatings Technology* **186**(1 – 2 *SPEC ISS*): 218 – 226 (2004).

Harle, J., H-W. Kim, N. Mordan, J.C. Knowles and V. Salih. Initial responses of human osteoblasts to sol-gel modified titanium with hydroxyapatite and titania composition. *Acta Biomaterialia* **2**(5): 547 – 556 (2006).

Hirschmugl, C.J. Frontiers in infrared spectroscopy at surfaces and interfaces. *Surface Science* **500**: 577 – 604 (2002).

Hole, B.B., J.A. Schwarz, J.L. Gilbert and B.L. Atkinson. A study of biologically active peptide sequences (P-15) on the surface of an ABM scaffold (PepGen P-15^{TM}) using AFM and FTIR. *Journal of Biomedical Materials Research—Part A* **74**(4): 712 – 721 (2005).

Hosaka, M., Y. Shibata and T. Miyazaki. Preliminary β-tricalcium phosphate coating prepared by discharging in a modified body fluid enhances collagen immobilization onto titanium. *Journal of Biomedical Materials Research—Part B Applied Biomaterials* **78**(2): 237 – 242 (2006).

Ishihara, K., J. Watanabe and Y. Iwasaki. Bioinspired polymer surfaces for prevention of bioresponse. *Materials Science Forum* **426 – 432**(4): 3171 – 3176 (2003).

Jackson, M. Fourier-transform infrared spectroscopic studies of Ca-binding proteins. *Biochemistry* **30**(40): 9681 – 9686 (1991).

Jardine, S. and J.I.B. Wilson. Plasma surface modification of ePTFE vascular grafts. *Plasma Processes and Polymers* **2**(4): 328 – 333 (2005).

Jena, B.P. and H. Hörber. *Atomic Force Microscopy in Cell Biology*. New York: Academic press (2002).

Kaladhar, K. and C.P. Sharma. Cell mimetic lateral stabilization of outer cell mimetic bilayer on polymer surfaces by peptide bonding and their blood compatibility. *Journal of Biomedical Materials Research—Part A* **79**(1): 23 – 35 (2006).

Kannan, R.Y., H.J. Salacinski, D.S. Vara, M. Odlyha and A.M. Seifalian. Review paper: Principles and applications of surface analytical techniques at the vascular interface. *Journal of Biomaterials Applications* **21**(1): 5 – 32 (2006).

Kazarian, S.G., Chan K.L. Andrew, V. Maquet and A.R. Boccaccini. Characterisation of bioactive and resorbable polylactide/Bioglass® composites by FTIR spectroscopic imaging. *Biomaterials* **25**(18): 3931 – 3938 (2004).

Klee, D., Z. Ademovic, A. Bosserhoff, H. Hoecker, G. Maziolis and H.J. Erli. Surface modification of poly(vinylidenefluoride) to improve the osteoblast adhesion. *Biomaterials* **24**(21): 3663 – 3670 (2003).

Ku, Y., C.P. Chung and J.H. Jang. The effect of the surface modification of titanium using a recombinant fragment of fibronectin and vitronectin on cell behavior. *Biomaterials* **26**(25): 5153 – 5157 (2005).

Kokubo, T. Design of bioactive bone substitutes based on biomineralization process. *Materials Science and Engineering C* **25**(2): 97 – 104 (2005).

Koenig, J.L. *Spectroscopy of Polymers*. 2nd edn. New York: Elsevier Science (1997).

Lee, K.B., S.J. Park, C.A. Mirkin, J.C. Smith and M. Mrksich. Protein Nanoarrays Generated by Dip-Pen Nanolithography. *Science* **295**(5560): 1702 – 1705 (2002).

Lenk, T.J., T.A. Horbett, B.D. Ratner and K.K. Chittur. Infrared spectroscopic studies of time-dependent changes in fibrinogen adsorbed to polyurethanes. *Langmuir* **7**(8): 1755 – 1764 (1991).

Lim, J.H., D.S. Ginger, K.B. Lee, J. Heo, J.M. Nam and C.A. Mirkin. Direct-Write Dip- Pen Nanolithography of Proteins on Modified Silicon Oxide Surfaces. *Angew. Chem. Int. Ed* **20**: 2411 – 2414 (2003).

McArthur, S.L. Applications of XPS in bioengineering. *Surface and Interface Analysis* **38**(11): 1380 – 1385 (2006).

Ma, Z., W. He, T. Yong and S. Ramakrishna. Grafting of gelatin on electrospun poly(caprolactone) nanofibers to improve endothelial cell spreading and proliferation and to control cell orientation. *Tissue Engineering* **11** (7 – 8): 1149 – 1158 (2005).

Mueller, M. *Fundamentals of Quantum Chemistry: Molecular Spectrocopy and Modern Electronic Structure Computations*. Kluwer Publishers (2001).

Ma, Z., M. Kotaki, T. Yong, W. He and S. Ramakrishna. Surface engineering of electrospun polyethylene terephthalate (PET) nanofibers towards development of a new material for blood vessel engineering. *Biomaterials* **26**(15): 2527 – 2536 (2005).

Mansur, H., R. Oréfice, M. Pereira, Z. Lobato, W. Vasconcelos and L. Machado. FTIR and UV-vis study of chemically engineered biomaterial surfaces for protein immobilization. *Spectroscopy* **16**(3 – 4): 351 – 360 (2002).

Mardilovich, A. and E. Kokkoli. Biomimetic peptide-amphiphiles for functional biomaterials: The role of GRGDSP and PHSRN Biomacromolecules. *Biomacromolecules* **5**(3): 950 – 957 (2004).

Morris, V.J., A.P. Gunning and A.R. Kirby. *Atomic Force Microscopy for Biologists*. Imperial College Press (1999).

Mori, H. and M. Tsukada. New silk protein: Modification of silk protein by gene engineering for production of biomaterials. *Reviews in Molecular Biotechnology* **74**(2): 95 – 103 (2000).

Morra, M. Biochemical modification of titanium surfaces: Peptides and ECM proteins. *European Cells and Materials* **12**: 1 – 15 (2006).

Morra, M. and V. Cassinelli. Biomaterials surface characterization and modification. *International Journal of Artificial Organs* **29**(9): 824 – 833 (2006).

Morra, M., C. Cassinelli, G. Cascardo, P. Cahalan, L. Cahalan, M. Fini and R. Giardino. Surface engineering of titanium by collagen immobilization Surface characterization and in vitro and in vivo studies. *Biomaterials* **24**(25): 4639 – 4654 (2003).

Morra, M., C. Cassinelli, G. Cascardo, L. Mazzucco, P. Borzini, M. Fini, G. Giavaresi and R. Giardino. Collagen I-coated titanium surfaces: Mesenchymal cell adhesion and in vivo evaluation in trabecular bone implants. *Journal of Biomedical Materials Research—Part A* **78**(3): 449 – 458 (2006).

Murayama, Y., M. Komatsu, K. Kuge and H. Hashimoto. Enhanced peptide molecular imaging using aqueous droplets. *Applied Surface Science* **252**(19): 6774 – 6776 (2006).

Mani, G., M.D. Feldman, D. Patel and C.M. Agrawal. Coronary stents: A materials perspective. *Biomaterials* **28**(9): 1689 – 1710 (2007).

Mwale, F., H.T. Wang, V. Nelea, L. Luo, J. Antoniou and M.R. Wertheimer. The effect of glow discharge plasma surface modification of polymers on the osteogenic differentiation of committed human mesenchymal stem cells. *Biomaterials* **27**(10): 2258 – 2264 (2006).

Nakamoto, N. *Infrared and Raman Spectra of Inorganic and Coordination Compounds*. John Wiley & Sons Inc. (1997).

Nakamoto, N. *Infrared and Raman Spectra of Inorganic and Coordination Compounds*. John Wiley & Sons Inc. (1997).

Ngiam, M., T.R. Hayes, S. Dhara and B. Su. Biomimetic apatite/polycaprolactone (PCL) nanofibres for bone tissue engineering scaffolds. *Key Engineering Materials* **330 – 332** II: 991 – 994 (2007).

Ni, G.X., W.W. Lu, B. Xu, K.Y. Chiu, C. Yang, Z.Y. Li, W.M. Lam and K.D.K. Luk. Interfacial behaviour of strontium-containing hydroxyapatite cement with cancellous and cortical bone. *Biomaterials* **27**(29): 5127 – 5133 (2006).

Ohri, R., S.K. Hahn, A.S. Hoffman, P.S. Stayton and C.M. Giachelli. Hyaluronic acid grafting mitigates calcification of glutaraldehyde-fixed bovine pericardium. *Journal of Biomedical Materials Research—Part A* **70**(2): 328 – 334 (2004).

Oyane, A., M. Uchida, Y. Yokoyama, C. Choong, J. Triffitt and A. Ito. Simple surface modification of poly(ε-caprolactone) to induce its apatite-forming ability. *Journal of Biomedical Materials Research—Part A* **75**(1): 138 – 145 (2005).

Peng, M.C., J.C. Lin, C.Y. Chen, J.J. Wu and X.Z. Lin. Studies of sulfonated polyethylene for biliary stent application. *Journal of Applied Polymer Science* **92**(4): 2450 – 2457 (2004).

Petrini, P., C.R. Arciola, I. Pezzali, S. Bozzini, L. Montanaro, M.C. Tanzi, P. Speziale and L. Visai. Antibacterial activity of zinc modified titanium oxide surface. *International Journal of Artificial Organs* **29**(4): 434 – 442 (2006).

Pier-Francesco, A., R.J. Adams, M.G.J. Waters and D.W. Williams. Titanium surface modification and its effect on the adherence of Porphyromonas gingivalis: An in vitro study. *Clinical Oral Implants Research* **17**(6): 633 – 637 (2006).

Poulin, S., M.C. Durrieu, S. Polizu and L.H. Yahia. Bioactive molecules for biomimetic materials: Identification of RGD peptide sequences by TOF-S-SIMS analysis. *Applied Surface Science* **252**: 6738 – 6741 (2006).

Park, G.E., M.A. Pattison, K. Park and T.J. Webster. Accelerated chondrocyte functions on NaOH-treated PLGA scaffolds. *Biomaterials* **26**(16): 3075 – 3082 (2005).

Pashkuleva, I., A.P. Marques, F. Vaz and R.L. Reis. Surface modification of starch based blends using potassium permanganate-nitric acid system and its effect on the adhesion and proliferation of osteoblast-like cells. *Journal of Materials Science: Materials in Medicine* **16**(1): 81 – 92 (2005).

Piner, R.D., J. Zhu, F. Xu, S. Hong and C.A. Mirkin. Dip Pen Nanolithography. *Science* **283**: 661 – 663 (1999).

Ratner, B.D. and S.J. Bryant. Biomaterials: Where we have been and where we are going. *Annual Review of Biomedical Engineering* **6**: 41 – 75 (2004).

Ratner, B.D., A. Hoffman, F.J. Schoen and J. Lemmons. *Biomaterials Science: An Introduction to materials in Medicine*. 2nd edn. San Diego: Elsevier Academic Press (2004).

Recum, A.V. *Handbook of Biomaterials Evaluation, 2nd edn.* Philadelphia Taylor Francis (1999).

Rosencwaig, A. and A. Gersho. Photoacoustic effect with solids: a theoretical treatment. *Science* **190**: 557 – 560 (1975).

Roach, P., D. Farrar and C.C. Perry. Surface tailoring for controlled protein adsorption: Effect of topography at the nanometer scale and chemistry. *Journal of the American Chemical Society* **128**(12): 3939 – 3945 (2006).

Rodolfa, K. T., A. Bruckbauer, D. Zhou, Y.E. Korchev and D. Klenerman. Two-component graded deposition of biomolecules with a double-barreled nanopipette. *Angew. Chem. Int.Edn.* **44**: 6854 – 6859 (2005).

Sagvolden, G., I. Giaever, E.O. Pettersen and J. Feder. Cell adhesion force microscopy. In: Proceedings of the National Academy of Sciences of the United States of America **96**(2): 471 – 476 (1999).

Salazar, R.B., A. Shovsky, H. Schonherr and G.J. Vancso. Dip-pen nanolithography on (bio)reactive monolayer and block-copolymer platforms: Deposition of lines of single macromolecules. *Small* **2** (11): 1274 – 1282 (2006).

Schuler, M., G.R.h. Owen, D.W. Hamilton, M. de Wild, M. Textor, D.M. Brunette and S.G.P. Tosatti. Biomimetic modification of titanium dental implant model surfaces using the RGDSP-peptide sequence: A cell morphology study. *Biomaterials* **27**(21): 4003 – 4015 (2006).

Servoli, E., D. Maniglio, A. Motta, R. Predazzer and C. Migliaresi. Surface properties of silk fibroin films and their interaction with fibroblasts. *Macromolecular Bioscience* **5**(12): 1175 – 1183 (2005).

Sharma, C.P. Surface modifications: Blood compatibility of cardiovascular devices. Transactions—7th World Biomaterials Congress, 2004. pp. 394.

M.A.M. Silva, A.E. Martinelli, C. Alves Jr. R.M. Nascimento, M.P. Távora and C.D. Vilar. Surface modification of Ti implants by plasma oxidation in hollow cathode discharge. *Surface and Coatings Technology* **200**(8): 2618 – 2626 (2006).

Speer, A.G., P.B. Cotton, J. Rode, A.M. Seddon, C.R. Neal, J. Holton and J.W. Costerton. Biliary stent blockage with bacterial biofilm A light and electron microscopy study. *Annals of Internal Medicine* **108**(4): 546 – 553 (1988).

Speranza, G., G. Gottardi, C. Pederzolli, L. Lunelli, R. Canteri, L. Pasquardini, E. Carli, A. Lui, D. Maniglio, M. Brugnara and M. Anderle. Role of chemical interactions in bacterial adhesion to polymer surfaces. *Biomaterials* **25**: 2029 – 2037 (2004).

Sul, Y.T., Y. Jeong, C. Johansson and T. Albrektsson. Oxidized bioactive implants are rapidly and strongly integrated in bone Part 1 - Experimental implants. *Clinical Oral Implants Research* **17**(5): 521 – 526 (2006).

Santiago, L.Y., R.W. Nowak, J.P. Rubin and K.G. Marra. Peptide-surface modification of poly(caprolactone) with laminin-derived sequences for adipose-derived stem cell applications. *Biomaterials* **27**(15): 2962 – 2969 (2006).

Smith, E., J. Yang, L. McGann, W. Sebald and H. Uludag. RGD-grafted thermoreversible polymers to facilitate attachment of BMP-2 responsive C2C12 cells. *Biomaterials* **26**(35): 7329 – 7338 (2005).

Taha, H., R.S. Marks, L.A. Gheber, I. Rousso, J. Newman, C. Sukenik and A. Lews. Protein printing with an atomic force sensing nanofountainpen. *Applied physics letter* **83**: 1041 – 1043 (2003).

Takai, E., K.D. Costa, A. Shaheen, C.T. Hung, X.E. Guo. Osteoblast elastic modulus measured by atomic force microscopy is substrate dependent. *Annals of Biomedical Engineering* **33**(7): 963 – 971 (2005).

Teixeira, A.I., P.F. Nealey and C.J. Murphy. Responses of human keratocytes to micro- and nanostructured substrates. *Journal of Biomedical Materials Research—Part A* **71**(3): 369 – 376 (2004).

Tsang, T.K., J. Pollack and H.B. Chodash. Inhibition of biliary endoprostheses occlusion by ampicillin-sulbactam in an in vitro model. *Journal of Laboratory and Clinical Medicine* **130**(6): 643 – 648 (1997).

Urban, M.W. *Vibrational Spectroscopy of Molecules and Macromolecules on Surfaces.* New York: Wiley-Interscience (1993).

Vanselow, R. and R. Howe. *Chemistry & Physics of Solid Surfaces*. Springer Publishers, (1982).

Vanzillotta, P.S., M.S. Sader, I.N. Bastos, Soares G. De Almeida (2006) Improvement of in vitro titanium bioactivity by three different surface treatments. *Dental Materials* **22**(3): 275 – 282 (2006).

Verma, D., K. Katti and D. Katti. Bioactivity in in situ hydroxyapatite-polycaprolactone composites. *Journal of Biomedical Materials Research—Part A* **78**(4): 772 – 780 (2006).

Verma, D., K. Katti and D. Katti. Experimental investigation of interfaces in hydroxyapatite/polyacrylic acid/polycaprolactone composites using photoacoustic FTIR spectroscopy. *Journal of Biomedical Materials Research—Part A* **77**(1): 59 – 66 (2006).

Vickerman, J.C. *Surface Analysis: The Principal Techniques*. Chichester: John Wiley and Sons (1997).

Wagner, M.S., T.A. Horbett and D.G. Castner. Characterizing multicomponent adsorbed protein films using electron spectroscopy for chemical analysis time-of-flight secondary ion mass spectrometry and radiolabeling: capabilities and limitations. *Biomaterials* **24**: 1897 – 1908 (2003).

Wang, J., X. Chen, M.L. Clarke and Z. Chen. Vibrational spectroscopic studies on fibrinogen adsorption at polystyrene/protein solution interfaces: Hydrophobic side chain and secondary structure changes. *Journal of Physical Chemistry* B **110**(10): 5017 – 5024 (2006).

Wang, M.S., L.B. Palmer, J.D. Schwartz and A. Razatos. Evaluating protein attraction and adhesion to biomaterials with the atomic force microscope. *Langmuir* **20**(18): 7753 – 7759 (2004).

Watt, J.F. and J. Wolstenholme. *An Introduction to Surface Analysis by XPS and AES.* Chichester John Wiley and Sons (2003).

Williams, D.F. Definitions in biomaterials. Proceedings of a Consensus Conference of the European Society of Biomaterials Chester England March 3 – 5 Vol. 4. New York: Elsevier (1987).

Winograd, N. Prospects for imaging TOF-SIMS: From fundamentals to biotechnology. *Applied Surface Science* **203 – 204**: 13 – 19 (2003).

Wolf-Brandstetter, C., A. Lode, T. Hanke, D. Scharnweber and H. Worch. Influence of modified extracellular matrices on Ti6AL4V implants on binding and release of VEGF. *Journal of Biomedical Materials Research—Part A* **79**(4): 882 – 894 (2006).

Wood, M.A., C.D.W. Wilkinson and A.S.G. Curtis. The effects of colloidal nanotopography on initial fibroblast adhesion and morphology. *IEEE Transactions on Nanobioscience* **5**(1): 20 – 31 (2006).

Wu, Y., B.C. Yang, C.L. Deng, Y.F. Tan and X.D. Zhang. The influence of surface bioactivated modification on titanium percutaneous implants anchored in bone. *International Journal of Artificial Organs* **29**(6): 630 – 638 (2006).

Xu, S. and G.Y. Liu. Nanometer-scale fabrication by simultaneous nanoshaving and molecular self-assembly. *Langmuir* **13**(2): 127 – 129 (1997).

Xu, S., S. Miller, P.E. Laibinis and G.Y. Liu. Fabrication of nanometer scale patterns within self-assembled monolayers by nanografting. *Langmuir* **15** (21): 7244 – 7251 (1999).

Yim, E.K.F., R.M. Reano, S.W. Pang, A.F. Yee, C.S. Chen and K.W. Leong. Nanopattern-induced changes in morphology and motility of smooth muscle cells. *Biomaterials* **26**(26): 5405 – 5413 (2005).

Yao, C., E.B. Slamovich and T.J. Webster. Increased osteoblast adhesion on nano-rough anodized titanium and CoCrMo. In: *NSTI Nanotechnology Conference and Trade Show - NSTI Nanotech , Technical Proceedings* **2**: 119 – 122 (2006).

Yao, C., E.B. Slamovich and T.J. Webster. Titanium nanosurface modification by anodization for orthopedic applications. In: Materials Research Society Symposium Proceedings **845**: 215 – 220 (2005).

Yoshinari, M., T. Hayakawa, K. Matsuzaka, T. Inoue, Y. Oda, M. Shimono, T. Ide and T. Tanaka. Oxygen plasma surface modification enhances immobilization of simvastatin acid. *Biomedical Research* **27**(1): 29 – 36 (2006).

Yu, J.J., Y.H. Tan, X. Li, P.K. Kuo and G.Y. Liu. A nanoengineering approach to regulate the lateral heterogeneity of self-assembled monolayers. *Journal of the American Chemical Society* **128**(35): 11,574 – 11,581 (2006).

Yuan, Y., F. Ai, X. Zang, W. Zhuang, J. Shen and S. Lin. Polyurethane vascular catheter surface grafted with zwitterionic sulfobetaine monomer activated by ozone. *Colloids and Surfaces B*: *Biointerfaces* **35**(1): 1 – 5 (2004).

Zhao, B.H., I-S. Lee, W. Bai, F.Z. Cui and H.L. Feng. Improvement of fibroblast adherence to titanium surface by calcium phosphate coating formed with IBAD. *Surface and Coatings Technology* **193**(1 – 3 SPEC ISS): 366 – 371 (2005).

Zhu, A.P., Z. Ming and S. Jian. Blood compatibility of chitosan/heparin complex surface modified PTFE vascular graft. *Applied Surface Science* **241:** 485 – 492 (2005).

Zreiqat, H., S.M. Valenzuela, B.B. Nissan, R. Roest, C. Knabe, R.J. Radlanski, H. Renz and P.J. Evans. The effect of surface chemistry modification of titanium alloy on signalling pathways in human osteoblasts. *Biomaterials* **26**(36): 7579 – 7586 (2005).

Zurlinden, K., M. Laub and H.P. Jennissen. Chemical functionalization of a hydroxyapatite based bone replacement material for the immobilization of proteins. *Materialwissenschaft und Werkstofftechnik* **36**(12): 820 – 827 (2005).

Zhao, M., Q.X. Zheng, X.D. Guo, D.P. Quan, J. Hao and Y.T. Wang. Study on biomimic mineralization of poly lactide-co-glycolide. *Chinese Journal of Biomedical Engineering* **24**(2): 145 – 149 (2005).

9 Carbon Nanotubes for Electrochemical and Electronic Biosensing Applications

Ningyi Liu[1], Qing Zhang[1], Mary B Chan-Park[2], Changming Li[2] and Peng Chen[2]

[1] Microelectronics Centre, School of Electrical and Electronic Engineering, Nanyang Technological University, Nanyang Avenue, Singapore 639798
[2] School of Chemical and Biomedical Engineering, Nanyang Technological University, Nanyang Avenue, Singapore 639798

Abstract The structure of carbon nanotubes (CNTs), a type of macromolecular systems, can be thought as rolling up a graphene sheet along certain directions. The unique properties of CNTs, such as very high surface/volume ratio, high chemical stability, high electro-catalytic activity and high charge transfer efficiency, make CNTs a very suitable material for biosensor applications. It is due to these advantages that a variety of CNT related biosensors have been developed since discovery of CNTs. In this chapter, recently reported CNT-based electrochemical and electronic biosensing applications are summarized.

9.1 Introduction

Biosensors, a subtype of sensor devices, are designed to characterize biological properties of various biomaterials from monitoring the physical and chemical signals in the biological materials. Biosensors, typically, consist of sensing elements and signal transducers. The elements selectively sense the analytes, while the transducers convert chemical and biological variations into appropriate physical signals, such as electrical and optical signals, whose change corresponds to the analyte concentration. Biosensors have two characteristics. One is that the sensing elements are attached with biological materials, such as single-strand DNA (ssDNA), proteins (enzymes, antibodies, etc.), cells and so on. The other is that biosensors are used to track the biological processes ((Balasubramanian and Burghard, 2006) and references therein).

Carbon nanotube (CNT) is a type of macromolecular systems. The structure of

(1) Corresponding e-mail: eqzhang@ntu.edu.sg

CNTs can be thought as rolling up a graphene sheet along certain directions. The unique properties of CNT have drawn a lot of research attention in various biosensor applications. For example, CNTs have a high surface/volume ratio. Thus, the surface area of CNT-modified electrodes for electrochemical detection would be increased. Moreover, it also exhibits very high chemical stability and hardly reacts with analytes. It has also been found that the CNT can enhance electro-catalytic activity and promote electron-transfer reactions for a wide range of electroactive species. CNT-modified electrodes can alleviate surface-fouling and immobilize important biomolecules. CNT has a 1-D structure that enables efficient charge transfer between the surface-anchored biomolecules and CNTs. Therefore, the conductivity of CNT, especially semiconducting SWNT, is found to be remarkably sensitive to the surface adsorbates. In addition, CNTs are easily functionalized with biorecognition layers which selectively react with bio-analytes. These properties make CNT a very suitable material for electrical biosensors, including electrochemical biosensor and electronic biosensor ((Katz and Willner, 2004; Wang, 2005b) and references therein).

The aim of this review is to cover recently reported applications integrating CNTs into electrical biosensing systems. This chapter is organized as follows. Various design principles of CNT based biosensors are described in the second section. In the third section, a collection of CNT-based electrochemical biosensors are presented, followed by the CNTFET-based electronic biosensors in the fourth section. Finally, the future prospects are discussed.

9.2 Design Principles of CNT-Based Biosensors

Biological species could be detected by a variety of classical methodologies, such as fluorescence and spectrometry with high sensitivity and selectivity. However, these techniques are of complicated systems and difficulties to miniaturize. These drawbacks could be overcome by electrical biosensing techniques. In last decade, CNTs have been utilized as electrodes or transducers to perform electrical biosensing. In the following discussion, we classify CNT-based biosensors into several categories according to different configurations.

9.2.1 CNTs as Modifiers of Electrode Surfaces

The common used electrodes in electrochemical biosensors included carbon electrodes (glassy carbon, graphite, activated carbon, etc.), metallic electrodes (Au, Pt and so on), conducting polymer electrodes, metal oxides electrodes, different composite electrodes, etc.. Some of these electrodes are of a poor sensitivity and stability, long response time and high overpotential for electron transfer reactions in electrochemical sensor applications. Some of them are very expensive such as noble metal electrodes. In contrast, CNTs, both non-oriented and oriented, with their fast electron transfer and anti-surface fouling properties, could overcome most of these disadvantages.

9.2.1.1 Non-Oriented Modification

Non-oriented modification means that CNTs on the electrode surface are randomly distributed. Casting a CNT suspension onto the support electrodes is the simplest and mostly used method. Because CNTs are insoluble in most solvents, the first step of processing CNTs into a thin films on electrodes is to get a homogeneous CNT suspension, some of which were prepared by dissolving CNTs in a solution of concentrated sulfuric acid (Musameh et al., 2002) or Nafion (Deo et al., 2005; Hocevar et al., 2005; Luong et al., 2005; Tsai et al., 2005; Wang et al., 2003a; Wu et al., 2006). The latter one has extra benefits like improved anti-interferent ability and mechanical strength due to the good cation exchange, discriminative and biocompatibility properties of Nafion, a perfluorosulfonated and negatively charged polymer. Moreover, with the aid of surfactants, such as dihexadecylphosphate (DHP) (Wu and Hu, 2003, 2006; Wu et al., 2006) and sodium dodecylbenzenesulfonate (SDBS) (Wu et al., 2006), CNTs were easily dispersed into the aqueous solution. In addition to aqueous media, other solvents such as *N*, *N*-dimethylformamide (DMF) (Liu and Lin, 2005, Wang et al., 2002; Wang et al., 2004, Wei et al., 2006; Zeng et al., 2006), chloroform (Zhang et al., 2006) and acetone (Jin et al., 2006; Wu et al., 2002) were also used to prepare CNT suspension. Further to this, oxidized CNTs after long-time acid treatment, however, could be directly stabilized in aqueous solution (Lawrence and Wang, 2006; Zhu et al., 2005) because of the electrostatic repulsion induced by the negatively charged chemical groups on MWNTs (Zhu et al., 2005). In the above processes, ultrasonication was usually used to assist effective dispersion of CNTs. After that, a small volume of CNT suspension was drop-casted on the polished glassy carbon electrode (GCE) or metallic electrodes.

Applying the chemical vapor deposition (CVD) method could also fabricate an electrode with non-oriented CNT modification (Tang et al., 2004). Another simple preparation method involves gently rubbing the electrode surfaces on filter papers coating with purified MWNTs (Salimi et al., 2005).

9.2.1.2 Oriented Modification

Assembling oriented CNTs on electrodes is another way to fabricate CNT-modified electrodes for electrochemical detections. Most of these modifications were originated from the CNT growth process, which not only improves the electrical contact between CNTs and the conducting electrodes, but also makes CNTs free of impurities caused by surfactants or binders.

Direct growth of vertically aligned CNT arrays on graphite or gold substrate could be immediately utilized for electrical biosensing (Tang et al., 2006; Ye et al., 2004). But some of such electrodes were further functionalized with biomaterials for biological detection (Roy et al., 2006; Wang et al., 2004).

To improve the signal-to-noise ratio and detection limits, nanoelectrode array (NEA) based on low-density aligned CNTs were developed for detecting of glucose (Lin et al., 2004) and DNA (Koehne et al., 2003; Koehne et al., 2004; Li et al., 2003). The CNTs were firstly grown on the substrate with controlled spacing and density (Fig. 9.1). Then CNT NEAs were insulated between each other with spin-coated epon epoxy resin or deposited SiO_2. Subsequently the protruding parts of CNT NEA were removed by polishing process. The exposed tips of CNT NEA were functionalized and covalently immobilized with GOx or probe ssDNA. In this setup, the aligned CNT NEA exhibited high elecrocatalytic activity and fast electron transfer rate (ETR) because the edges of the nanotubes are exposed (Li et al., 2002).

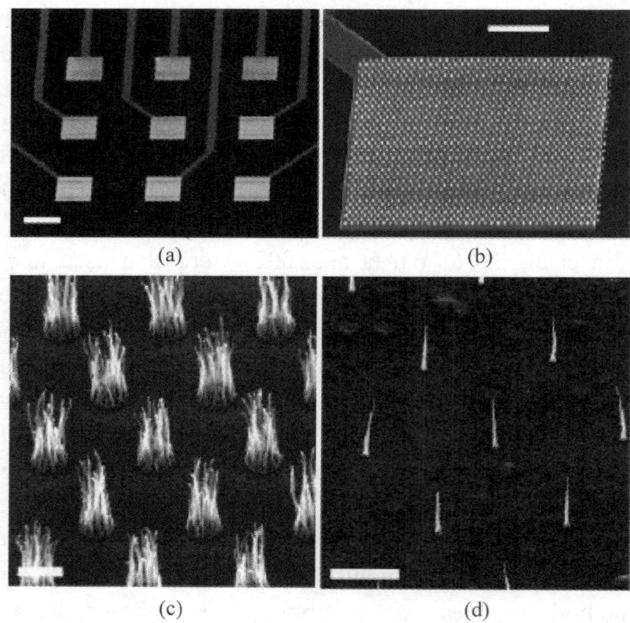

Figure 9.1 SEM images of CNT nanoelectrode array: (a) 3×3 electrode array. (b) array of CNT bundles on one of the electrode pads. (c) and (d) array of CNTs at UV-lithography and e-beam patterned Ni spots, respectively. The scale bars are 200, 50, 2 and 5 μm, respectively. Reprinted from (Li et al., 2003) with permission

Post-synthesization transfer of the CNT array method was also applied to fabricate oriented-CNT modified electrodes (Gao et al., 2003; Wang et al., 2003a; Wang et al., 2003b). Briefly speaking, a thin layer of metal (such as Au) was deposited on the top surface of as-synthesized aligned CNT array and then the substrate which supported the CNT to grow was etched away.

Another way to prepare vertically aligned CNT array was the self-assembly technique (Liu et al., 2005; Patolsky et al., 2004). The carboxylized CNTs generated from oxidative scission were covalently immobilized on a cysteamine monolayer coated gold electrodes via amide bond in a manner of perpendicular orientation.

9.2.2 CNT-Based Composite Electrodes

Carbon paste and composite electrodes, fabricated by mixing carbon powder with mineral oil or other binders, have been used in electrochemical detection for years. After the application of CNTs in this field, CNT-based composite electrodes could be prepared in a similar manner by mixing CNTs powder with a number of binders, e.g. mineral oil, bromoform, Teflon, polymers like Polypyrrole (PPy) and chitosan (CHIT) and so on. The CNT-based composite electrode was fabricated by casting the resulting composite on the top of a support substrate (Fig. 9.2(a)) (Zhang and Gorski, 2005a; Zhang and Gorski 2005b), or packing it into a glass capillary or a Teflon tube (Fig. 9.2(b)) (Luque et al., 2006; Wang and Musameh, 2003b; Yang et al., 2006).

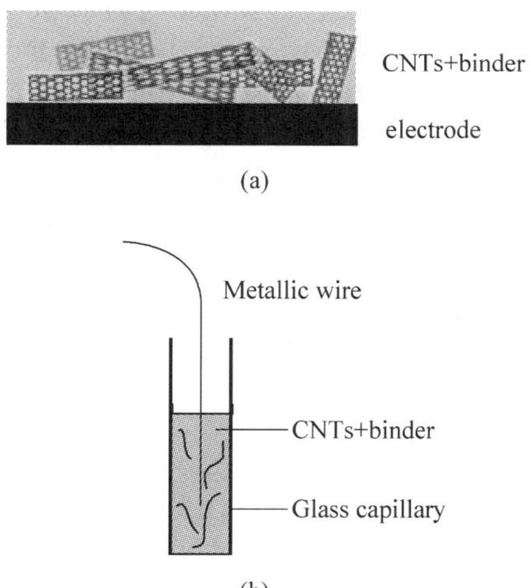

Figure 9.2 Schematic drawing of two types of CNT composite electrodes: (a) composite of CNTs and binder was casted on the top of a support electrode. (b) composite was packed into the electrode cavity of a glass capillary or a Teflon tube

The first CNT-based composite electrodes used bromoform as binder and then was packed into a glass tube (Britto et al., 1996). The CNTs are usually mixed with mineral oil at a certain ration of weight percentage to form CNT-based composite electrodes (Luque et al., 2006; Ly, 2006; Pedano and Rivas, 2004; Rubianes and Rivas, 2005). Similarly, the CNT/Teflon composite was prepared in dry state by hand-mixing CNTs and Teflon, and the resulted composite was then packed firmly into the cavity of a glass sleeve (Wang and Musameh, 2003b). Moreover, the composite electrode using PPy as the binder was made by cyclic voltammetry (CV) in the mixed solution of pyrrole and MWNTs (Cheng et al., 2005). CHIT was also used as a binder (Zhang and Gorski, 2005a, 2005b). The MWNTs were solubilized in the matrix of such hydrophilic ion-conducting biopolymer. In some biosensing applications mentioned above, the CNT based composite was further mixed with biological molecules (enzymes for example) to obtain biomolecule functionalized CNT-based composite electrodes (Luque et al., 2006; Ly, 2006, Rubianes and Rivas, 2005; Wang and Musameh 2003b).

Furthermore, a layer-by-layer (LBL) technique was another method to fabricate CNT-based composite electrode. It was reported that alternate drop casting of carboxylized MWNT suspension and electropolymerization of neutral red (NR) assembled five layers of homogeneous and stable MWNTs and poly(neutral red) (PNR) film on a GCE (Qu et al., 2006).

9.2.3 Nanoparticles Decorated CNT-Based Electrodes

Due to their unique size and shape, nanoparticles (NPs) frequently exhibit unusual physical and chemical properties, such as large surface-to-volumeratio and promotion of the electron transfer. Another important characteristic of some nanoparticles, such as Pt, is the bio-compatibility, which could preserve the biological activity of attached biological molecules. On the other hand, transition metals, especially noble metals, display high catalytic activities for many chemical reactions. Due to these reasons and easy miniaturization to nanoscale dimensions, metallic nanoparticles have been used for chemical/biochemical sensing applications. Further incorporation with CNTs, which have a large surface area, a high ETR and the electrocatalytic activity as well, makes the nanoparticle and CNT modified electrodes achieve a higher sensitivity.

The main techniques have been employed to immobilize metallic nanoparticles on CNT-modified electrodes including: direct adsorption of preformed nanoparticles (Hrapovic et al., 2004; Luque et al., 2006; Male et al., 2004; Wu and Hu, 2005; Yang et al., 2006), chemical deposition from metal salt solutions (Shi et al., 2005), or electrodeposition from metal salt solutions (Fej et al., 2005, Tang et al., 2004). Among them, electrodeposition method is much more efficient as it was capable to control the density and size of metallic nanoparticles through adjusting applied potential (Day et al., 2005, Tang et al., 2004).

In direct adsorption method, the Pt nanoparticles, which could rapidly oxidize H_2O_2 produced from enzymatic reaction, were prepared elsewhere. Subsequently they were dissolved in a Nafion solution (Hrapovic et al., 2004) or a silicate sol (Yang et al., 2006), which were then mixed with CNTs. In contrast, the chemical deposition and electrodeposition of Pt nanoparticles were normally fabricated by the reduction of H_2PtCl_6: after immersing the CNTs or CNT-modified electrodes in H_2PtCl_6 solution, a reductive chemical $Na_2S_2O_4$ (Shi et al., 2005), or a specific potential (Fei et al., 2005, Tang et al., 2004), was applied, respectively.

Cu nanoparticles prepared through the reduction of copper dodecyl sulfate ($Cu(DS)_2$), were embedded in Nafion and SWNTs composite on the surface of a Cu electrode as shown in Fig. 9.3 (Male et al., 2004). Moreover, a biosensor with Cu particles in the manner of direct adsorption was prepared by mixing enzyme, Cu particles and MWNTs with mineral oil to form a composite electrode for glucose detection (Luque et al., 2006). This glucose biosensor also used Ir particles, instead of Cu, for the preparation of the electrode in a similar manner.

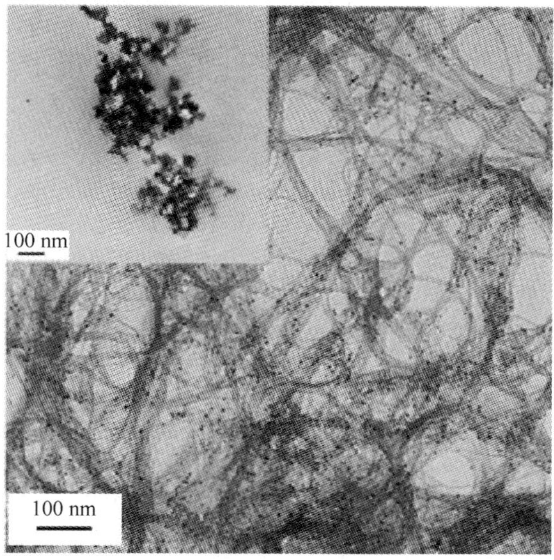

Figure 9.3 TEM image of SWNT decorated with Cu nanoparticles, prepared by reduction of $Cu(DS)_2$. (Inset) TEM image of Cu nanoparticles in the presence of Nafion. Reprinted from (Male et al., 2004) with permission

An MWNT modified Au electrode with Au-colloids adsorption was prepared by solubilizing MWNTs in the DHP which was dispersed in colloid Au aqueous solution for the determination of cytochrome c(Wu and Hu, 2005).

9.2.4 CNTs as Key Sensing Elements

So far, we have discussed using CNTs as the microelectrode modifier for electrochemical detection purpose. In these devices, CNTs mainly work as a role of transducer. However, CNTs, especially SWNTs, could also function as key sensing elements in the detectors with different structures.

Electronic biosensor with CNTFET structure, a type of CNT-based biosensors, has a similar configuration to MOSFET. However, in CNTFET, SWNTs are utilized as the conducting channel, instead of silicon channel. As the SWNT conducting channel of CNTFET is open to the environment, it is found to be very sensitive to the variation of environmental conditions. The SWNTs across the source and drain could be implemented through direct growth using CVD technique or AC dielectrophoresis technique (Li et al., 2004; Li et al., 2005). These SWNTs were individual semiconducting nanotube bundles (Besteman et al., 2003; Bradley et al., 2004; Star et al., 2003), or SWNT networks (Bradley et al., 2005; Star et al., 2006). For the detection purpose, SWNTs working as sensing part were exposed to detection species, while a back gate (silicon or gold) (Kojima et al., 2005; Star et al., 2003) or a liquid gate (Chen et al., 2003, 2004) was used to measure the device responses to detection species.

In order to achieve higher sensitivity for specific species, the SWNTs in most of CNTFETs were functionalized with biological molecules, such as antibodies for specific recognition, ssDNA array for detection of DNA hybridization and enzymes for the study of enzymatic reaction, etc. As shown in Fig. 9.4(a), these biological molecules were observed to non-covalent adsorb on the SWNTs (Bradley et al., 2005; Byon and Choi, 2006; Chen et al., 2004; Kojima et al., 2005; Star et al., 2004; Star et al., 2006; Tang et al., 2006) via weak interactions such as hydrophobic interaction between the nanotubes and hydrophobic domains of biological molecules (Shim et al., 2002). The immobilization of biological molecules could also be implemented through a linking layer, such as carbodiimidazole-activated Tween 20 (CDI-Tween) (Chen et al., 2003; So et al., 2005), polyethyleneimine/polyethyleneglycol (PEI/PEG) (Rouhanizadeh et al., 2005; Star et al., 2003), 1-pyrenebutanoic acid succinimidyl ester (Besteman et al., 2003; Li et al., 2005), which could be coated on the nanotubes prior to the functionalization (Fig. 9.4(b)). These linking molecules bound one end of their molecule chains to SWNTs through van der Waals interactions, while their other end attached to the biological molecules through amide bond formation.

It has been reported that the CNTFET could also be functionalized at the back gate region instead on SWNTs (Maehashi et al., 2004; Takeda et al., 2005), which might affect the effect potential around SWNTs during experiments (Fig. 9.4(c)).

9.2.5 CNT-Based Biosensors with Immobilized Biological Molecules

In order to improve the sensitivity and selectivity of CNT-based biosensors for detecting of some specific species, a broad spectrum of biological molecules, including DNA and proteins (enzymes and antibodies, etc.), were immobilized on these biosensors. These biosensors can be grouped into two main categories: electrochemical biosensors and CNTFET-based electronic biosensors. In the

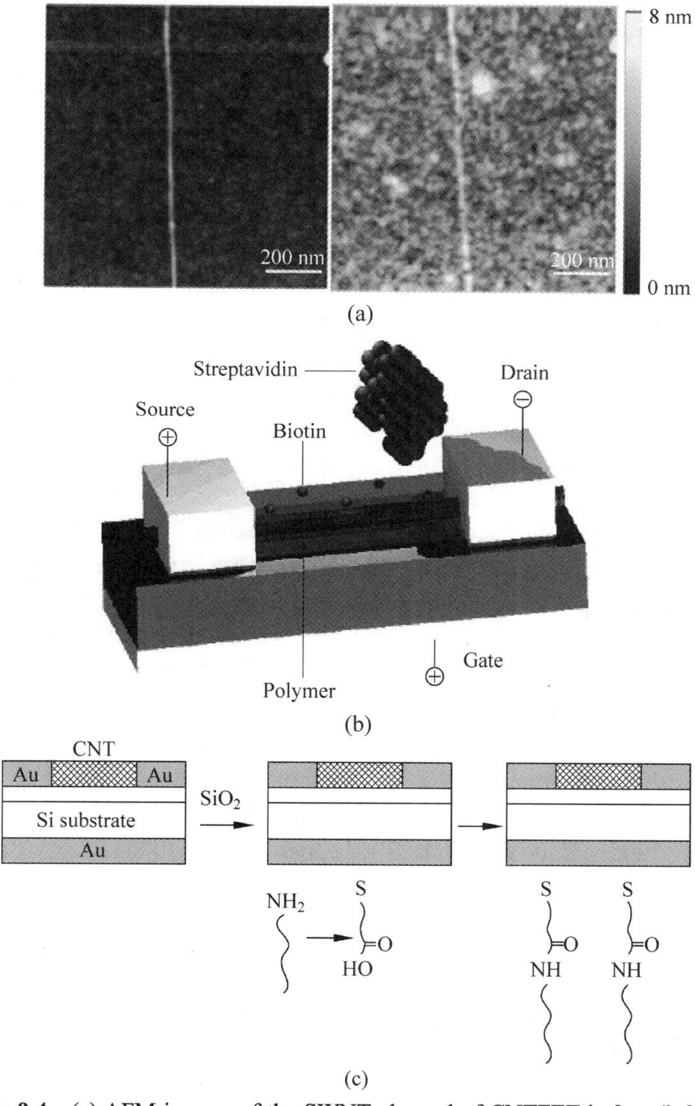

Figure 9.4 (a) AFM images of the SWNT channel of CNTFET before (left) and after (right) the direct adsorption of α-PSA. Reprinted from (Kojima et al., 2005) with permission. (b) Schematic of the CNTFET with a polymeric linking layer. A molecular receptor was used to functionalize such polymer for the recognition of a biomolecule. Reprinted from (Star et al., 2003) with permission. (c) Chemical modification scheme at the gold back gate region of CNTFET for the conjugation with biomolecules. Reprinted from (Maehashi et al., 2004) with permission

former one, CNTs mainly serves as transducer which converts the signals from the active biological molecules to the electrode substrate through electrochemical reactions. While in the latter as described in previous part, CNTs it plays a key role in sensing by a nanoscale transistor built by CNTs. Two techniques developed for immobilizing of probe molecules are covalent attachment and noncovalent attachment including direct adsorption and entrapment method. In the following, a brief overview of various immobilization techniques is given.

9.2.5.1 Direct Adsorption

Noncovalent functionalization of CNTs could be realized through weak interactions, e.g. hydrogen bonding, π-π stacking, electrostatic forces, van der Waals forces and hydrophobic interactions, which could be used to directly adsorb biological molecules on CNTs ((Trojanowicz, 2006) and references therein).

In electrochemical biosensors, pre-CNT-modification method, in other words, mixing CNT and biomolecules first and cast the electrode with the resulting mixture later, is a simple way for the direct adsorption of biological molecules on the electrode surface. A glucose biosensor was demonstrated by using a mixture of MWNTs, Nafion and Glucose Oxidase (Gox) as the GCE modifier (Tsai et al., 2005). A similar process could be seen from these biosensors based on CNT-composite electrode (Ly, 2006; Rubianes and Rivas, 2005). In addition, MWNT, Teflon and GOx were hand-mixed together in the dry state and the prepared composite electrode was used for glucose detection (Wang and Musameh, 2003b).

Biomolecules immobilization could also be achieved by post-CNT-modification, including incubation of the CNT-modified electrode in the biomolecules solution (Tang et al., 2004; Wang et al., 2003a; Wang et al., 2003b; Zhang et al., 2005), or drop cast small volume of the biomolecules solution on the CNT-modified electrode (Deo et al., 2005; Hrapovic et al., 2004; Joshi et al., 2005; Zhao et al., 2005). GOx/PtNP/CNT/graphite electrode for glucose detection was prepared by incubation the PtNP/CNT/graphite electrode in the enzyme GOx solution for 12 h, and then washed carefully with double-distilled water and dried (Tang et al., 2004). Another example was that an MWNT-modified electrode was dropped with 10 μL AChE solution for organophosphorus compound detection (Joshi et al., 2005).

In order to optimize performance of electrodes through adjusting controlled thickness, structural morphology, and biocatalyst loading, the LBL technique was also involved in direct adsorption of biomolecules on CNT-modified electrode. Alternate layers of GOx adsorbed MWNTs could be simply prepared by repeatedly immersing the electrode to MWNT solution and then GOx solution (Huang et al., 2006). This technique could also be applied to achieve alternate electrostatic adsorption of different charged components. MWNTs wrapped by positively charged poly(diallyldimethylammonium chloride) (PDDA) were assembled layer-by-layer with negatively charged GOx on a chemically functionalized Au electrode (Zhao and Ju, 2006) (Fig. 9.5). Similar structures were presented (Guo et al., 2004; Liu and Lin, 2006).

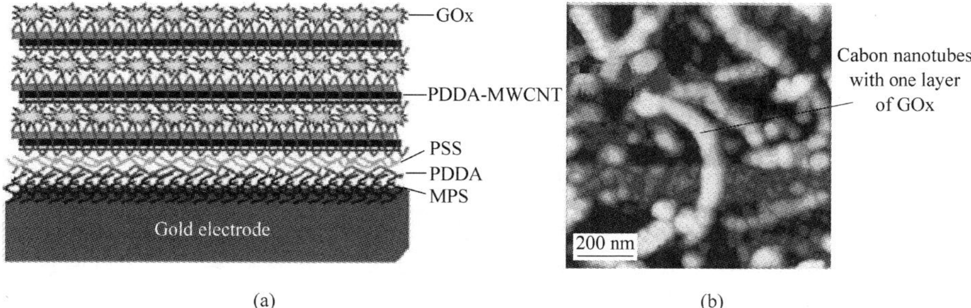

Figure 9.5 (a) Schematic of the multilayer membranes prepared by LBL technique. (b) AFM image of GOx-PDDA·MWNT (LBL)/PSS/PDDA/MPS membranes on gold electrode. Reprinted from (Zhao and Ju, 2006) with permission

Noncovalent adsorption of biological molecules could also be enhanced by using cross-linking molecules. After dropping the enzyme solution on Pt nanoparticle decorated SWNT/GCE, glutaraldehyde was applied on the resulting electrode to crosslink enzyme (Hrapovic et al., 2004). Similarly, GOx was immobilized onto PNR/MWNT multilayers modified GCE by crosslinking enzyme using glutaraldehyde (Qu et al., 2006). Moreover, prevention of the biological molecules from loss could also be implemented by covering a protective thin film say Nafion, which improved the anti-interferent ability of relevant electrodes simultaneously (Tang et al., 2004).

Switch intention to electronic biosensors based on CNTFET structure, biological molecules were found to directly adsorb on the SWNTs if a linking molecule layer was not introduced (Bradley et al., 2005; Byon and Choi, 2006; Chen et al., 2004; Kojima et al., 2005; Star et al., 2004; Star et al., 2006; Tang et al., 2006).

9.2.5.2 Entrapment

Biological molecule entrapment is other method to noncovalently immobilize biological molecules on the electrode surface. It can be achieved in two ways, i.e., encapsulation and electropolymerization.

In encapsulation methodology, biological molecules were immobilized within hydrogels or sol-gel materials while retained their native bioactivity. Hydrogel and sol-gel have excellent properties including high binding capacity with electrodes, large surface area, and an improvement in the electrical communication between electrodes and biological molecules, etc. These positive aspects enhance the sensor response. The encapsulation can be realized by pre-CNT-modification method, which incorporate biological molecules and CNTs into the hydrogel or the sol-gel matrix at first and subsequently casting this composite onto the support electrode (Fig. 9.6(a)) (Joshi et al., 2005). Two glucose biosensors were prepared in this scheme by encapsulating GOx, as well as CNTs, into a sol-gel matrix (Kandimalla et al., 2006; Yang et al., 2006). Alternatively, in post-CNT-modification method, biological molecules incubated in hydrogel or sol-gel matrix could be brought onto the CNT-modified electrodes (Fig. 9.6(b)), as suggested for a glucose biosensor (Salimi et al., 2004) and cholesterol biosensor (Shi et al., 2005).

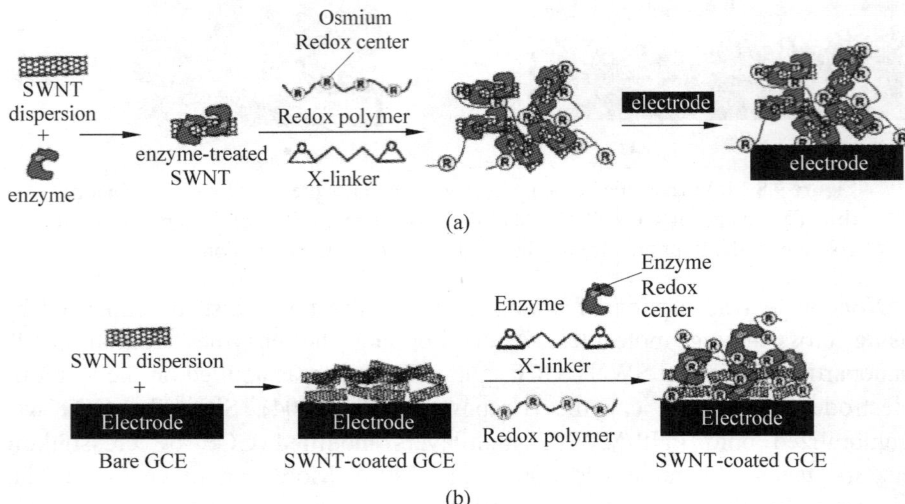

Figure 9.6 Schematic of biomolecules encapsulation with CNT: (a) fabrication of sensor via pre-CNT-modification method. CNTs were first incubated with an enzyme solution, and then the hydrogel or sol-gel was introduced to form a matrix, which is later brought on a substrate. (b) fabrication of sensor via post-CNT-modification method. A film of CNTs was first cast onto a support electrode. Subsequently, a hydrogel or sol-gel composite containing enzyme is casted on such a CNT-coated electrode. Reprinted from (Joshi et al., 2005) with permission

Biological molecules could also be embedded into a polymer matrix simply by mixing them with the monomer. The mixture is then electropolymerized on support electrode. The intimate contact between the biocomponent and polymer enable an efficient signal transduction. A highly sensitive glucose sensor was constructed on an MWNT modified electrode based on the entrapment of GOx on poly-*o*-aminophenol (POAP)-electropolymerized matrix (Ye et al., 2005). PPy was other polymer used for this purpose, since it can be electropolymerized at neutral pH and allow the entrapment of a wide range of biocatalysts. The pyrrole electropolymerization aided GOx immobilization could be performed not only on non-oriented CNT-modified electrode via mixing pyrrole, GOx and oxidized MWNTs (Wang and Musameh, 2005a), but also on aligned CNT arrays (Gao et al., 2003). Figure 9.7 shows SEM images of such a PPy-coated CNT array.

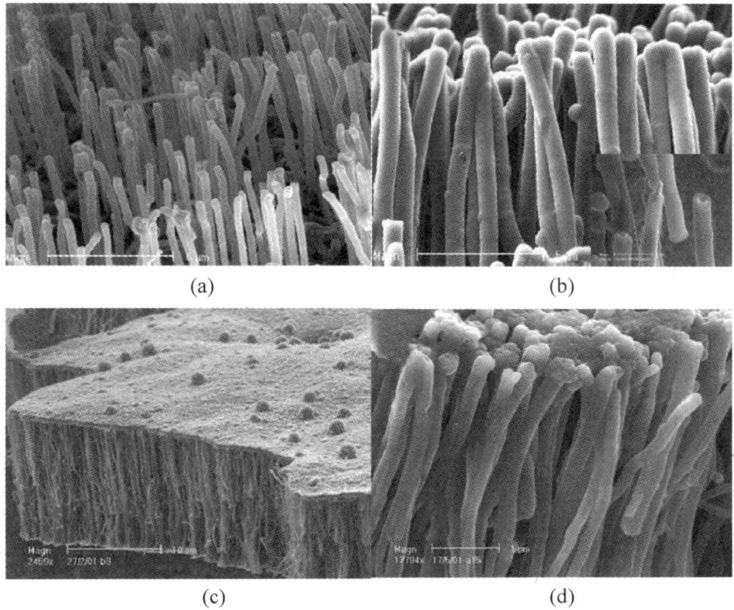

Figure 9.7 SEM images of: (a) pristine CNT array. (b) aligned PPy-CNT coaxial nanowires. (c) PPy only deposited on the top surface of CNTs due to the high density of tube array. (d) polymer formed on both walls and top surface of the CNT array. Reprinted from (Gao et al., 2003) with permission

9.2.5.3 Covalent Attachment

Typically, the biological molecules are randomly distributed on the electrode surface if noncovalent immobilization method is utilized. In addition, the direct adsorption may be not strong so that some biological molecules may loss during analysis. In contrast, covalent attachment method could produce a robust immobilization of biological molecules. And the distribution of biological molecules could also be somewhat controlled by using CNTs as framework. For instance, enzyme GOx was found to covalently attach to the broken tips of vertically aligned MWNTs via amide linkages between amine residues on GOx and carboxylic groups on the MWNT tips in the presence of coupling agents 1-ethyl-3-(3-dimethylaminopropyl)carbodiimide (EDC) (Lin et al., 2004). Through amide linkage, it has been confirmed that flavin adenine dinucleotide (FAD) covalently bound to the tips of self-assembled MWNT arrays and then apo-GOx was reconstituted on the FAD units. This structure can enhance direct electron transfer between electrode and redox active center of GOx (Liu et al., 2005; Patolsky et al., 2004). Figure 9.8 illustrates the fabrication scheme and relevant AFM images of such an electrode.

In comparison, researchers did not immobilize biological molecules directly on SWNTs through covalent bond in CNTFET-based electronic biosensors. Because they believed that oxidation of SWNTs broke up the aromaticity of benzene units

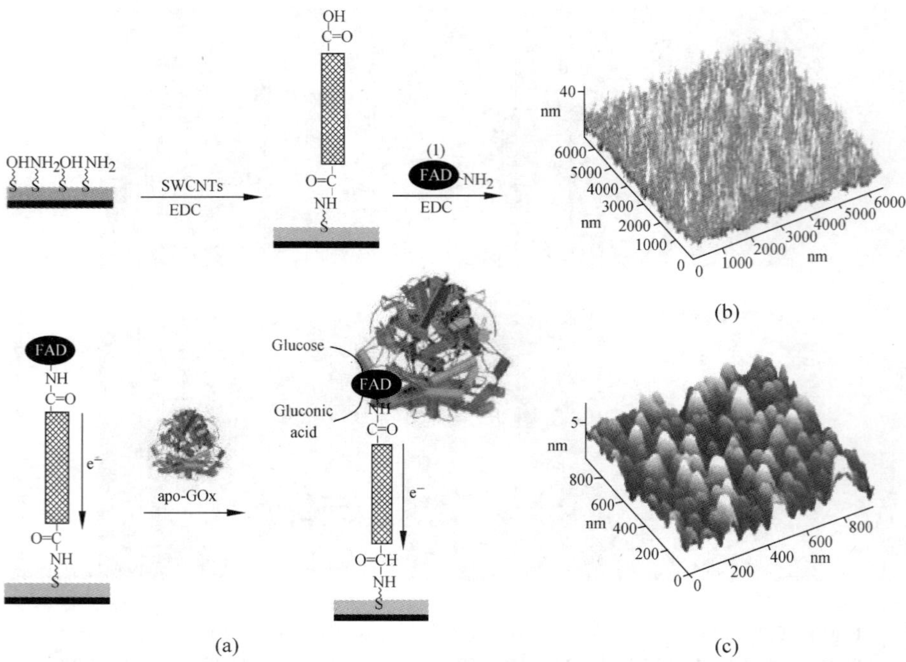

Figure 9.8 (a) Schematic of self-assembled SWNT array and then covalent binding with Gox; (b) AFM image of self-assembled SWNT array through covalently linking to a cystamine/2-thioethanol monolayer functionalized Au electrode after 90 min of coupling; (c) AFM image of the GOx reconstituted on the FAD-functionalized CNTs array. Reprinted from (Patolsky et al., 2004) with permission

of SWNTs and imparted carboxyl and ether substituents on sidewall of SWNTs, which may affect the intrinsic electronic property of SWNT. Instead, biological molecules were covalently attached to the SWNTs via linking molecules, of which other end bound to SWNTs through van der Waals interactions or π-π stacking (Besteman et al., 2003; Chen et al., 2003; Li et al., 2005; Maehashi et al., 2004; Rouhanizadeh et al., 2006; So et al., 2005; Star et al., 2003; Takeda et al., 2005).

9.3 Electrochemical Detection of Biomolecules

Electrochemical techniques of detecting biomaterials in solutions are attractive because of their simplicity and low-cost. In this section we discuss various electrochemical biosensors based on CNTs. In the first part we discuss the assessment criteria for different biosensors. We will present a large number of biosensors to detect various biomolecules in the second part. We also compile glucose biosensors modified by CNT in Table 9.1, and CNT-modified DNA biosensor in Table 9.2. Other biomolecule-functionalized electrochemical biosensors are summarized in Table 9.3. Biosensors without biomolecule-functionalization are summarized in Table 9.4.

Table 9.1 Summary of CNT-based electrochemical glucose biosensors and their important parameters

No. & Ref. evence	Electrodes	Design principles	Sensitivity $[(mmol/L)^{-1}]$	Linear range [mmol/L]	Res-ponse time [s]	Stability
G1 (Male et al., 2004)	CuNP-SWNT-Nafion/ GCE and CuNP-SWNT-Nafion/Cu	Nanoparticle decoration	256 μA	$2.5 \times 10^{-4} - 0.5$	10	
G2 (Tang et al., 2004)	Nafion/Gox/PtNP/CNT/ graphite	Nanoparticle decoration, direct adsorption	14 μA	0.1 – 13.5	<5	73.5% after 22 days
G3 (Hrapovic et al., 2004)	Gox/PtNP-SWNT-Nafion/ GCE	Nanoparticle decoration, direct adsorption	2.11 μA	0.0005 – 5	3	
G4 (Wang et al., 2003b)	Gox/MWNT-array/Au	Oriented modification, direct adsorption	1.75 μA	0.05 – 13	<16	96.3% after 1 month, 94.4% after 2 month, and 91.2% after 3 month
G5 (Yang et al., 2006)	Gox/PtNP-Silicate-SGC-MWNTPE	Nanoparticle decoration, direct adsorption	1.11 μA	1 – 25	<15	90% after 3 days, and 80% after 1 month
G6 (Ye et al., 2005)	POAP-Gox/FePc-MWNT/ GCE	Entrapment	0.735 μA	0.0005 – 4	<8	120 days
G7 (Qu et al., 2006)	Gox/PNR-cMWNT (LBL)/GCE	Direct adsorption	0.6 μA	0.05 – 10	<10	Constant in first 17 days, and 85% after 1 month
G8 (Tsai et al., 2005)	Gox-MWNT-Nafion/GCE	Entrapment	0.33 μA	0.025 – 2	<3	
G9 (Gao et al., 2003)	Gox-Ppy/MWNT-array/Au	Oriented modification, Entrapment	0.31 μA	2.5 – 20		70% after 3 days
G10 (Ye et al., 2004)	MWNT-array/GCE	Oriented modification	0.22 μA	0.002 – 11	<10	

Continued

No. & Ref. evence	Electrodes	Design principles	Sensitivity $[(mmol/L)^{-1}]$	Linear range [mmol/L]	Res-ponse time [s]	Stability
G11 (Salimi et al., 2004)	Gox-SGC/MWNT/BPPG	Entrapment	0.196 μA	0.2 – 20	<5	3 weeks
G12 (Wang and Musameh, 2003b)	Gox/Teflon-MWNT	CNT composite electrode, direct adsorption	0.14 μA	2 – 12	25	
G13 (Zhao and Ju, 2006)	Gox-PDDA·MWNT(LBL)/ PSS/PDDA/MPS/Au	Entrapment	44 nA	0.058 – 5	<8	82% after 5 weeks
G14 (Huang et al., 2006)	Gox-MWNT(LBL)/graphite	Entrapment	39 nA	0.5 – 15	6.7	
G15 (Kandimalla et al., 2006)	Gox-FMC-BSA-MWNT-SGC/GCE	Entrapment	18 nA	0.05 – 20	25	96% after 110 days
G16 (Luque et al., 2006)	Gox-CuNP-MWNTPE, Gox-IrNP-MWNTPE	CNT composite electrode, nanoparticle decoration, direct adsorption	8.3 nA (Cu), 7.1 nA (Ir)	1.8 – 12 (Cu), 0 – 20 (Ir)	10 (Cu), 12 (Ir)	Constant in 2 months, and 24% after 6 months
G17 (Lin et al., 2004)	Gox-cMWNT-array/Si	Oriented modification, covalent attachment	~2.5 nA	0.08 – 30	20 – 30	
G18 (Wang and Musameh, 2005a)	Ppy-Gox-cMWNT/GCE	Entrapment	2.33 nA	0.2 – 50	15	

The blanks in the columns indicate that these data were not available in corresponding references. If not indicating 'oriented modification' in the column of 'Design priciples', 'non-oriented modification' is a default design principle.

C carbozylized, BPPG basal plane pyrolytic graphite, BSA bovine serum albumin, FePc iron phthalocyanine, FMC ferrocenemonocarboxylic acid, GCE glassy carbon electrode, Gox glucose Oxidase, LBL layer-by-layer technique, MPS 3-mercapto-1-propanesulfonic-acid, NP Nanoparticle, PDDA poly(dimethyldiallylammonium chloride), MWNTPE MWNTpaste electrode, PNR poly(neutral red), POAP poly-*o*-aminophenol, Ppy polypyrrole, PSS poly(sodium 4-styrenesulfonate), SGC sol-gel composite.

Table 9.2 Summary of CNT-based electrochemical DNA biosensors

Objective	No.	Sensors	Design Principles	Ref.
DNA hybridization	D1	DNR; ssDNA-cMWNT/GCE	Covalent attachment	(Cai et al., 2003a)
	D2	ssDNA-Ppy/cMWNT/GCE	Entrapment	(Cai et al., 2003b)
	D3	$Ru(bpy)_3^{2+}$; ssDNA-cMWNT-array-SiO_2/Si	Oriented modification, covalent attachment	(Koehne et al., 2003; Koehne et al., 2004; Li et al., 2003)
	D4	ssDNA/cMWNT-DNA/CPE	Covalent attachment	(Kerman et al., 2004)
	D5	DNR; cMWNT-Ppy/GCE; ssDNA/RSH/MNP	CNT composite electrode	(Cheng et al., 2005)
	D6	MWNT/GCE; probe-ssDNA-MNP; target-ssDNA-ALP		(Wang et al., 2004b)
	D7	MB; ssDNA-cMWNT-array/Au	Oriented modification, covalent attachment	(Wang et al., 2004)
	D8	DNR; ssDNA-cMWNT-PtNP-Nafion/GCE	Covalent attachment	(Zhu et al., 2005)
	D9	MWNT/GCE; probe-ssDNA1-cCNT-ALP; probe-ssDNA2-MNP		(Wang et al., 2004a)
	D10	MWNT/GCE; probe-ssDNA1/PSS/ALP-PDDA (LBL)/SWNT; probe-ssDNA2-MNP		(Munge et al., 2005)
DNA and nucleic acids	D11	SWNT/GCE		(Wang et al., 2004)
	D12	MWNTPE	CNT composite electrode	(Pedano and Rivas, 2004)
	D13	MB; DNA/MWNT-chitosan/graphite	Direct adsorption	(Li et al., 2005)

If not indicating 'oriented modification' in the column of 'Design priciples', 'non-oriented modification' is a default design principle.

c carbozylized, ALP alkaline phosphatase, CPE carbon paste electrode, DNR daunomycin, GCE glassy carbon electrode, LBL layer-by-layer technique, MB methylene blue, MNP magnetite nanoparticle, MWNTPE MWNTpaste electrode, NP nanoparticle, PDDA poly(diallyldimethylammoniumchloride), PPy polypyrrole, PSS poly(sodium 4-styrenesulfonate), RSH mercapatoacetic acid, ssDNA single-stranded DNA.

Table 9.3 Summary of biomolecules-functionalized CNT-based biosensors

Analyte	Occurrence	Biomolecule functionzlied on electrode	Electrodes	Design Principles	Ref. No.
Cholesterol	Blood	Cholesterol oxidase (ChOx)	PDDA-ChOx(LBL)/ cMWNTs/Au	Entrapment	(Guo et al., 2004)
			ChOx/MWNT/SPE	Direct adsorption	(Li et al., 2005)
			ChOx-SGC/PtNP/ CNT/graphite	Nanoparticle decoration, entrapment	(Shi et al., 2005)
			ChOx/PVA/MWNT-array/Si	Oriented modification, direct adsorption	(Roy et al., 2006)
Choline	Tissues	Choline oxidase (ChOx)	ChOx-SGC/MWNT/ Pt	Entrapment	(Song et al., 2006)
Dopamine	Brain tissue, blood	DNA	DNA/CNTPE	CNT composite electrode	(Ly, 2006)
DNA	Bioassays	ssDNA	See Table 9.2		
Glucose	Blood, body fluids	Glucose oxidase (GOx)	See Table 9.1		
Lactate	Human sweat	Lactate oxidase (LOx)	LOx/cSWNT/GCE LOx/cSWNT/Si/ITO	Direct adsorption	(Weber et al., 2006)
			LOx/CNTPE	CNT composite electrode, direct adsorption	(Rubianes and Rivas, 2005)
Organophos-phate compounds	Agriculture, environment	Acteylcholin-esterase (AChE)	AChE/MWNT/SPE	Direct adsorption	(Joshi et al., 2005)
			PDDA-AChE(LBL) /MWNT/GCE	Entrapment	(Liu and Lin, 2006)
		Organophos-p horus hydrolase (OPH)	OPH/MWNT-Nafion/GCE	Direct adsorption	(Deo et al., 2005)
Phenolic compounds	Water, food products	Polyphenol oxidase (PPOx)	PPOx/CNTPE	Direct adsorption	(Rubianes and Rivas, 2005)
		Tyrosinase (Ty)	Nafion/Ty/SWNT/ GCE	Direct adsorption	(Zhao et al., 2005)
Putrescine	Tissue, pharmacy	Putrescine oxidase (POx)	Glutaraldehyde/ POx/APTES-MWNT-Nafion/GCE	Entrapment	(Luong et al., 2005)

If not indicating 'oriented modification' in the column of 'Design priciples', 'non-oriented modification' is a default design principle.

c carbozylized, APTES γ–aminopropyltriethoxysilane, CNTPE CNT paste electrode, GCE glassy carbon electrode, ITO indium tin oxide, LBL layer-by-layer technique, NP nanoparticle, PDDA poly(diallyldimethylammoniumchloride), PVA polyvinyl alcohol, SGC sol-gel composite, SPE screen-printed electrode.

Table 9.4 Summary of biomolecule-free CNT-based biosensors for various biological molecules

Analyte	Occurrence	Electrodes	Ref. No.
L-Cysteine	Biological system	Pt/CNT/graphite	(Fei et al., 2005)
Cytochrome *c*	Biological system	aSWNT/GCE	(Wang et al., 2002)
		AuNP/MWNT/DHP/Au	(Wu and Hu, 2005)
Dopamine	Brain tissue, blood	CNT/bromoform/glass-tube	(Britto et al., 1996)
		MWNT-Nafion/CFE	(Hocevar et al., 2005)
		PSS/SWNT/GCE	(Zhang et al., 2006)
Folic acid	Tissue, food products	MWNT/Au	(Wei et al., 2006)
Glutathione	Biological system	CNT-array	(Tang et al., 2006)
Indole-3-acetic acid	Plant cells	MWNT/GCE	(Wu et al., 2003)
Lincomycin	Pharmacy	MWNT-DHP/GCE MWNT-SDBS/GCE MWNT-Nafion/GCE	(Wu et al., 2006)
Morphine	Blood, body fluids	MWNT/GCE	(Salimi et al., 2005)
NADH	Living cells	MWNT/GCE	(Musameh et al., 2002)
		TB/MWNT/BPPG AC/MWNT/BPPG	(Lawrence and Wang, 2006)
		TBO-CHIT-MWNT/GCE	(Zhang and Gorski, 2005b)
		AZU-CHIT/MWNT/GCE	(Zhang and Gorski, 2005a)
		CNTEC	(Pumera et al., 2006)
Nitric oxide	Biological system	Nafion/MWNT/GCE	(Wu et al., 2002)
		Myb/MWNT/GCE	(Zhang et al., 2005)
Phenolic compounds	Water, food products	MWNT-Nafion/GCE	(Wang et al., 2003a)
Procaine	Pharmacy	MWNT/GCE	(Wu et al., 2006)
Theophylline	Pharmacy	cMWNT/GCE	(Zhu et al., 2005)
Quercetin	Flavor, pharmacy	MWNT/Ch/graphite	(Jin et al., 2006)
Rutin	Plants	MWNT- β-CD/GCE	(He et al., 2006)
		SWNT/Au	(Zeng et al., 2006)
Thiocholine	Environment	CNT/GCE	(Liu et al., 2005)

a actived, AC azure C, AZU Azure dye, BPPG basal plane pyrolytic graphite, CD cyclodextrin, CFE carbon fiber electrode, Ch choline, CHIT chitosan, CNTEC CNT-epoxy composite, DHP dihexadecylphosphate, GCE glassy carbon electrode, Myb myoglobin, NP nanoparticle, PSS poly(styrene sulfonic acid) sodium salt, SDBS sodium dodecylbenzenesulfonate, TB toluidine blue, TBO toluidine Blue O.

9.3.1 Assessment Criteria of Sensors

When designing various CNT-based biosensors for practical application, several measurement parameters are of importance. Detection range is the most essential one, which determines the sensitivity, specificity and dynamic range required by the sensors. For example, normal level of glucose in human vein is 3.89 – 6.11 mmol/L and thus the fasting plasma glucose level at or above 7.0 mmol/L is diagnosed as diabetes. Because of this, a practical glucose sensor should cover a detection range from a few μmol/L to 15 mmol/L. A cholesterol sensor should be sensitive in the range of 50 – 400 mg/dL (1.3 – 10.4 mmol/L), because the desirable level of LDL cholesterol is considered to be less than 100 mg/dL (2.6 mmol/L) and a patient who has a level of larger than 240 mg/dL (>6.2 mmol/L) of cholesterol is running a high risk of heart disease. As some biomolecules, like enzymes, degrade during storage, a biosensor with high stability is a vital characteristic. Of course, specificity, sensitivity, accuracy, response time and reproducibility, etc, are also very critical to electrochemical sensors.

9.3.2 Electrochemical Biosensors

9.3.2.1 Glucose

Glucose is the principal circulating sugar in the blood and the major energy source of the body. A high fasting blood sugar level is an indication of prediabetic and diabetic conditions. As a result, a tight monitoring of blood glucose level is one of the most frequently performed routine analyses in clinics and hospitals.

Conventionally, enzyme GOx is used in biosensors to detect the concentration of glucose. GOx catalyzes the oxidation of β-D-glucose into D-glucono-1,5-lactone, while oxygen (O_2) acts as final electron acceptor and then is reduced as hydrogen peroxide (H_2O_2), which is electrochemically detectable. The concentration of glucose is determined by monitoring the resulting charge and current through enzyme.

We compiled the design principles and performance characteristics of reported CNT-based biosensors in a descent order of sensitivity in Table 9.1, where the performance of a variety CNT-based glucose sensor are listed. One should note that the total electrode current was referred in comparison of the sensitivities because the surface area of electrodes was seldom reported in most of papers.

One can see that four of the top five most sensitive glucose biosensors were decorated with metallic nanoparticles. The sensor with Cu Nanoparticle (G1) exhibited a highest sensitivity of 256 $\mu A/(mmol \cdot L^{-1})$ as shown in Fig. 9.9(a). But the linear range from 2.5×10^{-4} to 0.5 mmol/L, was much lower than clinical detection level of glucose. Pt nanoparticle-decorated sensor G2, G3, and G5 showed preferable linear detecting range. Figure 9.9(b) illustrated the response of sensor G5 to glucose with and without Pt nanoparticle attachment. In addition, both G2 and G3 used a pre-selective membrane Nafion to improve the selectivity of such sensors. The difference is that G3 utilized Nafion as solubilizing agent of CNTs, while a thin Nafion layer was coated on the surface of CNT-modified electrode in G2. Compared with another nanoparticles decorated CNT-based glucose biosensors (G1, G3, G5 and G16), G2 showed a superior performance with relatively high sensitivity and clinically compatible detection range.

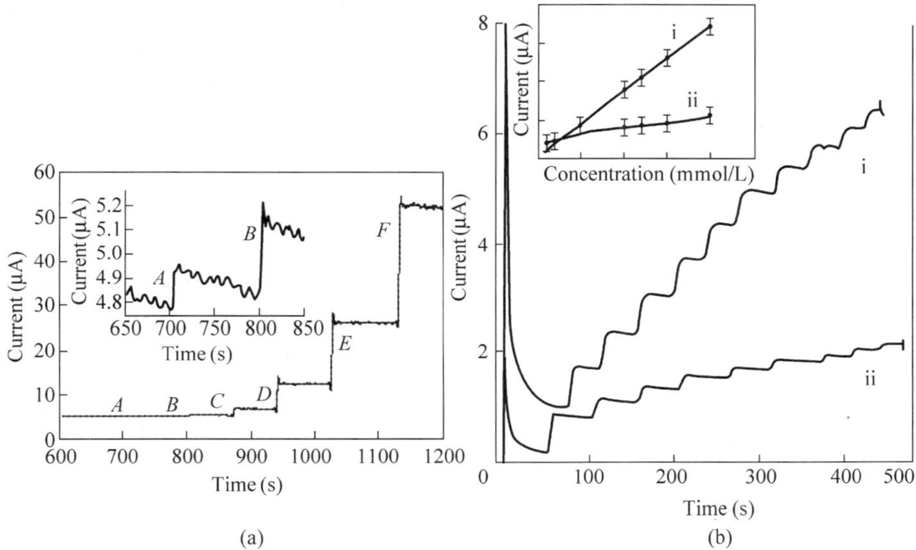

Figure 9.9 (a) The performance of sensor G1 with CuNP-SWNT-Nafion/GCE (refer to Table 9.1) in amperometrically detecting glucose of different concentrations, 0.5, 1.0, 5, 20, 50, 100 μmol/L at 0.65 V vs. Ag/AgCl (3 mol/L NaCl). (Inset) addition of 0.5 μmol/L and 1.0 μmol/L of glucose, respectively. Reprinted from (Male et al., 2004) with permission. (b) Real-time monitor of successive addition of 2 mmol/L glucose at the biosensors (i) with Pt nanoparticles and (ii) without Pt nanoparticles measured at 0.1 V vs. SCE. (Inset) the calibration curve for the glucose addition. Reprinted from (Yang et al., 2006) with permission

Immobilization of GOx on the electrode surface using entrapment methods (electropolymerization and encapsulation) was also commonly adopted. G6 immobilized GOx on a poly-*o*-aminophenol (POAP) electropolymerized electrode surface. GOx was immobilized in a Nafion matrix in G8. Both G9 and G18 entrapped GOx within an electropolymerized PPy film, but G18 exhibited a much lower sensitivity. This could be attributed to the fact that the MWNTs were in direct contact with the substrate of G9, while the CNTs are just suspended and loosely contacted with the substrate of G18. G11 and G15 both encapsulated GOx into a sol-gel composite, and the resulted sensitivities were 196 and 18 nA, respectively. In G13 and G14, LBL technique was utilized to entrap GOx with CNTs at the surface of the electrode. In this category of sensors, G11 is more practical for clinical application.

In term of the response time, Pt Nanoparticle-decorated sensors S2 and S3 demonstrated the fastest response of less that 5 s with high sensitivity. Some biosensors prepared by entrapment of GOx, say G8 and G11, also showed a fast response. However, the sensors without GOx, such as G1 and G10, had relatively slow response.

9.3.2.2 Cholesterol

Cholesterol is a fatty lipid that is a primary component of the cell membranes and a precursor to steroid hormones. Cholesterol is also found in the blood circulation of humans. Its concentration in the blood plasma can influence the pathogenesis of some conditions, such as the development of atherosclerotic plaque and coronary artery disease. In this sense, the determination of cholesterol concentration in clinical diagnosis is essential. To prepare amperometric cholesterol biosensor, Guo and coworkers utilized LBL technique to deposit cholesterol oxidase (ChOx) onto carboxylized-MWNTs/Au electrode (Guo et al., 2004). The device detection range for cholesterol measurement was from 0.2 up to 6 mmol/L. A biosensor based on MWNTs/screen-printed-carbon electrodes was also used to detect cholesterol in the range of 100 – 400 mg/dL (Li et al., 2005). Moreover, by immobilizing ChOx with sol-gel on Pt nanoparticles decorated CNT/graphite electrodes, Shi et al. developed a sensor for the detection ranging from 4 to 100 μmol/L (Shi et al., 2005). In addition, vertically-aligned MWNTs modified with polyvinyl alcohol (PVA) was reported to detect cholesterol (Roy et al., 2006).

9.3.2.3 Choline

Choline, often classified in the vitamin B complex, is a natural amine and essential for cardiovascular and brain function and for cellular membrane composition and repair. An amperometric sensor for choline detection has been demonstrated by immobilization of choline oxidase within aqueous sol-gel-based composites on an MWNTs coated Pt electrode (Song et al., 2006). The choline sensor exhibited a wide measurement range (5 – 100 μmol/L), fast response (< 8 s) and low detection limit (0.1 μmol/L).

9.3.2.4 L-Cysteine

Cysteine is one of the 20 amino acids commonly found in animal proteins. Its L-stereoisomer participates in the biosynthesis of mammalian protein. Cysteine is often used to produce of various flavors. Therefore, determination of L-cysteine is very important in food, pharmaceutical and personal care industries. But due to slow electron transfer, conventional electrodes are not satisfactory. In contrast, Pt decorated MWNT/graphite electrodes were capable of sensing L-cysteine with a large detection range of 0.5 – 100 μmol/L (Fei et al., 2005).

9.3.2.5 Cytochrome *c*

Cytochrome *c*, or cyt *c*, is a highly conserved protein, can be found in plants, animals, and many unicellular organisms. It is also a small heme protein found loosely associated with the inner membrane of the mitochondrion. However, detection of cyt *c* always faces difficulty because of the non-effective detection attributed to the protein denaturation at electrode surface and subsequently extremely slow electron-transfer kinetics. A CNT based cyt *c* sensor was demonstrated with activated SWNTs film modified GCE (Wang et al., 2002). The peak current of such sensor increased linearly with the concentration of cyt *c* in the range of from 30 to 700 μmol/L. In addition, colloid Au (diameter of 20 nm) immobilized MWNTs/Au electrode was prepared for the same purpose (Wu and Hu, 2005).

9.3.2.6 Dopamine

Dopamine is a kind of chemicals naturally produced in the body. In human brain, dopamine functions as a neurotransmitter and a neurohormone. Thus it is essential to the normal functioning of the central nervous system. Dopamine is also used as a medication that acts on the sympathetic nervous system, producing effects such as increased heart rate and blood pressure. Obviously, precise determination of dopamine in brain tissues is demanded in clinical diagnoses. The first reported biosensor using CNTs modified electrode was a dopamine biosensor by Britto et al. (Britto et al., 1996). Figure 9.10(a) depicts the differential pulse voltammetry (DPV) response of this sensor for various concentrations of dopamine. In addition to this, CNT-modified electrodes, combined with negatively charged pre-selective membrane, including Nafion (Hocevar et al., 2005) and poly(styrene sulfonic acid) (PSS) (Zhang et al., 2006), were used to detect dopamine in the presence ascorbate and ascorbic acid. Hocevar et al. invented a disposable dopamine microsensor utilizing MWNT and Nafion modified carbon fiber microelectrode to achieve a linear detection range from 2 to 20 μmol/L and a detection limit of 70 nmol/L towards dopamine (Hocevar et al., 2005). The dopamine sensor based on PSS/ SWNT/GCE exhibited good performance, such as a large determination range (16 nmol/L – 600 μmol/L) and a low detection limit (8 nmol/L) (Zhang et al., 2006). Moreover, a DNA immobilized CNT composite electrode was used to detect dopamine with an ultra small detection limit of 0.021 nmol/L (Ly, 2006) (Fig. 9.10(b)). Polyphenol oxidase (PPOx)-modified CNTPE was also used to detect dopamine with a detection limit 1 μmol/L (Rubianes and Rivas, 2005).

9.3.2.7 Folic acid

Folic acid (FA) is one of forms of a water-soluble vitamin B that is important for the formation of red and white blood cells. It occurs naturally in food and can also be taken as supplements. An FA sensor with MWNTs/Au electrodes was developed by Wei and coworkers (Wei et al., 2006). Under optimized conditions, the voltammetric sensor responded linearly to the concentration of FA from 0.02 – 1 μmol/L.

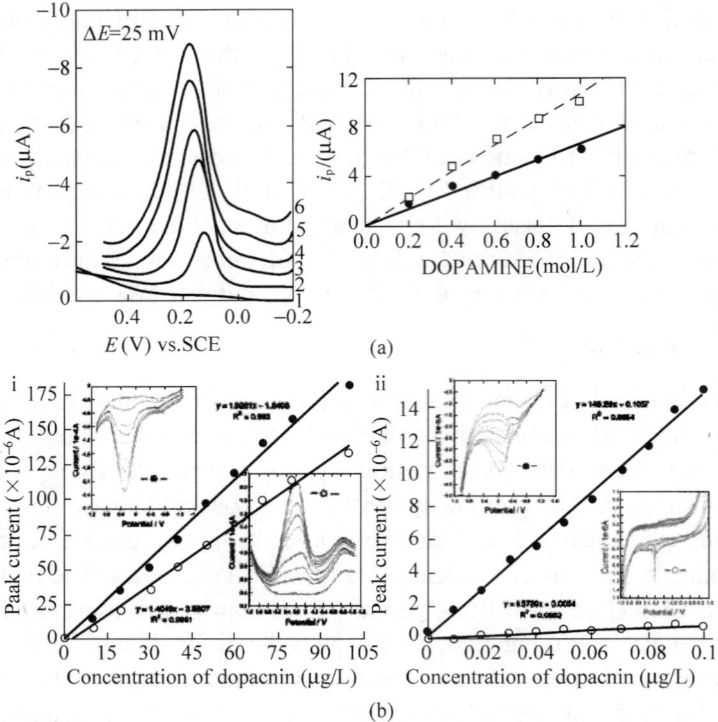

Figure 9.10 (a) DPV responses (left) and the corresponding calibration plot (right) of dopamine in PBS at a MWNT composite electrode. Marks from No. 1 to 6 corresponded to 0, 200, 400, 600, 800, 1000 mmol/L addition of dopamine. Reprinted from (Britto et al., 1996) with permission. (b) the calibration curve of square-wave (SW) stripping voltammetry of dopamine at various concentrations: (i) 0, 10, 20, 30, 40, 50, 60, 70, 80 and 100 mg/L; and (ii) 0, 0.01, 0.02, 0.03, 0.04, 0.05, 0.06, 0.07, 0.08, 0.09, 0.1 and 0.11 μg/L at optimum conditions. (Inset) (i) anodic and cathodic SW stripping voltammograms; (ii) SW anodic and CV voltammograms. Reprinted from (Ly, 2006) with permission

9.3.2.8 Glutathione

Glutathione (GSH) is a tripeptide of the amino acids glycine, cystine, and glutamic acid existing widely in plants and animal tissues and constructing reduced and oxidized forms in biological oxidation-reduction reactions. A well-aligned CNT arrays grown directly on graphite substrate was used as working electrode to detect GSH (Tang et al., 2006). It had excellent electrochemical activity and good anti-fouling property for direct electrochemical oxidation of GSH, with a response time of 5 s, a low detection limit of 0.2 μmol/L and a high sensitivity of 254.8 nA/(μmol $\cdot$ L^{-1} $\cdot$ cm^2).

9.3.2.9 Indole-3-acetic acid

Indole-3-acetic acid, also known as IAA, is generally considered to be the most important native auxin, promoting elongation of stems and roots. An amperometric sensor for IAA was prepared by coating MWNTs onto GCE (Wu et al., 2003). The linear response with the concentration of IAA and the detection limit was 0.1 – 50 μmol/L and 0.02 μmol/L, respectively.

9.3.2.10 Lactate

Lactate is constantly produced during normal metabolism and exercise. It is one of several molecules and ions in human sweat. Thus determination of lactate would help us to monitor human physiological conditions. GCE and silicon/indium tin oxide (Si/ITO) substrate modified with lactate oxidase (LOx)-immobilized carboxylized SWNTs was used to detect lactate respectively (Weber et al., 2006). It had a linear response in the range of 1 – 4 mmol/L and 10 – 50 mmol/L, respectively. Lactate could also be detected using LOx modified CNT paste electrodes with a detection limit of 300 μmol/L (Rubianes and Rivas, 2005).

9.3.2.11 Lincomycin

Lincomycin is an antibiotic derived from cultures of the bacterium *Streptomyces lincolnensis,* used in the treatment of certain penicillin-resistant infections. The detection of lincomycin by GCE modified with MWNTs, which were stabilized by DHP, SDBS and Nafion, respectively, was demonstrated. (Wu et al., 2006). The MWNT-DHP/GCE was found to have a linear response from 0.45 to 150 μmol/L and a detection limit of 0.2 μmol/L.

9.3.2.12 Morphine

Morphine is an extremely powerful opiate analgesic drug and the principal active agent in opium. Determination of morphine in biological samples is meaningful to monitor drug concentration and therapeutic level in humans. An MWNT/GCE based morphine electrochemical sensor with a linear detection range of 0.5 – 150 μmol/L, a calculated detection limit of 0.2 μmol/L, and a sensitivity of 10 nA/(μmol/L) has been reported (Salimi et al., 2005).

9.3.2.13 NADH

β-Nicotinamide adenine dinucleotide (NADH) is of importance in living cells because NAD^+/NADH couple is a cofactor system for several hundreds of dehydrogenase enzymes. Conventional electrodes determining oxidation of NADH, however, are highly irreversible and poorly stable because of a large overpotential and surface fouling by the reaction products. These problems were overcome by utilizing MWNT/GCE sensors (Musameh et al., 2002). The overvoltage of NADH oxidation was lower by ~0.5 V compared to a bare GCE, and more that 90% initial activity remained after 60 min stirring in NADH solution. Furthermore, the synergistic effects of CNTs and redox mediators (RM) towards the NADH oxidation were reported in several papers (Lawrence and Wang, 2006, Zhang and

Gorski, 2005a, 2005b). Zhang and Gorski. covalently attached RM Toluidine Blue O (TBO) and Zure dye (AZU) to polysaccharide chain of chitosan (CHIT) and interspersed with MWNTs. Such TBO-CHIT-MWNT and AZU-CHIT-MWNT film electrode decreased the overpotential for the mediated process, while amplified the NADH current by several tens of times and reducing the response time to ~5 s (Zhang and Gorski, 2005a, 2005b). Lawrence and Wang. adsorbed the phenothiazine dyes (toluidine blue and azure C) on the MWNTs modified basal plane pyrolytic graphite (BPPG) electrode, which promoted low potential, sensitive and stable determination of NADH (Lawrence and Wang, 2006). An MWNTs-epoxy composite electrode was also found to have a better performance toward NADH than graphite composites electrode (Pumera et al., 2006).

9.3.2.14 Nitric oxide

Nitric oxide (NO) is an important signaling molecule in the body of mammals including humans. Its biological functions at low concentrations are as signals in many diverse physiological processes such as blood pressure control, neuro-transmission, learning and memory. Applying Nafion/MWNTs/GCE, the NO could be detected linearly in the range of $2\times10^{-7}-1.5\times10^{-4}$ mol/L with a detection limit of 8.0×10^{-8} mol/L (Wu et al., 2002). The Nafion thin film was used to eliminate the interference from anions, especially nitrite. The same group also reported to utilize myoglobin (Myb) functionalized MWNTs/GCE for the same purpose (Zhang et al., 2005). Such a sensor was based on the electrochemical reduction of NO, hence avoided the possible interference of oxidizable substance in solution. The performance of Myb/MWNTs/GC based biosensor was nearly the same with previous one.

9.3.2.15 Organophosphate compounds

Organophosphate (OP) compounds are a diverse group of chemicals used in domestic and industrial settings, including insecticides, nerve gases, etc. Accordingly, early and rapid detection of these toxic agents in food and environment is on a growing demand in homeland security and healthcare. During the past decade, biosensors based on inhibition of acetylcholine esterase (AChE) were widely used for detecting OP compounds. For instance, a disposable biosensor for OPs was developed based on the enzyme AChE functionalized MWNTs modified screen-printed electrodes (SPE) (Joshi et al., 2005). The mechanism of the OP sensor is to evaluate the inhabitation of the AChE by OP compounds, which was determined by measuring the electro-oxidation current of thiocholine generated by the AChE catalyzed hydrolysis of acteylthiocholine (ATCh). MWNTs acted as physical immobilization matrix for enzyme, while exhibited electro-catalytic activity toward thiocholine. The overpotential for thiocholine oxidation was found to be as low as 0.2 V without using a mediating redox species, and the detection limit for paraoxon is 0.5 nmol/L (0.145 ppb). Moreover, utilizing the direct biosensing route of enzyme organophosphorus hydrolase (OPH), which catalyzed the hydrolysis of OP compounds, an OPH-functionalized MWNT-Nafion/GCE was developed to detect OP compounds amperometrically (Deo et al., 2005). Such sensor could detect as low as 0.15 μmol/L paraoxon and 0.8 μmol/L methyl parathion with sensitivities of 25 and 6 nA/(μmol · L^{-1}), respectively. Recently, Liu et al. demonstrated a self-assembled AChE-functionalized MWNT/GCE to detect OP compounds (Liu and Lin, 2006). AChE was kept bioactively in a sandwich-like structure, where AChE molecules were embedded in two PDDA layers on the surface of MWNTs. Low oxidation overvoltage (+0.15 V) and detection limit as low as 0.4 pmol/L paraoxon with a 6-min inhibition time was achieved by such CNTs-modified electrode.

9.3.2.16 Phenolic compounds

Phenolic compounds are the hydroxy derivatives of benzene and its condensed aromatic systems. Not only are they naturally occurring compounds distributed in many plants, vegetables and food products, but also some of them are toxic. Unfortunately the detection of phenolic compounds using traditional solid electrodes were challenged by surface fouling attributed to the polymeric oxidation products. Wang and coworkers have overcome the problem by using MWNT-Nafion/GCE (Wang et al., 2003a). The stability of this sensor was largely enhanced with 85% of initial activity remaining after 30 mins. in phenol solution, compared to complete inhibition of the redox process within 6 mins at the bare surface. Enzyme was also utilized in some CNT-modified biosensors. For example, SWNTs were used as supporting material of enzyme tyrosinase in an amperometric sensor (Zhao et al., 2005). The electrode detected the catalyzed oxidation of phenolic compounds in the presence of oxygen, with a sensitivity of 155 μA/(mmol · L^{-1}) for phenol. The sensor was also used to detect benzoic acid with a linear response in the range of 2.5 μmol/L – 12.4 μmol/L. In addition, Polyphenol oxidase (PPOx) was reported to functionalize a CNTPE-based sensor to detect various phenolic compounds, including phenol, catequeine, etc. (Rubianes and Rivas, 2005).

9.3.2.17 Procaine

Procaine is the first injectable man-made local anesthetic drug. Although procaine is rarely used today, procaine has the advantage of reducing bleeding without leading to the euphoric and addictive qualities, unlike other local anesthetics. Wu et al. utilized MWNT-film modified GCE for voltammetrical procaine detection (Wu et al., 2006). The reporeted detection limit is 200 nmol/L.

9.3.2.18 Putrescine

Putrescine is a foul-smelling ptomaine produced in decaying animal tissue by decarboxylation of ornithine. It can be used for many analytical and clinical applications, such as cancer marker, bacterial diagnosis and etc. An amperometric biosensor was constructed on a γ-Aminopropyltriethoxysilane (APTES)-modified MWNT/GCE (Luong et al., 2005). Compared to classical electrodes, direct electron transfer between putrescine oxidase (POx) and the MWNTs modified GCE surface without using mediators was achieved in such a biosensor, where APTES was not only used to assist to solubilize MWNTs, but also served as an immobilization matrix for POx. The sensor exhibited a detecting range of 0.5 – 250 μmol/L.

9.3.2.19 Theophyllin

Theophylline (TP) is used to prevent and treat wheezing, shortness of breath, and difficulty breathing caused by asthma, etc. AGCE casted with carboxylic MWNTs was utilized to detect TP (Zhu et al., 2005). The biosensor showed a linear response to the TP concentration in the range $3\times10^{-7}-1.0\times10^{-5}$ mol/L with an estimated detection limit of 0.05 μmol/L.

9.3.2.20 Quercetin

Quercetin, one kind of flavonoids, forms the 'backbone' for many other flavonoids such as the citrus flavonoids rutin and hesperidin. Quercetin has significant anti-inflammatory activity because of direct inhibition of several initial processes of inflammation. In addition, quercetin shows various positive effects to human health in combating or helping to prevent cancer, prostatitis, heart disease, etc.. Thus monitoring quercetin concentration is of interest in many aspects. Jin et al. applied MWNTs-modified paraffin-impregnated graphite disk using choline (Ch) bond and catalyzer (MWNT/Ch/WGE) to detect quercetin (Jin et al., 2006). Under the optimum conditions, the sensor showed sensitivity up to 40 μmol/L with a detection limit of 4.8 nmol/L and a signal lose of 20% after two month storage.

9.3.2.21 Rutin

Rutin is a citrus bioflavonoid found in many plants, especially in black tea and apple peels. In humans, rutin can attach to the to the iron ion Fe^{2+}, which prevents Fe^{2+} from binding to H_2O_2 and creating a highly reactive free radical which may cause cell damage. Therefore, rapid, sensitive and reliable methods are welcomed to determine rutin in drug analysis. Combining GCE with β-cyclodextrin (β-CD) incorporated MWNTs, He et al. reported to obtain a detection range of rutin form $4.0\times10^{-7}-1.0\times10^{-3}$ mol/L and estimated the detection limit to be 2.0×10^{-7} mol/L (He et al., 2006). Electrochemical behavior of rutin was investigated voltammetrically at a SWNTs modified gold electrode. The sensor exhibited a linear response in the range of $2.0\times10^{-8}-5.0\times10^{-6}$ mol/L with a detection limit as low as 1.0×10^{-8} mol/L (Zeng et al., 2006).

9.3.2.22 Thiocholine

Thiocholine (TCh) is one of the products in acetylcholinesterase (AChE) catalyzed hydrolysis of thiocholine ester (AChE). It is used to monitoring the AChE inhabitation, which is a biomarker for the toxic effect of some pesticides, such as organophosphorus compounds (OPs). Thus, the analysis of TCh is demanded for pollute control monitoring. The major drawbacks of using GC, CP, and bulk metal electrodes for TCh detection is the high oxidation overpotential, which leads to cause high background current and interference from other electroactive compounds. However, using an MWNT modified GCE (Liu et al., 2005), the enzymatically generated TCh was detected at lower oxidation overpotential (0.15 V) and higher sensitivity. Under optimal batch condition, the detection limit was 5×10^{-6} mol/L. Furthermore, by applying constant-potential flow injection analysis, the detection limit was greatly improved to 3×10^{-7} mol/L.

9.3.2.23 DNA

DNA is a genetic material in cells that holds the inherited instructions for growth, development, and cellular functioning. The development of an effective DNA-sensing system, therefore, is vital in these studies. Besides traditional DNA detection techniques such as fluorescent, radiochemical and chemiluminscent methods, electrochemical methods are attractive for their simple and low-cost solutions to DNA analysis ((Gooding 2002) and references within).

The use of CNT in electrochemical DNA sensors has recently attracted many researchers. A range of sensors in the literature are compiled in Table 9.2. These CNT-modified sensors are utilized to detect DNA (Li et al., 2005; Pedano and Rivas, 2004; Wang et al., 2004) and DNA hybridization (Cai et al., 2003a, 2003b; Cheng et al., 2005, Kerman et al., 2004; Koehne et al., 2003, 2004; Li et al., 2003; Munge et al., 2005; Wang et al., 2004a; Wang et al., 2004b; Wang et al., 2004; Zhu et al., 2005), respectively.

One of commonly used methods to prepare CNT-modified sensors for DNA hybridization detection was to attach ssDNA onto carboxylized CNT-modified electrode (including D1-D4, D7, D8), which was allowed to monitor a current signal when the complementary sequence (target) hybridizes with the immobilized ssDNA (probe). The first reported such sensor (D1) was based on a ssDNA-modified MWNT/GCE. A 24-based complementary ssDNA was detected using DPV in the presence of the electroactive intercalator daunomycin (DNR). The average anodic current of DNR was linear with the concentration of complementary ssDNA in the range of 0.2 nmol/L to 50 nmol/L with a detection limit of 0.1 nmol/L. The sensor D1 also exhibited a good selectivity towards the oligonucleotide sequences with a mismatch of a few bases. The hybridization of less than 10^6 DNA targets can be measured by combining the MWNT nanoelectrode array (MWNTNEA) electrodes (D3) with $Ru(byp)_3^{2+}$ mediated guanine oxidation (Li et al., 2003). When detecting the long single-stranded PCR amplicon with a large number of inherent guanine bases, the detection limit was further lowered to under ~1000 target DNAs (Koehne et al., 2003). Sensor D8 utilized CNTs to promote electro-transfer reactions and platinum nanoparticles for its high catalytic activities, achieving a detection limit of 0.01 nmol/L for target DNA, while employing DNR as an indicator (Fig. 9.11). Moreover, using methylene blue (MB) as a redox indicator, a DNA-hybridization sensor (D7) was fabricated on self-assembled MWNTs with covalently attached probe DNA, as shown in Fig. 9.12.

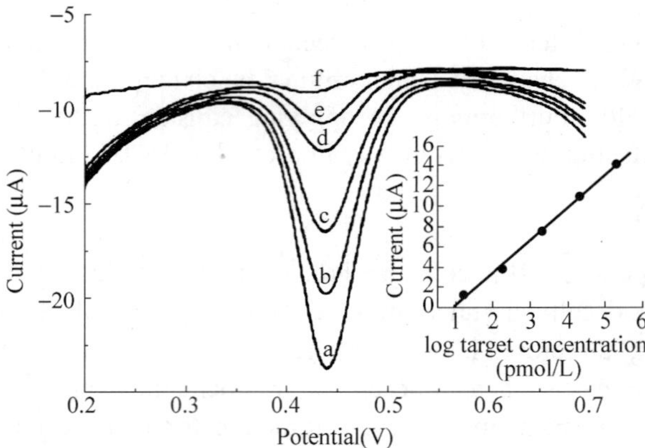

Figure 9.11 DPV voltammograms of Pt nanoparticles decorated ssDNA-MWNT/GC electrodes for different concentrations of target DNA: (a) 2.25×10^5 pmol/L; (b) 2.25×10^4 pmol/L; (c) 2.25×10^3 pmol/L; (d) 2.25×10^2 pmol/L; (e) 2.25×10^1 pmol/L; (f) 0.0 pmol/L. (Inset) the corresponding logarithmic calibration plot. Reprinted from (Zhu et al., 2005) with permission

Furthermore, DNA-hybridization sensors fabricated with previous method were also developed in the absence of indicator. D2 detected DNA sequences on a complementary DNA-doped PPy film on MWNT/GCE with by AC impedance measurement. When hybridization occurred, a decrease of impedance value was observed. D4 attached carboxylized MWNTs onto a CPE using a hybridization assay, and the probe DNA was further covalently adsorbed on the MWNTs. Such sensor provided a larger surface area for DNA immobilization and consequently exhibited a detection limit down to 10 pg/mL.

Magnetite nanoparticle (MNP) modified CNT-based sensors were prepared for DNA hybridization detection. In D5, A MWNT/PPy-modified GCE detected the DNA hybridization by capping the ssDNA probe on mercapatoacetic acid (RSH)-coated MNPs, which exhibits unique hybridization selectivity and effective discrimination ability in mismatched DNA sequences. The degree of hybridization corresponded to the reduction peak current of the indicator DNR. The detective limit of target DNA was as low as 2.3×10^{-14} mol/L. Wang and his group also developed enzyme-based electrochemical sensors (D6, D9, and D10) for the purpose. The DNA hybridization applied enzyme alkaline phosphatase (ALP) as tag and MNP as the collector for specific DNA sequences in D6. The hybridization information could be acquired from the enzymatically liberated product on a MWNT/GCE. Furthermore, CNTs played a dual-amplication role in both recognition and transduction events in sensors D9 and D10. The CNTs were not only loaded

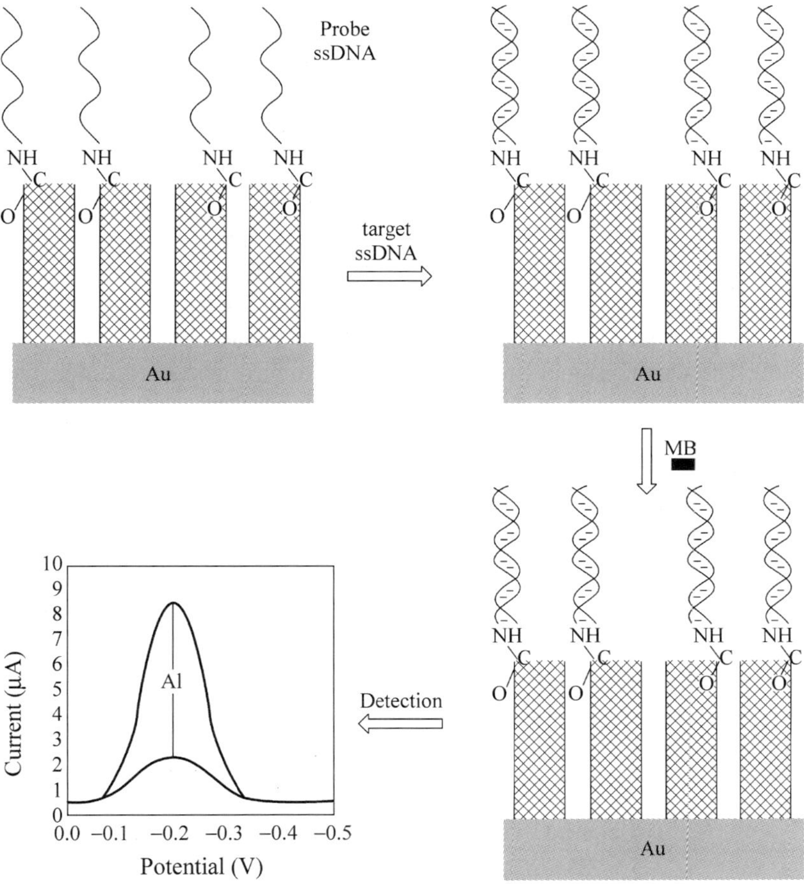

Figure 9.12 Schematic of the preparation of ssDNA-MWNT-array modified Au electrodes and the detection of target ssDNA sequences in the presence of an indicator, methylene blue (MB). Reprinted from (Wang et al., 2004) with permission

with various enzyme ALP tags and used as DNA labels during hybridization detection, but also used to modify the GCE and accumulate the product of the enzymatic reaction. Such sensor could detect DNA down to 80 copies (5.4 amol/L). The difference between D9 and D10 was that the ALP tracer was immobilized on CNTs by LBL method in D10.

The DNA could be detected on CNT modified electrodes, involving SWNT/GCE (D11), MWNTPE (D12), and DNA/MWNT-chitosan/graphite electrode (D13).

9.3.2.24 Others

Other species detected with the aid of CNT-modified electrodes include uric acid and norepinephrine (simultaneous detection by a chitosan-MWNT modified GCE (Lu et al., 2005)), cholera toxin (CT) (with anti-CT-immobilized, liposome-and-ploy(3,4-ethylenedioxythiophene)-coated-MWNT-Nafion/GCE (Viswanathan et al., 2006)) .

9.4 Field-Effect Transistors Based on SWNTs

Field-effect transistors (FETs) fabricated with SWNTs as active part of the device have been intensely studied since SWNTs are prospective candidates in molecule electronics. Because the most sensitive elements, pristine or specifically functionalized SWNTs, are worked as exposed conducing channel, the electronic properties of CNTFETs are sensitive to attached specific molecules and its surrounding environment. Therefore, CNTFETs were not only used for various chemical gases, such as NO_2, NH_3, etc. (Bradley et al., 2003, Qi et al., 2003, Zhang et al., 2006), but also sensitive to biorecognition events, biocatalytic processes and so on. The sensing signal from CNTFETs due to these species could be obtained

Table 9.5 Summary of the biosensors based on CNTFETs

Objective	Biomolecule functionzlied on SWNTs	With a linker layer (Y/N)	References
Protein recognition	Biotin, SpA, U1A	Y	(Chen et al., 2003)
	Biotin	Y	(Star et al., 2003)
	hCG	N	(Chen et al., 2004)
	HA	Y	(Takeda et al., 2005)
	α-PSA	N	(Kojima et al., 2005)
	Anti-copper oxLDL	Y	(Rouhanizadeh et al., 2006)
	Thrombin aptamer	Y	(So et al., 2005)
	PSA-AB	Y	(Li et al., 2005)
	SpA, hCG	N	(Byon and Choi, 2006)
DNA hybridization	PNA	Y	(Maehashi et al., 2004)
	ssDNA	N	(Star et al., 2006)
	ssDNA	N	(Tang et al., 2006)
Enzymatic study	GOx	Y	(Besteman et al., 2003)
	Starch	N	(Star et al., 2004)
Protein adsorption	Cytc	N	(Boussaad et al., 2003)
	SA	N	(Bradley et al., 2004)
	SA, IgG	N	(Atashbar et al., 2006)
Others	Cell membrane	N	(Bradley et al., 2005)

α-PSA anti-pig serum albumin, cytc cytochrome c, GOx glucose oxidas, hCG human chorionic gonadotropin, IgG immunoglobulin G, oxLDL oxidized low density lipoprotein, PNA peptide nucleic acid, PSA-AB anti-prostate-specific antigen monoclonal antibody, SA streptavidin, SpA staphylococcal protein A, ssDNA single-stranded DNA.

from two different ways. One is the chemiresistor configuration by monitoring real-time conductance change of CNT during analytes addition. The other way is to monitor the field-effect modulated conductance after introduction of the analytes. This kind of sensors sometimes is referred as chemFET.

In the following, we enumerate various papers utilizing CNTFET in biosensing applications, and also compile these biosensors and some of their aspects in Table 9.5.

9.4.1 Protein Recognition

Some proteins, especially antibodies, that are specific to corresponding antigens, have been utilized as recognition receptors in CNTFET biosensors. Most of exploited biological applications of CNTFETs are to recognize specific protein.

Chen et al. firstly reported to used CNTFET in such application (Chen et al., 2003). They found the Tween-coated SWNTs exhibited excellence resistance to the non-specific binding (NSB) of various proteins. Thus CNTFETs coated with biotinylated Tween, staphylococcal protein A (SpA)-Tween and U1A antigen-Tween could real-timely monitor the specific binding of streptavidin, IgG and 10E3 down to 1 nmol/L, respectively. The interferences from the NSB of other proteins could be eliminated. Response of such device to 10E3 could be seen in Fig. 9.13(a). Similarly, Star and his coworkers also applied CNTFET devices to detect specific protein binding (Star et al., 2003). Alternatively, a PEI/PEG polymer coating layer had been used as the prohibitor for NSB of proteins and linking molecules between SWNTs and molecular receptor, biotin. The biotin-streptavidin binding events could be observed from the shift of transfer characteristics of the CNTFETs (Fig. 9.13(b)). Another example for label-free detection of biomolecules was to differentiate low density lipoprotein (LDL) cholesterol between the reduced (native LDL) and the oxidized state (oxLDL) on an anti-copper oxLDL antibody conjugated CNT network-based FET, in which a PEI/PEG layer was appeared as the linker (Rouhanizadeh et al., 2006). Furthermore, complementary detection of prostate-specific antigen (PSA) was achieved by utilizing p-type CNTFETs and *n*-type In_2O_3 nanowire based FETs both anchored with anti-PSA monoclonalantibody (PSA-AB) via linking molecules (Li et al., 2005).

The antibody, anti-pig serum albumin (α-PSA), was directly immobilized on SWNTs through NSB without linking molecules (Kojima et al., 2005). Subsequently, the adsorption of antigen, PSA, was investigated from the real-time detection and characteristics change of CNTFETs.

Considering their high specificity, relatively inexpensive and capability of reversible denaturation, aptamers, which are artificial oligonucleotides, were used as an alternative to protein-based sensing elements (So et al., 2005). 15-mer ssDNA aptamer bound to CNTFET via CDI-Tween could specifically attach to blood-clotting factor thrombin, and the detection limit to aptamer of the biosensor was around 10 nmol/L.

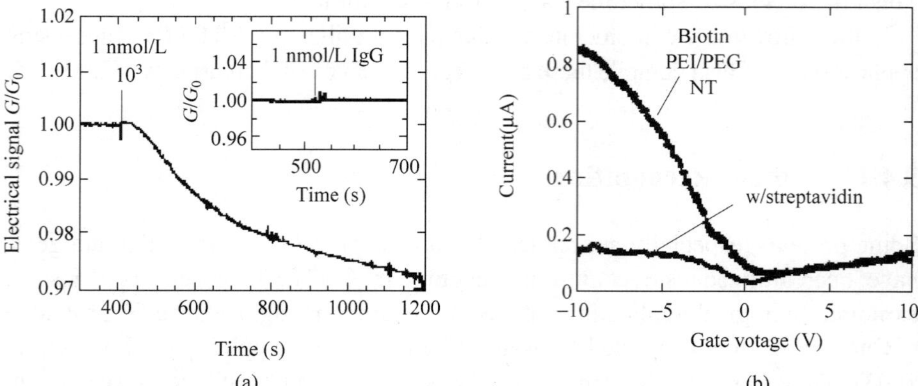

Figure 9.13 (a) The Conductance vs. time curve shown that a recombinant human autoantigen functionalized CNTFET exhibited specific response to ≤ 1 nmol/L 10^3 mAbs. (Inset) the same device shown selectivity that reject the interference polyclonal IgG at a much larger concentration of 1 μmol/L (Inset). Reprinted from (Chen et al., 2003) with permission. (b) Transfer characteristic change of a biotinylated polymer-coated CNTFET before and after exposing to streptavidin. Reprinted from (Star et al., 2003) with permission

In order to further understand the biosensing mechanism of the specific protein recognition by CNTFET, Chen et al. conducted a series of control experiments to block selected areas of the devices, including only contacts between SWNTs and metallic electrodes, both contacts and exposed SWNTs, or none of such two regions (Chen et al., 2004). These devices were subsequently used for protein recognition. The results revealed that electronic effects occurring at the contacts due to the protein adsorption induced Schottky barrier modulation dominated the electronic biosensing signal. And the contribution from the exposed SWNTs was negligible if the adsorbed species were not highly charged. With this knowledge in mind, Byon and Choi purposefully modified the device geometry to increase the Schottky contact area (Byon and Choi, 2006). This modification was implemented by evaporating metallic source/drain electrode at a tilted angle using a shadow mask. In comparison with the detection limit in the sensing of proteins or protein-protein interactions in previous works (Chen et al., 2003, Chen et al., 2004), which is ca. 100 pmol/L to 100 nmol/L, devices with increased Schottky area could detect proteins as low as 1 pmol/L concentrations.

Alternatively, a different architecture, in which protein receptor hemagglutinins (HA) was immobilized on the back-gate side of CNTFET via linking molecules instead of SWNTs channel, was prepared to detect anti-HA binding (Takeda et al., 2005). The detection limit of anti-HA was estimated to be 5×10^{-8} mg/mL, and was better than enzyme-linked immunosorbent assay (ELISA) system.

9.4.2 DNA Hybridization

Nowadays, the development of genome diagnosis has been a subject with great interest, in which label-free electronic methods, including CNTFET based biosensors, are believed to be a potential way for sensitive, selective and low cost detection of DNA hybridization (Fig. 9.14). The first SWNT transistor used for this purpose was developed in association with covalently immobilized amino modified peptide nucleic acid (PNA) oligonucleotides onto Au surface of the back gate via a self-assembled monolayer (SAM) (Maehashi et al., 2004). This device could effectively detect the complementary DNA with a concentration as low as 6.8 fmol/L. Moreover, Star et al. also utilized CNT network FETs as selective detectors for DNA immobilization and hybridization (Star et al., 2006). The probe DNA was non-covalently adsorbed on the SWNT network instead of the back gate region as reported in ref. (Maehashi et al., 2004). The devices were further used for the label-free detection of DNA hybridization at picomolar to micromolar concentrations. It was also found that the addition of Mg^{2+} during hybridization could improve the sensitivity of DNA detection probably by increasing the extent and overall efficiency of DNA hybridization on SWNTs. The mechanism of DNA detection using CNTFET devices, however, is still under argument. Star et al. suggested a charge-based mechanism (Star et al., 2006). In contrast, Tang and his coworkers demonstrated that DNA hybridization on the contact regions of the CNTFET caused a more significant contribution to the acute electrical conductance change, probably due to the modulation of energy level alignment between SWNTs and Au electrodes (Tang et al., 2006). More experiments are still needed to clarify such issue.

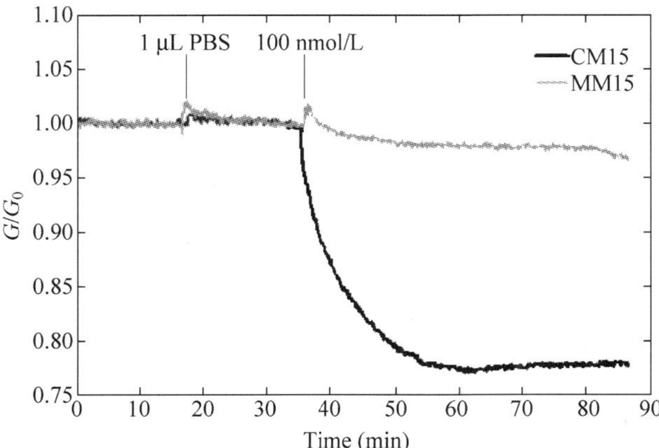

Figure 9.14 Real-time monitoring of 15mer DNA hybridization in PBS on a ssDNA functionalized CNTFET. Two liquid cells were used in parallel for simultaneous drop adding 5 μL of complementary (blue) and mismatched (green) target oligo solutions to 500 μL of buffer. Reprinted from (Tang et al., 2006) with permission

9.4.3 Enzymatic Study

With GOx attached to the nanotube sidewall through linking molecules, a liquid-gated FET device could be used for the detection of glucose (Fig. 9.15) (Besteman et al., 2003). It was observed that the immobilization of GOx induced the transfer characteristics negative gate voltage shift, which was probably due to a change in the capacitance of the tube. Subsequently, the addition of 0.1 mmol/L glucose solution increased the conductance of enzyme functionalized CNTFETs, but the exact mechanism was not explained. Furthermore, an alternative approach was used to detect the enzymatic degradation of starch on CNTFET (Star et al., 2004). Instead of enzyme, the substrate of an enzymatic reaction, starch, was attached to the devices surface directly, leading to a shift in the transfer characteristics of devices. After incubation of these devices in aqueous buffer solutions of enzyme amyloglucosidase (AMG), the I_d - V_g curve almost completely recovered to the trace record before the starch deposition, suggesting that nearly all the starch were hydrolyzed to glucose and then washed away by buffer solution, because the AMG along would not affect the device characteristics and the adsorbed starch could not be washed off by buffer solution along.

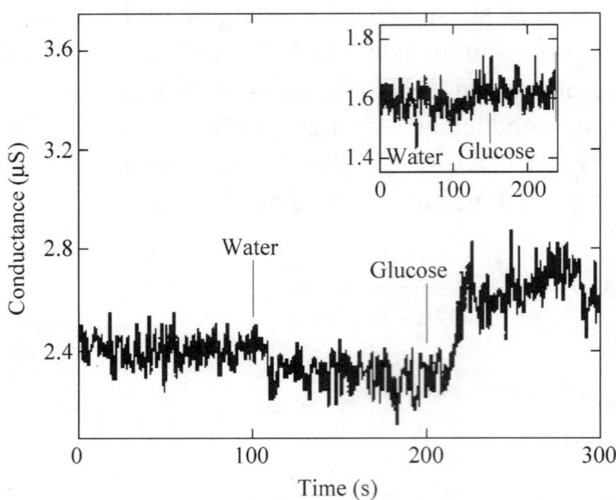

Figure 9.15 Real-time monitoring of the GOx functionalized CNTFET to glucose. Arrows showed the addition of 2 μL milli-Q water and 2 μL 0.1 mmol/L glucose to the device. (Inset) the same measurement on a control CNTFET without GOx. Reprinted from (Besteman et al., 2003) with permission

9.4.4 Protein Adsorption

Noncovalent adsorption of proteins, such as cytochrome *c* (Boussaad et al., 2003) and streptavidin (Atashbar et al., 2006, Bradley et al., 2004), IgG immunoglobulin

G (IgG) (Atashbar et al., 2006), could also be simply detected by SWNT or SWNT-network based FET devices. Such NSB on bare unmodified SWNTs could alter the electrical characteristics of devices. Charge transfer between proteins and the SWNTs may be responsible to the detection process.

9.4.5 Others

Bradley et al. integrated a complex biological system, the cell membrane of Halobacterium salinarum, with CNTFET device, and found that both of them were preserved their properties and functions (Bradley et al., 2005). On the same time, the charge distribution in this biological system was investigated.

9.5 Conclusions and Future Prospects

We have summarized recent advances in the applications of CNTs for biosensing, in which electrochemical biosensing and electronic biosensing were emphasized. The large surface/volume ratio, bio-compatibility and high electrical sensing sensitivity of CNTs are the key advantages for biosensing applications. The marked electrocatalytic reactivity and efficient electron transfer, coupled with the resistance to surface fouling and hence to high stability, pave the way for the construction of a wide range of electrochemical and electronic biosensors with many attractive analytical characteristics.

However, the exploitation of CNTs in the applications of biosensors is still in its infancy. Future efforts should aim at a more in-depth understanding the chemical and physical properties of CNT and new configurations of CNT-based biosensors. More work is needed to settle the dilemma whether the oxygen-containing surface groups on CNTs after oxidants treatment could improve the electrocatalytic ability of CNTs (Day et al., 2004, Musameh et al., 2005). To fabricate CNT NEA in large-scale through vertically aligned CNTs at a low density could have promising potentials as interstitial space between nanoelectrodes could be filled with a passivation layer and only the tips of CNTs are exposed for electrochemical detection in order to minimize the background current (Koehne et al., 2003, Koehne et al., 2004, Li et al., 2003, Lin et al., 2004, Tu et al., 2005). In addition, the open ends and defects in CNTs were found to have similar properties with edge planes of highly ordered pyrolytic graphite (HOPG) and acted as electro-catalytically active sites (Banks and Compton, 2005, Gooding et al., 2003, Nugent et al., 2001). This discovery could be further utilized to improve the electrochemical activity and sensitivity of CNT-modified electrodes. Furthermore, the role of contact between CNTs and the metallic electrodes is believed to play an important role in the CNT transistors and should also be further investigated, since it was suggested that the modulation of the Schottky barrier might dominate in the response of CNTFET-based biosensor to analyte (Chen et al., 2004, Tang et al., 2006). Due to integrate of biological cell membranes with CNTFETs for monitoring charge distribution in the cell membrane (Bradley et al., 2005), one also needs to study the cytotoxity of CNTs towards biological species. These directions of development could bring a bright prospect to the new generation of CNT-based biosensors for a variety of applications.

Acknowledgement

We acknowledge generous support of this work by the Agency for Science, Technology and Research (A-STAR) (Project No. 0421140041) and MOE AcRF Tier 2 Funding (ARC17/07, T207B1203).

Reference

Atashbar, M. Z., B. E. Bejcek and S. Singamaneni. *IEEE Sensors Journal* **6**: 524 – 528 (2006).

Balasubramanian, K. and M. Burghard. *Anal. Bioanal. Chem.* **385**: 452 – 468 (2006).

Banks, C. E. and R. G. Compton. *Analyst* **130**: 1232 (2005).

Besteman, K., J.-O. Lee, F. G. M. Wiertz, H. A. Heering and C. Dekker. *Nano Lett.* **3**: 727 – 730 (2003).

Boussaad, S., N. J. Tao, R. Zhang, T. Hopson and L. A. Nagahara. *Chem. Commun.* 1502 – 1503 (2003).

Bradley, K., J.-C. P. Gabriel, M. Briman, A. Star and G. Gruner. *Phy. Rev. Lett.* **91**: 218,301 (2003).

Bradley, K., M. Briman, A. Star and G. Gru1ner. *Nano Lett.* **4**: 253 – 256 (2004).

Bradley, K., A. Davis, J.-C. P. Gabriel and G. Gruner. *Nano Lett.* **5**: 841 – 845 (2005).

Britto, P. J., K. S. V. Santhanam and P. M. Ajayan. *Bioelectrochemistry and Bioenergetics* **41**: 121 – 125 (1996).

Byon, H. R. and H. C. Choi. *J. Am. Chem. Soc.* **128**: 2188 – 2189 (2006).

Cai, H., X. Cao, Y. Jiang, P. He and Y. Fang. *Anal. Bioanal. Chem.* **375**: 287 – 293 (2003a).

Cai, H., Y. Xu, P. He and Y. Fang. *Electroanalysis* **15**: 1864 – 1870 (2003b).

Chen, R. J., S. Bangsaruntip, K. A. Drouvalakis, N. W. S. Kam, M. Shim, Y. Li, W. Kim, P. J. Utz and H. Dai. *Proc. Natl. Acad. Sci. USA*. **100**: 4984 – 4989 (2003).

Chen, R. J., H. C. Choi, S. Bangsaruntip, E. Yenilmez, X. Tang, Q. Wang, Y.-L. Chang and H. Dai. *J. Am. Chem. Soc.* **126**: 1563 – 1568 (2004).

Cheng, G., J. Zhao, Y. Tu, P. He and Y. Fang. *Analytica Chimica Acta* **533**: 11 – 16 (2005).

Day, T. M., N. Wilson and J. V. Macpherson. *J. Am. Chem. Soc.* **126**: 16,724 (2004).

Day, T. M., P. R. Unwin, N. R. Wilson and J. V. Macpherson. *J. Am. Chem. Soc.* **127**: 10,639 – 10,647 (2005).

Deo, R. P., J. Wang, I. Block, A. Mulchandani, K. A. Joshi, M. Trojanowicz, F. Scholz, W. Chen and Y. Lin. *Analytica Chimica Acta* **530**: 185 – 189 (2005).

Fei, S., J. Chen, S. Yao, G. Deng, D. He and Y. Kuang. *Analytical Biochemistry* **339**: 29 – 35 (2005).

Gao, M., L. Dai and G. G. Wallace. *Electroanalysis* **15**: 1089 – 1094 (2003).

Gooding, J. J. *Electroanalysis* **14**: 1149 – 1156 (2002).

Gooding, J. J., R. Wibowo, J. Liu, W. Yang, D. Losic, S. Orbons, F. J. Mearns, J. G. Shapter and D. B. Hibbert. *J. Am. Chem. Soc.* **125**: 9006 (2003).

Guo, M., J. Chen, J. Li, L. Nie and S. Yao. *Electroanalysis* **16**: 1992 – 1998 (2004).

He, J., Y. Yang, X. Yang, Y. Liu, Z. Liu, G. Shen and R. Yu. *Sensors and Actuators* B **114**: 94 – 100 (2006).

Hocevar, S. B., J. Wang, R. P. Deo, M. Musameh and B. Ogorevc. *Electroanalysis* **17**: 417 – 422 (2005).

Hrapovic, S., Y. Liu, K. B. Male and J. H. T. Luong. *Anal. Chem.* **76**: 1083 – 1088 (2004).

Huang, J., Y. Yang, H. Shi, Z. Song, Z. Zhao, J.-i. Anzai, T. Osa and Q. Chen. *Materials Science and Engineering C* **26**: 113 – 117 (2006).

Jin, G., J. He, Z. Rui and F. Meng. *Electrochimica Acta* **51**: 4341 – 4346 (2006).

Joshi, K. A., J. Tang, R. Haddon, J. Wang, W. Chen and A. Mulchandania. *Electroanalysis* **17**: 54 – 58 (2005).

Joshi, P. P., S. A. Merchant, Y. Wang and D. W. Schmidtke. **77**: 3183 – 3188 (2005).

Kandimalla, V. B., V. S. Tripathi and H. Ju. *Biomaterials* **27**: 1167 – 1174 (2006).

Katz, E. and I. Willner. *Chem. Phys. Chem* **5**: 1084 (2004).

Kerman, K., Y. Morita, Y. Takamura, M. Ozsoz and E. Tamiya. *Electroanalysis* **16**: 1667 – 1672 (2004).

Koehne, J., H. Chen, J. Li, A. M. Cassell, Q. Ye, H. T. Ng, J. Han and M. Meyyappan. *Nanotechnology* **14**: 1239 – 1245 (2003).

Koehne, J., J. Li, A. M. Cassell, H. Chen, Q. Ye, H. T. Ng, J. Han and M. Meyyappan. *Journal of Materials Chemistry* **14**: 676 – 684 (2004).

Kojima, A., C. K. Hyon, T. Kamimura, M. Maeda and K. Matsumoto. *Jpn. J. Appl. Phys.* **44**: 1596 – 1598 (2005).

Lawrence, N. S. and J. Wang. *Electrochemistry Communications* **8**: 71 – 76 (2006).

Li, C., M. Curreli, H. Lin, B. Lei, F. N. Ishikawa, R. Datar, R. J. Cote, M. E. Thompson and C. Zhou. *J. Am. Chem. Soc.* **127**: 12,484 – 12,485 (2005).

Li, G., J. M. Liao, G. Q. Hua, N. Z. Ma and P. J. Wu. *Biosensors and Bioelectronics* **20**: 2140 – 2144 (2005).

Li, J., A. Cassell, L. Delzeit, J. Han and M. Meyyappan. *J. Phys. Chem. B* **106**: 9299 – 9305 (2002).

Li, J., H. T. Ng, A. Cassell, W. Fan, H. Chen, Q. Ye, J. Koehne, J. Han and M. Meyyappan, *Nano Letters* **3**: 597 – 602 (2003).

Li, J., Q. Zhang, D. Yang and J. Tian. *Carbon* **42**: 2263 – 2267 (2004).

Li, J., Q. Liu, Y. Liu, S. Liu and S. Yao. *Analytical Biochemistry* **246**: 107 – 114 (2005).

Li, J., Q. Zhang, N. Peng and Q. Zhu. *Applied Physics Letters* **86**: 153,116 (2005).

Lin, Y., F. Lu, Y. Tu and Z. Ren. *Nano Letter* **4**: 191 – 195 (2004).

Liu, G., S. L. Riechers, M. C. Mellen and Y. Lin. *Electrochemistry Communications* **7**: 1163 – 1169 (2005).

Liu, G. and Y. Lin. *Anal. Chem.* **78**: 835 – 843 (2006).

Liu, J., A. Chou, W. Rahmat, M. N. Paddon-Row and J. J. Gooding. *Electroanalysis* **17**: 38 – 46 (2005).

Lu, G., L. Jiang, F. Song, C. Liu and L. Jiang. *Electroanalysis* **17**: 901 – 905 (2005).

Luong, J. H. T., S. Hrapovic and D. Wang. *Electroanalysis* **17**: 47 – 53 (2005).

Luque, G. L., N. F. Ferreyra and G. A. Rivas. *Microchim Acta* **152**: 277 – 283 (2006).

Ly, S. Y. *Bioelectrochemistry* **68**: 227 – 231 (2006).

Maehashi, K., K. Matsumoto, K. Kerman, Y. Takamura and E. Tamiya. *Japanese Journal of Applied Physics* **43**: L1558 – L1560 (2004).

Male, K. B., S. Hrapovic, Y. Liu, D. Wang and J. H. T. Luong. *Analytica Chimica Acta* **516**: 35 – 41 (2004).

Munge, B., G. Liu, G. Collins and J. Wang. *Anal. Chem.* **77**: 4662 – 4666 (2005).

Musameh, M., J. Wang, A. Merkoci and Y. Lin. *Electrochemistry Communications* **4**: 743 – 746 (2002).

Musameh, M., N. S. Lawrence and J. Wang. *Electrochem. Commun.* **7**: 14 (2005).

Nugent, J. M., K. S. V. Santhanam, A. Rubio and P. M. Ajayan. *Nano Lett.* **1**: 87 (2001).

Patolsky, F., Y. Weizmann and I. Willner. *Angew. Chem. Int. Ed.* **43**: 2113 – 2117 (2004).

Pedano, M. L. and G. A. Rivas. *Electrochemistry Communications* **6**: 10 – 16 (2004).

Pumera, M., A. Merkoc and S. Alegret. *Sensors and Actuators B* **113**: 617 – 622 (2006).

Qi, P., O. Vermesh, M. Grecu, A. Javey, Q. Wang, H. Dai, S. Peng and K. J. Cho. *Nano Lett.* **3**: 347 – 351 (2003).

Qu, F., M. Yang, J. Chen, G. Shen and R. Yu. *Analytical Letters* **39**: 1785 – 1799 (2006).

Rouhanizadeh, M., T. Tang, C. Li, J. Hwang, C. Zhou and T. K. Hsiai. *Sensors and Actuators B* **114**: 788 – 798 (2005).

Rouhanizadeh, M., T. Tang, C. Li, J. Hwang, C. Zhou and T. K. Hsiai. *Sensors and Actuators B* **114**: 788 – 798 (2006).

Roy, S., H. Vedala and W. Choi. *Nanotechnology* **17**: S14 – S18 (2006).

Rubianes, M. D. and G. A. Rivas. *Electroanalysis* **17**: 73 – 78 (2005).

Salimi, A., R. G. Compton and R. Hallaj. *Analytical Biochemistry* **333**: 49 – 56 (2004).

Salimi, A., R. Hallaj and G.-R. Khayatian. *Electroanalysis* **17**: 873 – 879 (2005).

Shi, Q., T. Peng, Y. Zhu and C. F. Yang. *Electroanalysis* **17**: 857 – 861 (2005).

Shim, M., N. W. S. Kam, R. J. Chen, Y. Li and H. Dai. *Nano Lett.* **2**: 285 – 288 (2002).

So, H.-M., K. Won, Y. H. Kim, B.-K. Kim, B. H. Ryu, P. S. Na, H. Kim and J.-O. Lee. *J. Am. Chem. Soc.* **127**: 11,906 – 11,907 (2005).

Song, Z., J. Huang, B. Wu, H. Shi, J.-I. Anzai and Q. Chen. *Sensors and Actuators B* **115**: 626 – 633 (2006).

Star, A., J.-C. P. Gabriel, K. Bradley and G. Gruner. *Nano Lett.* **3**: 459 – 463 (2003).

Star, A., V. Joshi, T.-R. Han, M. V. P. Altoe, G. Gruner and J. F. Stoddart. *Organic Letters* **6**: 2089 – 2092 (2004).

Star, A., E. Tu, J. Niemann, J.-C. P. Gabriel, C. S. Joiner and C. Valcke. *Proc. Natl. Acad. Sci. USA*. **103**: 921 – 926 (2006).

Takeda, S., A. Sbagyo, Y. Sakoda, A. Ishii, M. Sawamura, K. Sueoka, H. Kida, K. Mukasa and K. Matsumoto. *Biosensors and Bioelectronics* **21**: 201 – 205 (2005).

Tang, H., J. Chen, S. Yao, L. Nie, G. Deng and Y. Kuang. *Analytical Biochemistry* **331**: 89 – 97 (2004).

Tang, H., J. Chen, L. Nie, S. Yao and Y. Kuang. *Electrochimica Acta* **51**: 3046 – 3051 (2006).

Tang, X., S. Bansaruntip, N. Nakayama, E. Yenilmez, Y.-l. Chang and Q. Wang. *Nano Lett.* **6**: 1632 – 1636 (2006).

Trojanowicz, M. *Trends in Analytical Chemistry* **25**: 480 (2006).

Tsai, Y., S. Li and J. Chen. *Langmuir* **21**: 3653 – 3658 (2005).

Tu, Y., Y. Lin, W. Yantasee and Z. Ren. *Electroanalysis* **17**: 79 (2005).

Viswanathan, S., L. Wu, M.-R. Huang and J.-a. A. Ho. *Anal. Chem.* **78**: 1115 – 1121 (2006).

Wang, J., M. Li, Z. Shi, N. Li and Z. Gu. *Anal. Chem.* **74**: 1993 – 1997 (2002).

Wang, J., R. P. Deo and M. Musameh. *Electroanalysis* **15**: 1830 – 1834 (2003a).

Wang, J. and M. Musameh. *Anal. Chem.* **75**: 2075 – 2079 (2003b).

Wang, J., M. Li, Z. Shi, N. Li and Z. Gua. *Electroanalysis* **16**: 140 – 144 (2004).

Wang, J., G. Liu and M. R. Jan. J. *Am. Chem. Soc.* **126**: 3010 – 3011 (2004a).

Wang, J., A.-N. Kawde and M. R. Jan. *Biosensors and Bioelectronics* **20**: 995 – 1000 (2004b).

Wang, J. and M. Musameh. *Analytica Chimica Acta* **539**: 209 – 213 (2005a).

Wang, J. Electroanalysis **17**: 7 – 14 (2005b).

Wang, S. G., Q. Zhang, R. Wang and S. F. Yoon, *Biochemical and Biophysical Research Communications* **311**: 572 – 576 (2003a).

Wang, S. G., Q. Zhang, R. Wang, S. F. Yoon, J. Ahn, D. J. Yang, J. Z. Tian, J. Q. Li and Q. Zhou. *Electrochemistry Communications* **5**: 800 – 803 (2003b).

Wang, S. G., R. Wang, P. J. Sellin and Q. Zhang. *Biochemical and Biophysical Research Communications* **325**: 1433 – 1437 (2004).

Weber, J., A. Kumar, A. Kumar and S. Bhansali. *Sensors and Actuators B* **117**: 308 – 313 (2006).

Wei, S., F. Zhao, Z. Xu and B. Zeng. *Microchim Acta* **152**: 285 – 290 (2006).

Wu, F., G. Zhao and X. Wei. *Electrochemistry Communications* **4**: 690 – 694 (2002).

Wu, K., Y. Sun and S. Hu. *Sensors and Actuators B* **96**: 658 – 662 (2003).

Wu, K., H. Wang, F. Chen and S. Hu. *Bioelectrochemistry* **68**: 144 – 149 (2006).

Wu, Y. and S. Hu. *Colloids and Surfaces B: Biointerfaces* **41**: 299 – 304 (2005).

Wu, Y., S. Ye and S. Hu. *Journal of Pharmaceutical and Biomedical Analysis* **41**: 820 – 824 (2006).

Yang, M., Y. Yang, Y. Liu, G. Shen and R. Yu. *Biosensors and Bioelectronics* **21**: 1125 – 1131 (2006).

Ye, J., Y. Wen, W. Zhang, L. M. Gan, G. Xu and F. Sheu. *Electrochemistry Communications* **6**: 66 – 70 (2004).

Ye, J., Y. Wen, W. Zhang, H. Cui, G. Xu and F.-S. Sheu. *Electroanalysis* **17**: 89 – 96 (2005).

Zeng, B., S. Wei, F. Xiao and F. Zhao. *Sensors and Actuators B* **115**: 240 – 246 (2006).

Zhang, J., A. Boyd, A. Tselev, M. Paranjape and P. Barbara. *Applied Physics Letters* **88**: 123,112 (2006).

Zhang, L., G. Zhao, X. Wei and Z. Yang. *Electroanalysis* **17**: 630 – 634 (2005).
Zhang, M. and W. Gorski. *Anal. Chem.* **77**: 3960 – 3965 (2005a).
Zhang, M. and W. Gorski. *J. Am. Chem.* Soc. **127**: 2058 – 2059 (2005b).
Zhang, Y., Y. Cai, and S. Su. *Analytical Biochemistry* **350**: 285 – 291 (2006).
Zhao, H. and H. Ju. *Analytical Biochemistry* **350**: 138 – 144 (2006).
Zhao, Q., L. Guan, Z. Gu and Q. Zhuang. *Electroanalysis* **17**: 85 – 88 (2005).
Zhu, N., Z. Chang, P. He and Y. Fang. *Analytica Chimica Acta* **545**: 21 – 26 (2005).
Zhu, Y., Z. Zhang and D. Pang. *Journal of Electroanalytical Chemistry* **581**: 303 – 309 (2005).

10 Heparin-Conjugated Nanointerfaces for Biomedical Applications

Ki Dong Park, Yoon Ki Joung, Jin Woo Bae, Dong Hyun Go

Dept. of Molecular Science and Technology, Ajou University, SUWON 443-749, Korea

Abstract This chapter describes some examples of heparin-conjugated nanointerfaces for biomedical applications in terms of both development and application. First, heparin-conjugated linear and star shaped poly(lactic acid) (PLA-Hep and sPLA-Hep) to improve blood compatibility and its related biocompatibility of degradable polymers were introduced. Second, a heparin-conjugated PM system that consists of Tetronic and poly(ε-caprolactone) (PCL) is described as an injectable vehicle for an effective long-term delivery of growth factors. Finally, the heparin-immobilized small intestinal submucosa (SIS) was investigated to observe the effect of heparin immobilization on blood compatibility, in vitro fibroblast attachment and in vivo calcification of SIS. All of these examples demonstrate that heparin-conjugated nanointerfaces might be a versatile and promising tool to achieve advanced biomaterials.

10.1 Introduction

Heparin, a sulfated polysaccharide belonging to the family of glycosaminoglycans, has numerous important biological activities that are associated with its interaction with diverse proteins. Heparin is widely used as an anticoagulant drug based on its ability to accelerate the rate at which antithrombin inhibits serine proteases in the blood coagulation cascade. Therefore, the incorporation of heparin to biomaterials has been studied by dispersing heparin within the biomaterial (Kito and Matsuda, 1996), by ionic binding or covalent immobilization of heparin (Bourin and Lindahl, 1993).

The biological activities of heparin primarily result from their interaction with hundreds of different proteins including enzymes (i.e. thrombin), lipoproteins, growth factors, chemokines, viral coat proteins, extracellular matrix proteins, etc. (Linhardt, 2003). Specific recognition between heparin and proteins also requires

(1) Corresponding e-mail: kdp@ajou.ac.kr

defined sequences within the heparin chain. Heparin predominantly exhibits linear helical secondary structures with sulfo and carboxyl groups displayed at defined intervals and in defined orientations along the polysaccharide backbone. Heparin-binding domain on a protein would, therefore, require a minimum number of saccharide residues within the heparin chain to appropriately display these charged groups to facilitate a tight and specific interaction (Capila and Linhardt, 2002).

The incorporation of heparin to biomaterials has been widely studied to improve the biocompatibility (blood and cell) of biomaterials. In particular, heparinized surfaces play crucial roles in biological phenomena as interfaces between biological environments (i.e. blood, tissues, etc.) and biomaterials for a variety of biomedical applications. Such surfaces have been mainly prepared and investigated by coating, self-assembling in aqueous solution, immobilization on existing natural (or synthetic) surfaces, and so on. As advancing in biomedical fields, however, bioactive surfaces with 'nano' size have lately attracted considerable remark, which can designate a novel term 'nanointerface'. The nanointerface has many advantages with various functionalities such as the immobilization of bioactive molecules to utilize it for biomedical applications. In this chapter, some examples of heparin-conjugated nanointerfaces for biomedical applications are introduced in terms of material and application.

The use of biodegradable polymers has been proposed recently for several applications including tissue engineering, gene therapy, novel drug delivery systems, implantable devices, and nanotechnology. Further applications of biodegradable polymers have been desired in blood-contacting situations such as vascular prosthesis where temporary reconstruction and/or stabilization of tissue and organs is needed, and intravascular stents that should maintain blood vessels open after balloon dilatation (Agrawal et al., 1992). However, thrombus formation and cell compatibility are still serious problems in the use of biodegradable polymers like polylactide (PLA) and investigations on properties of the materials that contact tissue are rarely found. Therefore, heparin-conjugated linear and star shaped PLAs (PLA-Hep and sPLA-Hep) to improve blood compatibility and its related biocompatibility of degradable polymers were investigated and introduced in this chapter.

Polymeric micelles (PMs), supramolecular assemblies of block copolymers, have been receiving intrinsic attention as colloidal carrier systems for delivery of poor absorbable hydrophobic drugs and proteins (Kakizawa and Kataoka, 2002). The micelles serve the segregated core which is shown to function as a reservoir for hydrophilic drugs such as proteins and peptides as well as the hydrophilic shell which pays an important role in absorption of drug carrier since it derives a well-dispersion property in aqueous environment (Kataoka et al., 2001). Over the past few decades, several technologies have been found to deliver growth factors by incorporating matrices (Wissink et al., 2001), microparticles (Perets et al., 2003) and etc. However, the bioavailability of growth factors is generally poor, since they are poorly absorbed and have a short half-life due to the enzymatic degradation and self-aggregation (Edelman, 1993). To overcome these limitations, heparin is a very promising molecule for introducing to the delivery system for growth factors. Of our studies, therefore, a heparin-conjugated PM system that consists of Tetronic® and poly(ε-caprolactone) (PCL) is described as an injectable vehicle for an effective long-term delivery of growth factor in this chapter.

Since artificial prosthetics such as synthetic polymers and metals were used in the field of cardiovascular surgery, biomaterials possessing essential characteristics of native tissues and organs which are to be replaced have been constantly required for the development of an ideal artificial substitute. Consequently, the use of xenograft and allograft tissues has been in the center of cardiovascular research (Hilbert et al., 1998). Small intestinal submucosa (SIS), a relatively acellular collagen-based matrix derived from porcine small intestine, has been extensively used as a cardiovascular bioprosthesis such as heart valve (Matheny et al., 2000), vascular graft (Roeder et al., 1999), and tissue patch for the repair of myocardial infarction (Badylak et al., 2003). Collagen-based biomaterial such as SIS has typically required chemical or physical pretreatment to enhance in vivo biochemical and mechanical properties. The heparin binding which led to the formation of bridge between adjacent fibrils reduced the calcium accumulation site. In this chapter, The SIS that is chemically modified with heparin is introduced. The heparin-immobilized SIS was investigated to observe the effect of heparin immobilization on blood compatibility, in vitro fibroblast attachment, and in vivo calcification of SIS.

10.2 Heparin-Bound Biodegradable Polymers for Biocompatible Interfaces

10.2.1 Heparin-Conjugated Polylactide (PLA-Hep)

10.2.1.1 Synthesis of PLA-Hep

PLA has been prepared by the method that previously reported (Ajioka et al., 1995). Briefly, L-lactide (10 g, 0.07 mol) was melted at 180℃ for 30 min. in a nitrogen atmosphere. Stannous octoate (0.1 wt% of L-lactide) was added to melted L-lactide solution. The mixture was degassed and stirred at 150℃ for 30 min. The product was dissolved in chloroform and then precipitated in excess methanol. The precipitate was filtered and dried overnight under vacuum.

PLA-Hep was prepared by direct coupling reaction using DCC/DMAP chemistry (Fig. 10.1). Heparin (1.8 g, 1×10^{-4} mol) and PLA (0.5 g, 0.5×10^{-4} mol) were first dissolved in the mixture of formamide (50 mL) and *N*,*N*-dimethylformamide (DMF, 50 mL). DCC (1×10^{-4} mol) and DMAP (1×10^{-4} mol) were added to heparin solution with stirring for 10 minutes. Then, PLA solution was dropped into the reaction solution with stirring at 50℃ for 12 h under nitrogen atmosphere. After the coupling reaction, the reaction solution was precipitated in excess methanol and then the precipitate was washed with distilled water. The washed precipitate was dissolved in chloroform and the solution was precipitated in excess methanol. After filtering, the precipitate was dried at 35℃ for 24 h in vacuo to eliminate the residual solvent.

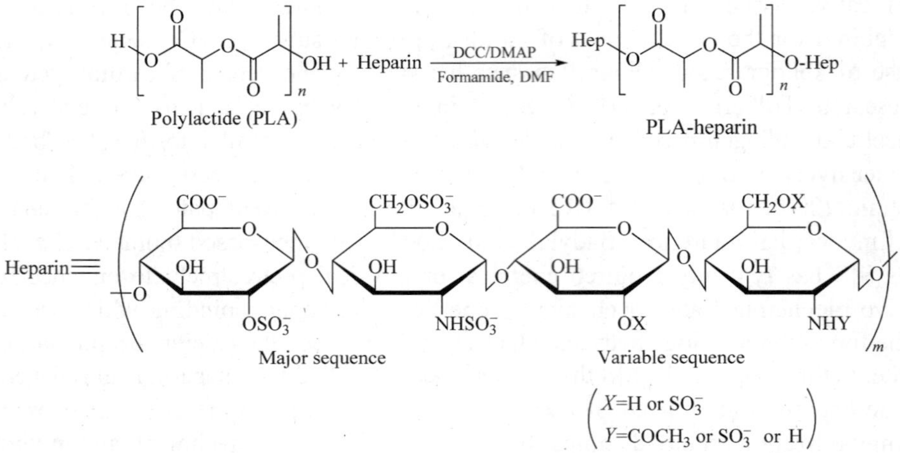

Figure 10.1 Scheme for the conjugation of heparin to PLA

Purified glass beads were coated with PLA and PLA-Hep solutions (0.1% *w*/*v* in chloroform), filtered through microfilter, and dried in vacuo at 25℃ for 24 h. Finally, the obtained beads were mechanically sieved to remove aggregation. Glass slides were also coated with PLA and PLA-Hep solutions (0.1% *w*/*v* in chloroform) by spin-coater (2000 r/min, 2 min), and then dried in vacuo for 24 h. The structure of the PLA-Hep was characterized by Fourier Transform Infrared Spectrophotometer (FT-IR, Nicolet, Magma-IR 550) and elemental analyzer (Fisons EA 1108, Italy). The wettability of the PLA and the PLA-Hep surface was characterized by static contact angle (SCA, GBX Instrumentation Scientificque, DGD fast/60). The contact angles were measured by putting sessile droplet of triple-distilled water on the PLA and PLA-Hep surfaces.

FT-IR was used to confirm the result of the synthesis. The unreacted hydroxyl groups of the PLA show a fairly sharp absorption near 3600 cm^{-1}, whereas there is a broader absorption in the 3300 – 3500 cm^{-1}, which can be identified by characteristic N-H bond stretching adsorption and/or hydrogen-bonded hydroxyl groups of the PLA-Hep. In addition, IR spectra of the PLA-Hep display the new absorption bands near 1250 and 1650 cm^{-1} compared to that of the PLA, which are characteristic adsorption peaks of sulfonyl group ($—SO_3$ stretching) and amino group (N—H bending) of conjugated heparin. These results indicate the formation of the PLA-Hep. The sulfur content of the PLA-Hep measured by elemental analyzer was determined to be 1.34% (calculated value was 2.70%).

The contact angle data of the PLA and PLA-Hep surfaces are summarized in Table 10.1. The static contact angle of the PLA-Hep was decreased by 14 degree as compared to the PLA, suggesting that the exposure of conjugated heparin on surface contribute to increased wettability of the PLA-Hep surface (decreased angle).

Table 10.1 Water contact angles of PLA and PLA-heparin

Substrate	Contact angle (deg.)
PLA	84.0 ± 0.5
PLA-Hep	70.3 ± 0.4

(mean ± standard deviation, $n = 5$)

Quantitative analysis of conjugated heparin. The content of conjugated heparin was analyzed by the toluidine blue colorimetric method (Smith et al., 1980). An aliquot of toluidine blue solution (0.05 g of toluidine blue was dissolved in 1 L of 0.01 mol/L HCl containing 0.2% NaCl) was pipetted into each of four test tubes. The 0.1 mL of heparin standard solution with various concentrations (0.1 – 2 μg/mL in 0.2% NaCl) was added to the toluidine blue solution. Hexane (1.0 mL) was added to each solution and the solutions were vortexed for 30 seconds and allowed for a phase separation. The absorbance of the aqueous layers was determined at 631 nm on a UV spectrophotometer. For direct quantitative determination of heparin, the dye-binding interactions with toluidine blue were utilized. The amount of surface exposed heparin associated with PLA-Hep was measured to be 0.067 $\mu g/cm^2$.

10.2.1.2 Blood Compatibility Test

Activated partial thromboplastin time (APTT) assay. The anticoagulant activity of PLA-Hep was determined by means of an APTT assay. In conjunction with incubated plasma, thromboplastin (Pathromtin®SL) enables the individual factors of the intrinsic coagulation system to be quantified and permits diagnosis of hemophilia. Calcium ions of calcium chloride trigger the coagulation process; the time for the formation of a fibrin clot is measured.

Briefly, the PLA and the PLA-Hep coated glass beads (0.01 g) were added into the test tube. Citrated standard plasma (100 μL) and Pathromtin®SL (100 μL) were then pipetted into a test tube pre-warmed to 37℃, and it was incubated for 3 minutes at 37℃. On adding the calcium chloride solution (100 μL, 0.025 mol/L) at 37℃, the timer on a fibrintimer (Behring Fibrintimer, Hamburg, Germany) starts to measure the clotting time. A calibration curve of clotting time was obtained by measuring the clotting time of heparin solution with various concentrations (0.05 – 3 μg/mL). Standard curve of clotting time was made using heparin as a reference. The anticoagulant activity of the PLA-Hep was calculated by the standard curve, which is compared with the activities of the PLA and free heparin.

In vitro heparin's bioactivity was determined by an APTT assay. The clotting time of the PLA-Hep conjugate measured by APTT was prolonged when compared with the PLA control, as summarized in Table 10.2. The activity of conjugated heparin was calculated to be 17.39 % as compared to free heparin (187 unit/mg). The unique anticoagulant property of heparin is that it binds to antithrombin (AT-III) present in the blood plasma (Linhardt, 2003), the major inhibitor of the coagulation cascade; thereby the complex formed readily reacts with thrombin to inhibit the formation of fibrin network which is an important step for the thrombosis (Jang et al., 1990). The conjugated heparin might inhibit the intrinsic coagulation factors, thus leading to a suppression of thrombin activity. Thus it is possible that PLA-Hep surface may bind AT-III from the plasma and are thus able to neutralize the activity of clotting factors generated at the blood-material interface.

Table 10.2 APTT data of PLA and PLA-Hep (mean ± standard deviation, $n = 5$)

Substrate	APTT (s)
PLA	31.8 ± 0.2
PLA-heparin	49.9 ± 0.1

In vitro protein adsorption. A bicinchoninic acid protein assay (Micro BCA^{TM}) was performed to determine the total amount of protein adsorbed onto the surfaces (Smith et al., 1985). After equilibrium with 0.1 mol/L PBS (pH = 7.4) for 12 h, the PLA and PLA-Hep coated glass slides (circular, diameter = 2 mm) were incubated in 24-well plates containing 2 mL of PPP at 37℃ for 5, 15, 30, 60, and 120 min, respectively. Each sample was then rinsed with PBS and incubated with 2 mL of PBS containing SDS solution (1.0 wt.% SDS + 1 m mol/L EDTA + 0.1 mol/L Tris, pH = 7.4) for 1 h to measure the amount of irreversibly adsorbed proteins on surfaces. The amount of adsorbed protein was measured with a BCA protein assay kit (Pierce Chemical Co., Rockford, IL).

When biomaterials are in contact with blood, proteins are first adsorbed instantaneously onto the surfaces and deformed. Then platelets are adhered to the surfaces, are activated and aggregated, so that platelets may play a major role in thrombus formation. Therefore, a study on protein adsorption and platelet adhesion is the important step in evaluating the blood compatibility of biomaterials.

Protein adsorption studies were performed with human PPP. As shown in Fig. 10.2, PLA-Hep surface demonstrated lower protein adsorption than untreated PLA surface. It is well known that the protein adsorption to polymer surface is regulated by ionic, hydrophilic and/or hydrophobic interactions and thus influenced by various factors, including surface compositions, wettability, surface charges,

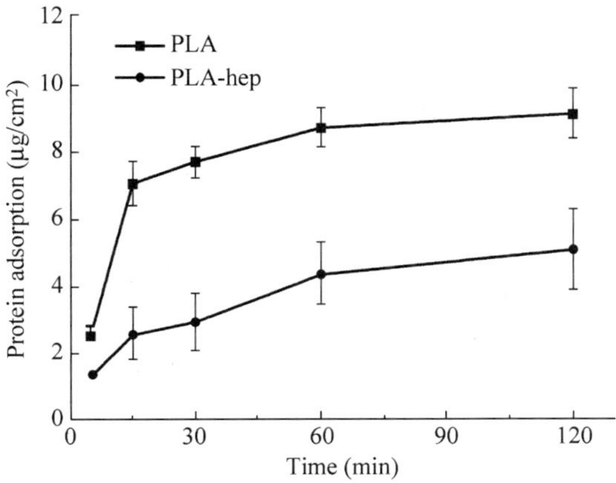

Figure 10.2 Protein adsorption on PLA and PLA-hep surfaces

and roughness. In general, fibrinogen as a major protein adsorbed among a number of proteins in blood, has been shown to adsorb at the lower level on the heparin-modified surface (Thomas et al., 2000). The protein adsorption results (Fig. 10.4) indicate that the change of surface properties including the enhanced hydrophilicity by conjugation of heparin sterically prevents proteins from closely approaching the surface. The adsorption behavior of single proteins (fibrinogen, albumin, gamma globulin) on the PLA-Hep surface is under investigation.

In vitro platelet adhesion. The PLA and the PLA-Hep coated glass beads (0.5 g) were carefully weighed into plastic disposable 5 mL syringes and equilibrated with 2 mL of phosphate-buffered saline (PBS, pH = 7.4, 0.15 mol/L) for overnight. Prior to adhesion studies, the buffer was removed from the syringe and then 2 mL of human PRP (platelet no. 139 ea/mL) was introduced into the syringe. The syringes were tapped to remove air bubbles, sealed, and rotated in a shaking incubator at 37℃ for adhesion times of 5, 15, 30, 60, and 120 min. At each time point, the syringes were quickly removed from the shaking incubator, and immediately counted for depleted platelets in the PRP with the hemacytometer. The amount of platelets that adhered upon the specimen was calculated by subtracting the number of unadhered platelets from the number of diluted platelets that were initially incubated.

Figure 10.3 shows the in-vitro adhesion behavior of platelets on the PLA-Hep. The amount of adhered platelets on the PLA-Hep was lower than control the PLA. Fibrinogen plays an important role in platelet-surface attachment. Platelet GPIIb/IIIa can only recognize the bound fibrinogen that has undergone appropriate conformational changes (Park et al., 1990). Thus it appears that the inhibitory effect of heparin-conjugated PLA on protein adsorption subsequently plays a passive role on platelet-surface attachment. Such depressed interaction of heparin-conjugated PLA with platelets was also explained by electrical repulsions between negatively charged groups of heparin and platelets.

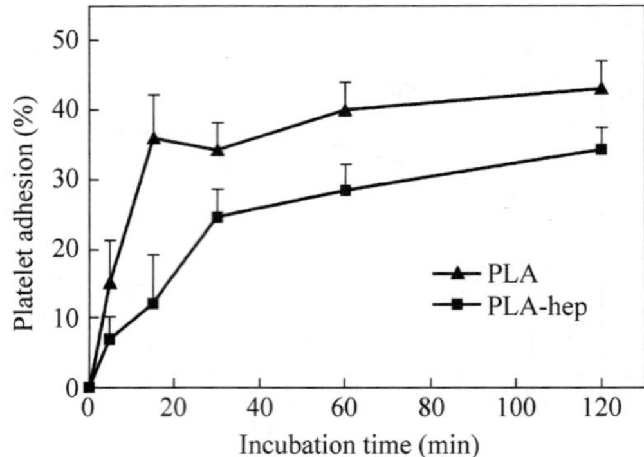

Figure 10.3 Platelet adhesion on PLA and PLA-Hep surfaces. (The data are expressed as percentage of the number of adhered platelet with respect to the total number of platelets)

10.2.2 Heparin-Conjugated Star-Shaped PLA (sPLA-Hep)

10.2.2.1 Synthesis of sPLA-Hep

Star-shaped PLA (sPLA) were synthesized by bulk ring-opening polymerization of L-lactide with pentaerythritol as a four-arm initiator and stannous octoate as a catalyst. Pure L-lactide (10 g, 69.4 mmol) and pentaerythritol (0.236 g, 1.7 mmol) were placed in a dried glass ampoule containing a teflon-coated magnetic stirring bar and the stannous octoate catalyst (0.141 g, 0.34 mmol) added as a solution in toluene. The reactants were dried under reduced pressure, at 60℃ for 30 min. The ampule was then sealed under vacuum, and the polymerization carried out at 130℃ for 6 h. After the reaction, the product was dissolved in chloroform, filtered through a 0.45 μm membrane filter, and precipitated in excess methanol two times. The precipitate was isolated and dried overnight under vacuum.

The sPLA-Hep conjugate was prepared by coupling heparin to sPLA using carbonyldiimidazole (CDI) chemistry as shown in Fig. 10.4. Hydroxyl groups of sPLA were activated by CDI for the reaction with the remained amino-terminal groups of heparin. CDI (2 equivalent to the hydroxyl group's mole of sPLA) in dry chloroform was added to the sPLA in chloroform and stirred for 6 hrs at room temperature under a nitrogen atmosphere. The reaction mixture was precipitated in diethyl ether and dried under vacuum, to give CDI-activated sPLA.

Heparin (3 g, 0.2 mmol) and the CDI-activated sPLA (0.5 g, 0.05 mmol) were first dissolved in the formamide (300 mL) and *N,N*-DMF 50 mL), respectively. Then, sPLA solution was dropped into heparin solution with stirring at 40℃ for 24 h under nitrogen atmosphere. After the coupling reaction, the reaction solution was precipitated in excess methanol and then the precipitate was washed in distilled water. The precipitate was dissolved in chloroform and the solution was precipitated in excess methanol. After filtering, the precipitate was dried at 35℃ for 24 h in vacuo to eliminate the residual solvent (Fig. 10.4).

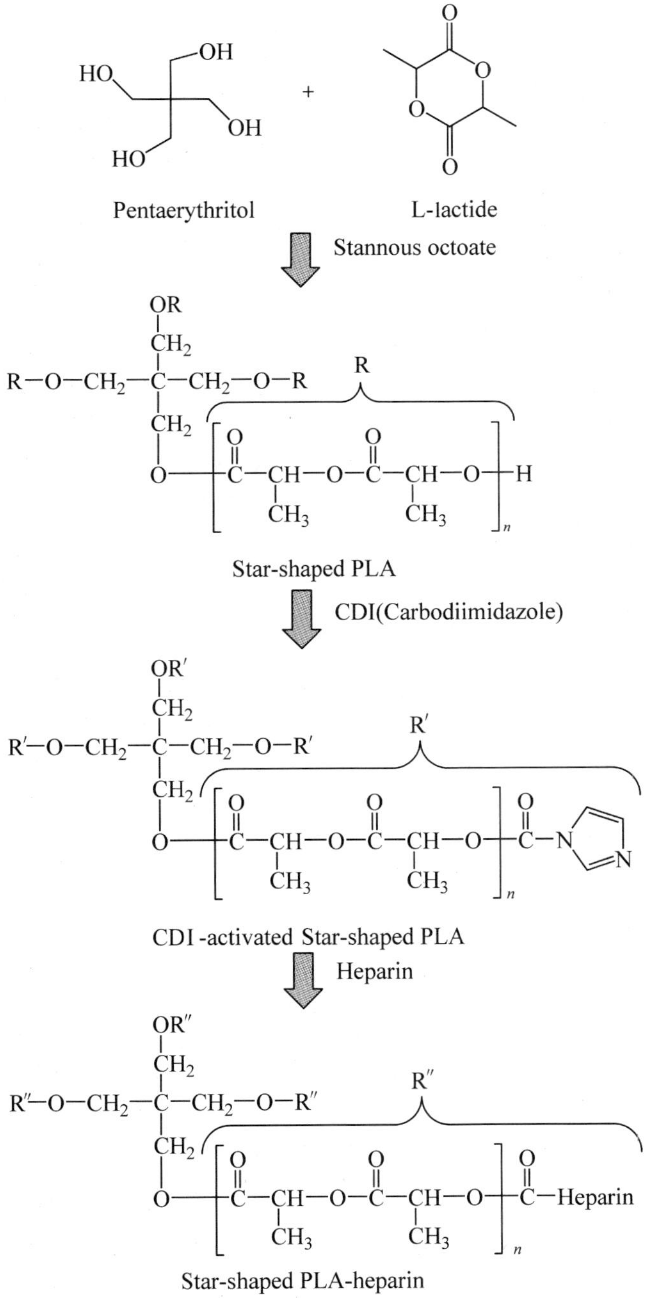
HO
OH
OH
HO
+
O
O
O
O
Pentaerythritol
L-lactide
Stannous octoate
OR
CH2
R—O—CH2—C—CH2—O—R
CH2
O
R
O
O
C—CH—O—C—CH—O
H
CH3
CH3
n
Star-shaped PLA
CDI(Carbodiimidazole)
OR′
R′—O—CH2—C—CH2—O—R′
R′
C—N
N
CDI -activated Star-shaped PLA
Heparin
OR″
R″—O—CH2—C—CH2—O—R″
R″
C—Heparin
Star-shaped PLA-heparin

Figure 10.4 Illustration for the synthesis of sPLA-Hep

Glass slides and glass beads (size: 150 – 210 μm, Sigma) were cleaned by soaking in chromic acid for 24 h and then washed with ethanol and distilled water. Purified glass beads were coated with the sPLA and the sPLA-Hep solutions (0.1% *w/v* in chloroform), filtered through microfilter, and dried in vacuo at 25℃ for 24 h. Finally, the obtained beads were mechanically sieved to remove aggregation. Glass slides were also coated with the sPLA and sPLA-Hep solutions (0.1% *w/v* in chloroform) by spin-coater (2000 r/min, 2 min), and then dried in vacuo for 24 h. The glass slides and glass beads were utilized for the measurement of static contact angle, activated partial thromboplastin assay (APTT) and the evaluation of in-vitro blood compatibility (platelet adhesion and protein adsorption test), respectively.

The molecular weight of the sPLA was measured by gel permeation chromatography equipped with 515 HPLC pump, 717 plus auto sampler and differential refractometer (Waters Co., USA). The structure of the PLA-heparin was characterized by Fourier Transform Infrared Spectrophotometer (FT-IR, Nicolet, and Magma-IR 550). The wettability of the sPLA and the sPLA-Hep surface was characterized by static contact angle measurement (SCA, GBX Instrumentation Scientificque, DGD fast/60). The contact angles were measured by putting sessile droplet of triple-distilled water on the sPLA and the sPLA-Hep surfaces.

The sPLA were synthesized by ring-opening polymerization in bulk. Stannous octoate was used as a catalyst because of its known low toxicity. The molecular weight of synthesized the sPLA measured by GPC was shown to be 10,676 (M_n), 11,678 (M_w) and 1.09 (PDI). The sPLA-Hep was prepared by coupling reaction using CDI, which utilizes the terminal hydroxyl groups of the sPLA and the amino groups of heparin molecules.

FT-IR spectra of the sPLA and the sPLA-Hep showed successful result for the synthesis as that of the PLA-Hep. The hydrophilicity of the surface was evaluated based on the water contact angle which was measured using a sessile drop method. The contact angles of the sPLA and the sPLA-Hep surfaces has been shown to be $(101.3 \pm 0.5)^\circ$ and $(87.2 \pm 0.4)^\circ$, respectively. The static contact angle of the sPLA-Hep was decreased by 14° as compared to the sPLA, suggesting that the exposure of conjugated heparin on surface contribute to increased wettability of the sPLA-Hep surface (decreased angle).

Quantitative analysis of heparin. The content of conjugated heparin was analyzed by the toluidine blue colorimetric method like the case of the PLA-Hep. The amount of surface exposed heparin associated with the sPLA-Hep surface was measured to be 1.432 μg/cm^2. Higher content of heparin on surface has been achieved by the sPLA-Hep when compared to linear sPLA-Hep surface (0.067 μg/cm^2).

10.2.2.2 Blood Compatibility Test

APTT assay. Briefly, the sPLA and the sPLA-Hep coated glass beads (0.01 g) were added into the test tube. Citrated standard plasma (100 μL) and Pathromtin®SL

(100 μL) were then pipetted into a test tube pre-warmed to 37℃, and it was incubated for 3 min at 37℃. On adding the calcium chloride solution (100 μL, 0.025 mol/L) at 37℃, the timer on a coagulation analyzer (SYSMEX CA 50, Kobe, Japan) starts to measure the clotting time. A calibration curve of clotting time was obtained by measuring the clotting time of heparin solution with various concentrations (0.005 – 10 μg/mL). The anticoagulant activity of sPLA-Hep was calculated by the standard curve, which is compared with the activities of sPLA and free heparin.

Covalent binding of heparin ingeneral result, in a loss of biological activity as compared to free heparin because of increased coupling of essential functional groups of heparin to the surface. Therefore, in vitro bioactivity of surface bonded heparin was determined by APTT assay. The clotting time of sPLA-Hep conjugate measured by APTT was prolonged when compared with sPLA control (sPLA; (34.90 ± 0.36)s, sPLA-Hep; (58.17 ± 3.00)s). The activity of conjugated heparin was estimated to be 38.6% as compared to free heparin (165 unit/mg). In our previous study on the APTT assay of Linear PLA-heparin conjugate, the heparin activity was evaluated to be 17.39%. The unique anticoagulant property of heparin is that it binds to antithrombin III (AT-III) present in the blood plasma (Linhardt, 2003), the major inhibitor of the coagulation cascade, thereby the complex formed readily reacts with thrombin to inhibit the formation of fibrin network which is an important step for the thrombosis (Jang et al., 1990). The conjugated heparin might inhibit the intrinsic coagulation factors, thus leading to a suppression of thrombin activity.

In vitro plasma protein adsorption. A bicinchoninic acid protein assay (Micro BCA^{TM}) was performed to determine the total amount of protein adsorbed onto the surface. After equilibrium with 0.1 mol/L PBS (pH = 7.4) for 12 h, the sPLA and the sPLA-Hep coated glass slides (circular, diameter: 12 mm) were incubated in 24-well plates containing 2 mL of platelet-poor plasma (PPP) at 37℃ for 60 min, respectively. Each sample was then rinsed with PBS and incubated with 2 mL of PBS containing sodium dodecylsulfate (SDS) solution (1.0 wt.% SDS + 1 mmol/L EDTA + 0.1 mol/L Tris, pH = 7.4) for 1 h to measure the amount of irreversibly adsorbed proteins on surface. It has been checked and confirmed that surface adsorbed proteins were completely removed after SDS treatment for 1 h. The amount of adsorbed protein was measured with a BCA protein assay kit (Product No. 23231, 23232, 23234, Pierce Chemical Co., Rockford, IL).

Proteins are adsorbed on the materials instantly when contacted with foreign materials and deformed to react further with blood or tissue components, and therefore, protein adsorption might regulate all the subsequent living system-material interactions. It is well known that the behavior of protein adsorption onto polymer surface depended significantly on the surface characteristics, such as ionic, hydrophilic and/or hydrophobic interactions and thus influenced by various factors, including surface compositions, wettability, surface charges, and roughness. After proteins are adsorbed, then platelets are adhered to the surface, and then the adhered platelet are activated and aggregated, so that platelets may play a major role in thrombus formation. Therefore, a study on protein adsorption and platelet adhesion is the important step in evaluating the blood compatibility of biomaterials.

Protein adsorption studies were performed with human PPP. As shown in Fig. 10.5, the sPLA-Hep surface demonstrated lower protein adsorption than control the sPLA surface. In general, fibrinogen as a major protein adsorbed among a number of proteins in blood, has been shown to adsorb at the lower level on the heparin-modified surface (Thomas et al., 2000). The protein adsorption indicates that the change of surface properties including the enhanced hydrophilicity by conjugation of heparin sterically prevents proteins from closely approaching the surface.

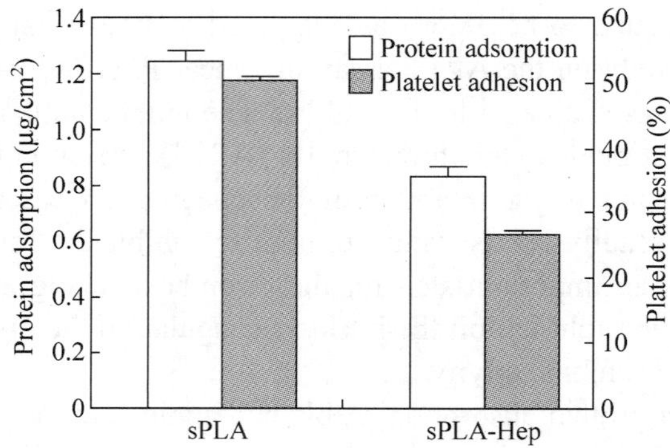

Figure 10.5 Protein adsorption and platelet adhesion after 60 min. incubation on the sPLA and the sPLA-Hep (The data are expressed as percentage of the number of adhered platelet with respect to the total number of platelets)

In vitro platelet adhesion. In vitro platelet adhesion was measured by the sPLA and the sPLA-Hep coated glass beads (0.5 g) were introduced into plastic disposable 5 mL syringes and hydrated with 2 mL of phosphate-buffered saline (PBS, pH = 7.4, 0.15 mol/L) for 1 day. Prior to adhesion studies, the buffer was removed from the syringe and then 2 mL of human Platelet Rich Plasma (PRP, platelet no. 139 ea/mL) was introduced into the syringe. The syringes were tapped to remove air bubbles, sealed, and rotated in a shaking incubator at 37℃ for adhesion times of 60 min. At each time interval, the syringes were quickly removed from the shaking incubator, and immediately counted depleted platelets in the PRP with the hemacytometer. The amount of platelets that adhered upon the specimen was calculated by subtracting the number of not-adhered platelets from the number of diluted platelets that were initially incubated.

Figure 10.5 shows the data of in vitro platelet adhesion of the sPLA-Hep. The amount of adhered platelets on sPLA-Hep was lower than the control sPLA. Fibrinogen plays an important role in platelet—surface attachment. Platelet

GPIIb/IIIa can only recognize the bound fibrinogen that has undergone appropriate conformational changes (Park et al., 1990). This might be contributed to decreased platelet adhesion on the sPLA-Hep as compared to the sPLA, although detailed mechanism is subject to further study. Such depressed interaction of the sPLA-Hep with platelets and proteins can be also explained by electrical repulsions between negatively charged groups of heparin and platelets.

10.2.2.3 In Vitro Assay for Cell Compatibility

1. In vitro Cell culture

Mouse fibroblasts were cultured to confluence in Dulbecco's modified Eagle's medium (DMEM) supplemented with 10% fetal bovine serum (FBS) and 1% penicillin/streptomycin. Cells were detached with 0.25% trypsin- EDTA. Cell culture media and reagents were purchased from Gibco (Invitrogen Corp. NY). Cells were counted by hemocytometer and seeded on the sPLA and the sPLA-Hep coated surface at a density of 10^4 cells per each glass. Cells on the each surface are cultured in 24-well tissue culture plate (Cornings Inc., Costar, NY) at 37℃ and 5% CO_2 incubator.

2. Cell growth assay (Actin staining)

In the fibroblast growth assay, the cells on the sPLA and sPLA-Hep coated surfaces were cultured for 5 days. After incubation, cells were washed with PBS and fixed with 4% paraformaldehyde (Sigma, MO) solution in PBS, incubated for 15 min at 37℃ under 5% CO_2 and permeabilized by 0.1% buffered Triton χ-100 solution for 15 min. And then cells were soaked in 4 drops of-Image iT signal enhancer (Molecular Probes, OR), incubated for 30 min at room temperature and rinsed thoroughly with PBS. Substrates were stained in 1 μmol/L Alexa Fluor 488 phalloidin (Molecular Probes, OR) for 1 h at 4℃. After substrates were washed by PBS five times, they were soaked with ProLong cold antifade reagent (Molecular Probes, OR), and covered with cover glass. Cell spreading area is analyzed by image analyzing software in Veiwan Analyzer program.

The cell culture experiments of the sPLA- and the sPLA-Hep-coated surface with mouse fibroblasts was utilized to illustrate the enhanced cell compatibility of the heparinized sPLA by specific protein interaction. The cells on the sPLA and the sPLA-Hep surfaces were cultured for 5 days, and actin filament of fibroblasts on the each surface was stained for cell growth assay. As shown in Fig. 10.6, the cell growth and differentiation characteristics on the sPLA-Hep coated surface were improved than the sPLA surface. In addition, Fig. 10.7 shows the wide cell spreading area of the sPLA-Hep surface by image analyzing software was also enhanced than the control sPLA surface.

The interactions of heparin with extracellular signaling molecules (growth factors and cytokines) have been discovered and many studies have performed to investigate the mechanism of the specific recognition between the proteins and heparin. Heparin predominantly exhibits linear helical secondary structures with

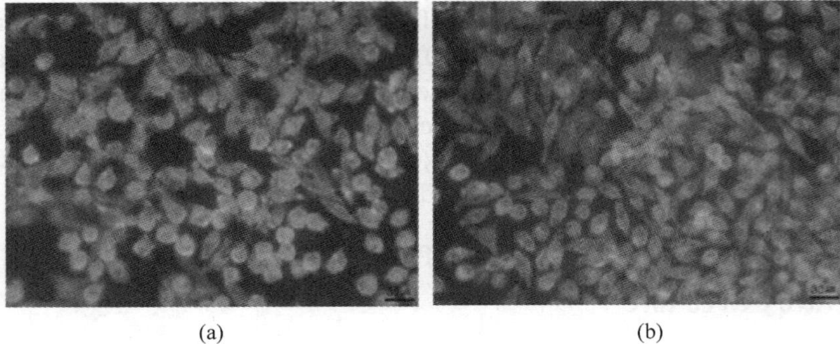

(a) (b)

Figure 10.6 Immunofluorescent staining of fibroblast cultured after 5 days on (a) the sPLA and (b) the sPLA-Hep surface

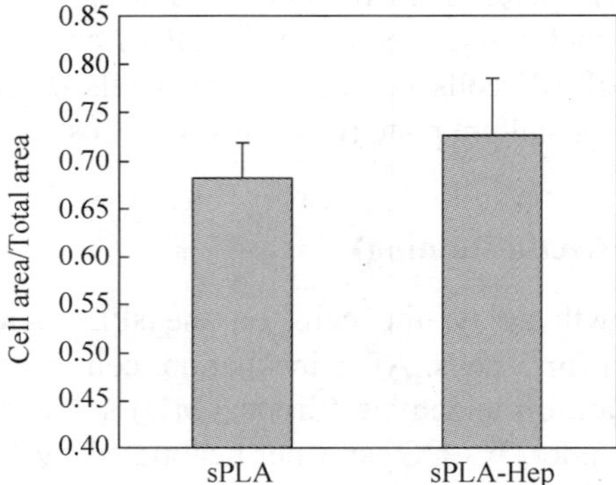

Figure 10.7 Cell spreading area of fibroblast cultured after 5 days on (a) the sPLA and (b) the sPLA-Hep surface

sulfo and carboxyl groups displayed at defined intervals and in defined orientations along the polysaccharide backbone. Because of this heparin structure, heparin can be showed specific recognition with extracellular signaling molecules and positive influence on the cell growth and differentiation. Therefore, heparin immobilized biomaterials have a lot of potential for tissue engineering.

10.3 Heparin-Conjugated Polymeric Micelles

10.3.1 Synthesis of Tetronic®-PCL-Heparin Conjugate

Tetronic®-PCL (TC) copolymer was synthesized by bulk ring-opening polymerization of ε-caprolactone with Tetronic® 1307 (Fig. 10.8) as a four-arm initiator and stannous octoate as a catalyst. Briefly, ε-caprolactone (6 mmol) and Tetronic® 1307 (0.6 mmol) were placed into the ampoule containing Sn-oct (0.17 mmol) and the reactants were dried under reduced pressure at 60℃ for 30 min. The ampoule was then sealed under vacuum and the polymerization was carried out at 110℃ for 20 h. The product was dissolved in chloroform, filtered through a 0.45 μm pore membrane filter, and precipitated in excess diethyl ether twice. Then the precipitate was filtered and dried overnight under vacuum (Choi et al., 1998).

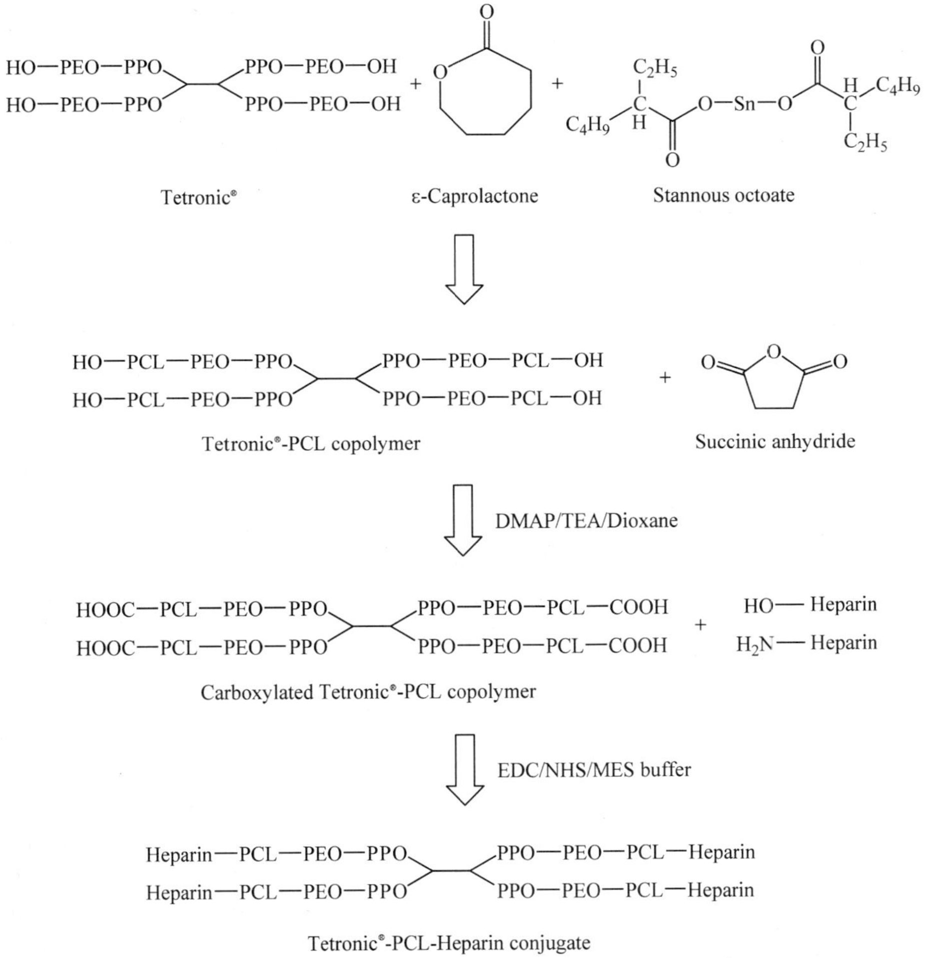

HO—PEO—PPO / HO—PEO—PPO — PPO—PEO—OH / PPO—PEO—OH + ε-Caprolactone + Stannous octoate (C_2H_5, C_4H_9, O—Sn—O)

Tetronic® ε-Caprolactone Stannous octoate

HO—PCL—PEO—PPO / HO—PCL—PEO—PPO — PPO—PEO—PCL—OH / PPO—PEO—PCL—OH + Succinic anhydride

Tetronic®-PCL copolymer Succinic anhydride

DMAP/TEA/Dioxane

HOOC—PCL—PEO—PPO / HOOC—PCL—PEO—PPO — PPO—PEO—PCL—COOH / PPO—PEO—PCL—COOH + HO— Heparin / H_2N— Heparin

Carboxylated Tetronic®-PCL copolymer

EDC/NHS/MES buffer

Heparin—PCL—PEO—PPO / Heparin—PCL—PEO—PPO — PPO—PEO—PCL—Heparin / PPO—PEO—PCL—Heparin

Tetronic®-PCL-Heparin conjugate

Figure 10.8 Total schematic procedure in preparation of Tetronic®-PCL-heparin

To carboxylate the end of TC, TC copolymer (10 g, 0.46 mmol), SA (0.25 g, 2.49 mmol), DMAP (0.244 g, 1.99 mmol), and TEA (0.203 g, 2 mmol) were dissolved in 300 mL anhydrous dioxane and stirred for 24 h at room temperature. The solvent was evaporated with a rotary evaporator. The residue was taken from in chloroform, filtered, and precipitated in ethyl ether twice. The precipitate was filtered and dried overnight under vacuum (Lee et al., 2001).

Tetronic®-PCL-heparin (TCH) conjugate was prepared by EDC/NHS methods (Chung et al., 2005). Carboxylated TC (4 g, 0.2 mmol) was coupled with heparin by EDC (0.156 g, 0.81 mmol) and NHS (0.047 g, 0.41 mmol) in MES buffer (0.05 mol/L, pH = 5.6) at room temperature for 24 h. After reaction, the product was dialyzed against distilled water using a membrane (molecular weight cut-off = 15,000) for 3 days and then lyophilized to result in the product.

The structure characterization of TC and TCH, the contents and activity of the conjugated heparin and the molecular weight of TC were previously reported (Lee et al., in press). The molecular weight of the synthesized TC sample was measured by GPC and it was 20,280 (M_n), 20,300 (M_w) and 1.00 (PDI), respectively. The FT-IR spectra of TCH showed that peaks appeared at 1755 cm^{-1} and 1650 cm^{-1} could be assigned to carbonyl stretching vibration of PCL and heparin, respectively. In addition, FT-IR spectra of TCH displayed the new broader absorption bands in 3300 – 3600 cm^{-1} which can be identified by hydroxyl groups of conjugated heparin. In the ^{1}H-NMR analysis, the chemical shifts of CH_2 of the PCL block main chain at 1.4, 1.6, 2.2, and 4.0 ppm, are found. And, the existence of a covalent bond between the Tetronic® and the PCL blocks is evident from a low-intensity multiplet at 4.15 ppm representing methylene protons of the acylated end unit of PEO chain. The typical peaks of heparin appeared at 1.9, 2.8, 3.2, 4.1, and 4.2 ppm (10^{-6}). These results indicated that the TCH conjugate had been well synthesized.

The amount of heparin associated with the TCH was 0.44 μg/μg. The activity of conjugated heparin measured by APTT assay was calculated as (43.6 ± 2.4)% as compared to free heparin (140 unit/mg). Even though the heparin activity for binding with proteins could not be predicted from APTT results that indicating the anticoagulant activity of heparin, the specific interaction with a protein (e.g. Antithrombin III) was indirectly confirmed.

10.3.2 Preparation of bFGF Loaded Polymeric Micelle

Polymeric micelle containing bFGF was prepared by the single emulsion and solvent evaporation method. To briefly describe, the TCH conjugate (20 mg/d H_2O 1 mL) was dissolved in methanol (1 mL) in a glass vial. The solution was stirred at 37℃ for 24 h and then dried at 50℃ overnight, allowing slow evaporation of methanol and formation of micelles. And the micelle solution was sonicated for 30 min using BRANSON 5510 sonicator (Branson ultrasonics, USA). The micelle solution was filtered with a syringe filter (pore size = 0.45 μm) and then filtered again through a millipore centrifugal filter fevice (MW cut-off= 100 kDa) for solution purification.

The TCH and bFGF (400 ng/mL) were stirred at 37℃ for 24 h, allowing interactions between immobilized heparin and bFGF. The unbound bFGF was removed using salting-out salt methods by adding 10 wt% PEO 0.1 mL (Ghosh, 2004). bFGF loaded micelle solution was sonicated for 30 min and finally lyophilized to give the resultant.

In order to estimate the CMC of the PMs in distilled water, the fluorescence measurement was carried out using pyrene as a probe (Wilhelm et al., 1991). The PM solutions were made with different concentration, ranging from 10^{-6} to 10^{2} mg/mL. Fluorescence excitation spectra were obtained with emission wavelengths of 390 nm as a function of the concentration of the PMs using spectrofluorometer (JASCO FP-6500, Japan). Excitation and emission bandwidths were 3.0 and 1.5 nm, respectively.

The size and distribution of micelle were measured by dynamic light scattering (DLS) using an argon ion laser system (Brookhaven Instruments BI200SM, UK) set at a wavelength of 633 nm laser source. The sample solutions passing through a 0.45-μm filter were transferred into the light scattering cells. The intensity autocorrelation was measured at a scattering angle 90° with a Brookhaven BI-9000AT autocorrelator at 25℃. The correlation function was accepted when the difference between the measured and the calculated baseline was less than 0.1%. CONTIN algorithms were used in the Laplace inversion of the autocorrelation function to obtain the size distribution of micelles (Antony et al., 1998). The morphology of TCH PMs was analyzed by high resolution transmission electron microscopy (JEOL 300 kV, USA). The TCH micelle solution with a concentration of 5.5 mg/ml was dropped on a 300 mesh copper grid coated with carbon. The samples were stained with 1% (*w*/*v*) phosphotungstic acid and dried at room temperature for 24 h.

Physical properties of the micelles. The TC showed the same value as compared with the CMC of Tetronic®, which indicates that the short PCL blocks on Tetronic® did not contribute to the micelle formation. However, the increased CMC after the conjugation of heparin represents that hydrophilic moiety like heparin significantly affects to the micelle formation of block copolymers. Depending on the molecular weight of the block copolymers with change in the composition, the sizes of PMs were varied. Accordingly, TC micelle size was slightly increased as compared with Tetronic and size of TCH micelle was greatly increased due to heparin which exists on the shell of micelles. All samples showed the narrow and unimodal distribution. TEM image of TCH micelles revealed the spherical shape and the dried diameters ranged from approximately 150 to 200 nm (Fig. 10.9).

The size of TCH and TC micelles after the bFGF addition was studied to confirm the specific affinity between heparin and bFGF. The diameter of TCH and TC micelles after the bFGF addition was longer than that of one before bFGF addition. Particularly, the TCH showed significant change due to the high amount of bFGF, which bFGF selectively interact with heparin on the outer shell of micelles. In bFGF loading efficiencies of micelles, TC micelles had the bFGF loading efficiency of 30% – 40% as well as the increment in the micelle size as shown in Table 10.3 and Table 10.4, which resulted from non-specific interactions with TC. However, higher bFGF loading of approximately 70% was obtained from heparin conjugated TC micelles. Therefore, these results support that heparin can bind with bFGF through the specific interaction.

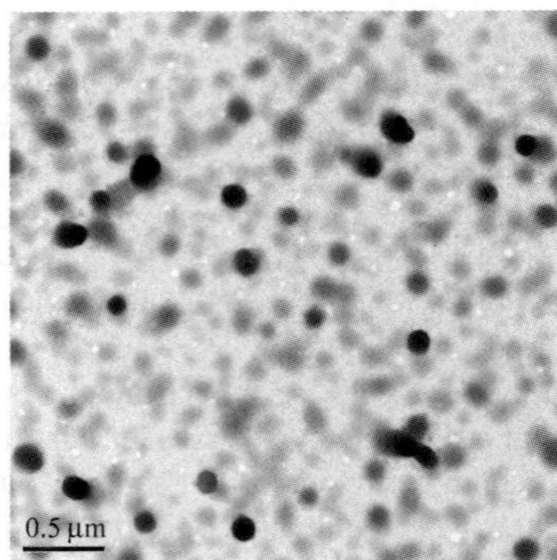

Figure 10.9 Representative TEM image of Tetronic®-PCL-heparin micelle. Panel shows a spherical aggregate with less than 200 nm diameter. Scale bar = 0.5 μm

Table 10.3 The CMC and diameter of micelles from Tetronic® derivatives

	Tetronic®	Tetronic®-PCL	Tetronic®-PCL-heparin
CMC (g/l)	0.03	0.03	0.11
Size (nm)[a]	16.9 ± 0.2	25.3 ± 0.5	114.1 ± 0.6
+ bFGF (nm)[b]	—	54.2 ± 0.2	193.2 ± 0.3

[a] The diameter of empty micelles ($n = 3$, mean ± S.D.)

[b] The diameter of bFGF-loaded micelles ($n = 3$, mean ± S.D.)

Table 10.4 bFGF loading efficiency of Tetronic® derivatives

	Tetronic®	Tetronic®-PCL	Tetronic®-PCL-heparin
LE (%)	39.7 ± 8.8	37.5 ± 4.3	70.5 ± 8.2

10.3.3 bFGF Release Study

The bFGF loading amount was investigated using a visible platelet reader (ELISA, Biotrak, UK) by measuring the UV absorbance at 540 nm from the readings at 450 nm. The bFGF loading efficiency (LE) was calculated by the weight ratio of bFGF to pre-weighed bFGF-loaded micelles. The bFGF quantitative assay was carried out using human FGF basic immunoassay kit (R&D systems).

In vitro release kinetics of bFGF from TCH micelles was performed using previously dried 20 mg of samples. The micelle solution (2 wt%) was placed into a dialysis bag, and then immersed into a large vial containing 49 mL of heated PBS (pH = 7.4, 37℃). At the appropriate time intervals, 5 mL of the released medium was collected from each sample and the medium was replaced by fresh medium.

In vitro bFGF release profiles from the PM are shown in Fig. 10.10. In all samples, no burst release was observed and bFGF was released slowly from the TCH micelle (Figs. 10.10 and 10.11). Interestingly, very small amounts of bFGF were released from the TC micelle, with total released percentage of 20%. This discontinuous release pattern might be caused by the intermolecular aggregation of bFGF in aqueous state (Wang, 1999). bFGF, which was weakly bound on TC micelles by non-specific interaction, could participate readily in the aggregation process with a neighboring bFGF. Eventually, bFGF aggregates could not escape from the dialysis membrane because of the size effect. In order to confirm this phenomenon related to bFGF aggregation, free heparin as the inhibitor for aggregation was added into TC micelle solution and their release behavior was investigated and shown in Fig. 10.10 (Wang, 2005). After heparin addition, bFGF was released, and passed through the membrane.

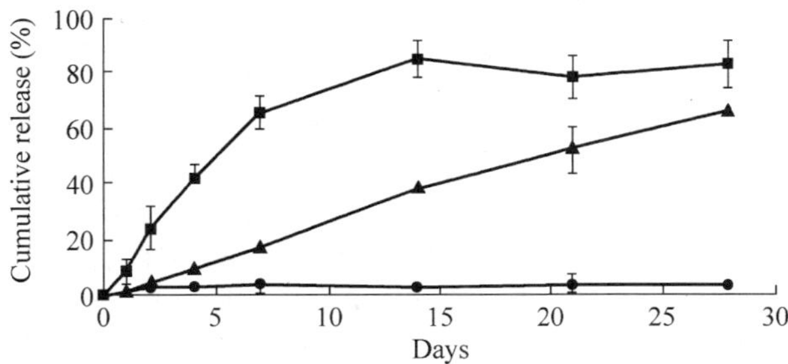

Figure 10.10 Cumulative bFGF release profiles of Tetronic® derivatives. In vitro pharmacokinetic studies are illustrated. Released bFGF from Tetronic®-PCL 0.40 mg/mL PBS solution (●), Tetronic®-PCL 0.40 mg/mL PBS solution + heparin 0.09 mg/mL (■), Tetronic®-PCL-heparin 0.40 mg/mL PBS solution (▲) ($n = 3$, mean ± S.D.)

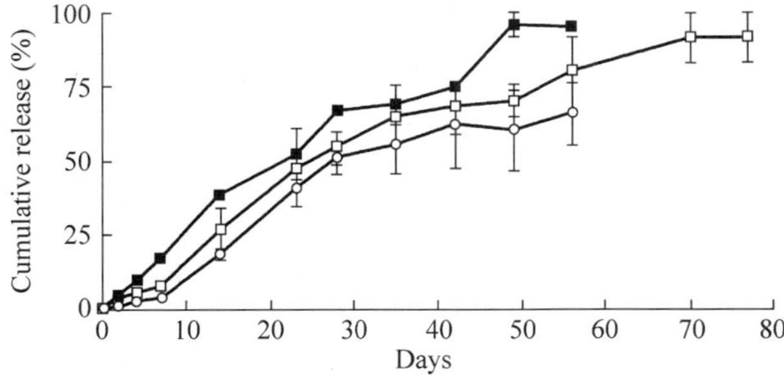

Figure 10.11 Cumulative bFGF release profile of Tetronic®-PCL-Heparin. Tetronic®-PCL-heparin 0.40 mg/mL PBS solution (■), Tetronic®-PCL-heparin 0.80 mg/mL PBS solution (□), and Tetronic®-PCL-heparin 2.40 mg/mL PBS solution (○) ($n = 3$, mean ± S.D.)

The number of micelle might influence the drug release kinetics. Figure 10.11 represents cumulative bFGF release profiles from the TCH micelle with different concentrations. As the content of the TCH micelle in PBS increases, the release rates of bFGF was decreased, which is likely based on the micelle packing mechanism (Jeong et al., 1999).

10.3.4 Bioactivity of the Released bFGF

Bioactivity of the released bFGFs was represented by circular dicroism (CD) spectra (Jasco 810 W, Japan). Measurements were performed in quartz cells of 1 mm path lengths. Spectra were recorded at 30℃ under conditions containing average of 10 scans between 190 and 260 nm, bandwidth of 1.0 nm, a scanning rate of 10 nm/min, a wavelength step of 0.2 nm and a time constant of 2 s. The native bFGF solutions with various concentrations and released bFGF solutions were prepared in 10 mmol/L sodium phosphate buffer (pH = 7.4). Cells with a shorter path length were used to record spectra of concentrated samples. Cells with a longer path length were used for dilute solutions. The CD band intensities were expressed as molar ellipticities, $[\theta]_M$, in $(°)\cdot cm^2\cdot dmol^{-1}$.

Although the bioactivity of growth factors released from the carrier is essential for their in vivo availability, their activity loss may occur through the structural change during the manufacturing process or storage. To verify bFGF activity, the structural changes for the released bFGF were monitored until 2 months by CD spectra, with the native bFGF at various concentrations from 0.5 to 500 ng. The simultaneous transition as well as the intensity in CD spectra yielded valuable information about the secondary structure of proteins, which means biological functions. As shown in Fig. 10.9, CD spectra of the released bFGF were very similar with native bFGF, indicating that the biological activity of bFGF was maintained by 2 months. In vivo bioactivity assay is under investigation.

10.4 Heparin-Immobilized Small Intestinal Submucosa (SIS)

10.4.1 Preparation of Heparin-Immobilized SIS

Fresh SIS was prepared as previously described in a report (Lindberg and Badylak, 2001). Briefly, freshly harvested porcine jejunum was obtained from a local slaughterhouse. It is inverted and the superficial layers of the tunica mucosa are removed by scrapping with a knife handle. The tissue is then reverted to its original orientation and the serosa and tunica muscularis are removed. The SIS sheets were rinsed extensively in water and sterilized by exposure to 0.1% (*v*/*v*) peracetic acid. Finally, the obtained SIS sheets were stored in Hank's balanced solution before use.

The SIS tissue was chemically modified as shown in Fig. 10.12. Heparin was immobilized onto SIS tissue by direct coupling of heparin containing amino groups after GA fixation. A series of control specimens was pretreated with 0.625% (*v*/*v*) GA solution for 10 days at 4℃ in PBS (pH = 7.4). GA-treated SIS was then incubated in 0.75% (*w*/*v*) heparin solution in PBS (pH = 11) at 4℃ for 5 days. The modified SIS tissues were rinsed with excess PBS and stabilized by treating them with 0.01 N sodium borohydride at 4℃ for 16 h.

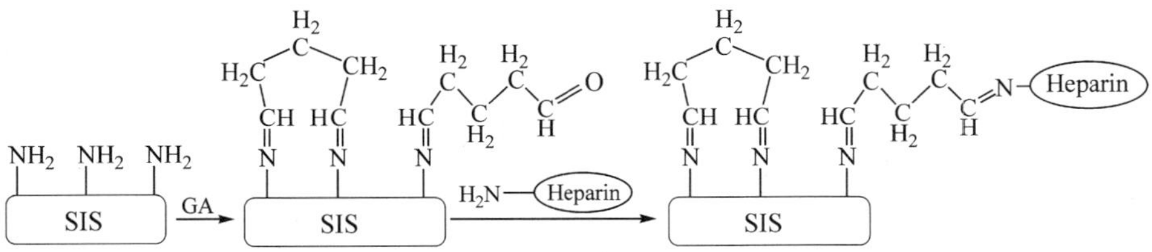

Figure 10.12 Scheme for heparin-immobilized SIS

GA was employed as a cross-linking agent to react with amino acid residues of collagen. After GA treatment, heparin was immobilized onto free aldehyde groups of GA already bound to SIS tissue. The chemical reaction between the residual aldehyde and amine groups occurs via Shiff base formation. The unstable Shiff bases were converted to stable secondary amines by $NaBH_4$. The amount and anticoagulant activity of heparin bound to the modified SIS was (0.40 ± 0.08) μg/cm^2 and 12.7%, respectively.

10.4.2 Blood Compatibility Test

In vitro plasma protein adsorption and platelet adhesion test were carried out with the modified SIS tissues (1 cm × 1 cm) which were equilibrated with PBS (pH = 7.4) for 12 h. The total amount of plasma proteins that were adsorbed onto the specimen was quantitatively analyzed by BCA kit and the number of adhered platelets was counted using a hemocytometer (Jee et al., 2004).

Figure 10.13(a) shows the adsorption of human plasma proteins onto the SIS tissues. The total amount of plasma proteins adsorbed onto the SIS-GA-heparin was 1.03 μg/cm^2, which was lower than that adsorbed onto fresh SIS. The amount of protein adsorbed onto SIS-GA was almost similar to that adsorbed onto SIS-GA-heparin. As shown in Fig. 10.13(b), indicating the number of platelets adhered to the modified SIS surface, the adhesion of platelets to SIS-GA-heparin was decreased. These results demonstrated that blood compatibility of the modified SIS was improved by heparin immobilization.

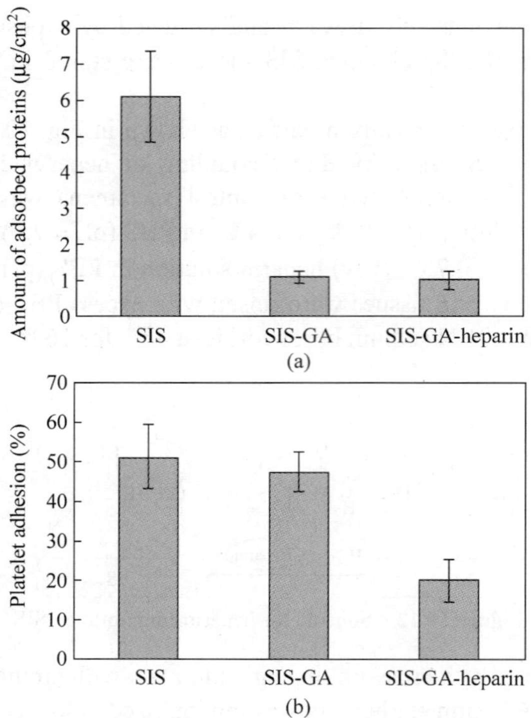

Figure 10.13 In vitro blood compatibility of the modified SIS tissues. Plasma protein adsorption (a) and platelet adhesion (b) after 1 h incubation. (mean ± S.D., $n = 4$)

Additionally, mechanical properties and enzymatic digestion with the modified SIS were investigated. The durability and resistance to collagenase digestion for SIS-GA-heparin was similar to those of SIS-GA.

10.4.3 In Vitro Fibroblast Attachment

Primary human dermal fibroblasts were maintained in DMEM supplemented with 10% FBS, penicillin (50 units/mL), and streptomycin (50 μg/mL) in a humidified environment at 37℃ and 5% CO_2. Cells were seeded at 1×10^3 cell/cm^2 by diluting the cell suspension. After incubation for 3 h at 37℃ in an atmosphere of 5% CO_2, each sample was washed twice with PBS at 37℃ in order to remove unattached cells. And the number of attached cells was assessed in a hexosaminidase reaction (Erokhina et al., 1994).

In vitro human dermal fibroblasts attachment on SIS-GA-heparin was significantly increased in comparison with fresh SIS (Fig. 10.14). Several cell culture studies demonstrated that the SIS construct as a bioscaffold, including various growth factors and ECM proteins, can promote cell growth (Badylak, 2004). Heparin has been known to regulate cellular behaviors by binding with a

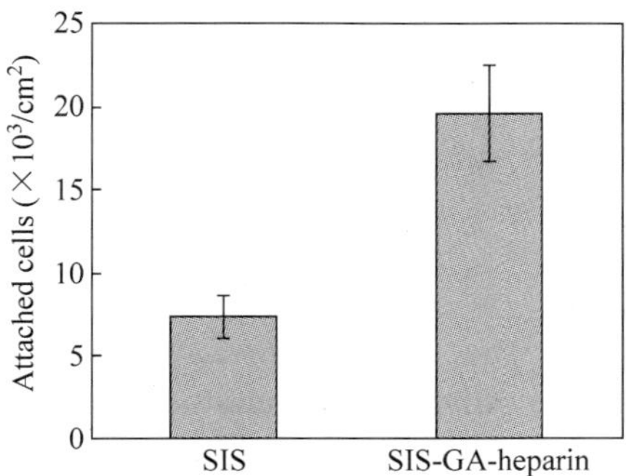

Figure 10.14 In vitro attachment of human dermal fibroblast on the modified SIS after 3 h incubation (mean ± S.D., $n = 4$)

number of biologically important proteins such as growth factors and ECM proteins (Capila and Linhardt, 2002). Therefore, this result supported that the heparin immobilized SIS can improve the attachment and proliferation of seeded cells. Also, this modified SIS can be reduced its cytotoxicity by removing the residual aldehyde groups, which are resulted from GA fixation.

10.4.4 In Vivo Calcification

In vivo calcification was studied using a rabbit subcutaneous implantation model. GA and heparin treated SIS tissues (1 cm× 1 cm) were implanted onto the subcutaneous muscle for the period of 8 weeks. After the retrieved tissues were rinsed with distilled water, lyophilized to constant weight, and the amount of calcium was determined by Inductively coupled plasma atomic emission spectrophotometer (ICP, 138 Ultrace, Jobin Yvon Co.) on 1.0 mol/L HCl hydrolysates of dried tissues.

From in vivo calcification, calcium contents of retrieved tissues are summarized in Table 10.5 When compared with the GA treated SIS, calcium deposition was significantly decreased in heparin immobilized SIS. Residual aldehyde groups after GA treatment can be further reacted with amine groups of materials. It may be hypothesized that, after the GA treatment, free aldehyde moieties on the surface of the implant undergo oxidation, followed by acid formation, and this acid may traps the host plasma calcium. The slow release of GA from the prosthesis promotes

Table 10.5 In vivo calcium deposition on the modified SISs

Sample	Ca	P
SIS-GA	194.8 ± 14.7	14.3 ± 0.9
SIS-GA-heparin	84.6 ± 9.7	2.9 ± 0.3

unit: μg/mg of tissue (mean ± S.D., $n = 4$)

the host-plasma calcium-acid bound complex (Chanda, 1995). Immobilization of heparin onto SIS tissue may fill the intertropocollagen spaces, blocks the potential binding sites, and thus makes the decreased calcium deposition.

10.5 Conclusions

Heparin was conjugated to polymers and another biomolecule to be utilized as functionalized interfaces for biomedical applications. The heparinized interfaces showed adequate biological properties of inherent heparin in addition to biomedical properties such as biodegradability, micelle formation, and inherent properties of natural materials. The detailed summaries are successively mentioned as follows:

Novel heparin-conjugated biodegradable polymers containing the PLA-Hep and the sPLA-Hep were investigated to improve blood and cell compatibility. In vitro studies indicate inhibitory effects of the biodegradable polymers on protein adsorption, platelet adhesion as well as enhanced anticoagulant activity and cell compatibility Therefore, the heparin-conjugated PLAs can be utilized as surfaces in blood-prosthesis applications such as temporary reconstruction, stabilization of tissue and organs, and especially scaffold materials for tissue engineering.

The TCH micelle was developed as an injectable drug carrier of nano-aggregate type. This micelle showed the ability to bind with bFGF as an example of HBGF. Furthermore, controlled long-term bFGF release with no loss of bioactivity was achieved and the inhibitory effect of heparin against bFGF aggregation was additionally verified. From these results, it is suggested that TCH micelles can be not only directly injected into the damaged tissue but also used after incorporation into other hydrogels or pre-formed matrices. Consequently, the heparinized micelle is expected to be useful as a novel growth factor delivery system for tissue regeneration.

Finally, the SIS-GA-heparin was evaluated with in vitro and in vivo assay to investigate the effect of modification. Such assay showed that the heparinized SIS surface has blood/cell compatibility and inhibitory effect against calcification. Based upon the obtained results, the SIS-GA-heparin can be useful for the development of calcification-resistant and biocompatible tissue patches, vascular graft, and heart valve for cardiovascular applications.

References

Agrawal, C.M., K.F. Haas, D.A. Leopold and H.G. Clark. *Biomaterials* **13**: 176 (1992).

Ajioka, M., K. Enomoto, K. Suzuki and A. Yamaguchi. *Bull. Chem. Soc. Jpn.* **68**: 2125 (1995).

Antony, T., A. Saxena, K.B. Royb and H.B. Bohidara. *J. Biochem. Biophys. Methods* **36**: 75 (1998).

Badylak, S., J. Obermiller, L. Geddes and R. Matheny. *Heart Surg. Forum* **6(2)**: E20 (2003).
Badylak, S. *Transpl. Immunol.* **12**: 367 (2004).
Bourin, M.C. and U. Lindahl. *Biochem. J.* **289**: 313 (1993).
Capila, I. and R.J. Linhardt. *Angew. Chem. Int. Ed.* **41**: 390 (2002).
Chanda, J. *Ann. Thorac. Surg.* **60**: S339 (1995).
Choi, Y.K., Y.H. Bae and S.W. Kim. *Macromolecules* **31**: 766 (1998).
Chung, H.J., D.H. Go, J.W. Bae, I.K. Jung, J.W. Lee and K.D. Park. *Curr. Appl. Phys.* **5**: 485 (2005).
Edelman, E.R., M.A. Nugent and M.J. Karnovsky. *Proc. Natl. Acad. Sci. USA* **90**: 1513 (1993).
Erokhina, M.V., A. A. Shtil, S. S. Shushanov, T. A. Sidorova, A. A. Stavrovskaya. *FEBS Lett.* **341**: 295 (1994).
Ghosh, R. J. *Membrane Sci.* **237**: 109 (2004).
Goldfarb, M. *Cytokine Growth Rev.* **7**: 311 (1996).
Hilbert, S. L., V. J. Ferrans and M. Jones. *Med. Prog. Technol.* **14**: 115 (1998).
Jang, I.K., H.K. Gold, A.A. Ziskind, R.C. Leinbach, J.F. Fallon and D. Collen. *Circulation* **81**: 219 (1990).
Jee, K.S., H.D. Park, K.D. Park, Y.H. Kim and J.W. Shin *Biomacromolecules* **5**: 1877 (2004).
Jeong, B., Y.H. Bae and S.W. Kim. *Macromolecules* **32**: 7064 (1999).
Kakizawa, Y. and K. Kataoka. *Adv. Drug Deliver. Rev.* **54**: 203 (2002).
Kataoka, K., A. Harada and Y. Nagasaki. *Adv. Drug Deliver. Rev.* **47**: 113 (2001).
Kito, H. and T.J. Matsuda. *Biomed. Mater. Res.* **30**: 321 (1996).
Lee, J.S., D.H. Go, J.W. Bae and K.D. Park. *Curr. Appl. Phys.* (in press)
Lee, S.H., S.H. Kim, Y.K. Han and Y.H. Kim. *J. Polym. Sci.* A **39**: 973 (2001).
Lindberg, K. and S. Badylak. *Burns* **27**: 254 (2001).
Linhardt, R.J. *J. Med. Chem.* **46**: 2551 (2003).
Matheny, R.G., M.L. Hutchison, P.E. Dryden, M.D. Hiles and C.J. Shaar. *J. Heart Valve Dis.* **9**: 769 (2000).
Park, K., F.W. Mao and H. Park. *Biomaterials* **11**: 24 (1990).
Perets, A., Y. Baruch, F. Weisbuch, G. Shoshany, G. Neufeld and S. Cohen. *J. Biomed. Mater. Res.* A **65A(4)**: 489 (2003).
Roeder R., J. Wolfe, N. Lianakis, T. Hinson, L.A. Geddes and J. Obermiller. *J. Biomed. Mater. Res.* **47**: 65 (1999).
Smith, P.K., R.I. Krohn, G.T. Hermanson, A.K. Mallia, F.H. Gartner, M.D. Provenzano, E.K. Fujimoto, N.M. Goeke, B.J. Olson and D.C. Klenk. *Anal. Biochem.* **150**: 76 (1985).
Smith, P.K., A.K. Mallia and G.T. Hermanson. *Anal. Biochem.* **109**: 466 (1980).
Thomas, C., S.D. Gladwin, F.W. Robert and H.R.R. Gundu. *Biomaterials* **21**: 699 (2000).
Wang, W. *Int. J. Pharm.* **185**: 129 (1999).
Wang, W. *Int. J. Pharm.* **289**: 1 (2005).
Wilhelm, M., C.L. Zhao, Y. Wang, R. Xu and M.A. Winnik. *Macromolecules* **24**: 1033 (1991).
Wissink, M.J.B., R. Beernink, J.S. Pieper, A.A. Poot, G.H.M. Engbers, T. Beugeling, W.G. vanAken and J. Feijen. *Biomaterials* **22**: 2291 (2001).

11 Inorganic Nanoparticles for Biomedical Applications

Mei Chee Tan[1], Gan Moog Chow[1], Lei Ren[2] and Qiqing Zhang[2]

[1] Department of Materials Science & Engineering, National University of Singapore, Singapore 119077

[2] Biomedical Engineering Research Center, Medical College, Xiamen University, Xiamen 361005, China

Abstract Polymer, lipid, metal, semiconductor, and hybrid composite nanoparticles with dimensions < 100 nm, have been developed extensively for potential biomedical applications like drug delivery systems, molecular sensing devices, and diagnostic imaging. In this overview, only inorganic nanoparticles for drug delivery will be addressed. Inorganic nanoparticles exhibit magnetic, electrical and optical properties that differed from their bulk counterparts. These physical properties could be tailored by controlling the size, shape, surface, and domain interactions in the nanoparticles. The incorporation of the unique properties of nanoparticles has expanded alternative platforms for drug delivery. The drug delivery systems highlighted in this overview include unguided, magnetically-guided, and optically-triggered delivery systems. These delivery systems are developed to enable improved localization and control of the drug's sphere of influence. This would potentially allow for more efficient therapy with lower dosages and reduced adverse side effects.

11.1 Introduction

Nanoparticles have driven the development of various biomedical applications, including drug delivery systems, diagnostic imaging, and molecular sensing devices (Jaspreet et al., 2005; West and Halas, 2000, 2003; Prasad, 2004; Holm et al., 2002). In this overview, only inorganic nanoparticles for drug delivery are addressed. Sustained release and targeted drug delivery systems are designed to optimize therapeutic efficiency of drugs and localize the drug's sphere of influence to regions of interest (Jaspreet et al., 2005; Brannon-Peppas and Blanchette, 2004;

---

(1) Corresponding e-mail: msecgm@nus.edu.sg

Kost and Langer, 2001). The optimal drug delivery system must not be removed too rapidly from either the systemic circulatory system or region of interest, and maintain a minimal drug leakage away from target site. Drugs released from the carriers should remain functionally active, and unloaded drug carriers should subsequently be cleared from systemic circulation (Petrak, 2006).

The characteristic dimensions of nanoparticles in the length scale of < 100 nm have driven interests for its applications in intravenous delivery, pulmonary delivery, and intracellular delivery. Using nanoparticles, an improved efficiency for pulmonary delivery was achieved (Chavanpatil et al., 2006; Hughes, 2005). For applications of nanoparticles in cancer therapy, liposomes and polymeric drug carriers of $\leqslant 100$ nm were reported to show increased permeability and localization at tumor sites. This was attributed to reduced diffusive barrier for nanoparticles given that gap junctions of the tumor vasculature were estimated to be ~100 – 600 nm (Allen, 2002; Panyam and Labhasetwar, 2003). Besides particle size, surface properties of nanoparticles would influence cellular uptake and distribution of nanoparticles (Moghimi et al., 2001). Nanoparticles with a more hydrophobic surface are taken up by cells to a greater extent through both endocytosis and phagocytosis than those with a hydrophilic surface.

Surface modification of nanoparticles is often required to improve its stability, compatibility, and functionality. Surface characteristics of nanoparticles have been engineered using surfactants that served as molecular linkers and improved particle stability (Kossovsky et al., 1994; Love et al., 2005; Caruso, 2002; Chan, 2006). Surfactants would reduce the surface energy of nanoparticles and enhance its stability by acting as a barrier to agglomeration through either steric hindrance or repulsive electrostatic forces. Functional groups on surfactants have enabled the coupling of nanoparticles with biomolecules such as drugs or antibodies (see Fig. 11.1). Subsequently, the surface functionalized nanoparticles would be able to serve as drug carriers, with potential for specific localization if particles were also modified with antibodies.

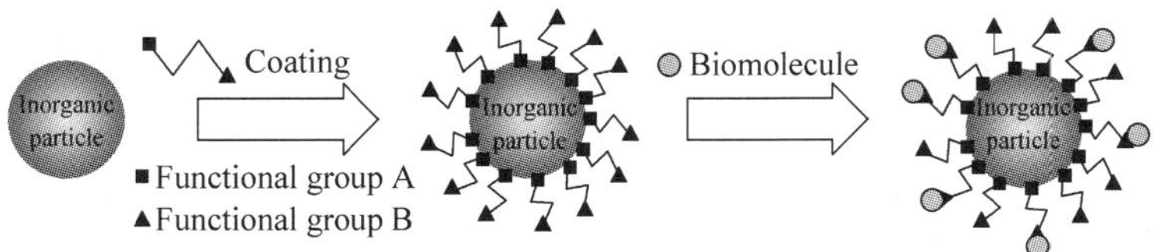

Figure 11.1 Schematic of surface functionalization of inorganic nanoparticles

Ceramics such as calcium phosphates (e.g. hydroxyapatite), silica, and titania are known to be biocompatible (Jin and Ye, 2007). The use of inorganic ceramic nanoparticles offers higher thermal and chemical stability than polymeric nanoparticles. Thus, encapsulation of drugs within ceramic particles would give better protection of labile agents against denaturation (Hasirci et al., 2006). In addition, with the increasing percentage of surface atoms and increasing separation between energy states (i.e. more discrete energy levels) with decreasing size, inorganic nanoparticles exhibit unique magnetic, electrical and optical properties that differ from its bulk counterparts (Kittel, 2005; Whitesides, 2005; Pitkethly, 2004). Properties of nanoparticles could be tailored by controlling the size, crystal structure, shape, surface, and domain interactions in nanoparticles. For instance, Au nanoparticles of $\leqslant$5 nm and bulk Au did not exhibit any absorption within the visible range, while Au nanoparticles with diameters of 5 – 100 nm showed a distinct size-dependent absorption band at 520 – 570 nm (Kreibig and Vollmer, 1995; Link and El-Sayed, 1999, 2000). In addition, optical properties of metallic nanoparticles could be modified by using different surfactants to tailor optical properties (Persson, 1993; Linnert et al., 1993; Hilger et al., 2000; Salgueiriño-Maceira et al., 2003; Pinchuk et al., 2004). Therefore, physical properties of inorganic nanoparticles could be exploited to enable local release at regions of interest with tunable sensitivity and responsiveness. Drug-loaded magnetic nanoparticles could be guided under an applied magnetic field to a specific area for subsequent release. Similarly, localized release could be achieved using light to trigger drug release from optically-active drug nanocarriers.

The drug delivery systems highlighted in this overview are unguided, magnetically-guided and optically-triggered delivery systems. An introduction to the different approaches adopted by each drug delivery system will be described. An overview of different chemical synthetic and surface functionalization methods for the different carriers are also presented. Besides some commonly used ceramic nanoparticles like hydroxyapatite, considering that most inorganic nanoparticles are non-resorbable and non-degradable with unknown in vivo clearance, significant nanoparticle accumulation within the systemic circulation may occur (Singh et al., 2006). With the increasing dominance of size and surface effects at the nanoscale, toxicity assessments of conventional bulk materials (U.S. Food and Drug Administration, 2000) and microparticles (Foster et al., 2001) may not be applicable. Thus, it would be crucial to evaluate cytotoxic effects of nanoparticles (Hood, 2004; Kagan et al., 2005; Barnard, 2006; Sayes et al., 2004; Kirchner et al., 2005). Cytotoxic properties of non-degradable magnetic and optically-active inorganic nanoparticles would be mentioned in this chapter.

11.2 Unguided Drug Delivery Systems

Ceramic nanoparticles have mostly been developed for sustained drug release systems to enhance delivery efficiency, reduce undesired systemic effects and improved convenience to patients. The most popular ceramic materials used in clinical applications are silica and calcium phosphate (e.g. hydroxyapatite). Besides non-viral gene delivery, their most significant contribution was found as substrates for tissue engineering, bone regeneration and bone repair (Vallet-Regi, 2006). In particular, calcium-based ceramic materials have an advantage over other polymeric materials for bone repair due to its better bonding to living bone and its ability to catalyze bone growth due to increased nucleation of apatite. For instance, hydroxyapatite is a ceramic similar to the mineral part of bone.

Biomolecules and therapeutic agents were combined with ceramic particles to develop materials that functioned as controlled release systems (Vallet-Regi, 2006; Gadre and Gouma, 2006). Performance of biodoped ceramics were governed by the chemical activity and functionality of attached biomolecules. Adsorption properties of ceramic materials are governed partly by pore size, matrix structure, and surface functional groups. Surface functional groups could be further modified using different chemical species to expand its ability to attach different biomolecules. The chemical activity of biomolecules would be influenced by interfacial interactions between biomolecules and ceramic matrix. An ideal biodoped ceramic would exhibit a good long term stability under potentially adverse conditions, high loading density for biomolecules that remains bioactive, and resistant to leaching of biomolecules (Vallet-Regi, 2006). Biodoped ceramic materials have been used either as a porous solid piece (e.g. implants) or in injectable form for development of non-invasive surgical applications (Vallet-Regi, 2006; Ben-Nissan, 2004; Hou et al., 2004; Temenoff and Mikos, 2000).

11.2.1 Chemical Synthesis of Ceramic Nanomaterials

Main chemical synthetic methods for ceramics include sol-gel processing and precipitation. The sol-gel technique typically involved hydrolysis of metal alkoxide, $M(OR)x$ precursors in the presence of alcohol as a co-solvent to form metal hydroxyls (Klein, 1996; Livage et al., 1998; Vioux, 1997; Oskam, 2006; Brinker and Sherrer, 1990; Niederberger and Garnweitner, 2006). This was followed by condensation of metal hydroxyl groups, where either water or alcohol as by product. Some processing parameters commonly used to control nucleation and growth kinetics were chain length of metal alkoxide precursors, surfactants, solvent (molecular weight of alcohol), temperature, pH, and mechanical agitation. As condensation continues, larger aggregates were formed and viscosity of sol increases resulting in subsequent formation of a gel. Capillary forces during solvent removal from the pores would lead to gel shrinkage. Using the Stöber method developed from sol-gel principles, silica particles with a range of different sizes was prepared (Green et al., 2003). Another common method, particularly for hydroxyapatite, is precipitation of metallic salt (calcium nitrates) with a base (ammonium phosphate) (Ahn et al., 2001; Kumta et al, 2005). The nucleation and growth kinetics were primarily governed by the pH of the starting solution (Ahn et al., 2001; Kumta et al., 2005). The degree of crystallization and prevention of growth of undesired secondary phases were controlled by using different aging temperatures.

11.2.2 Functionalization of Ceramic Nanomaterials

Silica nanoparticles without surface modification did not seem to condense and deliver DNA (Luo and Saltzman, 2006). For DNA delivery using nanoparticles, the extended long chain DNA molecules were condensed to reduce its occupied spatial volume. The presence of surface amino groups on silica nanoparticles upon modification with aminosilanes, would enable it to tightly bind with plasmid DNA and serve as a gene delivery carrier. Using silica nanoparticles as a gene delivery carrier would prevent DNA from being degraded by environmental enzymes. In addition, it was reported that DNA-loaded silica nanoparticles showed an enhanced cellular uptake when compared to other commercial DNA transfection vectors available. Silica nanoparticles were found to enhance the transfer efficiency of commercially available transfection vectors by a factor of 1 – 7 (Luo, 2005; Xu et al., 2006). Another commonly used non-viral gene delivery carrier is calcium phosphate (apatite, hydroxyapatite, and carbonated apatite) based materials. Calcium phosphate materials are suitable candidates as a gene delivery carrier due to its biocompatibility, biodegradability and known adsorptive capacity of DNA on bare calcium phosphate. Calcium phosphate gene carriers were prepared through the co-precipiation of calcium phosphate particles with DNA (Luo, 2005; Olton et al., 2007; Zhu et al., 2004). However, lower levels of gene expression in comparison to viral approaches were observed. This was associated with difficulties associated with endosomal escape, insufficient protection of DNA from nuclease degradation, and inefficient nuclear uptake.

Biomolecules were often encapsulated using a modified sol gel process with addition of amino acids, sugars, or cytoprotecting agents like glycerol or other polymer additives like polyethylene glycol (Avnir et al., 2006; Coradin and Livage, 2007). Protein encapsulation within rigid ceramic pores of similar dimensions offers protection against other denaturing forces in the presence of an organic solvent or extreme pH. Porous blocks of calcium hydroxyapatite and tricalcium phosphate were evaluated as sustained release system fro anticancer drugs, cisplatin, and methotrexate (Uchida et al., 1992; Itokazu et al., 1998). In addition, hybrids of ceramic and polymeric materials mixed with therapeutic agents (e.g. tissue growth factors or small molecule drugs) are often used. Polymeric-ceramic hybrids offer a combination of properties that were unique to either polymeric or ceramic materials alone. Properties of such polymeric-ceramic hybrids would depend on the percentage of each constitutive component present. A sustained release strategy developed was the use of a polymer (poly(lactic-*co*-glycolic acid)) with acidic degradation products to control the dissolution of a basic inorganic component (apatite) on which a therapeutic agent (e.g. bone morphogenetic proteins) were adsorbed (Yong et al., 2004; Yong, 2005). The release profile could be altered by changing variables that affect polymer degradation (type, molecular,and composition) and/or apatite dissolution (loading and particle size).

11.3 Magnetically-Guided Drug Delivery Systems

11.3.1 Magnetic Guiding

Magnetically-responsive delivery systems introduced into the systemic circulation are directed to regions of interest using an applied magnetic field. The external magnetic field of ~0.8 – 1.7 T, may be a magnet or an array of magnets placed near a lesion or tumor, either externally placed or implanted. (Hayden and Häfeli, 2006; Gould, 2006; Alexiou et al., 2006; Jurgons et al., 2006). Therapeutic agents were subsequently released using either another trigger such as ultrasonic waves or an alternating magnetic field (Kost and Langer, 2001; Tirelli, 2006; Frimpong et al., 2007). Magnetically modulated drug delivery systems prepared using large magnetic particles embedded in a polymer matrix, were shown to enhance drug release rates upon application of an oscillating magnetic field. Drug release rates were shown to be dependent on the characteristics of magnetic field (e.g. field strength, and amplitude) and polymer properties (e.g. rigidity of polymer matrix). When the holding magnets were removed, the particles would either redistribute into the blood supply to be eventually cleared by the reticuloendothelial system or remain within the region of interest to be cleared by extravasation.

Recent studies demonstrated successful localization of doxorubicin-loaded 200 nm Fe@C particles, and 80 nm to 2 μm silica-coated Fe_3O_4/γ-Fe_2O_3 particles using implanted Au-plated permanent magnets. The magnetic implants were Au-plated to improve chemical stability and biocompatibility. Though high particle concentrations were found in the liver, magnetic carriers were drawn to the left kidney close to an implanted magnet whereas no particles were observed in right kidneys of the rabbits tested. Similar studies using externally placed magnets showed successful localization of magnetic particles at the peritoneal cavity of mice. The efficacy and potential for pulmonary embolism of magnetically-guided drug delivery systems would be governed by physiological parameters, temporal localization kinetics, and microcirculatory flow (Lübbe et al., 1999).

11.3.2 Chemical Synthesis and Properties of Magnetic Nanostructures

Iron-based magnetic nanomaterials, particularly magnetite (Fe_3O_4) or maghemite (γ-Fe_2O_3) due to its better chemical stability and lower toxicity, are most commonly used compared to alternative cobalt- and nickel- based nanomaterials (Qiang et al., 2006). Magnetic nanoparticles have been prepared using several chemical methods to control nucleation and growth rates. The size, morphology, and composition of particles synthesized were governed by the nucleation and growth rates, whereas the size dispersion would depend on decoupling of nucleation and growth rates (Turkevich et al., 1951; Stokes and Evans, 1997; Sheludko, 1996; Davey and Garside, 2000; Huber, 2005). Base precipitation of iron salts from a surfactant-containing aqueous solution at low temperatures was a common chemical method for aqueous synthesis of magnetic nanoparticles (Chatterjee et al., 2003). Another synthetic method is the thermal decomposition of organometallic precursors in high-boiling solvents in the presence of stabilizing ligands, such as oleic acid or oleyl amine. Organometallic-based synthesis often resulted in magnetic nanoparticles with a narrow size distribution ($\sigma < 5\%$) and high degree of crystallinity (see Fig. 11.2) (Lin and Samia, 2006; Park et al., 2004; Behrens et al., 2006; Hyeon, 2003).

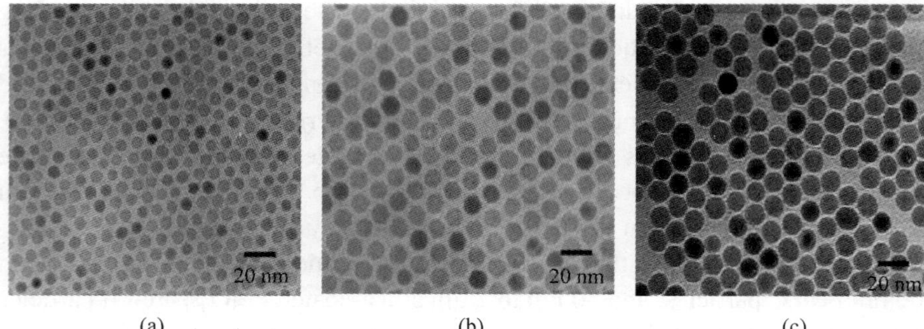

Figure 11.2 (a) 7 nm (b) 11 nm and (c) 13 nm γ-Fe_2O_3 nanoparticles synthesized using thermal decomposition of organometallic precursors (Hyeon, 2003; Hyeon et al., 2001). Adapted from (Hyeon, 2003). Reprinted with permission from (Hyeon et al., *J. Am. Chem. Soc.* 2001). Copyright (2001) American Chemical Society

The magnetic particles must exhibit high magnetization and superparamagnetic behavior at room temperature for guidance and immobilization to region of interest (Neuberger et al., 2005). Particles with high saturation magnetization would be localized more easily to a region using lower external magnetic fields. As the size decreases, thermal energy may be sufficient to give rise to fluctuations of magnetization directions. Thus, particles below a critical size (e.g. ~10 nm for Fe_3O_4 or γ-Fe_2O_3) would be magnetized by an applied magnetic field but retain no permanent magnetism upon removal of the applied field. Particles with this superparamagnetic behavior would have reduced tendency for agglomeration that was driven by magnetic attractive forces. While decreasing particle size would result in the desirable superparamagnetic behavior, a trade-off would be reduced saturation magnetization. Smaller particles with lower saturation magnetization may have less effective localization, while larger particles may have lower cellular uptake and higher chances for embolism.

11.3.3 Functionalization of Magnetic Nanoparticles

Surfaces of magnetic nanoparticles are modified with polymeric, metallic or oxide surface to improve either its stability against agglomeration, bioavailability and biomolecular functionalization (A.K. Gupta and M. Gupta, 2005; Berry and Gurtis, 2003). Particles were often surface functionalized with either an organic, polymeric or inorganic layer using either ligand exchange or encapsulation methods (Hong et al., 2005; Bruce and Sen, 2005; Templeton et al., 2000). Particles were coated with a layer of organic surfactants during chemical synthesis to prevent agglomeration. However, such surfactants might not provide the necessary chemical functionality needed for its eventual applications. Thus, surfactants covering the particles were replaced with other surfactants using various ligand exchange methods. Particles could be encapsulated by a polymeric coating by precipitation of inorganic salts in an aqueous polymer solution (Yu and Chow, 2004; Babes et al., 1999). For instance, Fe_3O_4 or γ-Fe_2O_3 particles were commonly encapsulated with dextran or starch for improved biocompatibility and solubility. It was also demonstrated that after surface modification, an anticancer drug (carboplatin) was bound to polymethyl metacrylic acid coated γ-Fe_2O_3 particles (Fig. 11.3) (Yu and Chow, 2004). Silica-coated particles provide enhanced stability and surface silanol groups for covalent coupling (Bruce and Sen, 2005). After hydrolysis and condensation of organosilanes that were deposited on the particle surface, a silica coating was formed. Characteristics of the final surface layer depended on reaction variables such as solvent type, temperature, or time, as well as on the catalyst and organosilane concentrations used.

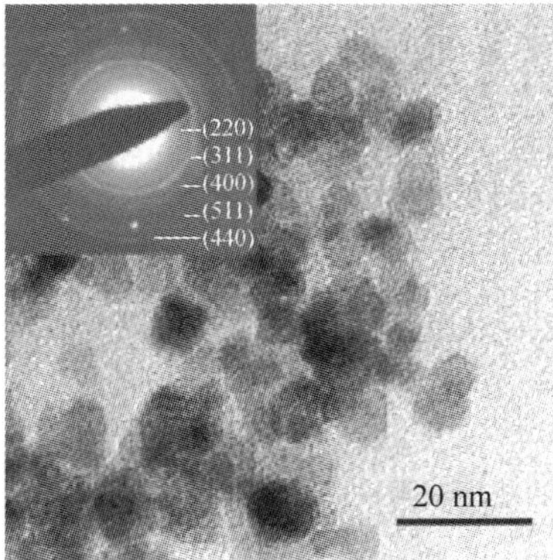

Figure 11.3 Transmission electron micrograph and corresponding electron diffraction pattern of polymethyl acrylic acid coated γ-Fe_2O_3 particles (Yu and Chow, 2004). —Reproduced by permission of The Royal Society of Chemistry

11.3.4 Biocompatibility of Magnetic Nanoparticles for Drug Delivery

It was reported that besides intrinsic size effects, the surface coating had an important role in the cytotoxicity of oleic acid coated nickel ferrite nanoparticles (Yin et al., 2005). It was found that particle size of uncoated nickel ferrite was not a significant factor on cytotoxicity when there were no 'toxic' functional groups on particle surface. In contrast, oleic acid-coated nickel ferrite particles of ~150 nm and ~10 nm were cytotoxic. If oleic acid molecules were present as monomer, they were not cytotoxic. However, if they developed micelles or coated on the ferrite particles, i.e. when their functional groups were spatially aligned, cytotoxicity was observed. Larger particles had a larger cytotoxic effect than smaller particles when one or two layers of oleic acid were deposited on particle surface. This could be related to surfactant reactivity and interfacial interaction areas that were dependent on particle size. The difference in surface energies with particle sizes may have affected surfactant conformation, which may alter the surfactant reactivity. Thus, the same surfactant may behave differently when it interacts with cells. Also, with a larger effective interaction area for a larger particle compared to that for a smaller particle as shown in Fig. 11.4, the larger particle will exert a larger localized stimulus on the cells. It was subsequently suggested in the report that that a single localized stimulus from a larger particle was stronger and more toxic than an equivalent sum of stimuli at different locations exerted by smaller particles.

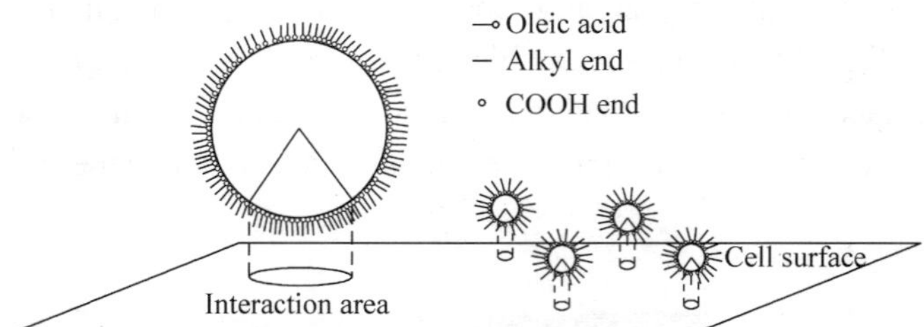

Figure 11.4 Sketch of the various interaction areas of individual particle with one layer oleic acid coating. A single large particle possessed larger interaction areas with more function groups. While, the big number of small particles increased number of interaction points, there were less functional groups at each interaction point (Yin et al., 2005). —Reprinted from H. Yin, H.P. Too and G.M. Chow. The effects of particle size and surface coating on the cytotoxicity of nickel ferrite. *Biomaterials*, 26: 5818 – 5826, Copyright (2005), with permission from Elsevier

11.4 Optically-Triggered Drug Delivery Systems

Near infrared (NIR) light ($\lambda = 650 - 1000$ nm), with its deep penetration in living tissues shown in and high signal-to-background ratio, has been exploited for biomedical imaging, photoablation and photodynamic therapy (Frangioni, 2003;

Sato et al., 2001; Dolmans et al., 2003). The extent of NIR light propagation would be governed by absorption and scattering properties of tissues (Waynant et al., 2001; Niemz, 2002; Vogel and Venugopalan, 2003). Major tissue absorbers of NIR light are hemoglobin, melanin, and water, while composition, size, and morphology of tissue components control the light scattering. The absorption and scattering properties would influence volumetric energy distribution induced by laser irradiation, and set the boundaries for localized NIR-activated drug release systems. NIR light was reported to travel through 10 cm of breast tissue and 4 cm of skull tissue using microwatt sources (Weissleder, 2001). A targeted drug delivery system that incorporated NIR-sensitive nanoparticles and tissue penetrative NIR light to trigger drug release was developed (Ren and Chow, 2003; Chow et al., 2006; Tan, 2006). This could potentially improve chemotherapy treatment by minimizing deleterious side effects and allowing minimally invasive treatment of surgically inoperable tumors.

11.4.1 Chemical Synthesis and Properties of NIR-Sensitive Nanoparticles

Metallic nanoparticles and metallic nanoshells with size-dependent optical properties, particularly chemically stable Au nanoparticles, have been utilized as molecular sensors (West and Halas, 2003; Prasad, 2004; Holm et al., 2002). As sensors, binding of molecules would give rise to either fluorescence enhancement or plasmon resonance shifts. NIR-sensitive metallic nanoshells (Oldenburg et al., 1998). with size and shell thickness dependent properties were investigated for applications in imaging (Loo et al., 2005), hyperthermia (Hirsch et al., 2003), temperature-responsive delivery systems (Sershen and West, 2006), and immunoassays (Hirsch et al., 2003, 2006). For the NIR-activated drug delivery system, the NIR-sensitive nanoparticles were synthesized by reduction of $HAuCl_4$ with Na_2S (Ren and Chow, 2003; Chow et al., 2006; Zhou et al., 1994; Averitt et al., 1997). These as-synthesized nanoparticles were chemically stable and exhibited two absorption bands at ~530 nm and in the NIR region of 650 – 1100 nm. The as-synthesized nanoparticles were composites of crystalline Au and amorphous Au_2S (Tan, 2006; Tan et al., Submitted). The NIR absorption was unique to as-synthesized nanoparticles, and was absent in either Au or Au_2S nanoparticles. There was no evidence that NIR absorption properties were related to a core-shell structure as suggested in earlier work in the literature. Therefore, NIR absorption was likely due to interfacial effects on particle polarization from introduction of amorphous Au_2S in a predominantly crystalline Au matrix (Tan, 2006; Tan et al., Submitted). The effects of concentration ratios for precursors used in the chemical synthesis of nanoparticles were correlated with the resultant NIR properties. Consequently, by varying concentration ratios of precursors, the optical properties of as-synthesized nanoparticles were tailored (Chow et al., 2006; Tan, 2006). This ability to tailor optical properties would advance potential use of as-synthesized nanoparticles for optically-activated drug delivery systems or other biomedical applications.

11.4.2 Functionalization of NIR-Sensitive Nanoparticles

Functionalization of NIR-sensitive Au-Au_2S nanoparticles with surfactants has facilitated the loading of anticancer drugs as shown in Fig. 11.5 (Chow et al., 2006; Tan, 2006). Surfactants of different hydrocarbon chain lengths were used to modify the nanoparticles, and subsequently altered interfacial interactions between nanoparticles and surfactants. The loading of anticancer drugs governed by surfactant interfacial interactions was correlated to the surfactant chain length. In addition, inorganic-organic interfacial interactions between nanoparticles and surfactants may be used to manipulate the optical properties of NIR sensitive drug delivery system. Drug release was triggered upon NIR laser irradiation using a Nd:YAG pulse laser at $\lambda = 1064$ nm (Ren and Chow, 2003). The structural and microstructural changes of Au-Au_2S nanoparticles upon NIR laser irradiation were studied. Insights to NIR triggered drug release process were elucidated from the estimated magnitude of thermal effects and structural and microstructural changes induced by NIR irradiation (Tan, 2006).

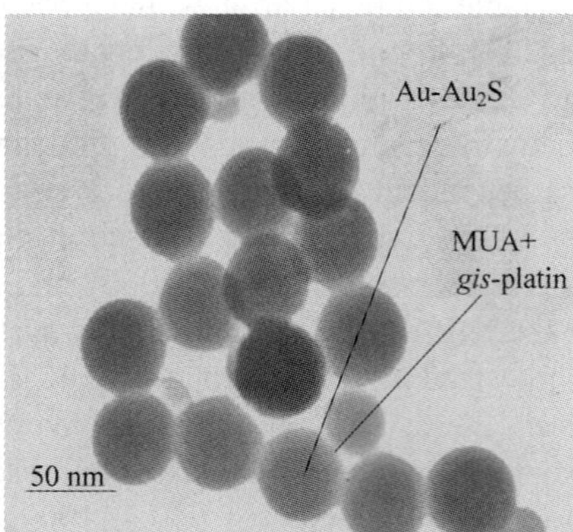

Figure 11.5 Cisplatin-loaded surface modified Au-Au_2S nanoparticles (Ren and Chow, 2003).—Reprinted from L. Ren and G.M. Chow. Synthesis of NIR-sensitive Au-Au_2S nanocolloids for drug delivery. *Materials Science and Engineering* C, 23: 113 – 116, Copyright (2003), with permission from Elsevier

11.4.3 Biocompatibility of NIR-Sensitive Nanoparticles for Drug Delivery

The in vitro cytotoxicity of the NIR-sensitive Au-Au_2S drug delivery system was assessed using breast cancer cells for its potential clinical application (Tan, 2006).

The in vitro cytotoxicity of surfactant-modified nanoparticles and drug-loaded-surfactant-modified nanoparticles were investigated. (Tan, 2006) It was found that the in vitro toxicity of drug-loaded-surfactant-modified nanoparticles depended on the surfactant used for drug adsorption. The in vitro cytotoxic effects of released drugs in the supernatant fraction collected after NIR irradiation of drug-loaded-surfactant-modified nanoparticles were evaluated. It was found that the released drug was chemically modified with increased toxicity. In addition, transmission electron microscopy (TEM) micrographs indicated that both Au-Au_2S nanoparticles and cisplatin-loaded Au-Au_2S nanoparticles were found associated with the plasma membrane or in small vesicles within cells. Studies on in vitro carcinogenicity of nanoparticles using a medium-term (25 days) NIH/3T3 cells transformation test was also conducted (Ren et al., submitted). Examination using light microscopy of the cells exposed to the Au-Au_2S NPs and cisplatin-loaded Au-Au_2S nanoparticles revealed morphological alterations when compared to that of control cells. However, no difference in cell morphology among cells exposed to cisplatin-loaded Au-Au_2S nanoparticles was observed. This indicated that cisplatin-loaded Au-Au_2S nanoparticles did not cause carcinogenicity in vitro below a maximum recommended dosage in the given system.

Similar in vivo biodistribution profiles (Fig. 11.6) of nanoparticles using both intra-tumor and tail vein injection administration routes were observed (Huang et al., submitted). Most particles accumulated in the reticulo-endothelial system, mainly liver and spleen. Small amounts of Au-Au_2S nanoparticles were found in the lung, probably due to embolism of agglomerated nanoparticles in lung capillaries. While the mass of Au-Au_2S NPs in the kidneys increased to 0.95 μg/g within 7 days, no Au-Au_2S NPs were deposited in other organs like brain, heart, muscle, bone, intestine, and blood. Using the tail vein injection for particle administration resulted in reduced concentration in the biodistribution profile

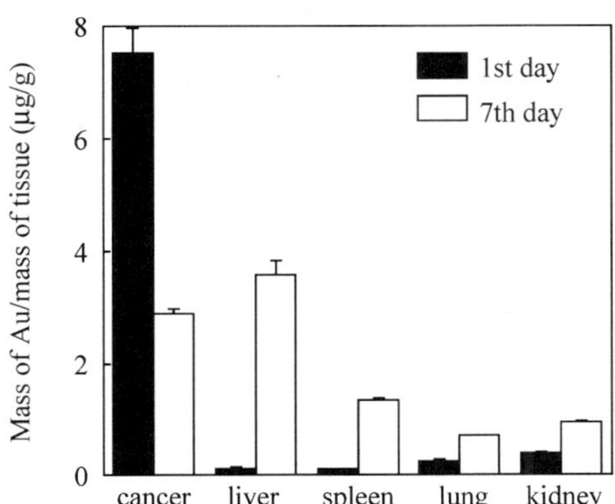

Figure 11.6 Biodistribution of Au-Au_2S NPs in KM mice treated by intra-tumor injection at different time points (Huang et al., submitted)

compared to that of using the intra-tumor route. This was due to the enhanced penetration and retention effect of tumors for particles of 50 – 100 nm. This suggested that intra- tumor injection may improve local tumor response and minimize any systemic side effects.

In summary, preliminary findings from the short and long-term in vitro suggested that cisplatin-loaded Au-Au_2S nanoparticles were non-toxic below a maximum recommended dosage. It remains premature to draw definitive conclusions about the toxicities, if any, of Au-Au_2S nanoparticles. Further work is required to evaluate if the unique physicochemical properties of Au-Au_2S nanoparticles would introduce other injurious mechanisms and pathological lesions.

11.5 Summary

The incorporation of the unique properties (chemical stability, magnetic and optical) of inorganic nanoparticles has expanded alternative platforms for drug delivery. These drug delivery systems were developed to enable improved localization and control of the drug's sphere of influence. This would potentially allow for more efficient therapy with lower dosages and reduced adverse side effects. A multidisciplinary approach would be needed for advancement of the delivery systems to its eventual applications. Optimization of chemical synthetic and functionalization methods to improve quality (distribution, loading capacities) of drug carrier would facilitate developmental progress of drug delivery systems. Further scientific development on understanding of release mechanisms for better engineering control of these drug delivery systems would be required. More detailed in vitro and in vivo work on the nanoparticle-cellular interfacial interactions and its implications on safety of inorganic nanoparticles would also be critical.

References

Ahn, E.S., N.J. Gleason, A. Nakahira and J.Y. Ying. Nanostructure processing of hydroxyapatite-based bioceramics, *Nano Letters* **1**: 149 (2001).

Alexiou C., et al. Targeting cancer cells: Magnetic nanoparticles as drug carriers. *Eur. Biophys. J.* **35**: 446 (2006).

Allen, T.M. Ligand-targeted therapeutics in anticancer therapy. *Nature Rev. Cancer* **2**: 750 (2002).

Averitt, R.D., D. Sarkar and N.J. Halas. Plasmon resonance shifts of Au-coated Au_2S nanoshells: Insight into multicomponent nanoparticle growth. *Phys. Rev. Lett.* **78**: 4217 (1997).

Avnir, D., T. Coradin, O. Lev and J. Livage. Recent bioapplications of sol-gel materials. *J. Mater. Chem.* **16**: 1013 (2006).

Babes, L., B. Denizot, G. Tanguy, J.J. Le Jeune and P. Jallet. Synthesis of iron oxide nanoparticles used as MRI contrast agents: A parametric study, *J. Colloid Interf. Sci.* **212**: 474 (1999).

Barnard, A.S. Nanohazards: Knowledge is our first defense. *Nat. Mat.* **5**: 245 (2006).

Behrens, S., et al. Surface engineering of Co and FeCo nanoparticles for biomedical applications. *J. Phys. Condens. Matter* **18**: 2543 (2006).

Ben-Nissan, B. Nanoceramics in biomedical applications. *MRS Bulletin* **1**: 28 (2004).

Berry, C.C. and A.S.G. Curtis. Functionalization of magnetic nanoparticles for applications in biomedicine. *J. Physics D* **36**: R198 (2003).

Brannon-Peppas, L., and J.O. Blanchette. Nanoparticle and targeted systems for cancer therapy. *Adv. Drug Del. Rev.* **56**: 1649 (2004).

Brinker, C.J. and G.W. Sherrer. *Sol-gel Science*, Academic Press, New York (1990).

Bruce, I.J. and T. Sen. Surface modification of magnetic nanoparticles with alkoxysilanes and their application in magnetic bioseparations. *Langmuir* **21**: 7029 (2005).

Caruso, F. Nanoengineering of particle surfaces. *Adv. Mater.* **13**: 11 (2002).

Chan, W.C.W. Bionanotechnology Progress and Advances. *Biol. Blood Marrow Transplant.* **12**: 87 (2006).

Chatterjee, J., Y. Haik and C.J. Chen. Size dependent magnetic properties of iron oxide nanoparticles. *J. Magnetism Mag. Mater.* **257**: 113 (2003).

Chavanpatil, M.D., A. Khdair and J. Panyam. Nanoparticles for cellular drug delivery: mechanisms and factors influencing delivery. *J Nanosci. Nanotech.* **6**: 2651 (2006).

Chow, G.M., M.C. Tan, L. Ren and J.Y. Ying. NIR-sensitive nanoparticles. *US patent application pending*. Publication Number 2006099146 (2006).

Coradin, T. and J. Livage. Aqueous silicates in biological sol-gel applications: New perspective for old precursors. *Acct. Chem. Res.* **40**: 819 (2007).

Davey, R.J., J. Garside. *From Molecules to Crystallizers*. Oxford University Press, Oxford, England (2000).

Dolmans, D.E.J.G.J., D. Fukumura and R.K. Jain. Timeline: Photodynamic therapy for cancer. *Nat. Rev. Cancer* **3**: 380 (2003).

Frangioni, J.V. In vivo near-infrared fluorescence imaging. *Curr. Opin. Chem. Biol.* **7**: 626 (2003).

Frimpong, R.A., S. Fraser and J.Z. Hilt. Synthesis and temperature response analysis of magnetic-hydrogel nanocomposites. *J. Biomed Mater. Res. A* **80**: 1 (2007).

Gadre, Y.S. and P.I. Gouma. Biodoped ceramics: Synthesis, properties and applications. *J. Ame. Ceram. Soc.* **89**: 2987 (2006).

Gould, P. Nanomagnetism shows in vivo potential. *Nanotoday* **1**: 34 (2006).

Green, D.L., J.S. Lin , Y. Lam, M.Z.C. Hu, D.W. Schaefer and M.T. Harris. Size, volume fraction, and nucleation of Stober silica nanoparticles. *J. Colloid Interf. Sci.* **266**: 346 (2003).

Gupta, A.K. and M. Gupta, Synthesis and surface engineering of iron oxide nanoparticles for biomedical applications. *Biomaterials* **26**: 3995 (2005).

Hasirci, V., E. Vrana, P. Zorlutuna, A. Ndreu, P. Yilgor, F.B. Basmanav and E. Aydin. Nanobiomaterials: A review of the existing science and technology, and new approaches. *J. Biomater. Sci. Polymer Edn.* **17**: 1241 (2006).

Hayden, M.E. and U.O. Häfeli. 'Magnetic bandages' for targeted delivery of therapeutic agents. *J. Phys.: Condens. Matter* **18**: S2877 (2006).

Hilger, A., N. Cüppers, M. Tenfelde and U. Kreibig. Surface and interface effects in the optical properties of silver nanoparticles. *Eur. Phys. J. D.* **10**: 115 (2000).

Hirsch, L.R. et al. Nanoshell-mediated near-infrared thermal therapy of tumors under magnetic resonance guidance. *Proc. Natl. Acad. Sci. USA* **100**: 13,549 (2003).

Hirsch, L.R., A.M. Gobin, A.R. Lowery, F. Tam, R.A. Drezek, N.J. Halas and J.L. West. Metal nanoshells. *Annals Biomed. Engin.* **34**: 15 (2006).

Hirsch, L.R., J.B. Jackson, A. Lee, N.J. Halas and J.L. West. A whole blood immunoassay using gold nanoshells. *Anal. Chem.* **75**: 2377 (2003).

Holm, B.A., et al. Nanotechnology in biomedical applications. *Mol. Cryst. Liq. Cryst.* **374**: 589 (2002).

Hong, R., N.O. Fischer, T. Emrick and V.M. Rotello. Surface PEGylation and ligand exchange chemistry of FePt nanoparticles for biological applications. *Chem. Mater.* **17**: 4617 (2005).

Hood, E. Nanotechnology: Looking as we leap. *Enviro. Health Persp.* **112**: A741 (2004).

Hou, Q., P.A. De Bank and K.M. Shakesheff. Injectable scaffolds for tissue regeneration. *J. Mater. Chem.* **14**: 1915 (2004).

Huang, X.L., B. Zhang, L. Ren, S.F. Ye, L.P. Sun, Q.Q. Zhang, M.C. Tan and G.M. Chow. In vivo toxic studies and biodistribution of NIR-Sensitive Au-Au_2S nanoparticles as potential drug delivery carriers. Submitted.

Huber, D.L. Synthesis, properties, and applications of iron nanoparticles. *Small* **1**: 482 (2005).

Hughes, G.A., Nanostructure-mediated drug delivery. *Nanomed.*: *Nanotech., Biol. Med.* **1**: 22 (2005).

Hyeon, T. Chemical synthesis of magnetic nanoparticles. *Chem. Comm.* 927 (2003).

Hyeon, T., S.S. Lee, J. Park, Y. Chung and H.B. Na. Synthesis of highly crystalline and monodisperse maghemite nanocrystallites without a size selection process. *J. Am. Chem. Soc.* **123**: 12,798 (2001).

Itokazu, M., T. Sugiyama, T. Ohno, E. Wada and Y. Katagiri. Development of porous apatite ceramic for local delivery of chemotherapeutic agents. *J. Biomed. Mater Res.* **39**: 536 (1998).

Jaspreet, K.V., M.K. Reddy, V.D. Labhasetwar, Nanosystems in drug targeting: opportunities and challenges. *Curr. Nanosci.* **1**: 47 (2005).

Jin, S. and K. Ye. Nanoparticle-mediated drug delivery and gene therapy. *Biotechnol Prog* **23**: 32 (2007).

Jurgons, R., C. Seliger, A. Hilpert, L. Trahms, S. Odenbach and C. Alexiou, Drug loaded magnetic nanoparticles for cancer therapy, *J. Phys.: Condens. Matter* **18**: S2893 (2006).

Foster, K.A., M. Yazdanian and K.L. Audus. Microparticulate uptake mechanisms of in vitro cell culture models of the respiratory epithelium. *J Pharmacy Pharmacology* **53**: 57 (2001). Kagan, V.E., H. Bayir and A.A. Shvedova. Nanomedicine and nanotoxicology: Two sides of the same coin. *Nanomedicine* **1**: 313 (2005).

Kirchner, C., et al. Cytotoxicity of colloidal CdSe and CdSe/ZnS nanoparticles, *Nano Lett.* **5**: 331 (2005).

Kittel C. *Introduction to Solid State Physics. 8th Ed.* Hoboken: John Wiley & Sons (2005).

Klein, L.C. Processing of nanostructured sol-gel materials. In: A.S. Edelstein and R.C. Cammarata. eds. *Nanomaterials*: *Synthesis, Properties and Applications*. Institute of Physics Publishing, Bristol and Philadelphia, pp. 147 (1996).

Kossovsky, N., et al. Surface-modified nanocrystalline ceramics for drug delivery applications. *Biomaterials* **15**: 1201 (1994).

Kost, J., R. Langer. Responsive polymeric delivery systems. *Adv. Drug Del. Rev.* **46**: 125 (2001).

Kreibig, U. and M. Vollmer. *Optical Properties of Metal Clusters*. Berlin: Springer (1995).

Kumta, P.N., C. Sfeir, D.H. Lee, D. Olton and D. Choi. Nanostructured calcium phosphates for biomedical applications: Novel synthesis and characterization. *Acta Biomat.* **1**: 65 (2005).

Lin, X.M. and C.S. Samia. Synthesis, assembly and physical properties of magnetic nanoparticles. *J. Magnetism Magnetic Mater.* **305**: 100 (2006).

Link, S. and M.A. El-Sayed. Shape and size dependence of radiative, non-radiative and photothermal properties of gold nanocrystals. *Int. Rev. Phys. Chem.* **19**: 409 (2000).

Link, S. and M.A. El-Sayed. Size and temperature dependence of the plasmon absorption of colloidal gold. *J. Phys. Chem. B* **103**: 4212 (1999).

Linnert, T., P. Mulvaney and A. Henglein. Surface chemistry of colloidal silver: Surface plasmon damping by chemisorbed I-, SH-, and C_6H_5S-. *J. Phys. Chem.* **97**: 679 (1993).

Livage, J., M. Henry and C. Sanchez. Sol-gel chemistry of transition metal oxides. *Prog. Solid State Chem.* **18**: 259 (1988).

Loo, C., A. Lowery, N. Halas, J. West and R. Drezek. Immunotargeted nanoshells for integrated cancer imaging and therapy. *Nano Lett.* **5**: 709 (2005).

Love, J.C., L.A. Estroff, J.K. Kriebel, R.G. Nuzzo and G.M. Whitesides. Self-assembled monolayers of thiolates on metals as a form of nanotechnology. *Chem. Rev.* **105**: 1103 (2005).

Lübbe, A.S., C. Bergemann, J. Brock and D.G. McClure. Physiological aspects in magnetic drug-targeting. *J. Magnetism Magnetic Mater.* **194**: 149 (1999).

Luo, D. and W.M. Saltzman. Thinking of silica. *Gene therapy* **13**: 585 (2006).

Luo, D. Nanotechnology and DNA Delivery. *MRS Bulletin* **30**: 654 (2005).

Moghimi, S.M., A.C. Hunter and J.C. Murray. Long-circulating and target-specific nanoparticles: Theory to practice. *Pharmacol. Rev.* **53**: 283 (2001).

Neuberger, T., B. Schopf, H. Hormann, M. Hofmann and B. von Rechenberg. Superparamagnetic nanoparticles for biomedical applications; Possibilities and limitations of a new drug delivery system. *J. Magnetism and Magnetic Mater* **293**: 483 (2005).

Niederberger, M. and G. Garnweitner. Organic reaction pathways in the nonaqueous synthesis of metal oxide nanoparticles. *Chem. Eur. J.* **12**: 7282 (2006).

Niemz, M.H. *Laser-Tissue Interactions: Fundamentals and Applications*. Springer-Verlag: Berlin (2002).

Oldenburg, S.J., R.D. Averitt, S.L. Westcott and N.J. Halas. Nanoengineering of optical resonances. *Chem. Phys. Lett.* **288**: 243 (1998).

Olton, D., J. Li, M.E. Wilson, T. Rogers, J. Close, L. Huang, P.N. Kumta and C. Sfeir. Nanostructured calcium phosphates for non-viral gene delivery: Influence of the synthesis parameters on transfection efficiency. *Biomaterials* **28**: 1267 (2007).

Oskam, G. Metal oxide nanoparticles: Synthesis, characterization and application. *J. Sol-Gel Sci. Technol.* **37**: 161 (2006).

Panyam, J. and V. Labhasetwar. Biodegradable nanoparticles for drug and gene delivery to cells and tissue. *Adv. Drug Del. Rev.* **55**: 329 (2003).

Park, J., et al. Ultra-large-scale synthesis of monodisperse nanocrystals. *Nature Mater.* **3**: 891 (2004).

Persson, B.N.J. Polarizability of small spherical metal particles influence of the matrix environment. *Surf. Sci.* **281**: 153 (1993).

Petrak, K., Nanotechnology and site-targeted drug delivery. *J. Biomater. Sci. Polymer Edn.* **17**: 1209 (2006).

Pinchuk, A., U. Kreibig and A. Hilger. Optical properties of metallic nanoparticles: Influence of interface effects and interband transitions. *Surf. Sci.* **557**: 269 (2004).

Pitkethly, M.J. Nanomaterials—the driving force. *NanoToday* **12**: 20 (2004).

Prasad, P.N., *Nanophotonics*. Hoboken, NJ: John Wiley & Sons (2004).

Qiang, Y., J. Antony, A. Sharma, J. Nutting, D. Sikes and D. Meyer. Iron/iron oxide core-shell nanoclusters for biomedical applications. *J. Nanoparticle Res* **8**: 489 (2006).

Ren, L. and G.M. Chow. Synthesis of NIR-sensitive Au-Au_2S nanocolloids for drug delivery. *Mater. Sci. Eng. C* **23**: 113 (2003).

Ren, L., X.L. Huang, B. Zhang, L.P. Sun, Q.Q. Zhang, M.C. Tan and G.M. Chow. Cisplatin loaded Au-Au_2S nanoparticles for potential cancer therapy: Cytotoxicity. in vitro Carcinogenicity, and cellular uptake. Submitted.

Salgueiriño-Maceira V., R. Caruso and L.M. Liz-Marzán. Coated colloids with tailored optical properties. *J. Phys. Chem. B* **107**: 10,990 (2003).

Sato, S., et al. Nanosecond, high-intensity pulsed laser ablation of myocardium tissue at the ultraviolet, visible, and near-infrared wavelengths: In-vitro study. *Lasers Surg. Med.* **29**: 464 (2001).

Sayes, C.M., et al. The differential cytotoxicity of water-soluble fullerenes. *Nano Lett.* **4**: 1881 (2004).

Sershen, S., J. West. Implantable, polymeric systems for modulated drug delivery. *Adv. Drug Del. Rev.* **54**: 1225 (2002).

Sheludko, A. *Colloid Chemistry*. Elsevier: Amsterdam (1966).

Singh, R., et al. Tissue biodistribution and blood clearance rates of intravenously administered carbon nanotube radiotracers. *Proc. Natl. Acad. Sci. USA.* **103**: 3357 (2006).

Stokes, R.J. and D.F. Evans. *Fundamentals of Interfacial Engineering*. New York: Wiley-VCH (1997).

Tan, M.C. NIR-sensitive nanoparticles for targeted drug delivery. PhD Thesis, (2006).

Tan, M.C., J.Y. Ying and G.M. Chow. Structure and microstructure of NIR-absorbing Au-Au_2S nanoparticles. Submitted.

Temenoff, J.S. and A.G. Mikos. Injectable biodegradable materials for orthopedic tissue engineering. *Biomaterials* **21**: 2405 (2000).

Templeton, A.C., W.P. Wuelfing and R.W. Murray. Monolayer-protected cluster molecules. *Acc. Chem. Res.* **33**: 27 (2000).

Tirelli, N. (Bio)responsive nanoparticles. *Curr. Opin. Coll. Interf. Sci.* **11**: 210 (2006).

Turkevich, J., P.C. Stevenson and J. Hillier. The nucleation and growth processes in the synthesis of colloidal gold. *Discuss. Faraday Soc.* **11**: 55 (1951).

U.S. Food and Drug Administration. http://www.cfsan.fda.gov/~redbook/red-toca.html, Toxicological Principles for the Safety Assessment of Food Ingredients, 2000.

Uchida, A., Y. Shinto, N. Araki and K. Ono. Slow release of anticancer drugs from porous calcium hydroxyapatite ceramic. *J. Orthop. Res.* **10**: 440 (1992).

Vallet-Regi, M. Ordered mesoporous materials in the context of drug delivery systems and bone tissue engineering. *Chem. Eur. J.* **12**: 5934 (2006).

Vallet-Regi, M. Revisiting ceramics for medical applications. *Dalton Trans.* **44**: 5211 (2006).

Vioux, A. Nonhydrolytic sol-gel routes to oxides. *Chem. Mater.* **9**: 2292 (1997).

Vogel, A. and V. Venugopalan. Mechanisms of pulsed laser ablation of biological tissues. *Chem. Rev.* **103**: 577 (2003).

Waynant, R.W., I.K. Ilev and I. Gannot. Mid-infrared laser applications in medicine and biology. *Philos. Trans. R. Soc. Lond. Ser. A-Math Phys. Eng. Sci.* **359**: 635 (2001).

Weissleder, R. A clearer vision for in vivo imaging. *Nat. Biotechnol.* **19**: 316 (2001).

West, J.L., N.J. Halas. Applications of nanotechnology to biotechnology. *Curr. Opin. Biotech.* **11**: 215 (2000).

West, J.L., N.J. Halas. Engineered nanomaterials for biophotonics applications: Improving sensing, imaging, and therapeutics. *Ann. Rev. Biomed. Eng.* **5**: 285 (2003).

Whitesides, G.M. Nanoscience, nanotechnology, and chemistry. *Small* **1**: 172 (2005).

Xu, Z.P., Q.H. Zeng, G.Q. Lu and A.B. Yu. Inorganic nanoparticles as carriers for efficient cellular delivery. *Chemical Engineering Science* **61**: 1027 (2006).

Yin, H., H.P. Too and G.M. Chow. The effects of particle size and surface coating on the cytotoxicity of nickel ferrite. *Biomaterials* **26**: 5818 (2005).

Yong, T.H., Apatite-polymer composites for the controlled delivery of bone morphogenetic proteins. PhD Thesis. MIT (2005).

Yong, T.H., E.A. Hager and J.Y. Ying. Apatite-polymer composite particles for controlled delivery of BMP-2. Singapore-MIT Alliance Symposium Proceedings (2004).

Yu, S. and G.M. Chow. Carboxyl group (—CO_2H) functionalized ferrimagnetic iron oxide nanoparticles for potential bio-applications. *J. Mater. Chem.* **14**: 2781 (2004).

Zhou, H.S., I. Honma and H. Komiyama. Controlled synthesis and quantum-size effect in gold-coated nanoparticles. *Phys. Rev. B* **50**: 12,052 (1994).

Zhu, S.H., et al. Hydroxyapatite nanoparticles as a novel gene carrier. *J. Nanoparticle Res.* **6**: 307 (2004).

12 Nano Metal Particles for Biomedical Applications

Kyung A. Kang, Bin Hong and Hanzhu Jin

Department of Chemical Engineering, University of Louisville
Louisville, KY 40292, USA

Abstract In the management of human health, nano-sized tools are usually more effective than larger ones because they can be incorporated into the systems more in a fundamental (cellular or molecular) level, causing less negative side effects. One of these nano tools that are currently getting much attention is nanometal particle (NMPs). NMPs have many unique properties that are not present in their bulk form. When these unique properties are positively utilized in biological systems they can be very effective for the diagnosis and/or treatment for various diseases. In this article, examples of various applications of NMPs in biomedical sciences and technology are reviewed and a few examples that are currently studied in our research group are demonstrated. It should be noted that, in this article, only a limited publications are cited out of the large volume of NMP related ones, and the readers should not assume that the examples listed in this article are representing all of the currently available NMP tools used in biomedical field. It should also be noted that the authors for this articles are not experts in nanotechnology but are bioengineers.

Keyword Nanometal particles, biosensing, bioimaging, diagnosis, treatment

12.1 NMPs as Contrast Agents for Bioimaging

Many disease diagnoses are done by a principle similar of 'systems identification method,' which has been extensively used for engineering systems for decades. The only difference is that the system, in this case, is a living system. An input signal is applied to, and disturbs the system of our interest, and its responses to the disturbance (i.e. output) is analyzed to understand the system's behavior. For biomedical application, it is highly desirable if the input signal application and the output signal retrieval can be done non- or minimally- invasively. Examples of these inputs for biomedical applications are lights (e.g., ultraviclet (UV), visible, near infrared, and infrared), ultrasound (e.g. sonogram), X-ray (e.g. mammography

(1) Corresponding e-mail: kakang01@louisville.edu

and computerized tomography (CT) scan), electromagnetic wave (e.g. magnetic reasorance spectroscopy (MRS) and magnetic reasonance image (MRI), positron (e.g., positron emission tomography (PET)), etc. The response (output) signal usually provides considerable information about the system but if it is not strong enough then early and/or accurate diagnosis is difficult. Contrast agents that can enhance the signal from the system can, therefore, be very useful especially for this type of situations.

Utilizing NMPs for enhancing the signal from the targeted living system has been attempted in various bio-tools. For MRI, magnetic NMPs are used for this purpose (Weissleder et al., 1990). Superparamagnetic, iron oxides (Fe_2O_3/Fe_3O_4; Feridex I.V.® or Endorem®; Advanced Magnetics, Cambridge, MA) are a few examples of currently used MRI contrast agents. When the surfac of these particles is treated with disease representing biomolecules (e.g. cancer cell specific hormones, antibodies, etc.), the particles can be accumulated much more specifically in the diseased areas, enhancing the contrast for the target and minimizing the negative effect of the particle accumulation in excrtory organs (Josephson et al., 1999; Leuschner et al., 2005).

Nanogold paricles (NGPs) have been extensively used as contrast agents for various imaging techniques. Gold colloids were observed by electron microscopy (Kraemer, 1942) and bio-molecules linked gold colloids were used as targeted contrast agent for this tool. NGPs are also excellent optical contrast agent and, with their inert nature, they can be used for cell and animal studies with less negative side effects than other metals. Figure 12.1(a) shows the optical contrast

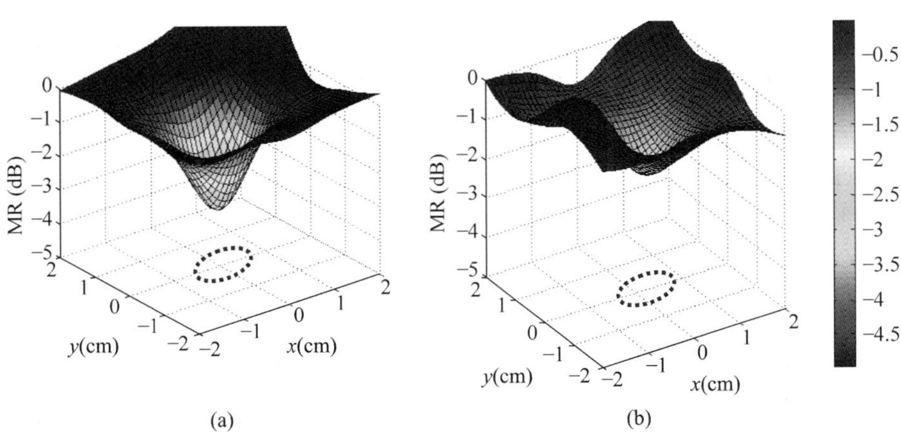

Figure 12.1 Optical contrasts created by an empty vitamin E capsules (oval shape with a dimension of 1.0 cm × 1.0 cm × 1.5 cm) filled with (a) 0.1wt% of 150 nm NGP and (b) 0.1wt% of 10 nm – 20 nm Fe_3O_4 particles, placed 1 cm deep in an experimental breast model whose optical property was adjusted to those of human breast tissue. Near infrared-time resolved spectroscopy (NIR-TRS) spectra, at the wavelength of 788 nm were obtained in transmittance and the spectra were transferred to frequency domain. The modulation frequency analyzed here is at 100 MHz. The black dashed ellipsoids indicate the tumor model size and position (Color Fig. 17)

generated by NGP particles for a near infrared (NIR) wavelength at 780 nm (Jin and Kang, 2007). An empty vitamin E capsule (1.0 cm× 1.0 cm× 1.5 cm) was filled with 0.01wt% NGPs (with the ingredient used for breast tissue model) and placed in an experimental model with the optical properties of human breast tissue. NGPs at a size of 150 nm generate significant optical contrast at a concentration as little as 0.01wt%. Optical contrast generated by Fe_3O_4 particles (10 – 20 nm for this study), which is usually used for MRI contrast and also used for cancer hyperthermia, was also tested for their optical contrast, and they were found to provide a very good optical contrast, although not as strong as NGPs. Loo et al. (2004, 2005) synthesized gold nanoshells filled with silica, which can control optical properties (absorption and scattering coefficients) of the target by the core/shell ratio and the overall size. These particles were conjugated with anti-cancer-antibody and tested for optical, molecular imaging and optical coherence tomography (OCT). With 10 nm gold nanoshells on 120 nm silica core, cancer cells were shown with a significantly increased scattering contrast.

12.2 Fluorescing NMPs

Approximately 50 years ago, Lawson et al. (1960) discovered that, when PbTe and PbSe were evaporated and formed small crystals, photoconductive layers were formed. Later, other researchers (Bergstresser and Cohen, 1967) also found that other semiconductor nanostructures showed excellent fluorescence (Larson et al., 2003). These nano-structures were later named as quantum dots (QDs). Exemplary materials showing these properties in a nano crystal form are CdTe, CdSe, ZnS, and ZnTe. Compared to fluorephores, QDs have advantages of higher quantum yield (QY) and better photo-stability. Since the excitation/emission wavelengths of QDs can be flexibly adjusted either by the size or composition, they can be used for multicolor labeling (Gao et al., 2004) for various biomarkers, which is highly beneficial for multi-biomarker sensing/imanging (Smith et al., 2006).

Recently, QDs has been extensively used for cellular and/or animal studies, although not extensively for human yet. QDs have been very useful for tracking cells and for studying vascular structures (Stroh et al., 2005) and imaging of normal and cancer cells (Kaul et al., 2003); peptide coated, ZnS-capped CdSe QDs showed their accumulating in the lung of mice after the intra venous injection, whereas two other peptide conjugated QDs were directed to blood vessels or lymphatic vessels in tumors (Akerman et al., 2002); Hama et al., (2006) used QDs of two different emission spectra for lymphatic imaging, by the two different size of the QDs. The QDs allowed simultaneous visualization of two separate, lymphatic flow drainages; Stroh et al., (2005) showed that QDs can be used for image and differentiating tumor vessels from the perivascular cells and the matrix. They also used QDs to study the effect of the particle size on the accessibility to the tumor. QD-labeled, bone marrow-derived precursor cells to the tumor vasculature were successfully monitored; QDs for near infrared (NIR) have been used during a major cancer surgery for mapping sentinel lymph nodes mapping as image guidance. Injection of only 400 pmol of NIR QDs permitted sentinel lymph nodes positioned 1 cm deep to be imaged easily in real time, using excitation fluence rates of only 5 mW/cm^2. Kim et al., (2004), Soltesz et al., (2005), and Gao et al., (2004), reported QD probes for tumor targeting and imaging in live animals. The surface of QDs was treated with the amphiphilic, triblock-copolymer, which then was linked to prostate tumor-targeting antibodies. The study results indicated that the QD probes can be accumulated at human prostate cancer sites in mice by both enhanced permeation and retention, and via the antibody against cancer-specific cell-surface biomarkers. Multicolor fluorescence imaging of cancer cells was achieved under in vivo conditions.

The biocompatibility and the safety of QDs for human use are still under investigation.

12.3 NMPs with High Plamon Field for Fluorescence Manipulation

Fluorephores have a unique property of absorbing a particular wavelength of light and emitting light at another wavelength. For decades, they have been extensively used as effective signal mediators for observing biological phenomena, especially disease related ones, via optical biosensing and bioimaging. As a signal mediator, a fluorophore emitting stronger fluorescence per molecule (i.e. per biomarker) provides a more sensitive tool. This effectiveness gage of a fluorephore is often expressed in terms of its quantum yield, which is the ratio of the number of photons generated for emission to the number of the photons absorbed by a fluorophore.

Many fluorophores have a molecular structure such that their excited electrons are often paired with lone pair electrons within their own molecular structure, without being used for fluorescence emission, which is often called 'self quenching' of fluorescence. A strong plasmon field on the surface of a certain type of NMPs can attract these lone pair electrons and alter their fluorescence emission. Good candidate metals possessing a strong plasmon field at their nano-size are gold, silver, and platinum, because of their special molecular nature of holding high electron density around them (Kang and Hong, 2006).

One of the mechanisms of altering fluorescence by these NMPs is as follows: when oscillating electrons in the surface plamon field of an NMP couple with excited electrons of a fluorophore, an instantaneous electron attraction or even an electron transfer occurs from the fluorophore to the NMP, causing the electrons involved in the fluorescence emission altered in their energy states. The level of this alteration depends upon the strength of the plasmon field where the fluorophore is placed. The plasmon field strength depends upon the metal type, the size of an NMP, from the distance and the nanoparticle (Ruppin, 1975; Geddes et al., 2003; Kang and Hong, 2006; Hong and Kong, 2006).

Placing a fluorophore (or light emitting entities in general, including QDs) around an NMP with high surface plasmon polariton field (SPPF) will result one of the following three scenarios (Fig. 12.2): (a) if the fluorophore is placed very close to the NMP and therefore, is inside an SPPF with a very high strength, then most electrons including the ones for fluorescence emission are attract to the NMP, resulting partial or total fluorescence quenching; (b) If the fluorophore is placed far away from the NMP (outside the plamson field), then there will be little change in the fluorescence; (c) if the fluorophore is at a particular distance from an NMP, where only the electrons that are normally participated in self-quenching are attracted to the SPPF, then the fluorescence is enhanced. In our studies, the spacing between a fluorophore and an NMP was artificially changed by immobilizing self assembled monolayer (SAM) on the surface of NMPs. To avoid the crowding fluorophores, which may result in inter-molecular queching, the fluorophore concentration to be tested was very carefully selected, after numerous tests, at the level much lower than the lower limit for this type of quenching.

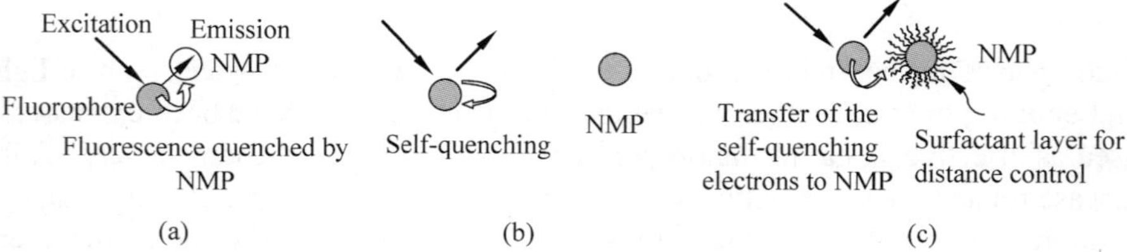

Figure 12.2 A schematic diagram illustrating the effect of the distance between a fluorophore and a nanogold particle on fluorescence: (a) too close—a fluorophore receives excitation light but the emission light is quenched, because the NGP attracts most of the electrons including the ones for fluorescence generation. (b) Too far—the plasmon field around the NGP does not reach the fluorophore. (c) At an appropriate distance—a fluorophore receives the excitation light and an NGP attracts the electrons normally used for self-quenching, resulting in more emission light

The mechanism of quenching and enhancing the fluorescence can be beneficially used, depending upon the specific needs.

12.3.1 NMPs Used for Fluorescence Quenching

As the way fluorescing is used as signal mediation of a biological reaction, quenching can also be used by turning off a steadily-on, fluorescing light or vice versa. Dubertret and his coworkers (2001) have used 1.5 nm nanogold particles to quench fluorescence of fluorephores by attaching an NGP to a single stranded, hairpin DNA (Fig. 12.3). When the probe encounters the target molecule, it forms a hybrid that is more stable than the hairpin. Then the NGP no longer quench the fluorescence of the fluorophore and fluorescence emit the light; In a slightly different application, Chang and his co-workers (2005) developed a QD with inherent signal amplification upon interaction with a targeted proteolytic enzyme, which is useful for imaging in much better target-specific cancer detection and diagnosis. In this system, QDs are bound to nanogold particles (NGPs) via a proteolytically (collagenase) degradable peptide sequence to suppress luminescence (Fig. 12.4). With the conjugation of NGPs to QDs, 71% reduction in luminescence was achieved. Release of NGPs by peptide cleavage restores radiative QD photoluminescence and, a 52% rise in luminescence over 47 h of exposure to 0.2 mg/mL collagenase.

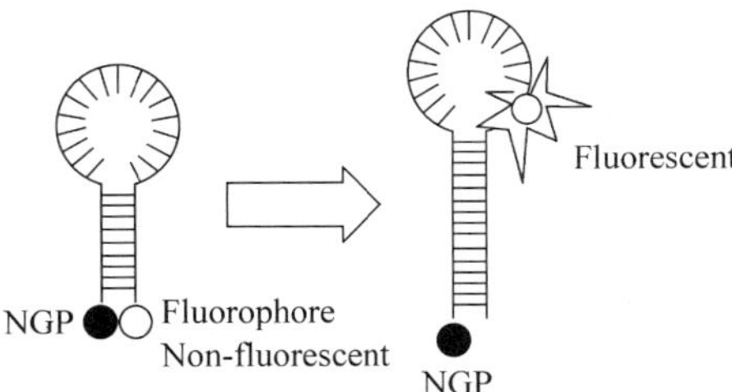

Figure 12.3 An illustration of an NGP quenching fluorescence at a close distance from a fluorophore in a hairpin shaped structure. A target molecule having stronger attraction to the fluorophore than the bond of the hairpin releases the fluorophore from the structure. Then the fluorescence is retrieved

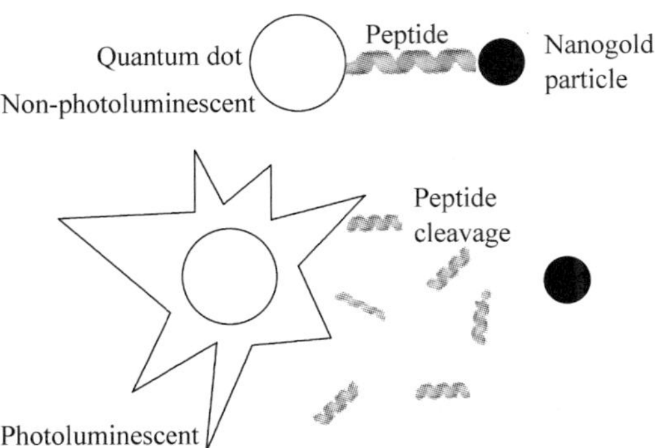

Figure 12.4 A schematic illustration of an NGP's quenching of flurescence of a QD. A protease representing the targeted disease digests the peptide which links the QD and the NGP. As the QD releases it emits intensive fluorescence

12.3.2 NMP for Fluorescence Enhancement in Biosensing

For the fluorescence enhancement by NMPs, here, our study results from the free form of fluorophores in solution (Fig. 12.5(a)) and from a fluorophore mediated, immuno-biosensing (Fig. 12.5(b)) are illustrated. The basic mechanism of this sensing system is an immuno-sandwich assay on the surface of an optical fiber. Briefly, one type of antibody 1° Mab, specific to the target molecule, is immobilized on the surface of an optical fiber and the fiber is incased in a chamber, forming an immuno-optical sensing unit. The sample is injected to the sensing chamber and the target molecule reacts with the antibody on the fiber surface. The sensor is then washed to remove the non-reacted molecules and another type of antibody linked with a fluorophore –2° Mab is applied to the chamber, to forma sandwich complex. Excitation light is applied to the sensor and then the emitted light is retrieved and correlated to the concentration of the target molecules in the sample. This tool is faster to complete the assay and more user friendly than enzyme linked immuno sorption assay (ELISA). The assay procedure is simpler and can be completed within minutes instead of hours, with the sensitivity as high as a pico molar level. In this article, only the qualitative experimental results are shown and more thorough, quantitative study is currently in progress.

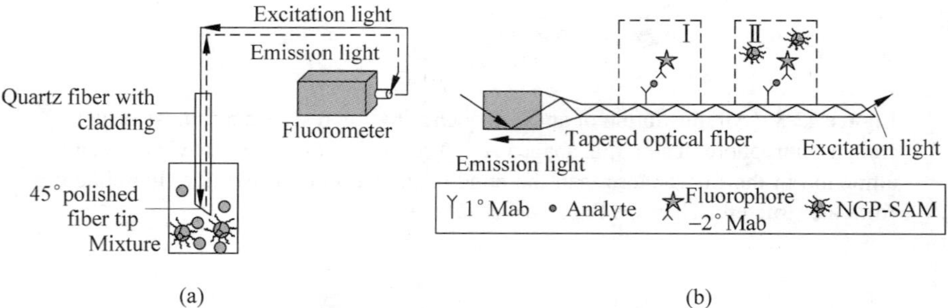

Figure 12.5 Schematic diagrams of fluorescence measurements for (a) free fluorophore and (b) the fluorophore mediated, fiber-optic biosensing

Our definition of enhancement in this study is the increase in the fluorescence divided by the fluorescence intensity without the enhancer (control).

As previously stated, an effectiveness of fluorescence enhancement by an NMP depends upon the strength of SPPF where the fluophore is placed and the SPPF strength around an NMP depends upon the metal type, the size of the NMP, and the distance from the NMP surface. The amount of the fluorescence that can be enhanced by NMPs is that of the normally self-quenched and, therefore, the maximum fluorescence that can be recovered is 1-QY.

To verify this mechanism of the instantaneous transfer of the lone pair electrons from the fluorophore to the NGP, we have performed a simple experiment using pyrrolidine and a fluorophore, Cy5. Pyrrolidine is a small, non-fluorescent molecule with the structure similar to a part of Cy5, which has the nitrogen atom with lone pair electrons. Figure 12.6 illustrates the structures of Cy5 and pyrrolidine, and also their possible interaction with an NGP. According to our theory, Cy5 self-quenches fluorescence by the intra molecular electron transfer (white ribbon arrow in the figure); Cy5 interacts with the SPPF of an NGP via INTER-molecular electron transfer, resulting in fluorescence enhancement (grey ribbon arrow); added pyrrolidine molecules compete with Cy5 for the interaction with the NGP (black ribbon arrow). Pyrrolidine does not fluoresce, has little steric hindrance because of its small size and therefore, if it is mixed in a solution with Cy5 and NGPs, it can react with NGPs more easyly than Cy5 can. Also, a small amount of pyrrolidine in the solution is not expected to affect chemical or physical properties of the solution (e.g. viscosity, polarity, hydrogen-bonding, etc.). For the experiment, first, Cy5 was dissolved in PBS buffer solution and 5 nm NGP (5 nm NGP) linked with 2 nm self assembled monolayer (SAM) (SAM 2 nm) were added at a molar ratio of Cy5 to NGP, 200: 1 and the fluorescence was measured. At this ratio, approximately 30% of fluorescence enhancement was observed (the initial fluorescence level; Fig. 12.7). Then, pyrrolidine was added to the solution little by little and the fluorescence started to decreased until it reached the fluorescence level of the Cy5 solution without NGPs (dotted line), confirming that NGPs, in fact, interact with the lone pair electrons of Cy5 molecules and cause the fluorescence enhancement.

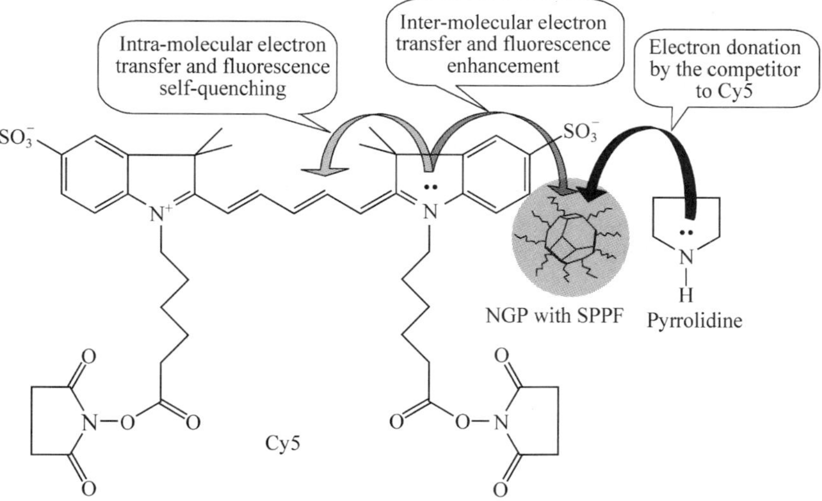

Figure 12.6 A schematic diagram of the interaction among Cy5, pyrrolidine, and an NGP. The white ribbon arrow donates the INTRA molecular electron transfer inside the Cy5. The grey ribbon arrow means the INTER molecular electron transfer between the Cy5 and the NGP. The black ribbon arrow shows the INTER molecular electron transfer between the pyrrolidine and the NGP. Lone pair electrons are shown as double black dots

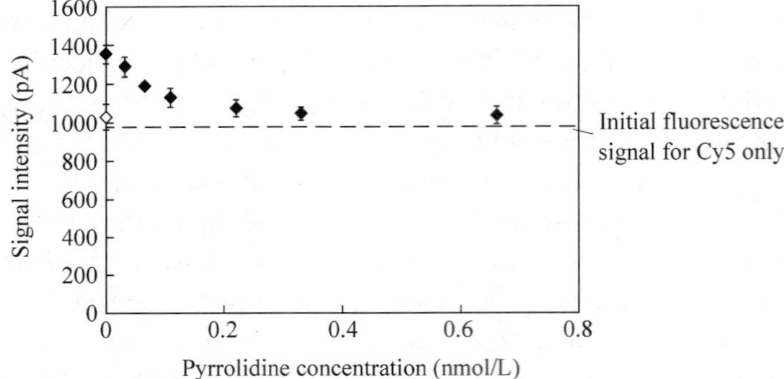

Figure 12.7 The effect of pyrrolidine concentration on the fluorescence enhancement of free Cy5 by NGPs. The signal intensity of Cy5 solution without NGPs was shown as the dotted line (Experimental conditions: Free Cy5 concentration, 66 nmol/L; 5 nm NGP-SAM 2 nm concentration, 0.33 nmol/L)

1. Metal Type

For this part of study, nanosilver particles (NSPs) and NGPs at a size of 20 nm were selected. 20 nm was chosen simply because, at the time of our study, it was the smallest size that was commercially available for NSP. These nanoparticles are sold with tannic acid (length, ~3 nm) as surfactant (SAM 3 nm) on their surface. These particles were tested in fluorophore mediated, sandwich immuno-sensing of a cardiac marker B-type natriuretic peptide (BNP) in human plasma at a concentration of 0.5 ng-BNP/mL-plasma (Fig. 12.8), while the nanoparticles are applied after the sandwich complex is formed on the senor surface (Fig. 12.5(b)). In this study, the particle concentration was set to be 0.2 nmol/L since it was the optimal NGP concentration with our biosensor studies. As can be seen in Fig. 12.8, NSPs showed the enhancement of 30%, and NGPs, 114%, illustrating the differences in plasmon strength for different metals.

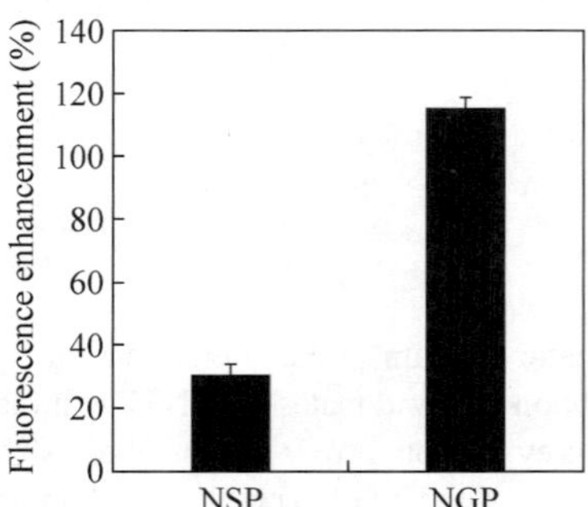

Figure 12.8 Fluorescence enhancement in BNP biosensing by 20 nm NSP-SAM 3 nm and 20 nm NGP-SAM 3 nm (Experimental conditions: fluorophore used, Cy5; sensor size, 1.5 cm; BNP concentration, 0.5 ng-BNP/mL-plasma, NGP-SAM concentration, 0.2 nmol/L)

2. Particle Size

The effect of the NMP size was studied using the NGPs at sizes of 2, 5, and 10 nm (commercially available ones). For this study, the thickness of a SAM remained to be 3 nm (SAM 3 nm; tannic acid). The measurement on the emitted fluorescence was both for a free Cy5 and for immuno-biosensing Fig. 12.9. The enhancement for the free Cy5 by 2, 5 and 10 nm NGPs were 42%, 30%, and 11%, respectively, showing a less enhancement with the greater NGP size, confirming the differences in the plasmon density for the NGPs at different sizes. For the biosensing, protein C (an anticoatulant in plasma) was used an analyte and, the enhancements were 115%, 102%, and 12%, respectively. There were similar trend in the enhancement for free Cy5 or Cy5 mediated sensors qualitatively, but the biosensing showed much higher enhancment. This may be because free fluorophores suspended in solution interact with the NGPs in a three-dimensional space, while the biosensing provides the surface-bound fluorophores, and therefore, the fluorescence retrieval is much more effective.

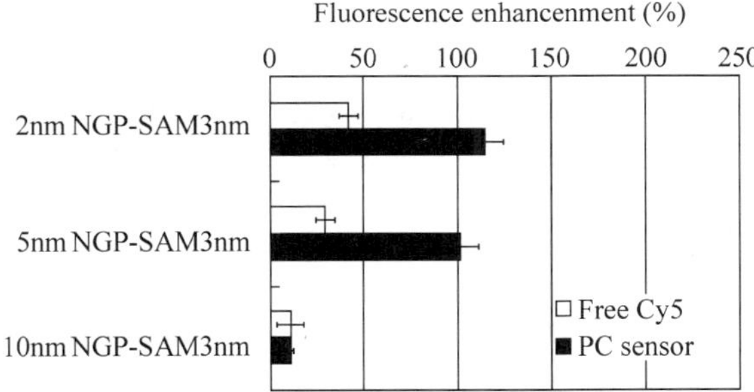

Figure 12.9 The effect of the NGP size on the fluorescence enhancement for the free Cy5 and the Cy5 mediated PC sensing (Experimental conditions: For free Cy5 measurement, the concentration of Cy5, 66 nmol/L; PC sensor size, 6 cm; PC sample, 1 μg-PC/mL-plasma; SAM thickness, 3 nm; NGP size used, 2, 5, and 10 nm)

3. Distance between a Fluorophore and an NMP

As previous stated, here, the spacing between a fluorophore and an NMP was artificially changed by immobilizing self assembled monolayer on the surface of NMPs. However, the SAM thickness here is not the actual distance but the minimum distance between a fluophore and an NGP because NGPs are floating in a solution. The SAMs at approximately 1, 2, and 3 nm (*L*-glutathione, 16-mercaptohexadecanoic acid, and tannic acid, respectively) were reacted with NGPs at a size of 5 nm (5 nm NGP). The 5 nm NGPs coated with SAMs (5 nm NGP-SAMs) were then applied to both the free Cy5 and the Cy5 mediated PC biosensor, and the level of enhancement was observed (Fig. 12.10). For both the free Cy5 and PC sensors, the SAM thickness of 2 nm (SAM 2 nm) demonstrated

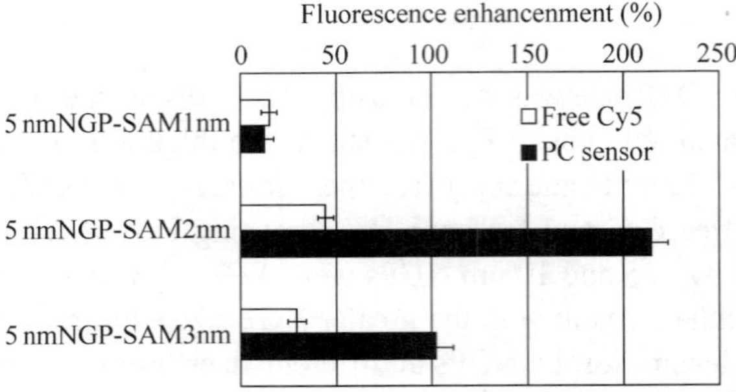

Figure 12.10 The effect of the SAM thickness on the fluorescence enhancement for the free Cy5 and the Cy5 mediated PC sensing (Experimental conditions: for free Cy5 measurement, the concentration of Cy5, 66 nmol/L; PC sensor size, 6 cm; PC as sample)

the greatest enhancements. Although there was enhancement, 1 nm may have been too close to prevent reduction in radiative emission, and 3 nm, too far to reroute the electrons for effective enhancement.

4. Quantum Yield of Fluorophore

As stated, the maximum amount of the enhanced (retrieved) fluorescence depends upon the QY of a fluorophore. In other words, if the quantum yield of a fluorophore is low due to the extensive self quenching, then the amount of fluorescence to be retrieved would be higher. To test this hypothesis, Alexa fluor™ 647, another fluorophore that has very similar maximum excitation and emission (Ex/Em) wavelengths with a QY different from that of Cy5, was selected. The QYs of Cy5 and AF647 are ~0.28 and ~0.56, respectively, and both have the excitation and emission maxima at or around 649 and 670 nm, respectively (Anderson and Nerurkar, 2002; Berlier et al. 2003). As can be seen in Fig. 12.11, for the free fluorophore, AF647 showed only a small enhancement and for the PC biosensing, it showed none, indirectly showing the effect of QY on the enhancement level.

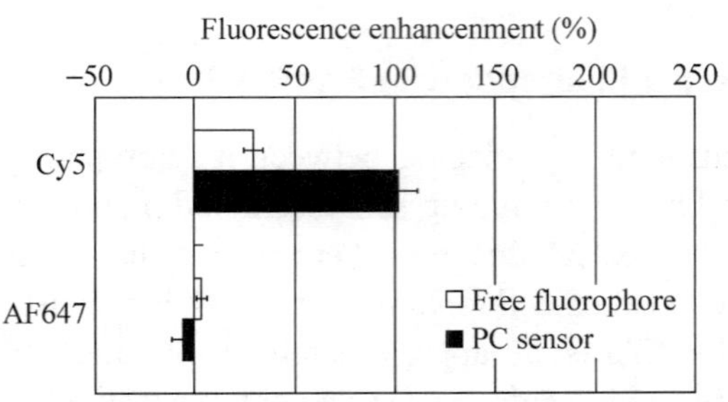

Figure 12.11 The effect of the fluorophore quantum yields on the fluorescence enhancement for the free fluorophore and the fluorophore mediated PC sensing (Experimental conditions: For the measurement of free fluorophores, the concentration of Cy5 and AF647, 66 nmol/L; PC sensor size, 6 cm; NGP-SAM used: 5 nm NGP-SAM 3 nm)

12.3.3 NMP for Fluorescence Enhancement in Bioimaging

When a fluorophore is used for in-vivo bio-imaging, unlike in ex-vivo biosensing or bioimaging, the fluorophore and the NMP may not be separately applied to the system. In bioimaging, fluorophores are usually designed to target specific bio-molecules in the cell or organelle and if these two entities are separately applied there is no guarantee that both would arrive together at the target site, although special manipulation may be designed to do so. Therefore, the fluorophore needs to be somehow immobilized to the NMP with a spacer appropriate for the enhancement. Indocyanine green (ICG; Cardio-green) is an FDA approved NIR contrast agent but a rather poor fluorophore, in terms of the quantum yield (QY = 0.032 in plasma; Licha et al., 2000). Maximal excietation and emission wavelengths for ICG are 780 and 830 nm, respectively. Since ICG does not have any side chain to react, Cypate, an ICG derivative with a carboxylic group was used (Achilefu et al., 2000). For this study, commercially available protein A (PA: 1 nm) or streptavidin (SA: 3 nm) linked 5 or 10 nm NGPs were used. Since multiple numbers of these protein molecules are immobilized on the surface of an NGP the resulting Cypate linked NGPs via these proteins would probably be as shown in Fig. 12.12. Cypate was linked to 5 or 10 nm NGP-PA and NPG-SA

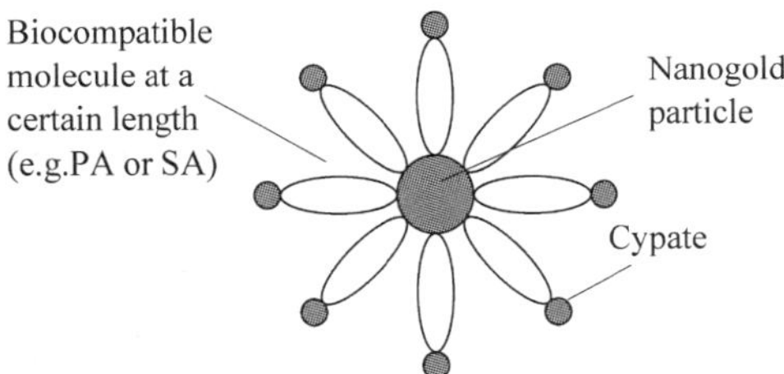

Figure 12.12 A schematic diagram of possible binding struture of Cypate and NGP via protein A (PA) and stepavidin (SA)

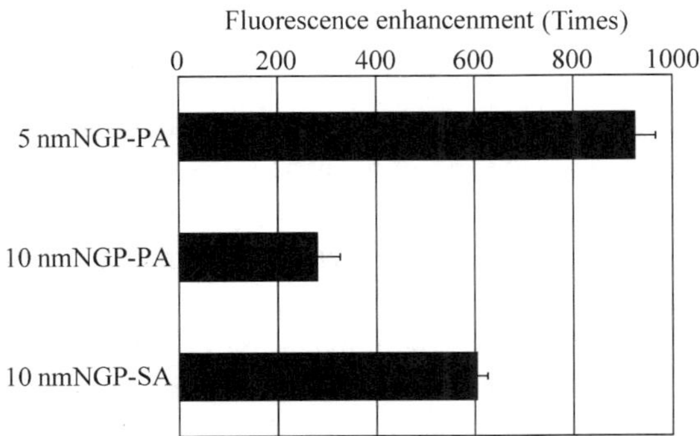

Figure 12.13 Fluorescence enhancement by Cypate linked, PA coated, 5 nm NGP (5 nm NGP-PA), PA coated 10 nm NGP (10 nm NGP-PA), or SA coated 10 nm NGP (10 nm NGP-SA) compared to Cypate alone (Experimental conditions: Cypate concentration, 30 μmol/L)

and the resulting fluorescence of Cypate-PA/SA-NGP was compared to that of Cypate only (Fig. 12.13). The fluorescence signal by Cypate linked 5 nm NGP, via PA spacer showed the best performance and the enhancement level was as high as 900 times. For the 10 nm NGP, 3 nm-spacer (SA) provided a higher enhancement than 1 nm-spacer (PA). This result shows that NMPs (in this case NGPs) with high biocompatibility, can be highly effective for enhancing the fluorescence of the fluorophores that can be used for bio-imaging of human.

12.4 Magnetic NMPs for Bioseparation

The size of the magnetic particles for bio-separation application is usually larger than the usual sense of 'nano' (equal or less than 100 nm), because the particle needs to be big enough to generate sufficient magnetic force, to be effective for the separation purpose. These particles are usually surface treated with anti-target molecules. The anti-target molecule on the surface of the particles reacts with the target molecule and the target molecule containing magnetic particles are then captured by a magnetic field or a type of particle separating systems. After the particles are washed to remove un-wanted/un-reacted materials from the surface and then the target molecule can be retrieved by releasing them from the anti-target molecule by changing the liquid condition where the particles are placed. After removing the target molecules, the particles can be used again. Here we are listing some of the application examples.

Coker et al. (1997) have used polyacrylamide/magnetite (PAM) composite beads in a magnetically stabilized fluidized bed (MSFB). The PAM beads were stable in most buffers from pH 1.1 to 10. This approach allowed MSFB operation at superficial velocities close to those used in high pressure liquid chromatography (HPLC) (~0.1 mm/s) with a magnetic field applied to stabilize the bed. The beads were used in affinity separation of chymotrypsin from the sample of a mixture with equal concentrations of trypsin and chymotrypsin. Although the adsorption capacity of the beads was less than that of other beads the purity of the product was higher; Magnetic agarose beads were used to separate angioI-TEM-ρ-lactamase from *E. coli* lysate and able to concentrate the target molecule without a centrifugation process (Abudabi and Beitle 1998). This method is especially good for separating biomolecules in a highly viscous fermentation broth with various lysates because particles in such a broth are not easily centrifuged, filtered, or separated by packed bed chromatography; Yang and his colleagues (2006) used magnetic poly methyl methacrylate (PMMA) beads coated with polyethylene glycol and functionalized with amine groups. *P*-aminobenzamidine was covalently immobilized onto magnetic beads for the purification of nattokinase directly from the purification broth. The purification process took only 40 minutes with a purifcation factor of 8.76 and a yield of 87%; Magnetic adsorbent (i.e.

ferro-carbon particle) has been used to adsorb toxic materials at low, medium and high molecular weights from blood stream (Torchilin and European 2000). A high gradient magnetic separator is used to remove the tonxin adsorbed, magnetic particles from the blood stream. Animal experiments have shown high effectiveness of the removal of low molecular weight toxins using this technique.

12.5 Magnetic NMPs for Biosensing

Most sensing techniques separate the target molecule from the mixture with other molecules in the sample, before the actual application of a signal mediator for sensing. As shown in the previous section, magnetic force can also be used for separating the target molecule utilizing anti-biomarker conjugated nano- (or micro-) sized superparamagnetic particles. For sensing, the target molecule bound on the particle surface is quantified by several different way: for examples, the change in the interference in magnetic field due to the particles, the chemical signal created by the reaction between the target molecule on the particle surface and another molecule that develops color, the change in the magnetic field strength by the magnetic particles reacted with the anti-target molecules, etc. Figs. 12.14 and 12.15 illustrate one of the elegantly designed sensing techniques using magnetic particles, which was developed by the Dr. C. H. Ahn research group at the University of Cincinnati (with the permission of Dr. Ahn; Choi et al., 2002). Figure 12.14 illustrates the procedure for their immunoassay using magnetic particles with a chemical detection system: First, magnetic beads coated with

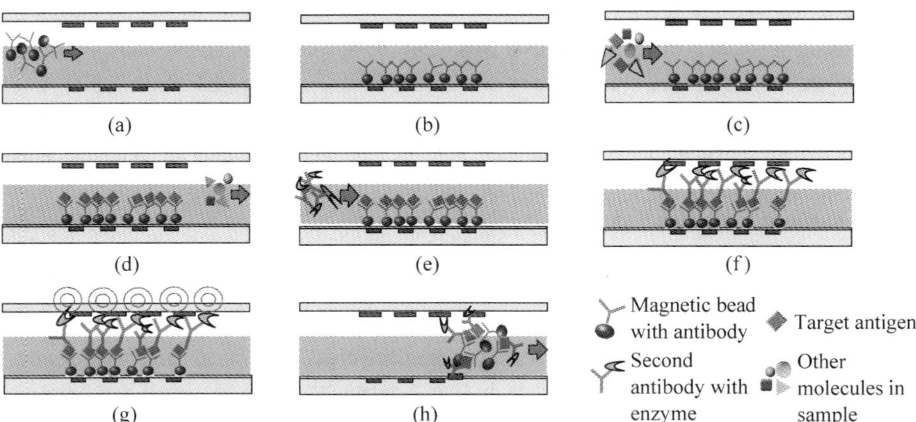

Figure 12.14 Schematic diagrams of the immunoassay using magnetic particles: (a) injection of magnetic beads conjugated with antibody to the chamber. (b) separation and holding of beads. (c) introduction of samples. (d) immuno-reaction with the target antigen. (e) second antibody application. (f) excess second antibody is washed away. (g) antigen sensing. (h) regeneration of the sensor (Provided by Dr. C. H. Chong at the University of Cincinnati)

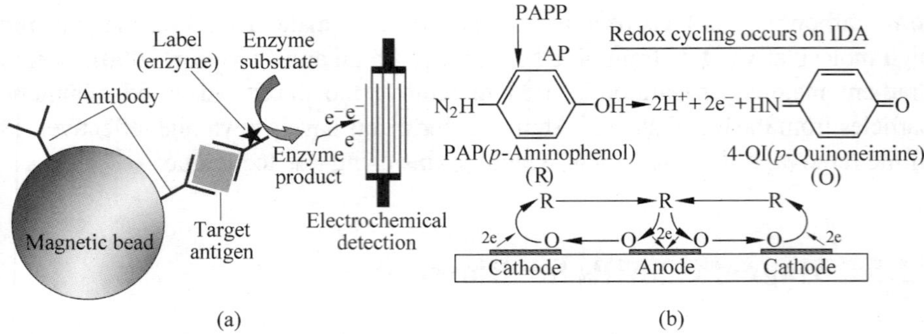

Figure 12.15 Schematic diagrams of the immunoassay with detection by electrochemistry: (a) magnetic particle-based immunoreaction and detection and (b) redox cycle electrochemical sensor combined with immunoreaction (Provided by Dr. C. H. Chong at the University of Cincinnati)

antibodies are injected into the sensing chamber and beads in the chamber are held by magnetic force on the wall of the sensing chamber. When the sample is introduced to the chamber, immunoreaction occurs between the antibody on the particle surface and the target antigen. After the magnetic particles are washed to remove unreacted biomolecules, the second antibody is applied and the antigen on the particle reacts with the second antibody. After this reacrtion, the excess antibody is washed away and the amount of antigen is quantified by an enzymatic reaction (Fig. 12.15(a)) between the second antibody and another molecules generating chemicals that can be quantified by electro- chemical sensing (Fig. 12.15(b)). After the assay, the magnetic field is removed and the particles are washed away and the sensing system is ready for a new assay, enabling continuous sensing.

Many other researchers have also used magnetic particles for sensing. Meyer, and his co-workers used magnetic beads labeled with antibodies against a cardiac marker c-reactive protein and pathogenic bacteria (Meyer et al., 2007a, 2007b, 2007c; in press-b), at a highly sensitive level. The mechanism of sensing is as follows: An immuno affinity chromatography column captures the target molecule in the sample and then magnetic particles coated with another type of antibody are run through the column. The antibodies on the surface of magnetic particle are captured by the target molecule in the column. When the magnetic force at a certain frequency is applied to the column, then the response from the column changes with the level of captured magnetic particles. By correlating this change and the concentration of the anlayte in the sample, they were able to accurately quantify/detect the target molecules in the sample; Bulte and his co-workers (1999, 2001) used 'magnetodendrimers' to track cell migration and myelination and also to track the stem cell migration; Varshney and Li (2007) have developed an impedance biosensor based on the integrated arrayed microelectrode coupled with magnetic nanoparticle–antibody conjugates, to detect *E. coli* in ground beef; Lermo, et al. (2007) used magnetic beads for DNA amplification directly with a novel magnetic primer. Their DNA biosensor was able to detect the changes at single nucleotide polymorphism level, when stringent hybridization conditions were used. The sensor was tested for *Salmonella spp.*; Gorschlüeter et al. (2002a; 2002b) developed analyte-labeled magnetic microparticles. Detection is achieved by measuring electrochemical current changes occurring when bead-labeled analyte molecules get specifically bound to microelectrodes. When the magnetic force exceeds the specific binding force of the analyte molecule, the bound microparticles are removed. Then a signal is generated, and a transducer measures the specific binding forces; Graham et al. (2003) used a micron sized sensors to detect the binding of single streptavidin functionalized, 2 μm magnetic microspheres on a biotinylated sensor surface; Connolly and St. Pierre (2001) developed a method based on the detection of shifts in the frequency-dependent magnetic susceptibility of magnetic colloids caused by the increase in hydrodynamic radius by the specific binding of biomolecules.

12.6 Magnetic NMPs for Cancer Hyperthermia

Hyperthermia for cancer treatment can be done either by ablating tumor with a high thermal energy or by applying low heat to keep the diseased tissue at 42 – 45℃. At this temperature the enzymes required for cell survival get deactivated and cells slowly die. The low heat hyperthermia is, therefore, a cancer treatment with a minimal damage to the normal tissue (Storm, 1983). Utilization of magnetic particles for hyperthermic therapy was first investigated by Gilchrist et al. (1957). They injected iron oxide particles into lymph nodes of dogs and observed temperature increases of approximately 5℃ after exposuing the animals to an alternating electro magnetic (AEM) field. Magnetic nanoparticles can be effectively heated in AEM field by hysterisis loss, Neel relaxation, or/and Brownian relaxation (Hergt et al., 1998). When magnetic materials with multi- domains are exposed to a magnetic field, the domain with the same direction of applied magnetic field grows and the other ones shrink. This domain replacement in the material along the AEM field produces heat by hysterisis loss. Neel Relaxation is due to the rotation of the internal magnetic dipole in the single-domain particles along the AEM field. When the carrier liquid for these particles has a sufficiently low viscosity, heat can also be generated by the physical rotation of the particles along the applied AEM field, which is called Brownian Relaxation. When these magnetic NMPs are placed in AEM, depending on the mean particle size and the properties of the medium where they are placed, one or multiple heating mechanisms may be involved (Andra and Nowak 2007; Hergt et al., 2002). One of the most frequently used particles for hyperthermia is Fe_3O_4 nanoparticle (Jordan et al., 1999; Bahadur and Giri 2003; Tartaj et al., 2003; Momet et al., 2004) or Fe_2O_3 particle (Yan et al., 2005). As previously stated, FDA has approved iron oxide based MRI contrast agents for human use.

These nanoparticles are often coated with biocompatible materials. Examples of these materials are dextran (Jozefczak and Skumiel 2007; Zhang et al., 2007), Polyethylene glycol (PEG; Acar et al., 2005; Shultz et al., 2007), liposome (Yanase et al., 1998; Hamaguchi et al., 2003; Matsuoka et al., 2004; Kawai et al., 2005; Tanaka et al., 2005), or other biocompatible polymers (Zhao et al., 2005). The coating makes the particles hydrophilic without immunogenic response when injected in vivo. Hilger et al. (2005) have applied dextran coated Fe_2O_3 and Fe_3O_4 particles at a size range of 10 – 20 nm for hyperthermia. After injecting these partides to mice, intra-tumorally (~22 mg-NMP/ 3 cm^3-tumor), by applying AEM at a frequency of 0.4 MHz and the field amplitude of 6.5 kA/m, for four minutes, the temperature at a center of the tumor was raised up to 71℃; Cancer-specific antibodies are also frequently linked to the coated layer for enhancing the tumor targeting ability (Shinkai et al., 2001; Gruttner et al., 2006).

The AEM applicator for hyperthermia can be usually either a coil shape or a pancake shape but for a non-invasive application of AEM to a large organ, the pancake shape may be more accommodating. Also, one can use more than one applicators for applying the AEM field properly to the magnetic particle accumulated, tumor site. Mathematical estimation of AEM field distribution can be helpful for designing an appropriate geometry of applicator(s). An example of simulated, AEM field strength distributions for a single and a double pancake type applicators is shown in Fig. 12.16. The level of brightness shows the density of the magnetic field. For the single pancake-shaped applicator, the field density seems to be distributed close to the surface of the applicator, with only a little depth penetration (Fig. 12.14(a)). For the two-pancake system with the same current flow directions for both, the magnetic density between two applicators are greatly enhanced, also increasing the penetration depth (Fig. 12.16(b)).

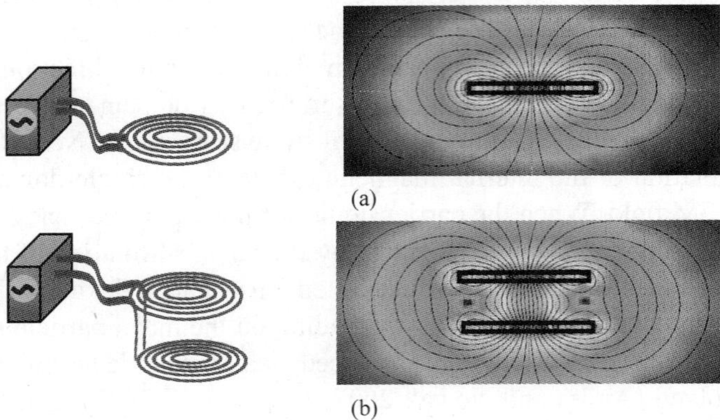

Figure 12.16 Schematic diagrams of (a) a single and (b) a double pancake-shaped AEM applicators and the simulation result of the magnetic field distribution (front view)

The AEM frequency at a giga hertz level is the microwave that we is used at home and at this frequency, dielectric heating occurs, which should be avoid in magnetic nanoparticle mediated hyperthermia. We have performed a study to select the proper AEM frequency range that can heat nanoparticles, without heating normal tissue (Jin and Kang, 2007). The samples that we tested were distilled water, bovine hemoglobin solution at a concentration of 0.14 g/mL-water (concentration in normal blood), NaCl solution at 0.9% (physiological concentration), and the ground beef. 4 ml of each sample in a glass tube was placed inside the solenoid shaped induction heater coil, at frequencies of 0.45, 5.4, and 9.2 MHz, at 5 kW for 2 minutes. The distilled water was not heated at all three frequencies. Hemoglobin was not heated at the frequencies tested, either. The NaCl solution was heated extensively at 5.4 and 9.2 MHz. The ground beef was also heated at 5.4 and 9.2 MHz, probably due to the salt content in the meat. The frequency of 0.45 MHz was, therefore, selected for the next studies.

The heating performance of various particle sizes was studied at 0.45 MHz and 5 kW (Fig. 12.17). The temperature increases in agar containing Fe_2O_3 or Fe_3O_4 nanoparticles at concentrations from 0.1wt% to 1wt% were measured after 2 min of exposure in a solenoid shaped AEM applicator. For all particles, the heating was linearly proportional to the particle concentration in the sample. For the samples containing Fe_3O_4 at 10 – 20 nm or 20 – 30 nm, the temperature increases were approximately at a rate of 35℃/wt% of particles. With Fe_3O_4 particles at 40 – 60 nm, however, it was 9℃/wt%, indicating that the heating capability of Fe_3O_4 nanoparticles depend on their particle sizes. For the sample containing 20 – 30 nm Fe_2O_3, the rate of temperature increase was 30℃/wt%, which was very close to the Fe_3O_4 particles at the size range of 10 – 30 nm. For the Feridex I.V.® (FDA approved MRI contrast agent) which are a 5 nm Fe_3O_4 particles, the rate of temperature increase was 3℃/wt%, lower than that for other sizes but, with increases in heating time, this slower heating rate can be compensated.

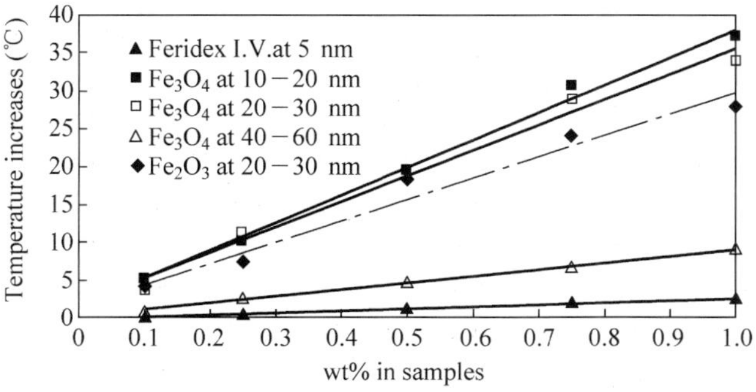

Figure 12.17 The effect of particle size on heating performance of iron oxide nanoparticles by AEM field The concentrations of iron oxide in the samples were 0.1wt% – 1wt%. The samples were heated at a 0.45 MHz frequency and 5 kW power for 2 min

12.7 Multi-Functional NMPs

The most desired method for managing disease is the detection/diagnosis at an earliest possible stage and also the treatment at the same time or immediately after the diagnosis. For this approach, researchers have been developing multifunctional entities with the three important properties—the biomarker targeting, the detection, and the treatment. Also, for each property, one may use multiple modalities for more accuracy. Liposomes (Saito et al., 2004), dendrimers (Majoros et al., 2005), and encapsulation (Reddy et al., 2006) may have been more frequently used methods for this purpose. For NMPs, QDs are starting to be used for this multifunctional approach (Sinha et al., 2006). Also, since many MRI contrast agents are based on Fe_3O_4 particles, researchers manipulate the particle to add more functions to them (Fortina et al., 2007). One good example for this multifunctional appoach is the study results by Dr. Naomi Halas's research group at the University of Rice. They have developed optically tunable nano gold shells filled with dielectric core, functionalized with cancer specific antibodies for cancer targeting. The scattering property of the particle was used for cancer detection and the optical heating was used for cancer therapy (Loo et al., 2005; Fortina et al., 2007).

Here, an example of the development of a multifunctional NMP studied in our research group is illustrated with more details. As shown in our previous study results above, Fe_3O_4 nanoparticles at size 5 – 60 nm are heated well, especially at the range of 10 – 30 nm, in the AEM field at a frequency of 0.45 MHz and a power of 5 kW, without heating any tissue components (see Section 12.6 in this article). Fe_3O_4 nanoparticles are reasonably good near infrared (NIR) absorbers (Fig. 12.1(b)). But NGPs at a size range of 10 – 250 nm are even stronger NIR absorbers (Fig. 12.1(a)). Gold has other advantageous properties, such as, the chemical inertness, the ability of easily conjugating biologicals, and also the property of quenching/enhancing fluorescence (see Section 12.3 in this article). Therefore, gold coated Fe_3O_4 nanoparticles (Jin and Kang, 2007) can act as good NIR absorber and highly effective fluorescent contrast agent with Cypate linkage for optical breast cancer detection (Jin and Kang, 2006), and also thermal guide for tumor hyperthermia. The gold coated Fe_3O_4 particles did not lose its heating capability (Jin and Kang, 2007) and the NIR absorption and also flurorescence enhancing property were excellent. For this particular example, the cancer targeting moiety was luteinizing hormone-releasing hormone (LHRH). Many cancer types including breast cancers express receptors for LHRH and most visceral organs do not express LHRH receptors, or express only at a low level (Kakar, 2003). LHRH is a peptide of 10 amino acids and spontaneously reacts with the surface of nanometal particles by its *N*-terminal amine group via its self-assembling nature. Also, as a cancer targeting agent, LHRH can be much more economical than humanized monoclonal antibodies. Researchers have demonstrated that the breast cancer cells can be targeted through their high affinity LHRH receptors present on the cell membrane (Leuschner et al., 2005; Kakar et al., 2008). As an initial test for using LHRH as a tumor targeting agent, LHRH was linked to NGPs or Fe_3O_4 nanoparticles (eventually LHRH will be linked to gold-coated Fe_3O_4 nanoparticles) (Fig. 12.18). The binding affinity of LHRH linked NGPs was studied using the mouse gonadotrope cell line (LβT2) expressing LHRH receptors. LHRH-linked NGPs showed a similar binding affinity (about 0.1 nmol/L) to the native LHRH peptide, suggesting that the LHRH conjugated NGP retains its binding affinity (Jin and Kang, 2008).

The ultimate goal of our study is to build a multi-fuctional nanoentity, LHRH and Cypate linked, gold coated Fe_3O_4 nanoparticle. These particle can provide the properties of cancer targeting, high NIR absorption and fluorescence, also possibly providing MRI contrast, for a minimally invasive, early cancer diagnosis, and minimally invasive hyperthermic treatment of cancer (Fig. 12.19).

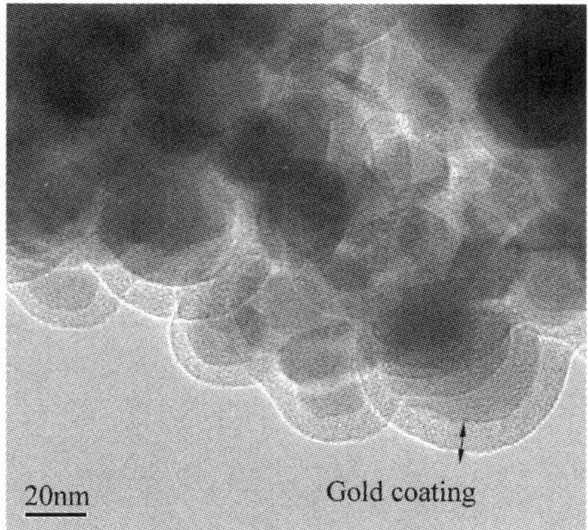

Figure 12.18 A TEM image of gold coated Fe_3O_4 nanoparticles

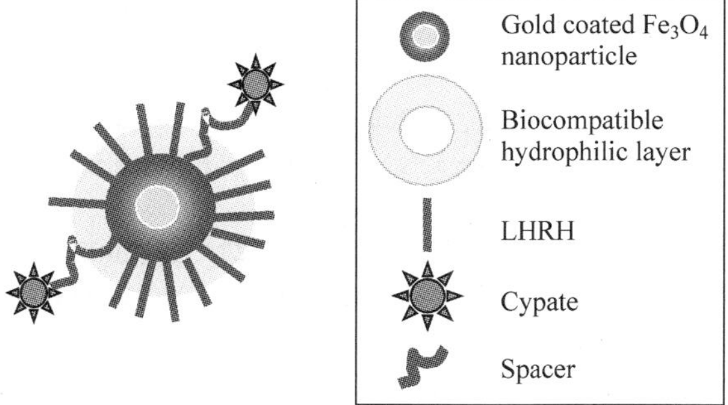

Figure 12.19 A multi-functional nano entity with the properties of cancer targeting, a high absorption/flurescnece/MRI contrasts and cancer hyperthermia by AEM energy

12.8 Conclusions

The biomedical applications of nanometal particles have been expanding rapidly and will be even more popular as time passes because of their numerous advantageous natures in the size and also the unique and beneficial properties of nano-sized metals, as described in the article. It is evident that the examples that are listed in this article are only a small portion of the currently used NMPs for biomedical applications. One task still remained to be seriously studied for the in-vivo application of these particles is the possible toxicity of metal particles in human body and also the accumulation in the excretoray organs. Also the clustering tendency of NMPs due to the unstable nature of nanosized materials needs to be overcome for more general use of these partilces. The active efforts by many multi-disciplinary scientists toward resolving these issues are expected to enable the utilization of NMPs for human being soon.

Acknowledgements

The authors acknowledge the Kentucky Science and Engineering Foundation for the financial support of the metallic nanoparticle study and the National Science Foundation (BES-0330075) for funding on Protein C and the cardiac marker biosensing system. The authors would also like to express thanks to Dr. Achilefu for supplying Cypate for our study. We appreciate Dr. C. H. Ahn at the University of Cincinnati for providing figures for their sensing system using magnetic particles and Dr. Donglu Shi at the University of Cincinnati for providing the gold coated Fe_3O_4 particles and the TEM images.

References

Abudabi, T. and R.R. Beitle, *J. Chromatogr.* A **795**: 211 (1998).

Acar, H., R.S. Garass, F. Syud, P. Bonitatebus and A.M. Kulkarni. *J. Magn. Magn. Mater.* **293**(1): 1 (2005).

Achilefu, S., R.B. Dorshow, J.E. Bugaj, R. Rajagopalan. *Invest Radiol.* **35**: 479 (2000).

Akerman M.E., W.C. Chan, P. Laakkonen, S.N. Bhatia and E. Ruoslahti. *Proc. Natl. Acad. Sci.* USA **99**: 12,617 (2002).

Anderson, G.P. and N.L. Nerurkar. *J. Immunol Methods.* **271**: 17 (2002).

Andra, W. and H. Nowak. *Magnetism in Medicine.* Berlin: Wiley-VCH (2007).

Bahadur, D. and J. Giri. *Sadhana* **28**(3&4): 639 (2003).

Berlier, J.E., A. Rothe, G. Buller, J. Bradford, D.R. Gray, B.J. Filanoski, W.G. Telford, S. Yue, J. Liu, C-Y Cheung, W. Chang, J.D. Hirsch, J.M. Beechem, R.P. Haugland and R.P. Haugland. *Journal of Histochemistry and Cytochemistry* **51**(12): 1699 (2003).

Bulte, J.W.M., S.C. Zhang, P. van Gelderen, V. Herynek, E.K. Jordan and I.D. Duncan. *Proc. Natl. Acad. Sci. USA* **96**(26): 15,256 – 15,261 (1999)

Bulte, W.M.J., T. Douglas, B. Witwer, S-C. Zhang, E. Strable, B.K. Lewis, H. Zywicke, B. Miller, P. van Gelderen, B.M. Moskowitz, I.D. Duncan and J.A. Frank. *Nat. Biotechnol.* **19**: 1141 (2001).

Chang, E., J.S. Miller, J. Sun, W.W. Yu, V.L. Colvin, R. Drezek and J.L. West. *Biochemical and Biophysical Research Communications* **334**(4): 1317 (2005).

Choi, J., K.W. Oh, J.H. Thomas, W.R.Heineman, H.B. Halsall, J.H. Nevin, A.J. Helmicki, H.T. Henderson, C.H. Ahn. *Lab Chip* **2**: 27 (2002).

Cocker, T. M., J.F. Conan and A.E. Rachel. *Biotechnol. Bioeng.* **53**: 79 (1997).

Connolly, J. and T.G. St Pierre. *J. Magn. Magn. Mater.* **225**: 156 (2001).

Dubertret, B., M. Calame, A.J. Libchaber. *Nat. Biotechnol.* **19**: 3659 (2001).

Gao, X.H., Y.Y. Cui, R.M. Levenson, L.W.K. Chung and S.M. Nie. *Nat. Biotechnol.* **22**: 969 (2004).

Geddes, C.D., A. Parfenov, D. Roll, M. J. Uddin, and J. R. Lakowicz. *Journal of Fluorescence* **13**(6): 453 (2003).

Fortina, P., L.J. Kricha, D.J. Graves, J. Park, T. Hyslop, F. Tam, N. Halas, S. Surrey, S.A. Waldman. *Trends Biotechnol.* **25**(4): 145 (2007).

Gilchrist, R.K., R. Medal, W.D. Shorey, R.C. Hanselman, J.C. Parrott and C.B. Taylor. *Ann Surg.* **146**(4): 596 (1957).

Gorschlüter, A., C. Sundermeier, B. Roß and M. Knoll. *Sens. Actuators* B **85**: 158 (2002a).

Gorschlüter, A., L.H. Mak, C. Sundermeier, B. Roß and M. Knoll. *Biomed. Tech.* **47**: 213 (2002b).

Graham, D.L., H.A. Ferreira, P.P. Freitas, and J.M.S. Cabral. *Biosensors and Bioelectronics.* **18**: 483 (2003).

Gruttner, C., K. Muller, J. Teller, F. Westphala, A. Foreman and R. Ivkovb. *J. Magn. Magn. Mater.* **311**: 181 (2007).

Hama, Y., Y. Koyama, Y. Urano, P.L. Choyke and H. Kobayashi. *Breast Cancer Res Treat.* **17**(6): 1426 (2006).

Hamaguchi, S., I. Tohnai, A. Ito, K. Mitsudo, T. Shigetomi, M. Ito, H. Honda, T. Kobayashi and M. Ueda. *Cancer Sci.* **94**(9): 834 (2003).

Harisinghani, M.G., S. Saini, R. Weissleder, P.F. Hanh, R.K. Yantiss, C. Tempany, B.J. Wood and P.R. Mueller. *Am. J. Roentgenol.* **172**: 1347 (1999).

Hergt, R., W. Andra, C.G. d'Ambly, I. Hilger, W.A. Kaiser, U. Richter, and H. Schmidt. *IEEE Trans. Magn.* **34**(5): 3745 (1998).

Hergt, R., R. Hiergeist, I. Hilger and W.A. Kaiser. *Recent Res. Dev. Mater. Sci.* **3**: 723 (2002).

Hilger, I., R. Hergt and W.A. Kaiser. *J. Magn. Magn. Mater.* **293**: 314 (2005).

Hirsch L.R., R.J. Stafford, J.A. Bankson, S.R. Sershen, B. Rivera, R.E. Price, J.D., Hazle, N.J., Halas, J.L. West. *Proc. Natl. Acad. Sci.* USA **100**(23): 13,549 (2003).

Hong, B. and K.A. Kang. *Biosensor and Bioelectronics* **21**: 1333 (2006).

Inoue, S., M. Goda, H. Du, M.D. Disney, B.L. Miller and T.D. Krauss. *Biol. Bull.* **201**: 231 (2001).

Jin, H. and K.A. Kang. *Advances in Experimental Medicine and Biology* **566**: 167 (2005).

Jin, H. and K.A. Kang. *Advances in Experimental Medicine and Biology*, **599**: 45 (2007).

Jin, H, B. Hong, S.S. Kakar and K.A. Kang. *Advances in Experimental Medicine and Biology*, **614**: 275 (2008).

Jozefczak, A. and A. Skumiel. *J. Magn. Magn. Mater.* **311**(1): 193 (2007).

Jordan, A., R. Scholz, P. Wust, H. Fahling and R. Felix. *J. Magn. Magn. Mater.* **201**: 413 (1999).

Josephson, L., C.H., Tung, A. Moore, R. Weissleder. *Bioconjuate Chem.* **10**: 186 (1999).

Kakar, S.S., S.J. Winters, W. Zacharias, D.M. Miller and S. Flynn. *Gene* **308**: 67 (2003).

Kakar, S.S, H. Jin, B. Hong, J.W. Eaton and K.A. Kang. Proceeding of the 2006 Annual Conference on the International Society of Oxygen Transport to Tissue, August 2006, Louisville, KY (Accepted).

Kang, K.A. and B. Hong, Critical Reviews™ in *Eukaryotic Gene Expression* **16**(1): 45 (2006).

Kaul, Z., T. Yaguchi, S.C. Kaul, T. Hirano, R. Wadhwa and K. Taira. *Cell. Res.* **13**: 503 (2003).

Kawai, N., A. Ito, Y. Nakahara, M. Futakuchi, T. Shirai, H. Honda, T. Kobayashi and K. Kohri. *The Prostate* **64**: 373 (2005).

Kim, S., Y.T. Lim, E.G. Soltesz, A.M. De Grand, J. Lee, A. Nakayama, J.A. Parker, T. Mihaljevic, R.G. Laurence, D.M. Dor, L.H. Cohn, M.G. Bawendi and J.V. Frangioni. *Nat. Biotechnol.* **22**: 93 (2004).

Larson D.R., W.R. Zipfel, R.M. Williams, S.W. Clark, M.P. Bruchez, F.W. Wise and W.W. Webb. *Science* **300**: 1434 (2003).

Lawson, W.D., F.A. Smith and A.S. Young. *J. Electrochem. Soci.* **107**: 206 (1960).

Lermo, A., S. Campoy, J. Barbé, S. Hernández, S. Alegret and M.I. Pividori. *Biosens. Bioelectro.* **22**(9 – 10): 2010 (2007).

Leuschner, C., C. Kumar, M.O. Urbina, J. Zhou, W. Soboyejo, W. Hansel and F. Hormes. Nanotech. Technical Proceedings for the 2005 NSTI Nanotechnolgy Conference and Trade Show, **1**: 5 (2005).

Licha, K., R. Riefke, V. Ntziachristos, A. Becker, B. Chance and W. Semmler. *Photochem. Photobiol.* **72**: 392 (2000).

Loo, C., A. Lin, L. Hirsch, M.H. Lee, J. Barton, N. Halas, J. West and R. Drezek. *Technology in Cancer Research and Treatment* **3**: 33 (2004).

Loo, C., A. Lowery, N. Halas, J. West and R. Drezek. *Nano Lett.* **5**: 709 (2005).

Majoros, J.J., T.P. Thomas, C.B. Mehta and J.R. Baker, Jr. *J. Med. Chem.* **48**(19): 5892 (2005).

Matsuoka, F., M. Shinkai, H. Honda, T. Kubo, T. Sugita and T. Kobayasi. *Biomagn. Res. Technol.* **2**(1): 3 (2004).

Meyer, H.F.M., M. Hartmann, H.-J. Krause, G. Blankenstein, B. Mueller-Chorus, J. Oster, P. Miethe and M. Keusgen, Biosensors and Bioelectronics **22**: 973, (2007a).

Meyer, H.F.M., H.-J. Krause, M. Hartmann, P. Miethe, J. Oster and M. Keusgen, Journal of Magnetism and Magnetic Materials, **68**(2): 218, (2007b).

Meyer, H.F.M., M. Stehr, S. Bhuju, H.-J. Krause, M. Hartmann, P. Miethe, M. Singh and M. Keusgen, Journal of Microbiological Methods, **311**(1): 259, (2007c).

Mornet, S., S. Vasseur, F. Grasset and E. Duguet. *J. Mater. Chem.* **14**: 2161(2004).

Reddy, G.R., M.S. Bhojani, P. McConville, J. Moody, B.A. Moffat, D.A., Haoo, G. Kim, Y-E L., Koo, M.J., Wooliscroft, J.V. Sugai, T.D., Johnson, M.A. Philbert, R. Kopelman, A. Rehemtulla and B.D. Ross. *Clin. Cancer Res.* **12**(22): 6677 (2006).

Ruppin R. *Phys Rev* B. **11**(8): 2871 (1975).

Saito, R., J.R. Bringas, T.R. McKnight, M.F. Wendland, C. Mamot, D.C. Drummond, D.B. Kirpotin, J.W., Park, M.S., Berger and K.S. Bankiewicz. *Cancer Res.* **64**(7): 2573 (2004).

Sinha, R., G.J. Kim, S. Nie and D.M. Shin. *Mol. Cancer Ther.* **5**(8): 1909 (2006).

Shinkai, M., L. Biao, H. Honda, K. Yoshikawa, K. Shimizu, S. Saga, T. Wakabayashi, J. Yoshida and T. Kobayashi. *Cancer Science* **92**(10): 1138 (2001).

Shultz, M.D, S. Calvin, P.P. Fatouros, S.A. Morrison and E.E. Carpenter. *J. Magn. Magn. Mater.* **311**(1): 464 (2007).

Smith, AM, S. Dave, S. Nie, L. True and X. Gao. *Expert Rev Mol Diagn.* **6**(2): 231 (2006).

Soltesz E.G., S. Kim, R.G. Laurence, A.M. DeGrand, C.P. Parungo, D.M. Dor, L.H. Cohn, M.G. Bawendi, J.V. Frangioni and T. Mihaljevic. *Ann. Thorac. Surg.* **79**(1): 269 (2005).

Storm, F.K. *Hyperthermia in Cancer Therapy*. Boston: G. K. Hall Medical Publishers (1983).

Stroh, M., J.P. Zimmer, D.G. Duda, T.S. Levchenko, K.S. Cohen, E.B. Brown, D.T. Scadden, V.P. Torchilin, M.G. Bawendi, D. Fukumura and R.K. Jain. *Nat. Med.* **11**: 678 (2005).

Tanaka, K., A. Ito, T. Kobayashi, T. Kawamura, S. Shimada, K. Matsumoto, T. Saida and H. Honda. *J. BioSci. Bioengr.* **100**(1): 112 (2005).

Tartaj, P., M.P. Morales, S. Veintemillas-Verdaguer, T. Gonźalez-Carreno and C.J. Serna. *J. Phys. D: Appl. Phys.* **36**: R182 (2003).

Torchilin, V.P., European. *J. Pharma. Sci.* **11**(Supplement 2): S81 (2000).

Varshney M. and Li, Y. *Biosensors and Bioelectronics*, **22**(11): 2408 (2007).

Weissleder R., G. Elizondo, J. Wittenberg, C.A. Babito, H.H. Bengele and L. Josephson. *Radiol.* **175**: 489 (1990).

Yan, S., D. Zhang, N. Gu, J. Zheng, A. Ding and Z. Wang. *J. Nanosci. Nanotechnol.* **5**(5): 1185 (2005).

Yanase, M., M. Shinkai, H. Honda, T. Wakabayashi, J. Yoshida and T. Kobayshi. *Jpn. J. Cancer Res.* **89**: 463 (1998).

Yang, C., J. Xing, Y. Guan and H. Liu. *Appl. Microbiolo and Biotechnol.* **72**(3): 616 (2006).

Zhang, L.Y., H.C. Gu and X.M. Wang. *J. Magn. Magn. Mater.* **311**: 228 (2007).

Zhao, A.J., P. Yao, C.S. Kang, X. Yuan, J. Chang and P. Pu. *J. Magn. Magn. Mater.* **295**(1): 37 (2005).

13 Micro- and Nanoscale Technologies in High-Throughput Biomedical Experimentation

Vikramaditya G. Yadav[1,2], Mark D. Brigham[3], Yibo Ling[3,4], Christopher Rivest[2], Utkan Demirci[4,5], Ali Khademhosseini[4,5]

[1] Department of Chemical Engineering, University of Waterloo, Waterloo, ON N2L 3G1, Canada

[2] Department of Chemical Engineering, Massachusetts Institute of Technology, Cambridge, MA 02139, USA

[3] Department of Electrical Engineering and Computer Science, Massachusetts Institute of Technology, Cambridge, MA 02139, USA

[4] Harvard-MIT Division of Health Sciences and Technology, Massachusetts Institute of Technology, Cambridge, MA 02139, USA

[5] Department of Medicine, Brigham and Women's Hospital, Harvard Medical School, Boston, MA 02139, USA

Abstract Biological systems are highly complex. To analyze the intricate workings of biological systems in an affordable and timely manner, a number of technologies have been developed to analyze biological systems in a highly parallel manner. Of these tools, micro- and nanoscale technologies have emerged as an effective tool because they can be used to automate, miniaturize, and multiplex biochemical assays to study biological functions at the cellular and genomic level at reduced experimentation costs. Herein, we provide a broad overview of several micro- and nanoscale technologies, as well as discuss their current and future applications. Our review primarily focuses on the microarray technologies and their applications to platforms such as DNA, cell, and protein arrays. We also provide a brief description of micro- and nanopatterning of substrates and scaffolds, and their effect on stem cell differentiation and cellular co-cultures. Additionally, augmentation of the microarray technology via integration with microfluidic technologies; and the application of microarrays as biochemical detection platforms are also discussed. Wherever appropriate, current limitations, suitable alternatives, and directions for future research have also been presented.

---

(1) Corresponding e-mail: alik@mit.edu

13.1 Introduction

Biological systems are inherently complex and regulated by simultaneous interactions between thousands of genes and genetic products in a temporally and spatially organized manner. Thus, to understand biological systems it is desirable to replicate the complexity observed within natural systems. As a consequence, there has been a recent rise in the demand for powerful tools to undertake highly-parallel experiments to enable rapid probing and quantification of nucleic acids, proteins, molecular signals and cells (Situma et al., 2006).

Microscale technologies (which can reach nanoscale resolution) have been used in the semiconductor and microelectronics industries for nearly half a century (Franssila, 2004; Khademhosseini et al., 2006). However, their widespread use in the biomedical sciences is a recent phenomenon. Micro- and nanoscale technologies offer the promise of automating, miniaturizing, and multiplexing biochemical assays to study biological functions at the cellular and genomic level at reduced experimentation costs (Palsson and Bhatia, 2004). Biochemical and cellular microarrays, microfluidic systems, and micro- and nanoengineered biochemical detection platforms constitute some prominent examples of the application of micro- and nanoscale technologies to high-throughput experimentation (Fig. 13.1). Microarrays enable the simultaneous analyses of thousands of nucleic acids, genes, proteins, and cells on a single chip. Such capacity for massively parallel biomolecular analysis is key to the high-throughput study and optimization of dynamic biological phenomena such as cell-matrix interactions. Although the exact molecular mechanisms that elicit cellular-fate processes remain imprecisely defined, microarrays can be effectively used to characterize cellular behavior in response to specific physiochemical changes and, in turn, may help elucidate the biochemical machinery of cell differentiation. Microfluidic gradient generation systems can also be used to perform high- throughput cell-based experiments. Microfluidic systems are cheap, minimize consumption of expensive reagents, and generally require low cell populations for experimentation. Microfluidic systems could potentially be used for performing rapid screening experiments, evaluating drug toxicity, and investigating optimal culture conditions for the facilitation of specific cellular-fate processes. Lastly, micro- and nanoengineered biochemical detection platforms are emerging as viable solutions for clinical, environmental, food, and chemical testing.

Libraries of molecules, candidate drugs, biomaterials, and cells will become more accessible and user-friendly in the years ahead. However, this increased availability of biological agents will be fruitless without high-throughput functional assays to verify their clinical or experimental value. Micro- and nanoscale technologies provide biomedical engineers with valuable tools for screening libraries and facilitate an unprecedented degree of control over the cellular microenvironment (Khade mhosseini et al., 2006; Palsson and Bhatia, 2004). As such, the advantages of using them for high-throughput biological experimentation to probe cellular behavior and genomic activity are manifold.

The fabrication of micro- and nanoscale devices is generally achieved using either a ‘bottom-up’ or ‘top-down’ approach. Bottom-up approaches generally involve the buildup of atoms or molecules in a controlled, thermodynamically-regulated manner to form nanostructures (Khademhosseini and Langer, 2006). An example of a bottom-up approach is atomic or molecular self-assembly. Contrastingly, top-down fabrication technologies include techniques such as photolithography, soft lithography, nanomoulding, dip-pen lithography, and micro- and nanofluidics (Khademhosseini and Langer, 2006).

Herein, we present a brief overview of the application of top-down micro- and nanoscale technologies in high-throughput biological experimentation by providing categorical examples while elaborating specific applications of each group of technologies. We initially review microarray technologies by discussing aspects such as fabrication, existing applications and emerging developments. Next, applications of microfluidic technologies in high-throughput experimentation will be presented. The automation and integration of microfluidics with other micro- and nanoscale technologies shall also be examined. Finally, novel micro- and nanoengineered detection methodologies will be introduced. We shall also discuss the current limitations of these technologies. Furthermore, directions for future research in the applications of micro- and nanoscale technologies to high-throughput biomedical experimentation will be presented (Fig. 13.1).

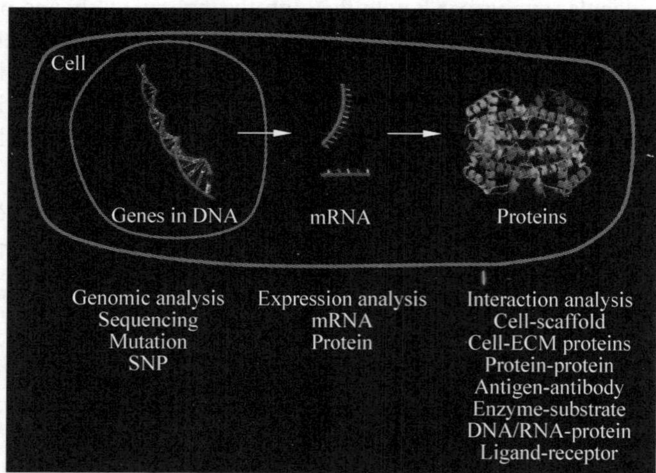

Figure 13.1 Applications of microscale and nanoscale technologies in high-throughput biological experimentation

13.2 Microarray Technologies

Microarrays tools are widely used in the analyses of biomolecules and tissues. They permit the parallel analyses of thousands of biological samples, thereby facilitating the rapid profiling of macromolecules and their physiological and pathological changes on a genome-wide scale (Stratowa and Abseher, 2005). In 2003, the total global market for microarrays was approximately \$596 million and it is expected to rise to \$1 billion by 2010 (Taylor, 2005).

Microarrays were first fabricated during the late 1980s. Early microarrays were simple arrangements of peptides and oligonucleotides on glass slides (Taylor, 2005). In the years that followed, complex cDNA arrays for gene expression analyses were also developed. The subsequent emergence of proteomics has created opportunities for the development of protein and antibody-based microarrays designed to aid in identifying protein products from gene expression. More recently, advances in micro- and nanofabrication have enabled the synthesis of cellular microarrays to investigate and direct cellular fate process activities such as growth, migration, and differentiation (Table 13.1).

Table 13.1 Types of microarrays and their applications (Stratowa and Abseher, 2005)

Probe	Array name	Domain	Profiling
DNA	Matrix CGH*	Genome	Genotypic
Oligonucleotide	Oligonucleotide array	Genome Transcriptome	Polymorphic Expression
CDNA	cDNA microarray	Transcriptome	Expression
Protein	Protein array Antibody array	Proteome Proteome	Expression/activity Expression
Tissue	Tissue microarray	Tissuome Organome	Histological Histological

*CGH: Comparative genomic hybridization

13.2.1 Evolution of Microarrays

A microarray generally consists of a substrate and an active layer of immobilized detection molecules. The active layer is comprised of oligonucleotides, DNA, RNA, antibodies, or other biomolecules that bind to specific analytes. In some cases, microarrays are designed with embedded optical or electrochemical transducers to detect binding events or reactions occurring between the active layer and analytes. In the absence of transducer elements within microarrays, receptor-analyte complex formation is detected via radioisotope, fluorometric or chemiluminescent scanning instruments.

From a technological standpoint, microarrays represent an evolution in biosensors (Taylor, 2005). Conventional biosensors can only measure a single analyte at a time. In contrast, microarrays have up to 10^6 detection sites/cm^2, and can perform simultaneous, multianalyte detection (Schultz and Taylor, 2005).

Both, biosensors and microarrays utilize a biospecific surface for affinity or indirect analyte capture, coupled with a transducer or detector for qualitative or quantitative detection (Taylor, 2005; Schultz and Taylor, 2005). While biosensor detection and data processing is built into the unit, microarrays require highly sophisticated scanners for detecting and reporting capture events (Table 13.2).

Table 13.2 Comparison between construction of biosensors and microarrays (Taylor, 2005)

Component/function	Biosensors	Microarrays
Substrates	Glass, membrane, polymer	Glass, membrane, polymer
Receptors	Antibodies, other proteins, oligonucleotides, DNA, RNA	Antibodies, other proteins, oligonucleotides, DNA, RNA
Transducers	Optical, electrochemical, piezoelectric, surface acoustic wave, thermal etc.	None
Detection	Transducer output	Radioactivity, fluorescence and chemiluminescene scanning
Data processing	Integrated software	Scanner software
Detection site density	1 detection site per device	10^6 detection sites/cm^2

13.2.2 Microarray Fabrication and Applications

As shown in Fig. 13.2, microarray fabrication is typically initiated by substrate activation via surface-treatment, followed by the binding of receptor molecules to the substrate to yield an array. Receptor molecules are applied to the activated substrate by one of two major methods: (1) direct spotting, and (2) in situ synthesis. A more recent approach, called polymeric embedding, involves entrapment of receptor molecules within a multilayered polymer matrix to generate inexpensive microarrays. Then, samples and controls are hybridized onto the array, fluorescently or radioisotopically labeled, and scanned. This is followed by data reduction and interpretation.

Generally, the desirable material properties of microarray substrates are high degree of surface smoothness, low background fluorescence, low coefficients of thermal expansion, low reflectivity, and high transmission. The most commonly used substrates for microarray fabrication include fused silica, borosilicate glass, aluminosilicates, and zinc titania (Taylor, 2005). Additionally, the successful use of porous materials such as nitrocellulose, nylon membranes, polyacrylamide gels, and block copolymers to fabricate microarrays for the study of receptor- target interactions in three-dimensions has also been reported (Timofeev et al., 1996).

The simplest approach to fabricate a microarray is the direct adsorption of receptor molecules onto a substrate. However, adsorption onto a substrate could

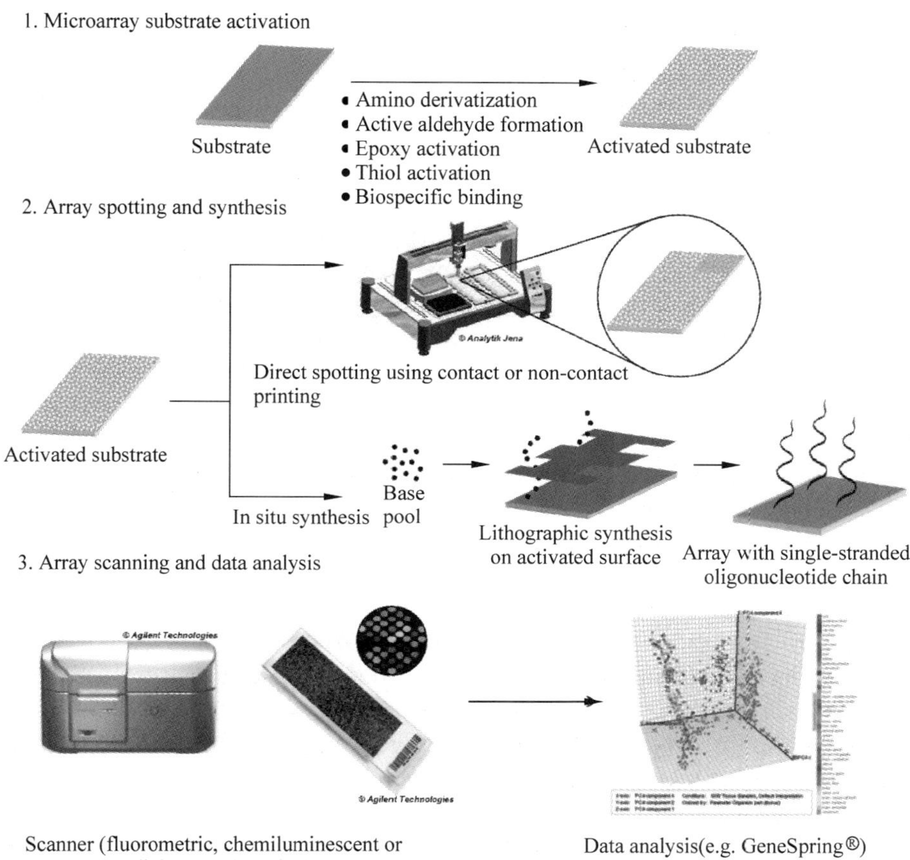

Figure 13.2 Common steps in the fabrication and use of a microarray

potentially result in inactivation of the biomolecules or blocking of its active binding sites. To prevent inactivation and blocking, substrates are first activated via chemical modification. Some common surface modification processes include amino derivatization of available hydroxyl groups on the surface; formation of highly-reactive, free aldehyde groups; epoxy activation; thiol activation; and biospecific binding by immobilization of biotin-containing biomacromolecules using avidin (Taylor, 2005). These functional groups bind to available groups in oligonucleotides, proteins, antibodies and on the cell-surface, and, by properly orienting the receptor molecule alleviate the problems associated with the direct electrostatic conjugation of biomolecules onto substrates.

Array spotting follows surface activation. Arrays are printed using either direct spotting or in situ synthesis. Both methods are capable of applying picoliter to nanoliter volumes of DNA, RNA or protein onto a substrate. Automated robotic spotting instruments perform direct spotting. Robotic spotters use either contact printing or non-contact piezoelectric ink-jet printing for reproducible generation of arrays. Direct spotting deposits $10 - 10^4$ picoliter of solution per reaction center, resulting in spot diameters ranging from 50 to 1000 μm (Taylor, 2005). Direct spotting is used to generate arrays that contain 100 – 10,000 reaction centers, although arrays with as high as 50,000 reaction centers have also been synthesized (Taylor, 2005).

On the other hand, in situ synthesis is predominantly used to generate oligonucleotide, DNA and cDNA microarrays. In situ synthesis is a photolithographic technique by which oligonucleotide reaction centers can be directly synthesized on the substrate itself. In situ synthesis involves the repeated addition of amino acids and nucleotides to a growing peptide or oligonucleotide chain via a step-wise synthesis using linkers containing photochemically removable protecting groups. At each addition step, photolithographic masks are used to direct the deprotection of specific chain end-groups, while monomers containing protecting groups on one of their two linker sites are linked to the deprotected end of the growing chain. This fabrication methodology, which yields high-density arrays with specifically-known oligonucleotide sequences, was first successfully commercialized by Affymetrix. The hallmark of this process is that it permits variation in the length of oligonucleotide chains at different reaction centers. In situ synthesis produces the highest density arrays possible, with some microarrays possessing hundreds of thousands of reaction centers (Taylor, 2005).

Following the application of receptor molecules to the surface of the substrates, samples, and control solutions are hybridized onto the active arrays. As intended, the analytes in the samples bind to the receptors. Post-hybridization, the receptor-analyte complexes are tagged with fluorescent, chemiluminescent or radioisotopic labels, and then detected and quantified using fluorometric, chemiluminescent or radioisotope scanners respectively. Fluorescent labeling is the method of choice for genomic and proteomic array analyses. Protein and immunoassay microarrays are occasionally analyzed using chemiluminescent scanners. Probe molecules are only labeled using radioactive isotopes when difficulties with conventional labeling techniques arise. Generally, proteins are labeled with ^{32}P to avoid the undirected, non-specific, multisite labeling generally observed during biotinylation (Taylor, 2005). Labels can be incorporated into the oligonucleotide chains tethered to the surface of the substrate by synthesizing the chains from labeled nucleotides or PCR primers. Some commonly used labels include the cyanine labels (Cy2, Cy3, Cy5, etc.), the Alexa fluorescent dyes (Alexa 488, 532, 546, 568, etc.), fluorescein, rhodamine 6 G and phycoerythrin.

Inside the microarray scanner, the fluorescent dyes and labels are excited with lasers or white light, and the subsequently emitted light is detected using a photomultiplier tube (PMT) or a charge-coupled device (CCD) camera. A PMT is capable of both, amplifying and measuring low levels of fluorescent emissions, whereas, CCD scanners/imagers utilize emission filters to focus the fluorescent light onto the CCD camera. Evidently, CCDs are less sensitive than PMTs, and most CCD detectors integrate emission signals over time, leading to longer scan and analysis times. Most commercially available scanners, such as the Affymetrix

GeneChip, have two lasers—at excitation wavelengths of 532 and 635 nm—and use a PMT detector to analyze microarrays. Such scanners can generate a pixel resolution between 1 – 10 μm (Taylor, 2005). More recently, Tecan and Perkin Elmer have manufactured microarray scanners that employ four lasers. The Tecan LS scanner is integrated with two PMTs, and can scan a variety of substrates, ranging from microarray glass slides to microtitreplates. Fluorometric scanners are able to detect receptor-target concentrations as low as a few attomoles (10^{-18} mol/L).

13.2.3 DNA and cDNA Microarrays

DNA and cDNA microarrays were among the first microarrays developed, and are primarily used in genomic and expression analysis, determination of the base sequence of DNA fragments, and defining genetic activity and function in samples (Hong et al., 2005). The principal objective of early experiments involving DNA and cDNA microarrays was to analyze whole and/or targeted segments of the genomes of humans, animals, plants, and microbes for drug discovery, diagnostics, and other bio-based products (Khademhosseini, 2005).

DNA and cDNA microarrays are extensively used in toxicological and pathological research. In fact, the ability to efficiently expedite biochemical assays has furthered the development of toxicogenomics—a scientific discipline that combines the emerging technologies of genomics and bioinformatics to identify and characterize biochemical mechanisms of action of known toxicants inside the bodies of animals and plants. In a toxicogenomic study, mRNA from healthy and diseased individuals are isolated, refined and then reverse-transcribed to obtain cDNA. Individual genes or genetic fragments from the DNA are analyzed for their expression levels, and differences between the healthy and diseased samples, called single nucleotide polymorphisms (SNPs) are determined. The result is collection of genes that genetically characterize a disease state. Gene family identification of this type would be unobtainable without high-throughput analysis by DNA microarrays. Affymetrix has successfully designed microarrays that host the entire genomes of humans as well as other organisms (Affymetrix, 2006). Such arrays can aid in the rapid analysis of the whole genome—subsequently enabling genome-wide SNP detection and diagnoses for diseases such as AIDS. Additionally, technologies such as Affymetrix's GeneChip the humanimmunodeficiency virus (HIV) PRT are also able to detect known mutations in the protease and reverse transcriptase enzymes of HIV-1—facilitating the development of effective therapeutic solutions for countering AIDS (Affymetrix, 2006).

Expression arrays are also being applied to pharmacogenomics to predict how a patient might respond to a specific drug, taking into account the mRNA and proteins produced by the patient; and the potential toxicity of a drug. For example, microarrays are now used to assess drug toxicity in the liver (Taylor,

2005). The method for elucidating drug toxicity mechanisms using microarrays is similar to the technique used for detecting SNPs. This is shown in Fig. 13.3. In addition to toxicological and pathological research, DNA microarrays are also successfully being used for drug discovery applications (Khademhosseini, 2005; Gerhold et al., 2001; Modden et al., 2000), and cancer (Brem et al., 2001; Gwssman, 2001; Graveel et al., 2001; Kalma et al., 2001; Monni et al., 2001; Okabe et al., 2001) and neuroscience research (Cavallaro et al., 2001; Geschwind, 2000; Zirlinger et al., 2001). Presently, considerable research is being directed towards improving the sensitivity of DNA and cDNA microarrays. Studies have demonstrated that sensitivity can be vastly improved by engineering surfaces with nanoscale features (Hong et al., 2005; Sunkara et al., 2006).

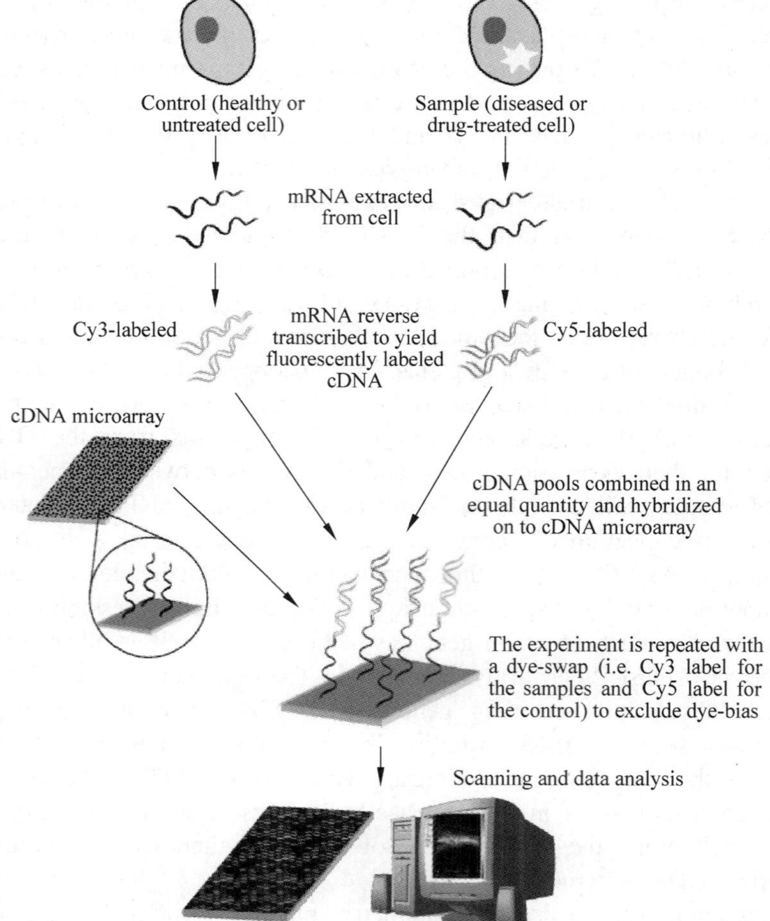

Figure 13.3 Steps for evaluating potential drug candidates and understanding the biological mechanisms of toxicants

13.2.4 Protein and Antibody-Based Microarrays

Although DNA microarrays can effectively determine RNA expression within a cell, they are inadequate for estimating levels of protein expression in cells. In 1999, nearly a decade after the fabrication of the first DNA microarrays, the need to accurately explain protein expression led to the development of protein microarrays (Haab et al., 2001). The primary goal of protein microarray technology is to determine the presence and quantify the proteins in cells or tissues. There are two types of protein microarrays: functional protein microarrays and antibody arrays. Functional protein microarrays are used to study the interaction of proteins with other molecules. On the other hand, antibody microarrays are miniaturized enzyme-linked immunosorbent assays (ELISAs), and can detect proteins with high sensitivity and selectivity.

Protein microarrays play an important role in proteomics—the analysis of total proteins expressed in a cell. Recent studies have successfully demonstrated the use of protein microarrays constructed from an entire cloned yeast proteome to study cellular structure and function within the organism (Zhu et al., 2001). Each of the nearly 5800 yeast proteins were produced, purified, and immobilized to glutaraldehyde-activated slides in duplicates. The chip was then used to investigate the specific binding of avidinfluorophone-labeled PI (a secondary messenger in transmembrane cellular communication) to the immobilized proteins. Following binding and washing, the bound PI was detected using fluorometry. Results suggested a differential binding of PI to the yeast membrane proteins—supporting the hypothesis that PI interacts with only specific membrane proteins. The study demonstrated a method for understanding a component of cell functionality based on spatial distribution of proteins in the cell and biomolecule adhesion quantified in a protein microarray. Similar studies are now being conducted to develop new drug therapies for treating dysfunctional cells and tissue; and characterizing novel functions for some well-studied proteins (Taylor, 2005; Zhu et al., 2001).

Protein microarrays are also being used to study phosphorylation mechanisms, as demonstrated by the studies aimed at understanding the binding of yeast protein kinases to large protein microarrays. Using data generated from protein-protein binding, protein-DNA binding and phosphorylation experiments, network maps containing information on intracellular interactions and regulatory pathways can been generated (Jansen et al., 2003; Luscombe et al., 2004). A better understanding of regulatory networks within the cells could potentially lead to the development of superior drug candidates (Ge, 2000; MacBeath et al., 1999).

In addition to drug discovery, protein microarrays have been used to detect and investigate autoimmune reactions in the body by incubating small volumes of the patient's serum onto antigen-immobilized arrays (Joos et al., 2000). By using a patient's serum as a test analyte, the antigen-marker complex bindings can be quantified. The degree of formation of such complexes characterizes the autoimmune reactions of the body. This method offers a highly-parallel, high-efficiency and high-throughput disease diagnosis and detection platform. Antibody and antigen microarrays have tremendous potential in cancer research as diagnosis and characterization tools. Recent studies have demonstrated that combining multiple serum markers in a single antibody microarray radically increases the number of proteins that can be simultaneously detected and quantified (Carpelan-Holmstrom et al., 2002; Louhimo et al., 2002). Antibody microarrays have also been used to detect protein expression levels in UV-irradiated neoplasial tissue (Knezevic et al., 2001). The recently developed ProteinChip assay is based on the protein microarray technology. The ProteinChip technology has already been shown to be extremely useful in the identification and analyses of protein markers in diseased cells and tumours (Snijders et al., 2001). It is hypothesized that the integration of protein microarrays with bioinformatics would aid the rapid and accurate discrimination of cancerous cells from non-cancerous ones, thereby exhibiting utility as a high-throughput screening tool. Enzyme-based microarrays have also been used in the study of peroxidases, phosphotases, and kinases (MacBeath and Schreiber, 2000; Zhu et al., 2007). Protein and antibody-based microarrays are also used in immunoassays, profiling of protein and protein complexes (e.g. proteoglycans and proteolipids), and detection of biological warfare agents (Taylor, 2005; Timofeev et al., 1996).

Several technical challenges hinder the widespread use of protein microarrays as a disease detection tool. Firstly, protein function is strongly dependent on its three-dimensional structure. Active-site inhibition by structural deformation on account of binding to substrates is a common stumbling block for this technology. Additionally, protein-protein interactions are complicated by the onset of post-translational modifications such phosphorylation and glycosylation. Therefore, protein arrays are now being fabricated with post-translationally modified proteins or specific antibodies in order to actively sense such interactions.

Most of the current research in protein microarrays is directed at further increasing the sensitivity and throughput of these assays, and minimizing false positives (Khademhosseini, 2005). One potential method for increasing the sensitivity of the assay is to enhance the functionality of the immobilized proteins by using spacer molecules that minimize non-specific protein adsorption through surface modification (Khademhosseini, 2005). Studies using biomimetic surfaces have successfully demonstrated a 6- to 50-fold increase in assay sensitivity. Additionally, the development of biomaterials that offer improved control over the attachment and density of proteins on the substrate could alleviate some of the problems associated with protein immobilization onto the microarrays. Recent studies focusing on the use of self-assembling monolayers (Houseman et al., 2002), three-dimensional microstructures (Kang et al., 2005), and immobilized proteins specially inserted with a histidine-tag onto glass slides containing a metal-chelating group (Zhu et al., 2001) have shown improvement in protein attachment to the microarray substrates.

13.2.5 Cell-Based Microarrays

The use of cell-based microarrays as high-throughput analytical platforms is a fairly recent phenomenon, and as such, the market for these technologies is still miniscule in comparison to the DNA and protein microarray markets. Generally, cell-based microarrays are used for biosensing and cell-screening applications, and studying the interactions between cells and biomaterials.

Characterizations of ligand-receptor interactions on cellular surfaces are of interest to a broad range of researchers in the biomedical sciences. In one application, microarrays of B cells derived from murine spleens and human blood were successfully developed (Yamamura et al., 2005). These microarrays contained nearly 2×10^5 microchambers, and used Ca^{2+} mobilization within activated cells to effectively profile ligand-receptor binding. The microchambers were designed such that each compartment can accommodate no more than a single cell. Using fluorometry, intracellular Ca^{2+} in the B cells was quantified prior to and following incubation of characteristic antigens on the microarray. Subsequently, signal transduction in ligand-receptor pathways was elucidated by estimating the change in intracellular Ca^{2+} levels in the pre- and post-antigen binding states of the B-cells. This approach to studying ligand-receptor interactions offers significant advantages over flow cytometry, which is unable to monitor individual cells. Similar single-cell arrays have also been fabricated by using poly (dimethylsiloxane) (PDMS) (Rettig and Folch, 2005) and polystyrene (Dusseiller et al., 2005) microwells to study the cellular microenvironment in three dimensions.

Cell microarrays have proved useful for investigating stem cell biology and cellular fate processes, two areas vital to the field of tissue engineering. In one such study, a modified cell microarray was utilized to characterize the differentiation of human embryonic stem (hES) cells on different substrates (Anderson et al., 2004; Anderson et al., 2005). Therein, numerous biomaterials were directly synthesized onto a glass slide and subsequently incubated with hES cells for six days. Cells were then characterized to reveal the influence of each biomaterial on stem cell differentiation. Using a similar approach, the differentiation of hES cells cultured on different combinations of natural extracellular matrices (ECMs) was also investigated (Flaim et al., 2005). Each of these approaches enables the simultaneous screening of thousands of cell-material interactions in a relatively inexpensive, efficient manner.

Cell-based microarrays have also been applied to guide stem cell fates in numerous ways (Chin et al., 2004). Cellular micropatterning has been used to control cell shape and cellular fate processes such as migration, proliferation, differentiation and apoptosis (Hong et al., 2005; Sunkara et al., 2006). Rapidly screening individual cells for specific chemical stimuli is another demonstrated area of application for cell microarrays to stem cell research (Love et al., 2006). For studying chemical stimuli, individual cells are first exposed to characteristic microenvironments in inverted microchambers, following which, antibodies secreted by each cell was captured and detected.

Also printed arrays of full-length open reading frames (ORFs) of the genes in expression vectors, along with lipid transfection reagents was used for parallel transfection of hundreds of genes in a microarray format, thereby enabling the analysis of phenotypic effects of various genes (Ziauddin et al., 2001). Using similar approaches, cell microarrays could also be used to test the repression or silencing of genes in a sequence-specific manner using small, single-stranded anti-sense oligonucleotides, or small interfering RNA (Khademhosseini, 2005). Cell array systems are also being used for studying cellular behavior (Chin et al., 2004; Tourovskaia et al., 2005), profiling cellular interaction with potential drug candidates, and evaluating phenotypic changes resulting from the expression of specific proteins within cells (Khademhosseini, 2005; Khademhosseini et al., 2003; Suh et al., 2004).

Cell-based microarrays have also been used as biosensing devices (Kim et al., 2006). For example, colonies of live T cells were immobilized into functionalized patterned hydrogel microwells and then cultured with a confluent layer of antigen-capturing B cells. Samples containing the peptide analytes were then exposed to the colonies of the B cells. The peptide analytes in the samples are delivered to the T cells on account of the dynamic interactions between T cells and B cells within the microwells. The T cells respond to the introduction of the peptides analyses by producing a fluorescently detectable calcium signal. Thus, by engineering T cells to detect and distinguish a suite of pathogen-derived peptides, such cell-based biosensing platforms could effectively serve as large-scale disease diagnostic tools. Current limitations of cell-based assays include the inability to test many variables simultaneously as well as maintaining proper cell function in culture. Microengineered systems can be used to solve these problems. For example, to enable the simultaneously testing of multiple chemicals whilst maintaining proper cellular phenotypes in culture microfluidic channels may be used while to enhance cell function in vitro. Additionally, patterned co-cultures and multiphenotype cell arrays could also be used. It is anticipated that future developments in cell-based microarrays will make this technology an invaluable resource for undertaking high-throughput functional cell-based bioassays.

13.2.6 Other Microarrays and Microarray-Based Diagnostics

Microarrays are also extensively used in tissue engineering research. Microarrays fabricated from biopolymers and proteins derived from the extracellular matrix (ECM) have also been used to test molecular libraries and the effect of extracellular processes on cellular behavior (Khademhosseini, 2005). High-throughput testing of molecular libraries has already yielded favorable candidates for inducing osteogenesis (Jansen et al., 2003) and cardiomyogenesis (Wu et al., 2002) from ES cells, as well as dedifferentiation of committed cells (Chen et al., 2004). Recently, synthetic arrays, fabricated from a host of biomaterials, were successfully used to test the interaction of stem cells with various extracellular signals, and investigate the effects of polymeric materials on the differentiation of hES cells (Anderson et al., 2004) and mesenchymal stem cells (Anderson et al., 2005). Combinatorial matrices of numerous ECM proteins were utilized to evaluate the ability of these proteins to induce hepatic differentiation from murine ES cells, and maintain function of the differentiated hepatocytes (Flaim et al., 2005).

The use of microarrays has also been extended to clinical, environmental, food, and chemical testing (Taylor, 2005). Microarrays offer many advantages such as multiplexing of assays on a single chip, increasing analytical throughput, and decreasing costs. Microarrays are now being developed to utilize existing human and veterinary diagnostic technologies. An example of this is the recently-developed AmpliChip CYP450 microarray which is able to detect genetic variations in the genes for cytochrome P450 isoenzymes 2D6 and 2C19 in a reliable and efficient manner (Taylor, 2005). Variations in the genes that encode cytochrome P450 and its expressed enzymes could potentially change the metabolic mechanisms within an individual, and consequently affect the toxicity and efficacy of specific drugs in that individual (Taylor, 2005).

Other emerging microarray technologies include patterned polysaccharide and bead arrays (Blixt et al., 2004). Polysaccharide arrays can be used to study the interaction of libraries of chemicals and/or drugs with polysaccharides. It is hoped that future developments in this technology would provide a fillip to the discovery of drugs capable of interacting with cell-surface polysaccharides, and perhaps, aid in the advancement of the nascent field of glycomics—the study of the interaction of sugars with other molecules (Khademhosseini, 2005).

Developments such as the AmpliChip microarray have led to an increased investment in microarray diagnostic technologies. It is postulated that microarrays able to diagnose infectious diseases, blood disorders, and cancer; identify blood proteins and cardiac markers; analyze miniscule concentrations of industrial effluents and chemical waste; examine the quality of food products; and detect the presence of chemical and biological warfare agents will soon be developed.

13.3 Micro- and Nanoengineering for Biomedical Experimentation

Micro- and nanoengineering can also be used to generate topographical features on cell culture substrates in order to direct cellular fate processes such as cell growth, migration, and differentiation (Thapa et al., 2003). Such techniques could potentially be extended to high-throughput microarray technologies. Micro- and nano-textured substrates have been shown to significantly influence cell alignment (Thakar et al., 2003), adhesion (Thapa et al., 2003; Deutsch et al., 2000; Stato and Webster, 2004), gene expression (den Braber et al., 1998; van kooten et al., 1998; Walboomers et al., 1999), metabolic activity(de Oliveira and Nanci, 2004), and migration (Teixeira et al., 2003). Textured nanotopography generated by chemical etching, anodization and embedding nanoscale objects within biomaterials has also been used to increase osteoblast adhesion while decreasing the adhesion of other cell types (Price et al., 2003). Nanoparticles have also been embedded within biomaterials to reduce cell adhesion (Webster, 2001; Webster et al., 1999, 2000, 2001), and control cell-surface interactions (Stevens and George, 2005).

The successful in vitro replication of in vivo cellular fate processes is highly dependent on the control and regulation of cell-cell and cell-substrate interactions in three dimensions. Dynamic co-cultures of different cell types on specially-designed, geometrically optimized two-dimensional patterns is one alternative for achieving this objective. Substrate patterning techniques have also shown to direct cellular fate processes. For example, variations in the size and shape of adhesive protein patterns on substrates can induce varied cytoskeletal reconfigurations, and have been shown to effect cell adhesion (Miller et al., 2004), proliferation, and apoptosis (Chen et al., 1997). Human mesenchymal stem cells (MSCs) cultured on micropatterns of different shapes have been shown to differentiate to either adipocytes or osteoblasts (McBeath et al., 2004). Dynamic cell patterning has also been achieved using photocrosslinkable gels (Elbert and Hubbell, 2001; Schutt et al., 2003), thermally-responsive polymer surfaces (Okano et al., 1995), and reversibly cracked substrates (Zhu et al., 2005). Such techniques could be potentially integrated with the microarray technology to explore the two-dimensional effects of planar patterns of various adsorbed or chemically-bound molecules in a high-throughput manner. Additionally, hepatocytes and endothelial cells have been shown to produce better differentiated phenotypes when co-cultured with each other, as compared to their individual cultures owing to higher hepatocyte spheroid induction and subsequent optimum albumin secretion in the co-culture (Fukuda et al., 2005). Micropatterned co-cultures have also been successfully used to control the degree of heterotypic and homotypic cell-cell interactions, and study cell-cell interactions between hepatocytes and non-parenchymal fibroblasts (Bhatia et al., 1998a, 1998b, 1999). Micropatterned co-cultures have also been generated using thermally-responsive polymers (Hirose et al., 2000; Yamato et al., 2001), layer-by-layer deposition of ionic polymers (Khademhosseini et al., 2004), microfluidic deposition (Chiu et al., 2000), and micromoulding hydrogels (Tang et al., 2003).

It is a well-known fact that cellular phenotypic expression and stem cell fates are affected by both, interactions with other cells and surfaces, and by the diffusional limitations introduced within cellular microenvironment by physically confining cells and cell aggregates within defined spaces and architectures.

Microwells and microplates have been previously used to generate cell arrays consisting of many different cell types to study the effects of culturing and co-culturing cell types within confined spaces (Khademhosseini et al., 2005). This physical confinement of cells and other biochemical entities such liposomes within microwells has also been effectively used in high-throughput microarray applications (Thakar et al., 2003; Kalyankar et al., 2006). Alternatives for alleviating this problem include passively depositing cells at controlled densities (Bratten et al., 1998; Inoue et al., 2001; Khademhosseini et al., 2004; Maher et al., 1999; Prace et al., 1989; You et al., 1997), or docking cells within the microwells using microfluidic channels (Khademhosseini et al., 2005). The advantage of the later approach is that multiple cell types can be docked within the microwell lanes in a high-throughput manner. This technique could also be extended to align a set of microfluidic channels parallel to the original lanes of microwells in order to enable simultaneous combinatorial deposition of different cell types, analogous to DNA and protein microarrays (Kanda et al., 2004; Situma et al., 2005).

Additionally, the sensitivity of microarrays can also be increased by using nanoporous silica nanotubes (Kang et al., 2005; Wu et al., 2004), microporous silicon (Ressine et al., 2003), and beds of microbeads (Sato et al., 2001) to immobilize analytes from the samples. Non-adhesive poly(ethylene glycol) (PEG) microwells have also been successfully used to induce the formation of aggregates of non-anchorage-dependent cells such as ES cells (Khademhosseini et al., 2004; Karp et al., Submitted). Evidently, the use of micro- and nanoengineering approaches to selectively adhere and culture cells presents several advantages over techniques such as hanging drop and suspension culture methods.

13.4 Microfluidics

Microfluidic systems are structures designed for the manipulation of fluids in features with micro or nanometer dimensions. Microfluidic devices can be fabricated with astonishing complexity (Thorsen et al., 2002) and are apt for high-throughput experimentation. In typical microarray applications, the interrogation of low analyte concentrations relies on probe saturation, which can take hours. In contrast, microfluidic channels have demonstrably reduced mass transport times on microarrays by enabling a continuous delivery of targets (Hashimoto et al., 2005; Pappaert et al., 2003) at variable shears (Noerholm et al., 2004; Pappaert et al., 2003) and velocities (Vanderhoeven et al., 2004). Their size of operation also speeds up conventional experimental techniques like electrophoresis (Chung et al., 2003) while using a much smaller volume of reagents and biological materials than traditionally required. The potential increase in speed and the lower quantity of reagents and samples used for experimentation translates to commensurate savings in cost, making high-throughput experimentation more practical.

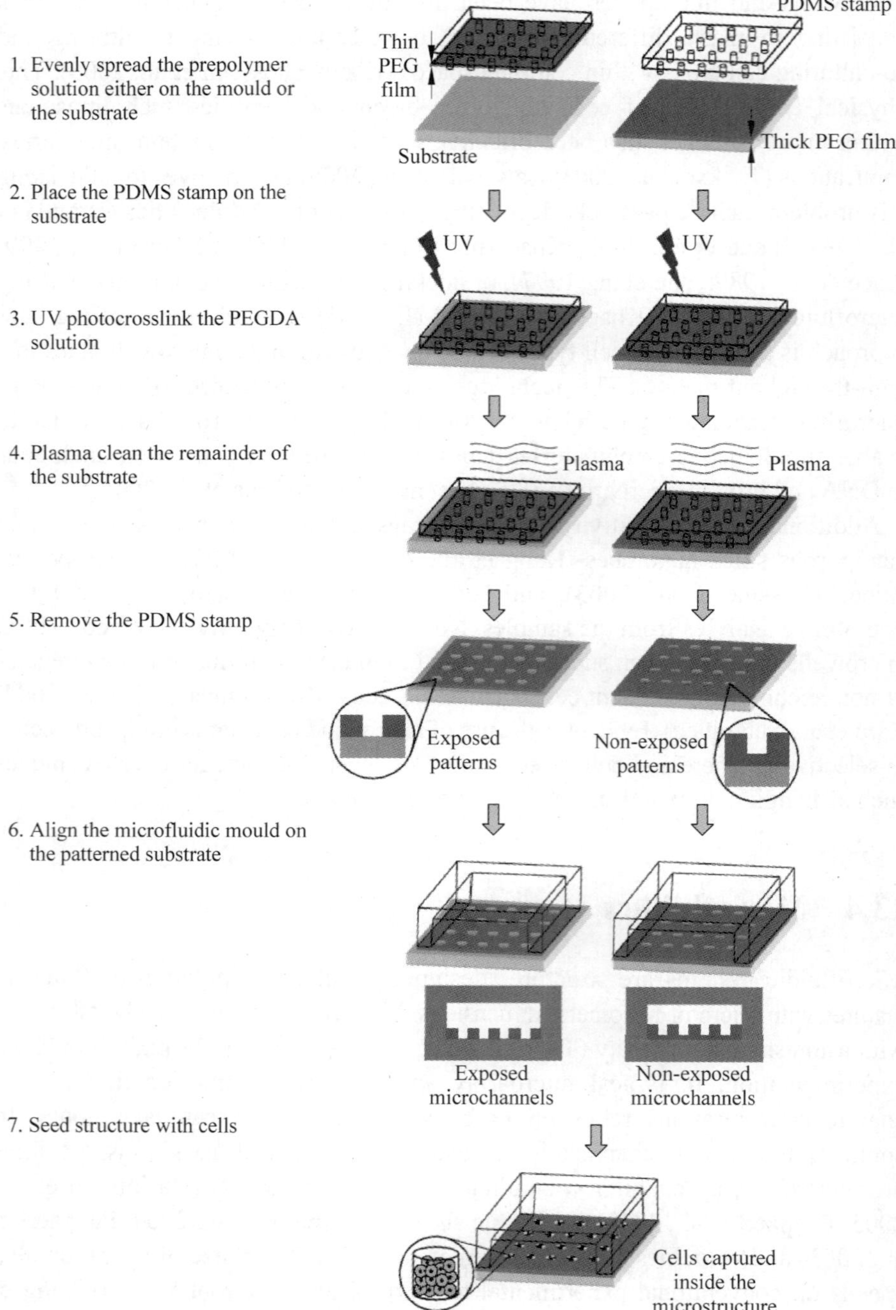

Figure 13.4 Schematic for fabrication of exposed and non-exposed microstructures inside microchannels. The final device combines the output of a microarray assay with the efficient analyte solution delivery provided by the microfluidic channel

The emergence of microfluidics has been facilitated by soft lithographic (Whitesides et al., 2001; Xia and Whitesides, 1998) techniques that were adopted from the semiconductor/microelectronics and micro-electro-mechanical systems (MEMS) industries. In soft lithography, elastomeric materials are cast and molded upon patterned planar surfaces generated through photolithography (Fig. 13.4). The resolution of molded patterns generated in soft lithography can range from tens of nanometers to hundreds of micrometers. This large range of resolution allows for a variety of feature sizes and shapes within the same microfluidic device. The variety of scales and functionality that can be incorporated into a single system makes microfluidics a powerful tool for the creation of automated, miniature biological experimentation devices. In a recently developed automated nucleic acid purification system (Hong et al., 2004), a small volume of cells was automatically isolated and lysed, and its DNA/mRNA purified and recovered with no pre- or post-sample treatments, all within a single microfluidics chip. Such devices substantially reduce the effort associated with more traditional biochemical analytical techniques. In the nucleic acid purification system mentioned above, approximately 0.4 nL of cell solution with reagent volumes of the same order of magnitude were used. The efficient use of expensive reagents and scarce samples could enable the cost effective, rapid analysis of small, cell populations. Even single-cell analysis is feasible on the volume scales of microfluidic devices. The automation potential has also been extended to perform parallel PCR (Auroux et al., 2004) and RT-PCR (Marcus et al., 2006) reactions as well as bioassays of human physiological fluids such as blood, serum, plasma, urine, and saliva (Srinivasan et al., 2004). One example of parallel analysis in microfluidics is the fully automated parallel screening of 32 high-affinity protein ligands synthesized through Click chemistry (Wang et al., 2006). High-throughput ELISA in which duplicate assays for 5 different proteins performed on 10 unique samples (Kartalov et al., 2006) have also been demonstrated.

In addition to providing an automated platform for performing established biochemical and molecular biology techniques and improving microarray throughput and efficiency, unique microscale fluid flow phenomena may be exploited to answer questions in fundamental biology in a high-throughput manner. Laminar flows found within microscale fluidic devices provide a unique tool for tuning the spatiotemporal cellular microenvironment to study the dynamic properties of biological systems in a high-throughput manner. In laminar flow regimes, convective mixing does not occur and transport between adjacent laminar streams is dominated by diffusive flux. This property has been harnessed to control the spatial positioning of soluble factors relative to cells (Takayama et al., 2001), pattern cells (Takayama et al., 2001), and etch microenvironments (Takayama et al., 2001). Additionally, diffusive flux properties have been exploited to generate well-defined gradients of soluble factors (Jeon et al., 2000), conjugated proteins (Takayama et al., 2001), and material crosslinking densities (Burdick et al., 2004). Such precise control of solution and, in turn, material properties provide opportunities to study fundamental biological questions regarding differential temperature or chemical treatment (Kartalov et al., 2006). Microfluidic gradient generation has been applied to investigations of cell migration, chemotaxis (Jeon et al., 2002; Hatch et al., 2001), axon extension (Dertinger et al., 2002; Taylor et al., 2005), and neural stem cell differentiation (Chung et al., 2006). Though these works were designed to establish basic principles and did not rely upon high-throughput methodologies, their eventual application to high-throughput systems is anticipated.

While the advantages of high-throughput microfluidic experimentation are widely noted, the practical problems of interfacing existing macroscale instrumentation with microfluidic devices has been an important obstacle in establishing microfluidic technology as a part of 'standard lab equipment' or for use within commercial devices. In particular, the precise actuation of nanoliter volumes of fluid flow is extremely challenging. Another challenge, the molecular detection of low concentrations within microfluidic channels, is discussed in Section 13.5. Though a number of solutions have been proposed, no standard methodology for engaging high-throughput applications exists. Previously, flow through arrays of microfluidic networks was controlled using syringe pumps (Hatch et al., 2001), gas-generation based pumps (Hong et al., 2003; Munyan et al., 2003), evaporation-based pumps (Walker and Beebe, 2002), gravity driven pumps (Cho et al., 2003), acoustic pumps (Nguyen and white, 1999), thermopneumatic pumps (Handique et al., 2001), and electrokinetic flow (Broyles et al., 2003; Emrich et al., 2002). Fluid actuation through these devices typically requires an external feeding tube and individual devices have not been shown to be ideal for the independent actuation of many pumps at once. Therefore, their practicality for potential high-throughput applications and complex microfluidic device actuation (such as the previously described nucleic acid purification systems that require the independent pumping of 10 or more fluid streams) is unclear.

For potential high-throughput applications, the pneumatic/hydraulic pressure-driven suite of pumps and valves developed by Fluidigm is promising (Unger et al., 2000). In this approach, pressurizable 'valve channels' aligned above or below reagent- or analyte-containing 'flow channels' are pressurized or depressurized to compress and close or decompress and open the flow channels. Sequential compression and decompression may be used to induce peristaltic pumping. An important advantage of this approach is that pressure-driven valve channels are capable of extending across multiple flow channels thereby enabling massive combinatorial actuation of fluid flow within many parallel microchannels. Although its sole high-throughput application has been in ELISA systems (Kartalov et al., 2006), this actuation approach has been extensively used to drive the previously mentioned nucleic acid purification (Hong et al., 2004), PCR (Auroux et al., 2004), and RT-PCR (Marcus et al., 2006) systems.

An alternative pumping/valving system that uses electronically-actuated pins of refreshable Braille systems also pumps using a peristaltic action (Gu et al.,

2004; Song et al., 2005). Specifically, Braille pins aligned along microfluidic channels can be programmed to push out and close elastomeric microchannels to either hold a channel shut (valve) or to push fluid along via peristaltic sequential depression. This approach is advantageous in that each pin may be independently computer controlled thereby enabling simultaneous actuation of each pumping/ valving mechanism independently. Braille pin actuation offers an advantage over pneumatic/hydraulic pressurized valve channels by eliminating the necessity for pressurizable tubing since actuation occurs 'on the chip'. An important consideration for high-throughput applications is that in contrast to pneumatic/hydraulic systems, Braille-based systems are not suitable for the combinatorial actuation of fluid flow within many parallel microchannels.

Microfluidic systems capable of combinatorial mixing (Neils et al., 2004) are highly scalable since numerous processes may be upscaled to run in parallel. The improvement in efficiency of microarray systems through the integration of microfluidics has been demonstrated, making improvements in microfluidic device design highly pertinent to microarray applications. Though many of the previously described applications of microfluidics were not performed in a high-throughput manner, the massive arraying of these processes is the predicted evolution of microfluidic technology.

13.5 Other Micro- and Nanoscale Technologies for Biological and Chemical Detection

In addition to microarray and microfluidic devices, a variety of novel micro and nanoengineered structures have recently been developed to augment existing methodologies for chemical and biological detection. Chemical and biological species have traditionally been detected through the use of fluorescently-tagged markers. Typically, a bound marker fluoresces at a well-defined spectrum of visible light under excitation with ultraviolet (UV) light. In high-throughput applications, traditional colorimetric assays suffer drawbacks such as rapid bleaching, narrow absorption spectrums, wide and asymmetric emission spectrums, and low detection sensitivity. The materialization of a suite of new nanomaterials such as quantum dots and nanowires hold promise for circumventing some of these problems.

Among other novel label-based biological and chemical detection schemes such as resin (Fenniri et al., 2001) or metallic barcoding (Nicewarner-Pena et al., 2004) and porous silicon photonic crystals (Cunin et al., 2002), the unique properties of quantom dots have enabled its quick emergence as a promising alternative to traditional fluorescent markers for high-throughput applications. These 10 – 20 nm fluorophores are composed of semiconductor nanocrystals that operate in a 'quantum confinement' size regime and allow for high resolution localization of proteins and cellular structures (Bruchez Jr. et al., 1998; Chan and Nie, 1998). The spectral emission properties of quantum dots can be finely tuned to emit light ranging from blue (450 nm) to near-infrared (900 nm) wavelengths at distinct and reproducible levels of intensity (Hotz, 2005). Furthermore, they exhibit a wide absorption band and a narrow (30 nm) and symmetric emission spectrum. These broad-absorption/narrow-emission properties make quantum dots especially suitable for high-throughput chemical and biological assays; quantum dots of many different colors and intensities may be simultaneously excited using a single light source, allowing for 'multiplexed' labeling and detection (Mattheakis et al., 2004; Han et al., 2001). In addition, whereas many traditional fluorescent markers quickly quench or bleed within seconds, quantum dots exhibit high photostability and may be continuously tracked for minutes or iteratively imaged over many hours. Quantum dots have already been used to image proteins (Olivos et al., 2003) and analyze cell receptor dynamics (Knezevic et al., 2001) such as signal transduction (Lidke et al., 2004; Rosenthal et al., 2002; Vu et al., 2005) and diffusion (Dahan et al., 2003) and their interface with high-throughput microfluidic and microarray devices is anticipated.

Alternatively, label-free nanotechnologies that may be useful for high-throughput applications are also being developed for detection. Over 30 years ago, modified planar semiconductors were shown to be capable of detecting the presence of biological and chemical species (Bergveld, 1972). In this approach, specific molecular receptors replaced the gate oxide of a field effect transistor (FET) resulting in charge accumulation/depletion upon analyte binding. The subsequent change in conductance of the material was monitored electrically. Recently, FET silicon nanowires were employed in an identical manner and the nanoscale size of the devices was shown to be advantageous in that the large surface area-to-volume ratio of the nanowires allowed charge accumulation in the entire bulk of the conducting material (rather than in a thin layer of much larger macroscale materials), resulting in extremely high detection sensitivity. Proof-of-concept nanowire sensors have been deployed to detect changes in ion concentration (Cui et al., 2003) as well as the presence of viruses (Cheng et al., 2006), ATP binding inhibitors (Wang et al., 2005), and cancer markers (Zheng et al., 2005). The hybridization of a nanowire and application to pH detection is shown in Fig. 13.5. While these nanowire sensors are still at an early stage of development, their size and sensitivity make them potentially suitable for interfacing with microarray and microfluidic high-throughput applications.

Silicon cantilevers are another label-free detection approach (Ziegler, 2004) that operate at the micron scale and which may be integrated into high-throughput devices. These cantilever beams detect molecules through the formation of surface stresses generated by the molecular adsorption of a specific ligand to the cantilever. Cantilever biosensing uses existing atomic force microscopy (AFM) technology to measure forces between cantilever and sample surfaces. Binding events stress the cantilever, causing it to bend and transduce this flexion for

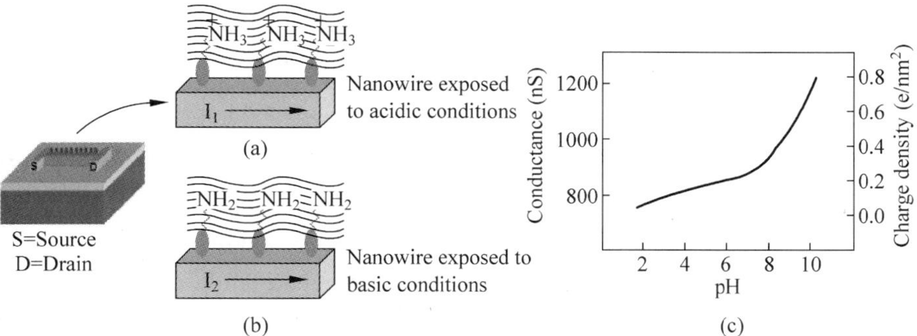

Figure 13.5 Application of a silicon nanowire in pH sensing. The silicon nanowire has been surface-treated to form pH-sensitive amino functional groups. The hybridized nanowire, when exposed to acidic solutions (a), assumes a net positive surface charge by formation of ammonium radicals. Conversely, when exposed to a basic solution (b), the ammonium groups deprotonate to form neutral surfaces. Variation in surface charge produces a change in conductance of the nanowire, which in turn is correlated to the pH of the solution (c)

detection. Cantilever bending may occur in response to one of three mechanisms: surface stress, mass loading, and temperature change. Surface stresses may be caused by the highly specific binding of analytes of interest to a single side of the cantilever. In contrast, the loading of a larger mass induces cantilever oscillation, which is transduced and can be detected. Rapid temperature shifts may also induce flexion of the cantilever. These specific detection mechanisms can be controlled through modulation of the cantilever material. Silicon, silicon nitride, and silicon oxide are currently most used in micro- and nano-scale cantilevers (Lavrik et al., 2004). Cantilever binding specificity is modulated through surface coating of the cantilever with the highly specific receptors also used in microarrays, including self-assembled monolayers, peptide sequences, DNA probes, or antibodies. Once a flexion mode/receptor combination has been characterized for a particular analyte, the bending caused by analyte binding is transductively measured and correlated with an analyte concentration. The transduction of cantilever bending can be detected through a number of techniques such as electric piezoresistive readouts, optical laser detection, piezoelectricity or capacitance changes. The piezoresistive method is compatible with cantilevers of a few hundred nanometers in length (Lavrik et al., 2004). Here, the resistance of silicon cantilevers doped in specific regions reflects the degree of deformation. Alternatively, optical beam deflection methods, though not amenable for nanometer-scale cantilevers offer high readout efficiencies. Piezoelectric methods use materials such as zinc oxide coated on the surface of the cantilever; the bending of the material generates a voltage, which can then be measured. Lastly, the capacitance method detects the capacitance between the cantilever beam and a substrate. The movement of the cantilever closer to the surface increases the capacitance while movement away decreases the capacitance, which can then be recorded and correlated to binding events. The small gap between cantilever and surface required for this latter method is an engineering challenge and therefore a disadvantage of this method.

13.6 Conclusions

Micro- and nanoscale technologies automate, miniaturize, and multiplex biochemical assays to study biological functions at the cellular and genomic level at reduced experimentation costs and in a high-throughput manner. Of these, the microarray technology is extensively used in the analysis and detection, of analytes—from whole cells and DNA, to environmental pollutants. Other microscale technologies such as microfluidic gradient generation systems successfully augment the applicability and functionality of the microarray platform. Presently, microarrays are moderately complex to use, and costly to manufacture. In the future, as this technology develops further, it is expected that microarrays will be routinely used, not only in the study of genes, genomes, and comparative genome hybridization, but also in nearly every single area necessitating high-throughput analysis and detection of analytes. Emerging disciplines such as pharmacogenomics, toxicogenomics, proteomics, as well as traditional fields such as clinical diagnostics, drug discovery, food and environmental analysis, and chemical and biological warfare defense will witness extensive use of the microarray technology. Microarrays have also spurred the development of inventive analytical devices and technologies such as MEMS and lab-on-a-chip, and accordingly, have revolutionized the amplification, separation, analysis, and detection of DNA via integration with microfluidics. Additionally, since microarrays and microfluidic technologies can perform experiments with higher sensitivity using less reagents, they present significant opportunities to increase the throughput and efficiency of DNA, RNA, oligonucleotides, proteins, polysaccharides, as well as cell-based assays. These technologies have also been applied in numerous diagnostic applications. A majority of the current research into micro- and nanoscale technologies focuses on increasing the sensitivity and speed of assays based on these technologies, while minimizing their size and cost. The union of microarrays and microfluidics promises previously unmatched throughput for diagnostics and screening applications.

Acknowledgements

The authors would like to acknowledge the funding received from the National Institute of Health, the MIT Institute for Soldier Nanotechnologies, the Coulter Foundation, the Center for Integration of Medicine and Innovative Technology (CIMIT), and the Draper Laboratory.

References

Affymetrix, I. Whole Genome Analysis (2006).

Anderson, D. G., D. Putnam, E. B. Lavik, T. A. Mahmood and R. Langer. Biomaterial microarrays: Rapid, microscale screening of polymer-cell interaction. *Biomaterials* **26**: 4892 – 4897 (2005).

Anderson, D. G., S. Levenberg and R. Langer. Nanoliter-scale synthesis of arrayed biomaterials and application to human embryonic stem cells. *Nat. Biotechnol.* **22**: 863 – 866 (2004).

Auroux, P. A., Y. Koc, A. deMello, A. Manz and P. J. Day. Miniaturised nucleic acid analysis. *Lab. Chip.* **4**: 534 – 546 (2004).

Bergveld, P. Development, operation, and application of the ion-sensitive field-effect transistor as a tool for electrophysiology. *IEEE Trans. Biomed. Eng.* **19**: 342 – 351 (1972).

Bhatia, S. N., M. L. Yarmush and M. Toner. Controlling cell interactions by micropatterning in co-cultures: Hepatocytes and 3T3 fibroblasts. *J. Biomed. Mater. Res.* **34**: 189 – 199 (1997).

Bhatia, S. N., U. J. Balis, M. L. Yarmush and M. Toner. Effect of cell-cell interactions in preservation of cellular phenotype: cocultivation of hepatocytes and nonparenchymal cells. *Faseb. J.* **13**: 1883 – 1900 (1999).

Bhatia, S. N., U. J. Balis, M. L. Yarmush and M. Toner. Microfabrication of hepatocyte/ fibroblast co-cultures: Role of homotypic cell interactions. *Biotechnol. Prog.* **14**: 378 – 387 (1998).

Bhatia, S. N., U. J. Balis, M. L. Yarmush and M. Toner. Probing heterotypic cell interactions: Hepatocyte function in microfabricated co-cultures. *J. Biomater. Sci. Polym. Ed.* **9**: 1137 – 1160 (1998).

Blixt, O., S. Head, T. Mondala, C. Scanlan, M. E. Huflejt, R. Alvarez, M. C. Bryan, F. Fazio, D. Calarese, J. Stevens, N. Razi, D. J. Stevens, J. J. Skehel, I. van Die, D. R. Burton, I. A. Wilson, R. Cummings, N. Bovin, C. H. Wong and J. C. Paulson. Printed covalent glycan array for ligand profiling of diverse glycan binding proteins. *Proc. Natl. Acad. Sci. USA* **101**: 17,033 – 17,038 (2004).

Bratten, C. D., P. H. Cobbold and J. M. Cooper. Single-cell measurements of purine release using a micromachined electroanalytical sensor. *Anal. Chem.* **70**: 1164 – 1170 (1998).

Brem, R., U. Certa, M. Neeb, A. P. Nair and C. Moroni. Global analysis of differential gene expression after transformation with the v-H-ras oncogene in a murine tumor model. *Oncogene* **20**: 2854 – 2858 (2001).

Broyles, B. S., S. C. Jacobson and J. M. Ramsey. Sample filtration, concentration, and separation integrated on microfluidic devices. *Anal. Chem.* **75**: 2761 – 2767 (2003).

Bruchez, M., Jr., M. Moronne, P. Gin, S. Weiss and A. P. Alivisatos. Semiconductor nanocrystals as fluorescent biological labels. *Science* **281**: 2013 – 2016 (1998).

Burdick, J. A., A. Khademhosseini and R. Langer. Fabrication of gradient hydrogels using a microfluidics/photopolymerization process. *Langmuir* **20**: 5153 – 5156 (2004).

Carpelan-Holmstrom, M., J. Louhimo, U. H. Stenman, H. Alfthan and C. Haglund. CEA, CA 19-9 and CA 72-4 improve the diagnostic accuracy in gastrointestinal cancers. *Anticancer Res.* **22**: 2311 – 2316 (2002).

Cavallaro, S., B. G. Schreurs, W. Zhao, V. D'Agata and D. L. Alkon. Gene expression profiles during long-term memory consolidation. *Eur. J. Neurosci.* **13**: 1809 – 1815 (2001).

Chan W. C. and S. Nie. Quantum dot bioconjugates for ultrasensitive nonisotopic detection. *Science* **281**: 2016 – 2018 (1998).

Chen, C. S., M. Mrksich, S. Huang, G. M. Whitesides and D. E. Ingber. Geometric control of cell life and death. *Science* **276**: 1425 – 1428 (1997).

Chen, S., Q. Zhang, X. Wu, P. G. Schultz and S. Ding. Dedifferentiation of lineage-committed cells by a small molecule. *J. Am. Chem. Soc.* **126**: 410 – 411 (2004).

Cheng, M. M., G. Cuda, Y. L. Bunimovich, M. Gaspari, J. R. Heath, H. D. Hill, C. A. Mirkin, A. J. Nijdam, R. Terracciano, T. Thundat and M. Ferrari. Nanotechnologies for biomolecular detection and medical diagnostics. *Curr. Opin. Chem. Biol.* **10**: 11 – 19 (2006).

Chin, V. I., P. Taupin, S. Sanga, J. Scheel, F. H. Gage and S. N. Bhatia. Microfabricated platform for studying stem cell fates. *Biotechnol. Bioeng.* **88**: 399 – 415 (2004).

Chiu, D. T., N. L. Jeon, S. Huang, R. S. Kane, C. J. Wargo, I. S. Choi, D. E. Ingber and G. M. Whitesides. Patterned deposition of cells and proteins onto surfaces by using three-dimensional microfluidic systems. *Proc. Natl. Acad. Sci. USA* **97**: 2408 – 2413 (2000).

Cho, B. S., T. G. Schuster, X. Zhu, D. Chang, G. D. Smith and S. Takayama. Passively driven integrated microfluidic system for separation of motile sperm. *Anal. Chem.* **75**: 1671 – 1675 (2003).

Chung, B. G., L. A. Flanagan, S. W. Rhee, P. H. Schwartz, A. P. Lee, E. S. Monuki and N. L. Jeon. Human neural stem cell growth and differentiation in a gradient-generating microfluidic device. *Lab. Chip* **5**: 401 – 406 (2005).

Chung, Y. C., Y. C. Lin, M. Z. Shiu and W. N. Chang. Microfluidic chip for fast nucleic acid hybridization. *Lab. Chip.* **3**: 228 – 233 (2003).

Cossman, J. Gene expression analysis of single neoplastic cells and the pathogenesis of Hodgkin's lymphoma. *J Histochem. Cytochem.* **49**: 799 – 800 (2001).

Cui, Y., Q. Wei, H. Park and C. M. Lieber. Nanowire nanosensors for highly sensitive and selective detection of biological and chemical species. *Science* **293**: 1289 – 1292 (2001).

Cunin, F., T. A. Schmedake, J. R. Link, Y. Y. Li, J. Koh, S. N. Bhatia, M. J. Sailor. Biomolecular screening with encoded porous-silicon photonic crystals. *Nat. Mater.* **1**: 39 – 41 (2002).

Dahan, M., S. Levi, C. Luccardini, P. Rostaing, B. Riveau and A. Triller. Diffusion dynamics of glycine receptors revealed by single-quantum dot tracking. *Science* **302**: 442 – 445 (2003).

de Oliveira P. T., A. Nanci. Nanotexturing of titanium-based surfaces upregulates expression of bone sialoprotein and osteopontin by cultured osteogenic cells. *Biomaterials* **25**: 403 – 413 (2004).

den Braber, E. T., J. E. de Ruijter, L. A. Ginsel, A. F. von Recum and J. A. Jansen. Orientation of ECM protein deposition, fibroblast cytoskeleton, and attachment complex components on silicone microgrooved surfaces. *J. Biomed. Mater. Res.* **40**: 291 – 300 (1998).

Dertinger, S. K., X. Jiang, Z. Li, V. N. Murthy and G. M. Whitesides. Gradients of substrate-bound laminin orient axonal specification of neurons. *Proc. Natl. Acad. Sci. USA* **99**: 12,542 – 12,547 (2002).

Deutsch, J., D. Motlagh, B. Russell and T. A. Desai. Fabrication of microtextured membranes for cardiac myocyte attachment and orientation. *J. Biomed. Mater. Res.* **53**: 267 – 275 (2000).

Dusseiller, M. R., D. Schlaepfer, M. Koch, R. Kroschewski and M. Textor. An inverted microcontact printing method on topographically structured polystyrene chips for arrayed micro-3-D culturing of single cells. *Biomaterials* **26**: 5917 – 5925 (2005).

Elbert D. L., J. A. Hubbell. Conjugate addition reactions combined with free-radical cross-linking for the design of materials for tissue engineering. *Biomacromolecules* **2**: 430 – 441 (2001).

Emrich, C. A., H. Tian, I. L. Medintz and R. A. Mathies. Microfabricated 384-lane capillary array electrophoresis bioanalyzer for ultrahigh-throughput genetic analysis. *Anal. Chem.* **74**: 5076 – 5083 (2002).

Fenniri, H., L. Ding, A. E. Ribbe and Y. Zyrianov. Barcoded resins: a new concept for polymer-supported combinatorial library self-deconvolution. *J. Am. Chem. Soc.* **123**: 8151 – 8152 (2001).

Flaim, C. J., S. Chien and S. N. Bhatia. An extracellular matrix microarray for probing cellular differentiation. *Nat. Methods*. **2**: 119 – 125 (2005).

Franssila, S. *Introduction to Microfabrication*. Chichester, West Sussex, England; Hoboken, NJ: J. Wiley (2004).

Fukuda, J., K. Okamura, K. Ishihara, H. Mizumoto, K. Nakazawa, H. Ijima, T. Kajiwara and K. Funatsu. Differentiation effects by the combination of spheroid formation and sodium butyrate treatment in human hepatoblastoma cell line (Hep G2): A possible cell source for hybrid artificial liver. *Cell Transplant* **14**: 819 – 827 (2005).

Ge, H. UPA, a universal protein array system for quantitative detection of protein-protein, protein-DNA, protein-RNA and protein-ligand interactions. *Nucleic. Acids. Res.* **28**: e3 (2000).

Gerhold, D., M. Lu, J. Xu, C. Austin, C. T. Caskey and T. Rushmore. Monitoring expression of genes involved in drug metabolism and toxicology using DNA microarrays. *Physiol Genomics* **5**: 161 – 170 (2001).

Geschwind, D. H. Mice, microarrays and the genetic diversity of the brain. *Proc. Natl. Acad. Sci. USA* **97**: 10,676 – 10,678 (2000).

Graveel, C. R., T. Jatkoe, S. J. Madore, A. L. Holt and P. J. Farnham. Expression profiling and identification of novel genes in hepatocellular carcinomas. *Oncogene* **20**: 2704 – 2712 (2001).

Gu, W., X. Zhu, N. Futai, B. S. Cho and S. Takayama. Computerized microfluidic cell culture using elastomeric channels and Braille displays. *Proc. Natl. Acad. Sci. USA* **101**: 15,861 – 15,866 (2004).

Haab, B. B., M. J. Dunham and P. O. Brown. Protein microarrays for highly parallel detection and quantitation of specific proteins and antibodies in complex solutions. *Genome. Biol.* **2**: RESEARCH0004 (2001).

Han, M., X. Gao, J. Z. Su and S. Nie. Quantum-dot-tagged microbeads for multiplexed optical coding of biomolecules. *Nat. Biotechnol.* **19**: 631 – 635 (2001).

Handique, K., D. T. Burke, C. H. Mastrangelo and M. A. Burns. On-chip thermopneumatic pressure for discrete drop pumping. *Anal. Chem.* **73**: 1831 – 1838 (2001).

Hashimoto, M., M. L. Hupert, M. C. Murphy, S. A. Soper, Y. W. Cheng and F. Barany. Ligase detection reaction/hybridization assays using three-dimensional microfluidic networks for the detection of low-abundant DNA point mutations. *Anal. Chem.* **77**: 3243 – 3255 (2005).

Hatch, A., A. E. Kamholz, K. R. Hawkins, M. S. Munson, E. A. Schilling, B. H. Weigl and P. Yager. A rapid diffusion immunoassay in a T-sensor. *Nat. Biotechnol.* **19**: 461 – 465 (2001).

Hirose, M., M. Yamato, O. H. Kwon, M. Harimoto, A. Kushida, T. Shimizu, A. Kikuchi and T. Okano. Temperature-Responsive surface for novel co-culture systems of hepatocytes with endothelial cells: 2-D patterned and double layered co-cultures. *Yonsei. Med. J.* **41**: 803 – 813 (2000).

Hong, B. J., V. Sunkara and J. W. Park. DNA microarrays on nanoscale-controlled surface. *Nucleic Acids Res.* **33**: e106 (2005).

Hong, C. C., S. Murugesan, S. Kim, G. Beaucage, J. W. Choi and C. H. Ahn. A functional on-chip pressure generator using solid chemical propellant for disposable lab-on-a-chip. *Lab. Chip.* **3**: 281 – 286 (2003).

Hong, J. W., V. Studer, G. Hang, W. F. Anderson and S. R. Quake. A nanoliter-scale nucleic acid processor with parallel architecture. *Nat. Biotechnol* **22**: 435 – 439 (2004).

Hotz, C. Z. Applications of quantum dots in biology: an overview. *Methods Mol. Biol.* **303**: 1 – 17 (2005).

Houseman, B. T., J. H. Huh, S. J. Kron and M. Mrksich. Peptide chips for the quantitative evaluation of protein kinase activity. *Nat. Biotechnol.* **20**: 270 – 274 (2002).

Inoue, I., Y. Wakamoto, H. Moriguchi, K. Okano and K. Yasuda. On-chip culture system for observation of isolated individual cells. *Lab. Chip.* **1**: 50 – 55 (2001).

Jansen, R., H. Yu, D. Greenbaum, Y. Kluger, N. J. Krogan, S. Chung, A. Emili, M. Snyder, J. F. Greenblatt and M. Gerstein. A Bayesian networks approach for predicting protein-protein interactions from genomic data. *Science* **302**: 449 – 453 (2003).

Jeon, N. L., H. Baskaran, S. K. W. Dertinger, G. M. Whitesides, L. Van De Water and M. Toner. Neutrophil chemotaxis in linear and complex gradients of interleukin-8 formed in a microfabricated device. *Nat. Biotechnol.* **20**: 826 – 830 (2002).

Jeon, N. L., S. K. W. Dertinger, D. T. Chiu, I. S. Choi, A. D. Stroock and G. M. Whitesides. Generation of solution and surface gradients using microfluidic systems. *Langmuir*. **16**(22): 8311 – 8316 (2000).

Joos, T. O., M. Schrenk, P. Hopfl, K. Kroger, U. Chowdhury, D. Stoll, D. Schorner, M. Durr, K. Herick, S. Rupp, K. Sohn and H. Hammerle. A microarray enzyme-linked immunosorbent assay for autoimmune diagnostics. *Electrophoresis* **21**: 2641 – 2650 (2000).

Kalma, Y., L. Marash, Y. Lamed and D. Ginsberg. Expression analysis using DNA microarrays demonstrates that E2F-1 up-regulates expression of DNA replication genes including replication protein A2. *Oncogene* **20**: 1379 – 1387 (2001).

Kalyankar, N. D., M. K. Sharma, S. V. Vaidya, D. Calhoun, C. Maldarelli, A. Couzis and L. Gilchrist. Arraying of intact liposomes into chemically functionalized microwells. *Langmuir* **22**: 5403 – 5411 (2006).

Kanda, V., J. K. Kariuki, D. J. Harrison and M. T. McDermott. Label-free reading of microarray-based immunoassays with surface plasmon resonance imaging. *Anal. Chem.* **76**: 7257 – 7262 (2004).

Kang, M., L. Trofin, M. O. Mota and C. R. Martin. Protein capture in silica nanotube membrane 3-D microwell arrays. *Anal. Chem.* **77**: 6243 – 6249 (2005).

Karp, J., J. Yeh, G. Eng, J. Fukuda, J. Blumling, K. Y. Suh, J. Cheng, J. Borenstein, R. Langer and A. Khademhosseini. Controlling size, shape and homogeneity of embryoid bodies using polymeric microwells. *Stem. Cells*. Submitted.

Kartalov, E. P., J. F. Zhong, A. Scherer, S. R. Quake, C. R. Taylor and W. F. Anderson. High-throughput multi-antigen microfluidic fluorescence immunoassays. *Biotechniques* **40**: 85 – 90 (2006).

Khademhosseini A., R. Langer. Nanobiotechnology for tissue engineering and drug delivery. *Chemical Engineering Progress* **102**: 38 – 42 (2006).

Khademhosseini, A. Chips to hits: microarray and microfluidic technologies for high-throughput analysis and drug discovery. September 12 – 15, 2005, MA, USA. *Expert. Rev. Mol. Diagn.* **5**: 843 – 846 (2005).

Khademhosseini, A., J. Yeh, G. Eng, J. Karp, H. Kaji, J. Borenstein, O. C. Farokhzad and R. Langer. Cell docking inside microwells within reversibly sealed microfluidic channels for fabricating multiphenotype cell arrays. *Lab. Chip*. **5**: 1380 – 1386 (2005).

Khademhosseini, A., J. Yeh, S. Jon, G. Eng, K. Y. Suh, J. A. Burdick and R. Langer. Molded polyethylene glycol microstructures for capturing cells within microfluidic channels. *Lab. Chip* **4**: 425 – 430 (2004).

Khademhosseini, A., K. Y. Suh, J. M. Yang, G. Eng, J. Yeh, S. Levenberg and R. Langer. Layer-by-layer deposition of hyaluronic acid and poly-*L*-lysine for patterned cell co-cultures. *Biomaterials* **25**: 3583 – 3592 (2004).

Khademhosseini, A., R. Langer, J. Borenstein and J. P. Vacanti. Microscale technologies for tissue engineering and biology. *Proc. Natl. Acad. Sci. USA* **103**: 2480 – 2487 (2006).

Khademhosseini, A., S. Jon, K. Y. Suh, T. N. Tran, G. Eng, J. Yeh, J. Seong and R. Langer. Direct patterning of protein- and cell-resistant polymeric monolayers and microstructures. *Adv. Mater.*. **15**: 1995 – 2000 (2003).

Kim, H., R. E. Cohen, P. T. Hammond and D. J. Irvine. Live lymphocyte arrays for biosensing. *Adv. Funct. Mater.* **16**: 1313 – 1323 (2006).

Knezevic, V., C. Leethanakul, V. E. Bichsel, J. M. Worth, V. V. Prabhu, J. S. Gutkind, L. A. Liotta, P. J. Munson, E. F. Petricoin and D. B. Krizman. Proteomic profiling of the cancer microenvironment by antibody arrays. *Proteomics* **1**: 1271 – 1278 (2001).

Lavrik, N. V., M. J. Sepaniak and P. G. Datskos. Cantilever transducers as a platform for chemical and biological sensors. *Review of Scientific Instruments* **75**: 2229 – 2253 (2004).

Lidke, D. S., P. Nagy, R. Heintzmann, D. J. Arndt-Jovin, J. N. Post, H. E. Grecco, E. A. Jares-Erijman and T. M. Jovin. Quantum dot ligands provide new insights into erbB/HER receptor-mediated signal transduction. *Nat. Biotechnol.* **22**: 198 – 203 (2004).

Louhimo, J., P. Finne, H. Alfthan, U. H. Stenman and C. Haglund. Combination of HCGbeta, CA 19-9 and CEA with logistic regression improves accuracy in gastrointestinal malignancies. *Anticancer Res.* **22**: 1759 – 1764 (2002).

Love, J. C., J. L. Ronan, G. M. Grotenbreg, A. G. van der Veen and H. L. Ploegh. A microengraving method for rapid selection of single cells producing antigen-specific antibodies. *Nat. Biotechnol.* **24**: 703 – 707 (2006).

Luscombe, N. M., M. M. Babu, H. Yu, M. Snyder, S. A. Teichmann and M. Gerstein. Genomic analysis of regulatory network dynamics reveals large topological changes. *Nature* **431**: 308 – 312 (2004).

MacBeath G., S. L. Schreiber. Printing proteins as microarrays for high-throughput function determination. *Science* **289**: 1760 – 1763 (2000).

MacBeath, G., A. N. Koehler and S. L. Schreiber. Printing small molecules as microarrays and detecting protein-ligand interactions en masse. *J. Am. Chem. Soc.* **121**: 7967 – 7968 (1999).

Madden, S. L., C. J. Wang and G. Landes. Serial analysis of gene expression: from gene discovery to target identification. *Drug. Discov. Today* **5**: 415 – 425 (2000).

Maher, M. P., J. Pine, J. Wright and Y. C. Tai. The neurochip: A new multielectrode device for stimulating and recording from cultured neurons. *J. Neurosci. Methods.* **87**: 45 – 56 (1999).

Marcus, J. S., W. F. Anderson and S. R. Quake. Parallel picoliter rt-PCR assays using microfluidics. *Anal. Chem.* **78**: 956 – 958 (2006).

Mattheakis, L. C., J. M. Dias, Y. J. Choi, J. Gong, M. P. Bruchez, J. Liu and E. Wang. Optical coding of mammalian cells using semiconductor quantum dots. *Anal. Biochem.* **327**: 200 – 208 (2004).

McBeath, R., D. M. Pirone, C. M. Nelson, K. Bhadriraju and C. S. Chen. Cell shape, cytoskeletal tension, and RhoA regulate stem cell lineage commitment. *Dev. Cell.* **6**: 483 – 495 (2004).

Miller, D. C., A. Thapa, K. M. Haberstroh and T. J. Webster. Endothelial and vascular smooth muscle cell function on poly (lactic-co-glycolic acid) with nano-structured surface features. *Biomaterials* **25**: 53 – 61 (2004).

Monni, O., M. Barlund, S. Mousses, J. Kononen, G. Sauter, M. Heiskanen, P. Paavola, K. Avela, Y. Chen, M. L. Bittner and A. Kallioniemi. Comprehensive copy number and gene expression profiling of the 17q23 amplicon in human breast cancer. *Proc. Natl. Acad. Sci. USA* **98**: 5711 – 5716 (2001).

Munyan, J. W., H. V. Fuentes, M. Draper, R. T. Kelly and A. T. Woolley. Electrically actuated, pressure-driven microfluidic pumps. *Lab. Chip* **3**: 217 – 220 (2003).

Neils, C., Z. Tyree, B. Finlayson and A. Folch. Combinatorial mixing of microfluidic streams. *Lab. Chip.* **4**: 342 – 350 (2004).

Nguyen N. T, R. M. White. Design and optimization of an ultrasonic flexural plate wave micropump using numerical simulation. *Sensors and Actuators A: Physical.* **77**: 229 – 236 (1999).

Nicewarner-Pena, S. R., R. G. Freeman, B. D. Reiss, L. He, D. J. Pena, I. D. Walton, R. Cromer, C. D. Keating and M. J. Natan. Submicrometer metallic barcodes. *Science* **294**: 137 – 141 (2001).

Noerholm, M., H. Bruus, M. H. Jakobsen, P. Telleman and N. B. Ramsing. Polymer microfluidic chip for online monitoring of microarray hybridizations. *Lab. Chip.* **4**: 28 – 37 (2004).

Okabe, H., S. Satoh, T. Kato, O. Kitahara, R. Yanagawa, Y. Yamaoka, T. Tsunoda, Y. Furukawa and Y. Nakamura. Genome-wide analysis of gene expression in human hepatocellular carcinomas using cDNA microarray: Identification of genes involved in viral carcinogenesis and tumor progression. *Cancer. Res.* **61**: 2129 – 2137 (2001).

Okano, T., N. Yamada, M. Okuhara, H. Sakai and Y. Sakurai. Mechanism of cell detachment from temperature-modulated, hydrophilic-hydrophobic polymer surfaces. *Biomaterials* **16**: 297 – 303 (1995).

Olivos, H. J., K. Bachhawat-Sikder and T. Kodadek. Quantum dots as a visual aid for screening bead-bound combinatorial libraries. *Chembiochem* **4**: 1242 – 1245 (2003).

Palsson, B, S. Bhatia. *Tissue Engineering*. Upper Saddle River, N.J.: Pearson Prentice Hall (2004).

Pappaert, K., J. Vanderhoeven, P. Van Hummelen, B. Dutta, D. Clicq, G. V. Baron and G. Desmet. Enhancement of DNA micro-array analysis using a shear-driven micro-channel flow system. *J. Chromatogr. A* **1014**: 1 – 9 (2003).

Parce, J. W., J. C. Owicki, K. M. Kercso, G. B. Sigal, H. G. Wada, V. C. Muir, L. J. Bousse, K. L. Ross, B. I. Sikic and H. M. McConnell. Detection of cell-affecting agents with a silicon biosensor. *Science* **246**: 243 – 247 (1989).

Price, R. L., M. C. Waid, K. M. Haberstroh and T. J. Webster. Selective bone cell adhesion on formulations containing carbon nanofibers. *Biomaterials* **24**: 1877 – 1887 (2003).

Ressine, A., S. Ekstrom, G. Marko-Varga and T. Laurell. Macro-/nanoporous silicon as a support for high-performance protein microarrays. *Anal. Chem.* **75**: 6968 – 6974 (2003).

Rettig J. R., A. Folch. Large-scale single-cell trapping and imaging using microwell arrays. *Anal. Chem.* **77**: 5628 – 5634 (2005).

Rosenthal, S. J., I. Tomlinson, E. M. Adkins, S. Schroeter, S. Adams, L. Swafford, J. McBride, Y. Wang, L. J. DeFelice and R. D. Blakely. Targeting cell surface receptors with ligand-conjugated nanocrystals. *J. Am. Chem. Soc.* **124**: 4586 – 4594 (2002).

Sato M., T. J. Webster. Nanobiotechnology: Implications for the future of nanotechnology in orthopedic applications. *Expert. Rev. Med. Devices.* **1**: 105 – 114 (2004).

Sato, K., M. Tokeshi, H. Kimura and T. Kitamori. Determination of carcinoembryonic antigen in human sera by integrated bead-bed immunoassay in a microchip for cancer diagnosis. *Anal. Chem.* **73**: 1213 – 1218 (2001).

Schultz, J. S., R. F. Taylor. *Handbook of chemical and biological sensors*. Bristol, England: IOP Publishing Ltd. (2005).

Schutt, M., S. S. Krupka, A. G. Milbradt, S. Deindl, E. K. Sinner, D. Oesterhelt, C. Renner and L. Moroder. Photocontrol of cell adhesion processes: model studies with cyclic azobenzene-RGD peptides. *Chem. Biol.* **10**: 487 – 490 (2003).

Situma, C., M. Hashimoto and S. A. Soper. Merging microfluidics with microarray-based bioassays. *Biomol. Eng.* **23**: 213 – 231 (2006).

Situma, C., Y. Wang, M. Hupert, F. Barany, R. L. McCarley and S. A. Soper. Fabrication of DNA microarrays onto poly(methyl methacrylate) with ultraviolet patterning and microfluidics for the detection of low-abundant point mutations. *Anal. Biochem.* **340**: 123 – 135 (2005).

Snijders, A. M., N. Nowak, R. Segraves, S. Blackwood, N. Brown, J. Conroy, G. Hamilton, A. K. Hindle, B. Huey, K. Kimura, S. Law, K. Myambo, J. Palmer, B. Ylstra, J. P. Yue, J. W. Gray, A. N. Jain, D. Pinkel and D. G. Albertson. Assembly of microarrays for genome-wide measurement of DNA copy number. *Nat. Genet.* **29**: 263 – 264 (2001).

Song, J. W., W. Gu, N. Futai, K. A. Warner, J. E. Nor and S. Takayama. Computer-controlled microcirculatory support system for endothelial cell culture and shearing. *Anal. Chem.* **77**: 3993 – 3999 (2005).

Srinivasan, V., V. K. Pamula and R. B. Fair. An integrated digital microfluidic lab-on-a-chip for clinical diagnostics on human physiological fluids. *Lab. Chip.* **4**: 310 – 315 (2004).

Stevens M. M. and J. H. George. Exploring and engineering the cell surface interface. *Science* **310**: 1135 – 1138 (2005).

Stratowa C., R. Abseher. Microarrays in disease and prognosis. In: *Encyclopedia of Life Sciences*. New York, NY: John Wiley & Sons Ltd. (2005).

Suh, K. Y., A. Khademhosseini, J. M. Yang, G. Eng and R. Langer. Soft lithgraphic patterning for long-term cell culture studies. *Adv. Mater*. **16**: 584 – 588 (2004).

Sunkara, V., B. J. Hong and J. W. Park. Sensitivity enhancement of DNA microarray on nano-scale controlled surface by using a streptavidin-fluorophore conjugate. *Biosens. Bioelectron.* 2006.

Takayama, S., E. Ostuni, P. LeDuc, K. Naruse, D. E. Ingber and G. M. Whitesides. Subcellular positioning of small molecules. *Nature* **411**: 1016 (2001).

Takayama, S., E. Ostuni, X. Qian, J. C. McDonald, X. Jiang, P. LeDuc, M.-H. Wu, D. Ingber and G. M. Whitesides. Topographical Micropatterning of Poly (dimethylsiloxane) Using Laminar Flows of Liquids in Capillaries. *Adv. Mater.* **13**: 570 – 574 (2001).

Takayama, S., J. C. McDonald, E. Ostuni, M. N. Liang, P. J. Kenis, R. F. Ismagilov and G. M. Whitesides. Patterning cells and their environments using multiple laminar fluid flows in capillary networks. *Proc. Natl. Acad. Sci. USA* **96**: 5545 – 5548 (1999).

Tang, M. D., A. P. Golden and J. Tien. Molding of three-dimensional microstructures of gels. *J. Am. Chem. Soc.* **125**: 12,988 – 12,989 (2003).

Taylor, A. M., M. Blurton-Jones, S. W. Rhee, D. H. Cribbs, C. W. Cotman and N. L. Jeon. A microfluidic culture platform for CNS axonal injury, regeneration and transport. *Nat. Methods*. **2**: 599 – 605 (2005).

Taylor, R. F. Microarrays. In: *Kirk-Othmer Encyclopedia of Chemical Technology*. vol. 16, pp. 380 – 394. New York, NY: John Wiley &Sons Ltd. (2005).

Teixeira, A. I., G. A. Abrams, P. J. Bertics, C. J. Murphy and P. F. Nealey. Epithelial contact guidance on well-defined micro- and nanostructured substrates. *J. Cell. Sci.* **116**: 1881 – 1892 (2003).

Thakar, R. G., F. Ho, N. F. Huang, D. Liepmann and S. Li. Regulation of vascular smooth muscle cells by micropatterning. *Biochem. Biophys. Res. Commun.* **307**: 883 – 890 (2003).

Thapa, A., T. J. Webster and K. M. Haberstroh. Polymers with nano-dimensional surface features enhance bladder smooth muscle cell adhesion. *J. Biomed. Mater. Res. A* **67**: 1374 – 1383 (2003).

Thorsen, T., S. J. Maerkl and S. R. Quake. Microfluidic large-scale integration. *Science* **298**: 580 – 584 (2002).

Timofeev, E., S. V. Kochetkova, A. D. Mirzabekov and V. L. Florentiev. Regioselective immobilization of short oligonucleotides to acrylic copolymer gels. *Nucleic Acids Res.* **24**: 3142 – 3148 (1996).

Tourovskaia, A., X. Figueroa-Masot and A. Folch. Differentiation-on-a-chip: A microfluidic platform for long-term cell culture studies. *Lab. Chip.* **5**: 14 – 29 (2005).

Unger, M. A., H. P. Chou, T. Thorsen, A. Scherer and S. R. Quake. Monolithic microfabricated valves and pumps by multilayer soft lithography. *Science* **288**: 113 – 116 (2000).

van Kooten, T. G., J. F. Whitesides and A. von Recum. Influence of silicone (PDMS) surface texture on human skin fibroblast proliferation as determined by cell cycle analysis. *J. Biomed. Mater. Res.* **43**: 1 – 14 (1998).

Vanderhoeven, J., K. Pappaert, B. Dutta, P. Vanhummelen, G. V. Baron and G. Desmet, Exploiting the benefits of miniaturization for the enhancement of DNA microarrays. *Electrophoresis* **25**: 3677 – 3686 (2004).

Vu, T. Q., R. Maddipati, T. A. Blute, B. J. Nehilla, L. Nusblat and T. A. Desai. Peptide-conjugated quantum dots activate neuronal receptors and initiate downstream signaling of neurite growth. *Nano. Lett.* **5**: 603 – 607 (2005).

Walboomers, X. F., H. J. Croes, L. A. Ginsel and J. A. Jansen. Contact guidance of rat fibroblasts on various implant materials. *J. Biomed. Mater. Res.* **47**: 204 – 212 (1999).

Walker G. M., D. J. Beebe. An evaporation-based microfluidic sample concentration method. *Lab. Chip* **2**: 57 – 61 (2002).

Wang, J., G. Sui, V. P. Mocharla, R. J. Lin, M. E. Phelps, H. C. Kolb and H. R. Tseng. Integrated microfluidics for parallel screening of an in situ click chemistry library. *Angew. Chem. Int. Ed. Engl.* **45**: 5276 – 5281 (2006).

Wang, W. U., C. Chen, K. H. Lin, Y. Fang and C. M. Lieber. Label-free detection of small-molecule-protein interactions by using nanowire nanosensors. *Proc. Natl. Acad. Sci. USA* **102**: 3208 – 3212 (2005).

Webster, T. J. Nanophase ceramics: The future orthopedic and dental implant material. In: *Nanostructured Materials*. New York, NY: Academic Press (2001).

Webster, T. J., C. Ergun, R. H. Doremus, R. W. Siegel and R. Bizios. Enhanced functions of osteoblasts on nanophase ceramics. *Biomaterials* **21**: 1803 – 1810 (2000).

Webster, T. J., C. Ergun, R. H. Doremus, R. W. Siegel and R. Bizios. Enhanced osteoclast-like cell functions on nanophase ceramics. *Biomaterials* **22**: 1327 – 1333 (2001).

Webster, T. J., R. W. Siegel and R. Bizios. Osteoblast adhesion on nanophase ceramics. *Biomaterials* **20**: 1221 – 1227 (1999).

Whitesides, G. M., E. Ostuni, S. Takayama, X. Jiang and D. E. Ingber. Soft lithography in biology and biochemistry. *Annu. Rev. Biomed. Eng.* **3**: 335 – 373 (2001).

Wu, X., S. Ding, Q. Ding, N. S. Gray and P. G. Schultz. A small molecule with osteogenesis-inducing activity in multipotent mesenchymal progenitor cells. *J. Am. Chem. Soc.* **124**: 14,520 – 14,521 (2002).

Wu, Y., P. de Kievit, L. Vahlkamp, D. Pijnenburg, M. Smit, M. Dankers, D. Melchers, M. Stax, P. J. Boender, C. Ingham, N. Bastiaensen, R. de Wijn, D. van Alewijk, H. van Damme, A. K. Raap, A. B. Chan and R. van Beuningen. Quantitative assessment of a novel flow-through porous microarray for the rapid analysis of gene expression profiles. *Nucleic. Acids. Res.* **32**: e123 (2004).

Xia Y. N. and G. M. Whitesides. Soft Lithography. *Angewandte Chemie-International Edition.* **37**: 550 – 575 (1998).

Yamamura, S., H. Kishi, Y. Tokimitsu, S. Kondo, R. Honda, S. R. Rao, M. Omori, E. Tamiya and A. Muraguchi. Single-cell microarray for analyzing cellular response. *Anal. Chem.* **77**: 8050 – 8056 (2005).

Yamato, M., M. Utsumi, A. Kushida, C. Konno, A. Kikuchi and T. Okano. Thermo-responsive culture dishes allow the intact harvest of multilayered keratinocyte sheets without dispase by reducing temperature. *Tissue Eng.* **7**: 473 – 480 (2001).

You, A. J., R. J. Jackman, G. M. Whitesides and S. L. Schreiber. A miniaturized arrayed assay format for detecting small molecule-protein interactions in cells. *Chem. Biol.* **4**: 969 – 975 (1997).

Zaari, N., S. K. Rajagopalan, S. K. Kim, A. J. Engler and J. Y. Wong. Photopolymerization in Microfluidic Gradient Generators: Microscale Control of Substrate Compliance to Manipulate Cell Response. *Adv. Mater.* 2133 – 2137 (2004).

Zheng, G., F. Patolsky, Y. Cui, W. U. Wang and C. M. Lieber. Multiplexed electrical detection of cancer markers with nanowire sensor arrays. *Nat. Biotechnol.* **23**: 1294 – 1301 (2005).

Zhu, H., J. F. Klemic, S. Chang, P. Bertone, A. Casamayor, K. G. Klemic, D. Smith, M. Gerstein, M. A. Reed and M. Snyder. Analysis of yeast protein kinases using protein chips. *Nat. Genet.* **26**: 283 – 289 (2000).

Zhu, H., M. Bilgin, R. Bangham, D. Hall, A. Casamayor, P. Bertone, N. Lan, R. Jansen, S. Bidlingmaier, T. Houfek, T. Mitchell, P. Miller, R. A. Dean, M. Gerstein and M. Snyder. Global analysis of protein activities using proteome chips. *Science* **293**: 2101 – 2105 (2001).

Zhu, X., K. L. Mills, P. R. Peters, J. H. Bahng, E. H. Liu, J. Shim, K. Naruse, M. E. Csete, M. D. Thouless and S. Takayama. Fabrication of reconfigurable protein matrices by cracking. *Nat. Mater.* **4**: 403 – 406 (2005).

Ziauddin J., D. M. Sabatini. Microarrays of cells expressing defined cDNAs. *Nature* **411**: 107 – 110 (2001).

Ziegler, C. Cantilever-based biosensors. *Anal. Bioanal. Chem.* **379**: 946 – 959 (2004).

Zirlinger, M., G. Kreiman and D. J. Anderson. Amygdala-enriched genes identified by microarray technology are restricted to specific amygdaloid subnuclei. *Proc. Natl. Acad. Sci. USA* **98**: 5270 – 5275 (2001).

14 Delivery System of Bioactive Molecules for Regenerative Medicine

Gilson Khang[1], Sun Jung Yoon[1], Soon Hee Kim[1],
Moon Suk Kim[2] and Hai Bang Lee[2]

[1] BK-21 Polymer BIN Fusion Res. Team, Chonbuk National University, Jeonju 561-756, Korea

[2] Nanobiomaterials Laboratory, Korea Research Institutes of Chemical Technology, Daejeon 305-606, Korea

Abstract It has been widely accepted that regenerative medicine as one part of nanomedicine offers an alternative technique to whole organ, tissue and cell transplantation for diseased, failed or malfunctioned body parts. To reconstruct a new tissue by regenerative medicine, triad components such as: (1) cells such as primary, adult and embryonic stem cell, (2) bioactive molecules such as hormone, cytokine, and growth factors and (3) delivery vehicles for cell and bioactive molecules must be needed.

Among of these three key components, the controlled release of bioactive molecule at molecular level from delivery vehicles might be played a very critical role in products of regenerative medicine. Especially, in order to differentiation of adult stem cell to specific cell and tissue, continuous release of bioactive vehicle can act to direct the growth of cells seeded within the porous structure of the delivery vehicle or of cells migrating from surrounding tissue, eventually mimicking a natural extracellular matrix. This chapter reviews the recent advances of (i) novel method of delivery system of bioactive molecule at molecular level, (ii) differentiation of adult stem cell using delivery system, and (iii) the effect of calcitriol with delivery vehicle as well as mesenchymal stem cells on bone formation in order to approach to a more natural three dimensional environment and support biological signals for tissue growth and reorganization.

14.1 Introduction

The nanomedicine may be broadly implicated as the comprehensive monitoring, control, construction, repair, defense, and improvement of all human biological

(1) Corresponding e-mail: gskhang@chonbuk.ac.kr

system, working from the molecular level using engineered devices, and nanostructures, ultimately to achieve medical benefit. Regenerative medicine as one of the most important part of nanomedicine was need to the materials to regulate cell signaling and differentiation and controlling morphogenesis resulting in helping to bring functional integration at molecular level (European Science Foundations, 2005). The goal of regenerative medicine as well as tissue engineering is to replace damaged or diseased tissue and organ with a biological substitute using triad components such as: (1) cells which are harvested and dissociated from the donor tissue including nerve, liver, pancreas, cartilage, and bone as well as precursor cells embryonic or adult stem cells, (2) bioactive molecules such as hormone, cytokine, and growth factor which are promoting cell adhesion, proliferation, migration, and differentiation by up-regulating the synthesis of protein, growth factors, and receptors, (3) delivery vehicles as scaffold substrates which could not only contain the cells but also provide constant and tailorable delivery of the bioactive molecules to the precise site where needed (Khang and Lee, 2001; Khang et al., 2006, 2007; Lee et al., 2003a).

Among of these three key components, the controlled release of bioactive molecules from delivery vehicles at the molecular level might be played a critical role in the development of biological substitutes on target (Baldwin and Saltzman, 1998; Tabata, 2000; Khang et al., 2003a). Especially, for the clinical application of adult stem cells, continuous release of bioactive molecules could act as chemoattractants to induce the differentiation of cells seeded within the porous structure of the implants or of cells migrating from surrounding tissue, eventually mimicking a natural extracelluar matrix (ECM) (Jorgensen et al., 2004; Khang et al., 2005; Kim et al., 2006; Krampera et al., 2006). This chapter reviews the recent advances of (1) novel method of delivery system of bioactive molecule at molecular level, (2) differentiation of adult stem cell using bioactive molecules delivery system, and (3) the effect of bone marrow-derived mesenchymal stem cell (BMSC) and calcitriol with delivery vehicle on bone formation in order to approach to a more natural three dimensional environment and support biological signals for tissue growth and reorganization.

14.2 Delivery Systems of Bioactive Molecules

14.2.1 Importance of Bioactive Molecules Release System for the Regenerative Medicine

Bioactive molecules including small and large molecules transmit signals to modulate cellular activity and tissue development such as cell patterning, motility, proliferation, aggregation, and gene expression. As in the development of the tissue engineered organs, regeneration of functional tissue requires maintenance of cell viability and differentiated function, encouragement of cell proliferation, modulation of the direction and speed of cell migration, and regulation of cellular adhesion. Table 14.1 listed typical bioactive molecules of potential application in regenerative medicine (Baldwin and Saltzman, 1998). For example, transforming growth factor-β_1 (TGF-β_1) might be required to induce cell proliferation as well as osteogenenic and chondrogenic differentiation of bone marrow derived stem cells (BMSCs), and brain-derivod neurotrophic (BDNF) can be enhanced to regenerate spinal cord injury. Also, Table 14.2 shows the typical formulations of bioactive molecules for stimuli with differentiation potential of BMSCs to desired cells to desired sites in the body such as adipogenesis, chondrogenesis, osteogenesis, tenogenesis, myogenesis, neurogenesis, and so on.

The common method for the delivery of bioactive molecules for the differentiation of stem cells is just formulation of chemical stimuli with nutrient media of cell culture dish. The most significant problem of the cocktail method of bioactive molecule in vitro and in vivo is the relatively short half-life, the relatively high molecular weight and size, very low tissue penetration, and potential toxicity of systemic level resulting in unwanted dedifferentiation of differentiated stem cell (Baldwin and Saltzman, 1998; Seal et al., 2001; Babensee et al., 2000; Tabata, 2000). One promising way of the improvement technique of their efficacy is the locally controlled release of bioactive molecules at the molecular level for desired release period by the impregnation into delivery vehicles using biomaterials. Through the impregnation into delivery vehicles, protein structure, and biological activity can be stabilized to a certain extent resulting in prolonging the release time at local site. The duration of bioactive molecules release from delivery

Table 14.1 Typical bioactive molecules of potential use in regenerative medicine (Baldwin and Saltzman, 1998)

Signaling to stem cell	Bioactive molecules	Half-life in blood plasma (min)	Potential use in regenerative medicine
Proliferation	Epidermal growth factor (EGF) Basic fibroblast growth factor (bFGF) TGF-β	2.32 1.5 11 – 160	Wound healing (Stimulation of cell growth)
Differentiation	nerve growth factor (NGF), BDNF bFGF	2.4 1.5	Maintenance of cell function
Migration	Formyl peptides NGF, BDNF	Varying 2.4	Inflammatory response Nerve regeneration
Aggregation	Antibodies HIV-1 Tat PEGylated peptide	Varying	Tissue formation

Table 14.2 Differentiation potential of bone marrow-derived mesenchymal stem cells (Khang et al., 2005)

Differentiation to:	Formulation of bioactive molecules of stimuli
Adipocytes	Dexamethasone + isobutylmethylxanthine Dexamethasone + isobutylmethylxanthine + indomethacin + insulin Dexamethasone + insulin
Chondrocytes	$TGF\beta_3$ + ascorbic acid $TGF\beta_1$ + ascorbic acid
Osteoblasts	Dexamethasone + β-glycerophosphate + ascorbic acid
Tenocytes	Bone morphogenetic protein-12 (BMP-12)
Hematopoietic Supporting stroma	Hydrocortisone + horse serum + hemopoietic stem cell
Skeletal muscle cell	5-Azacytidine
Smooth muscle cell	Platelet-derived growth factor-BB (PDGF-BB)
Cardiac muscle cell	bFGF
Astrocytes	Dimethylsulfoxide (DMSO) + dexamethasone
Oligodendrocytes Neurons	PDGF + EGF + linoleic acid

vehicles can be controlled by the types of biomaterials used, the loading amount of bioactive molecules, the formulation factors, and the fabrication process. The release mechanisms are largely divided to three categories such as (1) diffusion controlled, (2) degradation controlled, and (3) solvent controlled release mechanism through the selection of delivery vehicles. Mechanism of biodegradable delivery vehicles was controlled by degradation controlled, whereas that of nondegradable one was regulated by diffusion and/or solvent controlled. Desired release pattern such as constant, pulsatile, and time programmed behaviors along the specific site and the type of stem cell can be achieved by the appropriate combination of these mechanisms (Khang et al., 2003a). Also, release system of bioactive molecules might be designed in a variation with geometries and configurations such as scaffold, tube, nose, microsphere, injectable forms, micro- and nano-fiber, and so on (Gutowska et al., 2001; Qui and Park, 2001; Khang et al., 2003b).

Figures 14.1 and 14.2 show the typical example for the effect of delivery vehicles of bioactive molecules at molecular level. Figure 14.1 shows the successful neurogenesis of BMSCs using butylatehydroxyanisole (BHA) (Jang et al., 2005). One of significant drawback of cocktail methods was the dedifferentiation to original MSC due to short half life of bioactive molecules in in vitro and in vivo. However, Fig. 14.2 shows the neurogenesis of BMSC cell onto the BHA released poly (*L*-lactide-*co*-glycolide) (PLGA) film with various concentrations. We could observe that neuronal cell from stem cells were not dedifferentiated to original stem cell due to long acting released bioactivity from delivery vehicle. Table 14.3

lists delivery vehicles of various geometries loaded with different bioactive molecules for the application of regenerative medicine to various organs. Also, Table 14.4 lists the differentiation of MSC using delivery vehicles of various geometries loaded with different bioactive molecules.

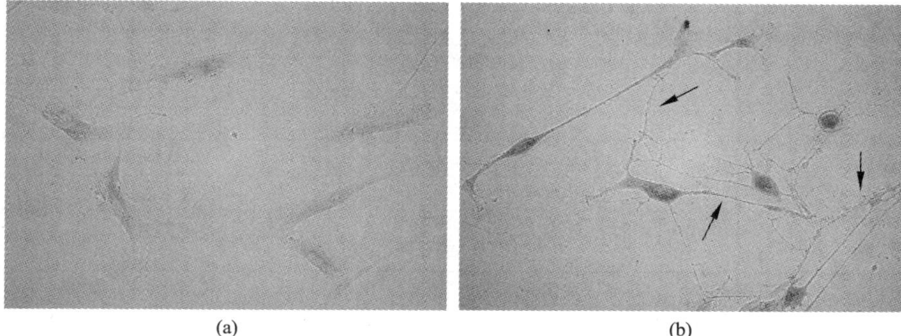

Figure 14.1 Neurogenesis of BMSCs using BHA in nutrient media. (a) Control and (b) 200 μmol/L BHA in DMEM after 2 h. Neuronal axon can be observed (arrow). Neuronal cells were stained by NSE. One of significant drawback of cocktail methods is the dedifferentiation to original BMSCs due to short half life of bioactive molecules in vitro and in vivo

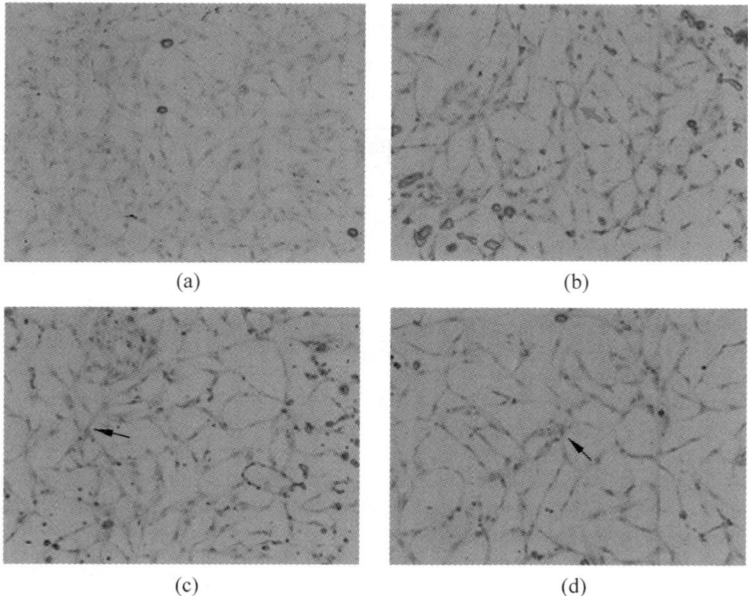

Figure 14.2 Neurogenesis of BMSCs onto the BHA released PLGA film. (a) Control, (b) 200 μmol/L, (c) 400 μmol/L and (d) 600 μmol/L BHA in PLGA (10 cm × 10 cm). Neuronal axon can be observed (arrow). Neuronal cells were stained by neurospecific enolase (NSE) at (b), (c) and (d), whereas (a) was not stained by NSE. Also, neurogenesis stem cells were not dedifferentiated to original stem cell due to long acting released bioactive molecule

Table 14.3 Delivery vehicles of various geometries loaded with different bioactive molecules for the application of regenerative medicine to various organs

Geometry	Matrix	Cytokine	Target organ	Reference
Scaffold	PLGA	BDNF	SCI	Kim et al., 2004 Kim et al., 2005a
	PPF/β-TCP	BMP-2	Bone	Chu et al., 2006
	PLGA	dexamethasone/ ascrobate-2-phosphate	Bone	Kim et al. 2005b
	PLGA	EGF	Liver	Mayer et al., 2000
	PLGA	VEGF		Sheridan et al., 2000
	Chitosan/ PLGA	PDGF-BB	Bone	Lee et al., 2002
	Chitosan	TGF-β_1	Cartilage	Kim et al., 2003
	Collagen	FGF-2	Enthothelialization	Côte et al., 2004
	Titanium fiber / Ca·P cement	TGF-β/BMP-2	Bone	Jansen et al., 2005
	PLLA	Bay K8644	Bone	Wood et al., 2006
Injectable gel	PLA-DX-PEG/ β-TCP	rh BMP-2	Bone	Yoneda et al., 2005
	Collagen	VEGF	Bone	Kleinheinz et al., 2005
	PNiPAAm	IGF-1, TGF-β_2	Catilage	Yasuda et al., 2006
	PLA-PEG-PLA	NT-3	SCI	Piantino et al., 2006
	Fibrin	NT-3	SCI	Taylor et al., 2006
	Fibirn	NT-3 (conjugate)	Endothelialization	Zisch et al., 2001
	Alginate	VEGF/bFGF	Cardiovascular	Lee et al., 2003
	OPF	TGF-β_1	Cartilage	Holland et al., 2005
	PEG-graft-chitosan	BSA		Bhattarai et al., 2005
	Fibrin	BFGF		Jeon et al., 2005
Microspheres	PLGA (PEG-diamine (gel))	TGF-β	Cartilage	DeFail et al., 2006
	PLGA	GDNF	CNS	Aubert-Pouëssel et al., 2004
	PLGA/PEG (POF:gel)	TP-508	Bone	Hedberg et al., 2002
	PLGA	EGF	SCI	Goraltchouk et al., 2006
Nanofiber	PLGA	PDGF-BB		Wei et al., 2006
	RADA16	4-PSA		Nagai et al., 2006

(1) PLA: poly (*L*-lactide); PLA: poly (lactide); DX: *p*-dioxanone; PEG: polyethylene glycol; SCI: Spinal cordinjury; VEGF: vascular endothelial cell growth factor; EGP: epithelial growth factor; PNiPAAm: poly (N-isopropylacrglamide); PPF: poly (propylene fumarate); β-TCP: β-tricalcium phosphate; IGF-I: insulin-like growth factor-1.

Table 14.4 Differentiation of MSCs using delivery vehicles of various geometries loaded with different bioactive molecules

Diffenentiation	Geometry	Matrix	Cytokine	Types of Stem cell	Reference
Osteogenesis	Hydrogel	Heparin-PEO	BMP-2	hMSC	Benoit et al., 2007
	Nanofiber	Nanosilk-fibrion	BMP-2	hBMSC	Li et al., 2006
	Hydrogel	MPEG-PCL	Dexamethasone	rBMSC	Kim et al., 2006
	Microspheres	PLGA	TGF-β_3	hMSC	Moioli et al., 2006
	Scaffold	SPCL	TGF-β_1, PPGF, BMP, IGF	rBMSC	Gomes et al., 2006
	Scaffold	CaP	TGF-β_1	rBMSC	Siebers et al., 2006
Osteogenesis Chondrogenesis	Scaffold	Collagen/GAG	Dexamethasone, ascorbate, β-glycerolphosphate	rMSC	Farrell et al., 2006
Chondrogenesis	Beads	Alginate/ collagen	TGF-β_1	BBMSC	Bosnakovski et al., 2006
	Microspheres	Alginate	TGF-β_1	hBMSC, hADASC	Mehlhorn et al., 2006
	Microspheres	Alginate/ chitosan	TGF-β_3 /Dexamethasone + ascorbate + ITX	hMSC	Pound et al., 2006
	Hydrogel	TGD-PEGDA		hESC	Hwang et al., 2006
Neurogenesis	Film	PLGA	BHA	rBMSC	Jang et al., 2005

(1) PEO: polyethyleneoxide; MPEG-PCL: methoxy(polyethyleneglycol)-poly(ε-caprolactone).

14.2.2 Scaffold System

A biodegradable and porous PLGA scaffold has been proposed for the application of bioactive molecule carrier and regeneration of spinal cord injury. BDNF loaded cylindrical PLGA scaffolds was prepared by ice-particle leaching method to control release from porous polymer scaffolds as shown in Fig. 14.3 (Kim et al., 2004; Kim et al., 2005a). The release amount of BDNF from BDNF loaded PLGA scaffold was observed over 4 weeks period in vitro at PBS, 37℃ and analyzed by ELISA. Prepared PLGA scaffold had uniform porosity and good interconnection between pores. Release amount of BDNF increased with increasing BDNF content as shown in Fig. 14.4. In in vivo animal experiment, a dramatically increased behavioral result has been observed using BDNF-loaded PLGA scaffolds with rBMSC in 3 mm cutting model for spinal cord injury. These results suggested that the release bioactive molecules can be useful for the nerve regeneration in the neural regenerative medicine area.

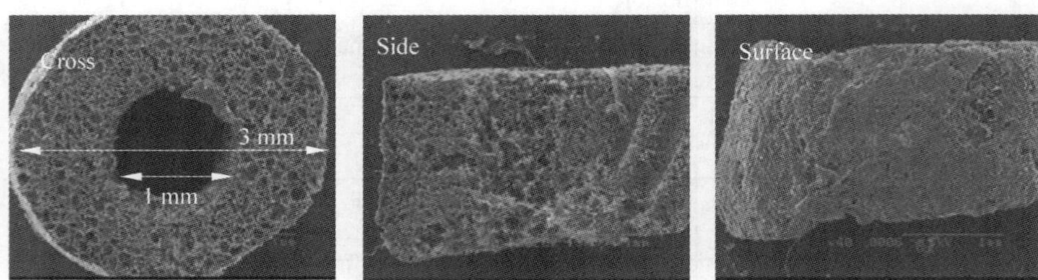

Figure 14.3 BDNF loaded PLGA scaffold as nerve conduit guidance. This nerve conduit guidance acts as delivery carrier of BDNF as well as undifferentiated stem cells to enhance the regeneration of spinal cord injury. Released BDNF induces and stimulates the neurogenesis of BMSCs

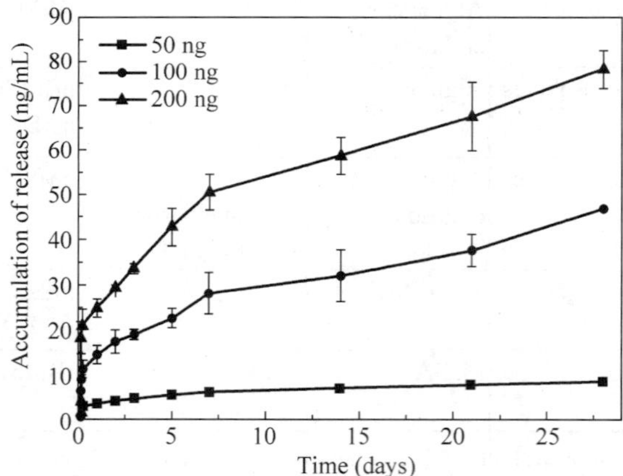

Figure 14.4 BDNF release from BDNF loaded PLGA scaffold with different loading amount of BDNF. Release of amount of bioactive molecules could be controlled by the loading amount

Chu et al., (2006) developed a tube-shaped composite scaffold made from PPF/TCP as structural component and dicalcium phosphate delyclrate (DCPD) mixture cement as bone morphogenetic protein (BMP) carrier. The scaffolds were implanted in 5 mm segmental bone defects in rat femur stabilized with a K-wire as intramedullary pin for 15 weeks with and without rhBMP-2. Results showed that the BMP loaded scaffolds had formed and bridged across the gap defect at 3 weeks, and restored the mechanical property of the rat femur after 15 weeks.

A porous PLGA scaffold contained dexamethasone and ascrobate-2-phosphate was prepared by solvent casting/salt leaching technique (Kim et al., 2005b). The fabricated scaffolds released dexamethasone and ascrobate-2-phosphate continuously over 3 months with almost zero-order release pattern. hMSCs in the scaffolds expressed high alkaline phosphatase and substantial mineralization was observed in the experimental scaffold with hMSCs in nude mouse model. There was no significant calcification at 9 weeks in control scaffolds and in the experimental scaffolds without hMSCs.

A woven polyethyleneterephtalate fabric was coated on one side with a biodegradable PLGA films impregnated with EGF in order to obtain a geometrically polarized scaffold structure for a bioartificial liver (Mayer et al., 2000). Hepatocyte culturing studies reveal that the formation of aggregates depends on mesh size and release patterns of EGF. VEGF was loaded in PLGA scaffold for the promotion of angiogenesis using a gas foaming processing approach with ~95% porosity (Sheridan et al., 2000). VEGF was subsequently incorporated into scaffold during the fabrication process and released in a controlled manner. Importantly, the released growth factor retains over 90% of its bioactivity. This study was successfully demonstrated a potential application for the bioactive molecules delivery vehicles for the neovascularization.

Lee et al. (2002) investigated new matrix based on chitosan/PLLA hybrid scaffold impregnated with PDGF-BB. Chitosan and PDGF-BB loaded PLLA scaffold induced increased osteoblast attachment as compared with intact PLLA. Results of this study demonstrated the usefulness of chitosan as drug releasing scaffolds and PDGF-BB as bioactive molecule to enhance tissue regeneration efficacy. For the regeneration of cartilage, Kim et al. (2003) attempted to design a novel type of porous chitosan scaffold containing TGF-β_1 to enhance chondrogenesis by emulsion method with 200 nm – 1.5 μm. The release rate of TGF-β_1 was much lower than that of bovine serum albumin over 10 days. It is obviously demonstrated from in vitro test that TGF-β_1 loaded scaffolds significantly augments the cell proliferation and production of ECM due to the long acting of TGF-β_1. These results suggest that the TGF-β_1 loaded chitosan delivery vehicle possesses a promising potential as an implant to cartilage defects.

A block copolymer of PLA-DX-PEG was used as an rhBMP-2 delivery vehicle for osteogenic materials (Yoneda et al., 2005). Three porous β-TCP cylinders were coated with the rhBMP-2/PLA-DX-PEG composite and then the prepared implants were studied in a critical-sized rabbit bone defect model. Bony union of the defect was recognized only in the BMP loaded group by radiography. The result of mechanical property of the repaired bone examined by the 3-point bending test was equivalent to the nonoperated-on femur at 24 weeks.

Denatured collagen scaffold has been demonstrated as a bioactive molecule delivery vehicle of FGF-2 for stimulation of angiogenesis (Côte et al., 2004). Titanium fiber mesh and porous CaP cement scaffolds were applied as delivery vehicle of rhTGF-β_1 and rhBMP-2 for bone regeneration (Jansen et al., 2005).

Quantification of the bone growth revealed that bone formation was increased significantly in all deliver vehicles by administration of rhTGF-β_1 and rhBMP-2. Also, Bay K8644 as calcium channel agonist released PLLA scaffold was developed for bone regeneration using perfusion-compression bioreactor resulting in the stable and maintaining of its bioactivity following culture of up to 28 days (Wood et al., 2006).

14.2.3 Injectable Hydrogel System

Injectable hydrogel system could be more convenient compared than scaffold system due to the delivery with minimal invasive operations. Collagen hydrogel system complexed with rhVEGF was manufactured to activate angiogenesis during cortical bone repair (Kleinheinz et al., 2005). Bicortical hole rabbit mandible was filled with optimized implants consisting of Type Ⅰ collagen matrix and rhVEGF$_{165}$. After 28 days, capillaries within regenerated bone and bone marrow were clearly shown and significant differences of bone density were found between control and study groups. This study showed that local release of rhVEGF165 enhanced angiogenesis in the defect area and thus improved osteogenesis.

The potential of a novel thermoreversible gelation polymer used by PNiPAAm was proposed to act as a three dimensional hydrogel scaffold and deliver both chondrocyte and growth factors (Yasuda el al., 2006). Chondrocytes suspended in chilled aqueous solutions of hydrogel in the presence or absence of the growth factors insulin-like growth factor-1 (IGF-1) and/or TGF-β_2. The cold cell/polymer suspensions were injected into a cylindrical silastic tube for molding and cultured at 37℃ for up to 16 weeks. The glycosaminoglycan and hydroxyproline contents in the specimens increased as a function of time and because of the presence of growth factors; those cultured with growth factors produced significantly more of these substances than those cultured without. Another thermosensitive hydrogel as PEG-grafted chitosan has been prepared to delivered protein drug for the application of regenerative medicine (Bhattarai et al., 2005).

Jain et al. (2006) demonstrated that BDNF loaded lipid microtubules and hydroethylated agarose was used to promote regeneration in the injured spinal cord. BDNF was loaded into lipid microtubules by incubating the BDNF solution with dehydrated microtubules. The results showed that the agarose gel not only conformed to the shape of the spinal cord cavity as it gelled in situ at 37.1℃, but also provided a carrier of microtubules loaded with BDNF. The degree of chondroitin sulfate proteoglycans and reactive astrocytes was reduced and the ability of regenerating fibers to enter the permissive hydrogel scaffold was enhanced with the delivery of BDNF to the lesion site after a dorsal over-hemisection injury in adult rats.

The degradable PEG hydrogels as a way to deliver nerotropin-3 (NT-3) that promote axon growth in the spinal cord injury model of adult rats has been attempted (Piantino et al., 2006). Hydrogel/NT-3-treated animals showed improved recovery in the locomotion tests compared to controls implanted with hydrogel alone. In the histological result, specimens with hydrogel/NT-3-treated animals showed increased axonal regeneration than controls in two major descending pathways for motor control, the corticospinal tract and the raphespinal tract. Fibrin as delivery carrier for NT-3 and vascular endothelial cell growth factor (VEGF) also applied to enhances neuronal fiber sprouting after spinal cord injury (Taylor et al., 2006) and endothelialization (Zisch et al., 2001), respectively. The kinetics of bFGF release from fibrin gel with various concentrations of fibrinogen, thrombin, and heparin was evaluated (Jeon et al., 2005). The rate of bFGF release from fibrin gel can be controlled and bFGF delivery carrier revealed therapeutic potential for angiogenesis on mouse ischemic limbs model.

Alginate injectable gel loaded with VEGF and bFGF on angiogenesis were compared (Lee et al., 2003b). This work suggested the utility of both VEGF and bFGF in promoting angiogenesis and VEGF is more appropriate for creating a dense bed of new blood vessels. Synthetic degradable oligo-PEG-fumarate hydrogel as a cell and bioactive molecules carriers for non-invasive means was tested for regeneration of cartilage (Holland et al., 2005). Dual growth factor as inhibitory leukemia factor-1 (ILF-1) and TGF-β_1 has been impregnated in synthetic hydrogel resulting in controllable release profile.

14.2.4 Microspheres System

Figure 14.5 shows the cultivation of human disc cell isolated from intervertebral discs on the TGF-β_1 impregnated PLGA microspheres for 3 days (Khang et al., submitted). Advantage of this method is able to mass culture due to large surface area and to inject using gage needle cell culture mass with noninvasive method.

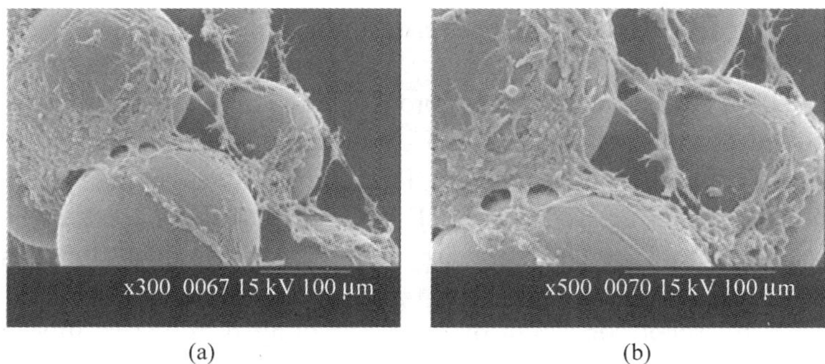

Figure 14.5 Attachment, expansion, and cell aggregation on TGF-β_1 impregnated PLGA microspheres cultured human disc cells: scanning electron microscope (SEM) at 3 days

DeFail et al. (2006) have encapsulated TGF-β_1 into PLGA microspheres, and subsequently incorporated the microspheres into biodegradable PEO-based hydrogels. The controlled release of TGF-β_1 encapsulated within microspheres embedded in scaffolds is better controlled when compared to delivery from microspheres alone and the burst release was decreased when the microspheres were embedded in the hydrogels. The concentration of TGF-β_1 released from the gels can be controlled by both the mass of microspheres embedded in the gel. These TGF-β_1 encapsulated microspheres embedded within biodegradable hydrogels could be applied to cartilage tissue formation.

GDNF releasing PLGA microsphere has been carried out (Aubert-Pouëssel et al., 2004). Various drugs, especially therapeutic proteins like neurotrophic factors such as NGF, CNTF and BDNF have been encapsulated in this type of brain delivery system. The release profile for the GDNF loaded microspheres was assessed in a low continuous flow system and showed a sustained release of effective GDNF doses over 56 days. Biodegradable GDNF releasing microspheres may represent an attractive alternative strategy in the treatment of pathologies such as Parkinson's disease.

PLGA/PEG blend microsphere loaded with osteogenic peptide TP508 were added to a mixture of PPF and sodium chloride for the fabrication of carrier that could allow for tissue ingrowth as well as for the controlled release kinetics of TP508 when implanted in an orthopedic defect site (Hedberg et al., 2002). These delivery vehicles could be applied to the formation of bone in vivo with various release kinetics and dosages. Goraltchouk et al. (2006) have been attempted the incorporation of bioactive molecule eluting PLGA microspheres into biodegradable nerve guidance channels for controlled release. EGF, co-encapsulated with PLGA microspheres in nerve guidance channel, was released for 56 days. Released EGF was found to be bioactive for at least 14 days as assessed by a neurosphere forming bioassay.

14.2.5 Nanofiber Scaffold System

Wei et al. (2006) have developed nanofibrous scaffold in a diameter of 50 – 500 nm for controlled delivery of rhPDGF-BB by means of the combination of phase separation and sugar leaching method. This diameter was similar size range to native collagen fiber. Released PDGF-BB was demonstrated to possess biological activity as evidenced by the stimulation of human gingival fibroblast DNA synthesis in vitro.

Biological hydrogel consisting of self-assembling peptide nanofibers can be used an excellent material in a broad range of biomedical and biological application ranging from three-dimensional scaffold matrix for regenerative medicine to bioactive molecules delivery vehicles (Zhang, 2003; Keyes-Baig et al., 2004;

Nagai et al., 2006). The individual nanofiber consists of ionic self-complementary peptides with 16 amino acids (RADA16) that are characterized by a stable β-sheet structure and undergo self-assembly into hydrogel containing ~ 99.5% *w*/*v* water. These nanofiber systems were well characterized and tested in a variety of regenerative medicine research application (Ellis-Behnke et al., 2006).

14.3 Differentiation of Adult Stem Cells Using Delivery System of Bioactive Molecules

Embryonic and adult mesnechymal stem cells are toti- and multi-potent cells, respectively. Among of these cells, MSCs can differentiate into mesenchyme-derived cell types such as an osteoblasts, chondorocytes, adipocytes and neuronal cells as discussed earlier (Figs. 14.1 and 14.2). The differentiation process of MSC may be stimulated by specific bioactive molecules, biophysical stimulation and appropriate and suitable three dimension environment as listed in Table 14.4.

14.3.1 Osteoegensis of MSC

Benoit et al. (2007) demonstrated the effect of heparin-functionalized PEG hydrogels impregnated with BMP2 and fibronectin on three dimensional hMSC osteogenic differentiation. BMP2 availability increased both ALP production and osteopontin gene expression, while fibronectin increased ALP production but not osteogenic gene expression. For the application to bone regeneration, BMP-2 loaded silk nanofibers prepared by electrospinning process were used from hMSC. hMSC were cultured for up 31 days under static condition in osteogenic media on functional scaffolds (Li et al., 2006). It could be observed electrospun nano-silk fibroin scaffolds supported hMSC growth and differentiation toward osteogenic outcomes.

MPEG-PCL diblock copolymer as thermo-sensitive hydrogels were synthesized (Kim et al., 2006). This gel mixed with rBMSC and dexamethasone was implanted in Sprague-Dawley rat. H&E and von Kossa staining were revealed that bone formation increased markedly with increasing dexamethasone concentration. It concluded that in situ gel carrier from synthetic hydrogel solution containing dexamethasone enable multipotent rBMSCs to produce viable bone when injected into rats.

TGF-β_3 loaded PLGA microspheres induced osteogenic differentiation from hMSC due to the controlled release of TGF-β_3 (Moioli et al., 2006). Farrell et al. (2006) reported a collagen-glycosaminoglycan scaffold system supported adult rMSC differentiation along osteogenic and chondrogenic routs. In this experiment, osteogenic factors were used as 10 nmol/L dexamethasone, 50 μmol/L ascorbic acid and 10 mmol/L β-glycerolphosphate. Osteogenesis was successfully performed by the analysis of the bone specific proteins, collagen I and osteocalcin and subsequent matrix mineralization.

Gomes et al. (2006) attempted in vitro localization of bone growth factors (TGF-β_1, PDGF, BMP and IGF) in construct of biodegradable scaffolds seeded with MSC and cultured in a flow perfusion reactor. Results showed that flow perfusion bioreactor culture of MSCs combined with the use of delivery vehicle may form bony structure. For the fabrication of TGF-β_1 release carrier, a porous β-TCP coating was deposited with electrostatic spray deposition method and 10 ng of TGF-β_1 was loaded on the substrate (Siebers et al., 2006). While proliferation of osteoblast-like cells was increased on TGF-β_1 loaded substrates, differentiation was inhibited or delayed. So, TGF-β_1 loaded porous β-TCP coating as a carrier materials is very useful for the controlled of differentiation of MSCs.

14.3.2 Chondrogenesis of MSCs

In order to investigate influence of collagen Type II ECM on MSC chondrogenesis, bovine MSCs were culture in two dimension as well as three dimension as alginate and collagen Type I and Type II hydrogel in both serum free medium and medium supplemented with TGF-β_1 (Bosnakovski et al., 2006). Differentiation was most prominent in cells cultured in collagen Type II hydrogel and it increased in a time-dependent manner. Additionally, the chondrogenesis influence of TGF-β_1 on MSCs cultured in collagen-incoporated ECM was analyzed. TGF-β_1 and dexamethasone treatment in the presence of collagen Type II provided more favorable conditions for expression of the chondrogenic phenotypes.

The differentiation expression pattern of ECM molecules in BMSC and adipose-derived adult system cells (ADASCs) following chondrogenic differentiation has been observed using TGF-β_1 loaded alginate microspheres (Mehlhorn et al., 2006). In response to TGF-β_1, collagen Type II and X were secreted more strongly by BMSCs than by ADASCs. BMSCs express a more mature phenotype than ADASCs after chondroinduction. TGF-β_1 induces alternative splicing of the α_1-procollagen Type II transcript in BMSCs, but not in ADASCs. This means that TGF-β_1 loaded alginate system acts to prevent hypertrophy in BMSCs or to promote chondrogenic maturation in ADASCs.

Another system using alginate/chitosan microcapsule impregnated with TGF-β_3 has been investigated for the promotion of chondrogenesis and osteogenesis from hBMSCs (Pound et al., 2006). Results demonstrated the important role of robust biomimicking nano-environment for the development of neoorgan. Human embryonic stem cell-derived cells in arginine-glycine-aspartale (RGD) modified poly(ethyleneglycol)-diacrylate (PEGDA) hydrogel was used for the possibility of chondrogenic differentiation (Hwang et al., 2006). In PEDGA hydrogels containing exogenous hyaluronic acid or Type Ⅰ collagen, no significant cell growth or matrix production was observed. In contrast, when these cells were encapsulated in RGD-modified PEDGA hydrogel, neocartilage with basophilic ECM deposition was observed within 3 weeks of culture, producing cartilage-specific gene up-regulation and ECM production. This result showed the importance for the three dimension environment of the tissue formation.

14.4 Repair of Diaphyseal Long Bone Defect with Calcitriol Released Delivery Vehicle and MSCs

Repairing large loaded bone defects using osteoconductive biomaterials alone remains a challenge because osteogenic cells are not likely to be recruited in the center of large defects without osteogenesity, and lack of absorbability, there remains significant obstacles to remodeling necessary to withstand repetitive mechanical loading (Khang et al., 2004, 2006). Therefore, biomaterials used to repair large loaded bone defects should not only have osteoconductive and osteoinductive properties, but also resorb completely without residual materials. Calcitriol loaded PLGA scaffolds and MSCs were used to prepare a fully absorbable, osteogenic biomaterial-cells complex for repairing loaded large bone defect as shown in Fig. 14.6. Calcitriol loaded PLGA scaffold was manufactured by solvent casting/salt leaching method, and MSCs seeded scaffolds were implanted

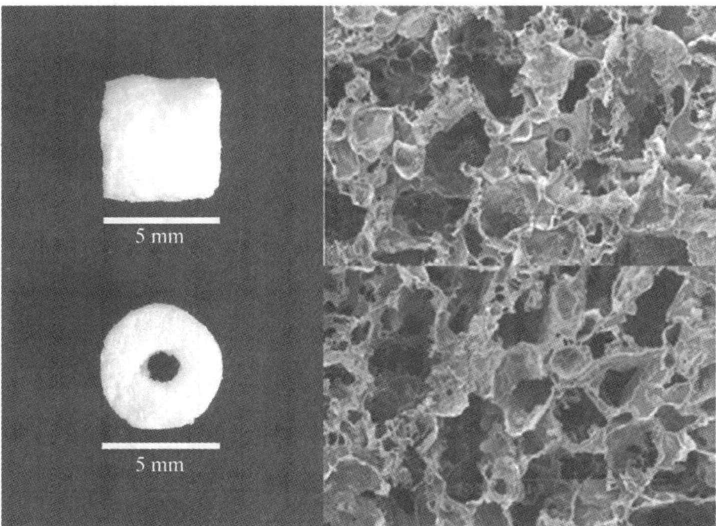

Figure 14.6 Macroscopic aspect of porous cylindrical calcitriol-loaded PLGA scaffold and SEM micrographs (original magnification × 100); images at left are axial and side views of the scaffold, and at right are SEM micrographs of surface (above) and cross section (below) of the scaffold

into critical sized diaphyseal defect of rabbit femur. The osteogenesity and degradability of the implants were confirmed by X-ray analysis, 3D-CT, RT-PCR, von Kossa and Masson's trichrome staining staining (Yoon et al., 2007a).

The calcitriol-loaded groups showed a time-dependent increase in callus more than 80% at 6 weeks, but the PLGA group without calcitriol showed only small amount of newly formed bone formation-less than 40% (Figs. 14.7 and 14.8). The 3-D CT image and frontal tomographic image of regenerated femurs showed that normal femur anatomy had been restored with cortical bone with no residual evidence of implanted PLGA scaffolds. Whereas calcitriol/PLGA with MSCs implants induced completely repair of entire cortex, calcitriol/PLGA without MSCs implants showed a partial cortical defect with incompletely regeneration of marrow cavity as shown in Fig. 14.9. In calcitriol-loaded groups, an abundance of new osteoid matrix on the inside of scaffold was observed at 2 weeks (Fig. 14.10). New bone formation was more evident in the calcitriol/PLGA/MSCs group.

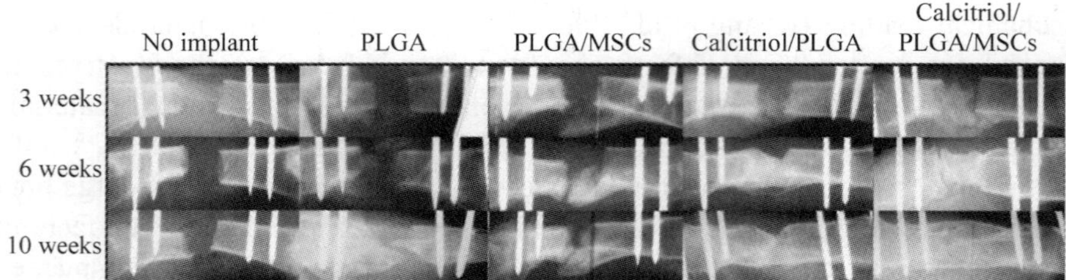

Figure 14.7 Representative femur radiographs. From left, critical size bone defect without implantation (sham surgery), implanted PLGA alone, calcitriol-loaded PLGA, PLGA/MSCs, calcitriol-loaded PLGA/MSCs. Sequential radiographs show bone repair at 3, 6, and 10 weeks after implantation

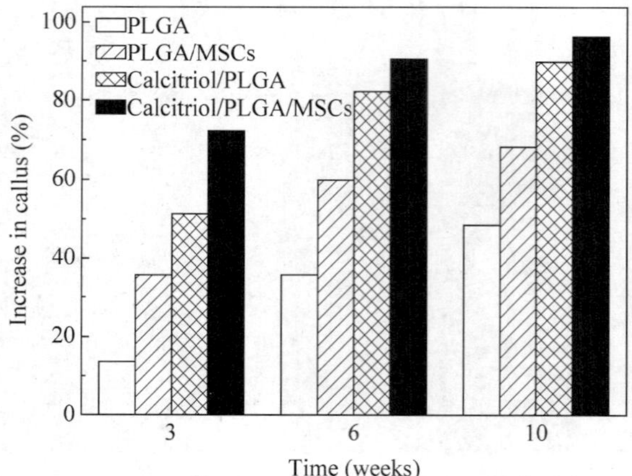

Figure 14.8 Calcitriol-loaded groups promoting a time-dependent increase in callus (nearly 100% at 10 weeks). The group PLGA combined MSCs promoted only small amount new bone formation

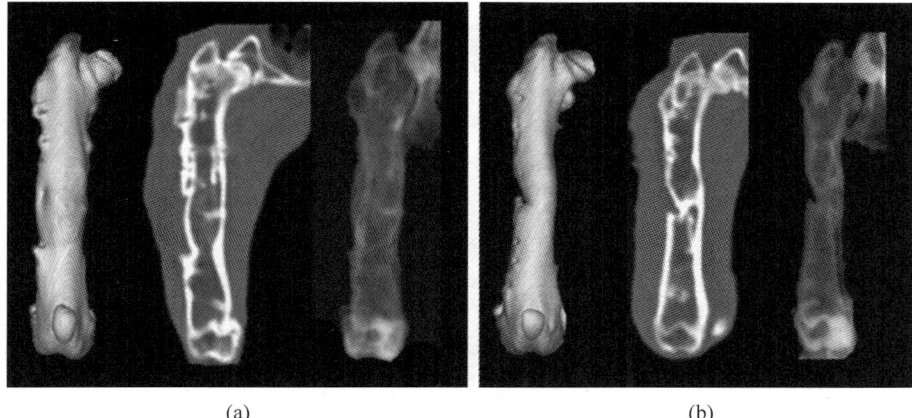

Figure 14.9 3D CT images of femur 20 weeks after surgery. The repaired defect with calcitriol-loaded scaffolds with MSCs is shown at left (a) and the implanted site with calcitriol-loaded scaffolds without MSCs is shown at right (b). The external fixator was removed 8 weeks after surgery. Note that PLGA was absorbed and cortical walls remodeled anatomically with the marrow cavity

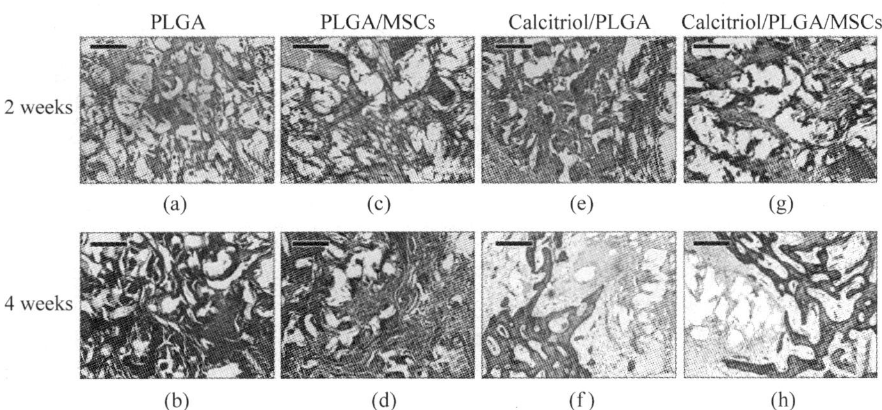

Figure 14.10 New bone deposition occurs at 14 days during healing of segmental bone defect filled with calcitriol-loaded PLGA groups compared to PLGA alone groups. Samples were analyzed at 2 weeks (a), (c), (e), (g) and 4 weeks (b), (d), (f), (h) postsurgery. (Scale bar = 200 μm)

Conversely, PLGA groups did not exhibit evidence of new osteoid matrix until postsurgical day 28. ALP upregulation of the calcitriol-loaded groups was detected at 10 day by RT-PCR compared to the calcitriol-unloaded groups, whether MSCs were seeded or not. Additionally, MSCs in calcitriol-loaded scaffold expressed an increased level of ALP, osteonectin and Type Ⅰ collagen mRNA as shown in Fig. 14.11. This experiment indicated that a slow-release mechanism of bioactive molecules play an important role to endow osteoinductivity to biomaterials and bioactive molecules loaded scaffold combined with MSCs might accelerate bone formation (Yoon et al., 2007b).

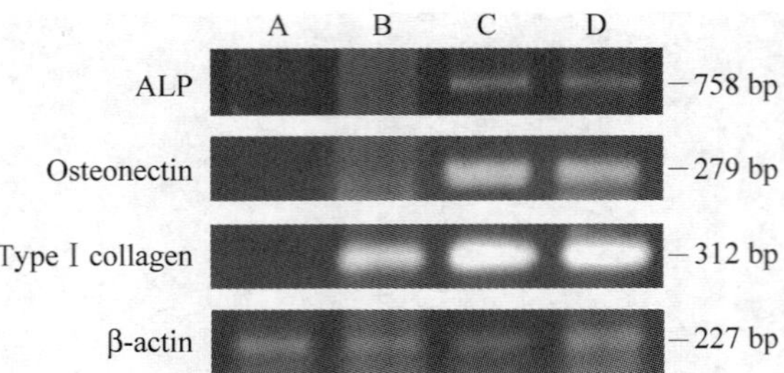

Figure 14.11 RT-PCR analysis of mRNA expression. RT-PCR analyses for markers of osteoblast differentiation were performed to evaluate osteoinductivity of the implanted scaffolds. Note the increase in the mRNA expression of ALP, osteonectin and type Ⅰ collagen of calcitriol-loaded groups (Ⅰ, Ⅲ). Representative agarose gels are shown. A: PLGA, B: PLGA/MSCs, C: Calcitriol/PLGA, and D: Calcitirol/PLGA/MSCs

14.5 Future Directions

Another available emerging technology is the tethering to the surface that is immobilization of protein on the surface of delivery vehicles. Immobilization of insulin and transferrin to the poly(methylmetacrylate) films stimulates the growth of fibroblast cell compared to same concentrations of soluble or physically adsorbed proteins (Griffith and Naughton, 2002; Ito et al., 1991). For the enhancement of bioactivity of bioactive molecules, PEO chain was applied as a short spacer between the surface of scaffold and the cytokine. Tethered EGF, immobilized to the scaffold through PEO chain, showed more improved DNA synthesis or cell rounding compared to the physically adsorbed EGF surface (Khul and Grriffith-Cima, 1996).

Conjugation of cytokine with inert carrier prolongs the short half-life of protein molecules. Inert carriers are albumin, gelatin, dextran, and PEG. Especially, PEGylation that means PEG conjugated bioactive molecules is most widely used for the release. It appears to decrease the rate of cytokine degradation, attenuate the immunological response, and reduce clearance by the kidneys (Hench and Polak, 2002; Duncan and Spreafico, 1994). Also, these PEGylated cytokine can be impregnated into delivery vehicle materials by physical entrapment for the sustained release. For example, NGF-conjugated dextran impregnated polymeric device was implanted directly into the brain of adult rats. Conjugated NGF could be penetrated into the brain tissue eight times than the unconjugated NGF. This conjugation method can be applied to the delivery of a proteins and peptides. Immobilized RGD and tyrosin-leucine-glycine-serine-arginine (YIGSR) which are typical ECM proteins onto the biomaterials can enhance cell viability, function and recombinant products in cell (Massia and Hubbell, 1990).

Gene-activating delivery vehicles are being designed to deliver to targeted gene resulting in the stimulation of specific cellular responses at the molecular level (Baldwin and Saltzman, 1998; Griffith and Naughton, 2002; Babensee et al., 2000). Modification of bioactive molecules with resorbable biomaterials systems obtains specific interactions with cell integrins resulting in cell activation. These bioactive bioglasses and macroporous delivery vehicles also can be designed to activate genes that stimulate regeneration of living tissue (Hench and Polak, 2002). Gene delivery would be accomplished by complexation with positively charged polymers, encapsulation, and gel by means of delivery vehicles structure (Gutowska et al., 2001). Methods of gene delivery for gene-activating delivery vehicles are almost same manner with those of protein, drug, and peptides.

14.6 Conclusion

Regenerative medicine is very important part of nanomedicine area. For the accomplishment of organ regeneration, cell delivery vehicles with controlled release system at molecular level and various geometries at sub-cell level must be needed for organ regeneration and tissue formation. Bioactive molecules released scaffolds are very effective for tissue formation. This effectiveness is amplified to incorporate with MSCs.

Acknowledgements

This work was supported by Stem Cell Research Center of Korea (SC3100).

References

Aubert-Pouëssel, A., M.C. Venier-Julienne, A. Clavreul, M. Sergent, C. Jollivet, C.N. Montero-Menei, E. Garcion, D.C. Bibby, P. Menei and J.P. Benoit. *J. Control. Release* **95**: 463 (2004).

Babensee, J.E, L.V. McIntire and A.G. Mikos. *Pharm. Res.* **17**: 497 (2000).

Baldwin, S.P., W.M. Saltzman. *Adv. Drug Deliv. Rev* **33**: 71 (1998).

Benoit, D.S.W., A.R. Durney and K.S. Anseth. *Biomaterials* **28**: 66 (2007).

Bhattarai, N., H.R. Ramay, J.Gunn, F.A. Matsen and M. Zhang. *J. Control. Release* **103**: 609 (2005).

Bosnakovski, D., M. Mizuno, G. Kim, S. Takagi, M. Okumura and T. Fujinaga. *Biotechnol. Bioeng.* **93**: 1152 (2006).

Chu, T.M., S.J. Warden, C.H. turner and R.L. Stewart. *Biomaterials* **28**: 459 (2007).

Côte, M.F., G. Laroche, E. Gagnon, P. Chevallier and C.F. Doillon. *J. Control. Release* **25**: 3761 (2004).

DeFail, A.J., C.R. Chu, N. Izzo and K. G. Marra. *Biomaterials* **27**: 1579 (2006).

Duncan, R. and F. Spreafico. *Clin. Pharmacokinet.* **27**: 290 (1994).

Ellis-Behnke, R., Y.X. Liang, S.W. You, D. Tay, S. Zhang, K.F. Seo, G. Schneider. *Proc. Natl. Acad. Sci.* USA. **103**: 5054 (2006).

European Science Foundation. Nanomedicine, An ESF-European Medical Research Council Forward Look Report. www.esf.org, 2005.

Farrell, E., F.J. O'Brien, P. Doyle, J. Fischer, I. Yannas, B.A. Harley, B. O'Connel, P.J. Prendergast and V.A. Campbell. *Tissue Eng.* **12**: 459 (2006).

Gomes, M.E, C.M. Bossano, C.M. Johnston, R.L. Reis and A.G. Mikos. *Tissue Eng.* **12**: 177 (2006).

Goraltchouk, A., V. Scanga, C.M. Morshead and M.S. Shoichet. *J. Control. Release* **110**: 400 (2006).

Griffith, L.G. and G. Naughton. *Science* **295**: 1009 (2002).

Gutowska, A., B. Jeong, M. Jasionowski. *Anat. Record* **263**: 342 (2001).

Hedberg, E.L., A. Tang, R.S. Crowther, D.H. Carney and A.G. Mikos. *J. Control. Release* **84**: 137 (2002).

Hench, L.L. and J.M. Polak. *Science* **295**: 1014 (2002).

Holland, T.A., Y. Tabata and A.G. Mikos. *J. Control. Release* **101**: 111 (2005).

Hwang, N.S., B.S.S. Varchese, A. Zhang and J. Elisseeff. *Tissue Eng.* **12**: 2695 (2006).

Ito, Y., S.Q. Lui and Y. Imanishi. *Biomaterials* **12**: 449 (1991).

Jain, A., Y.T. Kim, R.J. McKeo and R.V. Bellamkonda. *Biomaterials* **27**: 497 (2006).

Jang, W.Y., S.H. Kim, I. Lee, H.B. Lee and G. Khang. *Tissue Eng. Regen. Med.* **2**: 100 (2005).

Jansen, J.A., J.W.M. Vehof, P.Q. Ruhé, H. Kroeze-Deutman, Y. Kuboki, H. Takita, E.L. Hedgerg and A.G. Mikos. *J. Control. Release* **101**: 127 (2005).

Jeon, O., S.H. Ryu, J.H. Chung and B.S. Kim. *J. Control. Release* **105**: 249 (2005).

Jorgensen, C., J. Gordeladze and D. Noel. *Curr. Opin. Biotechnol.* **15**: 406 (2004).

Keyes-Baig, C., J. Duhamel, S.Y. Fung, J. Bezaire and P. Chen. *J. Am. Chem. Soc.* **126**: 7522 (2004).

Khang, G. and H.B. Lee. Cell-synthetic surface interaction: Physicochemical surface modification. In: A. Atala and R. Lanza, eds. *Methods of Tissue Engineering*. Academic Press, New York, p.771 (2001).

Khang, G., J.M. Rhee, J.K. Jeong, J.S. Lee, M.S. Kim, S.H. Cho and H.B. Lee. *Macromol. Res.* **11**: 207 (2003a).

Khang, G., E.K. Jeon, J.M. Rhee, I. Lee, S.J. Lee and H.B. Lee. *Macromol. Res.* **11**: 334 (2003b).

Khang, G., M.S. Kim, S.H. Cho, I. Lee, J.M. Rhee and H.B. Lee. *Tissue Eng. Regen. Med.* **1**: 9 (2004).

Khang G., K.D. Hong, S.H. Kim, S.K. Kim, M.S. Lee, M.S. Kim, I. Lee, J.M. Rhee and H.B. Lee. *Tissue Eng. Regen. Med.* **2**: 264 (2005).

Khang, G., S.J. Lee, M.S. Kim and H.B. Lee. Biomaterials: Tissue-Engineering and Scaffolds, In: S. Webster, ed. *Encyclopedia of Medical Devices and Instrumentation.* 2nd eds. John & Wiley Press, NY, p. 366 (2006).

Khang, G., S.H. Kim, M.S. Kim and H.B. Lee. Hybrid, Composite, and Complex Biomaterials for Scaffolds, In: A. Atala, R. Lanza, J.A. Thomson, and R.M. Nerem, eds. *Principles of Regenerative Medicine*, Elsevier, San Diego (2007).

Khul, P.R. and L.G. Grriffith-Cima. *Nature Med.* **2**: 1022 (1996).

Kim, S.E., J.H. Park, Y.W. Cho, H. Chung, S.Y. Jeong, E.H. Bae and I.C. Kwon. *J. Control. Release* **91**: 365 (2003).

Kim, S.K., K.D. Hong, J.W. Jang, S.J. Lee, M.S. Kim, G. Khang, I. Lee and H.B. Lee. *Tissue Eng. Regen. Med.* **1**: 149 (2004).

Kim, S.K., S.H. Kim, H.R. Lee, M.H. Cho, M.S. Kim, G. Khang and H.B. Lee. *Tissue Eng. Regen. Med.* **2**: 388 (2005a).

Kim, H., H. Suh, S. Jo, H. Kim, J. Lee, E. Kim, Y. Reinwald, S. Park, B. Min, I. Jo Biochem. *Biophys. Res. Commun.* **332**: 1053 (2005b).

Kim, M.S., S.K. Kim, S.H. Kim, H. Hyun, G. Khang and H.B. Lee. *Tissue Eng.* **12**: 2863 (2006).

Kleinheinz, J., U. Stratmann, U. Joos and H.P. Wiesmann. *J. Oral. Maxillofac Surg.* **63**: 1310 (2005).

Krampera, M., G. Pizzolo, G. Aprili and M. Franchini. *Bone* **39**: 678 (2006).

Lee, J.Y., S.H. Nam, S.Y. Im, Y.J. Park, Y.M. Lee, Y.J. Seol, C.P. Chung and S.J. Lee. *J. Control. Release* **78**: 187 (2002).

Lee, H.B., G. Khang and J.H. Lee. Polymeric Biomaterials. In: J.B. Park and J.D. Bronzino, eds. *Biomaterials:Principles and Application.* CRC Press, Boca Raton, FL, p.55 (2003a).

Lee, K.Y., M.C. Peters and D.J. Mooney. *J. Control. Release* **87**: 49 (2003b).

Li, C., C. Vepari, H.J. Jin, H.J. Kim and D.L. Kaplan. *Biomaterials* **27**: 3115 (2006).

Mayer, J., E. Karamuk, T. Alkaike and E. Wintermantel. *J. Control. Release* **64**: 81 (2000).

Massia, S.P. and J.A. Hubbell. *Anal. Biochem.* **187**: 292 (1990).

Mehlhorn, A.T., P. Niemeyer, S. Kaiser, G. Finkenzeller, G.B. Stark, N.P. Südkamp and H. Schmal. *Tissue Eng.* **12**: 2853 (2006).

Moioli, E.K., L. Hong, J. Guardado, P.A. Clark and J. Mao. *Tissue Eng.* **12**: 537 (2006).

Nagai, Y., L.D. Unsworth, S. Koutsopoulos, S. Zhang. *J. Control. Release* **115**: 18 (2000).

Piantino, J., J.A. Burdick, D. Goldberg, R. Langer and L.I. Benowitz. *Exp. Neurol.* **201**: 359 (2006).

Pound, J.C., D.W. Green, J.B. Chaudhuri, S. Mann, H.I. Roach and R.O.C. Oreffo. *Tissue Eng.* **12**: 2789 (2006).

Qui, Y. and K. Park. *Adv. Drug Deliv. Rev.* **53**: 321 (2001).

Seal, B. L., T. C. Otero and A. Panitch. *Mater. Sci. Eng.* **34**: 147 (2001).

Sheridan, M.H., L.D. Shea, M.C. Peters and D.J. Mooney. *J. Control. Release* **64**: 91 (2000).

Siebers, M.C., S.F. Walboomers, C.G. Sander, J.C.G. Wolke, O.C. Boerman and J.A. Jansen. *Tissue Eng.* **12**: 2449 (2006).

Tabata, Y. *PSTT* **3**: 80 (2000).

Taylor, S., E.S. Rosenzweig, J.W. McDonald III and S.E. Sakiyama-Elbert. *J. Control. Release* **113**: 226 (2006).

Wang, B., Y. Zhao, H. Lin, B. Chen, J. Zhang, J. Zhang, X. Wang, W. Zhao and J. Dai. *Neurosci. Lett.* **401**: 65 (2006).

Wei, G., Q. Jin, W.V. Giannobile and P.X. Ma. *J. Control. Release* **112**: 103 (2006).

Wood, M.A., S. Hughes, Y. Yang and A.J. El Haj. *J. Control. Release* **112**: 96 (2006).

Yasuda, A., K. Kojima, K.W. Tinsley, H. Yoshioka, Y. Mori and C.A. Vacanti. *Tissue Eng.* **12**: 1237 (2006).

Yoneda, M., J. Terai, Y. Imai, T. Okada, K. Nozaki, H. Inoue, S. Miyamoto and K. Takaoka. *Biomaterials* **26**: 5145 (2005).

Yoon, S.J., K.S. Park, M.S. Kim, J.M. Rhee, G. Khang and H.B. Lee. *Tissue Eng.* **13**: 1125 (2007a).

Yoon, S.J., K.S. Park, B.S. Choi, G. Khang, M.S. Kim, J.M. Rhee and H.B. Lee. *Key Materials Eng.* **342** – **343**: 161 (2007b).

Zhang, S. Nat. *Biotechnology* **21**: 1171 (2003).

Zisch, A.H., U. Schenk, J.C. Schense and S.E. Sakiyama-Elbert. *J. Control. Release* **72**: 101 (2001).

15 Modification of Nano-sized Materials for Drug Delivery

Tao Xu[1,2], Heather L. Nichols[1], Ning Zhang[1,3] and Xuejun Wen[1,3,4]

[1] Department of Bioengineering, Clemson University, Charleston, SC 29425, USA
[2] Wake Forest Institute for Regenerative Medicine, Wake Forest University School of Medicine, Winston-Salem, NC 27157, USA
[3] Department of Cell Biology and Anatomy, Medical University of South Carolina, Charleston, SC 29425, USA
[4] Department of Orthopedic Surgery, Medical University of South Carolina, Charleston, SC 29425, USA

Abstract As the field of nanotechnology advances, many nano-sized materials have been successfully used in drug delivery systems. However, recent practices in offering drugs with long circulation time and efficient targeting, and/or developing new therapeutic strategies are challenging nano-sized drug delivery carriers with more defined biological properties and functionalities. Most nano-sized delivery vehicles and materials currently being used cannot completely fulfill these requirements. To address these issues, syntheses of new carrier materials and modification of existing nano-sized materials with tunable properties are considered to be two effective strategies thus far. In this review article, we will focus on the latter. It is thought that through modification one can control and tailor the properties of nano-sized materials in a predictable manner, as well as provide them with precise properties and functionalities. These modifications can bring new and unique capabilities to many drug delivery systems. Recent progress on drug delivery applications for modified and functionalized nano-sized materials will be highlighted, after the methods used to modify nano-sized materials are discussed briefly.

15.1 Introduction

Throughout various fields of science and technology, a push towards the use of nano-scale technology is on the move. One area where nano-scale work is already well underway is within the field of drug delivery. In drug delivery, nanoparticles

(1) Corresponding e-mail: xjwen@clemson.edu

are fabricated in order to entrap and deliver specific pharmaceutical agents to various target locations within the body.

Traditional strategies for the delivery of therapeutic agents have relied upon oral and/or intravenous routes of administration. Both of these methods typically result in uneven distribution of the agent. Oral delivery requires larger doses due to exposure of the drug to the metabolic processes of the body. Systemic injectable drugs often have a low specificity; hence, large amounts of the drug need to be administered, creating a high concentration of the drug in the blood stream, potentially leading to toxic side effects. Nano-sized drug delivery systems as well as utilizing degradable and absorbable polymers provide a more efficient solution to many drug delivery obstacles.

Nano-sized materials refer to materials with structures ranging in size of 1 – 100 nm. At such small scale, unique physical, chemical, and biological properties and phenomena can be expected, since materials smaller than nanometer size are not governed by gravity but by the laws of quantum mechanics(Whitesides, 2003). Most drug delivery components, such as target sites (cell membrane, organelle, etc.), payloaded drugs (enzyme, proteins, DNA, etc.), or delivery pathways (gap junction, membrane pores and channels, etc.), involve some aspect of nano-dimenstionality, so this does not come as a surprise considering that nano-sized particles are capable of adapting and integrating into existing drug delivery systems (Cui and Gao, 2003; Laval et al. and Mazeran, 1999). Rapid developments of nano-sized materials have been made in site-specific drug delivery systems (Bauer et al., 2004; Mazzola, 2003). Recent studies show that nanoscale assemblies and particles have demonstrated enhanced delivery efficiency to specific host sites, when compared with their microscale counterparts (Moghimi and Szebeni, 2003; Muller et al., 2001; Takeuchi et al., 2001). The main reason for the significant efficiency improvement can be accounted for by size effects and the nonspecific scavengining of the carrier system in the reticuloendothelial system (part of immune system within the body). It is known that carrier systems larger than 400 nm in diameter are easily and rapidly captured by the reticuloendothelial system (Owens and Peppas, 2006). Therefore, larger carrier systems, like microscale particulates, exhibit poor delivery performance, since they cannot circulate in the bloodstream for a long enough time to deliver efficient amounts of drug to therapeutic targets.

With the further development of drug delivery systems, improved properties and functions of the carriers, such as prolonged circulation time, overcoming of body barriers, targeting delivery, are needed in modern drug carriers. Moreover, many new strategies and theories used for specific therapeutic purposes have been developed in clinical practices, and require drug delivery vehicles and materials with appropriate features (Sengupta et al., 2005). To further improve and optimize the properties of existing nano-sized materials to better suit the needs of drug delivery developments, modifications of nano-sized materials are essential (Moghimi et al., 2001; Moghimi and Szebeni, 2003; Niemeyer, 2001;

Oyewumi and Mumper, 2003; Pankhurst et al., 2003; Takeuchi et al., 2001).

Despite significant progress in this direction over the past decade, many fundamental problems remain unclear. In the following paper we will review some of these recent progresses in nano-based drug delivery systems after briefly summarizing available methods to modify these nano-sized systems.

15.2 Available Methods to Modify Nano-Sized Materials for Drug Delivery

Different therapeutic applications require special properties and functions of materials; therefore, methods to modify nano-sized materials to meet the needs of different drug delivery systems vary. With reviews on the fundamentals and principles of the modifications of nano-sized materials published elsewhere (Lin et al., 2004; Moghimi and Szebeni, 2003; Otsuka et al., 2003; Sun et al., 2002), this review will focus on the basic methods and technologies used to modify nano-sized materials for drug delivery. The methods are categorized according to the sites and structures of the modifications on nano-sized materials.

15.2.1 Surface Modification

Some reagents used in drug delivery applications need to be soluble and stable, as well as evenly distributed in aqueous media. However, most nano-sized materials lack adequate solubility in aqueous milieus and are not evenly distributed in solution. Nanoparticles often also show instability in suspensions and readily form agglomerations as a result of their large surface-to-volume ratio. When nanoparticles agglomerate, they lose their intended functionality and are usually cleared rapidly from biological systems (Kohler et al., 2004). One way to decrease agglomeration is to modify the surface properties of the nanoparticles. The surfaces of nano-sized materials can be modified with different reagents using various physical, chemical, and biological methods. These modifications often enhance solubility and stability of the nano-sized materials in aqueous media, and even offer new biological functions and properties.

15.2.1.1 Physical Modification

Physical methods, such as molecular coating (or adsorption) and surface entrapment have emerged as leading strategies for surface modifications of nano-sized materials. Through physical modifications, functional molecules and entities, varying charges, or active chemical groups can be introduced onto the surfaces of nano-sized materials, leading to the functionalization and/or activation of the surfaces of materials. Advantages of physical modifications include ease of handling and mild interactions with biomolecules through little or no damage to their bioactivities. These methods have certain disadvantages, which include physical linkages formed between substrates and coatings that are considered weak when compared to covalent bonds. Functional molecules may, therefore, detach from the surface when challenged by certain serum compounds for active binding sites (Langer et al., 2000).

Different non-covalent mechanisms, such as hydrophobic interactions (Neal et al., 1998; Park, 2003; Redhead et al., 2001), ionic interactions (Hrapovic et al., 2004; Lin et al., 2004) and π-π interactions (Artyukhin et al., 2004; Islam et al., 2003; Lin et al., 2004; Nakashima et al., 2002) are involved in the adsorptions of functional molecules and entities onto the surfaces of nano-sized materials. Here we use hydrophobic interactions as an example.

Hydrophobic interactions enhance adsorption ability and are easily produced by most proteins and enzymes. A variety of nonionic polymers with hydrophobic moieties or hydrophobic segments have been developed and coated onto nanoparticle surfaces through hydrophobic reactions (Gulyaev et al., 1999; Kreuter et al., 2003; Neal et al., 1998; Park et al., 2003; Redhead et al., 2001). The polyethylene oxide-polypropylene oxide (PEO-PPO) copolymer, which contains hydrophilic (PEO) and hydrophobic (PPO) moieties, is one example. The copolymers are absorbed onto the nanoparticle hydrophobic surfaces from an aqueous solution via hydrophobic interactions of the hydrophobic moiety (the anchor block) with the particle surface. The hydrophilic blocks extend into the aqueous medium to form a hydrophilic layer (Redhead et al., 2001). Nanoparticles of poly (D, L-lactide-*co*-glycolide) (PLGA) (Neal et al., 1998; Park et al., 2003; Redhead et al., 2001) and poly (lactic acid) (PLA) (Dunn et al., 1997; Rouzes et al., 2000; Younghoon Kim et al., 2005) can be modified using this approach. In addition, polysorbates, including polysorbate 20, 40, 60, and 80, are other examples of nonionic surfactants that have also been shown to absorb on nanoparticle surfaces through hydrophobic interactions (Gulyaev et al., 1999; Kreuter et al., 2003; Schroder and Sabel 1996; Sun et al., 2004).

Hydrophilic polysaccharides, such as dextran, do not readily absorb on nanoparticle surfaces through hydrophobic interactions. Through modification with a hydrophobic molecule, such as phenoxy groups (Rouzes et al., 2000), however, dextran derivatives (e.g. DexP conjugates) have been shown to be amphiphilic and produce stable suspensions of PLGA or PLA nanoparticles. In such cases, the hydrophobic phenoxy segments provide the anchor to the nanoparticle shell while the hydrophilic dextran chains protrude into solution (Coombes et al., 1997).

15.2.1.2 Chemical Modification

Functional molecules can covalently bond to the surfaces of nano-sized materials through particular chemical reactions. Compared with most physical modification, chemical modifications of nano-sized materials can activate the surfaces of the material for longer periods while linking molecules with material surfaces through stronger and more stable chemical bonds. However, certain limitations, such as denaturing of biomolecules, incompatibility, and even toxicity to biological systems of some cross-linkers, have restricted their use. Different chemical reagents and methods can be used in chemical modifications of nano-sized materials. For example, poly (acrylic acid)-based systems can be cross-linked by the addition of a diamine under conditions also used in peptide chemistry (Zhang, 1999).

1. Carbodiimide and Glutaraaldehyde Coupling Chemistry

Carbodiimide, glutaraaldehyde and their derivatives are covalent linkers that can tether functional molecules onto the surfaces of nano-sized materials via a covalent reaction with active chemical groups and sites, such as —NH_3, —COOH, and —SH, exhibited on the surfaces of the materials. These coupling linkers have been widely used in the surface modification of nano-sized materials in order to conjugate diverse functional molecules, including proteins, enzymes, peptides, DNA, and receptor ligands, with nano-sized materials (Chang et al., 2002; Davis et al., 2003; Haes et al., 2004; Huet al., 2004; Kikuchi et al., 2004; Kikuchi et al., 2002; Qhobosheane et al., 2001; Taylor et al., 2004).

2. PEG Chemistry

Nanoparticle surface functionalization using poly (ethylene glycol) (PEG) can effectively prevent nanoparticle agglomerations (colloidal stability) and protein adsorption, resulting in a longer circulation times of nanoparticles. Copolymerization of PEG with bulk materials is often used to couple PEG onto nanoparticles in order to form PEGylated nanoparticle systems (Moghimi et al., 2001; Otsuka et al., 2003). Several researchers have examined the applications of PEGylated nanoparticle systems such as PLA (Gref et al., 2000; Gref et al., 1994; Gref et al., 2001; Mosqueira et al., 2001a, 2001b; Quellec et al., 1998; Zambaux et al., 2001), polycyanoacrylate (Brigger et al., 2002; Calvo et al., 2002; Peracchia et al., 1997), human serum albumin (Lin et al., 1997; Lin et al.,2001; Lin et al., 1999), silica (Xu et al., 2003), and polystyrene (Taylor et al., 2004) nanoparticles. Resulting copolymers of PEGylated nanoparticles are often amphiphilic, i.e. the hydrophobic block is able to form a solid phase (particle core), while the hydrophilic part remains exposed on the surface. This hydrophilic coating is protective with the ability to reduce natural blood opsonization in physiological conditions and increase circulation time (Calvo et al., 2002), which is critical for drug delivery carriers. Heterobifunctional PEGs have also been used for nanoparticles to introduce reactive groups for further immobilization of ligand molecules (Kohler et al., 2004). The linked heterobifunctional PEGs contain both mercapto terminal groups and acetal terminal groups, which can be readily transformed into a reactive aldehyde group using a dilute acid (Otsuka et al., 2001).

15.2.1.3 Bio-Specific Modification

In order for a nanoparticle to be functional and biocompatible, bio-specific modification of the nanoparticle's surface is often necessary. Chemical and/or physical modification approaches allow biospecific molecules to be conjugated to nanoparticles, offering biospecific sites for further immobilization of specific ligands. These ligands are immobilized using biologically-specific reactions, including antibody-antigen (Zhang et al., 2003), receptor-ligand (Cui et al., 2003; Oyewumi and Mumper, 2003; Zhang et al., 2003; Zhang et al., 2002), avidin (or streptavidin)-biotin (Langer et al., 2000; Qhobosheane et al., 2001; Vinogradov et al., 2002), and DNA-DNA hybridization (Cai et al., 2003; Moghaddam et al., 2004). For example, surface modification of nanoparticles with folic acid (Oyewumi and Mumper, 2003), a biosepcific ligand to folate receptors often exhibited and overexpressed by human cancer cells (Wang and Low, 1998), has been accomplished. Cancer cells were shown to efficiently internalize the biologically modified nanoparticles due to the very high affinity of folic acid for folate receptors found at the cancer cell surfaces (Oyewumi and Mumper, 2003; Oyewumi et al., 2004; Zhang et al., 2002).

15.2.2 Shell-Core Modification

Fabricating drug carriers with certain shell-core structure is also an effective approach to modify nano-sized materials in drug delivery systems. Different therapeutic agents can be loaded in different layers of the shell and the core, and the sequential delivery of different drugs can be used in some specific therapeutic methods and strategies (Hood et al., 2002). In preparing the shell-core nano-sized carriers, the solid polymeric nanoparticles (the core) are usually added into aqueous lipid resuspension buffers, thus resulting in a lipid envelope (the shell) coated on the nanoparticles (Hood et al., 2002).

15.2.3 Bulk Modifications

Modifying the bulk of nano-sized materials by altering compositions and microstructures, i.e., addition of active components or formation of 3-D cross-linked networks, allows for fine tuning of material properties and can potentially change a material's function. Here we use nano gel as an example.

By entrapping nano-sized materials into the gel, a three-dimensional cross-linked polymer network immersed in fluid (Vinogradov et al., 2002), the properties can be tailored to meet specific needs of certain delivery systems. Nanogels, which are nano-sized flexible hydrophilic polymer gels (Lemieux et al., 2000; Vinogradov et al., 2002), are one example of a type of gel used as a drug delivery carrier. Kabanov and co-workers have synthesized cationic nanogels consisting of covalently cross-linked PEG and polyethylenimine (PEI) chains, nano-PEG-cross-PEI. Through ionic interactions, these nanogels can bind and encapsulate negatively charged oligonucleotide drugs spontaneously. One of the main advantages of nanogels is that they have a high carrying capacity for macromolecules, up to 50 wt%, which is a challenge for most conventional nano drug carriers (Vinogradov et al., 2004).

15.3 Applications for Drug Delivery of Modified Nano Sized Biomaterials

Nanoparticulate systems, including polymeric nanoparticles and polymeric self-assemblies can potentially revolutionize disease treatment through spatially and temporally controlled drug delivery (Kawashima, 2001). Two basic properties of nanoparticulates result in their advantageous use in drug delivery. First, nanoparticulates, due to their small size, can penetrate small capillaries and be taken up by cells, which allows for efficient drug accumulation at target sites in the body. Second, the use of biodegradable materials for nanoparticulate preparation allows for sustained drug release within the target over a period of days or even weeks after administration (Vinogradov et al., 2002). Using nano-sized elements in drug delivery has improved solubility, target ability and adhesion to specific tissues, as well as provided the ability to convert poorly soluble, poorly absorbable, and predisposed biologically active substances into promising drugs (Kawashima, 2001). However, some technical problems still exist, such as relatively short blood circulation times, low accessibility to physiological barriers of target sites (blood bran barrier, etc.) and low efficiency of gene transfection, limiting the clinical applications of nano-sized drug delivery systems. Suitable and effective modifications of these nanoparticle materials are necessary in order to overcome these obstacles.

15.3.1 Long Circulating Delivery

After intravenous administration, conventional nano-sized carriers tend to dramatically interact with opsonin proteins present in the blood serum. These proteins quickly bind to conventional non-stealth nanoparticles (opsonization), allowing macrophages of the mononuclear phagocytic system (MPS) to easily recognize and remove these drug delivery devices (usually within minutes) from the body. This opsonization and subsequent clearance by macrophages render these conventional nano-sized carriers ineffective as site-specific drug delivery devices (Owens and Peppas, 2006). Improving circulation time is still the main concern for nanoparticulate drug carriers. Numerous approaches for design and engineering of long circulating time carries have been developed (Moghimi et al., 2001; Moghimi and Szebeni, 2003). Among them, modifying the surfaces of nanoparticles by PEG and PEG derivatives has shown to be the most promising approach for prolonging circulation time (Moghimi et al., 2001; Moghimi and Szebeni, 2003).

15.3.1.1 Stealth Nanoparticles Surface Adsorped Amphipathic Multiblock Copolymers

The macrophages from MRS, which recognize and remove the nanoparticles in drug delivery systems are typically Kupffer cells, or macrophages of the liver. These cells cannot directly identify the nanoparticles themselves, but rather recognize specific opsonin proteins bound to the surface of the particles (Owens and Peppas, 2006). Therefore, one effective strategy to avoid phagocytic recognition and clearance of nanoparticles from the blood stream is by trying to stop or block the initial opsonization of nanoparticles. Although there are no absolute rules or methods available to completely and effectively block the opsonization of particles, research over the last decades has found some trends and methods that can be effective at slowing this process. It is found that the opsonization of hydrophobic particles, as compared to hydrophilic particles, has been shown to occur more quickly due the enhanced adsorbability of blood serum proteins on these surfaces (Owens and Peppas, 2006). Coating the nanoparticles with hydrophilic layers shows promise in preventing opsonization, thus leading to a prolonged circulation time of nanoparticles.

Amphipathic PEG containing copolymers, such as PEO-PPO type multi-block copolymers (commercially available as poloxamer and poloxamine surfactants), have been suggested for this purpose. These polymers are amphiphilic block copolymers consisting of blocks of ethylene oxide (EO) and propylene oxide (PO) monomer units, which are typically formed by anionic polymerization. These copolymers can adsorb efficiently onto the hydrophobic nanoparticle surface via hydrophobic PPO center blocks, while the PEO side-arms of the copolymers extend outward from the particle's surface, thus providing a hydrophilic barrier, as well as stability in suspension (Moghimi et al., 2001). Nanoparticulate materials, such as polystyrene, poly (methyl methacrylate) and poly (butyl 2-cyanoacrylate), when coated with PEO-PPO copolymers, have demonstrated increased circulation times and reduced liver accumulation after intravenous administration (Moghimi et al., 2001). Furthermore, improved drug sustained release profiles have lead investigators to focus on biodegradable nanoparticle system surfaces modified with PEO-PPO copolymers. Biodegradable PLGA, PLA, and poly (phosphazene) nanoparticles were surface treated with PEO-PPO copolymers and their derivatives. When loaded with model drug or therapeutic proteins (Zambaux et al., 2001), dramatically improved circulation and biodistribution behaviors of these biodegradable particles were observed (Neal et al., 1998; Vandorpe et al., 1997).

Factors such as chemical structure of the copolymer and the charge density were also shown to affect biological behaviors of the nanoparticles modified with PEO-PPO copolymers. For example, Neal et al. observed that aminiation of poloxamers and poloxamines significantly affected the biological properties of surface modified polystyrene nanospheres (Neal et al., 1998). The presence of protonated amine end groups induced by the aminiation of poloxamer 407 significantly reduced circulation time and increased liver uptake of the resulting nanospheres, compared to those coated with non-aminiated P-407. However, the negative effects of modified P-407 can be overcome if the charged amine groups are capped via acetylation. Neal et al. also suggested that there are certain factors other than steric stabilization that probably contribute to the enhanced circulation time and biodistribution behaviors of these nanospheres, such as chemical structures and surface charges of sterically stabilizing copolymers (Neal et al., 1998).

15.3.1.2 Stealth Nanoparticles Surface Chemically Grafting of PEG Chains and Its Derivatives

Another important method of drug delivery is to modify the non-stealth nanoparticles by covalently grafting of PEG chains and its derivatives (Moghimi et al., 2001). Numerous investigators have reported that, when compared to un-modified nanoparticles and those absorbed with Poloxamers or Poloxamines, PEG-chemically surface grafted nanoparticle systems allow reduced protein adsorption and complement activation, as well as increased circulation time. Poloxamer and Poloxamine have poor adsorptions onto hydrophilic nanoparticles (e.g. albumin) and desorption in circulation (Mosqueira et al., 2001). In PEG grafted nanoparticles, PEG density, chain length, and confirmation of the polymer on the surfaces of the modified nanoparticles directly effect desopsonization and circulation time. A drastic increase in blood circulation time has been observed with increasing molecular weight (MW) of PEG blocks in diblock PEG-PLGA copolymers (PEG chain length at the particle surface), and increasing PEG content in the particle (PEG chain density at the surface of the particles).

The mechanisms involved in prolonged circulation time of nanoparticles' surface modified with PEO-PPO or PEG polymers are still not well understood. Opsonization suppression by steric repulsion of PEO or PEG hydrated barriers is thought to be responsible for the increased residency of nanoparticles in the blood. The concept of 'steric hinderance' has been used to explain the roles of PEG and its derivatives in blocking and delaying the first step in the opsonization process. However, growing evidence suggests that prolonged lifetimes of sterically protected nanoparticles in circulation may not be directly related to reduced opsonizaiton. A combination of responsible mechanisms have been suggested, including the interface between sterically protected nanoparticles and various blood proteins, macrophage cell surface receptors, complement activation, and the physiological state of macrophages (Moghimi and Szebeni, 2003).

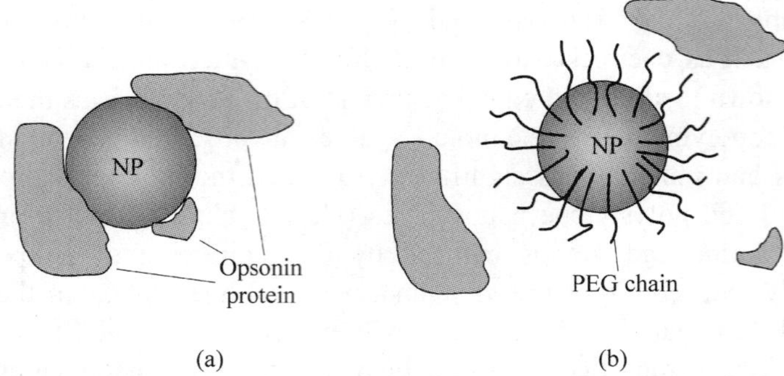

Figure 15.1 Schematic diagram of opsonization process of nanoparticles: (a) most opsonin proteins in blood serum tend to quickly bind to conventional non-stealth nanoparticles by hydrophobic interactions; (b) in PEG surface modified nanoparticles, PEG molecules provide a hydrophilic protective layer around the nanoparticles that is able to repel the absorption of opsonin proteins via steric repulsion forces, thereby blocking and delaying the opsonization process

15.3.2 Targeting Delivery

Drug targeting refers to selective drug delivery to specific physiological sites, organs, tissues, or cells where a drug's pharmacological activities are required. In addition to having enhanced circulation properties, most drug delivery systems need to target specific cells and tissues in the body in order to increase therapeutic efficiency, as well as decrease systemic side effects.

15.3.2.1 Brain Targeting and Blood-Brain Barrier

Any attempt to develop a new therapy for brain disease must deal with a vexing impediment. The blood brain barrier (BBB) is a stubbornly real obstacle for potential drugs against many disorders of the central nervous system (CNS). It is located at the level of the brain capillaries, where there is a convergence of different cell types: endothelial cells, pericytes, astrocytes, and microglias (perivascular macrophages). The brain microvessel endothelial cells (BMEC) that form the BBB display important morphological characteristics such as the presence of tight junctions between the cells, the absence of fenestrations and diminished pinocytic activity, that together help to restrict the passage of compounds from the blood into the extracellular environment of the brain. Also, tight junctions provide significant transendothelial electrical resistance (TEER) to BMEC and impede the penetration of potential therapeutic agents such as oligonucleotides, antibodies, peptides and proteins (Garcia-Garcia et al., 2005). Only nonionized, lipophilic and low molecular weight compounds were found to have the ability to cross the BBB by diffusion mechanisms (Schroder and Sabel, 1996). Consequently, the therapeutic value of many promising drugs is diminished significantly, thus limiting pharmacological treatment for neurological and psychiatric disorders.

Osmostic opening of the barrier is one of the earliest techniques to circumvent the barrier for therapeutic purposes and also the first to be used in humans (Begley, 2004). Osmotic agents, such as sugar, is infused into a carotic artery. The resulting high sugar concentration in brain capillaries sucks water out of the endothelial cells, shrinking them and opening gaps between cells. This treatment opens the barrier rapidly and it remains open for up to 30 min. Other techniques, such as blood-brain barrier disruption (BBBD) using by a receptor associated mechanism, biochemical modulation by employing vasoactive molecules such as bradykinin, leukotriene C4 and cereport to increase the permeability of brain tumor capillaries, and direct brain drug delivery (e.g. intracerebral delivery), have also been used in brain drug delivery. However, most conventional invasive procedures are unacceptably risky, since disrupting the barrier, even for brief periods, leaves the brain vulnerable to infection and damage from toxins. Even substances that circulate harmlessly through the peripheral bloodstream, such as albumin, can have deleterious effects if they enter the brain (Begley, 2004).

Looking for another entryway into the brain, researchers have found that polymer nanoparticles can be used to sneak drugs across the barrier. The use of nano-carriers, such as solid polymeric or lipid nanoparticles may be advantageous over the current strategies. These nano-carriers can not only mask the BBB limiting characteristics of the therapeutic drug molecule, but may also protect the drug from chemical/enzymatic degradation, and additionally provide the opportunity for sustained release characteristics. Reduction of toxicity to peripheral organs can also be achieved with these nano-carriers.

1. Coated Nanoparticles

Poly (butyl cyanoacrylate) (PBCA) nanoparticles were the first nanoparticles that were used for in-vivo drug delivery to the brain (Kreuter, 2001). Various surface modifications have been employed to increase the efficacy of these nanoparticles across the BBB. The most widely investigated has been overcoating the nanoparticles with polysorbate 80 (Kreuter, 2001). By using polysorbate 80 overcoated PBCA nanoparticles, hexapeptide dalargin was the first drug to cross the BBB and be successfully delivered to the brain via nanoparticles (Alyautdin et al., 1995). After intravenous injection, the nanoparticles loaded with dalargin demonstrated antinociceptive activity (the relief of the receptive neuron-related pain) (Alyautdin et al., 1995; Kreuter et al., 1995), while uncoated dalagrin nanoparticles exhibited no antinociceptive effect. Overcoatng with polysorbate 20, 40, and 60 led to antinociceptive effects similar to those of polysorbate 80, whereas other surfactants such as poloxamers 184, 188, 338, 407, and poloxamine 908 had no such effects (Kreuter et al., 1997). Other antinociceptive agents, such as the dipeptide kytorphin and loperamide were also tested and effects similar to those of dalargin were observed (Kreuter, 2001). Furthermore, polysorbate 80 coated PBCA nanoparticles were also used to deliver doxorubicin, an important anticancer drug, to the brain (Gulyaev et al., 1999). The brain concentration of systemically administered doxorubicin can be enhanced more than 60-fold as compared to free doxorubicin delivery through the use of nanoparticles.

How polysorbate coated nanoparticles cross the barrier is a matter of some debate. Studies from Olivier et al. (1999) suggested that the detergent coated nanoparticles could open the tight junctions between endothelial cells in the brain microvasculature, thus creating a paracellular pathway for nanoparticle translocation. However, both in vivo and in vitro studies performed by Kreuter et al. (2003) did not demonstrate any disruption of the BBB by the presence of polysorbate-80 (PS-80) coated nanoparticles since the permeability of the extracellular markers (sucrose and insulin) was not modified in the presence of 10 or 20 μg/mL of PBCA nanoparticles with and without polysorbate-80. This indicates, contrary to what was hypothesized by Olivier (Pardridge, 2002), no facilitation of the paracellular route by disruption of tight junctions due to nanoparticles. The enhancement of drug transport through the BBB by the coated nanoparticles may be explained by different mechanisms: (1) the binding of nanoparticles to the inner endothelial lining of the brain capillaries could provide a drug concentration gradient, thus improving passive diffusion and (2) brain endothelial cell uptake of nanoparticles may occur through endocytosis or transcytosis (Garcia-Garcia et al., 2005).

2. PEGylated Nanoparticles

Chemical surface modification of nanoparticles with PEG is another method to enhance drug delivery to the brain (Brigger et al., 2002; Calvo et al., 2002; Vinogradov et al., 2004). PEGylated nanoparticles have been shown to increase in concentration in the brain and spinal cord when compared to conventional non-PEGylated nanoparticles (Calvo et al., 2002). PEG grafted poly (hexadecyl-cyanoacrylate) (PEG-PHDCA) is an example. The preparation of the PEG-PHDCA copolymer was achieved by the synthesis of a cyanoacrylate monomer substituted with PEG and its co-polymerization with hexadecylcyanoacrylate. In this technology, the PEG is covalently attached to the hydrophobic block, rather than adsorbed, which seems to be the better choice to avoid the possibility of PEG desorption. PEG-PHDCA nanoparticles have been shown to penetrate into the brain to a greater extent than all the other nanoparticle formulations tested, including the above discussion of PS-80 nanoparticles. PEG containing nanogels have also been synthesized for the delivery of oligonucleotides as potential diagnostic and therapeutic agents for brain cancer and neurodegenerative disorders (Vinogradov et al., 2004). The accumulation of phosphorothioate oligodeoxynucleotides (ODN) in the brain of mice was shown to increase more than 15-fold after incorporation into nanogels when compared to free ODN after intravenous injection. It is thought that PEG modified nanoparticles could reach the brain by two mechanisms: passive diffusion due to the increase of BBB permeability and transport by nanoparticles-containing macrophages which infiltrate these inflammatory tissues (Garcia-Garcia et al., 2005).

15.3.2.2 Cell Targeting and Tumor Delivery of Drugs

Tumor cell-targeted drug delivery can significantly reduce drug toxicity, while increasing the drugs therapeutic effects (Bergey et al., 2002; Oyewumi and Mumper, 2003). The conjugation of antibodies, hormones, or other biospecific ligands with nanoparticles has been carried out for this purpose. These nanoparticles modified with certain cell-specific bio-ligands can bind and deliver drugs to specific cells. For example, cancer cells often over-express the folate receptor on its surface, therefore, folid acid, a low molecular weight targeting agent, can be used to target cancer cells (Lee and Huang, 1996; Lee and Low, 1995; Weitman et al., 1992). Folic acid binds to the folate receptor at cell surfaces and is internalized by receptor-mediated endocytosis (Antony, 1992; Lee and Huang, 1996; Lee and Low, 1995). Zhang and co-workers recently cultured human breast cancer cells with superparamagnetic magnetite nanoparticles surface-modified with biospecific ligands of folic acid (Zhang et al., 2002). They found that, when compared to unmodified nanoparticles, nanoparticles modified with the folic acid ligands increased the amount of nanoparticle uptake into breast cancer cells (Zhang et al., 2002). Furthermore, hyperthermia treatment, the use of magnetic nanoparticle temperature increase after exposure to certain magnetic fields for tumor specific drug delivery is providing a new method to treat cancer (Pankhurst et al., 2003; Wust et al., 2002). By controlling the frequency and strength of alternating magnetic fields, heat is generated in magnetic nanoparticles and conducted into immediately surrounding diseased tissue. When the temperature is maintained above the therapeutic threshold of 42° for 30 min or more, the cancer tissue is destroyed (Pankhurst et al., 2003).

Another form of cancer therapy involves the use of folic acid based nanoparticles with a nuclear medicine called neutron capture therapy (NCT). NCT delivers a stable (non-radioactive) nuclide to tumor cells, upon which irradiation by thermal or epithermal neutrons produces localized cytotoxic radiation (Oyewumi et al., 2004). Folate ligands have been found to be conjugated efficiently on gadolinium nanoparticle surface (Oyewumi and Mumper, 2003; Oyewumi et al., 2004). It was also demonstrated that cell uptake and tumor retention of folate-coated nanoparticles were significantly enhanced over nanoparticles coated with other molecules, such as PEG (Oyewumi et al., 2004).

Hepatocyte-specific targeting materials can perform liver-specific drug delivery of nanoparticles. One example is a galactose-carrying polymer. The galactose ligands can be recognized by the asialoglycoprotein receptors of hepatocytes (Hirabayashi et al., 1996; Kobayashi et al., 1986). Poly (vinyl benzyl lactonamide), a galactose-carrying polymer, was used to coat PLA nanoparticles in order to develop a biodegradable nanoparticle carrier system for liver-specific drug delivery (Cho et al., 2001a, 2001b). Studies demonstrated an increase in the internalization rate of the modified nanoparticles by the hepatocytes when compared to unmodified controls. The internalization process was suggested to be due to a receptor-mediated mechanism (Cho et al., 2001a, 2001b).

15.3.3 New Therapy and Drug Carriers

The drug delivery system is required to fit in the needs of clinical therapy. With the development of new therapeutic methods and strategies, drug carrier or delivery systems with specific functions and properties are needed accordingly. Recently, a serial combination of several different therapies and strategies have been developed to deal with serious tumor conditions (Chen and Zhang, 2006; Sengupta et al., 2005). Among them, the combination of traditional chemotherapy and new anti-angiogenic treatment is very promising. In the new therapy, a specific shell-core structure of the nanoparticle is developed to carry different therapeutic drugs. In the following, it is used as an example to explain the role of modification of nanoparticles in new therapy strategies.

Traditional chemotherapeutic agents kill all rapidly growing cells in the body—both cancer cells and other cells that divide quickly. This leads to the distressing side effects of chemotherapy and limits the practical dose and frequency of application of the drugs. One tactic to avoid these effects is to target the drug specifically to the tumor. On the other hand, anti-angiogenic treatment is a new concept in cancer therapy, in which the progression of cancer might be halted by preventing tumors from recruiting new blood vessels. It is obvious that simultaneous delivery of chemotherapeutic and anti-angiogenic drugs is beneficial. As an emerging model for tumor treatment, the combination of traditional chemotherapy with anti-angiogenesis agents has been proposed recently. However, the implementation of this strategy has faced two major obstacles. First, the long-term shutdown of tumor blood vessels by the anti-angiogenesis agent can prevent the tumor from receiving a therapeutic concentration of the chemotherapy agent. Second, inhibiting blood supply drives the intra-tumoral accumulation of hypoxia-inducible factor-1a (HIF1-a); overexpression of HIF1-a is correlated with increased tumor invasiveness and resistance to chemotherapy.

To address these issues, Sengupta et al. (2005), and Chen and Zhang (2006) have designed a novel drug delivery vehicle, termed a nanocell, which can sequentially release an anti-angiogenic drug and a traditional chemotherapeutic drug at high concentrations specifically into a tumor. Shell-core structure is incorporated into the delivery vehicle. The solid nanoparticles were fabricated from PLGA. Doxorubicin (traditional chemotherapeutic drug) was conjugated to PLGA to achieve a slow release profile. The solid PLGA nanoparticle cores were coated and nucleated inside a nanoscale phospholipid block-copolymer envelope composed of 2k-Da PEG- distearoylphosphatidylethanolamine (DSPE), phosphatidylcholine and cholesterol,in an optimal ratio entrapped with combretastatin (anti-angiogenesis agent). The size of the nanocells ranged between 180 and 200 nm in diameter. With the unique design, the nanocell enables a temporal release of two drugs. First, the disruption of this envelope inside a tumor would result in a rapid deployment of the anti-angiogenesis agent, leading to

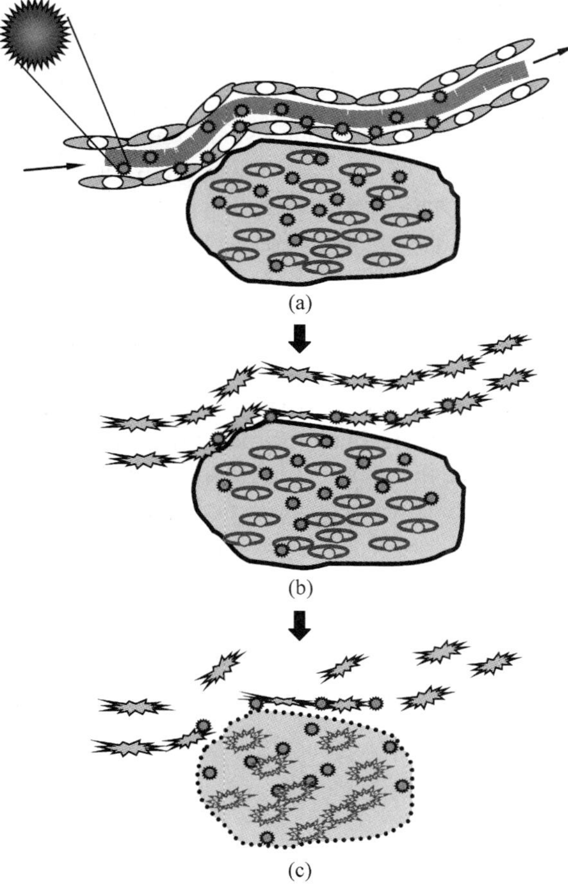

Figure 15.2 Schematic diagram of a new tumor therapy of the combination of conventional chemotherapy and anti-angiogenic treatment. (a) Novel shell-core structured nanoparticles are injected into bloodstream and selectively taken up by tumor tissue. The nanoparticles are composed of a nuclear PLGA nanoparticle within an extranuclear pegylated-lipid envelope, and chemotherapeutical and anti-angiogenic agents are loaded in the core and the shell layers, respectively. (b) The outer envelope first releases an anti-angiogenesis agent, causing a vascular shutdown. (c) The inner core of nanoparticles, which is trapped inside the tumor, gradually releases a chemotherapeutic drug to destroy the cancer cells, finally slowing the tumor growth

vascularcollapse and the intra-tumoral trapping of the nanoparticles. The inner nanoparticle, which is trapped inside the tumor, then releases a chemotherapy agent, should then kill the tumor cells. Sengupta et al. (2005) examined the effects of the delivery drugs on two types of tumor in mice and found the shell-core modified nano-sized delivery system can slow tumor growth more than either single drug delivered by conventional PLGA nanoparticles or two drugs delivered at the same time (Chen and Zhang, 2006).

15.4 Conclusions

The race to find effective strategies to improve the properties of existing nano-sized materials and enhance drug delivery is underway. Although great progress has been made in modifying nano-sized materials for drug delivery, many challenges and technical barriers still remain. For example, the biocompatibility and bio-functionality of nanoparticles need to be further improved and long-term clinical evaluations of these modified nanoparticles in vivo need to be performed. Precise and multi-site modifications of nanoparticles, especially asymmetrical nanoparticles, have not yet been investigated. Also, inefficiencies of nanoparticles modified with macromolecules due to steric hindrances need to be overcome. With the development of nanotechnology, medicine, and biomedical engineering, all of these problems have the potential to be solved, as well as the development of more nano-sized materials with enhanced biological properties and functions.

Acknowledgements

This publication was made possible by AO Research Fund (04-W55), Switzerland.

References

Alyautdin, R., D. Gothier et al. *European Journal of Pharmaceutics and Biopharmaceutics* **41**: 44 – 48 (1995).

Antony, A. C. *Blood* **79**: 2807 – 2820 (1992).

Artyukhin, A. B., O. Bakajin et al. *Langmuir* **20**: 1442 – 1448 (2004).

Bauer, L. A., N. S. Birenbaum et al. *Journal of Materials Chemistry* **14**: 517 – 526 (2004).

Begley, D. J. *Pharmacology & Therapeutics* **104**: 29 – 45 (2004).

Bergey, E. J., L. Levy et al. *Biomedical Microdevices* **4**: 293 – 299 (2002).

Brigger, I., J. Morizet et al. *Journal of Pharmacology and Experimental Therapeutics* **303**: 928 – 936 (2002).

Cai, H., Y. Xu et al. *Electroanalysis* **15**: 1864 – 1870 (2003).

Calvo, P., B. Gouritin et al. *European Journal of Neuroscience* **15**: 1317 – 1326 (2002).

Chang, M. C., T. Ikoma et al. *Journal of Materials Science-Materials in Medicine* **13**: 993 – 997 (2002).

Chen, W. and J. Zhang. *Journal of Nanoscience and Nanotechnology* **6**: 1159 – 1166 (2006).

Cho, C. S., K. Y. Cho et al. *Journal of Controlled Release* **77**: 7 – 15 (2001a).

Cho, C. S., A. Kobayashi et al. *Biomaterials* **22**: 45 – 51 (2001b).

Coombes, A. G. A., S. Tasker et al. *Biomaterials* **18**: 1153 – 1161 (1997).

Cui, D. X. and H. J. Gao. *Biotechnology Progress* **19**: 683 – 692 (2003).

Cui, Z. R., C. H. Hsu et al. *Drug Development and Industrial Pharmacy* **29**: 689 – 700 (2003).

Davis, J. J., K. S. Coleman et al. *Chemistry-a European Journal* **9**: 3732 – 3739 (2003).

Dunn, S. E., A. G. A. Coombes et al. *Journal of Controlled Release* **44**: 65 – 76 (1997).

Garcia-Garcia, E., K. Andrieux et al. *International Journal of Pharmaceutics* **298**: 274 – 292 (2005).

Gref, R., M. Luck et al. *Colloids and Surfaces B-Biointerfaces* **18**: 301 – 313 (2000).

Gref, R., Y. Minamitake et al. *Science* **263**: 1600 – 1603 (1994).

Gref, R., P. Quellec et al. *European Journal of Pharmaceutics and Biopharmaceutics* **51**: 111 – 118 (2001).

Gulyaev, A. E., S. E. Gelperina et al. *Pharmaceutical Research* **16**: 1564 – 1569 (1999).

Haes, A. J., W. P. Hall et al. *Nano Letters* **4**: 1029 – 1034 (2004).

Hirabayashi, H., M. Nishikawa et al. *Pharmaceutical Research* **13**: 880 – 884 (1996).

Hood, J. D., M. Bednarski et al. *Science* **296**: 2404 – 2407 (2002).

Hrapovic, S., Y. L. Liu et al. *Analytical Chemistry* **76**: 1083 – 1088 (2004).

Hu, H., Y. C. Ni et al. *Nano Letters* **4**: 507 – 511 (2004).

Islam, M. F., E. Rojas et al. *Nano Letters* **3**: 269 – 273 (2003).

K.S. Murthy, Q. M., C.G. Clark Jr. E.E. Remsen, K.L. Wooley. *Chem. Commun.* **773**: 74 (2001).

Kawashima, Y. *Advanced Drug Delivery Reviews* **47**: 1 – 2 (2001).

Kikuchi, M., H. N. Matsumoto et al. *Biomaterials* **25**: 63 – 69 (2004).

Kikuchi, M., T. Taguchi et al. In: *Bioceramics* **14**, ed., 449 – 452 (2002).

Kobayashi, A., T. Akaike et al. *Makromolekulare Chemie-Rapid Communications* **7**: 645 – 650 (1986).

Kohler, N., G. E. Fryxell et al. *Journal of the American Chemical Society* **126**: 7206 – 7211 (2004).

Kreuter, J. *Advanced Drug Delivery Reviews* **47**: 65 – 81 (2001).

Kreuter, J., R. N. Alyautdin et al. *Brain Research* **674**: 171 – 174 (1995).

Kreuter, J., V. E. Petrov et al. *Journal of Controlled Release* **49**: 81 – 87 (1997).

Kreuter, J., P. Ramge et al. *Pharmaceutical Research* **20**: 409 – 416 (2003).

Langer, K., C. Coester et al. *European Journal of Pharmaceutics and Biopharmaceutics* **49**: 303 – 307 (2000).

Laval, J. M., P. E. Mazeran et al. *Analyst* **125**: 29 – 33 (1999).

Lee, R. J. and L. Huang. *Journal of Biological Chemistry* **271**: 8481 – 8487 (1996).

Lee, R. J. and P. S. Low. *Biochimica Et Biophysica Acta-Biomembranes* **1233**: 134 – 144 (1995).

Lemieux, P., S. V. Vinogradov et al. *Journal of Drug Targeting* **8**: 91 – 105 (2000).

Lin, W., M. C. Garnett et al. *Biomaterials* **18**: 559 – 565 (1997).

Lin, W., M. C. Garnett et al. *Journal of Controlled Release* **71**: 117 – 126 (2001).
Lin, W., M. C. Garnett et al. *International Journal of Pharmaceutics* **189**: 161 – 170 (1999).
Lin, Y., S. Taylor et al. *Journal of Materials Chemistry* **14**: 527 – 541 (2004).
Lin, Y. H., F. Lu et al. *Nano Letters* **4**: 191 – 195 (2004).
Mazzola, L. *Nature Biotechnology* **21**: 1137 – 1143 (2003).
Moghaddam, M. J., S. Taylor et al. *Nano Letters* **4**: 89 – 93 (2004).
Moghimi, S. M., A. C. Hunter et al. *Pharmacological Reviews* **53**: 283 – 318 (2001).
Moghimi, S. M. and J. Szebeni. *Progress in Lipid Research* **42**: 463 – 478 (2003).
Mosqueira, V. C. F., P. Legrand et al. *Biomaterials* **22**: 2967 – 2979 (2001b).
Mosqueira, V. C. F., P. Legrand et al. *Pharmaceutical Research* **18**: 1411 – 1419 (2001a).
Muller, R. H., C. Jacobs et al. *Advanced Drug Delivery Reviews* **47**: 3 – 19 (2001).
Nakashima, N., Y. Tomonari et al. *Chemistry Letters*, 638 – 639 (2002).
Neal, J. C., S. Stolnik et al. *Pharmaceutical Research* **15**: 318 – 324 (1998).
Niemeyer, C. M. *Angewandte Chemie-International Edition* **40**: 4128 – 4158 (2001).
Olivier, J. C., L. Fenart et al. *Pharmaceutical Research* **16**: 1836 – 1842 (1999).
Otsuka, H., Y. Akiyama et al. *Journal of the American Chemical Society* **123**: 8226 – 8230 (2001).
Otsuka, H., Y. Nagasaki et al. *Advanced Drug Delivery Reviews* **55**: 403 – 419 (2003).
Owens, D. E. and N. A. Peppas. *International Journal of Pharmaceutics* **307**: 93 – 102 (2006).
Oyewumi, M. O. and R. J. Mumper. *International Journal of Pharmaceutics* **251**: 85 – 97 (2003).
Oyewumi, M. O., R. A. Yokel et al. *Journal of Controlled Release* **95**: 613 – 626 (2004).
Pankhurst, Q. A., J. Connolly et al. *Journal of Physics D-Applied Physics* **36**: R167 – R181 (2003).
Pardridge, W. M. In: *Molecular and Cellular Biology of Neuroprotection in the Cns*, A. Christian ed. New York: Plenum, 2002 397 – 430.
Park, Y. J., S. H. Nah et al. *Journal of Biomedical Materials Research* Part A **67A**: 751 – 760 (2003).
Peracchia, M. T., C. Vauthier et al. *Life Sciences* **61**: 749 – 761 (1997).
Q. Zhang, K. L. W. *Polym. Prepr.* **42**: 986 – 987 (1999).
Qhobosheane, M., S. Santra et al. *Analyst* **126**: 1274 – 1278 (2001).
Quellec, P., R. Gref et al. *Journal of Biomedical Materials Research* **42**: 45 – 54 (1998).
Redhead, H. M., S. S. Davis et al. *Journal of Controlled Release* **70**: 353 – 363 (2001).
Rouzes, C., R. Gref et al. *Journal of Biomedical Materials Research* **50**: 557 – 565 (2000).
Schroder, U. and B. A. Sabel. *Brain Research* **710**: 121 – 124 (1996).
Sengupta, S., D. Eavarone et al. *Nature* **436**: 568 – 572 (2005).
Sun, W. Q., C. S. Xie et al. *Biomaterials* **25**: 3065 – 3071 (2004).
Sun, Y. P., K. F. Fu et al. *Accounts of Chemical Research* **35**: 1096 – 1104 (2002).
Takeuchi, H., H. Yamamoto et al. *Advanced Drug Delivery Reviews* **47**: 39 – 54 (2001).
Taylor, S., L. W. Qu et al. *Biomacromolecules* **5**: 245 – 248 (2004).
Vandorpe, J., E. Schacht et al. *Biomaterials* **18**: 1147 – 1152 (1997).
Vinogradov, S. V., E. V. Batrakova et al. *Bioconjugate Chemistry* **15**: 50 – 60 (2004).
Vinogradov, S. V., T. K. Bronich et al. *Advanced Drug Delivery Reviews* **54**: 135 – 147 (2002).
Wang, S. and P. S. Low. *Journal of Controlled Release* **53**: 39 – 48 (1998).
Weitman, S. D., R. H. Lark et al. *Cancer Research* **52**: 3396 – 3401 (1992).

Whitesides, G. M. *Nature Biotechnology* **21**: 1161 – 1165 (2003).
Wust, P., B. Hildebrandt et al. *Lancet Oncology* **3**: 487 – 497 (2002).
Xu, H., F. Yan et al. *Journal of Biomedical Materials Research.* Part A **66A**: 870 – 879 (2003).
Younghoon Kim, P. D., David A Christian and D. E. Discher. *Nanotechnology* **16**: S484 – 491 (2005).
Zambaux, M. F., F. Bonneaux et al. *International Journal of Pharmaceutics* **212**: 1 – 9 (2001).
Zhang, C. X., Y. Zhang et al. *Analytical Biochemistry* **320**: 136 – 140 (2003).
Zhang, Y., N. Kohler et al. *Biomaterials* **23**: 1553 – 1561 (2002).

16 Polymeric Nano Micelles as a Drug Carrier

Moon Suk Kim[1], Hyun Hoon[1,2], Gilson Khang[2] and Hai Bang Lee[1]

[1] Fusion Biotechnology Research Center, Korea Research Institutes of Chemical Technology, Daejeon 305-606, Korea

[2] BK-21 Polymer BIN Fusion Research Team, Chonbuk National University, Jeonju 561-756, Korea

Abstract Over recent decades there has been increasing interest in developing drug delivery systems using polymeric micelles with nano size. Major challenges in drug delivery systems associated with nano micelles include achievement of a prolonged blood circulation and controlling appropriate drug release at target sites. The amphiphilic block copolymers show self-assembly behavior in aqueous media leading to micellar systems. Thus, the polymeric micelles formed in aqueous media from amphiphilic block copolymers are currently recognized as one of the most promising modalities of drug carriers. We will focus on the polymeric micelles as drug carrier. First, self-assembly of block copolymers in aqueous to form stable polymeric micelles will be discussed. The basic principles of self-assembly and micellization of block copolymers will be then given. Finally, we will concentrate on polymeric micelles, showing promise as long circulating carriers for drug delivery.

Keyword Nano, Micelle, Drug, Carrier

16.1 Introduction

Polymeric-nano carrier systems consist of small particles of nano diameter. They show promise as drug carrier in drug delivery systems (DDS) (Harada and Kataoka, 2006). When developing these systems, the goal is to obtain carriers with optimized drug loading and release properties, as well as long shelf life and low toxicity.

Self-assembly of macromolecules provides an efficient and rapid pathway for the preparation of polymeric drug carrier systems in the nanometer range (Nakashima and Bahadur, 2006; Disher and Eisenberg, 2002; Liu et al., 2001). Among the

(1) Corresponding e-mail: mskim@krict.re.kr

various aggregation processes, the most extensive study pertain to the self-assembly of block or graft copolymers (Gaucher et al., 2005; Signori et al., 2005). Block copolymers consist of two- or more- covalently bonded blocks with different physical and chemical properties (Riess et al., 1985). The increasing interest in block copolymers arises mainly from their unique and associative properties as a consequence of their molecular structure (Riess et al., 2003). One special class of block copolymers are so-called amphiphilic block copolymers with hydrophilic and hydrophobic moieties and thus with affinities for two different environments (Price et al., 1982; Piirma et al., 1992; Tuzar and Kratochvil, 1993; Alexandridis et al., 1996; Nace et al., 1996; Webber et al., 1996; Hamley et al., 1998; Xie and Xie, 1999; Alexandridis et al., 2000; Riess et al., 2002). Various kinds of amphiphilic block copolymers composed of a variety of hydrophilic and hydrophobic segments have so far been synthesized. The self-assemble characteristics of amphiphilic block copolymers are directly related to their segmental incompatibility. Their self-assembly behavior in aqueous media leading to micellar systems has been studied intensively from the physicochemical viewpoint. Thus, the polymeric micelles formed in aqueous media from amphiphilic block copolymers is one of the most intensively studied topics in the developing field of nano carrier for drug delivery.

Polymeric micelles with several formulations are currently recognized as one of the most promising modalities of drug carriers (Nishiyama and Kataoka, 2006). Therefore, polymeric micelles using amphiphilic block copolymers with unique properties have lent a strong impetus to biomedical applications as functional drug carriers in clinical trials.

In this chapter, we will focus on the polymeric micelles as drug carrier. First, self-assembly of amphiphilic block copolymers in aqueous to form stable polymeric micelles will be discussed. The basic principles of self-assembly and micellization of amphiphilic block copolymers will be then given. Finally, we will concentrate on polymeric micelles, showing promise as long circulating drug carrier.

16.2 Self-Assembly and Micellization of Amphiphilic Block Copolymers

16.2.1 Amphiphilic Block Copolymers

Amphiphilic block copolymers consist of hydrophilic and hydrophobic block segments (Rodriguez-Hernandez et al., 2005). The two blocks are not only incompatible, but they interact very differently with their environment depending on their chemical nature and relative molecular characteristics. This phenomenon can induce microphase separation of amphiphilic block copolymers, not only in aqueous media but also in organic solvents.

There are many kinds of amphiphilic block copolymers composed of a variety of hydrophilic and hydrophobic segments (Riess et al., 1985; Quirk et al., 1989; Chu and Zhou, 1996; Riess et al., 2002, 2003; Kim et al., 2004a, 2004b, 2005a, 2005b, 2006a, 2006b; Hyun et al. 2006). Hydrophilic block in amphiphilic block copolymers contains, though in most cases poly(ethylene oxide) constitutes the hydrophilic block which is uncharged (Nace et al., 1996; Xie et al., 1999), hydrophilic functional group with charged polymer salts such as ether, carboxyl, hydroxyl, amine, phosphate, and sulphate groups. The hydrophobic block could be polyester (ex. polycaprolactone, polylactide, and polyglycolide), polyamino acid (ex. polyaspartic acid and poly(gamma-benzyl-L-glutamate)), polyamine (ex. poly(L-lysine) and polyspermine), poly(propylene oxide), poly(butylene oxide), poly(styrene oxide), polyethylene, polystyrene, polybutadiene, etc. Besides different hydrophobic and hydrophilic blocks, the possibilities of large variations in total molecular weight and block composition provide copolymers with a wide range of hydrophilic-hydrophobic balance (HLB) which is limited in case of conventional surfactants.

16.2.2 Micellization of Amphiphilic Block Copolymers

Amphiphilic block copolymer behaves distinctively not only in aqueous media but also in organic solvents (Forster et al., 2002). In fact when an amphiphilic block copolymer is dissolved in aqueous that is a thermodynamical good solvent for hydrophilic block segment and a precipitant for the hydrophobic block segment (Fig. 16.1), the block copolymer chains spontaneously assemble into polymeric micelles with a diameter of several tens of nanometers in aqueous media (Klok and Lecommandoux, 2001).

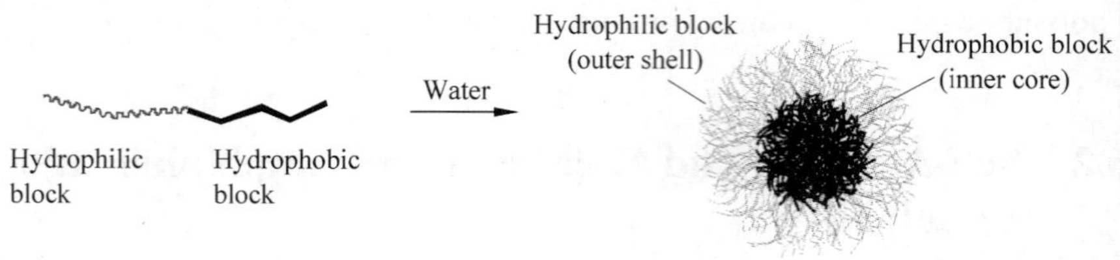

Figure 16.1 Formation of polymeric micelles from amphiphilic block copolymer

General procedures can be followed for the preparation of polymeric micelles (Munk, 1996). The first approach is to introduce the copolymer in a nonselective solvent, i.e., a common solvent for both blocks. In a second step, the subsequent addition of aqueous media as selective solvent, into a previously prepared solution from a common solvent, is followed. In next step, the common solvent is removed from the solution, usually via dialysis, or followed by ultrasonic stirring.

The micellization process of block copolymers in aqueous depends on the critical micelle concentration (CMC) (Moffitt et al., 1996; Hamley, 1998; Lodge,

2003; Hadjichristidis et al., 2003). If the CMC are not reached, self-assembly of amphiphilic block copolymers will not occur, and the block copolymer will behave in the aqueous as a unimer. On the contrary, if micelle formation is triggered, the micelles will be in thermodynamic equilibrium with unimers. In order to characterize a micellar system, several parameters have to be considered, including the equilibrium constant, CMC, the overall molar mass M_w of the micelle, its aggregation number Z and its morphology (Linse and Malmsten, 1992; Linse, 1994; Aranda-Espinoza et al., 2001). The shape and the size of the micelle aggregates after micellization of amphiphilic block copolymers are controlled by a variety of parameters that affect the balance between three major forces acting over the system: (1) the extent of constraints between the blocks forming the core (the block will be more or less stretched), (2) the interaction between chains forming the shell, and (3) the surface energy between the aqueous and the core of the micelle.

16.2.3 Polymeric Micelle Shape

From a theoretical point of view, the description of the micelle shape requires that the thermodynamic parameters of self-assembly be accounted for as well as the intra-micelle forces generated between the macromolecules inside the micelles (Rodriguez-Hernandez et al., 2005). These two factors (thermodynamics and intra-micelle forces) combined with the interactions between different micelles (inter-micelle forces) determine the type of self-assembled structure formed at equilibrium. It is then essential to understand the fundamentals that govern the interdependence between morphology and size of the polymeric micelles obtained by self-assembly, including decisive factors such as concentration, temperature, composition, block length, and amphiphilic block copolymer architecture.

The polymeric micelles are illustrated in Fig. 16.2. Polymeric micelles are generally spherical with narrow size distribution. Spherical micelles have the so-called 'core-shell' structure, in which an inner core is surrounded by an outer shell of hydrophilic polymers (Chu and Zhou, 1996). The hydrophilic block will be oriented towards the continuous aqueous medium and become the shell of the micelle formed, whereas the hydrophobic block will be shielded from the aqueous medium in the core of the structure. Formation of spherical micelles via self-assembly of block copolymers is directed by an entropically driven association mechanism.

But polymeric micelles may change in shape under certain conditions (Daoud and Cotton, 1982; Halperin, 1987; Shusharina et al., 1996; Wu and Gao, 2000; Shusharina et al., 2003). Micellar structures can be distinguished for block copolymers, depending on the relative length of the blocks. If the hydrophilic block is larger than the hydrophobic block, the micelles formed consist of a small core and a very large corona, and are thus called 'star-micelles'. By contrast, micelles having a large insoluble segment with a short soluble corona are referred to as 'crew-cut micelles' (Moffitt et al., 1996).

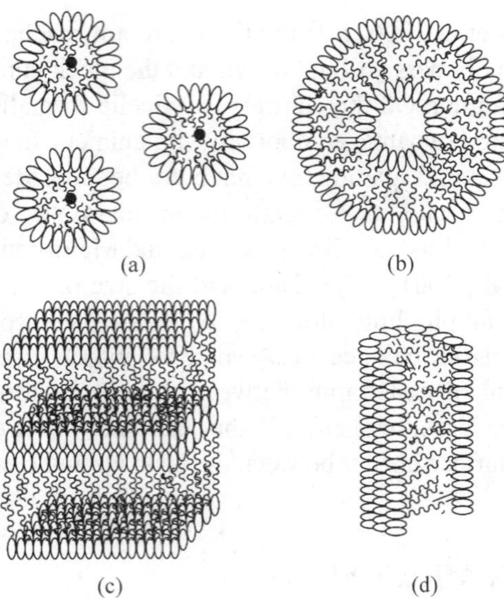

Figure 16.2 Structure of polymeric micelles (a) direct micelles, (b) vesicles, (c) lamellar, and (d) cylindrical micelles

Under specially circumstances, the polymeric micelles can be classified into several types with morphologies varying from spherical to vesicular or other less common structures (Chen and Jenekhe, 2000; Disher et al., 2000; Burke et al., 2001; Lee et al., 2001; Stoenescua and Meier, 2002; Soo and Eisenberg, 2004). Vesicles are nanometer-sized 'bags' whose double-layer outer membrane encloses an inner volume. They include uniform common vesicles, large polydisperse vesicles, entrapped vesicles, or hollow concentric vesicles. Because of the double layer, that recalls the structure of lipids in membrane cells, vesicles are also called polymersomes (polymer-based liposomes). In some aspects, polymersomes can be considered as 'giant nonbiological liposomes'. Amphiphilic block copolymers can form various vesicular architectures in solution.

In addition to common spherical micelles and vesicles, there are other more complex structures/morphologies, such as bilayers or cylinders, based on amphiphilic block copolymers. Cylindrical structure is prepared by a specifically designed amphiphilic block copolymers (Liu et al., 1996; Liu, 1997; Yu and Eisenberg, 1998a, 1998b; Stewart and Liu, 1999; Stewart et al., 2000).

16.2.4 Characterization of Polymeric Micelle Size

When an amphiphilic block copolymer is dissolved in aqueous, polymeric micelles is formed at ranging with a diameter of several tens of nanometers. Several techniques have been utilized for characterization of typical micelle size. Depending on the method of analysis employed, a variety of information about polymeric micelles can be determined (Hamley, 1998; Tuzar, 1996; Munk, 1996; Chu amd Zhou, 1996; Webber, 1996; Mortensen, 2000; Zana, 2000).

The most important are the scattering methods (Zhou and Chu, 1988a, 1988b; Brown et al., 1991, Schillen et al., 1993; Nolan et al., 1997; Burchard, 1983; Fukumine et al., 2000; de Banez et al., 2000; Imae et al., 2000). Dynamic (or quasi-elastic) light scattering (DLS) can be mainly used to estimate the hydrodynamic radius (R_H) of polymeric micelles from the determination of its diffusion coefficient (Fig. 16.3), in addition, the sensitivity and versatility of DLS allow changes in the micelle equilibrium due to variations of temperature, or other parameters to be monitored. Static light scattering (SLS) is a powerful technique to estimate average molar masses of self-assembled structures and their CMC. In addition, if scattering from the core and the shell of the micellar system is not very different, radius gyration (R_G) of polymeric micelles can be also calculated.

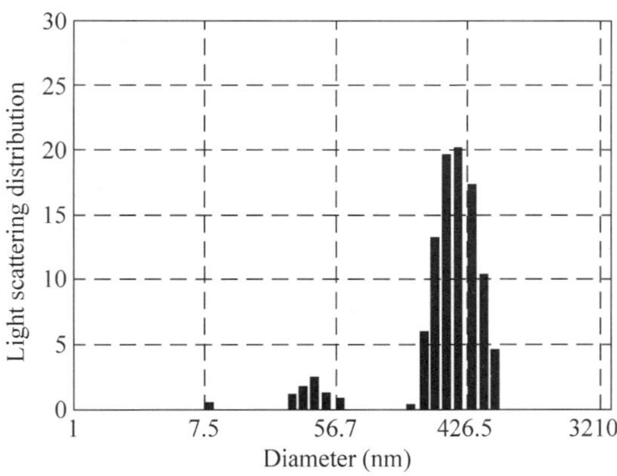

Figure 16.3 Dynamic light scattering (DLS) of polymeric micelles

Small-angle X-ray scattering (SAXS) in the analysis of polymeric micelle solutions has been also employed to obtain overall and internal sizes from differences in electron density of the aqueous and the polymeric micelles (Glatter et al., 1994; Wells et al., 2001). Finally, small-angle neutron scattering (SANS) gives information not only about the size, but also the cross-section (Mortensen and Pedersen, 1993). Other non-scattering methods such as transmission electron microscopy (TEM) and atomic force microscopy (AFM) provide images whereby size, shape or internal structure of the polymeric micelles can be confirmed.

16.2.5 CMC Determination of Polymeric Micelles

Micelle formation, or micellization, can be viewed as an alternative mechanism to adsorption at the interfaces for removing hydrophobic block from contact with water, thereby reducing the free energy of the system. The concentration at which micelles start to form is called CMC, and is an important characteristic of amphiphilic block copolymers.

The use of fluorescent probes is the most used method for the determination of the CMC (Kalyanasundaram and Thomas, 1977; Dong and Winnik, 1982; Calderara et al., 1994; Kim et al., 2005c). Pyrene is the preferred fluorescent probe because of its strong fluorescence in nonpolar domains and its weak radiation in polar media. Pyrene, a hydrophobic molecule, was preferentially distributed in the micelle core, causing changes in the photophysical properties. When the micelles are formed in an aqueous phase, pyrene molecules preferably locate inside or close to the hydrophobic microdomain of micelles, and consequently their photophysical characteristics change compared to pyrene molecules in water. The characteristic shift feature of pyrene excitation spectra from 335 to 338 nm is observed, indicating partitioning of pyrene into the hydrophobic micellar core. This shift was utilized to determine the CMC values. Figure 16.4 shows the fluorescence intensity ratio (I_{338}/I_{335}) of pyrene excitation spectra vs logarithm of amphiphilic block copolymer concentrations. A substantial increase of the intensity ratio begins above a certain concentration, indicating the onset of micelle formation. Therefore, the interception of two straight lines in the low concentration range is determined as CMC.

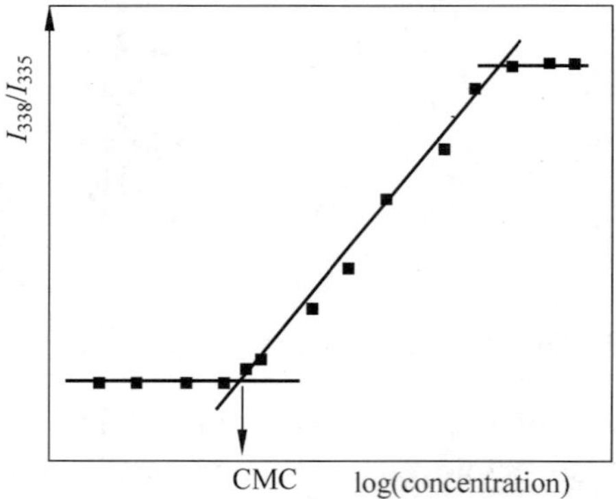

Figure 16.4 Experimental determination of CMC from fluorescence measurements with pyrene as a probe. Increasing intensity corresponds to encapsulation of pyrene in a hydrophobic environment and hence with micelle formation

UV-absorption spectroscopy has also been reported as a powerful technique for the determination of the CMC (Dominguez et al., 1997). This method is based on the tautomerism of 1-phenyl-1,3-butadione between keto and enol forms that possess different absorption maxima: 312 nm for the enolic form and 250 nm for the keto form, the former appearing in nonpolar solvents like cyclohexane and the latter in polar solvents, where H-bonding is destabilized in favor of the keto configuration.

Other methods, mainly scattering methods such as SLS, DLS or SAXS, extensively used for small surfactants, can in principle be used for polymeric micelles. However, they have found only limited application because of the very low signal intensity due to the much lower CMC's in block copolymers in comparison with low molar mass surfactants (Hamley et al., 1998).

16.3 Drug Loaded Polymeric Micelles

The formation of polymeric micelles by self-assemblies of amphiphilic block copolymers are unique structural characteristics described above. The structural characteristics of polymeric micelles, their mesoscopic size and core–shell structure, have some similarities to natural carriers such as viruses and lipoproteins. Polymeric micelles may play very important roles in a drug formulation as carriers for various drugs (Riess and Bahadur, 1985; Nace, 1996; Alexandridis and Lindman, 2000). The incorporation of drugs into the core of the micelle results in increased solubility, metabolic stability and circulation time for the drug (Prochazka et al., 1996; Kabanov and Alakhov, 2000; Liu et al., 2000; Malmsten, 2000; Tsitsilianis et al., 2000; Kataoka et al., 2001; Torchilin, 2001; Arshady, 2002; Kabanov et al., 2002). In addition, a hydrophilic shell has advantages in long-circulating of drugs, e.g. lowered uptake by reticuloendthelial systems and effective prevention of non-specific adsorption of proteins (Hawley et al., 1995; Stolnik et al., 1995; Torchilin, 1998; Ishida et al., 1999; Schiffelers et al., 1999; Kong et al., 2000). In this section, the focus is related to the application of self-assemblies of amphiphilic block copolymer as a drug carrier in DDS.

16.3.1 Drug Incorporation in Polymeric Micelles

The simplest ways of preparing drug-containing micelles is to solubilize solid drug or inject a small volume of a drug solution, in a water-miscible organic solvent, into micellar solutions in water (Kabanov, 1989; Kabanov et al., 1992; Milton-Harris, 1997; Benahmed et al., 2001). Depending on the type of drug used, activity of the drug and route of administration, the desired concentration of the drug in a pharmaceutical formulation may vary (Couvreur, 1988; Cammas-Marion et al., 2000; Kim et al., 2000; Liu et al., 2000). Quite often, for example, a relatively high concentration of drug in formulation (usually, several mg/mL) is needed for injection. In these cases, techniques that facilitate formation of equilibrium dispersions can be used. For example, drug and amphiphilic block copolymer are first dissolved in a common organic solvent and then the phases are reversed by slow addition of the aqueous media (Allen et al., 1999). The residual organic solvent is removed by dialysis or evaporation. Another technique involves evaporation of the solvent from a common organic solution of the drug and block copolymer, usually obtaining a dry film from the component mixture, which is then re-dispersed in the aqueous media.

16.3.2 Drug Solubilization Capacity of the Polymeric Micelles

Development of drug formulations in polymeric micelles quite faces limitations to the solubilization capacity of the micelles with respect to certain hydrophobic drugs. Obviously, the actual space available for incorporation of the drug in the core limits the solubilization capacity. Significant variation between the solubilization capacity of micelles formed by the same block copolymer with respect to various drugs is explained by differences in the structure of drug (Nagarajan, 1999). Many studies have indicated that the most important factor related to the drug solubilization capacity is the compatibility between the hydrophobic drugs and the core-forming block (Hurter et al., 1993; Gadelle et al., 1995; Nagarajan and Ganesh, 1996; Xing and Mattice, 1997). The amount of the incorporated hydrophobic drugs increases as the molecular volume of the hydrophobic drugs decreases. Furthermore, the solubilization capacity is greater when the core block-hydrophobic drugs interactions are favorable and the hydrophobic drugs-water surface tension is lower. As a result, for example, aromatic hydrocarbons are incorporated in polymeric micelles to a greater extent than aliphatic hydrocarbons. Overall, compared to conventional low molecular weight surfactants, amphiphilic block copolymers have relatively higher solubilization capacities and are more selective towards aromatic and heterocyclic compounds than towards aliphatic molecules. Since many drug molecules contain aromatic and heterocyclic groups, polymeric micelles appear to be particularly suited for the preparation of pharmaceutical formulations of such drug.

16.3.3 Drug Partitioning in Polymeric Micelles

In every micellar system containing hydrophobic drugs, there is always a dynamic exchange between the drugs incorporated in the micelle and those dissolved in the external solution, a process called 'partitioning'. If the rate of transfer of the drugs from micelles to aqueous equals the rate of the transfer from the aqueous to micelles, i.e., equilibrium is reached, then the partitioning is characterized by a thermodynamic constant, called the 'partition coefficient', P (Leo et al., 1971). By definition, the partition coefficient stands for the ratio:

$$P = \frac{[S_{\mathrm{m}}]}{[S_{\mathrm{w}}]}$$

where $[S_{\mathrm{m}}]$ and $[S_{\mathrm{w}}]$ are the drug concentrations in the micelle and aqueous microphase phase, respectively.

Conditions of equilibrium partitioning are rarely realized in the body. However, partitioning coefficient can be useful, as first estimation, to determine the amount of the drug, which is incorporated in the micelles in the formulation administered to the patient, as well as of the amount of the drug, which can be released upon dilution of this formulation in the body fluids.

Several methods have been proposed for determining the partition coefficients of drug in the polymeric micelles. Fluorescence technique is one convenient method that allows determination of the partition coefficients of drugs in polymeric micelles (Wilhelm et al., 1991; Kabanov et al., 1995). In the case of non-fluorescent drugs that contain chromophor groups, a method for partition coefficient determination is based on measuring the electronic spectra of these drugs. An alternative method for determination of the partition coefficients involves measuring the rates of diffusion of the drug from polymeric micelles through a semi-permeable membrane (Saito et al., 1996; Melik-Nubarov and Kozlov, 1998). The fluorescence- and diffusion-based techniques revealed that the partition coefficient values obtained by these two methods are in very good agreement with each other.

16.3.4 Drug Release from Polymeric Micelles

Beside incorporation of drugs into polymeric micelles, their release kinetics are also important aspects of polymeric micelles because this information is directly related to the design of drug delivery systems (Fig. 16.5). It can be considered in terms of the equilibrium behavior ('thermodynamic stability') and the dynamic behavior ('kinetic stability') (Alakhov et al., 1998). The CMC and the partition coefficient are the major thermodynamic constants determining the drug stability inside polymeric micelles and the drug release from polymeric micelles. The dilution of the polymeric micelles, for example, in the body fluids, results in a decrease in the portion of the drug-incorporated micelle. Furthermore, if the system is diluted below the CMC, the polymeric micelles are completely disintegrated and the drug is completely released in the external media. Thus, the CMC values can be characterized as 'from moderately stable to relatively unstable micelles'. In addition, polymeric micelles may exhibit high kinetic stability due to long lasting relaxation processes that result in a slow dissociation of the micelles after dilution to concentrations below the CMC.

The stability of drug-incorporated micelle correlated with drug release from polymeric micelles (Yokoyama et al., 1993; Kwon et al., 1995). If polymer micelles are formed by block copolymers containing higher hydrophobicity, the molecular motion of the chains in the core of such micelles is strongly physically attached to each other, resulting in particular stability of polymeric micelles (Allen et al., 1999). The drug release rates in such micelles are low due to slow diffusion of the drug through the core. Block copolymers of this type offer high blood circulation times combined with slow release of the free drug in the body. However, direct characterization of the drug stability and drug release in polymeric micelles, particularly, in the context of the determining of whether the polymeric

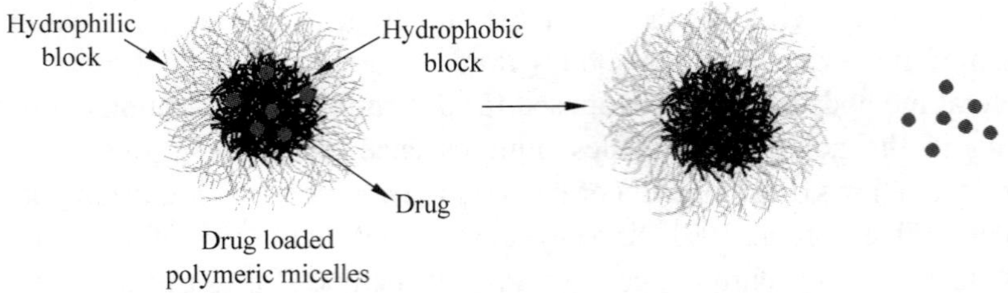

Figure 16.5 Drug release from the polymeric micelles

micelles formed in vitro are preserved in vivo, is technically difficult. Nevertheless, some attempts have been trying to address the drug stability and drug release of polymeric micelles in the presence of selected blood components, such as serum proteins (Kabanov et al., 1995; Kabanov and Alakhov, 2000).

16.4 Biological Applications of Polymeric Micelles

16.4.1 Biodistribution

A major objective of using polymeric micelles as a drug carrier is to modulate drug disposition in the body directed toward better therapeutic efficacy. For successful drug targeting, the achievement of a prolonged blood circulation of polymeric micelles might be of primary importance, because they are delivered to the target tissue through the bloodstream, and the extravasation process is generally considered to be slow and in a passive manner. However, there are several obstacles to the long circulation of polymeric micelles, which include glomerular excretion by the kidney and recognition by the reticuloendothelial system (RES) located in the liver, spleen and lung (Kataoka, 1996). The glomerular excretion can be avoided by using polymeric micelles with a larger molecular weight than its threshold value, which is 42 – 50 kDa for water-soluble polymers (Seymour et al., 1987). On the other hand, RES recognition may be avoidable by designing polymeric micelles to have a size smaller than 200 nm as well as an excellent biocompatibility (Stolnik et al., 1995; Mosqueria et al., 2001). It is known that non-biocompatible nanoparticles are recognized by the RES via the complement activation, followed by elimination from the circulation; however, the surface modification of nanoparticles with hydrophilic and biocompatible polymers, such as PEG with an effective protein-resistant property due to its steric repulsion effect (Jeon et al., 1991), can impair or even avoid RES recognition (Stolnik et al., 1995; Mosqueria et al., 2001). Therefore, it is likely that polymeric micelles covered with a high density of PEG shells might circumvent the aforementioned obstacles, thus showing a stealth property during blood circulation.

Polymeric micelles may not necessarily dissociate immediately after extreme dilution following intravenous injection into the body and their dissociation is kinetically slow. This property allows the micelles to circulate in the bloodstream until accumulation at target tissues. The distribution volume in the blood and plasma-to-blood ratio of the micelles is calculated to be nearly equivalent to the blood volume and the plasma space value, respectively, suggesting that polymeric micelles might distribute only to the blood compartment and hardly interact with blood cells immediately after their administration.

When the polymeric micelle in the liver and spleen have low values of tissue-to-blood concentration ratios comparable to those obtained from long-circulating liposomes (Allen and Hansen, 1991; Woodle et al., 1992), the polymeric micelle avoided the RES recognition as well as the entrapment by hepatic sinusoidal capillaries characterized by large interendothelial junctions (~100 nm) and the absence of the basement membranes. Furthermore, the constituent block copolymers might be finally excreted into the urine if their molecular weight is lower than the threshold of glomerular filtration. This suggests the safety of polymeric micelles with a low risk of chronic accumulation in the body.

16.4.2 Accumulation in Target Solid Tumors

Long-circulating polymeric carriers can preferentially and effectively accumulate in target tissue such as solid tumors. This phenomenon is explained by the microvascular hyperpermeability to circulating macromolecules and their impaired lymphatic drainage in solid tumors, and is termed the 'Enhanced Permeability and Retention (EPR) effect' (Matsumura and Maeda, 1986; Maeda, 2001). Polymeric micelles can show an enhanced accumulation in various types of solid tumors, which is most probably due to EPR effect (Kwon et al., 1994; Yokoyama et al., 1999; Nishiyama et al., 2003; Hamaguchi et al., 2005). The EPR effect appears to be a phenomenon universally observed in malignant tumors. The vascular cut-off sizes is ranging between 380 and 780 nm for human or murine tumors including mammary and colorectal carcinomas, hepatoma, glioma, and sarcoma (Hobbs et al., 1998; Jain, 2001). Hence, the vascular pore cut-off sizes of tumors are unlikely to be a significant obstacle to transvascular transport of polymeric micelles with a relatively small size (i.e. less than 100 nm). Thus, the EPR effect is a strategic basis for designing polymeric micelles for successful tumor-targeted therapy.

16.5 Conclusions and Outlook

Self-assemblies of amphiphilic block copolymers have many interesting features from both fundamental and applied viewpoints. In particular, polymeric micelles formed from amphiphilic block copolymers in aqueous, have been extensively investigated as typical self-assemblies. In this chapter, we focused on polymeric micelles with amphiphilic block copolymers in aqueous media by employing systematic method. The basic principles for the formation of polymeric micelles through the organization of block copolymers in aqueous and the physicochemical properties of drug loaded polymeric micelles have been briefly described. In addition, biological application of polymeric micelles has been given in last section.

Without any doubt, the primary reason for using polymeric systems is the ease and simplicity with which they can form ordered nanoscale structures in aqueous via self-assembly, meaning that expected shapes and sizes can be obtained without an additional trigger. In conclusion, we believe that control of the property of such polymeric nano-micelles as drug carrier is addressable challenges even though the use of these polymeric micelles is still in its infancy for practical clinical applications. Therefore, this research field provides opportunities for chemists, physicists and biochemists, etc. to develop systems that may eventually match in sophistication and precision biological structures elaborated by nature.

References

Alakhov, V.Y. and A.V. Kabanov. *Expert. Opin. Invest. Drugs* **7**: 1453 (1998).

Alexandridis, P. and T.A. *Hatton. Block Copolymers. Polymer Materials Encyclopedia 1*. Boca Raton: CRC Press, p.43 (1996).

Alexandridis, P. and B. Lindman. *Amphiphilic Block Copolymers: Self Assembly and Applications.* Amsterdam: Elsevier p. 1 (2000).

Allen, C., D. Maysinger and A. Eisenberg. *Colloids Surfaces B Biointerfaces* **16**: 3 (1999).

Allen, T.M. and C. Hansen. *Biochim. Biophys. Acta* **1068**: 133 (1991).

Aranda-Espinoza, H., H. Bermudez, F.S. Bates and D.E. Disher. *Phys. Rev. Lett.* **87**: 20,8301/1(2001).

Arshady, R., ed. *Polymers in Medicine and Biotechnology. The PMB Series, Vols 1 and 2.* London: Citus Books (2002).

Banez, M.V., K.L. Robinson and S.P. Armes. *Macromolecules* **33**: 451 (2000).

Benahmed, A., M. Ranger and J.C. Leroux. *Pharma. Res.***18**: 323 (2001).

Brown, W., K. Schillen, M. Almgren, S. Hvidt and P. Bahadur. *J. Phys. Chem.* **95**: 1850 (1991).

Burchard, W. *Adv. Polym. Sci.* **48**: 1 (1983).

Burke, S., H. Shen and A. Eisenberg. *Macromol. Symp.* **175**: 273 (2001).

Calderara, F., Z. Hruska, G. Hurtrez, J.P. Lerch, T. Nugay and G. Riess. *Macromolecules* **27**: 1210 (1994).

Cammas-Marion, S., M.M. Bear, A. Harada, Ph. Guerin and K. Kataoka. *Macromol. Chem. Phys.* **201**: 355 (2000).

Chu, B. and Z. Zhou. Physical chemistry of poly(oxyalkylene) block copolymer surfactants. In: V.N. Nace, ed. *Non-ionic Surfactants: Polyoxyalkylene Block Copolymers*, Vol. 60. New York: Marcel Dekker (1996).

Chen, X.L. and S.A. Jenekhe. *Macromolecules* **33**: 4610 (2000).

Couvreur, P. *Crit. Rev. Ther. Drug Carrier Syst.* **5**: 1 (1988).

Daoud, M. and J.P. Cotton. *J. Phys.* **43**: 531 (1982).

Disher, B.M., D.A. Hammer, F.S. Bates and D.E. Disher. *Curr. Opin. Colloid Interface Sci* **5**: 125 (2000).

Disher, D.E. and A. Eisenberg. *Polymer vesicles. Science* **297**: 967 (2002).

Dominguez, A., A. Fernandez, N. Gonzalez, E. Iglesias and L. Montenegro. *J. Chem. Education* **74**: 1227 (1997).

Dong, D.C. and M.A. Winnik. *Photochem. Photobiol.* **35**: 17(1982).

Fukumine, Y., K. Inomata, A. Takano and T. Nose. *Polymer* **41**: 5367 (2000).

Forster, S. and T. Plantenberg. *Angew. Chem. Int. Ed.* **41**: 688 (2002).

Gadelle, F., W.J. Koros and R.S. Schechter. *Macromolecules* **28**: 4883(1995).

Gaucher, G., M. Dufresne, V.P. Sant, N. Kang, D. Maysinger and J.-C. Leroux. *J. Control. Release* **109**: 169 (2005).

Glatter, G., K. S. Scherf and W. Brown. *Macromolecules* **27**: 6046 (1994).

Hadjichristidis, N., S. Pispas and G.A. Floudas. *Block Copolymers: Synthetic Strategies, Physical Properties, and Applications*. New York: Wiley (2003).

Hamaguchi, T., Y. Mastumura, M. Suzuki, K. Shimizu, R. Goda and I. Nakamura. *Br. J. Cancer* **92**: 1240 (2005).

Hamley, I,W. *The Physics of Block Copolymers*. Oxford: Oxford University Press (1998).

Halperin, A. Macromolecules **20**: 2943 (1987).

Hawley, A.E., S.S. Davis and L. Illum. *Adv. Drug Deliv. Rev.* **17**: 129 (1995).

Hamley, I.W. In: I.W. Hamley, ed. *The Physics of Block Copolymers.* Oxford Science Publication, p. 131 (1998).

Harada, A. and K. Kataoka. *Prog. Polym. Sci.* **31**: 949 (2006).

Hobbs, S.K., W.L. Monsky, F. Yuan, W.G. Roberts, L. Griffith and V.P. Torchilin. *Proc. Natl. Acad. Sci. USA* **95**: 4607 (1998).

Hurter, P.N., J.M.H.M. Scheutjens and T.A. Hatton. *Macromolecules* **26**. 5592 (1993).

Hyun, H., M.S. Kim, G. Khang and H.B. Lee. *J. Polym. Sci. Part A: Polym. Chem.* **44**: 4235 (2006).

Imae, T., H. Tabuchi, K. Funayama, A. Sato, T. Nakamura and N. Amaya. *Colloid Surf. A: Physicochem Engng. Aspects* **167**: 73 (2000).

Ishida, O., K. Maruyama, K. Sasaki and M. Iwatsuru. *Int. J. Pharm.* **190**: 49 (1999).

Jain, R.K. *Adv. Drug Deliv. Rev.* **46**: 149 (2001).

Jeon, S.I., J.H. Lee, J.D. Andrade and P.G. De Gennes. *J. Colloid Interface Sci.* **142**: 149 (1991).

Kabanov, A.V., et al. *FEBS Lett.* **258**: 343 (1989).

Kabanov, A.V., V.I. Slepnev, L.E. Kuznetsova, E.V. Batrakova, V.Y. Alakhov, N.S. Melik-Nubarov, P.G. Sveshnikov and V.A. Kabanov. *Biochem. Int.* **26**: 1035 (1992).

Kabanov, A.V., I.R. Nazarova, I.V. Astafieva, E.V. Batrakova, V.Y. Alakhov, A.A. Yaroslavov and V.A. Kabanov. *Macromolecules* **28**: 2303 (1995).

Kabanov, A.V. and V.Y. Alakhov. Micelles of amphiphilic block copolymers as vehicles for drug delivery. In: P. Alexandridis and B. Lindman, ed. *Amphiphilic Block Copolymers: Self-Assembly and Applications.* Amsterdam: Elsevier, p. 347 (2000).

Kabanov, A.V., E.V. Batrakova and V.Y. Alakhov. *J. Control. Release* **82**: 189 (2002).

Kakizawa, Y. and K. Kataoka. *Adv, Drug Deliv. Rev.* **54**: 203 (2002).

Kalyanasundaram, K. and J.K. Thomas. *J. Am. Chem. Soc.* **99**: 2039 (1977).

Kataoka, K. Targetable polymeric drugs (Chap. 4). In: K. Park, ed. *Controlled Drug Delivery: The Next Generation.* ACS, Washington DC (1996).

Kataoka, K., A. Harada and Y. Nagasaki. *Adv. Drug Deliv. Rev.* **47**: 113 (2001).

Kim, M.S., K.S. Seo, G. Khang, S.H. Cho and H.B. Lee, *J. Biomed. Mater. Res.* **70A**: 154 (2004a).

Kim, M.S., K.S. Seo, G. Khang, S.H. Cho and H.B. Lee. *J. Polym. Sci. Part A: Polym. Chem.* **42**: 5784 (2004b).

Kim, M.S., K.S. Seo, G. Khang and H.B. Lee. *Macromol. Rapid Commun.* **26**: 643 (2005a).

Kim, M.S., K.S. Seo, H. Hyun, G. Khang and H.B. Lee. *Int. J. Pharm.* **304**: 165 (2005b).

Kim, M.S., H. Hyun, Y.H. Cho, K.S. Seo, W.Y. Jang, S.K. Kim, G. Khang and H.B. Lee. *Poly. Bull.* **55**: 149 (2005c).

Kim, M.S., H. Hyun, G. Khang and H.B. Lee. *Macromolecules* **39**: 3099 (2006a).

Kim, M.S., H. Hyun, K.S. Seo, Y.H. Cho, G. Khang and H.B. Lee. *J. Polym. Sci. Part A: Polym. Chem.* **44**: 5413 (2006b).

Kim, S.Y., J.C. Ha and M.J. Lee. *J. Control. Release* **65**: 345 (2000).

Klok, H.-A. and S. Lecommandoux. *Adv. Mater.* **13**: 1217 (2001).

Kong, G., R.D. Braun and M.W. Dewhirst. *Cancer Res.* **60**: 4440 (2000).

Kwon, G.S., S. Suwa, M. Yokoyama, T. Okano, Y. Sakurai and K. Kataoka. *J. Control. Release* **29**: 17 (1994).

Kwon, G.S., M. Natio, M. Yokoyama, T. Okano, Y. Sakurai and K. Kataoka. *Pharm. Res.* **12**: 192 (1995).

Lee, J.C.-M., H. Bermudez, B.M. Discher, M.A. Sheehan, Y.Y. Won, F.S. Bates, et al. *Biotechnol. Bioeng.* **73**: 135 (2001).

Leo, A., C. Hansch and D. Elkins. *Chem. Rev.* **71**: 525 (1971).

Linse, P. and M. Malmsten. *Macromolecules* **25**: 5434 (1992).

Linse, P. *Macromolecules* **27**: 6404 (1994).

Liu, G., L. Qiao and A. Guo. *Macromolecules* **29**: 5508 (1996).

Liu, G. *Adv Nanofibers Mater.* **9**: 437 (1997).

Liu, S., H. Zhu, H. Zhao, M. Jiang and C. Wu. *Langmuir* **16**: 3712 (2000).

Liu, J.Q., Q. Zhang, E.E. Remsen and K.L. Wooley. *Biomacromolecules* **3**: 362 (2001).

Lodge, T.P. *Macromol. Chem. Phys.* **204**: 265 (2003).

Maeda, H. *Adv. Drug Deliv. Rev.* **46**: 169 (2001).

Malmsten, M. Block copolymers in pharmaceutics. In: P. Alexandridis and B. Lindman, eds. *Amphiphilic Block Copolymers: Self Assembly and Applications*. Amsterdam: Elsevier, p. 319 (2000).

Matsumura, Y. and H. Maeda. *Cancer. Res.* **46**: 6387 (1986).

Melik-Nubarov, N.S. and M.Y. Kozlov. *Colloid Polym. Sci.* **276**: 381 (1998).

Milton-Harris, J. *ACS Polym Prepr* (*Div. Polym. Chem*). **38**: 520 (1997).

Moffitt, M., K. Khougaz and A. Eisenberg. *Acc. Chem. Res.* **29**: 95 (1996).

Mortensen, K. and J.S. Pedersen. *Macromolecules* **26**: 805 (1993).

Mortensen, K. Small angle scattering studies of block copolymer micelles, micellar mesophases and networks. In: P. Alexandridis and B. Lindman, eds. *Amphiphilic Block Copolymers: Self assembly and Applications.* Amsterdam: Elsevier, p. 191 (2000).

Mosqueria, V.C.F., P. Legrand, A. Gulik, O. Bourdon, R. Gref and D. Labarre, et al. *Biomaterials* **22**: 2967 (2001).

Munk, P. Equilibrium and nonequilibrium polymer micelles. In: S.E. Webber, P. Munk and Z. Tuzar, eds. *Solvents and Selforganization of Polymer. NATO ASI Series, Serie E: Applied Sciences.* Vol. 327. Dordrecht: Kluwer Academic Publisher (1996).

Nagarajan, R. and K. Ganesh. *J. Colloid Interface Sci.* **184**: 489 (1996).

Nagarajan, R. *Colloids Surfaces B Biointerfaces* **16**: 55 (1999).

Nakashima, K. and P. Bahadur. *Adv. Colloid Interface Sci.* **123 – 126**: 75 (2006).

Nace, V.M. *Nonionic Surfactants: Polyoxyalkylene Block Copolymers. Surfactant Science Series 60.* New York: Marcel Dekker, p. 1 (1996).

Nishiyama, N., S. Okazaki, H. Cabral, M. Miyamoto, Y. Kato and Y. Sugiyama et al. *Cancer Res.* **63**: 8977 (2003).

Nishiyama, N. and K. Kataoka. *Pharmacology & Therapeutics* **112**: 630 (2006).

Nolan, S.L., R.J. Phillips, P.M. Cotts and S.R. Dungan. *J. Colloid Interface Sci.* **191**: 291 (1997).

Piirma, I. *Polymeric Surfactants. Surfactant Science Series 42.* New York: Marcel Dekker, p. 1 (1992).

Price, C. Colloidal properties of block copolymers. In: I. Goodman. *Developments in Block Copolymers 1.* London: Applied Science, p. 39 (1982).

Prochazka, K., T.J. Martin, S.E. Webber and P. Munk. *Macromolecules* **29**: 6526 (1996).

Quirk, R.P., D.J. Kinning and L.J. Fetters. *Block Copolymers. Comprehensive Polymer Science 7.* Oxford: Pergamon Press, p. 1 (1989).

Riess, G., G. Hurtrez and P. Bahadur. *Block copolymers. 2nd ed. Encyclopedia of Polymer Science and Engineering,* Vol. 2. New York: Wiley, p. 324 (1985).

Riess, G., Ph. Dumas and G. Hurtrez. *Block Copolymer Micelles and Assemblies. MML Series 5.* London: Citus Books, p. 69 (2002).

Riess, G. *Prog. Polym. Sci.* **28**: 1107 (2003).

Rodriguez-Hernandez, J., F. Checot, Y. Gnanou and S. Lecommandoux. *Prog. Polym. Sci.* **30**: 691 (2005).

Piirma, I. *Polymeric Surfactants. Surfactant Science Series 42.* Marcel Dekker: New York, p. 1 (1992).

Prochazka, K., T.J. Martin, S.E. Webber and P. Munk. *Macromolecules* **29**: 6526 (1996).

Price, C. Colloidal properties of block copolymers. In: I. Goodman, ed. *Developments in Block Copolymers 1.* London: Applied Science, p. 39 (1982).

Saito, Y., K. Miura, Y. Tokuoka, Y. Kondo, M. Abe and T. Sato. *J. Dispersion Sci. Technol.* **17**: 567 (1996).

Schiffelers, R.M., I.A. Bakker-Woudenberg, S.V. Snijders and G. Storm. *Biochim. Biophys. Acta* **1421**: 329 (1999).

Schillen, K., O. Glatter and W. Brown. *Prog. Colloid Polym. Sci.* **93**: 66 (1993).

Seymour, L.W., R. Duncan, J. Strohalm and J. Kopecek. *J. Biomed. Mater. Res.* **21**: 1341 (1987).

Shusharina, N.P., I.A. Nyrkova and A.R. Khoklov. *Macromolecules* **29**: 3167 (1996).

Shusharina, N.P., P. Alexandridis, P. Linse, S. Balijepalli and H.J.M. Gruenbauer. *Eur. Phys. J.* **10**: 45 (2003).

Soo, P.L., and A. Eisenberg, J. Polym. Sci. Part B, Poly. Phys. **42**: 923(2004).

Signori, F., F. Chiellini and R. Solaro. *Polymer* **46**: 9642 (2005).

Stewart, S. and G. Liu. *Chem. Mater.* **11**: 1048 (1999).

Stewart, S. and G. Liu. *Angew. Chem. Int. Ed.* **39**: 340 (2000).

Stolnik, S., L. Illum and S.S. Davis. *Adv. Drug Deliv. Rev.* **16**: 195 (1995).

Stoenescua, R. and W. Meier. *Chem. Commun.* **24**: 3016 (2002).

Torchilin, V.P. *J. Control. Release* **73**: 137 (2001).

Torchilin, V.P. In vitro and in vivo availability of liposomes. In: A.V. Kabanov, P.L. Felgner and L.W. Seymour, eds. *Self-assembling Complexes for Gene Delivery: From Laboratory to Clinical Trial.* Chichester, UK: Wiley, p. 277 (1998).

Tsitsilianis, C., D. Voulgaris, M. Stepanek, K. Podhajecka, K. Prochazka, Z. Tuzar and W. Brown. *Langmuir* **16**: 6868 (2000).

Tuzar, Z. and P. Kratochvil. Micelles of block and graft copolymers in solution. In: E. Matijevic, ed. *Surface and colloid science,* Vol. 15. Chapter 1. New York: Plenum Press, p. (1993).

Tuzar, Z. Overview of polymer micelles. In: S.E. Webber, P. Munk and Z. Tuzar, eds. *Solvents and Self-Organization of Polymer. NATO ASI Series, Serie E: Applied Sciences,* Vol. 327. Dordrecht : Kluwer Academic Publisher, p. 1 (1996).

Webber, S.E. Use of fluorescence methods to characterize the interior of polymer micelles. In: S.E. Webber, P. Munk and Z. Tuzar, eds. *Solvents and Self-Organization of Polymer. NATO ASI Series, Serie E: Applied Sciences,* Vol. 327. Dordrecht: Kluwer Academic Publisher (1996).

Wells, S., D. Taylor, M. Adam, J.M. De Simone and B. Farago. *Macromolecules* **34**: 6161 (2001).

Wilhelm, M., C.L. Zhao, Y. Wang, R. Xu, M.A. Winnik, J.L. Mura, G. Riess and M.D. Croucher. *Macromolecules* **24**: 1033 (1991). Woodle, M.C., K.K. Matthay, M.S. Newman, J.E. Hidayat, L.R. Collins and C. Redemann, et al. *Biochim. Biophys. Acta.* **1105**: 193 (1992).

Woodle, M.C., G. Storm, M.S. Newman, J.J. Jekot, L.R. Collins, F.J. Martin and F.C. Jr. Szoka. Pharm Res. **9**: 260 (1992).

Wu, C. and J. Gao. *Macromolecules* **33**: 645 (2000).

Xie, H.Q. and D. Xie. *Prog. Polym. Sci.* **24**: 275 (1999).

Xing, L. and W.L. Mattice. *Macromolecules* **30**: 1711 (1997).

Yokoyama, M., T. Sugiyama, T. Okano, Y. Sakurai, M. Naito and K. Kataoka. *Pharm. Res.* **10**: 895 (1999).

Yu, K.E. and A. Eisenberg. *Macromolecules* **31**: 3509 (1998a).

Yu, K.E. and A. Eisenberg. *Macromolecules* **31**: 5546 (1998b).

Zana, R. Fluorescence studies of amphiphilic block copolymers in solution. In: P. Alexandridis and B. Lindman, eds. *Amphiphilic Block Copolymers: Self Assembly and Applications.* Amsterdam: Elsevier, p. 221 (2000).

Zhou, Z. and B. Chu. *J. Colloid Interface Sci.* **126**: 171 (1988a).

Zhou, Z. and B. Chu. *Macromolecules* **21**: 2548 (1988b).

17 DNA Nanotechnology

Junping Zhang and Roger J. Narayan

Joint Department of Biomedical Engineering,
University of North Carolina and North Carolina State University
Chapel Hill, NC 27599-7575, USA

Abstract DNA, besides its function as a carrier of genetic information, is a promising biomolecule that can be patterned into two-dimensional or three-dimensional structures on the nanometer scale. It has been recently used as a template or a scaffold for the assembly of a wide variety of materials into periodic arrays and other patterned structures. These novel nanoscale materials demonstrate valuable functional, chemical, mechanical, electronic, and biological properties. DNA nanotechnology has a large number of potential applications, including use in molecular diagnostics, biosensors, therapeutics, and nanoelectronic circuitry.

17.1 Introduction

A major objective in the growing field of nanoscience is the creation of ordered nanostructures for executing complex operations. Deoxyribonucleic acid (DNA) is a very promising biological molecule for use in these structures because of its unique selective self-assembly, programmability, and synthesis properties. DNA can be directly incorporated within two-dimensional or three-dimensional nanoscale structures. In addition, it may be used as template or scaffold for the assembly of other materials into periodic nanoscale arrays.

These structures have large number of potential applications in molecular diagnostics, biosensors, therapeutics, nanoelectronic circuitry, and many other applications. For example, DNA sequences can be used to detect the synthesis of molecules as well as identify complementary molecules at very low concentrations. In addition, DNA molecule motors have unique abilities for releasing, capturing, and controlling molecules. Structures formed from DNA strands can be functionalized to organize as well as detect other materials. This chapter presents an overview

(1) Corresponding e-mail: roger_narayan@unc.edu

of the recent progress that has been made in DNA-based nanotechnology.

17.2 Basic Features of DNA

The major properties of DNA for the self-assembly of functional nanostructures include the following: (1) the base-pairing rules of nucleotides, (2) the ability of a single strand of DNA to bind a complementary sequence of DNA with high affinity, (3) the stability of DNA over a wide range of environmental conditions, and (4) hybridization of DNA is reversible and can be controlled by temperature. The double helix structure of DNA was discovered by Watson and Crick in 1953 (Watson et al., 1953). The unique functions of DNA result from its composition, structure, physical properties, and chemical properties. Deoxyribonucleic acid contains the four nucleotides, each of which is made up of a five-carbon sugar (deoxyribose), a heterocyclic base, and a phosphate group. Nucleotides include two purine molecules, adenine (A) and guanine (G), as well as two pyrimidine molecules, cytosine (C), and thymine (T). In DNA, two antiparallel polynucleotide strands are held together in a double helix by hydrogen bonds. The double helix is a nanoscale material, with a diameter of ~2 nm and a helical repeat of ~10 – 10.5 nucleotide pairs, resulting in a pitch of ~3.4 – 3.6 nm (Van Holde, 1989). DNA is relatively stiff, with a persistence length of 50 nm, which corresponds to ~15 double helical turns (Hagerman, 1988). Three hydrogen bonds form between cytosine and guanine molecules, and two hydrogen bonds form between adenine and thymine molecules; these nucleotide-nucleotide units are referred to as base pairs (Butler, 2001). DNA base pairing is the basis for the fabrication of many DNA-based nanostructures.

Hydrogen bonding between two complementary single DNA strands to form a double helix is called hybridization. When double-stranded DNA is heated to a sufficiently high temperature, the DNA will denature. The two strands will start to dehybridize and dissociate to single strands. If this denatured DNA is then cooled, the two single stands will rehybridize and reform a double helix structure at locations where complementary sequences exist. The melting temperature (T_m) is defined as the temperature at which 50% of the DNA species form a stable double helix and the other 50% have been separated to single strands (Santa Lucia, 1998). This value depends on both the length and the nucleotide sequence composition of the specific DNA molecule. DNA patterns and motifs may be constructed using Watson-Crick interactions and double-strand formation mechanisms. These materials may be used as building blocks for the assembly of larger two-dimensional and three-dimensional nanostructures. As a result of these unique properties, the DNA double helix is an ideal material for controlling the assembly of nanostructures.

17.3 Self-Assembly of DNA Aanostructures

17.3.1 Basic Concepts

In recent years, many research groups have developed novel approaches for controlling the formation and assembly of nanostructured materials. DNA has demonstrated significant promise for algorithmic assembly of materials, because DNA self-assembly processes are straightforward and programmable. One use of DNA involves forming stable Holliday junctions, which are branched DNA molecules with complex motifs. These structures can then be self-assembled to form well-defined nanometer-scale or micrometer-scale structures.

Seeman and his coworkers were the first to exploit the Watson-Crick base pairing to create stable branched DNA structures (Seeman, 1982; Mao et al., 1997; Seeman, 1991; Zhang and Seeman, 1992, 1994). It is possible to construct a quadrilateral structure by directing a branched motif to associate with other branched motifs by means of complementary sticky ends (Seeman, 2003a). There are four sticky ends, in which X is complementary to X' and Y is complementary to Y'. The quadrilateral structure maintains open valences on the available outside sticky ends. These sticky ends could be extended by adding additional monomers in order to produce a lattice in two dimensions or three dimensions. The square-like quadrilateral structure anticipated from interaction among four-arm junction structures is based on the assumption that the four-arm branched junctions are rigid and retain their cruciform shapes. In fact, the branched junctions are flexible to a certain extent, which may destroy the periodicity of the resulting material (Churchill et al., 1988; Lilley and Clegg, 1993). In order to resolve this issue, Seeman and co-workers constructed branched complexes known as double-crossover molecules (DX). These structures are created by joining two double helixes together by an exchange of strands (Li et al., 1996; Seeman, 2003b; Fu and Seeman, 1993). Double-crossover molecules are classified as either parallel (DP) or antiparallel (DA) by the relative orientation of their strands. Antiparallel molecules are often used in self-assembly due to their superior mechanical properties. These molecules are divided into two types according to the number of DNA strands per complex and the number of helical turns between the crossover points. DAO double crossover molecules exhibit antiparallel strand orientation and possess an odd (O) number of half-turns between crossover sites. On the other hand, DAE molecules have an even (E) number of half-turns between crossover sites. Both DAO and DAE tiles are approximately twice as rigid as linear duplex DNA (Sa-Ardyen et al., 2003). As a result, these structures are much stiffer than simple branched junctions. The first two-dimensional periodic arrays containing double-crossover molecules were described by Winfree et al. (1998). These relatively rigid arrays were formed using double-crossover molecules that contained appropriate sticky-ends.

17.3.2 Two-Dimensional DNA Array Structures

17.3.2.1 DNA Lattice Structures

Recent studies have described the use of rigid DNA tile structures for forming two-dimensional arrays. For example, LaBean et al. extended the double crossover motif to create triple-crossover (TX) molecules that could be assembled into larger two-dimensional structures (LaBean et al., 2000). Mao et al. (1999) utilized four Holliday junctions to construct a parallelogram DNA junction. Interactions among sticky-ended cohesions on several parallelograms can be used to produce periodic, cavity-containing arrays. Yan et al. (2003) created four-by-four tiles, which can assemble into two-dimensional nanogrids. Other helix tiles are also capable of assembling into two-dimensional arrays (Liu et al., 2004a; Mathieu et al., 2005; Park et al., 2005a; Wei et al., 2005). Another novel structure involves the fabrication of DNA nanotriangles using a tensegrity strategy. This novel process has expanded the number of possible DNA nanostructures that may be created (Ding et al., 2004; Liu et al., 2004b). Figure 17.1 gives some representative images of the DNA tiles and their corresponding two-dimensional periodic arrays. The assembly of a DNA nanotriangle from three four-arm junctions is shown in Fig. 17.1(a) (Liu et al., 2004b). Each single four-arm junction contains four helical arms, which stack into two duplexes. When two pairs of complementary sticky-ends are added to these two duplexes, the nanotriangles assemble into two-dimensional arrays. The three-component duplexes extend in three directions; as a result, the duplexes guide DNA array growth and enable three-dimensional self-assembly processes. Chelyapov et al. designed different triangular complexes and assembled them into a single hexagonal structure (Chelyapov et al., 2005). These equilateral triangles could not attach to themselves but could attach to other triangles (Fig. 17.1(b)). He et al. constructed a three-point-star DNA motif, which consisted of seven single strands that were organized in three interconnected four-arm junctions (He et al., 2005). In this structure, one T3 loop was located at the center. When proper sticky ends were added, the three-point-star motif self-assembled into hexagonal, porous two-dimensional arrays (Fig. 17.1(c)). These two-dimensional arrays can reach lengths of 1 mm. Recently, Liu and co-workers reported a strategy for producing DNA arrays with finite sizes (Liu et al., 2005a). In their process, DNA tile structures with asymmetric sticky ends were assembled into symmetric, finite-size arrays. For example, five-by-five nanogrids (Fig. 17.1(d)) may be constructed from seven unique cross-shaped tiles with *C*4 symmetry, instead of twenty-five. This strategy not only reduces the number of unique strands that are needed, but it also simplifies the sequence design process. The design time and the sample preparation time may be dramatically reduced. Fixed-size DNA tiling nanostructures also may be used as templates for fabrication of functionalized nanowires, nanocircuits, quantum cellular automata, and spintronic devices. Reishus et al. designed a double-double crossover (DDX) structure, which consists of four DNA double helices that are connected using a total of six reciprocal exchanges (Reishus et al., 2005). These DDX tiles can be self-assembled to form high-density, doubly-connected, planar structures (Fig. 17.1(e)). By adding sticky-ends to connect the left-most and right-most helices of the DX tiles, four-helix bundle tile may be constructed. These bundle tiles may be used to form even larger three-dimensional constructs. One long-term goal of self-assembly processes is the fabrication of complex two-dimensional patterns. For example, Barish et al. have demonstrated the creation of complex nanoscale patterns by algorithmic self-assembly technology (Barish et al., 2005). These algorithmically-defined patterns were formed by crystallizing four DNA tiles in a binary counting pattern on a polymer nucleating scaffold strand (Fig. 17.1(f)).

17.3.2.2 DNA Origami Structures

Rothemund recently developed a novel process known as 'scaffolded DNA origami', in which any arbitrary, complex, two-dimensional shape can be fabricated using a long, single-stranded DNA from a virus with a known genetic sequence (Rothemund, 2006). For example, Rothemund chose a 7 kilobase circular genomic DNA from the virus M13mp18 as a scaffold material. In order to hold the scaffold in place, hundreds of short (30 – 70 nucleotide long) 'staple' DNA strands were used to attach multiple parts of the long scaffold strand. Each 'staple' strand has two arms, which have independently complimentary bases to two different sequences of the long scaffold strand. As a result, these strands may be used to fold the long scaffold strand back and forth into any desired shape. Each of the short 'staple' strands can serve as a 6 nm pixel for representing part of a complex pattern in two-dimensional space. As a result, complex patterns, including words or images, may be formed. Rothemund has created a variety of two-dimensional shapes using one type of long virus genome strand and different units of 'staple' strands, including a square, a rectangle, a triangle, a five-pointed star, and a smiley face. Once a shape has been created, any desired pattern may be added in a straightforward manner. For example, he has created structures in the form of the letters 'D', 'N', and 'A', as well as a square representation of a map of the western hemisphere. These shapes and patterns demonstrate dimensions in the ~100 nm range, and exhibit much more complex than any previously constructed DNA objects. The individually patterned structures can also be further programmed to form larger lattices, such as a 30 MDa hexagon of triangles.

The method for fabricating custom DNA origami is simple to implement, high in yield (>90%), and low in cost. At this point, only two-dimensional shapes and structures have been created using this process; however, three-dimensional structures may be fabricated using a straightforward adaptation of the raster fill method. As a result, scientists from diverse fields may create a variety of desired complex patterns using the DNA origami method. For example, molecular electronic or plasmonic circuits can be created by attaching quantum dots, nanowires, nanotubes, or nanoparticles to origami structures. In addition, biologists can use DNA origami structures as templates for creating complex protein patterns.

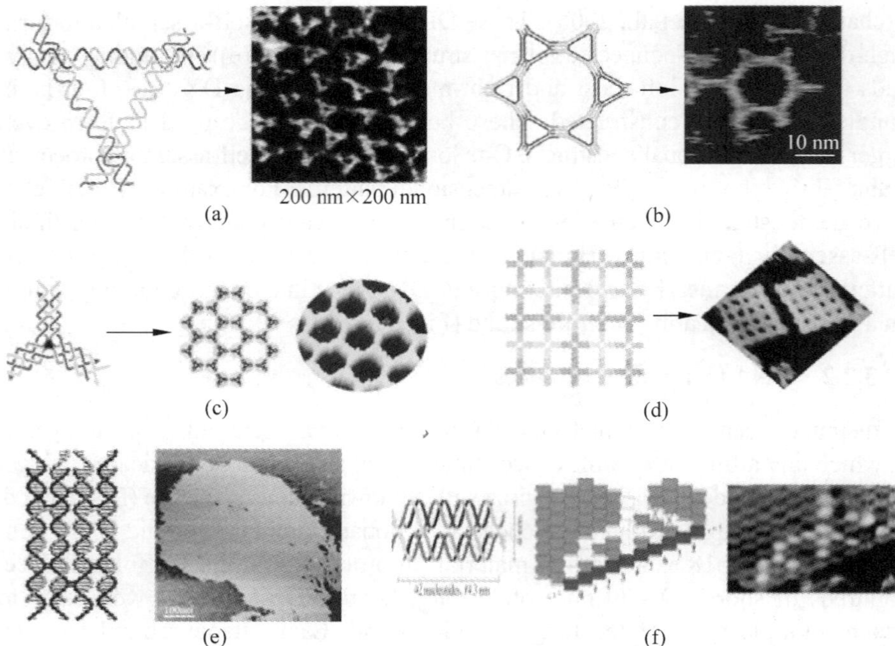

Figure 17.1 Schematic drawings of DNA tiles and atomic force micrographs of two-dimensional periodic arrays that were fabricated using these tiles (Color Fig. 18). (a) A DNA triangle tile that is composed of three four-arm junctions is shown on the left, and a two-dimensional array that was formed by self-assembly of these DNA triangles is shown on the right. (b) Schematic drawing and atomic force micrograph of a single hexagonal structure composed of six equilateral triangle complexes that are attached to one another. (c) A three-pointed star DNA motif is shown on the left, and hexagonal two-dimensional DNA lattices that were formed by self-assembly of three-point-star motifs with sticky ends are shown on the right. (d) Schematic drawing and atomic force micrograph of a 5×5 fixed-size array that was assembled from a cross-shaped tile structure with *C*4 symmetry. (e) A diagram of DNA double-double crossover tiles, which consist of eight strands that form four double helices, is shown on the left. These helices are connected by six reciprocal exchanges. Planar structures fabricated using the DNA double-double crossover structures are shown on the right. (f) A diagram of a binary pattern formed from rule tiles on a linear scaffold is shown in blue. Red crosses indicate tiles that exhibit mismatch with their neighbors. A corresponding atomic force micrograph is shown on the right. Figure (a) reprinted with permission from Liu, D., M.S. Wang, Z.X. Deng, R. Walulu and C.D. Mao. *J. Am. Chem. Soc.* 126: 2324 (2004). Copyright 2004 American Chemical Society. Figure (b) reprinted with permission from Chelyapov, N., Y. Brun, M. Gopalkrishnan, D. Reishus, B. Shaw and L. Adleman. *J. Am. Chem. Soc.* 126: 13,924 (2005). Copyright 2005 American Chemical Society. Figure (c) reprinted with permission from He, Y., Y. Chen, H. Liu, A. E. Ribbe and C. Mao. *J. Am. Chem. Soc.* 127: 12,202 (2005). Copyright 2005 American Chemical Society. Figure (d) reprinted with permission from Liu, Y., Y.G. Ke and H. Yan. *J. Am. Chem. Soc.* 127: 17,140 (2005). Copyright 2005 American Chemical Society. Figure (e) reprinted with permission from Reishus, D., B. Shaw, Y. Brun, N. Chelyapov and L. Adleman. *J. Am. Chem. Soc.* 127: 17,590 (2005). Copyright 2005 American Chemical Society. Figure (f) reprinted with permission from Barish, R.D., P.W.K. Rothemund and E. Winfree. *Nano Lett.* 5: 2586 (2005). Copyright 2005 American Chemical Society

17.3.2.3 DNA Nanotube Structures

DNA nanotubes are a promising template for biomimicry. For example nanotubes be used for the reproduction of microtubules, which serve as structural components within cells. In earlier studies involving self-assembly of double crossover tiles, triple crossover tiles, or four-by-four cross-shaped tiles, several μm-long ribbons or 20 – 100 nm wide, many μm-long tubes were observed (Ekani-Nkodo et al., 2004; O'Neill et al., 2006; Rothemund et al., 2004; Mitchell et al., 2004; Liu et al., 2004a; Yan et al., 2003). O'Neill et al. have described the self-assembly of DNA nanotubes from a single DAE-E tile (O'Neill et al., 2006). This tile contains a double crossover, antiparallel orientation of the strands through crossover locations as well as an even number of half-turns for both intramolecular distance and intermolecular distance between crossover locations (Rothemund et al., 2004). The DAE-E tile contains five DNA strands that hybridize into a rigid rectangular core, in which there is a single-stranded five-base long sticky end at each corner (Fig. 17.2). Liu et al. reported the growth of uniform DNA nanotube superstructures from types of two DNA triple-crossover tile building blocks, a triple-crossover (TAO) tile (tile A) and a TAO+2J tile (tile B) (Liu et al., 2004a). The B tile contains two extra dsDNA stems, and is modified by the replacement of the loop on one protruding stem with two thiol groups. Sticky ends located at the tile corners have been programmed such that A tiles attach to B tiles and B tiles attach to A tiles. In the proposed nanotube structure, B tile layers alternate with A tile layers. These triple-crossover nanotubes are very uniform, with a constant diameter of ~25 nm and lengths up to 20 μm. Ke et al. studied the formation and morphology of DNA tubes created using four-, eight-, and twelve-helix DNA tiles (Ke et al., 2006). They investigated nine assembly structures through the combination of three above different tiles and three sticky end association strategies (Fig. 17.3). Figure 17.4 contains the atomic force microscopy images of the lattices self-assembled from four-, eight-, and twelve-helix DNA nanostructures using the three different sticky end connection strategies. In order to investigate the effects of tile sizes, sticky-end strength, and flexibility on the formation of DNA tubes, three different sticky-ends were placed on the four corners of each tile. As shown in Fig. 17.4(a), 1SE refers to one single-helix sticky-end connection between two neighboring tiles that all face in the same direction, 1SE-C refers to one single helix sticky-end connection between two tiles in which one tile is rotated by 180° (corrugated design), and 2SE-C refers to two-helix sticky-end connections with corrugated design. Figure 17.4(b) show the characteristic DNA structures formed using four-helix, eight-helix, and twelve-helix structures with the three different sticky end connection strategies. Using 1SE connections, four-helix tiles can develop narrow tubes and eight-helix tiles can develop wide tubes as well as two-dimensional arrays. Twelve-helix tiles can develop open tubes using these connections. Using 1SE-C connections, no tube was fabricated using eight-helix tiles. The four-helix, eight-helix, and twelve-helix tiles can construct tubes using 2SE-C connections, which vary in width. However, the tube structures created using twelve-helix tiles with any of the three sticky-end connections are easily opened and destroyed. Analysis of the nine assembly structures created using a combination of sticky-end connections suggests that dimensional anisotropy of the DNA tile plays an interesting role in the self-assembly process. In addition, the orientation of the tiles, flexibility of the tiles, strength of the connection points, and the flexibility of the connection points also influence the self-assembly process of DNA tube structures. Rothemund et al. also suggested that tiles characteristics affect tube size and tube morphology (Rothemund et al., 2004). Fabrication of different patterns or the addition of decorations to the tile sets does not have significant influence on tube formation. On the other hand, modifications of the tiles (e.g. bulky hairpin groups located in the interior or at the interstices of the tube) disrupt stacking at the sticky-end contacts. In addition, alterations the intertile helix by more than one base pair may affect tube formation.

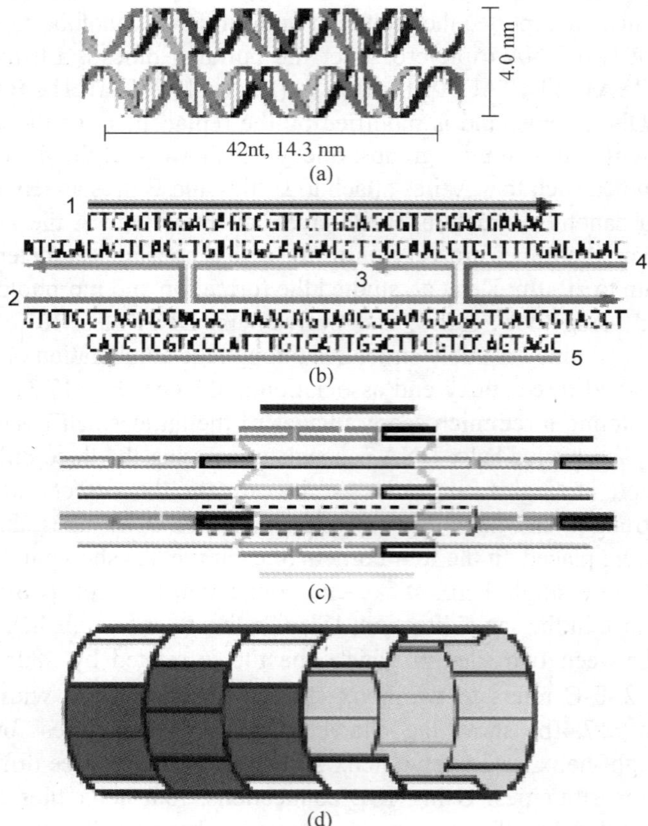

Figure 17.2 Schematic of DNA nanotube structure (Color Fig. 19). Reprinted with permission from Rothemund, P.W. K., A. Ekani-Nkodo, N. Papadakis, A. Kumar, D. K. Fygenson and E. Winfree. *J. Am. Chem. Soc.* 126: 16,344(2004). Copyright 2004 American Chemical Society

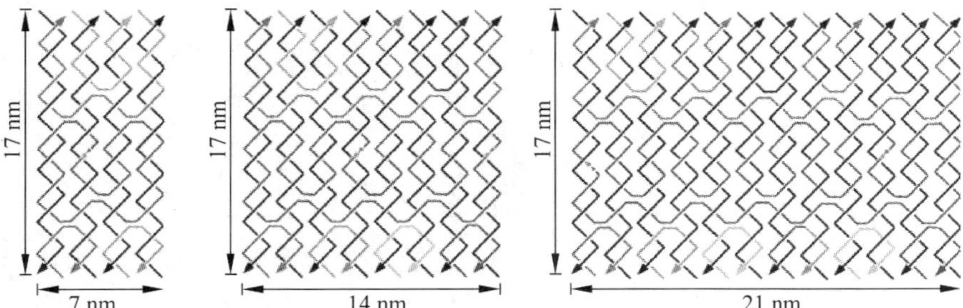

Figure 17.3 Schematics of (a) 4-helix tile, (b) 8-helix tile, and (c) 12-helix tile (Color Fig. 20). Reprinted with permission from Ke, Y.G., Y. Liu, J.P. Zhang, H. Yan. *J. Am. Chem. Soc.* 128: 4414 (2006). Copyright 2006 American Chemical Society

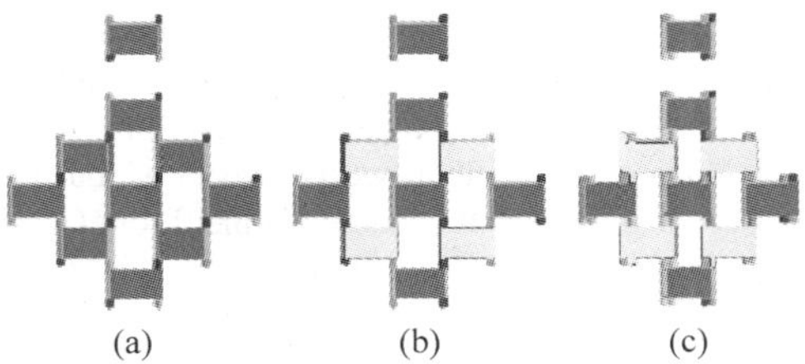

Figure 17.4 Schematics of three sticky end connections for each tile (Color Fig. 21). (a) 1SE. (b) 1SE-C. (c) 2SE-C. Sticky ends with identical colors are complementary to one another. Sticky ends with different colors contain tiles with opposite planes. Reprinted with permission from Ke, Y.G., Y. Liu, J.P. Zhang, and H. Yan. *J. Am. Chem. Soc.* 128: 4414 (2006). Copyright 2006 American Chemical Society

17.3.3 Three-Dimensional DNA Nanostructures

One major effort in the area of DNA nanotechnology involves the fabrication of three-dimensional structures using deoxyribonucleic acid. DNA is an ideal molecule for fabrication of rigid three-dimensional nanostructures because assembly can be controlled by base pairing and fabrication processes are relatively inexpensive. Goodman et al. constructed a family of rigid three-dimensional DNA tetrahedra, which possessed edge lengths of 10 nm (Goodman et al., 2005). These structures self-assembled in seconds, and could be connected by programmable DNA linkers (Fig. 17.5(a)). Each tetrahedron was formed from four short single DNA stands, which were designed to favor the construction of tetrahedron edges in a hierarchical molecular model (Fig. 17.5(b)). Atomic force microscopy images of the tetrahedral show that these structures have three 30-base pair (bp) edges meeting at one vertex and three 20-bp edges meeting on the opposite face. The three upper edges of individual tetrahedral exhibit sharp tips (Fig. 17.5(c)).

Shih et al. have demonstrated an elegant design for a DNA octahedron (Shih et al., 2004). A 1669-nucleotide DNA molecule was folded up with five 40-nucleotide

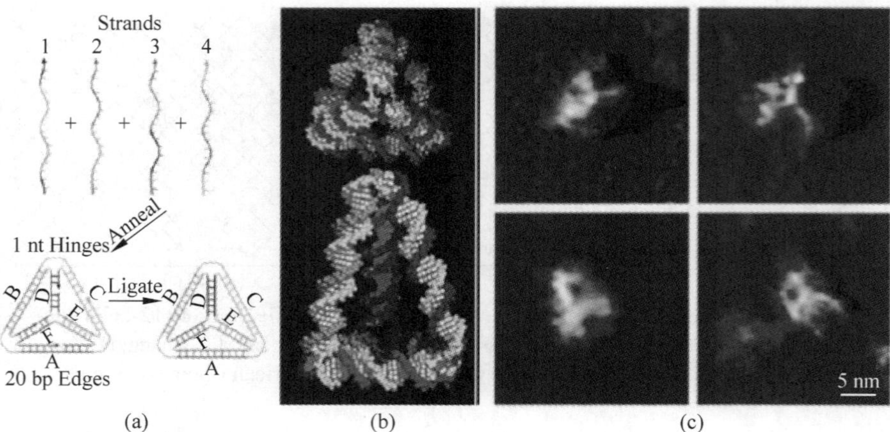

Figure 17.5 (a) Schematic depicting formation of DNA tetrahedron from four oligonucleotides (Color Fig. 22). The colored complementary subsequences underwent hybridization to form the edges of the tetrahedron structure. (b) Schematics of the DNA tetrahedron. (c) Atomic force microscopy images of four tetrahedra. In these images, three upper edges of the tetrahedra are visible. From Goodman, R.P., I.A.T. Schaap, C.F. Tardin, C.M. Erben, R.M. Berry, C.F. Schmidt, A.J. Turberfield. *Science* 310: 1661 (2005). Reprinted with permission from AAAS

synthetic oligodeoxynucleotides by a simple denaturation-renaturation process. The resulting octahedral structure exhibited a central cavity capable of holding a 14 nm sphere. The triangular opening on each face of the octahedron allows entry of a sphere up to 8 nm larger. These three-dimensional DNA octahedral structures could be used as cages to trap molecules and protect them from the outside environment. For example, DNA cages may be programmed to release specific molecules in response to a given signal.

17.4 Self-Assembly Properties of DNA Nanostructures

The development of assembly systems for the programmable placement of materials at the molecular scale has been an objective of DNA nanotechnology. The programmable self-assembly of DNA nanostructures is an exciting way to construct well-defined nm-scale and μm-scale structures. These materials may be used as programmable scaffolds for organization of nanomaterials. Several materials, including metal nanoparticles, semiconductor nanoparticles, polymer particles, and carbon nanotubes can be conjugated with DNA in order to prepare self-assembled nanostructures (Elghanian et al., 1997; Alivisatos et al., 1996; Mirkin et al., 1996, 1998; Loweth et al., 1999; Coffer et al., 1992, 1996; Pathak et al., 2001; Bigham and Coffer, 1995; Cassell et al., 1998; Torimoto et al., 1999; Mitchell et al., 1999; Nielsen et al., 1991; Dwyer et al., 2002; Li et al., 2005; Chen et al., 2001; Shim et al., 2002; Guo et al., 1998; Williams et al., 2002; Nguyen et al., 2002;

Xu et al., 2004; Fogleman et al., 2002; Abdalla et al., 2004). Recent studies have shown that DNA is a unique template for positioning and orienting other functional molecules with nanometer-scale precision.

17.4.1 DNA Templated Self-Assembly of Biological Molecules

17.4.1.1 DNA Cages for Trapping and Crystallization of Biological Molecules

The initial motivation for the creation of DNA-based nanostructures was for crystallography studies. Seeman et al. have suggested the construction of three-dimensional DNA crystalline cages for orienting biological molecules and complexing these molecules into periodic arrays (Seeman et al., 1982). Biological molecules organized within three-dimensional DNA lattices may be used to facilitate crystallographic structure determination studies. Crystalline arrays may also be utilized to position and orient materials within molecular electronic devices, nanorobotic devices, and other nanoscale devices.

17.4.1.2 DNA Scaffolds for Protein Arrays

Several advances have been made in assembly of biological molecules on DNA arrays in recent years. For example, complex DNA tile structures have been used to organize biological molecules into nanoscale and microscale patterns. Many current research efforts involve using self-assembling DNA nanostructures as scaffolds to construct and position biological molecules in programmed patterns. Aptamers constitute a versatile platform for nanoscale patterning of proteins and synthetic molecules. Liu et al. have recently demonstrated the use of selective DNA aptamer binding for attaching thrombin proteins to locations on a DNA array that was self-assembled from a triple-crossover DNA tile (Liu et al., 2005b). Aptamers are deoxyribonucleic acid or ribonucleic acid molecules that demonstrate an in vivo capability for binding ligands, including organic compounds, inorganic compounds, peptides, proteins, or even entire organisms (Ellington and Szostak, 1990, 1992). These unusual structures are usually less than 100 nucleotides in length. Aptamers are similar to antibodies in that they both have excellent affinity and specificity characteristics for target molecules (Murphy et al., 2003). Thrombin is a coagulation protein that has multiple effects on the coagulation cascade. It is a serine protease, which can recognize multiple macromolecules (Poort et al., 1996). It is possible to generate a virtually unlimited number of thrombin-aptamer pairs on a complex patterned DNA structure, because of the high affinity nature of aptamer-thrombin interaction.

Liu et al. examined a molecule known as thrombin-binding aptamer (TBA), a 15-base DNA aptamer with a d(GGTTGGTGTGGTTGG) sequence that binds thrombin with nanomolar affinity (Macaya et al., 1993). Figure 17.6 shows that TX DNA tiles may be used as templates to organize thrombin into one-dimensional periodic arrays. This TX tile has two DNA hairpin loops, which both protrude outward in the plane of the tile. One of the hairpin loops contains an aptamer sequence at the end of the stem. The other hairpin loop does not contain an aptamer sequence and serves as a control. The length of the stem can be modified such that the target binding molecules can be organized in any desired position and rotational orientation.

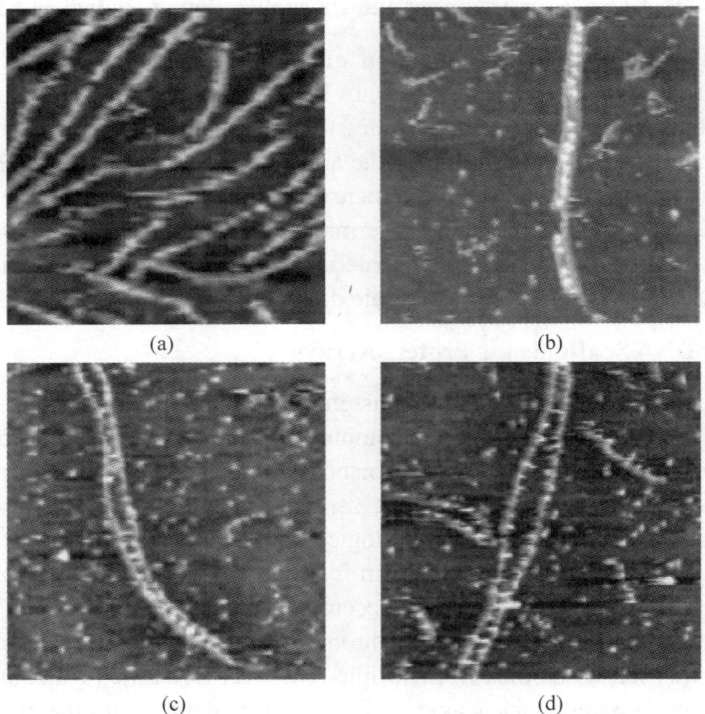

Figure 17.6 Atomic force microscopy images of aptamer-directed self-assembly of thrombin protein nanoarrays on a triple crossover DNA tile. (a) Triple crossover tiles with apatamer sequences. (b) – (d) Triple crossover tiles with thrombin protein nanoarrays. Reprinted from Liu, Y., C.X. Lin, H.Y. Li and H. Yan. *Angew. Chem. Int. Ed.* 44: 4333 (2005b) with permission of the publisher

Niemeyer et al. have demonstrated DNA-programmed assembly on surfaces using nucleotide-streptavidin conjugates (Niemeyer et al., 1994). Streptavidin can be conjugated with oligonucleotides by means of covalent linkages. These molecules can be arrayed at specific positions on oligonucleotide templates (Niemeyer et al., 1998; Niemeyer, 2002a). Biotin-labelled oligonucleotides also may be used to fabricate nanostructures (Park et al., 2001). The streptavidin-biotin pair has one of the largest free energies of association for noncovalent binding of a protein and a small ligand in solution. Niemeyer have made use of biotin-labeled dsDNA sequences in order to fabricate DNA-streptavidin networks (Niemeyer et al., 1999; 2000, 2001). More complex ligand-DNA structures have also been used to organize streptavidin molecules into specific spatial patterns. For example, two-dimensional DNA lattices with large cavity sizes can be self-assembled from four-by-four cross tiles. These structures are ideal templates for organizing biological molecules. For example, Yan et al. have assembled evenly-spaced streptavidin molecules on four-by-four DNA lattices using same cross-shaped tiles (Yan et al., 2003). The central strands of the cross tiles were functionalized with biotin molecules, which were then able to bind streptavidin molecules (Fig. 17.7). Individual streptavidin proteins are observed in the atomic force microscopy images of these structures. Park et al. also used four-by-four lattices that were self-assembled from two different cross-shaped tiles (tile A and tile B) as templates for arraying streptavidin into periodic two-dimensional patterns (Park et al., 2005b). In these structures, only the central strands of A tiles were modified with biotin groups. These results have shown that periodic, symmetric and partial addressable patterns can be obtained using two-tile DNA systems.

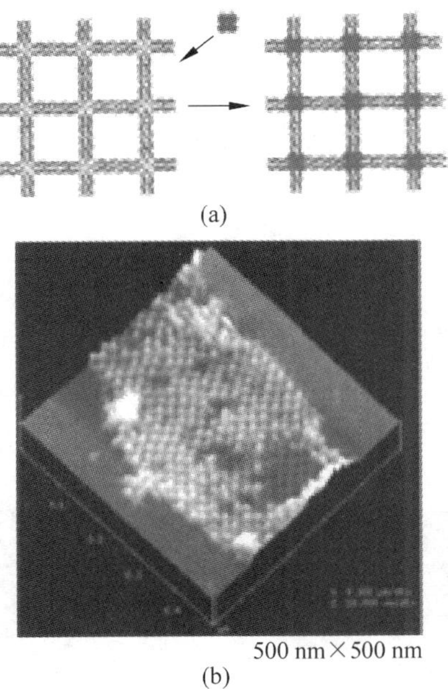

Figure 17.7 Schematic and atomic force micrograph depicting programmable assembly of protein arrays using biotin-streptavidin interaction on a DNA lattice. From Yan, H., S.H. Park, G. Ginkelstein, J.H. Reif and T.H. LaBean. *Science* 301: 1882 (2003). Reprinted with permission from AAAS

Highly sensitive and specific sensing (e.g. single-molecule detection) has recently been accomplished using DNA-templated protein arrays. For example, Lund et al. recently demonstrated assembly of finite-sized three-by-three DNA nanostructures from nine different tiles (Lund et al., 2005). In these structures, the distance between two tiles was ~18 nm. By adding an extra tile to the nine-tile array at zero position, index numbers could be assigned to each tile in the array (Fig. 17.8(a)). Biotin-functionalized strands complementary to probe sequences were located at the 'nine', 'five', and 'eight' positions, respectively (Fig. 17.8(b)). These biotinylated target strands were hybridized with nine-tile arrays and other biotinylated strands that were not complementary to the original probe sequences. Biotinylated nanostructures were incubated with streptavidin, which attached to biotin with a high degree of specificity. Streptavidin was used as a maker to detect probe strands that were complementary to the biotinylated target strands. Atomic force microscopy images demonstrated detection of probes at the 'nine', 'five', and 'eight' positions (Fig. 17.8(c)). Bright spots indicate the locations of the biotinylated target probe strands that were hybridized with streptavidin. Fully-addressable, finite-size sixteen-tile DNA arrays were assembled using a stepwise hierarchical assembly technique. These arrays were decorated with protein patterns that exhibited the shapes of the letters 'D', 'N', and 'A' (Fig. 17.9) (Park et al., 2006). Assembly of protein molecules on DNA templates may be used for biomimetic materials, biochips, immunoassays, biosensors, and a variety of other nanoscale patterned materials.

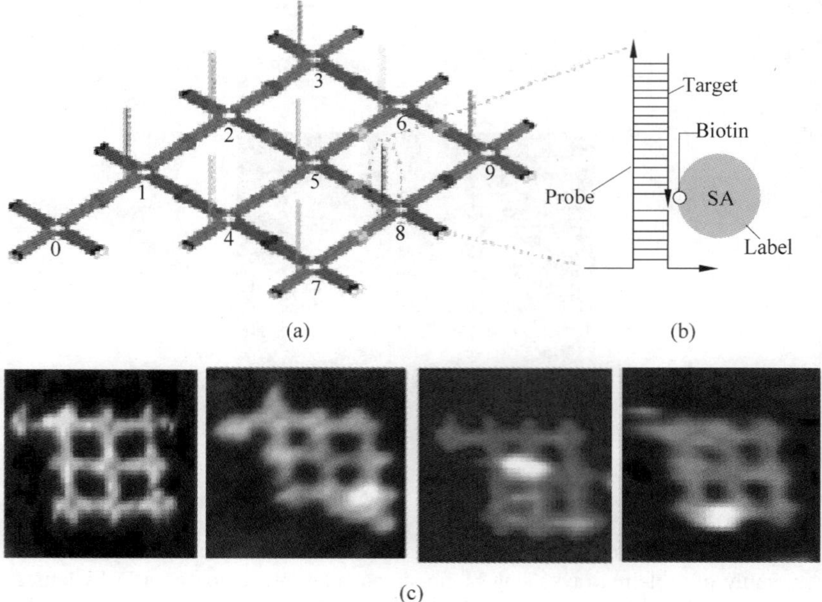

Figure 17.8 (a) Schematic of nine tile structure. (b) Schematic of probe strand. The probe strand is complementary to the biotinylated target strand, which is used for streptavidin hybridization. (c) Atomic force microscopy images of pure nine tile structures. Bright spots indicate the locations of the biotinylated target probe strands that were hybridized with streptavidin. Reprinted with permission from Lund, K., Y. Liu, S. Lindsay, H. Yan. *J. Am. Chem. Soc.* 127: 17,606(2005). Copyright 2005 American Chemical Society

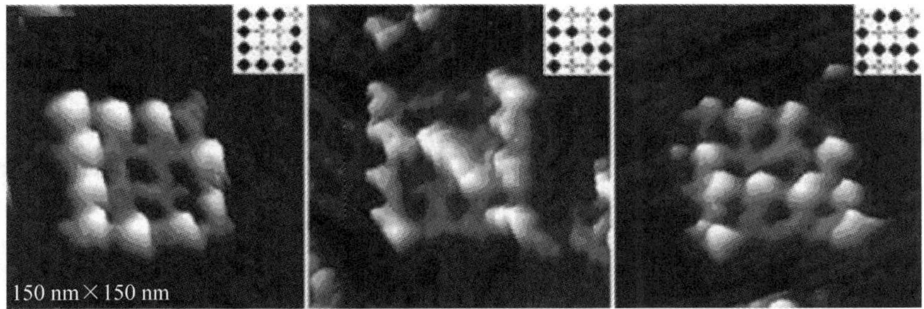

Figure 17.9 Atomic force microscopy images of protein patterns depicting the letters D, N and A on self-assembled sixteen-tile arrays. Reprinted from Park, S.H., C. Pistol, S.J. Ahn, J.H. Reif, A.R. Lebeck, C. Dwyer, T.H. LaBean. *Angew. Chem. Int. Ed.* 45: 735 (2006) with permission of the publisher

17.4.2 DNA-Templated Self-Assembly of Nanoscale Devices

Nanoparticles have unique size, optical, electronic, chemical and physical properties and have been considered for use in bottom-up assembly of high-density electronics and other functional devices (Mann et al., 2000; Lazarides and Schatz, 2000; Zhang et al., 2004). Many methods have been developed for assembling nanoparticles, but many of these are nonspecific and nonselective (Hermanson et al., 2001; Huang et al., 2001; Genov et al., 2004; Kim and Wei, 2001; Whang et al., 2001; Cui et al., 2004). Several investigators have shown that DNA is an ideal template material for the selective assembly of nanoparticles. In 1996, Mirkin and co-workers first reported using DNA as a linker to assemble colloidal gold nanoparticles into macroscopic aggregates (Mirkin et al., 1996, Elghanian et al., 1997). 13 nm gold nanoparticles were functionalized using noncomplementary 3'-thiol-linked oligonucleotides sequences and 5'-thiol-linked oligonucleotides sequences. A solution containing both of these molecules was prepared. When strands complementary to 3'-thiol-linked oligonucleotide sequence and the 5'-thiol-linked oligonucleotide sequence were added to this solution, the nanoparticles self-assembled into aggregates and the color of the solution changed. Niemeyer et al. have also described functionalization of gold nanoparticles with different thiolated oligonucleotide sequences for detection of various target sequences (Niemeyer et al., 2003).

17.5 Application of DNA-Based Nanotechnology

Several recent studies have shown that DNA nanostructures may be used as templates for creating arrays of proteins and nanoparticles. Alivisatos et al. and Loweth et al. have demonstrated functionalization of gold nanoparticles and organization of these structures into dimers, trimers, and other discrete structures

(Alivisatos et al., 1996; Loweth et al., 1995). In their work, gold particles were attached to either the 3' end or 5' end of long single-stranded DNA molecules using thiol interactions. By annealing two or three DNA – nanoparticle conjugates using a DNA template, homodimer or homotrimer structures can be assembled. Gold particles can be placed at well-defined positions by selecting an appropriate number of DNA strands (Fig. 17.10).

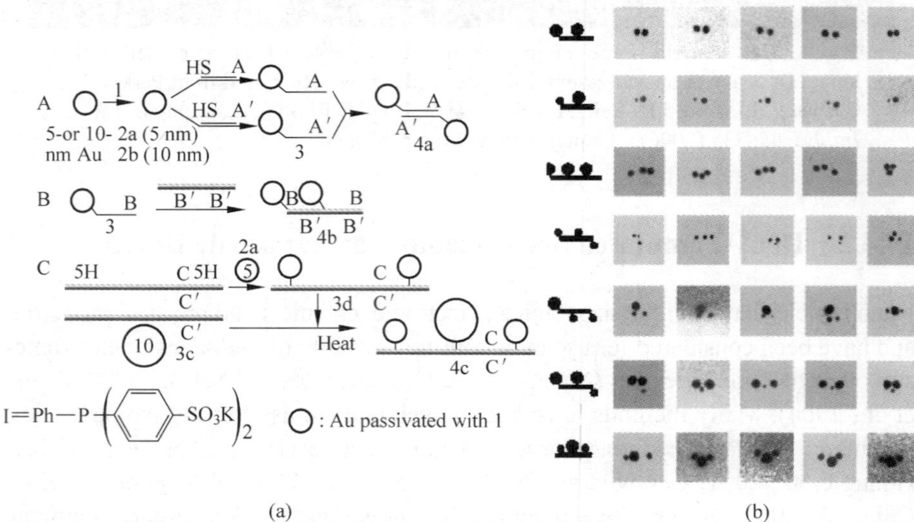

Figure 17.10 (a) Synthesis strategies for assembly of heterodimeric and heterotrimeric nanocrystal molecules. (b) Transmission electron micrographs of nanocrystal molecules that correspond to the strategies shown in (a). Reprinted from Loweth, C.J., W.B. Caldwell, X. Peng, A.P. Alivisatos, P.G. Schultz. *Angew. Chem. Int. Ed.* 38: 1808 (1999) with permission of the publisher

Bottom-up assembly of nanomaterials may be achieved through the use of self-assembled nanomaterials. For example, Zhang et al. recently reported two-dimensional assembly of 5 nm gold nanoparticles on four-by-four DNA tile structures (Zhang et al., 2006). Two tiles (A and B) composed of four-armed DNA branch junction self-assembled into two-dimensional structures, which contain a large number of periodic cavities (Fig. 17.11). The A tiles were modified with a short DNA single strand, which contained an A15 base sequence. This strand protrudes out of the two-dimensional tile face. The B tiles were functionalized with multiple T15 strands (average size = 16 strands), which were complementary to the A15 strands on the A tiles. When the modified gold nanoparticles were added to the surfaces of the two-dimensional nanogrids, the T15 strands hybridized with the A15 strands. Figure 17.12 contains atomic force microscopy images of a gold nanoparticle array templated by two-dimensional DNA nanogrids. A highly regular square pattern was observed, in which one gold nanoparticle was consistently missing from each center of each square. The absence of a gold nanoparticle at the center of each square results from the high density of T15 strands on the gold nanoparticle surfaces, which not only increase the particle diameter but also make the gold nanoparticle surface highly negatively charged. The particles repel each other if they are located too close together. As a result, a gold nanoparticle situated at the center of the square would violate this limit.

Using a similar strategy, Pinto et al. selectively self-assembled different-sized gold nanoparticles into parallel rows on a two-dimensional DX lattice (Pinto et al., 2005). The two-dimensional DX lattice is constructed from four different double-crossover tiles: A, B, C, and D (Fig. 17.13(a)). The B tiles and the D tiles have

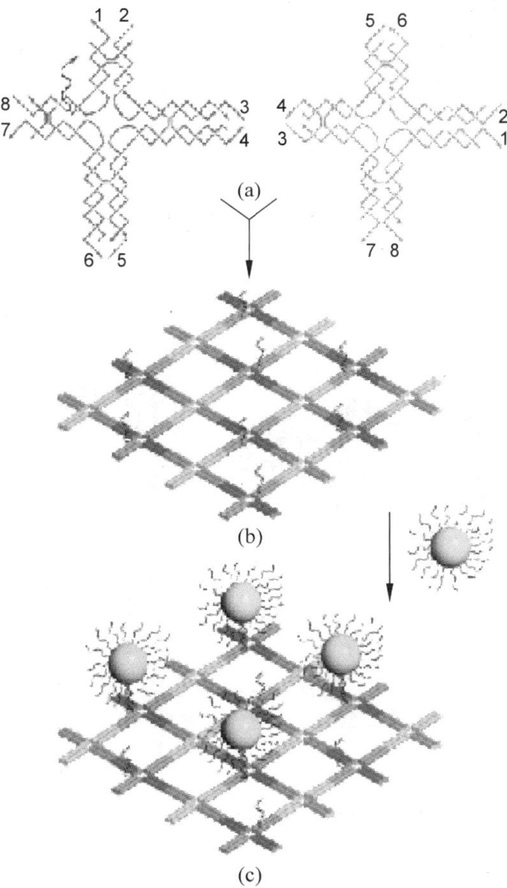

Figure 17.11 Mechanism for arraying gold nanoparticles on DNA nanogrids (Color Fig. 23). (a) In this figure, tile A is blue, and tile B is orange. The short strand A15 on tile A serves as a hybridization site for gold nanoparticles. (b) A DNA nanogrid formed from cross-shaped tiles. (c) Assembly of 5 nm gold particles on DNA nanogrids. Reprinted with permission from Zhang, J.P., Y. Liu, Y.G. Ke, H. Yan. *Nano. Lett.* 6: 248 (2006). Copyright 2006 American Chemical Society

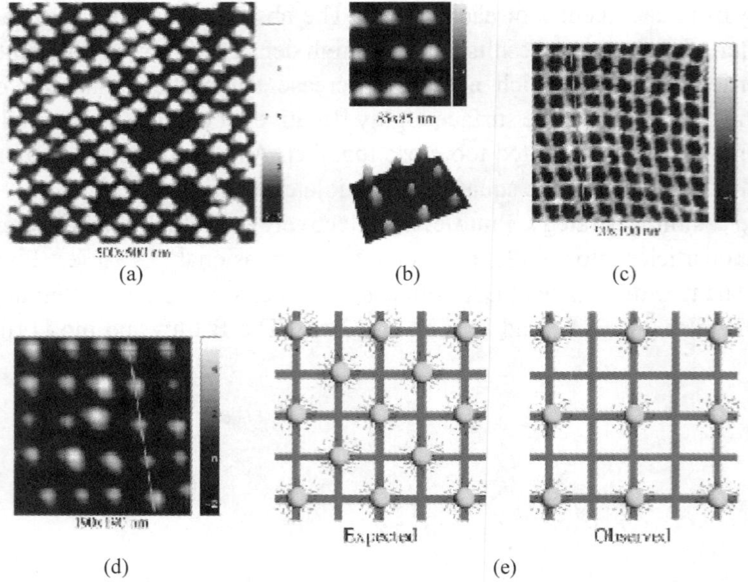

Figure 17.12 Atomic force micrographs showing gold nanoparticles assembled on two-dimensional DNA grids (Color Fig. 24). Reprinted with permission from Zhang, J.P., Y. Liu, Y.G. Ke, H. Yan. *Nano. Lett.* 6: 248 (2006). Copyright 2006 American Chemical Society

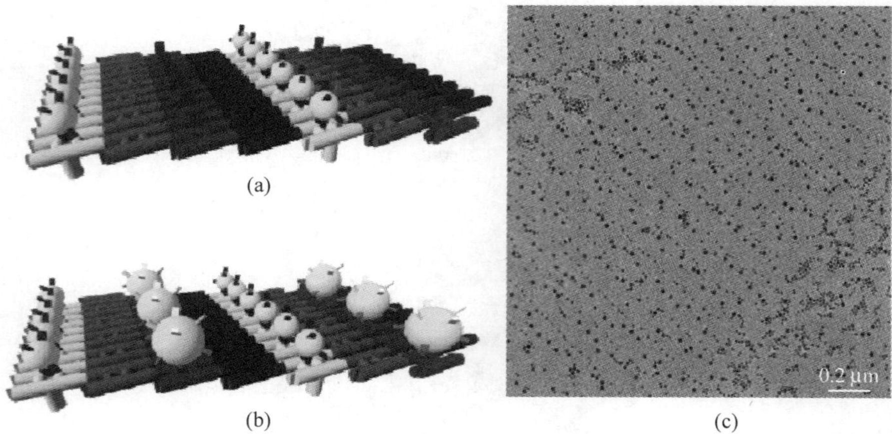

Figure 17.13 (a) A diagram of a two-dimensional lattice fabricated from four different double-crossover tiles, in which 5 nm gold particles are occupying the D tiling rows. (b) A diagram of a two-dimensional lattice fabricated from four different double-crossover tiles, in which 5 nm gold particles are occupying the D tiling rows and 10 nm gold particles are occupying the B tiling rows. (c) Transmission electron micrograph of array containing 5 nm gold particles and 10 nm gold particles (Color Fig. 25). Reprinted with permission from Pinto, Y.Y., J.D. Le, N.C. Seeman, K. Musier-Forsyth, T.A. Taton, R.A. Kiehl. *Nano Lett.* 5: 2399(2005). Copyright 2005 American Chemical Society

two different single-strand sequences that protrude out of the tile surfaces, which are used as hybridization sites for gold nanoparticles. 5 nm gold particles occupy the D tiling rows and 10 nm gold particles occupy the B tiling rows. The inter-row distance (e.g. the distance between two tiling rows) is ~32 nm. 5 nm gold nanoparticles and 10 nm gold nanoparticles were functionalized with thiol-modified DNA single strands, which were complementary to hybridization sites on the double-crossover tiles. 5 nm gold particles became attached to open hybridization sites on D tiles, and 10 nm gold particles became attached to open hybridization sites on B tiles (Fig. 17.13(b)). Figure 17.13(c) contains a transmission electron micrograph that shows an array of two gold particles with different sizes. In this figure, the parallel small gold particle lines and large gold particle lines are shown to alternate.

DNA-based systems can be used to build artificial systems that emulate cellular functions. Polymer-DNA complexes and liposome-DNA complexes have been used for gene delivery (Xu et al., 2002). Benenson et al. designed a DNA-based structure, which can be used for both sensing and drug release (Benenson et al., 2001). For example, Dittmer et al. have described the development of a DNA-based system with aptamers that can bind and release thrombin in a controlled manner (Dittmer et al., 2004). A DNA sequence containing aptamers has been used to construct a thrombin-binding G-quartet structure. This aptamer can bind thrombin and has sticky ends. When a complementary DNA strand is added to this system, it hybridizes with the sticky end of aptamer and destroys the G-quartet structure of the thrombin aptamer. As a result, thrombin is released from this structure. Niemeyer et al. have prepared nanoscale circles using streptavidin-DNA conjugations that can be used as building blocks for the development of novel immunological reagents (Niemeyer et al., 2000). Niemeyer has also demonstrated that streptavidin-DNA structures can be used for ultrasensitive trace analysis of proteins and other antigens. These structures can also be used for the development of complex biomolecular templates, which can be used for fabrication of nanometer-scale inorganic devices (Niemeyer, 2002b). DNA-directed self-assembly nanostructures can be used as diagnostic tools for analysis of biological molecules (Niemeyer, 2004).

17.6 Conclusions and Outlook

In the coming decades, the use of deoxyribonucleic acid for self-assembly of complex nanostructures and for templating other functional materials will become more significant. Two-dimensional DNA-based nanostructures, three-dimensional DNA-based nanostructures, and DNA-programmed assembly of materials have several potential applications. Significant progress has been made in the construction of complex DNA nanostructures for use in nanoscale computers, nanobiomotors, biosensors, and drug delivery devices. There are several issues that must be resolved for these novel materials to become significant components in next generation biomedical devices. Some of the challenges include extending two-dimensional structures to three-dimensional structures, achieving additional functional self-assembly capabilities, and exploring additional applications for DNA-based nanostructures.

References

Abdalla, M.A., J. Bayer, J.O. Raedler and K. Muellen. *Angew. Chem. Int. Ed.* **43**: 3967 (2004).

Alivisatos, A.P., K.P. Johnsson, X. Peng, T.E. Wilson, C.J. Loweth, M.P. Bruchez and P.G. Schultz. *Nature* **382**: 609 (1996).

Barish, R.D., P.W.K. Rothemund and E. Winfree. *Nano Lett.* **5**: 2586 (2005).

Benenson, Y., T. Paz-Elizur, R. Adar, E. Keinan, Z. Livneh and E. Shapiro. *Nature* **414**: 430 (2001).

Bigham, S.R. and J.L. Coffer. *Colloids Surfaces* A **95**: 211 (1995).

Butler, J. M. *Forensic DNA Typing*. New York: Elsevier, p. 14 (2001).

Cassell, A.M., W.A. Scrivens and J.M. Tour. *Angew. Chem. Int. Ed.* **37**: 1528 (1998).

Chelyapov, N., Y. Brun, M. Gopalkrishnan, D. Reishus, B. Shaw and L. Adleman. *J. Am. Chem. Soc.* **126**: 13,924 (2005).

Chen, R.J., Y. Zhang, D. Wang and H. Dai. *J. Am. Chem. Soc.* **123**: 3838 (2001).

Churchill, M.E.A., T.D. Tullius, N.R. Kallen and N.C. Seeman. *Proc. Natl. Acad. Sci.* USA **85**: 4653 (1988).

Coffer, J.L., S.R. Bigham, R.F. Pinizzotto and H. Yang. *Nanotechnol.* **3**: 69 (1992).

Coffer, J.L., S.R. Bigham, X. Li, R.F. Pinizzotto, Y.G. Rho, R.M. Pirtle and I.L. Pirtle. *Appl. Phys. Lett.* **69**: 3851 (1996).

Cui, Y., M.T. Bjork, J.A. Liddle, C. Sonnichsen, B. Boussert and A.P. Alivisatos. *Nano Lett.* **4**: 1093 (2004).

Ding, B.Q., R.J. Sha and N.C. Seeman. *J. Am. Chem. Soc.* **126**: 10,230 (2004).

Dittmer, W.U., A. Reuter and F. C. Simmel. *Angew. Chem. Int. Ed.* **43**: 3550 (2004).

Dwyer, C., M. Guthold, M. Falvo, S. Washburn, R. Superfine and D. Erie. *Nanotechnol* **13**: 601 (2002).

Ekani-Nkodo, A., A. Kumar and D.K. Fygenson. *Phys. Rev. Lett.* **93**: 268,301 (2004).

Elghanian, R., J.J. Storhoff, R.C. Mucic, R.L. Letsinger and C.A. Mirkin. *Scienc.* **277**: 1078 (1997).

Ellington, A.D. and J.W. Szostak. *Nature* **346**: 818 (1990).

Ellington, A.D. and J.W. Szostak. *Nature* **355**: 850 (1992).

Fogleman, E.A, W.C. Yount, J. Xu and S.L. Craig. *Angew. Chem. Int. Ed.* **41**: 4026 (2002).

Fu, T.J., and N.C. Seeman. *Biochemistry* **32**: 3211(1993)

Genov, D.A., A.K. Sarychev, V.M. Shalaev and A. Wei. *Nano Lett.* **4**: 153 (2004).

Gil, B., U. Ben-Dor, R. Adar and E. Shapiro. *Nature* **429**: 423 (2004).

Goodman, R.P., I.A.T. Schaap, C.F. Tardin, C.M. Erben, R.M. Berry, C.F. Schmidt and A.J. Turberfield. *Science* **310**: 1661 (2005).

Guo, Z., P.J. Sadler and S.C. Tsang. *Adv. Mater.* **10**: 701 (1998).

Hagerman, P.J. *Ann. Rev. Biophys. Biophys. Chem.* **17**: 265 (1988).

He, Y., Y. Chen, H. Liu, A. E. Ribbe and C. Mao. *J. Am. Chem. Soc.* **127**: 12,202 (2005).

Hermanson, K.D., S.O. Lumsdon, J.P. Williams, E.W. Kaler and O.D. Velev. *Science* **294**: 1082 (2001).

Huang, Y., X. Duan, Y. Cui, L.J. Lauhon, K. Kim and C.M. Lieber. *Science* **294**: 1313 (2001).

Ke, Y.G., Y. Liu, J.P. Zhang and H. Yan. *J. Am. Chem. Soc.* **128**: 4414 (2006).

Kim, B., S.L. Tripp and A. Wei. *J. Am. Chem. Soc.* **123**: 7955 (2001).

LaBean, T.H., H. Yan, J. Kopatsch, F.R. Liu, E. Winfree, J.H. Reif and N.C. Seeman. *J. Am. Chem. Soc.* **122**: 1848 (2000).

Lazarides, A.A., and G.C. Schatz. *J. Phys. Chem.* B **104**: 460 (2000).

Li, S., P. He, J. Dong, Z. Guo and L. Dai. *J. Am. Chem. Soc.* **127**: 14 (2005).

Li, X.J., X.P. Yang, J. Qi and N.C. Seeman. *J. Am. Chem. Soc.* **118**: 6131 (1996).

Lilley, D.M.J, and R.M. Clegg. *Annu. Rev. Biophys. Biomol. Struct* **22**: 299 (1993).

Liu, D., S.H. Park, J.H. Reif and T.H. LaBean. *Proc. Natl. Acad. Sci.* USA **101**: 717 (2004a).

Liu, D., M.S. Wang, Z.X. Deng, R. Walulu and C.D. Mao. *J. Am. Chem. Soc.* **126**: 2324 (2004b).

Liu, Y., Y.G. Ke and H. Yan. *J. Am. Chem. Soc.* **127**: 17,140 (2005a).

Liu, Y., C.X. Lin, H.Y. Li and H. Yan. *Angew. Chem. Int. Ed.* **44**: 4333 (2005b).

Loweth, C.J., W.B. Caldwell, X. Peng, A.P. Alivisatos and P.G. Schultz. *Angew. Chem. Int. Ed.* **38**: 1808 (1999).

Lund, K., Y. Liu, S. Lindsay and H. Yan. *J. Am. Chem. Soc.* **127**: 17,606 (2005).

Macaya, R.F., P. Schultze, F.W. Smith, J.A. Roe and J. Feigon. *Proc. Natl. Acad. Sci.* USA **90**: 3745 (1993).

Mann, B.S., W. Shenton and M. Li. *Adv. Mater.* **12**: 147 (2000).

Mao, C., W. Sun and N.C. Seeman. *Nature* **386**: 137 (1997).

Mao, C., W. Sun and N.C. Seeman. *J. Am. Chem. Soc.* **121**: 5437 (1999).

Mathieu, F., S.P. Liao, J. Kopatscht, T. Wang, C.D. Mao and N.C. Seeman. *Nano Lett.* **5**: 661 (2005).

Mirkin, C.A., R.L. Letsinger, R.C. Mucic and J.J. Storhoff. *Nature* **382**: 607 (1996).

Mirkin, R.C., J.J. Storhoff, C.A. Mirkin and R.L. Letsinger. *J. Am. Chem. Soc.* **120**: 12,674 (1998).

Mitchell, G.P., C.A. Mirkin and R.L. Letsinger. *J. Am. Chem. Soc.* **121**: 8122 (1999).

Mitchell, J.C., J.R. Harris, J. Malo, J. Bath and A.J. Turberfield. *J. Am. Chem. Soc.* **126**: 16,342 (2004).

Mucic, R.C., J.J. Storhoff, D.A. Mirkin and R.L. Letsinger. *J. Am. Chem. Soc.* **120**: 12,674 (1998).

Murphy, M.B., S.T. Fuller, P.M. Richardson and S.A. Doyle. *Nucleic Acids Res.* **31**: e110 (2003).

Nguyen, C.V., L. Delzeit, A.M. Cassell, J. Li, J. Han and M. Meyyappan. *Nano Lett.* **2**: 1079 (2002).

Nielsen, P.E.,mM. Engholm, R.H. Berg and O. Buchardt. *Science* **254**: 1497 (1991).

Niemeyer, C.M., T. Sano, C.L. Smith and C.R. Cantor. *Nucleic Acids Res.* **22**: 5530 (1994).

Niemeyer, C.M., W. Buerger and J. Peplies. *Angew. Chem. Int. Ed.* **37**: 2265 (1998).

Niemeyer, C.M., M. Adler, B. Pignataro, S. Lenhert, S. Gao, L. Chi, H. Fuchs and D. Blohm. *Nucleic Acids Res.* **27**: 4553 (1999).

Niemeyer, C.M., M. Adler, S. Gao and L. Chi. *Angew. Chem. Int. Ed.* **39**: 3055 (2000).

Niemeyer, C.M., M. Adler, S. Lenhert, S. Gao, H. Fuchs and L.F. Chi. *Europ. Chembiochem* **2**: 260 (2001).

Niemeyer, C.M. *Trends Biotechnol.* **9**: 395 (2002a).

Niemeyer, C.M. *Science* **297**: 62 (2002b).

Niemeyer, C.M., B. Ceyhan and P. Hazarika. *Angew. Chem. Int. Ed.* **42**: 5766 (2003).

Niemeyer, C.M. *Biochem. Soc. Trans.* **32**: 51 (2004).

O'Neill, P., P.W.K. Rothemund and D.K. Fygenson. *Nano Lett.* **6**: 1379 (2006).

Park, S.H., R. Barish, H.Y. Li, J.H. Reif, G. Finkelstein, H. Yan and T.H. LaBean. *Nano Lett.* **5**: 693 (2005a).

Park, S.H., P. Yin, Y. Liu, J.H. Reif, T.H. LaBean and H. Yan. *Nano Lett.* **5**: 729 (2005b).

Park, S.H., C. Pistol, S.J. Ahn, J.H. Reif, A.R. Lebeck, C. Dwyer and T.H. LaBean. *Angew. Chem. Int. Ed.* **45**: 735 (2006).

Park, S. J., A.A. Lazarides, C.A.Mirkin and R.L. Letsinger. *Angew. Chem. Int. Ed.* **40**: 2909 (2001).

Pathak, S., S.K. Choi, N. Arnheim and M. E. Thompson. *J. Am. Chem. Soc.* **123**: 4103 (2001).

Pinto, Y.Y., J.D. Le, N.C. Seeman, K. Musier-Forsyth, T.A. Taton and R.A. Kiehl. *Nano Lett.* **5**: 2399 (2005).

Poort S.R., F.R. Rosendaal, P.H. Reitsma and R.M. Bertina. *Blood* **88**: 3698 (1996).

Reynolds III, R.A., C.A. Mirkin and R.L. Letsinger. *J. Am. Chem. Soc.* **122**: 3795 (2000).

Reishus, D., B. Shaw, Y. Brun, N. Chelyapov and L. Adleman. *J. Am. Chem. Soc.* **127**: 17,590 (2005).

Rothemund, P.W. K., A. Ekani-Nkodo, N. Papadakis, A. Kumar, D. K. Fygenson and E. Winfree. *J. Am. Chem. Soc.* **126**: 16,344 (2004).

Rothemund, P.W. K. *Nature* **440**: 297 (2006).

Sa-Ardyen, P., A.V. Vologodskii and N.C. Seeman. *Biophys.* J. **84**: 3829 (2003).

Santa Lucia, J. *Proc. Natl. Acad. Sci.* USA **95**: 1460 (1998).

Seeman, N.C. *J. Theor. Biol.* **99**: 237 (1982).

Seeman, N.C. *DNA Cell Biol.* **10**: 475 (1991).

Seeman, N.C. *Chem. Biol.* **10**: 1151 (2003a).

Seeman, N.C. *Biochemistry* **42**: 7259 (2003b).

Shih, M. W., J. D. Quispe and G. F. Joyce. *Nature* **427**: 618 (2004).

Shim, M. ,N. W. S. Kam, R. J. Chen, Y. Li. and H. Dai. *Nano. Lett.* **2**: 285 (2002).

Torimoto, T., M. Yamashita, S. Kuwabata, T. Sakata, H. Mori and H. Yoneyama. *J. Phys. Chem.* B **103**: 42 (1999).

Van Holde, K.E. *Chromatin*. New York: Springer Verlag, p.111 (1989).

Watson, J.D. and F. H. Crick. *Nature* **171**: 737 (1953).

Wei, B. and Y. L. Mi. *Biomacromolecules* **6**: 2528 (2005).

Whang, D., S. Jin and C.M. Lieber. *Nano Lett.* **3**: 951 (2003).

Williams, K.A., P.T.M. Veenhuizen, B.G. de la Torre, R. Eritja and G. Dekker. *Nature* **420**: 761 (2002).

Winfree, E., F. Liu, L.A. Wenzler and N.C. Seeman. *Nature* **394**: 539 (1998).
Xu, J., E.A. Fogleman and S.L. Craig. *Macromolecules* **37**: 1863 (2004).
Xu, L., P. Frederik and K.F. Pirollo. *Hum. Gene Ther.* **13**: 469 (2002).
Yan, H., S.H. Park, G. Ginkelstein, J.H. Reif and T.H. LaBean. *Science* **301**: 1882 (2003).
Zhang J.P., X.J. Hu and P. Chen. *Appl. Catal.* A **226**: 49 (2004).
Zhang, J.P., Y. Liu, Y.G. Ke and H. Yan. *Nano. Lett.* **6**: 248 (2006).
Zhang, Y. and N.C. Seeman. *J. Am. Chem. Soc.* **114**: 2656 (1992).
Zhang Y. and N. C. Seeman. *J. Am. Chem. Soc.* **116**: 1661 (1994).

18 Nanoscale Bioactive Surfaces and Endosseous Implantology

Yunzhi Yang[1], Yongxing Liu[1], Sangwon Park[2], Hyunseung Kim[2], Kwangmin Lee[3] and Jeongtae Koh[4]

[1] Department of Biomedical Engineering and Bioimaging, College of Medicine, University of Tennessee Health Science Center, Memphis, TN 38163, USA

[2] Department of Prosthodontics, College of Dentistry, Chonnam National University, Gwangju 504-190, Korea

[3] Department of Materials Science and Engineering, College of Engineering, Chonnam National University, Gwangju 500-757, Korea

[4] Department of Phamacology and Dental Therapeutics, Chonnam National University, Gwangju 504-190, Korea

Abstract Titanium dental and orthopedic implant devices have been successfully used to restore function of patients' degenerative teeth, hips, and knees due to disease, injury, or aging. The clinical success of the dental and orthopedic implant devices is dependent on initial fixation, which is a result of osseointegration, a direct intimate contact between the implant device and surrounded bone tissue. However, the limited lifetimes of the load-bearing dental and orthopedic implant devices causes severe eco-social problems due to the loss of osseointegration. Currently, nanotechnology shows promise to enhance osseointegration. This chapter briefly introduces basic information regarding peri-implant endosseous healing, discusses effect of implant surface characteristics on osseointegration, and presents some recent progress in nanotechnology on osseointegration.

Keywords implant devices, osseointegration, nanotechnology

18.1 Introduction

With an increasing lifespan there will be an increasingly aged population. More people will suffer from age-related degenerative diseases in the near future. Functional losses can be partially or fully restored with the placement of artificial

(1) Corresponding e-mail: yyang19@utmem.edu

implant devices. For example, almost a million titanium (Ti) dental implant procedures are now conducted worldwide annually to restore the teeth function (Davies, 2003). The economic value of the US dental implant market exceeded half a billion dollars in 2005 (Davidoff, 2000). In addition, the years 2002 – 2011 are officially the 'Bone and Joint Decade', as recognized by President George W. Bush in 2002 because America's 'baby boom' generation is at the highest risk for orthopedic disease and injury in this decade. Currently, musculoskeletal diseases and injuries affect 43 million U.S. adults as the number one cause for disability in America, and the prevalence is growing. The disability due to bone and joint diseases can be restored by orthopedic implant devices, whose sales totaled approximately 3.43 billion dollars annually. This number has been steadily growing. For example, the number of total hip arthroplasty (THA) is projected to grow 174% by 2030. For knees, a growth of 673% is expected (Kurtz et al., 2006).

Dental and orthopedic endosseous implant devices have been successfully used in clinics for decades. Their success is believed to be based on osseointegration, which is defined as the direct histological bone-implant contact (Branemark et al., 1997, 1998; Albreektsson et al., 1981) which allows anchorage of the implants in bone tissue and their functional loading (Adell et al., 1981; Nevins and Langer, 1993). However, there are still many aspects of peri-implant bone healing that remains unclear. Studies have demonstrated success rates of Ti dental implants of 78% in the maxilla and 86% in the mandible after 15 years (National Institute of Health, 2005). Revisions of orthopedic implants, which are replacements or repairs made to already-inserted implants, will grow with the increasing human lifespan considering a fact that the lifespan of the orthopedic implant devices are no more than 12 – 15 years (Bares, 2006). In other words, the patients with THA surgery will need more than one procedure during their lifetime when they live a longer life.

A better understanding of peri-implant bone healing and interaction at the bone-implant interface as well as application of novel nanotechnology are expected to help to improve the success rate. The purpose of this chapter is to briefly discuss the mechanisms that comprise the biological cascade of early peri-implant bone healing and how the nanoscale bioactive surfaces potentially enhance osseointegration with respects of topography and chemistry.

18.2 Peri-implant Endosseous Healing and Osseointegration

18.2.1 Peri-Implant Endosseous Healing

In terms of the interaction between implant surface and bone, it is crucial to understand the biological cascade of new bone formation surrounding the implant towards osseointegration. Several excellent reviews have summarized the peri-implant bone healing (Davies, 2003; Franchi et al., 2005a, 2005b).

Briefly, the initial host response after implantation is similar to a common bone wound healing modified by the presence of the implant (Davies, 1990, 1996, 1998, 2003; Franchi et al., 2004a, 2004b, 2005a, 2005b; Jeroen et al., 2005; Puleo, 1999; Fini et al., 2004; Yang et al., 2006a). When an implant is inserted into a pre-drilled cavity, the blood and tissue fluid first come into contact with the implant surfaces. Water molecules, ions, and proteins adsorb and coat the implant surfaces, and then blood clot forms and fills the gap between the implant and pre-existing injured bone. Tissue healing around the implant starts with an inflammatory response. During the period of inflammation, all kinds of mediators and cytokines are released, including vasodilators, chemoattractants and platelet-derived growth factors (PDGF) and transforming growth factor-beta (TGF-β). These released substances initiate and regulate recruitment of inflammatory and other cells, the development of new blood vessels (angiogenesis), and overall cell response. Among the cells the macrophage is considered to govern the wound healing process. In addition to phagocytosis of cell debris and potential pathogens, macrophages secrete all kinds of mediators that regulate the responses and functions of many other cell types, thereby orchestrating the healing. Within the first few days after implantation, mesenchymal cells, pre-osteoblasts, and osteoblasts migrate to colonize the implant surface through clot and within the damaged area to produce extracellular matrix, start mineralization, and regenerate new bone. The new bone is formed by two mechanisms: intramembranous and endochondral ossification (Davies, 1996). Then the newly formed, immature bone is gradually remodeled to mature bone tissue by bone resorbing osteoclasts and bone forming osteoblasts. Compared with the relative short period of inflammatory and regenerative phase, the remodeling phase at the implantation sites may last for several years. It is worth noting that the remodeling of bone tissue not only exists at the implantation sites, but also occurs throughout life to remodel and repair bone.

In summary, the temporal peri-implant bone healing can be divided to three overlapping phases: inflammation, new bone formation, and bone remodeling (Jeroen et al., 2005; Yang et al., 2006; Cooper et al., 1987; Kienafel et al., 1999). Spatially, the peri-implant bone healing consists of three categories of osteogenesis: at the implant surface (contact osteogenesis), within the surgical microgap at sites of neovasculization, and the surgical host bone margin (distance osteogenesis) (Yang et al., 2006a, Cooper et al., 1989; Kenafel et al., 1999). Three unique environments for the osteoblastic cell can be envisioned; each environment may confer different biologic behavior to the cells (Ohtsu et al., 1997; Brunski et al., 2000). In other words, the new bone formation can proceed both from the host bone to the implant surface and from the implant surface to the host bone, thereby gradually sealing the gap and causing device integration.

As a combination of temporal and spatial bone healing, Davies claims three phases as follows (Davies, 2003): osteoconduction, denovo bone formation and bone remodeling. Here, osteoconduction phase includes the recruitment and migration of differentiating osteogenic cells to the implant surfaces, which is initiated by platelet activation as well as platelet derived growth factor release. Davies emphasized that the recruitment of differentiating osteogenic cells to the implant surface and subsequent bone formation is the key to maximize contact osteogenesis and provide implant stability (Davies, 2003). As such, implant features that may influence any or all of these rates of bone formation temporally and spatially will have the potential to enhance osseointegration.

18.2.2 Effect of Implant Surface Characteristics on Osseointegration

Osseointegration, the histological direct bone-implant contact, is critical for initial fixation, and has been considered the prerequisite for implant loading and long-term clinical success of endosseous dental and orthopedic implants. (Franchi et al., 2005a; Jeroen et al., 2005; Ohtsu et al., 1997; Brunski et al., 2000; Branemark et al., 1969; Zubery et al., 1999; Hui et al., 2001; Lorenzoni et al., 2003; Klinger et al., 1998; Carlsson et al., 2004) In order to achieve secure osseointegration, four equally important categories of factors must be recognized: (1) biocompatibility of implant devices; (2) surgical approach; (3) condition of the patient; (4) time.

Biocompatibility of implant devices include implant design; implant bulk properties such as elastic modulus, yield stress, ultimate stress, and fatigue stress; implant surface such as chemistry, topography, and crystal structure. The implant design, bulk, and surface properties will influence biomechanical status at the implantation sites. It is worth noting that the biocompatibility of implant devices is dependent on the applications. The biocompatibility definitions for cardiovascular and dental implants are significantly different. This book chapter will focus on the endosseous implant devices and the effect of implant surface characteristics on osseointegration.

Before we can discuss the effect of implant characteristics on peri-implant bone healing, we need to understand how the cells and implant surfaces communicate and interact with each other. Table 18.1 simplifies the cell-implant communication and influence factors. First, cells are able to communicate with implant directly via exchanges of ionic products released from the implants through biodegradation or/and dissolution. Second, cells also indirectly interact with the implant surfaces via adsorbed or circulating proteins through cell receptors. As such, all the factors that influence the biodegradation, dissolution, and protein adsorption will influence the cell—implant interaction and the biocompatibility of implant devices. The surface characteristics include surface chemistry, topography, wettability, charge, surface energy, crystal structure and crystallinity, and roughness. A crucial characteristic is the wettability and free surface energy of an implant surface.

Table 18.1 Communications between cells and implant surface

Cell-implant communication	Biocompatibility of implant	Characteristics of implant surface
Direct interaction through ion exchange	Biodegradation or/and dissolution, by which the released ionic products in vivo will change local concentration of soluble species and local pH	Surface chemistry and topography, wettability, surface energy, charge, crystal structure and crystallinity, roughness, surface area
Indirect interaction between cell receptors—circulating and adsorbed proteins (mediators)—implant surfaces	Protein adsorption, by which the adsorbed proteins, and entrapped growth factors will regulate cell adhesion, cell geometry, cell migration, proliferation, differentiation and function.	

When an implant is placed into the body, it will immediately surrounded by an aqueous liquid such as blood and biofluid. The primary component in the aqueous liquid is the water molecules, which will adsorb onto the implant surface and form a water monolayer or bilayer (Vogler, 1998). The structure and properties of water molecule layers depends on the implant surface properties at the atomic scale and is completely different from that of liquid water (Vogler, 1998). And then the ions and proteins within the surrounding liquid will incorporate into the layer of adsorbed and well-structured water molecules, which will determine the subsequent cell adhesion and its response. The ion species and concentrations will experience exchange between the surrounding liquid and the implant surface via dissolution or/and biodegradation which is related to chemistry, topography, roughness, surface area, crystal structure and crystallinity. The adsorbed protein types, concentration and conformation will depend on the implant surface chemistry, topography, charge, surface area, crystal structure and crystallinity; and not necessarily reflect the amount and ratio of the proteins in the surrounding liquid (Jeroen et al., 2005; Vogler, 1998; Horbert and Klumb, 1996; Steele et al., 1995; Yang et al., 2003).

18.2.3 Potential Advantage of Nanoscale Surfaces

It is well known that microscale features can exert control over cellular behavior (Flemming et al., 1999; Stevens and George, 2005; Discher et al., 2005; Curtis, 2004). Using micropatterned substrates, human and bovine capillary endothelial cells were switched from growth to apoptosis by decreasing texture size to progressively restrict cell extension (Chen et al., 1997). It has suggested that the surface topography regulates cell shape to govern cell fate with life and death (Chen et al., 1997). The recently emerging field of nanotechnology targets on controlling the material structures of nanoscale size in at least one dimension (*x*, *y* or *z*) (Jeroen et al., 2005; Malsch, 2005; Kumar et al., 2005; Greco et al., 2005; Wilson et al., 2005; Bronzino, 2006). The nanotechnology is expected to create a powerful tool to precisely control the nanoscale structure of an implant surface. For example, one promising application on the implant surface will be well able to regulate the specific protein adsorption and their conformation, thereby inducing desirable reaction with the biological environment.

Nanoscale biomaterials have been proposed as the next generation of endosseous implants by improving surface properties to create a more conducive environment for osteoblast function and bone ingrowth (Tasker et al., 2006; Christenson et al., 2006; Hasirci et al., 2006). The rationale is based on the natural three-dimensional nanoscale topographical cues of extracellular matrix (ECM) which generates significant effects upon cellular behaviors such as adhesion, orientation, migration, proliferation, differentiation and mineralization (Flemming et al., 1999; Stevens and George, 2005; Curtis, 2004, 2005; Discher et al., 2005; Tasker et al., 2006; Christenson et al., 2006; Hasirci et al., 2006; Kaplan et al., 1994; Schwartz and Boyan, 1994; Brauker et al., 1995; Douglas and Devaid, 1992; Webster et al., 2004; de Oliveria and Nanci, 2004). Also, natural bone itself has numerous nanometer features reflected by the mineral component hydroxyapatite (HA) which is between 2 and 5 nm wide and 50 nm long whereas the incorporated Type 1 collagen is a triple helix approximately 300 nm long (Curtis, 2005). In fact, many researches have advocated the efficacy of micro-/nanotopography to regulate cell behaviors (Flemming et al., 1999; Stevens and George, 2005; Curtis, 2004, 2005; Discher et al., 2005; Tasker et al., 2006; Christenson et al., 2006; Hasirci et al., 2006; Kaplan et al., 1994; Schwartz and Boyan, 1994; Brauker et al., 1995; Douglas and Devaid, 1992; Webster et al., 2004; de Oliveria and Nanci, 2004), signifying a great potential in controlling the in vivo performance of the implant when the surface was especially fabricated with appropriate structures. In contrast, untreated titanium implant surfaces that are smooth at the nanoscale do not provide such biological inspiration (Webster et al., 2004). Surfaces with designed nanostructures were evidenced to encourage initial cellular interactions and promote bone ingrowth (Christenson et al., 2006; de Oliveria and Nanci, 2004). Unfortunately, various research groups also reported contradictory results in terms of the benefits of nanoscale implant surfaces (Brunette and Chehroudi, 1999; Parker et al., 2002). One possible explanation is that the nanoscale surface changes the surface properties, but the nanoscale surface properties change with time. Figure 18.1(a) shows the sputtered nanoscale titania surface significantly reduces the water contact angle compared to microscale polished titanium surface, suggesting the increase in hydrophilicity. However, Fig. 18.1(b) shows the water contact angle on the surface of the sputtered nanoscale titania significantly increases with time. The significant differences in the surface wettability are believed to lead to different cell responses at the interface.

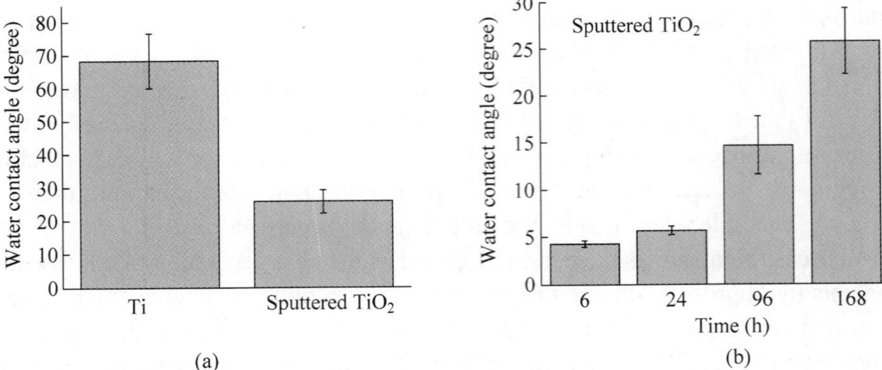

Figure 18.1 Water contact angles on titanium surface and sputtered titania (TiO_2) coating: (a) the sputtered titania coating exhibited significantly lower water contact angle compared to Ti control. (b) the water contact angle on the sputtered TiO_2 coating significantly increased with time

18.3 Nanoscale Bioactive Surfaces

18.3.1 Nanoscale Textured Surface

There are two strategies for fabrication of nanoscale structures: top-down (the miniaturization of higher scale structures) and bottom-up (the assembly of nanoscale structures from smaller structures) (Malsch, 2005; Kumar et al., 2005; Greco et al., 2005; Wilson et al., 2002; Bronzino, 2006; Tasker et al., 2006). Nanostructured features can be created on implants by using various techniques. The state-of-the-art techniques such as laser holography and X-ray lithography (Clark et al., 1991; Webb et al., 1996), and ion-beam lithography (Terris et al., 1996) are the well-controlled way to fabricate nanoscale features. Many other approaches were also developed including sputtering (Yang et al., 2005, 2006a, 2006b; Zhang et al., 2006), anodization (Geng et al., 2001; Oh et al., 2005), and glass phase topotaxy growth (solid state interfacial reaction) (Liu et al., 2004a, 2004b, 2004c, 2006; Hayakawa et al., 2005), and direct sintering (Webster et al., 1999; Price et al., 2003).

Sputtering techniques were known in the 1950s (Warner and Stockbridge, 1963) and then developed into a technique for depositing thin films (Chopra, 1969), which generally involves physical removal of target materials and then deposition of the removals onto adjacent surface to form a thin film in a vacuum environment. Figure 18.2 shows the schematic drawing of the sputtering deposition. During the sputtering deposition, the eroded target substances deposit on the substrate on an atom-by-atom basis, thereby allowing reconstruction and rebuilding a nanoscale coating in terms of grain and thickness.

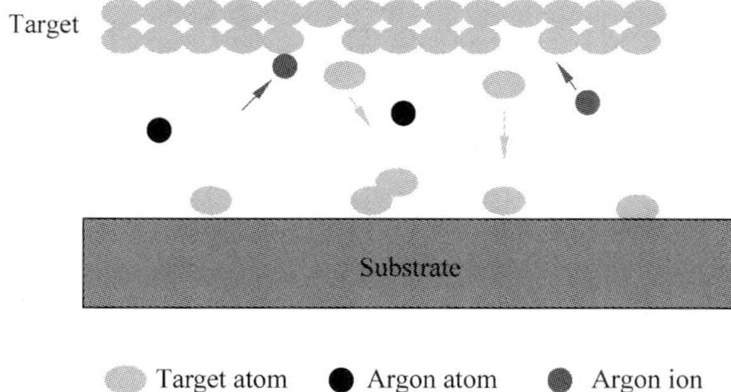

Figure 18.2 Schematic drawing of sputtering deposition. The energized argon ions bombard the target surfaces, and the eroded target atoms are deposited onto the substrates on an atom-by-atom basis. The film can be regulated by sputtering power, working gas type and pressure, deposition temperature, deposition time, and targets

Previously, we fabricated the dense nanoscale coating using sputtering deposition and characterized the coatings and biologically evaluated them using in vitro cell culture and in vivo animal study. Figure 18.3 shows the various dense sputtered coatings with nano-grain structures. The average crystal sizes for as-deposited TiO_2 coating and 600℃ heat-treated TiO_2 coating were observed approximately 20 nm and 80 nm compared to smooth surface on titanium control. These nanostructured

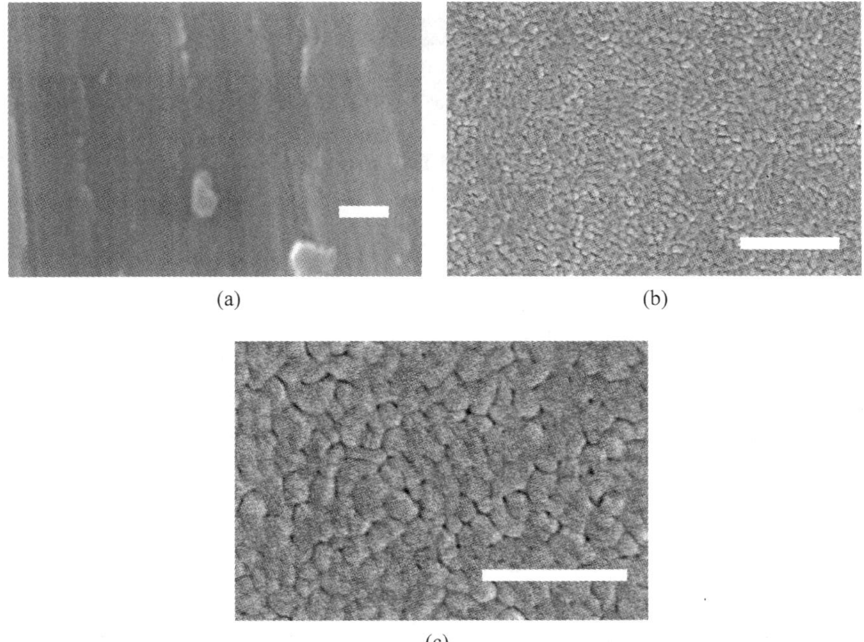

Figure 18.3 High resolution SEM pictures of Ti substrate and sputtered TiO_2 coatings (Yang et al., 2006a): (a) machined Ti substrate. (b) as-sputtered TiO_2 coating. (c) 600℃ post-deposition heat-treated sputtered TiO_2 coating. Bars = 500 nm

coatings significantly enhanced cell adhesion compared to control (Yang et al., 2003). No significant differences in cell proliferation and differentiation were observed between the dense nanoscale and polished Ti controls (Yang et al., 2003a, 2003b, 2004). We used dog femur model to evaluate the effect of nanoscale dense TiO_2 coating on osseointegration at 4 and 8 weeks after implantation (Yang et al., Submission). We compared Ti machined dental implants with the same dental implants sputtering coated with TiO_2 and postdeposition heat-treated TiO_2 coatings (Fig. 18.4). Reverse torque, histology, and scanning electron microscope (SEM) were used to characterize the osseointegration. The dense nanoscale titania coated machined Ti implant was not observed to improve the interfacial strength compared to the non-coated machined Ti implants (Fig. 18.5). The histology pictures show that both nanoscale TiO_2 coated implants and microscale machined

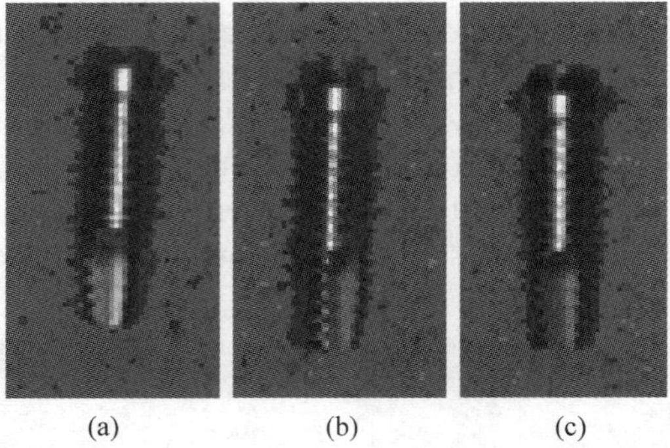

Figure 18.4 Dental implant pictures. (a) machined dental implant. (b) machined dental implant coated with as-sputtered TiO_2 coating. (c) machined dental implant coated with 600℃ heat-treated sputtered TiO_2 coating

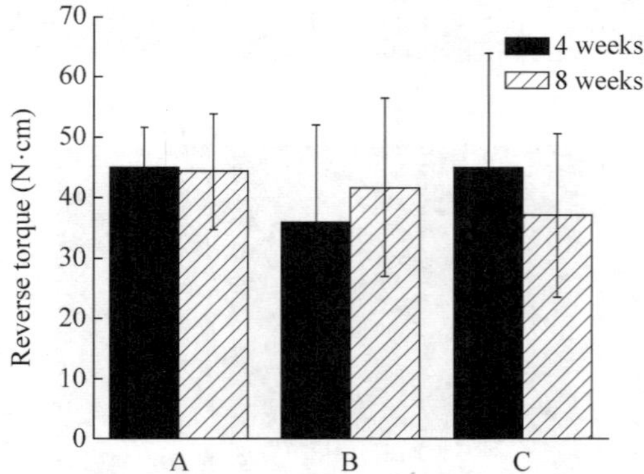

Figure 18.5 Interfacial strength between bone and dental implants evaluated by reverse torque measurement. (Yang et al., 2008) (a) machined dental implant. (b) machined dental implant coated with as-sputtered TiO_2 coating. (c) machined dental implant coated with 600℃ heat-treated sputtered TiO_2 coating

Ti implants formed osseointegration between implant and bone. There is no fibrous tissue at the interface (Fig. 18.6). SEM observation shows that bone debris still attached onto the extracted implants, suggesting the strong adhesion (Fig. 18.7).

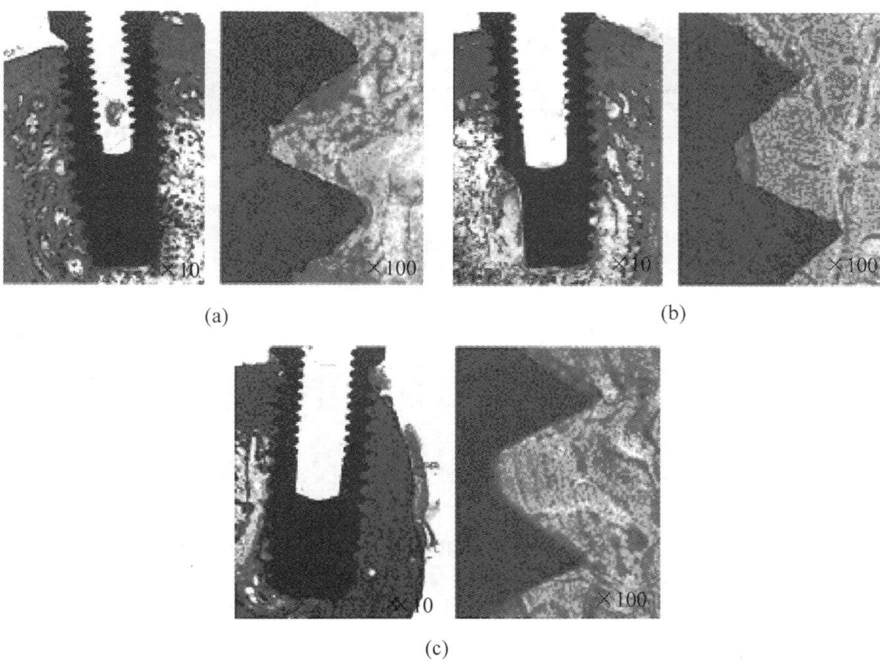

Figure 18.6 Histological interfaces between bone and dental implants. The samples were stained with hematoxylin and eosins. Osseointegration at all the interfaces were observed: (a) machined dental implant (Yang et al., 2008). (b) machined dental implant coated with as-sputtered TiO_2 coating. (c) machined dental implant coated with 600℃heat-treated sputtered TiO_2 coating. The left panel is with low magnification, × 10; and the right panel is with higher magnification, × 100

In addition to dense nanostructures, nanoporous surfaces were also developed by various methods. Anodization is also proposed as a promising nano-modification technique of titanium implants (Yao and Webster, 2006; Webster and Ahn, 2007). The well-aligned and high-density arrays of titanium oxide nanotubes (diameter: 25 to 65 nm) were produced in an aqueous solution containing 0.5 to 3.5 wt% hydrofluoric acid (Gong et al., 2001). After treatment with strong NaOH solution, the titanium oxide transformed to bioactive sodium titanate which induced the growth of nano-dimensioned HA phase after immersion in a simulated body fluid (Oh et al., 2005). In vitro culture of MC3T3-E1 cells on these titanium oxide nanotubes displayed significantly increased proliferation and differentiation compare to untreated titanium control (Oh et al., 2006). We treated different Ti surfaces using anodizing and obtained similar nanotube surfaces. Figure 18.8(a) shows a representative nanotube surface of titanium implant with 100 nm diameter

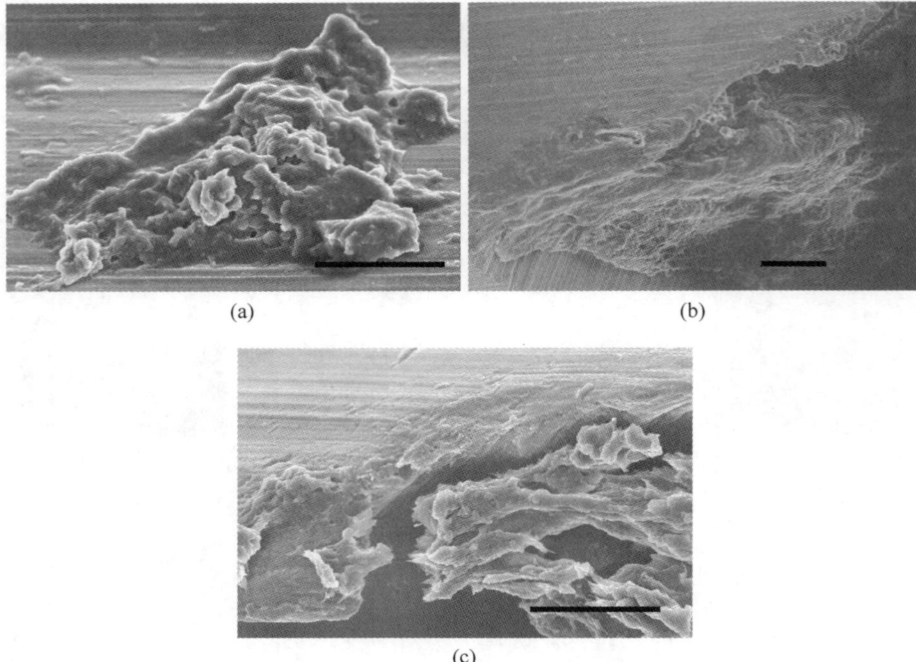

(a) (b)

(c)

Figure 18.7 The SEM observation of the extracted dental implants after reverse torque measurement (Yang, et al., 2008). (a) machined dental implant. (b) machined dental implant coated with as-sputtered TiO_2 coating. and (c) machined dental implant coated with 600℃ heat-treated sputtered TiO_2 coating. Bars = 50 μm

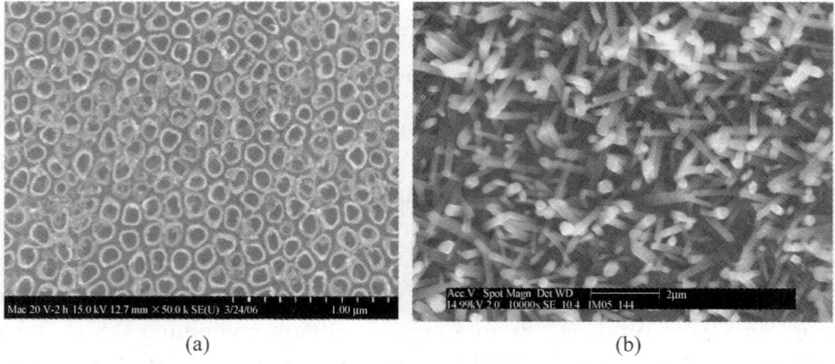

(a) (b)

Figure 18.8 High resolution SEM pictures of Nanostructures fabricated on titanium surfaces (Liu et al., 2004a, 2004b, 2005c, 2006; Hayakawa et al., 2005): (a) nanotubes derived from anodization. (b) nano rods derived from interfacial reaction

nanotubes. In addition, we recently developed a novel approach to produce nanorod array of titanium oxide on titanium substrates through a solid state interfacial reaction between a glass coating and titanium substrate (Fig. 18.8(b)) (Liu et al., 2004a, 2004b, 2004c, 2006; Hayakawa et al., 2005). The width of titanium oxide rods varied from < 100 nm to 1 – 2 μm by controlling the glass chemistry, reaction temperature and dwelling time. Shear strength of the rod-array layer on titanium substrate measured as high as 13 MPa. The as-obtained nanorod array displayed high in vitro bioactivity by depositing bone-like apatite in simulated body solutions (Liu et al., 2004c; Hayakawa et al., 2005). In vitro culture of mesenchymal cells indicated preliminarily positive responses compared to untreated control (Liu et al., 2004a, 2004b, 2006). Webster et al. (Webster et al., 1999; Price et al., 2003; Palin et al., 2005) reported that nanophase alumina and titania increase in osteoblast adhesion and the osteoblasts on nanostructured titanium surface produced three times more calcium deposition compared with microstructured (conventional) titanium (Webster et al., 1999; Price et al., 2003; Palin et al., 2005). All these above examples demonstrated that nanophase biomaterials have the potential for improving the efficacy of implants and for promoting osseointegration of implants. Nanophase materials deserve more attention in improving dental and orthopaedic implant performance.

18.3.2 Nanoscale Biological Molecules

In addition to nanoscale topographical cues, chemical modifications of implant surface by immobilizing and assembling nanoscale biological molecules are used to induce specific cell and tissue responses. These biological molecules include nanoscale peptides (Matsuura et al., 2000; Okamoto et al., 1998; Dee et al., 1998; Rezania and Healy, 1999), proteins, particularly, growth factors (Endo, 1995; Ito et al., 1998; Ong et al., 1997; Puleo et al., 2002), deoxyribonucleic acid (DNA) (van den Beucken et al., 2006a, 2006b), and antibiotics (Bunetel et al., 2001). These biological molecules are expected to control both the extent and type of cellular interactions and the cellular signal pathways in the early stages of osseointegration, thereby achieving a fast and more stable long-term integration of titanium implants. Excellent reviews of this topic outline the promising applications in the future (Jeroen et al., 2005; Hersel et al., 2003; LeBaron and Athanasiou, 2000).

The challenge of immobilization of nanoscale biological molecules is to retain the biological molecules onto the implant surface and enable their bioactivity in vivo as designed. There are three major mechanisms for the immobilization of biological molecules onto surfaces: (1) physical adsorption via van der waals or electrostatic interactions; (2) physical entrapment via use of a barrier; and (3) covalent bonding (Jeroen et al., 2005). The chemical bonding agents, such as organosilanes (Linsebigler et al., 1995; Iwasaki and Saito, 2003), photosensitive chemicals (Advincula et al., 2005), are able to form strong chemical bonds with the titanium oxide layer, other than self-assembly (Müller et al., 2006; Bumgardner et al., 2003), and direct immobilization (Kasemo, 1983; Klinger et al., 1997). The latter technologies exploit physical adsorption via van der Waals and electrostatic forces. Titanium is always covered with a thin TiO_2 layer when exposed to ambient and physiological environment, which has high dielectric constant and thus undergoes further modifications upon adsorption of various surrounding ions particularly proton in aqueous environment. The result is the adsorption of negatively charged OH^- radicals on the surface; the negatively charged surface the may electrostatically adsorb other positively charged ions and also biological agents (Weiskopf et al., 2007; Bessho et al., 1999). For instance, chondrotin sulphate (CS), which is a predominant type of glycosaminoglycans (GAGs) playing important roles in bone for cell adhesion, mineralization and other functions, was immobilized on titanium surfaces via calcium ions which electrostatically bridged the hydroxyl groups on titanium surface and carboxyl groups of CS. In vitro culture of osteoblast progenitor cells displayed a significantly faster initial cell attaching rate on the CS grafted titanium substrates compared to controls (Yang et al., 2004d). In fact, most of the above mentioned approaches reported encouraging in vitro effects. Particularly, bone morphogenetic proteins (BMPs) were immobilized on the surface of Ti-6Al-4V and reported to induce remarkable osteoinductivity. In an in vitro study involving immobilized BMPs, a significant enhancement of mesenchymal cell differentiation into osteoblasts was observed (Puleo et al., 2002). In an in vivo study involving BMP, bone-implant bonding strength and bone contact length were significantly improved when BMP was placed at the implant site in a canine model (Bessho et al., 1999).

18.3.3 Nanoscale Bioactive Calcium Phosphate Coating

Since the late 1960s biological fixation of load-bearing implants through bioactive ceramics coatings, typically calcium phosphates (CaP) and bioactive glasses, has been proposed as an alternative to cemented fixation (Yang et al., 2004d, 2006, 2007). Calcium phosphate coatings have largely demonstrated their success in promoting bone-implant integration. Calcium phosphates, particularly in the form of hydroxyapatite (HA, the main mineral phase of bone) and tricalcium phosphate (TCP) are important bio-inorganic materials well known of their excellent osteoconductive properties. The requirements for HA coatings have been described minimally in the Food and Drug Administration guidelines as well as in the ISO standards (Sun et al., 2001; FDA, 1992; ISO, 1996). Although the commercially plasma sprayed HA coated endosseous implant devices have been widely used in clinics for decades, there are some concerns in terms of variation or poor coating-substrate adhesion strength, non-uniformity in coating density and porosity, variation in structural and chemical properties due to coating process, and non-uniformity in coating properties between vendors (Cheang and Khor, 1996; Ducheyne and Cuckler, 1992; Lemons, 1988; Lacefield, 1988). In order to improve the adhesion strength between HA coating and Ti substrate, a functionally graded HA-Ti coating was fabricated using plasma spraying, where the Ti composition gradually reduced and HA composition gradually increased along the Ti substrate to the HA top layer. However, the adhesion strength of functionally graded coatings decreased compared to HA coated Ti (Table 18.2). The plasma spraying introduced a lot of pores reducing the contact area between layers, thereby reducing the cohesion and adhesion strength. However, using nanotechnology such as sputtering, it is feasible to achieve dense nanoscale functionally graded coatings to substantially improve the adhesion strength. In another study, a functionally graded stainless steel-diamond like carbon on artificial mechanical heart valve was fabricated using a two-target co-sputtering. A gradual change in composition was observed using X-ray photoelectron spectroscopy (XPS) depth analysis (Fig. 18.9), and the adhesion strength was significantly improved (Yang et al., 1997).

Table 18.2 Adhesive strength of different coatings to Ti substrates (Yang et al., 2006a; Liu et al., 2007)

Surfaces	Adhesive strength (MPa)
HA coating on Ti substrate	32.50 ± 3.56
Ti coating on Ti substrate	54.10 ± 1.33
HA coating on porous Ti-coated Ti substrate	21.40 ± 1.02

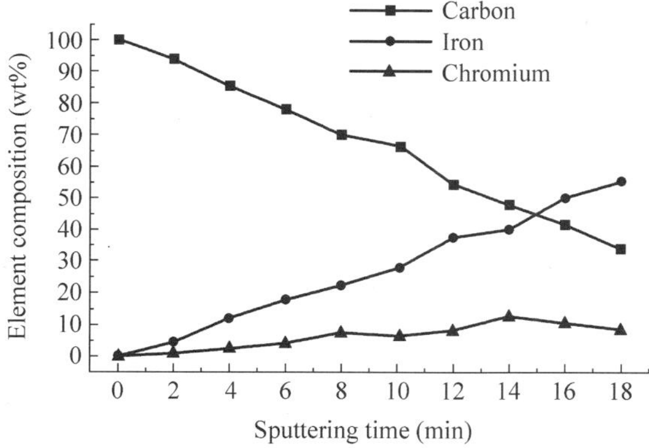

Figure 18.9 Elemental composition distribution of the diamond-like carbon-stainless steel functionally graded coating on the artificial mechanical heart valve (Yang et al., 1997). The distribution was evaluated by XPS depth analysis. Within the functionally graded coating, the carbon concentration reduced, and the iron and chromium concentrations increased along the direction of carbon outermost surface to stainless steel substrate (Yang et al., 1997)

There are controversies about the HA properties in terms of osteoconductivity and osteoinductivity. First is whether the osteoconductivity of HA is determined by its chemistry or topography. It is well known that the HA can readily adsorb proteins to their surface and form direct bone bonding at the HA-bone interface. However, Davies's group claimed that it is surface topography of the calcium phosphate, rather than the presence of calcium phosphate ions in the surface of materials that trigger the positive bone healing on calcium phosphate surfaces (Davies, 2003). They also argued that the excellent clinical outcome of plasma sprayed HA coating can not deconvolute the effects of surface chemical composition from those of the changes in surface topography (Gittlander et al., 1997). In another in vivo model study to compare the relative contribution of topography and chemistry to the osseointegration of HA-coated implant surface, it was found that the topography is a determining factor compared to chemistry in bone apposition (Hackingk et al., 2002). The second controversy is whether the HA is osteoinductive. Some studies reported HA scaffolds or spheres induced ectopic bone formation in animal models such as monkey and rabbits (Ripamonti, 1996; Yuan et al., 1999). The argument is that the HA contains a lot of micro/nano pores and possess very big surface area. Also, the HA has high affinity to growth factors such as BMP. It is possible that such the HA with a lot of micro/nano pores and surface area entraps enough growth factors to reach the threshold concentration to trigger the ectopic osteogenesis (Ripamonti, 1996; Yuan et al., 1799). However, no matter what debates there exist, it is very clear that the topography with different level of scales does be critical to not only the generation of contact osteogenesis, but also whether the surrounding bone matrix will bond to that surface.

Although there exists controversy about the chemistry role of the HA, the nanoscale HA in the forms of particle, coating, and scaffold and composite exhibit promising results in bone cell response using in vitro and in vivo models. In an in vitro study, human monocyte-derived macrophages and human osteoblast-like (HOB) cell models have been used to study the biocompatibility of nano-HA coatings (Huang et al., 2004). The nano-HA coating on glass substrates prepared by electrospraying was observed to support the attachment and the spread of HOB cells and does not trigger inflammatory response indicated by the release of lactate dehydrogenase (LDH) and tumor necrosis factor alpha (TNF-α) from cells (Huang et al., 2004). In another study, periosteal-derived osteoblast (POB) from the periosteum of 4-month human embryos could fully attach to and extend on porous nano-HA scaffolds, and formed extracellular matrix. Moreover, the presence of nano-HA scaffolds in cell culture could promote cell proliferation as compared to tissue culture plate ($p < 0.05$) (Zhang et al., 2004). In another separate study, a three-dimensional scaffold was prepared by rolling a porous nano-HA/collagen composite sheet. Bone-derived mesenchymal cells from neonatal Wistar rats were observed to continuously proliferate and migrate throughout the network of the coil. Eventually, three-dimensional polygonal cells and new bone matrix were observed within the composite scaffolds (Du et al., 1999). In a comparison study between nano-HA filler and micron-HA filler using a rat calvarial defect model, histological analysis and mechanical evaluation showed a more advanced bone formation and a more rapid increase in stiffness in the defects with the nano-HA augmented poly(propylene glycol-co-fumaric acid), suggesting an improved biological response to the nano-HA particles (Doherty et al., 2003). In another study, the tissue response to a nano-HA/collagen composite was investigated using a New Zealand rabbit femur model. The nano-HA/collagen composite was implanted in a marrow cavity. The process of implant degradation and bone substitution was observed during bone remodeling, suggesting that the composite can be involved in bone metabolism. In addition, the composite exhibited an isotropic mechanical behavior and similar microhardness with the femur compacta (Du et al., 1998). The advantage of the nanoscale HA may be due to the fact that the synthesized nano-HA is expected to be recognized as belonging to the body (Driessens et al., 2000). In other words, the synthesized nano-HA could be directly involved in the natural bone remodeling process, rather than being phagocytized like polymer debris (Driessens et al., 2000).

Like the dense nanoscale sputtered titania coatings, the dense nanoscale calcium phosphate coatings can be prepared by sputtering. The as-sputtered CaP coating typically consists of 100 – 200 nm grains. The as-sputtered CaP coating is usually amorphous phase (Ding et al., 1999; Wolke et al., 1994; Yang et al., 2003a, 2003b). Post-deposition heat-treatments at various temperatures with or without a humidified environment were capable of conversing the amorphous phases to crystalline phases forming an apatite-type phases. In addition, the crystallinity of the sputtered coatings can be well controlled by varying the post-deposition heat treatments (Ding et al., 1999; Wolke et al., 1994; Yang et al., 2003a, 2003b). The post-deposition heat treatment not only changes the crystal structure and crystallinity, but also changes the surface topography and composition (Ong et al., 1995, 1997; Yang et al., 2003c; Hulshoff et al., 1998).

As a result, the nanoscale HA coatings with different crystallinity, composition and surface morphology lead to different dissolution rate. For instance, the CaP coating heated at 400℃ (1.9% crystallinity) was observed to release more phosphorus ions as compared to that heated at 600℃ (1.9% crystallinity), whereas the as-sputtered CaP coatings (amorphous) were observed to have the greatest amount of phosphorus ions released (Yang et al., 2003c; Han et al., 2001; Sergo et al., 1997; Perozzollo et al., 2001). The nanoscale surface topography together with dissolution rates influenced cell adhesion and subsequent fate such as cytotoxicity and apoptosis (Hulshoff et al., 1998; Maxian et al., 1998; Maxian et al., 1993; Ong et al., 1999; Villarreal et al., 1998; Yang et al., 2003c). Integrin expression during the initial cell-material interactions was not affected by the surface chemistry in either sputtered CaP coating or titanium surfaces (ter Brugge, 2002). The nanoscale HA coating significantly increased the cell adhesion compared to Ti controls (Hulshoff et al., 1998). However, no significant differences in cell proliferation and differentiation were observed between nanoscale HA coating and Ti controls. We used the in vivo dog femur model to evaluate the effect of nanoscale HA coated Ti dental implant on its osseointegration. Although the osseointegration was histologically observed on both the nanoscale HA coated Ti dental implants and the machined Ti dental implants, the preliminary results did not exhibit significant differences in terms of interfacial strength. Other animal studies of the sputtered coatings have indicated an equivalent bone-implant contact length in the long term when compared to plasma-sprayed surfaces (Ong et al., 2002).

18.4 Summary

Nanotechnology is still in its infancy. Nanostructures on biomaterial surfaces and its effect on implantology will continue to be explored in the future. Many research of this topic is still in concept stage. With the development of top-down and bottom-up fabrication technology, precise control of surface topography at the nanoscale level on different substrates such as titanium and metal-ceramic composite will be available. Two fundamental questions need to be addressed: first, if the in vitro and in vivo cell response can be regulated by an implant surface with a precise control topographic and chemical cues; second, if the available regulation can vertically exert the impact on the therapy outcome and the evolution of nanotechnology itself. The continuing effort to extensively evaluate the nanoscale surface of an implant device in vitro and in vivo and the great potential for clinical applications will shape the science, healthcare and society in the future.

Acknowledgements

Part of the studies presented in this chapter was funded by grants from the Implant Dentistry Research and Education Foundation, March of Dimes Birth Defect Foundation, Wallace H. Coulter Foundation Early Career Translational Research Award, and International Collaboration Fund.

References

Adell, R., U. Lekholm, B. Rockler, P.I. Branemark. *Intl. J. Oral Surg.* **10**: 387 (1981).

Advincula, M., X. Fan, J. Lemons, R. Advincula. *Colloid. Surf.* B **42**(1): 29 (2005).

Albrektsson, T., P.I. Branemark, H.A. Hansson, J. Lindstrom. *Acta Orthop. Scand.* **52**: 155 (1981).

Bares,S. Memphis Bioworks Newsletter, **4** (2006).

Bessho, K., D.L. Carnes, R. Cavin, H.Y. Chen, J.L. Ong. *Clinical Oral. Implants Res.* **10**: 212 (1999).

Branemark, P.I., B.O. Hansson, R. Adell, U. Breine, J. Lindstrom, J. Hallen, J. Scand. *Plastic and Reconst. Surg.* **16**: 1 (1977).

Branemark, P.I., G.A. Zarb, T. Albrektsson. Tissue integrated prostheses. In: *Osseointegration in Clinical Dentistry*. Chicago: Quintessence, p. 11 (1985).

Branemark, P.I., R. Adell, U. Breine, B.O. Hansson, J. Lindstrom, O. Hallen, A. Ohman. *Scand. J. Plastic Reconst. Surg.* **3**: 81 (1969).

Brauker, J.H., V. E. Carr-Brendel, L. A. Martinson, J. Crudele, W. D. Johnston, R. D. Johnson. Neovascularization of synthetic membranes directed by membrane microarchitechture. *J. Biomed. Mater. Res.* **29**: 1517 – 1524 (1995).

Bronzino, J.D. Tissue Engineering and Artificial Organs. In: *The Biomedical Engineering Handbook.* 3rd ed. Boca Raton, FL: CRC Press, Inc. (2006).

Brunette, D.M., B. Chehroudi. *J. Biomed. Eng.* **121**: 49 (1999).

Brunski, J.B., D.A. Puleo, A. Nanci. *Int. J. Oral Maxillofac. Implants* **15**: 15 (2000).

Bumgardner, J.D., Jouett R, Y. Yang, J.L. Ong. *Journal of Biomaterials Science-Polymer Edition* 14: 1401 (2003).

Bunetel, L., J. Guérin, G. Agnani, S. Piel, H. Pinsard, J. C. Corbel and M. Bonnaure-Mallet. *Biomaterials* **22**: 3067 – 3072 (2001).

Carlsson, L.V., W. Macdonald, C.M. Jacobsson, T. Albrektsson. In: M.J. Yaszemski, D.J. Trantolo, K-U. Lewandrowski, V. Hasirci, D.E. Altobelli and D.L .Wise ed. *Biomaterials in Orthopedics*. New York: Marcel Dekker, Inc. p. 223 (2004).

Cheang, P., K.A. Khor. *Biomaterials* **17**: 537 (1996).

Chen, C.S., M. Mrksich, S. Huang, G.M. Whitesides, D.E. Ingber. *Science* **276**: 1425 (1997).

Chopra, K.L., *Thin Film Phenomena.* McGraw-Hill, New York (1969).

Christenson, E.M., K.S. Anseth., J.J.J.P. van den Beucken, C.K. Chan , B. Ercan, J.A. Jansen, C.T. Laurencin, W.-J. Li, R. Murugan, L.S. Nair, S. Ramakrishna, R.S. Tuan, T.J. Webster, A.G. Mikos. Nanobiomaterial applications in orthopedics. *J. Ortho. Res.* **25**: 11 (2006).

Clark, P., P. Connolly, A.S.G. Curtis, A.S.Gm J.A.T. Dow, C.D.W. Wilkinson. *J. Cell. Sci.* **99**: 73 (1991).

Cooper, L.F., T. Albreksson, B. Albreksson. *Acta Orthop. Scand.* **58**: 567 (1987).

Curtis, A. *Expery. Rev. Med. Devices* **2**(3): 293 (2005).

Curtis, A. *IEEE Transactions on Nanobioscience* **3**(4): 293 (2004).

Davidoff, S. R. Implant Dentistry **9**(3) (2000) www.dental-implants.com/executive_summary.html.

Davies, J.E. *Anatomical Record* **245**: 426 (1996).

Davies, J.E. *Intl. J. Prosthodontics* **11**: 391 (1998).

Davies, J.E. *J. Dent. Edu.* **67**(8): 932 (2003).

Davies, J.E., B. Lowenberg, A. Shiga. *J. Biomed. Mater. Res.* **24**: 1289 (1990).

de Oliveria, PT. Nanci. A. *Biomaterials* **25**: 403 (2004).

Dee, K.C., T.T. Andersen, R. Bizios. *J. Biomed. Mater. Res.* **40**: 371 (1998).

Ding, S., C. Ju, J. C. Lin. *J. Biomed. Mater. Res.* **44**: 266 (1999).

Discher, D. E., P. Janmey, Y. Wang. *Science* **310**: 1139 (2005).

Doherty, S.A., D.D. Hile, D.L. Wise, J.Y. Ying, S.T. Sonis, D.J. Trantolo. *Materials Research Society Symposium—Proceedings* **735**: 75 (2003).

Douglas, K., G. Devaid. MA/ Clark. Transfer of biologically derived nanometer-scale patterns to smooth substrates. *Science.* **257**: 642 – 644 (1992).

Driessens, F.C.M., M.G. Boltong, I. Khairoun, E.A.P. De Maeyer, M.P. Ginebra, R. wenz, J.A. Planell, R.M.H. Verbeeck. In: D.L. Wise, D.J. Trantolo, K.U. Lewandrowski, M.V. Gresser, M.J. Yaszemski. *Biomaterials Engineering and Devices. Human Applications.* Vol 2. New Jersey: Humana Press, p. 253 (2000).

Du, C., F.Z. Cui, X.D. Zhu, K. de Groot. *J. Biomed Mater. Res.* **44**: 407 (1999).

Du, C., F.Z. Cui, X.D. Zhu, K. de Groot. *J. Biomed. Mater. Res.* **42**: 540 (1998).

Ducheyne, P., J.M. Cuckler. *Clin. Orthop. Rel. Res.* **276**: 102 (1992).

Endo, K., *Dent. Mater. J.* **14**: 185 (1995).

FDA. Calcium Phosphate (Ca-P) Poating Draft Guidance for Preparation of FDA Submissions for Orthopedic and Dental Endosseous Implants. Washington, DC: Food and Drug Administration, p. 1 – 14 (1992).

Fini, M., G. Giavaresi, P. Torricelli, V. Corsari, R. Giardino, A. Nicolini, A. Carpi. *Biomedicine and Pharmacotherapy* **58**: 487 (2004).

Flemming, R.G., C.J. Murphy, G.A. Abrams, S.L. Goodman, P.F. Nealey. *Biomaterials* **20**: 573 (1999).

Franchi, M., B. Bacchelli, D. Martini, V. De Pasquale, E. Orsini, V. Ottani, M. Fini, G. Giavaresi, R. Giardino, A. Ruggeri. *Biomaterials* **25**: 2239 (2004a).

Franchi, M., E. Orsini, A. Trire, M. Quaranta, D. Martini, G. Giuliani, A. Ruggeri, V. Ottani. *Sci. World J.* **4**: 1083 (2004b).

Franchi, M., M. Fini, D. Martini, E. Orsini, L. Leonardi, A. Ruggeri, G. Giavaresi, V. Ottani. *Micron* **36**: 665 (2005b).

Franchi, M., M. Fini, G. Giavaresi, V. Ottani. *Micron* **36**: 630 (2005a).

Gittlander, M., G.B. Johansson, A. Wennerberg, T. Albrektsson, S. Radin, P. Ducheyne. *Biomaterials* **18**(7): 551 (1997).

Gong, D., C.A. Grimes, O,K. Varghese, W. Hu, R. S. Singh, Z. Chen, E.C. Dickey. *J. Mater. Res.* **16**: 3331 (2001).

Greco, R.S., F.B. Prinz, R.L. Smith. *Nanoscale Technology in Biological Systems.*Boca Raton: CRC Press (2005).

Hacking, S.A., M. Tanzer, E.J. Harvey, J.J. Krygier, J.D. Bobyn. *Clin. Orthop.* **133**: 24 (2002).

Han, Y., K. Xu, J. Lu. *J. Biomed. Mater. Res.* **55**: 596 (2001).

Hasirci, V., E. Vrana, P. Zorlutuna, A. Ndreu, P. Yilgor, F.B. Basmanav, E. Aydin. *J. Biomatere Sci. Polym. Ed.* **17**(11): 1241 (2006).

Hayakawa, S., Y. Liu, K. Okamoto, K. Tsuru, A. Osaka. Formation of titania submicro-scale rod arrays on titanium substrate and in vitro biocompatibility. In: *Nanoscale Materials Science in Biology and Medicine.* (Mater. Res. Soc. Symp. Proc. 845, Warrendale, PA, 2005) AA6.9

Hersel, U., C. Dahmen, H. Kessler. *Biomaterials* **24**: 4385 (2003).

Horbett, T.A., L.A. Klumb. In: W.P. Brash, ed. *Interfacial phenomena and bioproducts.* New York: Marcel Dekker (1996).

Huang, J., S.M. Best, W. Bonfield, R.A. Brooks, N. Rushton, S.N. Jayasinghe, M.J. Edirisinghe. *J. Mater. Sci: Mater. in Med.* **15**: 441 (2004).

Hui, E., J. Chow, D. Li, J. Liu, P. Wat, H. Law. *Clin. Oral Implant Dent. Rel. Res.* **3**(2): 79 (2001).

Hulshoff, J.E.G., K. van DijK, J.E. de Ruijte, F.J. R. Rietveld, L.A. Ginsel, J.A. Jansen. *J. Biomed. Mater. Res.* **40**: 464 (1998).

ISO. Implants for surgery: coating for hydroxyapatite ceramics. ISO; 1996, pp. 1 – 8.

Ito, Y., G. Chen, Y. Imanishi. *Bioconjug. Chem.* **9**: 277 (1998).

Iwasaki Y., N. Saito. *Colloid. Surf.* B **32**: 77 (2003).

Jeroen, J.J.P., V.D. Beucken, X.F. Walboomers, J.A. Jansen. In: N.H. Malsch. *Biomedical Nanotechnology.* Taylor & Francis, Boca Raton, p. 41 (2005).

Kaplan, F.S., W.C. Hayes, T.M. Keaveny, A. Boskey, T.A. Einhorn, J.P. Iannotti. Form and function of bone. In: Simon SP, ed. *Orthopedic Basic Science.* Rosemont, IL: American Academy of Orthopaedic Surgery pp. 127 – 184 (1994).

Kasemo, B. *J. Prosthet. Dent.* **49**: 832 (1983).

Kienafel, H., C. Sprey, A. Wilke, P. Griss. *J. Arthroplasty* **14**(3): 355 (1999).

Klinger, A., D. Steinberg, D. Kohavi, M. N. Sela. *J. Biomed. Mater. Res.* **36**: 387 (1997).

Klinger, M.M., F. Rahemtulla, C.W. Prince, L.C. Lucas, J.E. Lemons. *Crit. Rev. Oral. Biol. Med.* **9**(4): 449 (1998).

Kumar, C. S.S.R., J. Hormes, C. Leuschner. *Nanofabrication Towards Biomedical Applications. Techniques, Tools, Applications, and Impact.* Weinheim: wiley-VCH Verlag GmbH & Co. (2005).

Kurtz SM, Lau E, Zhao K, et al. The future burden of hip and knee revisions: U.S. projections from 2005 to 2030. Presented at the American Academy of Orthopedic Surgeons 73rd Annual meeting. March 22 – 26, 2006. Chicago.

Lacefield, W.R., In: P. Ducheyne, J.E. Lemons eds. *Bioceramics: Material Characteristics versus in vivo Behavior.* New York: The New York Academy of Science p. 72 (1988).

Lampin, M., C. Warocquier, C. Legris, M. Degrange and M. F. Sigot-Luizard. *J. Biomed. Mater. Res.* **36**(1): 99 (1997).

LeBaron, R.G., K.A. Athanasiou. *Tissue Eng.* **6**: 85 (2000).

Lemons, J.E., *Clin. Orthp. Rel. Res.* **235**: 220 (1988).

Linsebigler, A.L., G. Lu and Y. Yates, Jr. Chem. Rev. **95**: 735 (1995).

Liu, Y., K. Tsuru, S. Hayakawa, A. Osaka. *J. Ceram. Soc. Japan* **112**: 567 – 571 (2004a).

Liu, Y., K. Tsuru, S. Hayakawa, A. Osaka. *J. Ceram. Soc. Japan* **112**: 453 – 458 (2004b).

Liu, Y., K. Tsuru, S. Hayakawa, A. Osaka. *J. Ceram. Soc. Japan* **112**: 634 – 640 (2004c).

Liu, Y., S. Park, H. Kim, K. Lee, J. Koh, S. K. Nishimoto, J. Bumgardner, W. Haggard, Y. Yang. Osseointegration and titanium implant surface. In: W. Ahmed, N. Ali, eds. *Biomaterials and Biomedical Engineering.* Trans Tech Publishers (2007).

Liu, Y., W. Chen, Y. Yang, J. Ong, W. Haggard, J. Bumgardner. Fabrication of TiO_2 rod array and evaluation for cell attachment, The ADEA/AADR/CADR Meeting & Exhibition, March 8 – 11, 2006, Orlando, Florida, USA.

Lorenzoni, M., C. Pertl, K. Zhang, G. Wimmer, W.A. Wegscheider. *Clinical Oral Implants Research* **14**(2): 180 (2003).

Malsch, N.H. *Biomedical Nanotechnology*. Boca Raton: Taylor & Francis (2005).

Matsuura, T., R. Hosokawa, K. Okamoto, T. Kimoto and Y. Akagawa. *Biomaterials* **21**: 1121 (2000).

Maxia, S.H., J.P. Zawadsky, M.G. Dunn. *J. Biomed. Mater. Res.* **27**: 111 (1993).

Maxian, S.H., T. Di Stefano, M.C. Melican, M.L. Tiku, J.P. Zawadsky. *J. Biomed. Mater. Res.* **40**: 171 (1998).

Müller, R., J. Abke, E. Schnell, D. Scharnweber, R. Kujat, C. Englert, D. Taheri, M. Nerlich, M.Angele Pnagai, T. Hayakawa, A. Fukatsu, M. Yamamoto, M. Fukumoto, F. Nagahama. *Biomaterials* **27**: 4059 (2006).

National Institutes of Health, Department of Health and Human Services, Bethesda, MD; http://grants.nih.gov/grants/guide/rfa-files/RFA-DE-06-007.html. (accessed in August 2005)

Nevins, M., B. Langer. *Intl. J. Oral Maxillofac. Implants* **8**: 423 (1993).

Oh, S., C. Daraio, L.-H. Chen, T. R. Pisanic, R. R. Finones, S. Jin S. *J. Biomed. Mater. Res.* **78**A: 97 (2006).

Oh, S., R.R. Finones, C. Daraio, L. Chen, S. Jin. *Biomaterials.* **26**: 4938 (2005).

Ohtsu, A., H. Kusakari, T. Maeda, Y. Takano. *J Periodontol.* **68**: 270 (1997).

Okamoto, K., T. Matsuura, R. Hosokawa, Y. Akagawa. *J. Dent. Res.* **77**: 481 (1998).

Ong, J.L., D.L. Carnes, A. Sogal. *Interl. J. Oral. Maxillofac. Implants* **12**: 217 (1999).

Ong, J.L., G.N. Raikar, T. M. Smoot. *Biomaterials* **18**: 1271 (1997).

Ong, J.L., H.L. Cardenas, R. Cavin, D.L. Carnes. *Int. J. Oral Maxillofac. Implants* **12**: 649 (1997).

Ong, J.L., K. Bessho, D. Carnes. *Int. J. Oral. and Maxillofac Implants* **17**: 581 (2002).

Ong, J.L., L.C. Lucas, G.N. Raikar, C.W. Prince. In: D.L. Wise, D.E. Altobelli, E.R. Schwartz, M. Yaszemski, J.D. Gresser and D.J. Trantolo, eds. *Encyclopedia of Biomaterials and Bioengineering Materials, Part A: Materials*, Volume 2. Marcel Dekker, Inc., New York, p. 1565 (1995).

Palin, E., H. Liu, T. J. Webster. *Nanotechnology* **16**: 1828 (2005).

Parker, J.A., X.F. Walboomers, J.W. Von den Hiff, J.C. Maltha, J.A. Jansen. *J. Biomed. Mater. Res.* **61**: 91 (2002).

Perozzollo, D., W.R. Lacefiled, D.M. Brunette. *J. Biomed. Mater. Res.* **56**: 494 (2001).

Price, R.L., L. G. Gutwein, L. Kaledin, F. Tepper, T. J. Webster. *J. Biomed. Mater. Res.* **67**A:, 1284 – 1293 (2003).

Puleo, D.A., A. Nanci. *Biomaterials* **20**: 2311 (1999).

Puleo, D.A., R.A. Kissling and M.-S. Sheu. *Biomaterials* **23**: 2079 – 2087 (2002).

Rezania, A., K.E. Healy. *Biotechnol. Prog.* **15**: 19 (1999).

Ripamonti, U. *Biomaterials* **17**: 31 (1996).

Schwartz, Z., B. D. Boyan. Underlying mechanism at the bone-biomaterial interface. *J. Cell. Biochem.* **56**: 340 – 347 (1994).

Sergo, V., O. Sbaizero, D.R. Clarke. *Biomaterials* **18**: 477 (1997).

Steele, J.G., B.A. Dalton, G. Johnson, P.A. Underwood. *Biomaterials* **16**: 1057 (1995).

Stevens, M.M., J.H. George. *Science* **310**: 1135 (2005).

Sun, L., C.C. Berndt, K.A. Gross, A. Kucuk. *J. Biomed. Mater. Res.* (*Apply Biomater.*), **58**: 570 (2001).

Tasker, L. H., G. J. Sparey-Taylor and L. D. M. Nokes. CLIN ORTHOP, 1 (2006).

ter Brugge, P. J., J.A. Jansen. *Biomaterials* **23**: 3269 (2002).

Terris, B.D., H.J. Mamin, M.E. Best, J. A. Logan, D. Rugar. *Appl. Phys. Lett.* **69**: 4262 (1996).

van den Beucken, J.J.J., M.R.J. Vos, R.C. Thune, T. Hayakawa, T. Fukushima, Y. Okahata, X.F. Walboomers, N.A.J.M. Sommerdijk, R.J.M. Nolte, J.A. Jansen. *Biomaterials* **27**: 691 – 701 (2006b).

van den Beucken, J.J.J.P., X.F. Walboomers, M.R.J. Vos, N.A.J.M. Sommerdijk, R.J.M. Nolte, J.A. Jansen. *J. Biomed. Mater. Res.* **77**A: 202 – 211 (2006a).

Villarreal, D.R., A. Sogal, J.L. Ong. *J. Oral. Implantology* **29**: 67 (1998).

Vogler, E.A. Adv. *Colloid Interface Sci.* **74**: 69 (1998).

Warner, A. W., C. D. Stockbridge. *J. appl. Phys.* **34**: 437 (1963).

Webb, A., P. Clark, J. Skepper, A. Compston. A. Wood. *J. Cell. Sci.* **108**: 2747 (1995).

Webster, T.J., E.S. Ahn. *Adv. Biochem. Eng. Biotechnol.* **103**: 275 (2007).

Webster, T.J., M.C. Waid, J.L. McKenzie, R.L. Price, J.U. Ejiofor. *Nanotechnology* **15**: 48 (2004).

Webster, T.J., R.W. Siegel, R. Bizios. *Biomaterials* **20**: 1221 – 1227 (1999).

Weiskopf, S., Y. Liu, S. Kim, J.D. Bumgardner, W.O. Haggard, J. Ong and Y. Yang. Chondroitin Sulfate grafting on Titanium and Cell Attachment. IADR/AADR/CADR 85th General Session and Exhibition, New Orleans, LA March 21 – 24 (2007).

Wilson, M., K. Kannangara, G. Smith, M. Simmons, B. Raguse. *Nanotechnology Basic Science and Emerging Technologies*. Boca Raton: Chapman & Hall/CRC (2002).

Wolke, J.G. C., K. van Dijk, H.G. Schaeken, K. de Groot, J.A. Jansen. *J. Biomed. Mater. Res.* **28**: 1477 (1994).

Yang, Y. , N. Oh, Y. Liu, et al. *J.O.M.* **58**: 71 (2006a).

Yang, Y., C.M. Agrawal, K-H. Kim, H. Martin, K. Schulz, J. D. Bumgardner, J. L. Ong JL. *J. Oral. Implantology* **29**: 270 (2003c).

Yang, Y., D. Carnes, C.M. Agrawal and J.L. Ong. *J. Dent. Res. Spec.* A, **83** (2004).

Yang, Y., J. Ran and C. Zheng. Preparation of DLC / stainless steel gradient film materials using magnetron sputtering plasma method. In: C. Wu ed. 13th International Symposium on Plasma Chemistry, Symposium Proceedings. Vol. III, p. 1232 – 1237. Beijing, China: Peking University Press (1997).

Yang, Y., J.D. Bumgardner, R. Cavin, D.L. Carnes, J. L. Ong. *J. Dent. Res.* **82**: 449 (2003).

Yang, Y., J.D. Bumgardner, R. Cavin, D.L. Carnes, J.L. Ong. Osteoblast precursor cell attachment on heat-treated calcium phosphate coatings. *Journal of Dental Research* **82**(6): 449 – 453 (2003).

Yang, Y., K. Bessho, J.L. Ong. Hydroxyapatite Coatings. In: G. Wnek and G. Bowlin, eds. *Encyclopedia of Biomaterials and Biomedical Engineering (EBBE)*. NY: Marcel Dekker, Inc. p. 1 (2006).

Yang, Y., K. Bessho, J.L. Ong. In: M.J. Yaszemski, D.J. Trantolo, K.U. Lewandrowski, V. Hasirci, D.E. Altobelli and D.L. Wise ed. *Biomaterials in Orthopedics*. New York: Marcel Dekker, Inc. p. 401 (2004d).

Yang, Y., K. Kim, J.L. Ong. *Biomaterials* **26**: 327 (2005).

Yang, Y., K.H. Kim, C.M. Agrawal, J. L. Ong. *Biomaterials* **24**: 5131 (2003a).

Yang, Y., K.H. Kim, C.M. Agrawal, J. L. Ong. *J. Dent. Res.* **82**: 833 (2003b).

Yang, Y., Park, S., Lee, K., et al. (2008).

Yang, Y., R. Cavin, J.L. *Ong. J. Biomed. Mater. Res.* **67**A: 344 (2003).

Yang, Y., R. Glover, J.L. Ong. Protein adsorption and cell attachment on calcium phosphate coating of different heat treatment. *Transactions of the Society for Biomaterials*, 698 (2003).

Yao, C., T.J. Webster. *J. Nanosci. Nanotechnol.* **6**(9 – 10): 2682 (2006).

Yuan, H., K. Kurashina, J. D. de Bruijn, Y. Li, K. de Groot and X. Zhang. *Biomaterials* **20**(19): 1799 (1999).

Zhang, Q., S. Zhao, Z. Guo, Y. Dong, P. Lin, Y. Pu. *J. Southeast Uni.* (*Natural Science Edition*) **34**: 219 (2004).

Zhang, Z., Y. Yang, J.L. Ong. Nano-hydroxyapatite for biomedical applications. Tissue engineering and artificial organs. In: J.D. Bronzino, ed. *The Biomedical Engineering Handbook.* 3rd ed. CRC Press, Inc., Boca Raton, FL (2006).

Zubery, Y., N. Bichacho, O. Moses, H. Tal. *Intl. J. Periodont. Rest. Dent.* **19**(4): 343 (1999).

19 Carbon Nanotube Smart Materials for Biology and Medicine

Yeo Heung Yun[1], Vesselin N. Shanov[2], Adam Bange[3], William R. Heineman[3], H. Brian Halsall[3], Gautam Seth[1], Sarah K. Pixley[4], Michael Behbehani[4], Amit Bhattacharya[4], Zhongyun Dong[4], Sergey Yarmolenko[5], Inpil Kang[6] and Mark J. Schulz[1]

[1] Department of Mechanical Engineering University of Cincinnati, Cincinnati, OH 45221, USA

[2] Department of Chemical and Materials Engineering University of Cincinnati, Cincinnati, OH 45221, USA

[3] Department of Chemistry University of Cincinnati, Cincinnati, OH 45221, USA

[4] College of Medicine University of Cincinnati, Cincinnati, OH 45221, USA

[5] Department of Chemical and Mechanical Engineering, North Carolina A&T SU, Greensboro, NC 27411, USA

[6] Artificial Muscle Institute, Seoul 156-700, Korea

Abstract This chapter is an overview of potential applications of carbon nanotube smart materials in biology and medicine. Carbon nanotube arrays are forests of aligned nanotubes prepared on a substrate. The nanotubes have multifunctional properties that include high strength, sensing, actuation, and electronic properties. Several prototype smart material devices using nanotube arrays or nanotubes from the array are being developed by various groups that are co-authors of this chapter. The new devices include a biosensor, electrochemical actuator, nanotube probes, and a concept for a future in-body biosensor. Recently, aligned multi-wall carbon nanotube arrays over 1 cm tall were synthesized on large area substrates using a chemical vapor deposition process. The technique for growing nanotubes on large area substrates will open the door for low cost manufacturing of novel sensors, actuators, and devices for biology and medicine.

19.1 Introduction

Engineering materials have limitations in their physical or mechanical properties and biocompatibility for use in biomedical applications. Nanoengineering of

(1) Corresponding e-mail: yunyg@email.cu.edu

smart materials is one approach to address the need for improved materials for biomedical applications. Nanoengineering can be described as the process of synthesizing (Louchev et al., 2002; Vinciguerra et al., 2003; Vajtai et al., 2004; Hata et al., 2004; Yarmolenko et al., 2005; Schulz et al., 2006; Tu et al., 2002, 2003;Shanov et al., 2006) unique almost defect-free multifunctional material systems and machines starting from the nanoscale up. Nanoengineering is a new frontier that mimics the chemical and evolutionary processes found in nature to develop new generations of smart materials and intelligent systems that can sense and respond to their environments. The research described in this chapter is based on recent advances in manufacturing high density multi-wall carbon nanotube (MWCNT) arrays of parallel nanotubes. The many potential applications for nanotubes have accelerated research into techniques for their synthesis and processing, and the fabrication of devices build using carbon nanotubes (CNT). CNT growth, for example, has recently been improved with the help of intensive research and material characterization (Hata et al., 2004).

CNT are an exciting and versatile material. Electrical conductance, high mechanical stiffness, light weight, electron-spin resonance, electrochemical actuation, transistor behavior, piezoresistance, contact resistance, coulomb drag power generation, thermal conductivity, luminescence, and the possibilities for functionalizing CNT to change their intrinsic properties are reasons for the excitement. Biomedical applications of nanotubes have an especially large and immediate potential. Three applications can be categorized as: (1) biomedical diagnostic techniques (e.g. a nanoelectrode to record electrical activities of neurons), (2) drug delivery, and (3) prostheses, implants (e.g. neuroprostheses), and scaffolds for cell culturing. Carbon nanotube arrays can be considered smart materials because nanotubes have high mechanical strength, electrical conductivity, and piezoresistive and electrochemical sensing and actuation properties. The small size of the nanotubes is also an advantage in many biological applications. Moreover, macroscale smart materials can be built using nanophase constituent materials. Different properties of nanotube arrays and intermediate forms of nanotubes, and their applications are discussed in this paper. The applications are all work in progress and are presented in hope of generating new ideas for processing and application of nanotubes that can benefit medicine. The basic properties of nanotubes are well covered in the literature and are not described here. Several near-term practical applications of nanotubes in biomedicine are also well covered in the literature. This chapter focuses more on advanced synthesis and potentially breakthrough and futuristic applications of nanotubes in medicine. Topics covered include synthesis of super long nanotubes and patterned nanotubes and large area arrays, hydrophobicity, surface tension-induced swelling behavior, actuation, and sensing properties, and beginning development of several devices based on nanotubes.

The benefit of all this nanotechnology in the end will be measured by its application. Development of smart materials based on nanotechnology is in the beginning stages and has the potential to improve the way we generate and measure motion, and probe biomaterials from the nano to the macro scale. This chapter provides ideas how nanotubes can be put into applications. As you will see, nanotechnology is very interdisciplinary. Therefore, a large number of collaborators have contributed to this paper. It is felt that intersecting different technologies and investigating multiple applications has a synergistic effect and has enabled a lot of the progress in the field of nanomedicine. For example, a problem in developing nanoparticle contrast agents for magnetic resonance imaging is that nanotubes contain metal catalyst which must be removed. Removing the catalyst is a very difficult process. Recently carbon nanosphere chains are being developed for structural and electrical applications. The nanospheres are synthesized by a condensation process and are almost catalyst free. Thus, the nanospheres are a new material that may greatly simplify building nanoparticle contrast agents. As a second example, different substrates were being developed to grow nanotube arrays for medical applications. One substrate approach produced very long nanotubes, not useful for the intended medical application. However, the long nanotubes were ideal for structural reinforcement applications. Important is that in the end, applications come out.

19.2 Carbon Nanotube Array Synthesis

A brief overview of CNT synthesis is given here. Our group previously reported the synthesis of carbon nanotube arrays using water assisted chemical vapor deposition (Schulz et al., 2006; Shanov et al., 2006). Briefly, an electron-beam evaporator was used to deposit a 10-nm thick Al film on a Si/SiO_2 wafer, and the film was oxidized to produce Al_2O_3. Then, a composite catalyst (patent pending) was deposited on the $Si/SiO_2/Al_2O_3$ substrate. The nanotube array was then synthesized by thermal chemical vapor deposition (CVD) in a horizontal 2-in furnace (the EasyTube™ ET1000 by First Nano) furnace or a horizontal 3-in furnace (the EasyTube™ ET3000 by First Nano). Argon, ethylene, water, and hydrogen were used for deposition of the carbon nanotubes at a 750℃ growth temperature. The synthesized CNT arrays were characterized by environmental scanning electron microscopy (ESEM).

19.2.1 Array Synthesis

Nanotube arrays synthesized using an ET3000 furnace are shown in Figs. 19.1 and 19.2. The arrays were synthesized by First Nano Inc. using a substrate prepared at the University of Cincinnati. One-half of a 4 inch diameter substrate was used as shown in Fig. 19.1. The nanotube growth was about 11 mm. On a smaller 5 mm square substrate shown in Fig. 19.2, using the same process conditions, the growth was 17 mm. Better gas diffusion may have caused the larger growth for the smaller substrate. These two examples demonstrate that nanotubes can be mass produced on large substrates and that long nanotubes can be grown. Furthermore, it is expected that both these results will be exceeded soon.

Figure 19.1 Nanotube large area (half of 4 inch dia wafer) array synthesized by First Nano Inc. using a UC prepared substrate and the EasyTube™ ET3000 Nanofurnace produced by First Nano

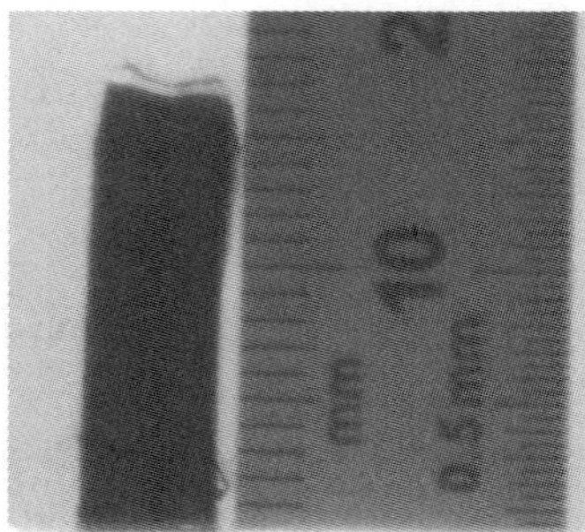

Figure 19.2 Nanotube long array synthesized by First Nano Inc. using a UC prepared substrate and the EasyTube™ ET3000 nanofurnace produced by First Nano

19.2.2 Synthesis of Carbon Nanotube Towers

Carbon nanotube towers are more convenient than bulk arrays for use in making biosensors and actuators. Our group previously reported the synthesis of carbon nanotube arrays using water assisted chemical vapor deposition process (Schulz et al., 2006). Briefly, an electron-beam evaporator was used to deposit a 10-nm thick Al film on a Si/SiO_2 wafer, before the film was oxidized to produce Al_2O_3. Then, iron catalyst was deposited through a shadow mask on the $Si/SiO_2/Al_2O_3$ substrate (Fig. 19.3). The nanotube array was then synthesized by thermal chemical vapor deposition in a horizontal 2-in EasyTubeTM (ET1000, FirstNano) furnace. Argon, ethylene, water, and hydrogen were used for deposition of the carbon nanotubes. Our group (Shanov et al., 2006) reported the influence of the intermediate buffer layer, Al_2O_3(10 nm) on the growth of MWCNT arrays with Fe used as the active catalyst, which is an effective way to grow long high density MWCNT arrays. SiO_2 on Si helps to prevent chemical reactions since pure Si can react with various catalysts, and the C in the catalyst might form silicates and C-silicate. Therefore, a chemically inert layer like SiO_2 helps to grow longer MWCNT arrays with high purity. The synthesized CNT arrays were characterized by environmental scanning electron microscopy.

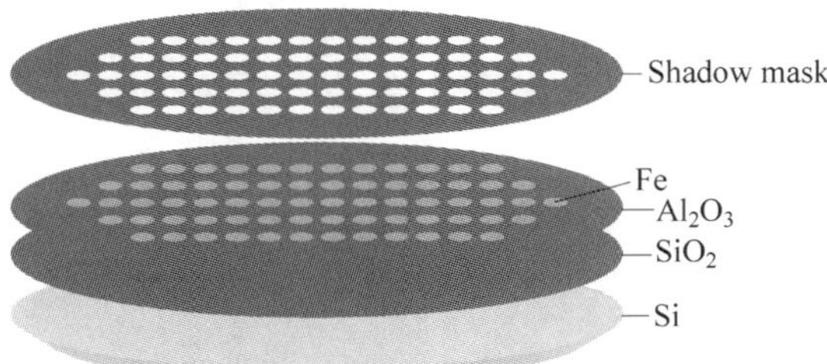

Figure 19.3 Patterned substrate preparation for nanotube array growth

Figures 19.4(a) – (c) show results of nanotube growth. Different magnifications are used in the images. Water vapor is used in the reaction to remove amorphous carbon. The $Fe/Al_2O_3/SiO_2/Si$ substrate is cut into 5 mm squares from one wafer and catalyst is patterned on 1 mm circles with 1 mm spacing between the circles. With the increase of growth time, the length of the CNT arrays increases for up to 10 hours. The goal is to grow nanotube towers in the mm length range. The mm-long nanotube posts are easy to handle to form devices.

The MWCNT array has high density without many impurities, which is ideal for further application development. Adhesion to the substrate is weak. One bundle of a MWCNT array block can be easily removed from the array using tweezers without damage. Figure 19.4(d) shows an 8 mm tall MWCNT patterned array on a Si wafer. Each tower (1 mm $\times$ 1 mm) of the patterned array contains around 1 billion nanotubes. The nanotube average diameter is 20 nm. The length to diameter aspect ratio is 200,000 : 1. The surface area of each tower (for an average 20 nm diameter, 4 mm length nanotube) is 2500 mm^2. In order to measure the resistivity of nanotube tower, epoxy was case into a nanotube tower. Both ends of the nanocomposite tower were polished and wired using conductive epoxy. The volume resistivity of the tower was 0.11 $\Omega \cdot cm$. The resistivity could be reduced by reducing the contact resistance of the wire to nanotube connection.

19.2.3 CNT Array Nanoskin and Nanostrands

Nanoskin and nanostrand fibers shown in Fig. 19.5(a),(b), respectively, are two other geometries of nanotubes that can be patterned on substrates. The nanoskin and nanostrands can improve the properties of composites that might be used in

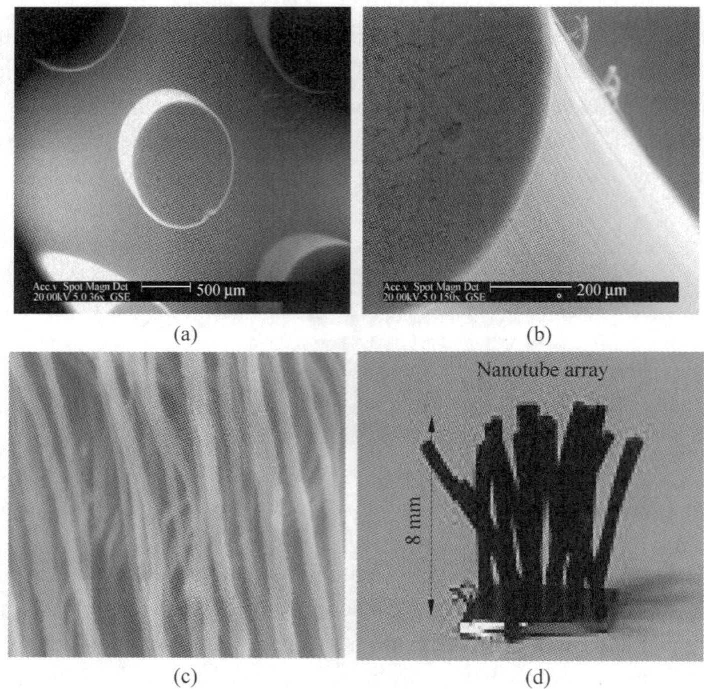

(a) (b)

(c) (d)

Figure 19.4 ESEM images of aligned multi-wall carbon nanotube patterned arrays: (a) one bundle of nanotubes called a tower. (b) top view of a nanotube tower. (c) high resolution side view of the nanotube tower. (d) picture of 8 mm tall MWCNT towers patterned on a Si wafer

biological applications, such as in prosthetics. CNT nanoskin can be strong, lightweight, absorb energy, reduce impact damage, and it can have electrical and thermal conductivity, and EMI shielding. The nanoskin can also be used for material health monitoring by sensing the electrochemical impedance of the material. The nanoskin can be filled with different polymer and elastomeric matrices, and the size of the nanotubes can be adjusted for use as a highly-compressible energy absorber. Tiles of nanotube arrays (Fig. 19.5(a)) can be formed into nanoskin for use on complex shapes.

CNT nanostrands (Fig. 19.5(b)) are micron diameter strands composed of millions of continuous multi-wall carbon nanotubes grown in a loose bundle by the chemical vapor deposition process on a silicon substrate. The nanostrands are similar to the nanotube towers but the strands are curved and longer than then towers. The nanostrands bend when as the length increases. The MWCNT forming the CNT nanostrands are 20 nm in outer diameter, 7 nm inner diameter, with about 15 concentric shells where the shells are separated by 0.34 nm. Potential applications of CNT nanostrands include polymer reinforcement, fibers for composite biomaterials, lightweight electrical wires, piezoresistive sensors for material health monitoring, sensors for biologic and haptic perception, and electrochemical biosensors. The microfibers can be filled with polymers, elastomers, conductive polymers, or ceramics to form nanocomposite biomaterials.

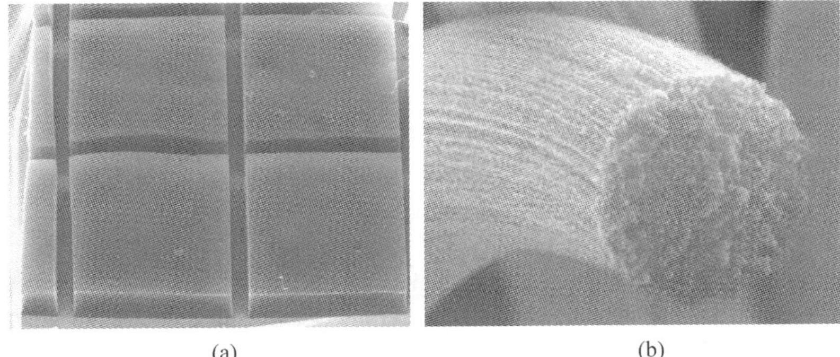

(a) (b)

Figure 19.5 Nanotube materials: (a) 1 mm square tiles of arrays. (b) 7 micron diameter nanostrand containing millions of MWCNT's

19.3 Properties of Carbon Nanotube Arrays

Different properties of CNT arrays that we consider to be smart material properties are discussed in this section. Smart materials possess multi-functional properties that can be used to sense or respond to their environment. Experimental studies of super-hydrophobicity and electro-wetting of nanotube carpet are important for processing the as-grown nanotubes, and to densify the carpet for some applications. The electro-wetting may also be used as an actuation property.

19.3.1 Hydrophobic Property

In Fig .19.6(a), a 10 μL drop of water is placed on the surface of a 1 mm long as-grown CNT array. The super-hydrophobic surface behavior is shown with an experimentally determined ($150° \pm 5°$) contact angle. The sliding angle was estimated as $20° \pm 5°$. The 1 mm long CNT carpet with about 10^8 CNT/cm^2 creates a large roughness resulting in the high contact angle. Shorter length CNT arrays had a lower contact angle. The CNT array can be chemically functionalized to make it more hydrophilic. It is first annealed at 500℃ for 5 h and immersed in concentrated 3 : 1 H_2SO_4/70% HNO_3 for acid treatment. HCl is added to the acid mixture to facilitate the termination of the opened ends and defects of the nanotube array with carboxylic acid groups. Then nanotube array is rinsed with NaOH solution to neutralize the sample. The final sample is washed with distilled water. Figure 19.6(b) shows the water drop wetting the functionalized array which has become hydrophilic. The hydrophobic property may be used to provide a synthetic material with selective interaction with biological materials.

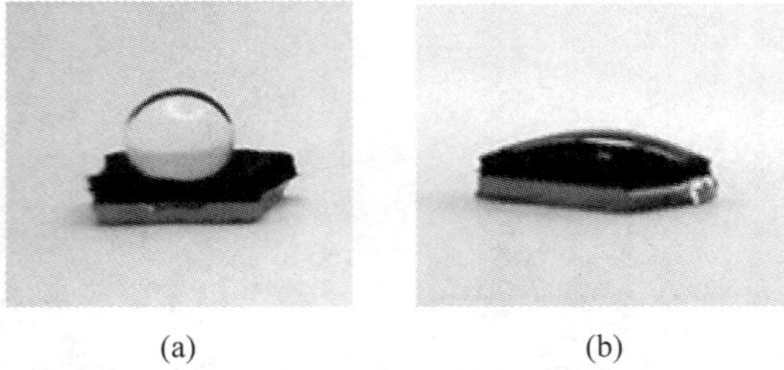

(a) (b)

Figure 19.6 Photo images of aligned multi-wall CNT array: (a) photo of a water droplet on a 1 mm long nanotube as grown array. (b) array after functionalization showing wetting of the surface

19.3.2 Electrowetting Property

Electrowetting is used for manipulating liquids on surfaces by applying small voltages. The electrostatic forces in electrowetting can reduce the contact angle and produce linear and oscillatory motion of entire droplets. It is demonstrated here that electrowetting can wet a CNT array that is hydrophobic. Figure 19.7 shows that a liquid drop, 10 μL of 1 mol/L NaCl, on a hydrophobic CNT array was made to wet the array by applying a small voltage (2 V) to the drop using a platinum wire. This experiment shows the potential to control the electrowetting property of the surface of a carbon nanotube array by connecting electrodes to the bottom of the nanotube array and applying a voltage. In this case, the nanotube electrode becomes permanently hydrophilic because the voltage caused the nanotube tips to be functionalized with hydroxyl or carboxyl groups. Reversing the electrowetting to re-form the droplet might be achieved by coating the carpet with parylene. Electrowetting gives freedom of water shedding design. This might be useful for example in biological implants and for body surfaces where control of the motion of fluid films is critical.

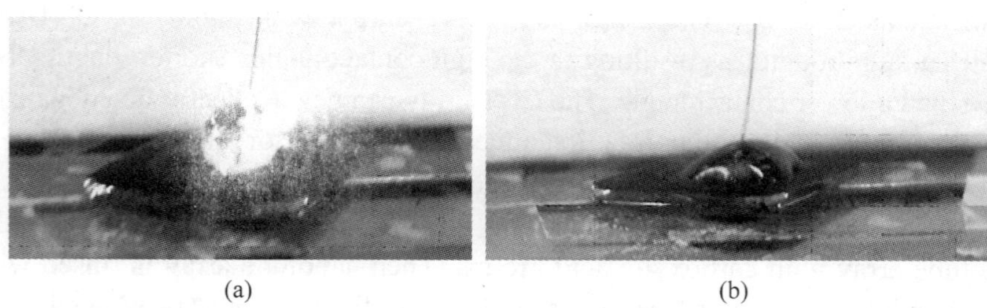

(a) (b)

Figure 19.7 Electrowetting on a CNT array: (a) platinum wire in the water drop at zero V. (b) with 2 V applied

19.3.3 Capillarity Property

Figures 19.8(a) – (c) show side-walls of an aligned nanotube array peeled off the Si wafer with 1 mm × 1 mm × 1 mm dimension. Even though it looks like the nanotube array is highly aligned at low magnification shown in Fig. 19.8(a), high resolution images in Figs. 19.8(b), (c) show the array has loosely oriented nanotubes with low density. In particular, the 1 mm long nanotube array behaves like a porous structure such as a sponge. Figures 19.8(d) – (f) show the dense structure obtained by infiltrating water into the array and evaporating the water. Since there is no holding force, the freestanding nanotube array shrinks freely without the generation of a crack when the water evaporates. The narrow spacing between the individual nanotubes creates a large surface tension. The huge surface area causes a large force and the array shrinks. Using acid instead of water and evaporating the liquid also causes the array to shrink.

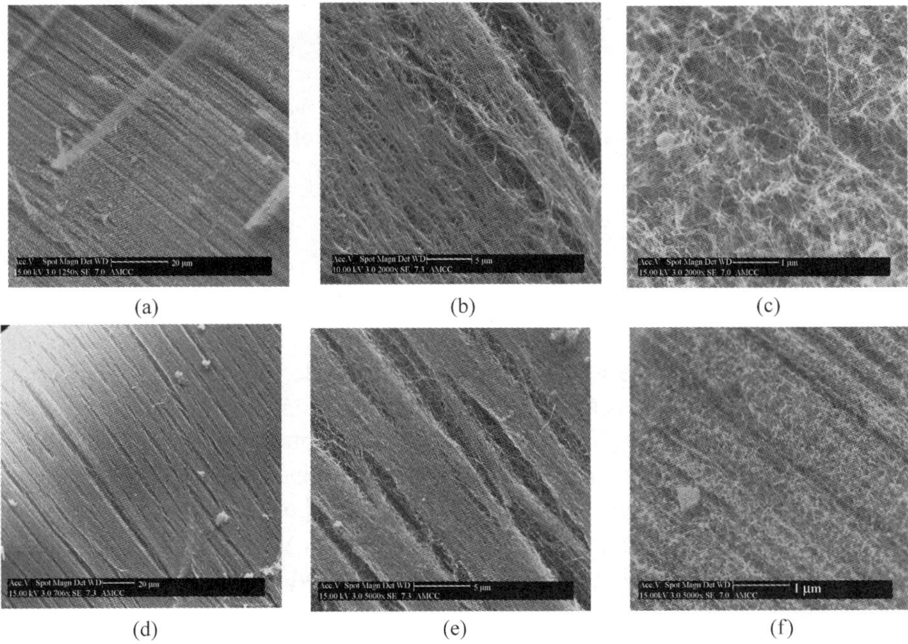

Figure 19.8 ESEM images of the side view of a CNT array as grown: (a) low magnification to (b),(c) high magnification. Filling the array with water or acid and evaporating the liquid causes the array to shrink. (d) low magnification to (f) high magnification

Figure 19.9 shows other views of the shrinking behavior of nanotube array. Even though adhesion between nanotube array and substrate creates a resistance to shrinking, overall, the capillarity force causes shrinking and creates a highly aligned nanotube array with high density. Compared to previous short nanotube arrays, the long nanotube array creates a large surface tension resulting in a highly dense nanotube array. These results are very reversible for more than 20 times from the wet to the dry state. This self-assembly method is one approach to improve the alignment and increase the density of the CNT array. The expansion property based on the re-wetting mechanism may be explored to develop a new volume expansion-type of actuator that might be used in the body.

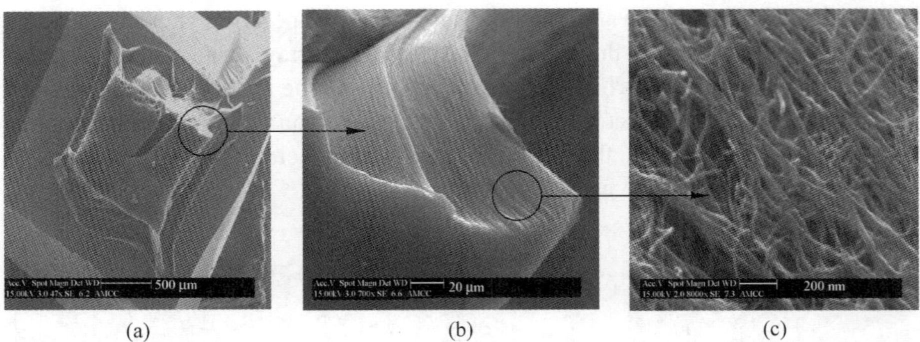

Figure 19.9 Dense CNT array on a Si wafer: (a) low magnification showing the shrinking of the array on the substrate, (b) structure of the array, and (c) high magnification showing individual nanotubes in the array

19.3.4 Nanotube Array Actuator

Based on the CNT towers which were synthesized, Fig. 19.10(a) shows the fabrication steps to make a nanotube tower electrode. First, the CNT tower is peeled off from the Si substrate by tweezers. One drop of preheated conductive epoxy is deposited on the glass substrate, and the nanotube tower is placed on the glass. A copper wire is connected to the conducting epoxy and cured in an oven at 80℃ for 1 h, as shown in Fig .19.10(b). The exposed conducting epoxy is sealed by Epon Resin 862 and EPICURE curing agent W at 120℃ for 4 h. Glass bead tape is pasted on the top of nanotube tower to reflect the laser displacement sensor optical signal.

The displacement of the nanotube tower actuator with applied voltage was measured using a laser displacement sensor (Keyence, LC-2400 Series) and a specially built test cell for characterizing the electrochemical properties of nanotubes, as shown in Fig. 19.10(c). Square wave potentials were applied between the working and counter electrodes using a National Instruments PCI board through a custom designed operational amplifier. Various square wave amplitudes are applied with frequencies ranging from 0.2 to 20 Hz. In order to supply enough power from the NI board, a voltage follower using a noninverting amplifier was designed using an operational amplifier with a gain of 10:1.

An electrochemical impedance spectroscopy (EIS) analysis was performed using a three-electrode cell, with the nanotube tower actuator as the working electrode, a Ag/AgCl used as the reference electrode, and a platinum plate as the counter electrode. EIS measurements were performed using a Gamry Potentiostat (Model: PCI4/750) coupled with the EIS (Gamry, EIS300) software. The cell was equilibrated for several hours after each step. A 2 mol/L NaCl electrolyte solution is used for the experiments.

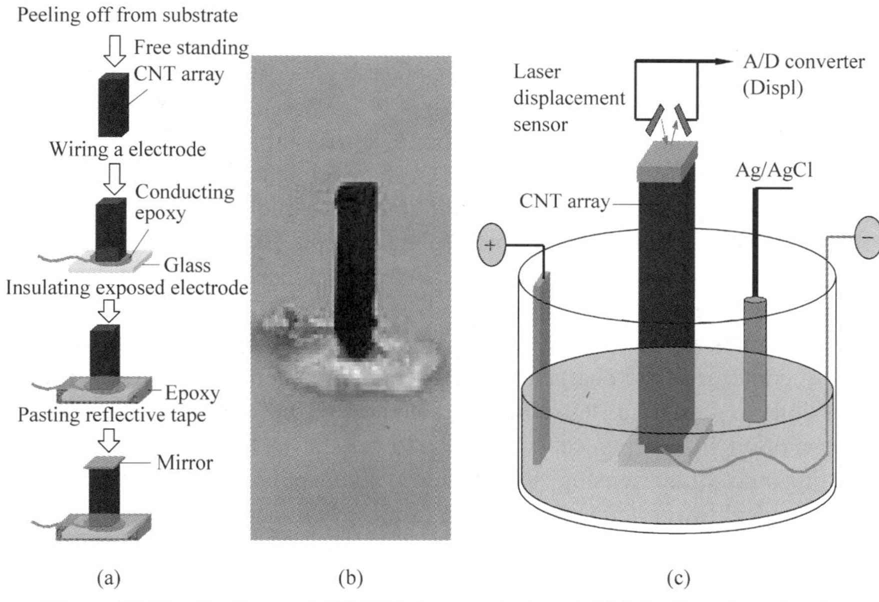

Figure 19.10 Testing an MWCNT tower actuator: (a) fabrication steps for the nanotube tower actuator. (b) the final fabricated actuator. and (c) the electrochemical analysis setup for testing the nanotube tower actuator, consisting of one nanotube tower which is fixed on a glass substrate, an Ag/AgCl reference electrode, and a Pt counter electrode

Figures 19.11(a),(b) show the relationship between the strain and the voltage applied to the nanotube tower actuator. As shown in Fig. 19.11(a), there is a non-uniform strain response with the square wave input. This problem would be solved by depositing an electrode layer on the top of the nanotube tower to bind the CNT electrodes to provide a higher voltage and uniform displacement. Strain of the nanotube tower closely follows the applied square wave potential of $\pm$ 2 V. With the increase of frequency, strain of the nanotube array decreases as shown in Fig. 19.11(b). The exact actuation behavior of the MWCNT needs further study to determine if the strain is uniform along the length and if only the outer surface of the nanotubes are expanding and actuating. If all the shells of the MWCNT could be made to actuate, the force would be the greatest possible. The results herein verified the actuation effect and that increasing the magnitude of the applied potential increases the strain. Probably the higher potential increases the charge accumulation at the nanotube tower/electrolyte interface and causes the faster response. However, too high of voltage would cause electrolysis of water and generate the bubbles on the surface of nanotube tower. This would decrease the lifetime of the actuator. Therefore, there is some limitation to increasing voltage to achieve high strain. A maximum strain of 2% has been predicted (Baughman et al., 1999) based on basal plane theory, but actual strains are up to 0.1% based on film-type single wall carbon nanotube actuators. The nanotube tower actuator shows strain up to 0.15%. Probably the straight aligned nanotube tower is the reason for higher strain comparing to entangled nanotube-film actuators. Excellent mechanical properties and good strain generation of the nanotube tower actuator might provide a solution for a new actuator material. Compared to the best-known ferroelectric, electrostrictive, and magnetostrictive materials, the low driving voltage of the CNT tower actuator is an advantage for various future applications such as smart structures, multi-link active catheters, artificial muscle, micro-pumps, molecular motors, or nano-robots. Another advantage is direct conversion of electrical energy to mechanical energy resulting in high strain generation. The high strength and high elastic modulus of nanotubes potentially might generate large forces during actuation. Since faradaic actuators basically come from the charge-discharge-charge method like a battery, it might be possible to design a self-powered actuator which means this device can actuate motion by storing capacitive charge in the nanotube structure. Power harvesting and strain sensing are other possible applications of the nanotube electrochemical tower. One other consideration when making the actuator is that the individual nanotubes are very long and winding and would buckle under a small load. Stabilizing nanotubes against buckling while still allowing access to the electrolyte is an area of further research. Smart materials using nanoscale particles are discussed.

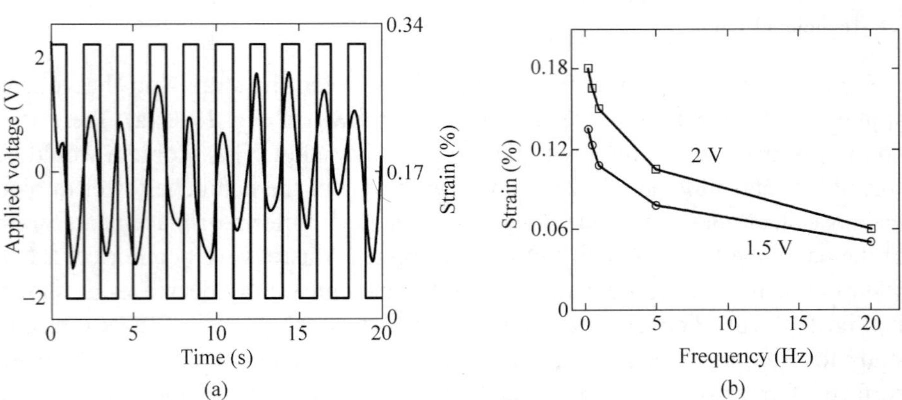

Figure 19.11 Strain of the nanotube tower: (a) at excitation frequency of 0.5 Hz, and (b) strain as a function of frequency and applied square wave voltage

19.4 Potential Applications of Nanotube Arrays In Biology and Medicine

The morphology and some of the properties of nanotubes were described. Now areas where CNT arrays and CNT can be put into applications in biology and medicine are described. An area of great interest across the world is nanoengineering of electronic devices that can detect disease in vitro using samples of blood, serum, or tissue. A more futurist area is to develop devices that can go inside the body to repair, monitor, and control biological systems. Overall, there is great opportunity to develop nanoscale smart materials for biology and medicine because of the many possibilities to engineer devices that work at the scale of biological molecules (the nanoscale) or cells (the micro-scale). Smart nanoscale materials and their devices would need some of the following capabilities depending on their specific application and whether the application is in vivo or in vitro: (1) a safe biocompatible material used for tissue scaffolding, bone repair; (2) power and communication by RF, or magnetically, or by light; (3) propulsion by shape control or vibration or magnetism; (4) illumination and vision; (5) drug release; (6) a piezoelectric shape changing particle; (7) power harvesting in ionic fluid; (8) materials to repair bone and cells; (9) a device to sample fluids in the body and return to a docking station in the body; (10) a contrast agent material; (11) stents; (12) magnetic collection; (13) an electrode to measure potentials; (14) a voltage source to control calcium channel activation and membrane potential; (15) surgical tools; (16) biosensing to detect disease; (17) ultrasound to break up blood clots while circulating in the arteries; (18) RF hypethermia to ablate and kill cancer cells; (19) strong wear resistant composite prostheses, and there are other properties that can be thought of.

Surprisingly, significant progress has already been made toward developing several of these capabilities. Advances include nanotube impedance biosensors and nanoparticles dispersed in polymers or electrolytes to provide electrical properties that can be interrogated to detect disease, and concepts and initial design for in body biosensors. In the literature, testing of nanotube biosensors with high sensitivity (Yun et al., 2007a, 2007b, 2006, in press, accepted; Li et al., 2003; Koehne et al., 2004; Schulz et al., 2007), and concept designs for nanobots and devices are reported. Future sensing applications will require specialized nano-electro-mechanical-systems (NEMS) such as sensor-transponders that can detect growth of cancer cells or overexpression of cytokines in the human body. Smart materials may also harvest power, actuate, and communicate with computers remotely. Design of nanostructured smart materials, devices, and interfaces will also provide tools for making advances in synthetic biology and systems biology. Nanoscale electrodes and biosensors may provide dynamic responses of cell signaling than can help model and understand systems biology. The following sections outline some early applications of nanoscale smart materials.

19.4.1 Electronic Biosensors

There are an increasing number of studies to develop biosensors using CNT. There are also a few studies using EIS and CNT to develop a biosensor. This approach is promising because the small electrode is coupled with an impedance analysis which is more sensitive than typical cyclic voltammetry (CV) analyses. This section reports fabrication of a nanotube array electrode and the immobilization of anti-mouse IgG on the open-end of the nanotube. The EIS of the nanotube-based biosensor was then tested under different concentrations of mouse-IgG. Based on a simple equivalent circuit, the relationship between electron transfer resistance and concentration of IgG was studied.

Figure 19.12 shows the fabrication steps to construct the nanotube tower electrode. First, the CNT tower was peeled off the Si substrate by a pair of tweezers and the array was cast in epoxy. The bottom section of a CNT tower was then polished and conducting epoxy was used to connect a Cu wire to the CNT tower. Then, the conducting portion of the nanotube was insulated using nonconductive epoxy. The top section of the array was polished to expose the nano-electrode.

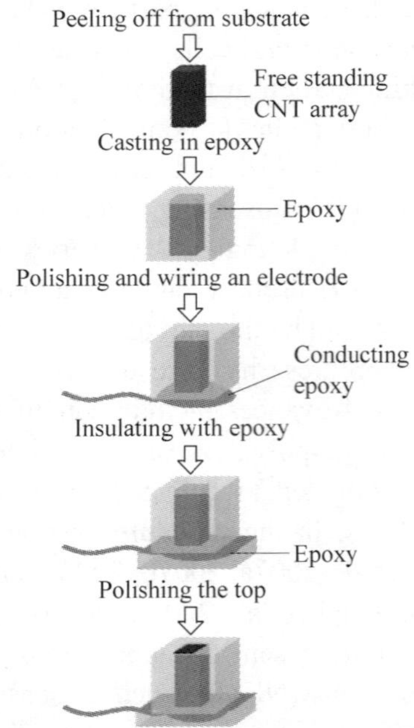

Figure 19.12 Tower electrode fabrication

Functionalization of the nanotube electrode is to attach special chemical groups to open-ended nanotubes that can act as receptors for other molecules. Electrochemical treatment at 1.5 V (versus Ag/AgCl) in 1.0 mol/L NaOH for 10 – 30 s was used to create carboxylic groups on the end of nanotube array. After functionalizing the nanotube electrodes with carboxylic groups, 1-Ethyl-3-

[3-dimethyalminopropyl] carbodimide hydrochloride (EDC) with sulfo-NHS was used to immobilize antibody to nanotube array. The electrode was immediately incubated for approximately 20 min with 10 mg EDC in 500 mL 2-(N-morpholio) ethanesulfonic acid (MES) buffer. Then the electrode was removed from EDC solution and immediately put into NHS solution (5 mg N-hydroxysuccinimide NHS in 500 μL MES buffer) for 20 min. The nanotube electrode was then immersed in 1% ethanol amine solution. Finally, the nanotube electrode was immersed in anti-mouse IgG solution (20 μL of donkey anti-mouse IgG in 1 mL PBS, pH 7.0) and incubated for 4 h. After rinsing with cold water, the sensor electrode was immersed into different concentrations of mouse IgG solution. Fig. 19.13(a) shows the final structure of the nanotube immunosensor. The EIS was performed using a three-electrode cell, with the nanotube electrode as the working electrode, an Ag/AgCl electrode used as the reference electrode, and a platinum wire as the counter electrode, as shown in Fig. 19.13(b). EIS measurements were performed using a Gamry Potentiostat (Model: PCI4/750) coupled with the EIS (Gamry, EIS300) software, Fig. 19.13(b). All testing was done at 0 V DC and 0.1 Hz to 300 kHz, and the sinusoidal potential magnitude is ± 20 mV in the redox probe 5 mmol/L $K_4[Fe(CN)_6]$, $K_3[Fe(CN)_6]$ with PBS (pH 7.0).

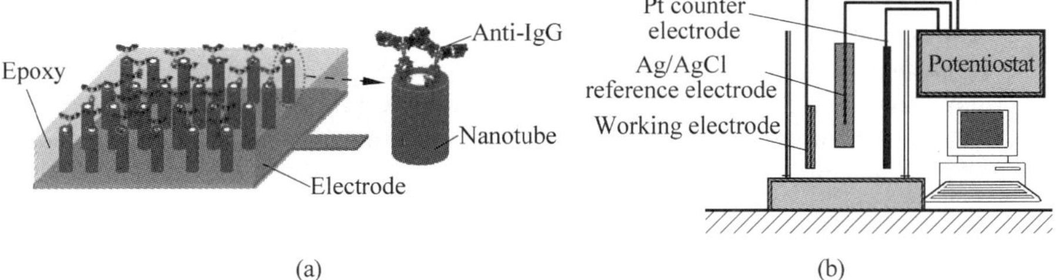

Figure 19.13 Nanotube array biosensor: (a) final structure of the nanotube immunosensor, and (b) test setup

Electron transfer of the redox couple is hindered by immobilization of the antibody and binding of the antigen. At the same time, the electron transfer resistance can be computed based on EIS measurements. Modeling the EIS response can be done using Randle's circuit. Randles circuit is an equivalent circuit representing each component at the interface and in the solution during an electrochemical reaction for comparison with the physical components; C_{dl}, the double layer capacitor; R_{et}, the electron transfer or polarization resistance; and R_s, the solution resistance. Randles circuit can be expressed as

$$Z(\omega) = R_{et} + \frac{R_{et}}{1+\omega^2 R_{et}^2 C_{dl}^2} - \frac{j\omega R_{et}^2 C_{dl}}{1+\omega^2 R_{et}^2 C_{dl}^2} = Z_{real} + jZ_{imag} \qquad (19.1)$$

The EIS response of Randle circuit is illustrated in Fig. 19.14(a). The diameter of the semicircle in the EIS Nyquist plot is called the electron transfer resistance,

R_{et}. The electron transfer resistance shows the electron transfer kinetics of the redox probe at the electrode diffusion layer. As shown in Fig. 19. 14(b), the electron transfer resistance, e.g., the diameter of semicircle, kept increasing after immobilization of the antibody and then the binding with the antigen. The EIS results show the typical Randles circuit response (Yun et al., 2007a, 2007b, 2006, in press, accepted; Li et al., 2003; Koehne et al., 2004; Schulz et al., 2007).

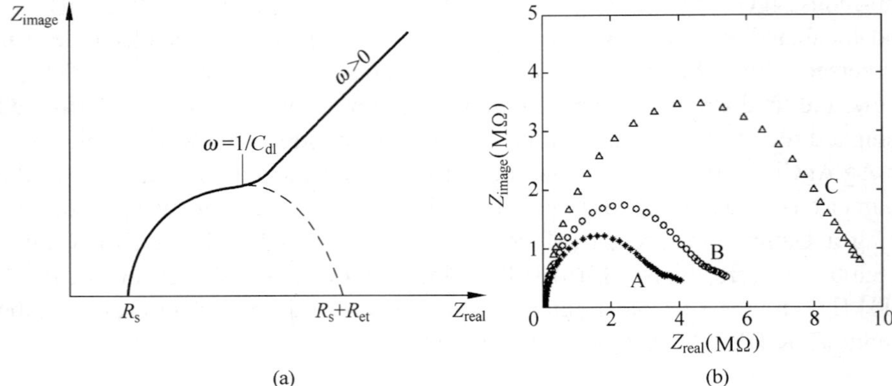

Figure 19.14 EIS theory and experimental result: (a) EIS Nyquist plot based on the theoretical Randles circuit; and (b) EIS for the nanotube electrode, after (a) functionalized nanotube array; (b) immobilized Donkey anti-mouse IgG; and (c) binding Mouse IgG. All experimental results are at a DC potential of 0 V, frequencies between 0.1 Hz and 300 kHz., and a sinusoidal potential magnitude of ± 20 mV in 5 mmol/L $K_4[Fe(CN)_6]$, $K_3[Fe(CN)_6]$ with PBS (pH 7.0)

Using the equivalent circuit model, the values of the curve fit parameters based on the experimental results in Fig. 19.14(b) are shown in Table 19. 1. Since the solution resistance represents the bulk properties of the electrolyte solution and diffusion of the applied redox probe, $[Fe(CN)_6]^{4-}/[Fe(CN)_6]^{3-}$, they are not affected much by the nanotube electrode chemical transformation. On the other hand, the double layer capacitance and electron transfer resistance represent the interface property of the electrode/electrolyte and will change due to insulating or coating the nanotube surface. As shown in Table 19.1, the double layer capacitance change is not as sensitive as the electron transfer resistance. The change in electron transfer resistance before and after adding the donkey anti-mouse IgG and the mouse IgG reaction is dramatically increased to 3500 kΩ. Therefore, the electron transfer resistance change, ΔR_{et} is chosen as the most sensitive parameter to indicate the detection of antibodies using the immunosensor. Future work is aimed at reducing the size of the electrode and to improve the sensitivity. The advantage of the electronic biosensor is that a fast result is obtained from a relatively simple test. This type of sensor may be useful to save time and reduce costs in clinical testing, for use as a portable at home test, and for use in remote regions such as Africa to check for disease.

Table 19.1 Estimated parameters for Randles equivalent circuit model

	R_{et}(MΩ)	C_{dl}(nF)	R_s(kΩ)
Bare electrode	2.9	2.5	6.4
Ab	4.0	2.0	7.2
Ab-Ag	7.5	2.7	7.7

19.4.2 Nanotube Electrodes for Biovoltage and Chemical Sensing

MWCNT arrays can be used as probes and needles. Figure 19.15(a) shows the experimental setup for welding nanotubes on a tungsten needle. An electronic micrometer was modified to hold two electrodes with one electrode fixed to a tungsten needle (Earnest F Fullam Inc.) for welding to nanotubes. The nanotube array is attached to the other electrode using carbon tape for holding scanning electron microscope samples. The nanotube welding is done by moving the needle toward the nanotube as shown in Fig. 19.15(b) and applying a voltage. High current makes the nanotube weld to the needle. Figure 9.15(c) shows welded nanotubes on tungsten tips. The nanotube tip diameters are about 200 nm. The welding is done in an inert atmosphere such as argon or nitrogen in a plastic glove box. Welding nanotubes to nanotubes is also being investigated. The nanotube probes can be used as a smaller biosensor to increase sensitivity for cancer detection, as electrodes for probing the neuronal response of cells in electrophysiology, for locating centers of epilepsy in the field of neurology, and for detecting chemical such as neurotransmitters. A variation on the nanotube electrode is do disperse nanotubes into eposy and for a needle. A nanotube composite microelectrode for monitoring dopamine levels using cyclic voltammetry and differential pulse voltammetry is discussed (Yun et al., in press).

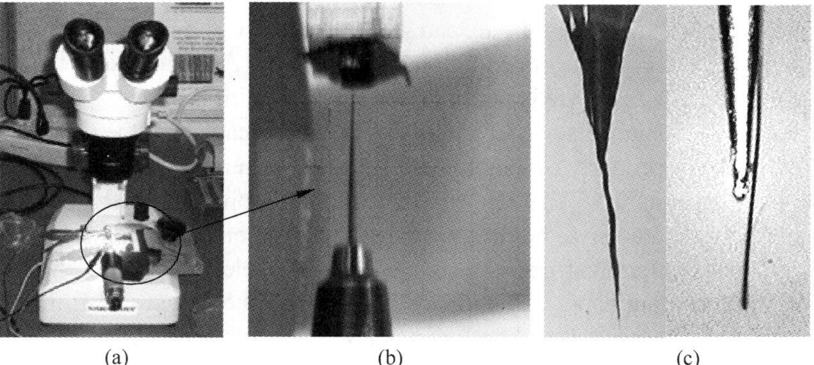

(a) (b) (c)

Figure 19.15 Experimental setup for welding CNT on a tungsten needle: (a) an optical stereo microscope. (b) probe tip positioned for welding to a nanotube array. (c) welded CNT bundles on tips of tungsten probes

19.4.3 Carbon Nanotube Sensor Film for Environmental Monitoring

Monitoring the environment for chemicals or biological agents may be done based on the biosensor using the EIS method. In this approach CNT film sensors are highly distributed on the surface of clothing to detect chemicals or biocides. An example of nanotube film (Kang et al., 2006a, 2006b) on a simple panel is shown in Fig. 19.16. CNT thread could be used in place of the film.

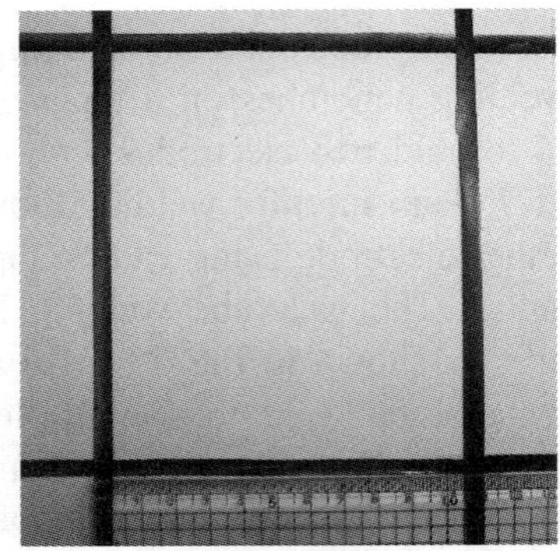

Figure 19.16 Spray-on carbon nanotube neurons in a grid pattern for environmental monitoring

The EIS system is a highly distributed network of CNT continuous film sensors that sense along their entire length and have a biomimetic architecture that allows coverage of large areas (Kang et al., 2006a). A 2 row and 2 column neuron prototype of the sensor is shown as a grid pattern in Fig. 19.16. The rows overlap the column neurons and are electrically insulated. The films can be independently connected or connected in series or parallel, or a combination of series and parallel depending on the sensitivity and coverage area desired. Chemicals or a liquid electrolyte can be detected by the film. The electrical impedance increases with concentration of the analyte. An example of the change in capacitance as electrolyte is put on a single sensor film is shown in Fig. 17. Up to a factor of 50 increase in capacitance occurs because of the double layer supercapacitance property of nanofibers. The change in resistance of the film due to the electrolyte is 6%. The electrical impedance properties of the sensor film can be used to characterize environmental contamination. Each contaminant may have a different electrical impedance spectrum. A table look up can be used to identify the contaminant. To improve selectivity, the nanotube film can be functionalized (chemically modified) to react with specific analytes, gases or liquids. The huge effective surface area of the film is an advantage for a gas sensor.

Using the electrical impedance (EI) analysis, long continuous sensors using spray-on nanotube film or embedded thread can be developed that significantly

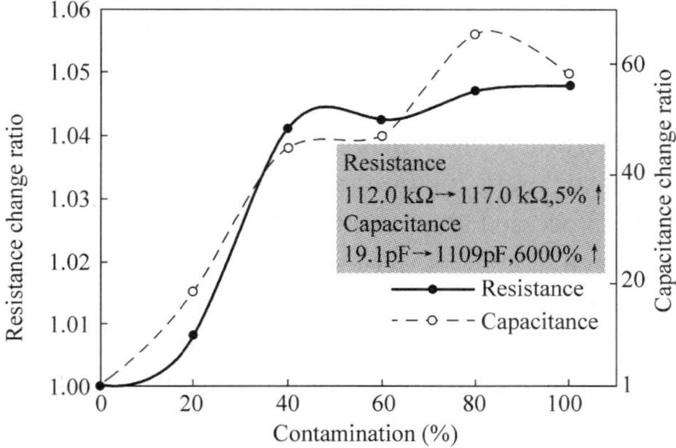

Figure 19.17 Electrolyte changes capacitance of the nanotube film, but resistance is almost constant

reduce the complexity and cost of environmental monitoring. A continuous sensor is a single long sensor that has one output signal. The electrochemical impedance of the thread is monitored continuously. An anomalous response from any section of the long sensor can be detected. Thus, a continuous sensor has only one output signal and can replace many individual sensors and still detect abnormal events. The thread will sense an electrolyte or gas. EIS based analysis at high frequency will be used to monitor the thread and to identify chemicals and ions in the environment or biological fluids. A Gamry Potentiostat is used for electrochemistry and impedance monitoring, as discussed in the sections on biosensing and actuation. The sensor can be modeled to represent EIS measurements using the Randles-Warburg model. Randles circuit is an equivalent circuit representing each component at the interface and in the thread during an electrochemical reaction for comparison with physical components. Randles Warburg parameters will be related to contamination in the environment.

19.4.4 Nanocomposite Materials for Biological Applications

Engineers face broad challenges in developing materials for biological applications like prosthetics. One attribute of smart materials is that they should be self-reliant which means they should be capable of resisting damage and continuously monitoring their condition. In some cases, the system or structure should also be capable of responding to its environment to improve performance or prevent degradation including self-repair of small damage. Materials with nanoscale features are important because almost all solid matter with nanoscale size has new or improved properties compared to bulk materials. These properties depend on the composition, size, and shape of the material, and include high specific strength and modulus, high electrical and thermal conductivity, a large surface area to volume ratio, nearly defect-free structure, and sensing and actuation properties. Carbon nanotube materials can form new composite materials (He et al., accepted; Shi et al., 2006; Kang et al., in press; Gao et al., 2006, 2007) that are strong and smart and thus may meet the requirements for biological applications. Composite materials for use in the body may consist of a nanoscale constituent material processed to an intermediate stage or combined with a matrix material to produce a durable macro-scale material that has multifunctional properties including sensing or actuation. Available nanoscale constituent materials include nanotubes, nanobelts, nanowires, and nanocoils made of carbon, silicon, nickel and other materials. The main advantage of nanostructured smart materials is that their mechanical, electronic, magnetic, optical, and thermal properties can be tailored to a specific bio application. Developing nanostructured smart materials for biology is a new area of research. To develop this area, three steps are suggested; (1) study the properties of nanoscale smart materials and develop a data base of the material properties and commercial availability of the materials, (2) use long nanotube materials to develop new intermediate forms of macro-scale smart materials such as thread, and (3) outline advantages that nanostructured smart materials would have in specific biological and medical applications.

Overall, this section proposes techniques for integrating nanoscale materials or intermediate components into polymers for use in advanced biological applications that can self-test and monitor their condition to provide enduring performance and safety. Materials that will be considered include super long carbon nanotubes, magnetic nickel nanowires (NW), and catalyst-free electrically conductive carbon nanosphere chains (CNSC). A take-home message from this chapter is that 'Nanoizing' materials is becoming a new technological science that should be put into widespread application by the bioengineering community.

19.4.4.1 Tailored Composites Using Carbon Nanotube Thread

A breakthrough application of long nanotubes is to spin thread. Long carbon nanotubes (CNT) called 'Black Cotton™' are being used to spin thread to provide reinforcement, sensing, and actuation simultaneously. An application example is using carbon nanotube thread/cloth to develop prosthetics with the desired properties in each direction. These structures will also evaluate and monitor their own integrity. Thread or rope/cables made from thread are the most basic structural elements that can be used alone as cables or muscle, or embedded in composite materials. Commercial scale quantities of the thread using the long carbon nanotubes grown in arrays may be available in 2008. The thread may provide the following properties for biological applications depending on the application: (1) reinforcement; (2) an antenna; (3) harvest a small amount of energy from ionic flow; (4) as a wet actuator; (5) chemical and biosensors; (6) a partial self-repair material; and (7) the nanotube thread can be used to reinforce polymers, elastomers, and possibly ceramics and powdered metals.

19.4.4.2 Smart Elastomer

New types of smart materials will be developed by loading CNT (Kang et al., 2006a, 2006c; Smart Materials Naon Lab at UC), CNT thread, CNSC, nickel nanowires or other nanoparticles into an elastomer such as polyurethane (PU) and forming a strain or magnetic sensor, actuator (to morph the material), or power harvester. A variation of this approach is to fill the grown long CNT arrays with PU. The smart elastomer will have electrical and thermal conduction, piezoresistive and piezomagnetic properties, and power harvesting properties. Initial experiments successfully integrated CNSC into PU. One application is to develop a sensor material that can be used in biomechanics studies. Forces generated in the material can be used to diagnose and predict several gait and safety problems, or to measure forces inside the body. The working principle of the smart material sensor considers forces generated in the material which are the normal force and shear force. Nanotube thread sensors are embedded in two directions in the elastomer, as shown in Fig. 19.18. The resistance of the thread changes with varying load. An analysis of the strains with two sensors embedded was performed. Red is the compressive strain sensor (vertical) and green is the shear strain sensor (at 45°). Stresses and forces can be computed knowing the strains. The normal compressive stress is $\sigma = E\varepsilon$, where E is the elastic modulus and ε is the normal strain. The shear stress is $\tau = G\gamma$, where G is the shear modulus and γ is the shear strain. The normal force is $N = \sigma A$, where A is the cross-sectional area. The horizontal shear force is $H = \tau A$. The coefficient of friction can also be computed as $\mu = H / N$. By measuring the normal and shear strains, the normal and shear forces can be determined and the minimum coefficient of friction computed. Slipping can be determined by monitoring the H and N forces and friction coefficient. Relationships between strains at the sensors and the x, y, and shear strains are

$$\varepsilon_{\theta_1} = \varepsilon_x \cos^2\theta_1 + \varepsilon_y \sin^2\theta_1 + \gamma_{xy} \sin\theta_1 \cos\theta_1,$$
$$\varepsilon_{\theta_2} = \varepsilon_x \cos^2\theta_2 + \varepsilon_y \sin^2\theta_2 + \gamma_{xy} \sin\theta_2 \cos\theta_2,$$
$$\varepsilon_{\theta_3} = \varepsilon_x \cos^2\theta_3 + \varepsilon_y \sin^2\theta_3 + \gamma_{xy} \sin\theta_3 \cos\theta_3.$$

These equations can be used to compute strains at any angle where the 'strain gage' threads are located. In the future, we envision adding an active friction modulator to the elastomer controlled by the friction sensor. Therefore, polymers and elastomers can be formed with CNT thread which reinforces the material and also acts as a sensor. Moreover, if the CNT thread is used in an electrolyte, it will have an actuation property. The effectiveness of the actuation is to be determined and is a good future research project.

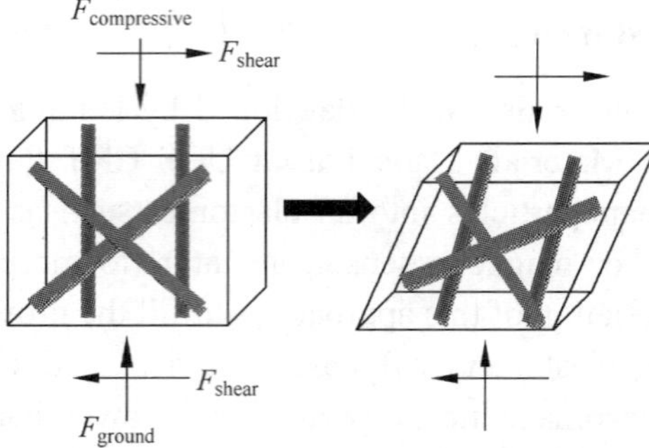

Figure 19.18 Nanotube thread sensors embedded in two directions in an elastomer

19.4.5 In-Body Biosensors: Optimistic Hopes and Wildest Outlook

This section gives ideas about producing biosensors that can go inside the body. This technology is futuristic but is becoming more feasible because of nanoscale materials. There are many compelling reasons for wanting to implant or temporarily put medical devices inside the body. Thus far, technologically, we have only been able to develop simple prosthetics that can go inside the body. But this is changing. Nanoscale materials are opening up the possibility to build revolutionary devices and tiny machines that can go inside the body and do what we want them to. This section describes a concept for an active biosensor that can go inside the body and detect disease early. Active biosensors perform electrochemical measurements and produce an electronic signal that is used to identify specific proteins, cells, ions or chemical species in body solutions. The active biosensor also has a feedback mechanism to increase its sensitivity or to activate a control function. The active biosensor is being designed and will be built using larger electronic components first, and finally pushed down in size using nanoscale materials.

Building small sensors and communicating with them is still an enormous technological problem. To attack this problem, nanoscale smart materials including nanotubes, nanowires, and nanobelts will be used to form nanostructured electronic components such as capacitors, inductors, solenoids, antennas, transistors, piezoresistive sensors, and electrochemical actuators. A four-arm nanomanipulator will be used for making prototype devices. The nanomanipulator operates under an environmental scanning electron microscope and can be used to assemble components into prototype biosensor devices. Bio-fouling and antenna design have been two long-standing obstacles to in-body sensor development and must be solved. Development of the In-Body Biosensor (IBB) will lay the framework to help to solve one of the grand challenges of medicine—putting medical devices in the body. The many possible applications for in-body sensors and medical devices include monitoring neurotransmitter signaling, wireless release of drugs in the sensor to kill cancer, sensor heating to kill cancer remotely, monitoring ions related to toxic metals, measuring temperature, pH, vibration due to blood clotting, and axonal responses. Many states in the body can be measured without using antibodies. But we may also consider using antibodies, aptamers, lectins, etc. The antibody has a limited lifetime and is not reusable, and this is a fundamental limitation for use with IBB.

19.4.5.1 Prior Art

Medical device manufacturers and researchers have been trying to put biosensors in the body and have prototype glucose sensors that have not been very accurate. Biofouling is the major obstacle. The sensor becomes covered with proteins and the sensitivity goes down. It is likely that the biofouling problem will require a solution other than through biochemistry, e.g. by poly-ethylene-glycol (PEG) or other coatings. An active biosensor is needed to mechanically overcome biofouling. Active biosensors are electromechanical devices that produce an electronic signal related to the concentration of analytes in body solutions. The active biosensor also uses feedback to improve sensitivity or activate a mechanical device that affects the analyte.

Biosensing has characteristically relied on standard sandwich bioaffinity assays (antibody-antigen) in connection with enzyme, fluorophore, or nanoparticle labels to detect disease-related proteins and toxins. The electronic biosensor proposed ideally would be non-functionalized (no antibody or binding reaction is used) and the sensor would respond directly to the analyte, which is required for long term in-body use. This type of biosensor for protein detection will be less sensitive and selective than conventional immunosensors. However, the in-body biosensor may detect ions, chemicals, and proteins in high concentrations. In some applications a low detection limit is not as important as detecting protein over-expression when it first occurs. In certain applications the biosensor will measure membrane potentials or nerve responses. The biosensor should be developed in stages; (1) first for in vitro use, (2) then for in vivo use. The active biosensor will be biocompatible and responsive to environmental and external stimuli, and will use electro-chemical impedance (EI) (Yun et al., 2007) to monitor the concentration of proteins, chemicals, and ions in the body, including Mg^{2+} and Ca^{2+}. A test bed should be set up to evaluate and compare biosensors to the gold standard Enzyme-linked Immunosorbent Assay (ELISA) method.

19.4.5.2 Sensor Initial Design

Impedance based biosensors are useful to identify chemicals and ions in biological fluids. Requirements for the sensors are high sensitivity, high selectivity, and fast response. The basic sensor platform we have been developing uses carbon nanotubes. Advantages of CNT electrodes for biosensors include high electrical conductivity, chemically inert, high mechanical modulus and strength, continuous measurements, and nano-scale size. A nanogap electrode is under development and will be used to obtain a high frequency impedance signature of ions in solution. A Gamry Potentiostat will be used for electrochemistry. LABVIEW will be use to develop the wireless control method.

The concept for an initial sensor design is briefly discussed. The sensor may be cylindrical with a coil antenna on the outside. The sensor receives an Radio frequency (RF) signal. Nanowires rectify the signal to charge nanotube capacitors. The circuit receives a high frequency signal and reflects it back. The frequency of the reflected signal depends on the impedance of the analyte thus detecting ion or protein concentrations. The sensor could also be used to measure axon potential, membrane potential, apply voltage or heat cells, deliver drugs, sample fluids, and do other tasks. The biosensor can go inside a living organism (plant and animal) and in particular the human body to detect disease and to understand cellular processes. The plan to develop the IBB has the following points: (1) Modeling. Develop a full electrical model of the sensor; (2) Large scale prototype. Build a cm size prototype of the sensor to demonstrate the principle; (3) Preliminary analyses for long-term development paths. This constitutes preliminary work for the eventual use of sensors in the body and includes: (a) test remote electrodes on the skin; (b) propagation of a biosignal through blood plasma; (c) nanocircuit analysis; (d) EIS modeling; (e) high frequency impedance; and (f) electrodes to prevent biofouling for long term in-body use; (4) Synthesis of nanoscale materials. Different appropriate processing techniques will be used for synthesis of the required nanoscale materials; (5) Nanostructured sensor design and fabrication. Nanoscale smart materials will be used to make a small sensor that will be tested in vitro.

This work will lay the groundwork for pushing down in size so the sensor could be used in the body (Schulz et al., 2007). A sensor may also be heated and used for destroying cancerous tissues. Doctors will be cautious about allowing nanosensors to float freely through the body. If sensors blocked a blood vessel it could cause a clot. Initially the sensors would be stationary in the body. Later they could circulate in blood when the size is small enough. Current within the biosensor would be induced much in the same way that a radio-frequency identification (RFID) chip works. Building small sensors and developing a way to communicate with these sensors is a large technological challenge. Approaches are also being considered to mass-produce the devices. A nanomanipulator (Fig. 19.19) can be used to develop a biosensor-transponder sensor. The sensor may also detect the growth of cancer cells or overexpression of cytokines in the human body. The sensor may also harvest power and communicate with a personal digital assistant (PDA) wirelessly.

It may be worthwhile to also consider the possibility of interfacing electronic devices with the human power and electrical system (muscles and neural system). Converting power in the body to electrical power may be more feasible than

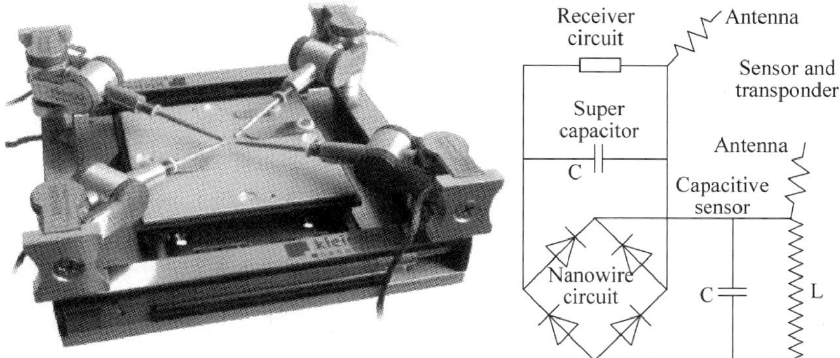

Figure 19.19 Nano-manipulator and initial sensor design

using RF or magnetic coupling of power to the biosensor. In the future, biosensors may interface with the biological neural system for in-messaging (control) and out-messaging (feedback). Use of biological material as a sensor to avoid the biocompatibility problem and to interface with the human neural system may also be considered.

19.4.6 Investigating Neuronal Activity and Function Using Nanotubes

Neurological disorders are thought to result from disruption of either normal neuronal function, which involves neuronal electrical activity, disruption of neuron or neuronal process migration that is necessary for regeneration after nerve injury, or disruption of developmental processes that occur during embryonic formation of the brain and spinal cord. To understand the mechanisms underlying these disruptions, there is an urgent need to better understand the biology of neurons. The unique properties of carbon nanotubes can be utilized to study neuronal function. First, the fact that the nanotubes conduct electricity can be exploited to; (1) detect and study neuronal electrical activity; and (2) to allow cross-talk between neurons when they are grown in vitro, thus duplicating the natural environment observed within the body. Second, the fact that the nanotubes are long, very thin structures can be used to duplicate the environment of migrating embryonic neurons or the outgrowth of regenerating neuronal processes. During development, neurons migrate along long, thin, radial glia to reach their final positions within the brain and spinal cord. When neuronal migration is disrupted during embryonic formation of the brain, the symptoms include mental retardation or epilepsy. Disorders that are thought to involve disruption of brain development (possibly neuronal migration) include autism and schizophrenia. Neuronal migration also occurs after tissue damage that results in cut nerves. The best substrates in normal tissue for successful nerve regeneration are long thin tubes or strings of glial cells. Thus, nanotubes are a novel substrate that strongly resembles natural substrates for neuronal migration. Nanotube arrays of different sizes and shapes and with different types of functionalization can be used to study key problems in neurobiology. Figure 19.20 illustrates the control over nanotube synthesis achieved by selectively growing aligned blocks of MWCNT on patterned silicon wafers. An e-beam writer is used to pattern the arrays.

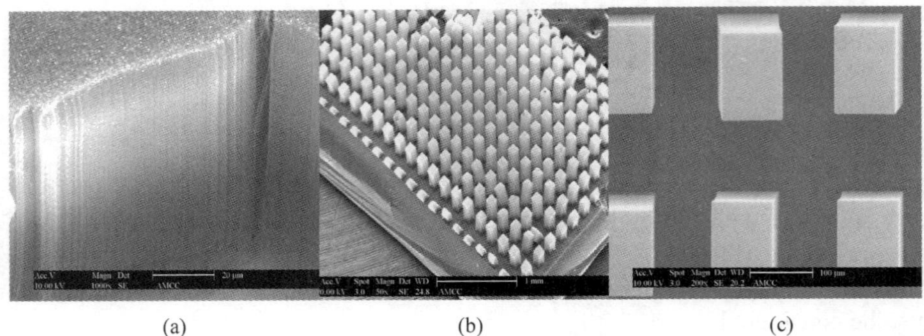

(a) (b) (c)

Figure 19.20 UC patterned nanotube arrays grown on Si wafers: (a) close-up view of side of array, (b) array of towers ~100 micron width, and (c) top view of towers each containing ~10^6 nanotubes

19.4.6.1 Goals of Neuron Research

The primary goal of this research is to design ways in which nanotubes or nanotube arrays can be used to study neuronal cell biology and function. Nanotube arrays can be developed that will: (1) allow the electrical recording of multiple neuron assemblies; and (2) promote the migration of neurons in a cell culture. We expect this work will encourage others in the neuroscience community to become interested in the use of nanotube technologies to study neuronal function. Conventional bioelectronic multi-electrode arrays (MEA) are relatively macroscale in size and are based on micro-electro-mechanical system (MEMS) technology. The sensitivity of the MEA is affected by global variables such as temperature, electrical noise, non-specific absorption, and the averaging of properties in the analyte. Our approach is to synthesize carbon nanotube arrays of the size scale of the cells, and to use a massively parallel array of millions of nanotube pairs to detect small electrical signals in the neural network. The nanoelectrode is actually becoming a key device in the field of electrophysiology and is expected to apply to neural diagnostics such as epilepsy and common neural-related diseases.

A carbon nanotube array-based sensor can effectively use the electrochemical properties of nanotubes as an electrophysiological analysis system. The nanotube-based array avoids the drawbacks of other electrode materials that include short life, unstable mechanical strength and low reliability. For electrophysiological measurement applications, carbon nanotubes have the advantages of small size, large surface area, sensitivity to electrolytes, fast response, and good reversibility at room temperature. At the same time, a carbon nanotube electrode system can be integrated with microelectronics and microfluids systems to gain advantages in miniaturization, multiplexing and automation. Multi-wall carbon nanotube arrays functionalized with special chemical groups can be used for enzyme immobilization and to form stabilizers and mediators used in cell culture research.

Carbon nanotubes whose length is on a multi-cellular scale will allow neuronal migration studies in cell culture. It is also possible to test the effects of coating nanotubes with proteins known to affect neuronal migration in vivo. If nanotubes promote neuronal migration in vitro, then their effects as implants can be explored to promote nerve regeneration in the intact animal.

19.4.6.2 Synthesis and Fabrication of Carbon Nanotube Array Electrodes

Nanotubes will be synthesized using patterned array growth to form electrodes. The design of the nanotube array will determine the sensitivity of the sensor. Figure 19.21 illustrates the sequential steps in the fabrication process, which will result in producing the nanotube array. Step 10 shows the array to be used as the neural sensor.

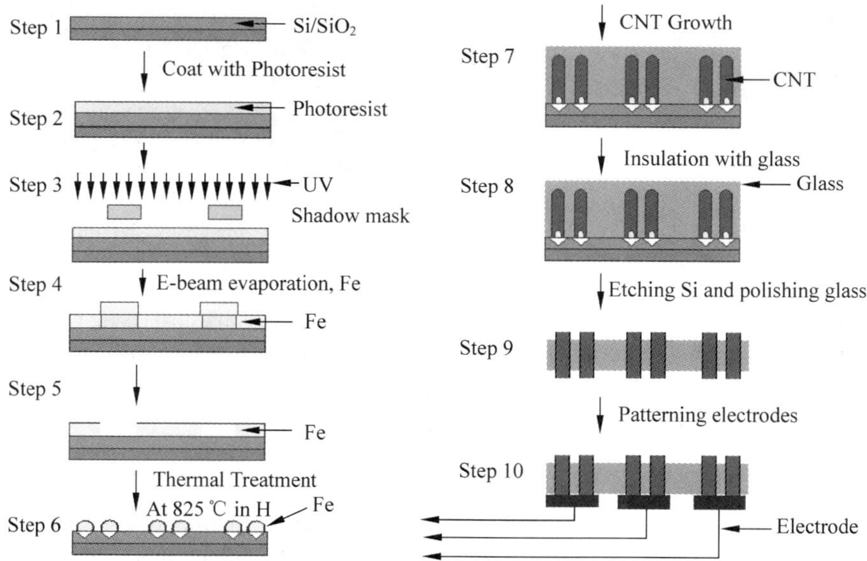

Figure 19.21 Fabrication steps for the vertically grown nanotube array (Color Fig. 26)

19.4.6.3 Culturing Cells on Nanotubes

Initial results growing cultured cells on carbon nanofibers (CNF) and nanotubes are shown in Fig. 19.22. The carbon nanofibers are a low cost lower performance analog to the multi-wall carbon nanotubes which will be used in later stages of testing. A detailed procedure for preparing nanotubes as a substrate for growing neurons is being developed. Experience gained has provided confidence that cells can be grown on nanotubes. We are at the stage of preparing different types of electrodes for cell growth and monitoring neuronal activity. Nanotubes will be spun into thread to make long conductors.

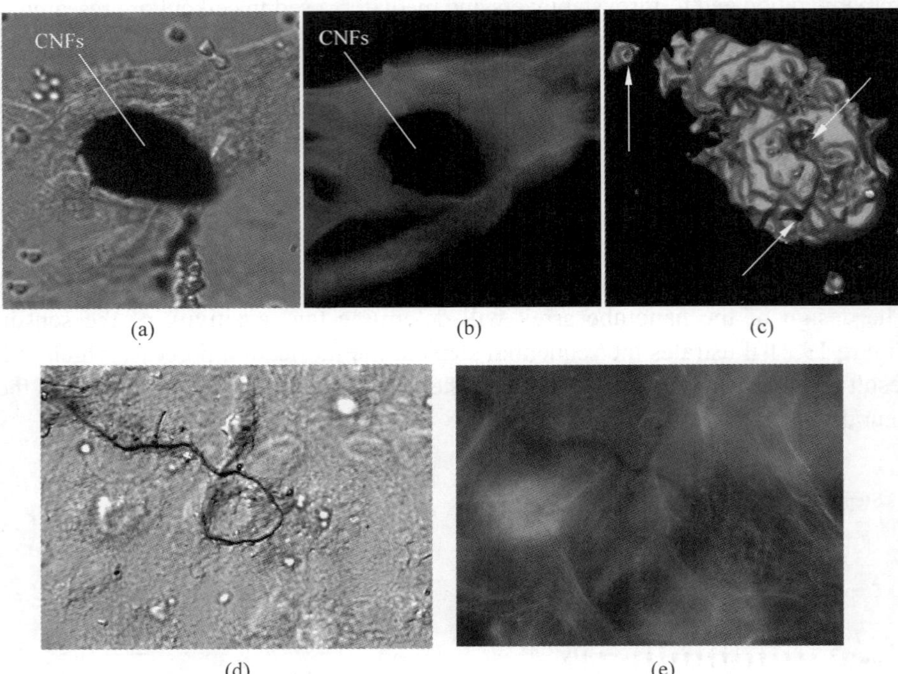

Figure 19.22 Cells cultured on nanofibers/nanotubes: (a) DIC image and (b) immuno-staining of microtubules in NIH 3T3 fibroblasts encircling CNF grown on a glass coverslip (olfactory cells grew similarly on CNFs, not shown). (c) Brain cell grown on top of a CNF array, on the vertical tips of CNFs, labeled with Cell Trakker Green, imaged on a confocal microscope, and viewed as a 3-D reconstruction. Arrows show indentations and holes made by tips of CNFs. (d) Fibroblast cell behavior with nanotubes—3T3 Cells and stained with α, β tubulin (microtubule)

19.4.6.4 Signal Analysis of a Neural Network

Neuronal signals can be measured using intracellular or extracellular recordings. An intracellular signal is known as a membrane potential, since the voltage signal is due to the electrical imbalance across the biological membrane. However, an extracellular signal arises from the electrical charge imbalance near the outside of the biological membrane. The extracellular potential is typically in the microvolt range, while the intracellular potential is measured in millivolts. The cell potential can be measured using a single channel recording device, like a patch-clamp electrode, which is now a standard and essential tool in any neuroscience research. However, to obtain a more complete picture of the neuronal network behavior, an experimental method to simultaneously record neuronal activity from many neurons is needed. A multi-electrode array in conjunction with multiple neurons in cell culture is a recent method to simultaneously record multi-neuronal activity and is based on MEMS technology. However, the MEMS Si-based micro size electrode arrays cannot provide electrochemical stability, mechanical strength, and long term multi-channel monitoring ability of spontaneous or evoked electrophysiological activity. The nanotube array is expected to overcome most of the problems of using Si.

From an experimental viewpoint, there are two approaches to the measurement of neuronal activity. The first is to grow dissociated neurons in vitro on the nanotube arrays and test them in vitro. Cells can be used either from established neuronal cell lines or prepared by dissociating neural tissue from a living system into individual cells (brain or olfactory sensory neurons). The second approach for neuronal sensing is to place a brain or olfactory tissue slice on the nanotube array. Both of these approaches should be evaluated. In both cases, to understand spatiotemporally coordinated activity in neural networks and the interaction between different areas or layers in tissue or cells, simultaneous multi-site nanoscale recording is a prerequisite. Thus, a nanoelectrode array (NEA) should be developed to provide ultrasensitive measurements of neuronal activity. A concept NEA is shown in Fig. 19.23. The following work is underway to develop a NEA: (1) design of a NEA to allow electrical recording from multiple neuron assemblies; (2) perform in vitro testing using the NEA. Using a tissue slice, the NEA will be used to monitor spikes and local field potentials and growth of the neurons. A goal would be to report for the first time recordings of single-unit spike activity with NEAs in acute slice preparations of neural tissues; (3) analyze neuronal activity and function. Analyze the neuronal activity and function, and the neuronal response to growth factors and electrical monitoring; (4) analyze neuronal migration. Using morphological measurements, analyze neuronal migration on NEAs or along the length of nanotubes coated with proteins known to affect neuronal migration in vivo; and (5) plan new medicine. Based on the analysis, propose new approaches to stimulate neuron growth and repair, and develop new concepts to treat neurological disorders.

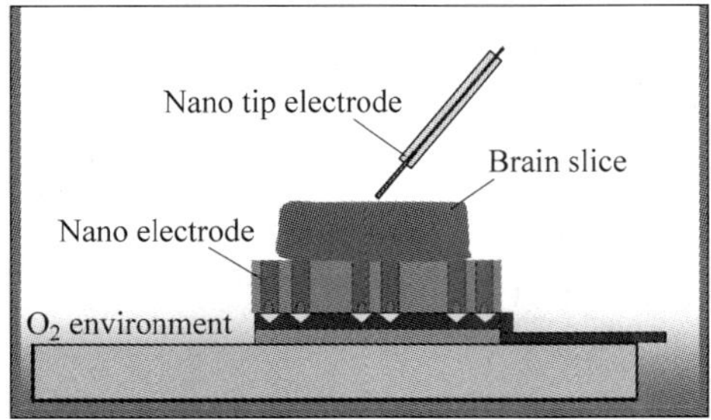

Figure 19.23 Concept nanotube electrode array

19.5 Conclusions

Multi-wall carbon nanotube arrays up to cm in length and with precise patterns were synthesized and used to develop several prototype smart materials devices. Overall, synthesis of the long multi-wall carbon nanotube arrays is opening the door for the development of new sensors, actuators, and multifunctional materials. Excellent mechanical properties, high electrochemical sensitivity, high strain generation of the nanotubes and electrically conductive probes will provide benefits for many applications in the area of nanomedicine. Several concepts were presented in the chapter to spur further thinking and research to use smart nanomaterials to benefit medicine.

Acknowledgement

This work was partly supported by Institute for Nanoscale Science and Technology at UC and NSF grant CMS-0510823. The instrumentation was partly provided by the Hayes Investment Fund through the state of Ohio, grant R117-030-L281-1290, and the Ohio Center for Aerospace Propulsion and Power at UC. This support is gratefully acknowledged

References

A.N. Kolmogorov, V.H. Crespi. Smoothest bearings: interlayer sliding in multiwalled carbon nanotubes. *Physical Review Letters*. **85** (22): 27 (2000).

Barisci, J.N., G.M. Spinks, G. Wallace, J.D. Madden and R.H. Baughman. Increased actuation rate of electromechanical carbon nanotube actuators using potential pulse with resistance compensation. *Smart Material Structure*. **12**: 549 – 555 (2003).

Baughman, R. H., Improved piezoelectric 0 – 3 ceramic particle/polymer composites. *Synthetic Metals*. **78**: 339 (1996).

Baughman, R.H., C. Cui, A. A. Zakhidov, Z. Iqbal, J. N. Barisci, G. M. Spinks, G. G. Wallace, A. Mazzoldi, D. Rossi, A. G. Rinzler, O. Jaschinski, S. Roth, M. Kertesz, Carbon nanotube actuators. *Science* **284** (3): 1340 (1999).

Cassie, A.B.D. and S. Baxter. Wettability of porous surfaces. *Transactions of the Faraday Society* **40**: 546 – 551 (1944).

Clean Technologies International Corp., http://www.cleantechnano.com/CleanTechNano/(2008).

Cumings J., P.G. Collins and A. Zettl. Peeling and sharpening multiwall nanotubes. *Nature* **406**: 586 (2000).

Cumings, J. and A. Zettl. Localization and nonlinear resistance in telescopically extended nanotubes. *Phys. Rev. Lett*. **93**: 086801 (2004).

Cumings, J., A. Zettl. resistance of telescoping nanotubes. In: Kuzmany, H. et al., eds. *Structural and Electronic Properties of Molecular Nanostructures*. American Inst. of Physics (2002).

Freitas, Robert A. *Nanomedicine, Vol. I: Basic Capabilities*, Landes Bioscience, 2001.

Gao, Yong, Peng He, Jie Lian, Lumin Wang, Dong Qian, Jian Zhao, Wei Wang, Mark J. Schulz, Ie Zhang, Xingping Zhou, Donglu Shi. Improving the mechanical properties of polycarbonate nanocomposites with plasma-modified carbon nanofibers. *Journal of Macromolecular Science, Part B, Physics*. 45:1 – 9 (2006).

Gao, Yong, Peng He, Jie Lian, Mark J. Schulz, Jiang Zhao, Wei Wang, Xiaqin Wang, Jing Zhang, Xingping Zhou, Donglu Shi. Effects of surface modification, carbon nanofiber concentration, and dispersion time on the mechanical properties of carbon-nanofiber -polycarbonate composites. *Journal of Applied Polymer Science* **103** (6): 3792 – 3797 (2007).

Gupta, S., M. Hughes, A.H. Windle, J. Robertson. Charge transfer in carbon nanotube actuators investigated using in situ Raman spectroscopy. Journal of Applied Physics. **95** (4): (2004).

Hata, K., Don N. Futaba, Kohei Mizuno, Tatsunori Namai, Motoo Yumura and Sumio Lijima. *Water-assisted highly efficient synthesis of impurity-free single-walled carbon Nanotubes*. **306**: 1362 – 1364 (2004).

He, Peng, Yong Gao, Jie Liang, Lumin Wang, Dong Qian, Jiang Zhao, Wei Wang, Mark J. Schulz, Xing Ping Zhou, Donglu Shi. Surface Modification and Ultrasonication Effect on the Mechanical Properties of Carbon Nanotube/Polycarbonate Composite. *Composites A*. accepted.

http://www.min.uc.edu/~mschulz/smartlab/smartlab.html, Smart Materials Nano Lab at UC (2007).

http://www.selfhealingmaterials.nl/index_eng.htm (2007).

http://www-g.eng.cam.ac.uk/edm/Publications/2007.html (2007).

Industrial Nano affiliated company; www.Blacklineascension.com. (2007).

Kang, Inpil, Gyung Rak Choi, Joo Yung Jung,Yong Hoon Chang, Yeon Sun Choi and Mark J. Schulz. A carbon nanotube film for power harvesting. *Key Engineering Materials* **326 – 328**: 1447 – 1450 (2006b).

Kang, Inpil, Joo Young Jung, Gyeong Rak Choi, Hyungki Park, Jong Won Lee, Kwang Joon Yoon, Yun Yeo-Heung, Vesselin Shanov and Mark J. Schulz. Developing of carbon nanotubes composite smart materials. Solid State Phenomena **119**: 207 – 210 (2007).

Kang, Inpil, Mark J. Schulz, Jong Won Lee, Gyeong Rak Choi and Yeon-Sun Choi. Strain sensors using carbon nanotube composites. Transactions of the Korean Society for Noise and Vibration Engineering. **16** (7): 762 – 768 (2006).

Kang, Inpil, Yun Yeo Heung, Jay H. Kim, Jong Won Lee Ramanand Gollapudi, Srinivas Subramaniam, Suhasini Narasimhadevara, Douglas Hurd, Goutham R. Kirikera, Vesselin Shanov, Mark J. Schulz, Donglu Shi, J.F. Boerio, Shankar Mall, Marina Ruggles-Wren. Introduction to carbon nanotube and nanofiber smart materials. *Composites B Journal*. **37**: (2006a).

Kang, Inpil, Yun Yeo Heung, Jay H. Kim, Jong Won Lee, Ramanand Gollapudi, Srinivas Subramaniam, Suhasini Narasimhadevara, Douglas Hurd, Goutham R. Kirikera, Vesselin

Shanov, Mark J. Schulz, Donglu Shi, J.F. Boerio, Shankar Mall, Marina Ruggles-Wren. Introduction to Carbon Nanotube and Nanofiber Smart Materials. (special issue) In press.

Kenneth, K. S. L., B. Jose, B. K. T. Kenneth, C. Manish, A. J. A. Gehan, I. M. William, H. M. Gareth and K. G. Karen. Superhydrophobic carbon nanotube.... Nano Letters **3** (12): 1701 – 1705 (2003).

Koehne, Jessica, Jun Li, Alan M. Cassell, Hua Chen, Qi Ye, Hou Tee Ng, Jie Han and M. Meyyappan. The fabrication and electrochemical characterization of carbon nanotube nanoelectrode arrays. *Journal of Material Chemistry*. **14**: 676 – 684 (2004).

Li, Jun, Hou Tee Ng, Alan Cassell, Wendy Fan, Hua Chen, Qi Ye, Jessica Koehne, Jie Han, and M. Meyyappan. Carbon nanotube nanoelectrode array for ultrasensitive DNA detection. *Nano Letters*. **3** (5): 597 – 602 (2003).

Liang Huinan, Wook Jun Nam, Stephen J Fonash. A self-contained nano-gap biomolecule impdeance sensor with fluidic control system. *Mater. Res. Symp. Proc*. Materials Research Society. 952 (2007)

Louchev, O.A., Yoichiro Sato Hisao Kanda. growth mechanism of carbon nanotube forests by chemical vapor deposition. *Applied Physics Letters*, Vol.80, No.15, pp. 2572 – 2575.

Lozovik, Y.E., A.M. Popov, A.V. Belikov, Classification of two-shell nanotubes with commensurate structures of shells. *Physics of the Solid State*. **45** (7): 1396 – 1402 (2003).

Lozovik, Y.E., A.V. Minogin, A.M. Popov. Possible nanomachines: nanotube walls as moveable elements. *Pis'ma v ZhETF*, **77**: (11): 759 – 763 (2003).

Nakalka, N., K. Watanabe. Quantum capacitances of molecules, fullerenes and carbon nanotubes by the partitioned real-space density functional method. *The European Physical Journal* **24**: 397 – 400 (2003).

Oh, E. van der waals interaction energies between non-planar bodies. *Korean J. Chem. Eng*. **21** (2): 494 – 503 (2004).

Pomorski, P., L. Pastewka, C. Roland, H. Guo, J. Wang. Capacitance, induced charges, and bound states of biased carbon nanotube systems. Physical Review B 69 (2004).

Roschier, L., J. Penttila, M. Martin, U. Tapper, C. Journet, P. Bernier, E.I. Kauppinen, P. Hakonen, M. Paalanen. Fabrication of single electron transistor using multiwalled carbon nanotube and scanning probe manipulation. Helsinki Univ. of Technology, Low Temperature Laboratory, FIN-02015, Finland.

Roth, S. R. H. Baughman. Actuators of individual carbon nanotubes. *Current Applied Physics*. **2**: 311 (2002).

Schulz, M.J., Ajit Kelkar, Mannur Sundaresan. *Nanoengineering of Structural, Functional and Smart Materials*. CRC Press.

Schulz, Mark J. YeoHeung Yun, Vesselin N. Shanov, Gautam Seth, Mitul Dadhania, Sergey Yarmolenko and Jag Sankar. Initial design of an in-body biosensor. abstract submitted, Third Annual Scientific Meeting of the American Academy of Nanomedicine (AANM), San Diego California (2007).

Shanov, V., Yeo-Heung Yun, Mark J. Schulz. Synthesis and characterization of carbon nanotube materials (Review). *Journal of the University of Chemical Technology and Metallurgy* **41** (4): 377 – 390 (2006).

Shanov, Vesselin, YeoHeung Yun, Mark J. Schulz, Ram Gollapudi, Sergey Yarmolenko, Sudhir Neralla, Jag Sankar, Yi Tu, Srinivas Subramaniam. A new intelligent material based on long carbon nanotube arrays. MRS Meeting, Boston (2005).

Shi, Donglu, Jie Lian, Peng He, L. M. Wang, Feng Xiao, Ling Yang, Mark J. Schulz, and David B. Mast. Plasma coating of carbon nanotubes for enhanced dispersion and interfacial bonding in polymer composites. Applied Physics Letters. **83**: 5301 (2003).

Tu Y., Yuehe Lin and Z. F. Ren, Nanoelectrode arrays based on low site density aligned carbon nanotube. *Nano Letters* **3** (1): 107 – 109 (2003).

Tu Y., Z. P. Huang, D.Z. Wang, J.G. Wen and Z. F. Ren. Growth of aligned carbon nanotubes with controlled site density. *Applied Physics Letters* **80** (21): 4018 (2002).

Vajtai, R., B. Q. Wei and P. M. Ajayan. Controlled Growth of Carbon Nanotubes. *Phil. Trans. R. Soc. Lon. A*. **362**: 2143 – 2160 (2004).

Verissimo-alves, M., B. Koiller, H. Chacham, R.B. Capaz. Electromechanical effects in carbon nanotubes. Instituto de Fisica, Universidade Federal de Rio de Janeriro, Brazil, July 5, 2004.

Vinciguerra V., Francesco Buonocore, Giuseppe Panzera and Luigi Occhipinti, Growth mechanisms in chemical vapour deposited carbon nanotubes. *Nanotechnology* **14**: 655 – 660 (2003).

Wang, J. and Mustafa Musameh. Carbon nanotube/teflon composite electrochemical sensors and biosensors. *Anal. Chem.* **75**: 2075 – 2079 (2003).

Yarmolenko, S., Sudheer Neralla, Jag Sankar, Vesselin Shanov, YeoHeung Yun, Mark J. Schulz. *The effect of substrate and catalyst properties on the growth of multi-wall carbon nanotube arrays*. Materials Research Society, Fall Meeting (2005).

Yeo-Heung, Yun, Atul Miskin, Phil Kang, Sachin Jain, Suhasini Narasimhadevara, Douglas Hurd, Mark J. Schulz; Vesselin Shanov, Tony He, F. James Boerio, Donglu Shi, Subrahmin Srivinas. Carbon nanofiber hybrid actuators, Part I: Liquid Electrolyte-Based. *Journal of Intelligent Material Systems and Structures*. **17** (2): 107 – 116 (2006).

Yoon H., Jining Xie, Jose K. Abraham, Vijay K. Varadan and Paul B. Ruffin. Passive wireless sensors using electrical transition of carbon nanotube junctions in polymer matrix. *Smart Mater. Struct.* **15**: S14 – S20 (2006).

Yun, YeoHeung, Adam Bange, Vesselin N. Shanov, William R. Heineman, H. Brian Halsall, Danny K. Wong, Michael Behbehani, Sarah Pixley, Amit Bhattacharya, Zhongyun Dong, Mark J. Schulz. A Nanotube composite microelectrode for monitoring dopamine levels using cyclic voltammetry and differential pulse voltammetry. Proceedings of the Institution of Mechanical Engineers, Part N, Journal of Nanoengineering and Nanosystems.

Yun, YeoHeung, Adam Bange, Vesselin N. Shanov, William R. Heineman, H. Brian Halsall, Zhongyun Dong, Abdul Jazieh, Yi Tu, Danny Wong, Sarah Pixley, Michael Behbehani, Mark J. Schulz. A carbon nanotube needle biosensor. *Journal of Nanoscience & Nanotechnology*. Accepted.

Yun, YeoHeung, Adam Bange, William R. Heineman, H. Brian Halsall, Vesselin N. Shanov, Zhongyun Dong, Sarah Pixley, Michael Behbehan, Abdul Jazieh, Yi Tu, Danny K.Y. Wong, Amit Bhattacharya, Mark J. Schulz. A nanotube array immunosensor for direct electrochemical detection of antigen-antibody binding. *Sens. Actuators B* **123**: 177 – 182: (2007a).

Yun, Yeo-Heung, Atul Miskin, Phil Kang, Sachin Jain, Suhasini Narasimhadevara, Douglas Hurd, Mark J. Schulz; Vesselin Shanov, Tony He, F. James Boerio, Donglu Shi, Subrahmin Srivinas. Carbon nanofiber hybrid actuators, Part II: solid electrolyte-based. *Journal of Intelligent Material Systems and Structures* **17** (3): 191 – 197.

Yun, Yeo-Heung, Ram Gollapudi, Vesselin Shanov, Mark J. Schulz, Zhongyun Dong, Abdul Jazieh, William Heineman, Brian Halsall, Danny Wong, Yi Tu, Srinivas Subramaniam. Carbon nanotubes grown on stainless steel to form plate and probe electrodes for chemical/biological sensing. *J. Nanosci. Nanotechnol.* **7**: 891 – 897 (2007b).

Yun, Yeo-Heung, Vesselin N. Shanov, Mark J. Schulz, Yi Tu, Sergey Yarmolenko, Sudhir Neralla. Carbon nanotube array smart materials. SPIE Smart Structures and NDE Conference. San Diego, CA (2006).

Yun, Yeo-Heung, Vesselin Shanov, Mark J Schulz, Suhasini Narasimhadevara1, Srinivas Subramaniam, Douglas Hurd, and F J Boerio. Development of novel single-wall carbon nanotube—epoxy composite ply actuators. *Smart Mater. Struct.* **14**: 1526 – 1532 (2005).

Yun, Yeo-Heung, Vesselin Shanov, Mark J. Schulz, Zhongyun Dong, Abdul Jazieh, William R. Heineman, H. Brian Halsall, Danny K. Y. Wong, Adam Bange, Yi Tu, Srinivas Subramaniam. High sensitivity carbon nanotube tower electrodes. *Sensors and Actuators* B **120**: 298 – 304 (2006).

Yun, Yeo-Heung, Vesselin Shanov, Yi Tu, Mark J. Schulz, Sergey Yarmolenko, Sudhir Neralla, Jag Sankar, Srinivas Subramaniam. A multi-wall carbon nanotube tower electrochemical actuator. *Nanoletters* **6** (4): (2006).

Zhao, Y., C-C. Ma, G. Chen, Q. Jiang. Energy dissipation mechanisms in carbon nanotube oscillators. Physical Review Letters **91** (17): (2003).

20 Microscopic Modeling of Phonon Modes in Semiconductor Nanocrystals

Wei Cheng[1,2], Shangfen Ren[1] and David T. Marx[1]

[1] Department of Physics, Illinois State Physics, Normal, IL 61790-4560, USA
[2] College of Nuclear Science and Technology, Beijing Normal University, Beijing 100875, China

Abstract Phonons of nanocrystals are quite different from those of the bulk. In this chapter, phonon modes of nanocrystals are calculated theoretically by a valence force field model. Group theory is employed and symmetry of each phonon modes is obtained. Raman intensity of phonon modes is calculated by bond polarizability approximation. Microscopic phonon modes are compared with macroscopic Lamb modes in spherical nanocrystals. Calculated Raman spectra are compared with experiments. Size effects of nanocrystals and their Raman spectra are discussed.

20.1 Introduction

Semiconductor nanocrystals (NCs) have attracted much research attention in recent years because of their importance toward fundamental understanding of physics on the nanoscale and potential applications in electronic devices, information processing, and non-linear optics (Yofee, 1993, 2001, 2002). A clear theoretical understanding of these properties requires a reliable description of phonon modes and electron-phonon interactions in NCs. Until now, most of the theoretical understanding of phonon modes in NCs is based on continuum dielectric models. Analytical expressions of the eigenfunctions for LO phonons (Klein, 1990) and surface optical phonons of small spherical (Duval, 1992; Klein et al., 1990; Frohlich, 1949; Fuchs and Kliewer, 1965; Ruppin and Englman, 1970; Trallero-Giner et al., 1992; Roca et al., 1994; Chamberlain, 1995; Trallero-Giner et al., 1998) and cylindrical (Li and Chen, 1997) NCs have been derived and the electron-phonon interactions have been calculated. The extended continuum dielectric model (Roca et al., 1994; Chamberlain et al., 1995; Trallero-Giner et al., 1998) coupling the mechanical vibrational amplitudes and the

(1) Corresponding e-mail: sf2004ren@yahoo.com

electrostatic potential has made major improvements over classical dielectric models in the study of phonon modes in NCs. One of the basic assumptions of all dielectric models is that the material is homogeneous and isotropic. However, that assumption is only valid in the long wavelength limit. When the NC size is small, in the range of a few nm, continuum dielectric models are intrinsically limited. On the other hand, one of the major difficulties of the microscopic modeling of phonon modes in NCs is its computational demands. For example, an 8-nm Ge NC has 11,855 atoms. Considering the three dimensional motion of each atom, the dynamic matrix contains 35,565 elements. This is an intimidating task even with the most advanced computers.

In recent years, we have developed a microscopic valence force field model (VFFM) (Ren et al., 2000, 2001; Ren, 2002a, 2002b, 2004; Qin and Ren, 2001, 2002a, 2002b; Qin and Ren, 2002; Cheng and Ren, 2002, 2003; 2003, 2005a, 2005b, 2005c). This model treats NCs as individual atoms, so sometimes we may refer to the VFFM as an atomic model, a microscopic model, or a lattice dynamics model. We have used the VFFM in two ways. The first way is to study phonon modes in NCs with symmetry by employing the projection operators of the irreducible representations of group theory to reduce the computational demand. For example, the matrix containing 35,565 elements for a spherical NCs with 11,855 atoms can be reduced to five matrices, with representations designated A_1, A_2, E, T_1, and T_2, with the sizes of 1592, 1368, 2960, 4335, and 4560, respectively (Ren et al., 2000). Therefore, the original problem is reduced to a problem that can be easily handled by most modern computers. Group theory also provides additional calculation versatility. Not only does it allow investigation of phonon modes in NCs with a much larger size, but also it allows the investigation of phonon modes in NCs with different symmetries. The second way to use the VFFM model is to treat semiconductor NCs without symmetry, such as alloy NCs with randomly distributed atoms. In this case, group theory is not employed and the dynamic matrix is solved directly (Ren et al., 2004).

Another advantage of the VFFM is that it allows us to treat NCs with various surface configurations involving a variety of relaxations and reconstructions. In general, we know that surface effects have always been one of the major concerns in investigations of properties of NCs because the smaller the size of NCs, the larger the ratio of surface states to bulk states. In our current investigations, we have only considered two different surfaces: (1) a free surface approximation (atomic bonds at the surfaces are truncated and atoms at surfaces are left with dangling bonds) and (2) a fixed surface (all atoms at the surface are bonded to fixed atoms at an outer shell). Real surfaces exist between these two limits. Nearly all microscopic modeling of phonon modes in NCs is carried out using the free surface approximation (Zi et al., 1996, 1998; Fu et al., 1999). In principle, surfaces with relaxations and reconstructions can be appropriately treated by the VFFM model as long as the surface configuration is known.

With this model, we have studied the size effects of phonon modes in semiconductor NCs, including monophase NCs, such as GaAs or InAs (Ren et al., 2000, 2001; Qin and Ren 2001), as well as NCs with a core of one material surrounded by a shell of another material, such as GaAs cores embedded in AlAs shells (Qin, 2002a, 2002b). We have also studied the effect of size on Raman intensities in Si NCs (Cheng and Ren, 2002) and the properties of Ge NCs with a fixed surface and compared them with those that have free surfaces (Ren and Cheng, 2002). Raman intensities of both Si and Ge NCs are calculated using the bond polarizability model (Bell, 1976).

Experimental techniques that can directly measure surface phonons in NC using either electrical or optical measurements have yet to be developed. In principle, a low-temperature, inelastic electron scanning tunneling microscope could be a sensitive technique for investigating surface phonon modes in NCs and their interaction with electrons. Until these experiments can be performed, low-frequency ($10 - 20\ cm^{-1}$) Raman spectroscopy is the only experimental technique available that can detect surface phonons and deduce the surface structures. Low-frequency Raman modes in spherical NC of various semiconductors embedded in glasses have been reported for Ge (Ovsyuk, 1988), CdS (Tanaka et al., 1993) embedded in GeO_2 glass, and CdSSe-doped silica-based glasses (Champagnon et al., 1991). One characteristic of these Raman modes is that their frequency scales linearly with the inverse of the diameter of the NC. They have typically been interpreted as spheroidal and torsional vibration modes of a continuum elastic sphere, the properties of which were calculated by Lamb (1882). According to Lamb's model, the frequencies of these spheroidal and torsional modes are quantized in terms of two quantum numbers: a branch number n and the angular momentum l. Since the model assumes the NC is an elastic continuum, it is expected to be valid only for large NC, but not for nm-sized NC containing fewer than 1000 atoms.

We have compared the computed Raman intensities of the phonon modes with the Raman selection rules of the Lamb modes. We found that for larger NC (i.e. d ~6.8 nm), the microscopic results agree well with the Raman selection rules of the continuum model based on group theory. However, for smaller NC (when $d < 4$ nm), the continuum model breaks down. Our results indicate that the identification of torsional modes in the Raman spectra of NC proposed by other authors is erroneous. Also, the spheroidal modes can be classified into primary spheroidal and primary transverse (Saviot and Murray, 2005).

The advance in semiconductor NC research is rapid. There are many important experimental and theoretical researches on the physical properties of semiconductor NCs. In this chapter of the book, our primary focus on our own investigations of the Raman intensities of phonon modes in semiconductor Si and Ge NCs by using the VFFM model. This chapter is organized as follows: first we describe the theory used to study phonons in Si or Ge NC systems; then we examine the results of Raman measurements of semiconductor NCs and discuss the correspondence of phonon properties in the microscopic and macroscopic models. We then conclude with a summary.

20.2 Theory

20.2.1 The Valence Force Field Model

The valence force field model (VFFM) that we have developed to investigate phonon modes in nanocrystals was originally used to study phonon modes in bulk materials (Harrison, 1980). In this model, the change of the total energy due to the lattice vibration is the sum of the change of the energy due to the short-range interactions and the change of the energy due to the long-range Coulomb interaction,

$$\Delta E = \Delta E_{\mathrm{s}} + \Delta E_{\mathrm{c}}$$

where the short-range interaction describes covalent bonding and the long-range Coulomb interactions are those typical of polar semiconductor compounds. For the short-range contributions, we use a VFFM with only two parameters and

$$\Delta E_{\mathrm{s}} = \sum_i \frac{1}{2} C_0 \left(\frac{\Delta d_i}{d_i} \right)^2 + \sum_j \frac{1}{2} C_1 (\Delta \theta_j)^2 \tag{20.1}$$

where C_0 and C_1 are two parameters describing the energy change due to a change in bond length and a change in bond angle, respectively. The summation runs over all bond lengths and bond angles. Because these two parameters have a simple and clear physical meaning, this model allows appropriate treatment of the interactions between atoms near and at the surface. It can be further used to treat the effects of surface relaxations and reconstructions on the vibrations when necessary.

For silicon or germanium NCs, the Coulomb interactions can be neglected; and only short range forces need consideration. As a result, only first and second neighbor interactions are included in the vibration Hamilton. As an example, we consider a Si lattice with three representative atoms A (0,0,0), $B\left(\frac{a}{4},\frac{a}{4},\frac{a}{4}\right)$ and $C\left(\frac{a}{2},0,\frac{a}{2}\right)$, where $a = 0.54325$ nm is the lattice constant. The energy related to bond AB stretching is

$$\begin{aligned} \Delta E_{AB} &= \left(\frac{1}{2}\right)\left(\frac{16}{3}\right) C_0 \left[\sqrt{\left(\frac{1}{4} + x_A - x_B\right)^2 + \left(\frac{1}{4} + y_A - y_B\right)^2 + \left(\frac{1}{4} + z_A - z_B\right)^2} - \frac{1}{4}\sqrt{3} \right]^2 \\ &\approx \left(\frac{1}{2}\right)\left(\frac{16}{3}\right) C_0 \left[(x_A - x_B)^2 + (y_A - y_B)^2 + (z_A - z_B)^2 \right] \end{aligned}$$

where x_A, y_A, z_A are the components of the displacement of atom A in units of a. The force matrices between the two atoms are

$$\frac{3}{16}\frac{2\Delta E_{AB}}{C_0} = (x_A, y_A, z_A)\begin{pmatrix}1 & 0 & 0\\ 0 & 1 & 0\\ 0 & 0 & 1\end{pmatrix}\begin{pmatrix}x_A\\ y_A\\ z_A\end{pmatrix} + (x_A, y_A, z_A)\begin{pmatrix}-2 & 0 & 0\\ 0 & -2 & 0\\ 0 & 0 & -2\end{pmatrix}\begin{pmatrix}x_B\\ y_B\\ z_B\end{pmatrix} +$$
$$(x_B, y_B, z_B)\begin{pmatrix}1 & 0 & 0\\ 0 & 1 & 0\\ 0 & 0 & 1\end{pmatrix}\begin{pmatrix}x_B\\ y_B\\ z_B\end{pmatrix}$$

where only first neighbors are included in this force field. The normal vector to plane ABC is

$$\boldsymbol{V}_{\perp} = \frac{\boldsymbol{BA}\times\boldsymbol{BC}}{|\boldsymbol{BA}||\boldsymbol{BC}|} = \frac{\sqrt{2}}{2}(-\boldsymbol{i}+\boldsymbol{k})$$

The vector perpendicular to bond AB and $\boldsymbol{V}_{\perp}$ is

$$\boldsymbol{V}_{pBA} = \frac{\boldsymbol{BA}\times\boldsymbol{V}_{\perp}}{|\boldsymbol{BA}|} = \frac{\sqrt{6}}{6}(-\boldsymbol{i}+2\boldsymbol{j}-\boldsymbol{k})$$

The vector perpendicular to bond BC and $\boldsymbol{V}_{\perp}$ is

$$\boldsymbol{V}_{pBC} = -\frac{\boldsymbol{BC}\times\boldsymbol{V}_{\perp}}{|\boldsymbol{BA}|} = \frac{\sqrt{6}}{6}(\boldsymbol{i}+2\boldsymbol{j}+\boldsymbol{k})$$

The energy related to a distortion of bond angle ABC is

$$\begin{aligned}\Delta E_{ABC} &\approx \left(\frac{1}{2}\right)\left(\frac{16}{3}\right)C_1\{[-(x_A-x_B)+2(y_A-y_B)-(z_A-z_B)]+\\ &\qquad [(x_C-x_B)+2(y_C-y_B)+(z_C-z_B)]\}^2\\ &= \left(\frac{1}{2}\right)\left(\frac{16}{3}\right)C_1(-x_A+x_C+2y_A-4y_B+2y_C-z_A+z_C)^2\end{aligned}$$

with force matrices

$$\frac{3}{16}\frac{2\Delta E_{ABC}}{C_1} = (x_A, y_A, z_A)\begin{pmatrix}1 & -2 & 1\\ -2 & 4 & -2\\ 1 & -2 & 1\end{pmatrix}\begin{pmatrix}x_A\\ y_A\\ z_A\end{pmatrix} + (x_A, y_A, z_A)\begin{pmatrix}0 & 4 & 0\\ 0 & -8 & 0\\ 0 & 4 & 0\end{pmatrix}\begin{pmatrix}x_B\\ y_B\\ z_B\end{pmatrix} +$$
$$(x_A, y_A, z_A)\begin{pmatrix}-1 & -2 & -1\\ 2 & 4 & 2\\ -1 & -2 & -1\end{pmatrix}\begin{pmatrix}x_C\\ y_C\\ z_C\end{pmatrix} + (x_B, y_B, z_B)\begin{pmatrix}0 & 0 & 0\\ 4 & -8 & 4\\ 0 & 0 & 0\end{pmatrix}\begin{pmatrix}x_A\\ y_A\\ z_A\end{pmatrix} +$$
$$(x_B, y_B, z_B)\begin{pmatrix}0 & 0 & 0\\ 0 & 16 & 0\\ 0 & 0 & 0\end{pmatrix}\begin{pmatrix}x_B\\ y_B\\ z_B\end{pmatrix} + (x_B, y_B, z_B)\begin{pmatrix}0 & 0 & 0\\ 4 & 8 & 4\\ 0 & 0 & 0\end{pmatrix}\begin{pmatrix}x_C\\ y_C\\ z_C\end{pmatrix} +$$

$$(x_C, y_C, z_C)\begin{pmatrix} -1 & 2 & -1 \\ -2 & 4 & -2 \\ -1 & 2 & -1 \end{pmatrix}\begin{pmatrix} x_A \\ y_A \\ z_A \end{pmatrix} + (x_C, y_C, z_C)\begin{pmatrix} 0 & 4 & 0 \\ 0 & 8 & 0 \\ 0 & 4 & 0 \end{pmatrix}\begin{pmatrix} x_B \\ y_B \\ z_B \end{pmatrix} + (x_C, y_C, z_C)\begin{pmatrix} 1 & 2 & 1 \\ 2 & 4 & 2 \\ 1 & 2 & 1 \end{pmatrix}\begin{pmatrix} x_C \\ y_C \\ z_C \end{pmatrix}$$

As shown in this example, second neighbor interactions exist in this force field. By use of these matrices, we can construct the vibrational dynamic matrix of phonons in the nanocrystal and obtain their eigenmodes and eigenfrequencies. When the NC is symmetric, the lattice dynamic matrix can be simplified. In this framework, special attention can be given to the interactions of the surface atoms. Generally speaking, internal atoms have four nearest neighbor atoms with 6 bond angles and 12 second nearest neighbor atoms with more bond angles involved. Surface atoms have less first and second neighbors and less bond angles involved accordingly.

20.2.2 Application of Group Theory to the Study of Nanocrystals

Group theory is widely used to calculate phonon as well as electronic properties of solids. By use of group theory, the large NCs (*d*~8.5 nm) can be calculated using the VFFM (Ren et al., 2001; Cheng and Ren, 2002). For Si or Ge NCs, the highest possible point group symmetry is T_d. A tetrahedron (*ABCD*) of T_d symmetry is shown in Fig. 20.1. There are many books discussing the T_d group (for example, Cotton, 1971). We list a few results below for convenience. The character table of T_d group is given in Table 20.1; and a set of irreducible representations is given in the Appendix A.1.

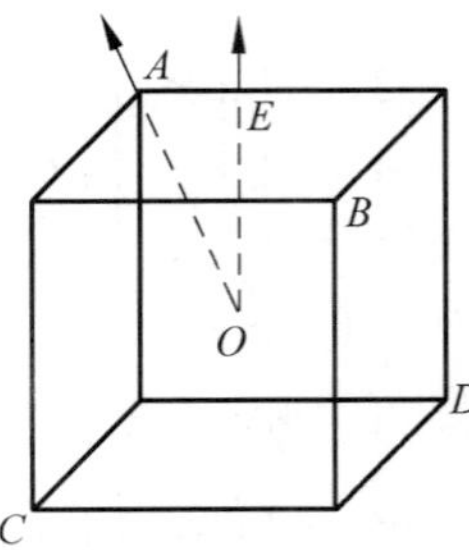

Figure 20.1 The symmetry of tetrahedron *ABCD* is T_d, which has five irreducible representations. The generation elements are the three-fold rotation element about *OA* ($\hat{C}_3$) and the two-fold rotation element about *OE* ($\hat{C}_2$), and a symmetry plane *OAB* ($\hat{\sigma}_d$)

There are two generation elements in the tetrahedral T group—one is the three-fold axis $\hat{C}_3$ and the other is the two-fold axis $\hat{C}_2$. Other group elements can be generated by products of these two. There are three generation elements in the T_d group. The extra generation element is $\hat{\sigma}_d$. Only the irreducible matrix of each is needed. For example, the three-fold rotation along OB can be expressed as $\hat{C}_2\hat{C}_3\hat{C}_2$. One set of irreducible representations is shown in the Appendix A.1. They are not unique; and any unitary transformations of them do not change the final results.

Projection operators of the irreducible representations of T_d group can be used for large NCs. The advantage of applying group theory to calculate phonon modes in different symmetries is even more obvious when calculating the Raman intensities for NCs with T_d symmetry. Because of the dependence of Raman intensity on symmetry, only phonon modes that are Raman active in that specific symmetry are necessary to consider. This further reduces the number of calculations required.

We assume an n-atom NC has T_d symmetry and that there are l nonequivalent wavefunctions. Then, all the wave functions of the NC can be written using group element notation as

$$\{|\hat{g}_v i\rangle; v = 1,2,\cdots,h(=24); i = 1,2,\cdots,l\}$$

where $\hat{g}_v$ is a group element in Table 20.1, i indicates one of the wave functions. The Hamilton equation for the NC system is

$$H\Psi^{(\alpha)} = E\Psi^{(\alpha)} \tag{20.2}$$

where $\alpha = A_1, A_2, E, T_1$, and T_2, the five irreducible representations shown in Table 20.1. The eigenfunctions $\Psi^{(\alpha)}$ can be obtained from the projection operators. We can also express them in a matrix form as

$$\Psi^{(\alpha)} = \sum_{j=1}^{l}\left[\frac{1}{\sqrt{h}}\sum_{v=1}^{h}\Gamma^{(\alpha)}(\hat{g}_v)|\hat{g}_v j\rangle\right]C_j \tag{20.3}$$

Table 20.1 Character table for the T_d symmetry group

T_d	$\hat{e}$	$8\hat{C}_3$	$3\hat{C}_2$	$6\hat{S}_4$	$6\hat{\sigma}_d$	Basis functions
A_1	1	1	1	1	1	$x^2+y^2+z^2$
A_2	1	1	1	−1	−1	
E	2	−1	2	0	0	$\left[\frac{\sqrt{3}}{3}(2z^2-x^2-y^2),(x^2-y^2)\right]$
T_1	3	0	−1	1	−1	
T_2	3	0	−1	−1	1	(x,y,z), (xy,yz,xz)

where h is the rank of group G, $\Gamma^{(\alpha)}(\hat{g}_v)$ is an irreducible representation matrix of group element $\hat{g}_v$ (shown in the Appendix A1), and C_j is a linear combination constant.

We then apply another matrix, $\frac{1}{\sqrt{h}}\sum_{u=1}^{h}\Gamma^{(\alpha)}(\hat{g}_u)^+\langle\hat{g}_u i|$ to left side of Eq. (20.2) to get the following determinant:

$$\left|H_{ij} - ES_{ij}\right| = 0 \tag{20.4}$$

where each element is a sub-matrix (a 3×3 for T_2) of the following form:

$$\begin{aligned} H_{ij}^{(\alpha)} &= \frac{1}{h}\sum_{u=1}^{h}\sum_{v=1}^{h}\langle\hat{g}_u i|H|\hat{g}_v j\rangle\Gamma^{(\alpha)}(\hat{g}_u)^+\Gamma^{(\alpha)}(\hat{g}_v) \\ &= \sum_{p=1}^{h}\langle i|H|\hat{g}_p j\rangle\Gamma^{(\alpha)}(\hat{g}_p) \end{aligned} \tag{20.5}$$

and

$$S_{ij}^{(\alpha)} = \sum_{p=1}^{h}\langle i|\hat{g}_p j\rangle\Gamma^{(\alpha)}(\hat{g}_p) \tag{20.6}$$

Let's calculate the total number of eigenvalues from Eq. (20.4). For the A_1 representation, it is a determinant equation of l-th order with l eigenvalues. For the T_2 representation, it is a determinant equation of $3l$-th order with $3l$ three-fold degenerate eigenvalues. Then, the total number of eigenvalues is

$$n = (l + l) + (2\times 2l) + (3\times 3l) + (3\times 3l) = 24l\,,$$

as expected.

There are many published works concerning electronic structure calculations using these formulas (for examples, Tang and Hang, 1995, 1996a, 1996b, 1997). Here, we will use Eq. (20.4) to solve the vibration problem.

As shown in Fig. 20.2, there are six bases (reference vectors): $|1\rangle$, $|2\rangle$, $|\hat{C}_3 1\rangle$, $|\hat{C}_3 2\rangle$, $|\hat{C}_3^{-1} 1\rangle$ and $|\hat{C}_3^{-1} 2\rangle$. The symmetry of this example is considered C_{3v}, D_{3v}, or perhaps even higher groups. The result can be more simplified. If the system is only of C_3 symmetry, the force field only contains simple bond stretching terms. If the virtual displacement along a vector $|V\rangle$ is denoted $\delta(V)$, then

$$\frac{2}{k}V_{\text{bond}} = \left[\delta a_1\cos\left(\frac{\pi}{6}\right) - \delta a_2\sin\left(\frac{\pi}{6}\right) + \delta(C_3 a_1)\cos\left(\frac{\pi}{6}\right) + \delta(C_3 a_2)\sin\left(\frac{\pi}{6}\right)\right]^2 +$$

$$\left[\delta(C_3 a_1)\cos\left(\frac{\pi}{6}\right) - \delta(C_3 a_2)\sin\left(\frac{\pi}{6}\right) + \delta(C_3 C_3 a_1)\cos\left(\frac{\pi}{6}\right) + \delta(C_3 C_3 a_2)\sin\left(\frac{\pi}{6}\right)\right]^2 +$$

$$\left[\delta(C_3^{-1}a_1)\cos\left(\frac{\pi}{6}\right)-\delta(C_3^{-1}a_2)\sin\left(\frac{\pi}{6}\right)+\delta(C_3^{-1}C_3a_1)\cos\left(\frac{\pi}{6}\right)+\delta(C_3^{-1}C_3a_2)\sin\left(\frac{\pi}{6}\right)\right]^2 \tag{20.7}$$

We note that the first term in Eq. (20.7) represents the virtual energy related to the left bond, the second term the bottom bond, and the third term the right bond. We only need to work out the first term from Fig. 20.2. For the other term, just use group theory, inserting group elements for each virtual displacement. We easily obtain the following matrix from Eq. (20.7):

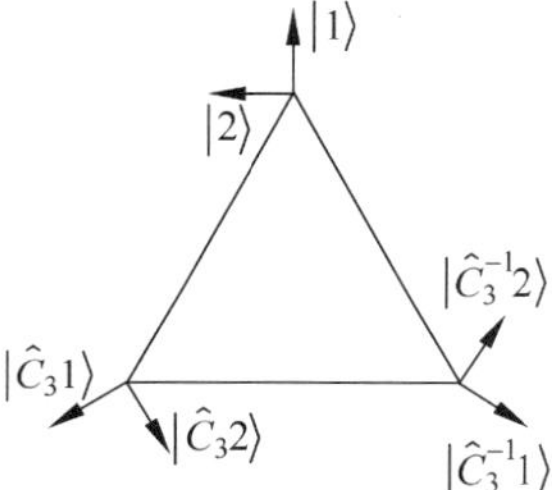

Figure 20.2 Bases of three atom in-plane vibration problem

$$\frac{2}{k}V_{\text{bond}}=\begin{pmatrix}\delta a_1 & \delta a_2\end{pmatrix}\begin{pmatrix}\frac{3}{2} & 0\\ 0 & \frac{1}{2}\end{pmatrix}\begin{pmatrix}\delta a_1\\ \delta a_2\end{pmatrix}+\begin{pmatrix}\delta a_1 & \delta a_2\end{pmatrix}\begin{pmatrix}\frac{3}{4} & \frac{\sqrt{3}}{4}\\ -\frac{\sqrt{3}}{4} & -\frac{1}{4}\end{pmatrix}\begin{pmatrix}\delta(C_3a_1)\\ \delta(C_3a_2)\end{pmatrix}+$$
$$\begin{pmatrix}\delta a_1 & \delta a_2\end{pmatrix}\begin{pmatrix}\frac{3}{4} & -\frac{\sqrt{3}}{4}\\ \frac{\sqrt{3}}{4} & -\frac{1}{4}\end{pmatrix}\begin{pmatrix}\delta(C_3^{-1}a_1)\\ \delta(C_3^{-1}a_2)\end{pmatrix}+\cdots \tag{20.8}$$

The additional terms may be neglected without any loss of information. The kinetic energy is

$$V_{\text{kinetic}}=\frac{1}{2}m\left[\frac{\mathrm{d}}{\mathrm{d}t}(\delta a_1)\right]^2+\frac{1}{2}m\left[\frac{\mathrm{d}}{\mathrm{d}t}(\delta a_2)\right]^2+\frac{1}{2}m\left[\frac{\mathrm{d}}{\mathrm{d}t}(C_3\delta a_1)\right]^2+\frac{1}{2}m\left[\frac{\mathrm{d}}{\mathrm{d}t}(C_3\delta a_2)\right]^2+$$
$$\frac{1}{2}m\left[\frac{\mathrm{d}}{\mathrm{d}t}(C_3^{-1}\delta a_1)\right]^2+\frac{1}{2}m\left[\frac{\mathrm{d}}{\mathrm{d}t}(C_3^{-1}\delta a_2)\right]^2$$
$$=\frac{1}{2}\begin{pmatrix}\frac{\mathrm{d}(\delta a_1)}{\mathrm{d}t} & \frac{\mathrm{d}(\delta a_2)}{\mathrm{d}t}\end{pmatrix}m\begin{pmatrix}1 & 0\\ 0 & 1\end{pmatrix}\begin{pmatrix}\frac{\mathrm{d}(\delta a_1)}{\mathrm{d}t}\\ \frac{\mathrm{d}(\delta a_2)}{\mathrm{d}t}\end{pmatrix}+\cdots \tag{20.9}$$

For the A modes, applying Eqs. (20.4), (20.8), (20.9) and matrices in Table 20.1, we get the following determinant:

$$\left| k\begin{pmatrix} \frac{3}{2} & 0 \\ 0 & \frac{1}{2} \end{pmatrix} + k\begin{pmatrix} \frac{3}{4} & \frac{\sqrt{3}}{4} \\ -\frac{\sqrt{3}}{4} & -\frac{1}{4} \end{pmatrix} + k\begin{pmatrix} \frac{3}{4} & -\frac{\sqrt{3}}{4} \\ \frac{\sqrt{3}}{4} & -\frac{1}{4} \end{pmatrix} - \omega^2 m \begin{pmatrix} 1 & 0 \\ 0 & 1 \end{pmatrix} \right| = 0$$

This is can be simplified to

$$\left| k\begin{pmatrix} 3 & 0 \\ 0 & 0 \end{pmatrix} - \omega^2 m \begin{pmatrix} 1 & 0 \\ 0 & 1 \end{pmatrix} \right| = 0$$

The solution is then:

$$\left|\Psi^{(A)}\right\rangle_1 = |1\rangle + |C_3 1\rangle + |C_3^{-1} 1\rangle, \omega_1^{(A)2} = \frac{3k}{m} \qquad \text{(breathing mode)}$$

$$\left|\Psi^{(A)}\right\rangle_2 = |2\rangle + |C_3 2\rangle + |C_3^{-1} 2\rangle, \omega_2^{(A)2} = 0 \qquad \text{(pure rotation)}$$

For the E modes, the calculation is a little more complicated. Applying Eqs. (20.4), (20.8), (20.9) and matrices in Table 20.1, we find,

$$\left| \begin{array}{l} k\begin{pmatrix} \frac{3}{2}\begin{pmatrix} 1 & 0 \\ 0 & 1 \end{pmatrix} & 0 \\ 0 & \frac{1}{2}\begin{pmatrix} 1 & 0 \\ 0 & 1 \end{pmatrix} \end{pmatrix} + k\begin{pmatrix} \frac{3}{4}\begin{pmatrix} -\frac{1}{2} & -\frac{\sqrt{3}}{2} \\ \frac{\sqrt{3}}{2} & -\frac{1}{2} \end{pmatrix} & \frac{\sqrt{3}}{4}\begin{pmatrix} -\frac{1}{2} & -\frac{\sqrt{3}}{2} \\ \frac{\sqrt{3}}{2} & -\frac{1}{2} \end{pmatrix} \\ -\frac{\sqrt{3}}{4}\begin{pmatrix} -\frac{1}{2} & -\frac{\sqrt{3}}{2} \\ \frac{\sqrt{3}}{2} & -\frac{1}{2} \end{pmatrix} & -\frac{1}{4}\begin{pmatrix} -\frac{1}{2} & -\frac{\sqrt{3}}{2} \\ \frac{\sqrt{3}}{2} & -\frac{1}{2} \end{pmatrix} \end{pmatrix} \\ +k\begin{pmatrix} \frac{3}{4}\begin{pmatrix} -\frac{1}{2} & \frac{\sqrt{3}}{2} \\ -\frac{\sqrt{3}}{2} & -\frac{1}{2} \end{pmatrix} & -\frac{\sqrt{3}}{4}\begin{pmatrix} -\frac{1}{2} & \frac{\sqrt{3}}{2} \\ -\frac{\sqrt{3}}{2} & -\frac{1}{2} \end{pmatrix} \\ \frac{\sqrt{3}}{2}\begin{pmatrix} -\frac{1}{2} & \frac{\sqrt{3}}{2} \\ -\frac{\sqrt{3}}{2} & -\frac{1}{2} \end{pmatrix} & -\frac{1}{4}\begin{pmatrix} -\frac{1}{2} & \frac{\sqrt{3}}{2} \\ -\frac{\sqrt{3}}{2} & -\frac{1}{2} \end{pmatrix} \end{pmatrix} - \omega^2 m \begin{pmatrix} \begin{pmatrix} 1 & 0 \\ 0 & 1 \end{pmatrix} & 0 \\ 0 & \begin{pmatrix} 1 & 0 \\ 0 & 1 \end{pmatrix} \end{pmatrix} \end{array} \right| = 0$$

It can be simplified as

$$\left| k\begin{pmatrix} \frac{3}{4}\begin{pmatrix}1 & 0\\ 0 & 1\end{pmatrix} & \frac{3}{4}\begin{pmatrix}0 & -1\\ 1 & 0\end{pmatrix} \\ \frac{3}{4}\begin{pmatrix}0 & 1\\ -1 & 0\end{pmatrix} & \frac{3}{4}\begin{pmatrix}1 & 0\\ 0 & 1\end{pmatrix}\end{pmatrix} - \omega^2 m \begin{pmatrix} \begin{pmatrix}1 & 0\\ 0 & 1\end{pmatrix} & 0 \\ 0 & \begin{pmatrix}1 & 0\\ 0 & 1\end{pmatrix}\end{pmatrix} \right| = 0 \qquad (20.10)$$

The reference eigenvectors can be chosen as projection operators $P_{11}, P_{12}, P_{21}, P_{22}$ times the bases and arranged in the following sequence:

$$\begin{pmatrix} |P_{11}1\rangle \\ |P_{12}1\rangle \\ |P_{11}2\rangle \\ |P_{12}2\rangle \end{pmatrix} \text{ or } \begin{pmatrix} |P_{21}1\rangle \\ |P_{22}1\rangle \\ |P_{21}2\rangle \\ |P_{22}2\rangle \end{pmatrix}.$$

Which are all equivalent in this case. If we choose the following matrix:

$$\Gamma^{(E)}(\hat{e}) = \begin{pmatrix}1 & 0\\ 0 & 1\end{pmatrix}, \Gamma^{(E)}(\hat{C}_3) = \begin{pmatrix} -\frac{1}{2} & -\frac{\sqrt{3}}{2} \\ \frac{\sqrt{3}}{2} & -\frac{1}{2} \end{pmatrix}, \Gamma^{(E)}(\hat{C}_3^{-1}) = \begin{pmatrix} -\frac{1}{2} & \frac{\sqrt{3}}{2} \\ -\frac{\sqrt{3}}{2} & -\frac{1}{2} \end{pmatrix},$$

the projected vectors are:

$$|P_{21}1\rangle = -|P_{12}1\rangle = \frac{\sqrt{3}}{2}|C_3 1\rangle - \frac{\sqrt{3}}{2}|C_3^{-1}1\rangle$$

$$|P_{21}2\rangle = -|P_{12}2\rangle = \frac{\sqrt{3}}{2}|C_3 2\rangle - \frac{\sqrt{3}}{2}|C_3^{-1}2\rangle$$

$$|P_{11}1\rangle = |P_{22}1\rangle = |1\rangle - \frac{1}{2}|C_3 1\rangle - \frac{1}{2}|C_3^{-1}1\rangle$$

$$|P_{11}2\rangle = |P_{22}2\rangle = |2\rangle - \frac{1}{2}|C_3 2\rangle - \frac{1}{2}|C_3^{-1}2\rangle$$

The result from Eq. (20.10) is then,

$$|\Psi^{(E)}\rangle_1 = |P_{11}1\rangle + |P_{12}2\rangle, \omega_1^{(E)2} = 0 \qquad \text{(translation)}$$

$$|\Psi^{(E)}\rangle_2 = |P_{12}1\rangle - |P_{11}2\rangle, \omega_2^{(E)2} = 0 \qquad \text{(translation)}$$

$$|\Psi^{(E)}\rangle_3 = |P_{12}1\rangle + |P_{11}2\rangle, \omega_1^{(E)2} = \frac{3k}{2m}$$

$$|\Psi^{(E)}\rangle_4 = |P_{11}1\rangle - |P_{12}2\rangle, \omega_2^{(E)2} = \frac{3k}{2m}$$

The normal modes are obtained by adding the amplitudes along the same basis vectors together.

20.2.3 The Bond Charge Approximation

Raman spectroscopy is a powerful tool to detect the structure of NCs. The Raman spectra selection rules may be obtained from group theory. However, the Raman scattering intensity cannot be predicted from group theory, but it can be calculated through the bond charge approximation (BPA). Calculations of phonon modes here are derived by the two parameter model (VFFM); and group theory is used to simply the calculations as described above. The BPA associates an axially-symmetric polarizability tensor with each bond (Bell, 1976; Cheng and Ren, 2002) as

$$\boldsymbol{P}(\boldsymbol{R}_{ij}) = \left\{ \alpha(R_{ij})\boldsymbol{I} + \gamma(R_{ij}) \left[\hat{\boldsymbol{R}}_{ij}\hat{\boldsymbol{R}}_{ij} - \frac{1}{3}\boldsymbol{I} \right] \right\} \tag{20.11}$$

where $\boldsymbol{I}$ is a unit matrix, $\alpha(R_{ij})$ is the mean polarizability, and $\gamma(R_{ij})$ describes the anisotropy of the polarizability. Here $\boldsymbol{R}_{ij}$ is the bond vector connecting atoms i and j. Both $\alpha(R_{ij})$ and $\gamma(R_{ij})$ are functions of bond length R_{ij}, but they are not direction dependent. R_{ij} is the length of $\boldsymbol{R}_{ij}$ and $\boldsymbol{R}_{ij} = \boldsymbol{R}_{ij} / R_{ij}$. When phonon vibrations are present, $\boldsymbol{R}_{ij} = \boldsymbol{r}_{ij} + \boldsymbol{u}_{ij} = \boldsymbol{r}_{ij} + \boldsymbol{u}_j - \boldsymbol{u}_i$, where $\boldsymbol{r}_{ij}$ is the bond vector at equilibrium, $\boldsymbol{u}_i$ is the displacement of atom i, and $\boldsymbol{u}_{ij}$ is the relative displacement of atoms j and i. For these vibrations, the condition $\boldsymbol{u}_{ij} \ll \boldsymbol{r}_{ij}$ always applies. Therefore, the polarizability tensor $\boldsymbol{P}(\boldsymbol{R}_{ij})$ can be expressed in terms of the displacements $\boldsymbol{u}_{ij}$ using a Taylor expansion. The constant term in this expansion can be ignored, since the total contribution to the Raman intensity from this term due all bonds vanishes. Retaining only the first order $\boldsymbol{u}_{ij}$ terms in the Taylor expansion, the polarizability tensor $\boldsymbol{P}(\boldsymbol{R}_{ij})$ can be simplified as the follows:

$$\begin{gathered} \boldsymbol{P}(\boldsymbol{R}_{ij}) \approx (\boldsymbol{u}_{ij} \cdot \hat{\boldsymbol{r}}_{ij}) \left[\alpha'(r_{ij})\boldsymbol{I} + \gamma'(r_{ij}) \left(\hat{\boldsymbol{r}}_{ij}\hat{\boldsymbol{r}}_{ij} - \frac{1}{3}\boldsymbol{I} \right) \right] + \\ r_{ij}^{-1}\gamma(r_{ij}) \left[\boldsymbol{u}_{ij}\hat{\boldsymbol{r}}_{ij} + \hat{\boldsymbol{r}}_{ij}\boldsymbol{u}_{ij} - 2(\boldsymbol{u}_{ij} \cdot \hat{\boldsymbol{r}}_{ij})\hat{\boldsymbol{r}}_{ij}\hat{\boldsymbol{r}}_{ij} \right] \end{gathered} \tag{20.12}$$

where $\alpha'(r_{ij})$ and $\gamma'(r_{ij})$ are derivatives of $\alpha(R_{ij})$ and $\gamma(R_{ij})$, respectively, with respect to $\boldsymbol{u}_{ij}$ evaluated at the equivalent bond vector $\boldsymbol{r}_{ij}$ and its unit vector $\boldsymbol{r}_{ij} = \boldsymbol{r}_{ij} / r_{ij}$.

In the diamond structure, there are two different kinds of local configurations. Below is one set of bond vectors using a Cartesian coordinate system. The other set is the inversion of the four vectors. The four bonds surrounding the atom at the origin are in the $\hat{r}_{01} = \frac{\sqrt{3}}{3}(1,-1,1)$, $\hat{r}_{02} = \frac{\sqrt{3}}{3}(-1,1,1)$, $\hat{r}_{03} = \frac{\sqrt{3}}{3}(1,1,-1)$, and $\hat{r}_{04} = \frac{\sqrt{3}}{3}(-1,-1,-1)$ directions. The four polarizations associated with the four bonds are:

$$\boldsymbol{P}(\boldsymbol{R}_{01}) = \frac{\sqrt{3}}{3}(u_{01,x} - u_{01,y} + u_{01,z})\left[\tilde{P}'_A\begin{pmatrix}1&0&0\\0&1&0\\0&0&1\end{pmatrix} + \frac{1}{3}\gamma'_A\begin{pmatrix}0&-1&1\\-1&0&-1\\1&-1&0\end{pmatrix}\right] +$$
$$\frac{\gamma_A\sqrt{3}}{9}\begin{pmatrix}4u_{01,x}+2u_{01,y}-2u_{01,z} & -u_{01,x}+u_{01,y}+2u_{01,z} & u_{01,x}+2u_{01,y}+u_{01,z}\\ -u_{01,x}+u_{01,y}+2u_{01,z} & -2u_{01,x}-4u_{01,y}-2u_{01,z} & 2u_{01,x}+u_{01,y}-u_{01,z}\\ u_{01,x}+2u_{01,y}+u_{01,z} & 2u_{01,x}+u_{01,y}-u_{01,z} & -2u_{01,x}+2u_{01,y}+4u_{01,z}\end{pmatrix}, \tag{20.13}$$

$$\boldsymbol{P}(\boldsymbol{R}_{02}) = \frac{\sqrt{3}}{3}(-u_{02,x} + u_{02,y} + u_{02,z})\left[\tilde{P}'_A\begin{pmatrix}1&0&0\\0&1&0\\0&0&1\end{pmatrix} + \frac{1}{3}\gamma'_A\begin{pmatrix}0&-1&-1\\-1&0&1\\-1&1&0\end{pmatrix}\right] +$$
$$\frac{\gamma_A\sqrt{3}}{9}\begin{pmatrix}-4u_{02,x}-2u_{02,y}-2u_{02,z} & u_{02,x}-u_{02,y}+2u_{02,z} & u_{02,x}+2u_{02,y}-u_{02,z}\\ u_{02,x}-u_{02,y}+2u_{02,z} & 2u_{02,x}+4u_{02,y}-2u_{02,z} & 2u_{02,x}+u_{02,y}+u_{02,z}\\ u_{02,x}+2u_{02,y}-u_{02,z} & 2u_{02,x}+u_{02,y}+u_{02,z} & 2u_{02,x}-2u_{02,y}+4u_{02,z}\end{pmatrix}, \tag{20.14}$$

$$\boldsymbol{P}(\boldsymbol{R}_{03}) = \frac{\sqrt{3}}{3}(u_{03,x} + u_{03,y} - u_{03,z})\left[\tilde{P}'_A\begin{pmatrix}1&0&0\\0&1&0\\0&0&1\end{pmatrix} + \frac{1}{3}\gamma'_A\begin{pmatrix}0&1&-1\\1&0&-1\\-1&-1&0\end{pmatrix}\right] +$$
$$\frac{\gamma_A\sqrt{3}}{9}\begin{pmatrix}4u_{03,x}-2u_{03,y}+2u_{03,z} & u_{03,x}+u_{03,y}+2u_{03,z} & -u_{03,x}+2u_{03,y}+u_{03,z}\\ u_{03,x}+u_{03,y}+2u_{03,z} & -2u_{03,x}+4u_{03,y}+2u_{03,z} & 2u_{03,x}-u_{03,y}+u_{03,z}\\ -u_{03,x}+2u_{03,y}+u_{03,z} & 2u_{03,x}-u_{03,y}+u_{03,z} & -2u_{03,x}-2u_{03,y}-4u_{03,z}\end{pmatrix}, \tag{20.15}$$

$$\boldsymbol{P}(\boldsymbol{R}_{04}) = \frac{\sqrt{3}}{3}(-u_{04,x} - u_{04,y} - u_{04,z})\left[\tilde{P}'_A\begin{pmatrix}1&0&0\\0&1&0\\0&0&1\end{pmatrix} + \frac{1}{3}\gamma'_A\begin{pmatrix}0&1&1\\1&0&1\\1&1&0\end{pmatrix}\right] +$$

$$\frac{\gamma_A\sqrt{3}}{9}\begin{pmatrix} -4u_{04,x}+2u_{04,y}+2u_{04,z} & -u_{04,x}-u_{04,y}+2u_{04,z} & -u_{04,x}+2u_{04,y}-u_{04,z} \\ -u_{04,x}-u_{04,y}+2u_{04,z} & 2u_{04,x}-4u_{04,y}+2u_{04,z} & 2u_{04,x}-u_{04,y}-u_{04,z} \\ -u_{04,x}+2u_{04,y}-u_{04,z} & 2u_{04,x}-u_{04,y}-u_{04,z} & 2u_{04,x}+2u_{04,y}-4u_{04,z} \end{pmatrix}. \tag{20.16}$$

We can then calculate the vibrational amplitudes of each mode for any NC. Using Eqs. (20.13) – (20.16), we sum the polarizability tensor of each bond to get the total scattering tensor $\boldsymbol{P}=\sum_{i<j}\boldsymbol{P}(\boldsymbol{R}_{ij})$. For unpolarized incident light scattered perpendicular to the direction of propagation, the intensities of Raman scattered components with frequencies $\Omega \pm \omega_l$ have the proportionality

$$I_{//}=\frac{\left(n_l+\frac{1}{2}\pm\frac{1}{2}\right)}{2\omega_l}\left[7G_l^2+45A_l^2\right]g(\omega_l)$$

$$I_{\perp}=\frac{\left(n_l+\frac{1}{2}\pm\frac{1}{2}\right)}{2\omega_l}\left(6G_l^2\right)g(\omega_l)$$

where

$$A_l=\frac{1}{3}(P_{11}^l+P_{22}^l+P_{33}^l) \tag{20.17}$$

and

$$G_l^2=\frac{1}{2}\left[(P_{11}^l-P_{22}^l)^2+(P_{22}^l-P_{33}^l)^2+(P_{33}^l-P_{11}^l)^2\right]+3\left[(P_{12}^l)^2+(P_{23}^l)^2+(P_{31}^l)^2\right] \tag{20.18}$$

are the invariants of the polarizability tensor.

20.2.4 Lamb Modes

In order to compare the NC phonon modes calculated by VFFM with the Lamb modes, we need to derive the analytical form of the displacements of the Lamb modes. Lamb's theory begins with the equation of a three dimensional elastic body (Lamb, 1982; Cheng et al., 2003):

$$\frac{\rho\partial^2\boldsymbol{D}}{\partial^2 t}=(\lambda+\mu)\nabla(\nabla\cdot\boldsymbol{D})+\mu\nabla^2\boldsymbol{D} \tag{20.19}$$

where $\boldsymbol{D}$ is the displacement vector and the two parameters λ and μ are Lamb constants related to the longitudinal and transverse sound velocity: $v_l = \sqrt{(\lambda + 2\mu)/\rho}$ and $v_\mathrm{t} = \sqrt{\mu/\rho}$.

For spheroidal modes, the displacements are

$$\boldsymbol{D}_{lu}^{(S)} = \nabla\phi_\mathrm{s} + \alpha\nabla\times\nabla\times\boldsymbol{A} \tag{20.20}$$

where l is angular momentum number; u denotes the different components and ranges from 1 to $2l+1$; and α is a constant determined by the stress-free boundary condition,

$$\phi_\mathrm{s} = j_l(hr)P_l^m(\cos\theta)\begin{Bmatrix}\cos m\varphi \\ \sin m\varphi\end{Bmatrix}\exp\{-\mathrm{i}\omega t\},$$

and

$$\boldsymbol{A} = (x\phi_V, y\phi_V, z\phi_V) \tag{20.21}$$

in Cartesian coordinates, and

$$\phi_V = j_l(kr)P_l^m(\cos\theta)\begin{Bmatrix}\cos m\varphi \\ \sin m\varphi\end{Bmatrix}\exp\{-\mathrm{i}\omega t\}.$$

In the above equations, h and k are related to the longitudinal and transverse sound velocity components: $h = \omega/v_\mathrm{l}$ and $k = \omega/v_\mathrm{t}$. In the free boundary condition, $\xi = hR$ and $\eta = kR$ satisfy the following relation for spheroidal modes:

$$\begin{aligned}&2\left\{\eta^2 + (l-1)(l+2)\left[\eta j_{l+1}(\eta)/j_l(\eta) - (l+1)\right]\right\}\xi j_{l+1}(\xi)/j_l(\xi) - 0.5\eta^4 + \\ &\quad (l-1)(2l+1)\eta^2 + \left[\eta^2 - 2l(l-1)(l+2)\right]\eta j_{l+1}(\eta)/j_l(\eta) = 0\end{aligned} \tag{20.22}$$

where R is the radius of the sphere and the η values depend on the ratio (v_l/v_t) in the spheroidal mode for the material. The η values for torsional modes do not depend on the material and are universal. For torsional modes, the displacements are

$$\boldsymbol{D}_{lu}^{(T)} = \nabla\times\boldsymbol{A}, \tag{20.23}$$

Under free boundary conditions, η satisfies the following torsional mode relation:

$$\frac{d\left(j_{l+1}(\eta)/j_l(\eta)\right)}{d\eta} = 0 \tag{20.24}$$

Because the η values are discrete within a free boundary condition, the ω values depend on a branch number $n(=0,1,2,\cdots)$ and an angular momentum number l. There are no $l = 0$ tosional modes. However, the eigenfrequencies for the $l = 0$ spheroidal modes are given by

$$4\frac{h^2}{k^2}\frac{j_1(\xi)}{\xi} - j_0(\xi) = 0 \tag{20.25}$$

Using Eqs. (20.20) – (20.22) and the averaged longitudinal and transverse speeds of sound for Ge, $v_l = 5.25 \times 10^3$ m/s and $v_t = 3.25 \times 10^3$ m/s, we have numerically obtained η values for different values of n and l. A few of these values are listed in Table 20.2; and these are also plotted for both spheroidal and torsional modes in Fig. 19.3. The points shown with a circle in Fig. 20.3 are Raman active modes.

Table 20.2 A few η values have been calculated, using Eqs. (20.22) and (20.23), along with the corresponding ω values for an NC with 7289 atoms ($r = 3.4$ nm) found by projection (to be discussed further in Section 20.4)

Lamb mode	Spheroidal				Torsional			
n	0	1	0	0	0	0	0	1
l	0	0	1	2	1	2	3	3
η	4.18	10.08	3.36	2.64	5.75	2.51	3.86	8.45
ω (cm^{-1})	19.6	48.1	14.8	12.9	27.2	11.7	16.3	38.9

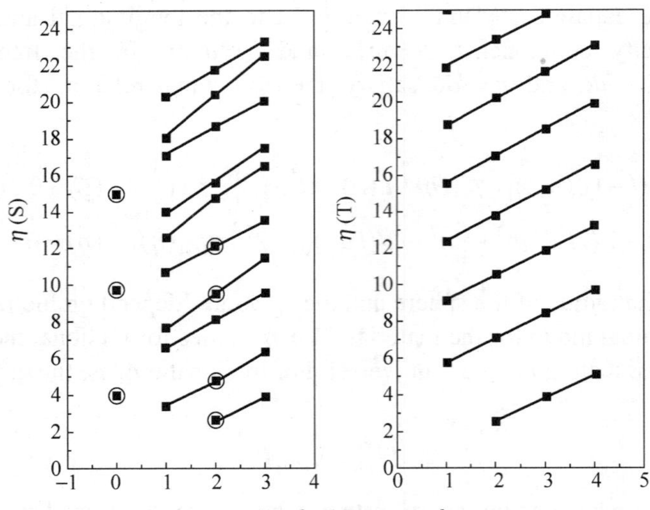

Figure 20.3 Calculated values of η for both spheroidal (S) and torsional (T) Lamb modes as a function of the angular momentum number l. The solid lines join $l \neq 0$ modes with the same branch number n (special case: join $l = 1$, n branch to $l = 2$, $n + 1$ branch). η increases with n in the sequence of $n = 0, 1, 2, \cdots$ Note that the values for the spheroidal mode are Ge specific, with the choice of transverse and longitudinal sound velocities given in the text. The modes indicated with circles are found to be Raman active by projection onto our 7289 Ge atom NC (to be discussed further in Section 20.4)

1. Displacements of the Spheroidal $l = 0$ mode

Neglecting constants and terms involving time, we have $\phi_S = j_0(hr)$ and $\phi_V = j_0(kr)$. From eq. (20.20), we obtain

$$\boldsymbol{D}_{01}^{(S)} = -h\frac{j_1(hr)}{r}(x\boldsymbol{e}_x + y\boldsymbol{e}_y + z\boldsymbol{e}_z) \tag{20.26}$$

This mode belongs to the A_1 representations in the T_d symmetry. Displacements of the spheroidal $l = 1$ and 2 modes are derived in Appendices A.2 and A.3.

2. Displacements of Torsional $l = 1$ Modes

There are three orthogonal torsional modes that form a complete set of bases, which can be calculated using the following approach. Neglecting constant and time-dependent terms, we have $\phi_V = xj_1(kr)/r$. From Eqs. (20.21) and (20.23):

$$\boldsymbol{D}_{11}^{(T)} = -z\frac{j_1(kr)}{r}\boldsymbol{e}_y + y\frac{j_1(kr)}{r}\boldsymbol{e}_z \tag{20.27}$$

Similarly, $\phi_V = yj_1(kr)/r$, and

$$\boldsymbol{D}_{12}^{(T)} = -x\frac{j_1(kr)}{r}\boldsymbol{e}_z + z\frac{j_1(kr)}{r}\boldsymbol{e}_x \tag{20.28}$$

and $\phi_V = zj_1(kr)/r$, and

$$\boldsymbol{D}_{13}^{(T)} = -y\frac{j_1(kr)}{r}\boldsymbol{e}_x + x\frac{j_1(kr)}{r}\boldsymbol{e}_y \tag{20.29}$$

These $l = 1$ Lamb modes with displacements $\boldsymbol{D}_{11}^{(T)}$, $\boldsymbol{D}_{12}^{(T)}$, and $\boldsymbol{D}_{13}^{(T)}$ belong to T_1 representations in T_d symmetry, and $\boldsymbol{D}_{11}^{(T)}$, $\boldsymbol{D}_{12}^{(T)}$, and $\boldsymbol{D}_{13}^{(T)}$ form a set of orthogonal complete bases,

$$\begin{aligned} &\iiint \boldsymbol{D}_{11}^{(T)} \cdot \boldsymbol{D}_{11}^{(T)}\mathrm{d}V = \iiint \boldsymbol{D}_{12}^{(T)} \cdot \boldsymbol{D}_{12}^{(T)}\mathrm{d}V = \iiint \boldsymbol{D}_{13}^{(T)} \cdot \boldsymbol{D}_{13}^{(T)}\mathrm{d}V \\ &\iiint \boldsymbol{D}_{11}^{(T)} \cdot \boldsymbol{D}_{12}^{(T)}\mathrm{d}V = \iiint \boldsymbol{D}_{12}^{(T)} \cdot \boldsymbol{D}_{13}^{(T)}\mathrm{d}V = \iiint \boldsymbol{D}_{11}^{(T)} \cdot \boldsymbol{D}_{13}^{(T)}\mathrm{d}V = 0 \end{aligned} \tag{20.30}$$

because the Lamb modes are vibrations of a continuous sphere. In order to compare the results with vibration amplitudes of a NC, the above integrals should be replaced by summations. In our calculations, we have selected the vibration amplitudes at the atomic positions and normalize them to one, similar to the normalized vibrational amplitudes of the NC in the VFFM. Displacements of torsional $l = 2$, 3, and 4 modes are derived in Appendices A.4 through A.6.

20.3 Results and Discussion

20.3.1 Phonon Density of States for Nanocrystals

We have calculated the phonon modes in Ge NCs (Ren and Qin, 2002) in the size range up to 7 nm in diameter with two different types of surfaces, free or fixed. The phonon density of states (PDOS) $D(\omega)$ is calculated with Lorentz broadening

$$D(\omega) = \frac{1}{\pi}\sum_i \frac{n_i \Gamma}{\Gamma^2 + (\omega - \omega_i)^2} \tag{20.31}$$

where the summation is over all phonon modes; ω_i is the eigenfrequency for phonon mode i; and n_i is the degeneracy number, which has a value of 1 for modes A_1 and A_2, a value of 2 for the E modes, and a value of 3 for the T_1 and T_2 modes; and Γ is the Lorentz half-width, which is 0.5 cm^{-1} in our calculations.

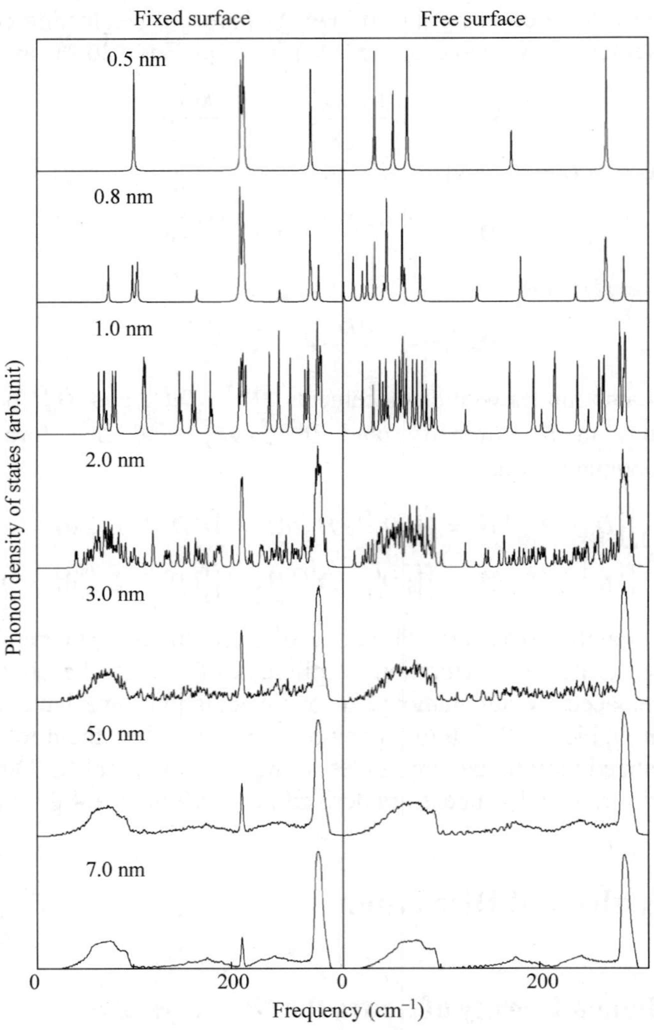

Figure 20.4 The total PDOS for Ge NCs with either fixed or free surfaces of various diameters has been calculated and is shown here

The PDOS of NCs with these two types of surfaces of a few sizes of NCs are shown in Fig. 20.4. The left panel is for NCs with fixed surface, and the right panel is for NCs with free surface. Comparing these results, we notice that there are more low frequency peaks in NCs with free surfaces than for NCs with fixed surfaces. This is particularly true when the size of the NCs is < 3 nm. As the size of NCs increases, the PDOS of NCs for both types of surfaces approach that of bulk. One major feature of phonons in NCs with fixed surface is that there is always a major peak at a frequency of approximately 211 cm^{-1}, which is within the frequency range between optical and acoustic phonons of the bulk Ge. This peak is due to interfacial phonons, which are still easily observed for NCs that are 7 nm in diameter, the maximum size of our present calculations.

Our results for NCs with the two types of surfaces are directly compared with the bulk phonon DOS in Fig. 20.5. The solid line is for the DOS of Ge bulk material, and the dashed and dotted lines are for NCs of 7.0 nm with fixed and free surfaces, respectively. The major difference of the PDOS of NCs with fixed surfaces is the existence of the interfacial phonon peak. The PDOS of NCs with free surfaces is obviously higher than that of Ge bulk material in the low frequency range. For the major optical peak, the PDOS of both types of NCs are lower than that of bulk with a slight red shift in the frequencies. This shift is particularly obvious for the NCs with free surfaces. Both the differences in the low frequency range and of the major optical peak indicate the influence of surface effects on phonon modes in the long wavelength range of the bulk material. The longer the wavelength, the greater is the effect of surface differences on the Raman spectrum. Some of these features will be further below.

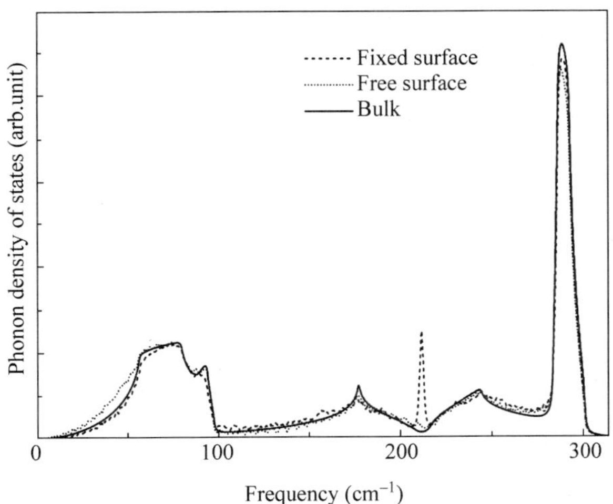

Figure 20.5 The calculated total PDOS is shown for bulk Ge material and for NCs with fixed or free surfaces with an approximate diameter of 7.0 nm

20.3.2 Raman Intensities

Raman intensities can be calculated using the bond charge approximation (BPA) as described in Section 20.2.3. Raman intensities for the phonon modes of NCs with two different types of surfaces with approximate diameters between 0.5 to 7.0 nm were calculated using the BPA. The total Raman intensity I is calculated by the Lorentz broadening

$$I = \frac{1}{\pi}\sum_{l} \frac{I_l \Gamma}{\Gamma^2 + (\omega - \omega_l)^2} \tag{20.32}$$

where I_l and ω_l are the scattering intensity and eigenfrequency of mode l, respectively, and Γ is the Lorentz half-width, which is 0.5 cm^{-1} in the calculations for Ge and 0.64 cm^{-1} in the Si calculations.

Raman intensities for the A_1, E, and T_2 modes for both Ge and Si NCs have been calculated and investigated. Our results indicate that even though the size effects on strength of Raman peaks of Ge NCs with free surfaces are very similar to those of Si NCs (Cheng and Ren, 2002), the size effects on strength of Raman peaks of NCs with fixed surface are obviously different. We have listed the related important data in Tables 20.3 and 20.4. In general, the Raman strengths of NCs with fixed surfaces are more similar to that of bulk material, but they also have some unique features. These will be discussed in detail below.

Table 20.3 The Raman intensities of the A_1, E, and T_2 modes for Si NCs with various sizes are given. The data listed are, in order: the diameters d of the NCs, the number N of atoms in the NCs, the intensity of the highest peak of the A_1 modes I_{A1}, the intensity of the highest peak of the E modes I_E, the intensity of the highest peak of the T_2 modes in the low-frequency range $I_{T2}(l)$, the intensity of the highest peak of the T_2 modes in the high-frequency range $I_{T2}(h)$, the frequency of the first peak of the A_1 modes ω_{A1}, the frequency of the first peak of the E modes ω_E, the frequency of the first peak of the T_2 modes in the low-frequency range $\omega_{T2}(l)$, and the frequency of the highest peak of the T_2 modes in the high-frequency range $\omega_{T2}(h)$. All the intensities listed are the Raman intensity per atom. All frequencies are given in the unit of cm^{-1}

d(nm)	N	I_{A1}	I_E	$I_{T2}(l)$	$I_{T2}(h)$	ω_{A1}	ω_E	$\omega_{T2}(l)$	$\omega_{T2}(h)$
1.411	87	7.65	9.70	10.99	9.88	129.8	46.7	58.8	506.4
1.939	191	5.88	5.58	6.61	9.60	98.4	35.2	46.9	511.2
2.474	417	3.55	3.53	4.79	9.47	83.3	27.2	37.5	514.3
2.975	705	2.69	2.76	3.66	9.22	69.0	23.3	31.2	515.6
3.467	1099	2.46	2.03	2.64	9.25	61.4	19.7	26.6	516.5
3.991	1707	1.84	1.51	1.97	9.24	53.2	16.9	22.9	517.1
5.000	3265	1.27	1.01	1.34	9.47	43.2	13.4	18.8	517.7
5.999	5707	0.91	0.72	0.93	9.67	36.0	10.9	15.5	518.1
6.997	9041	0.68	0.54	0.69	10.04	30.9	9.2	13.4	518.3
7.579	11489	0.58	0.46	0.59	10.26	28.6	8.6	12.4	518.3

Table 20.4 The Raman intensities of the T_2 modes for Ge NCs with two different surfaces, a free surface or a fixed surface are tabulated. The data listed, in order, are the diameter of the NC d, the number of atoms in the NC N, the frequency of the highest T_2 peak ω_{T2}(free), and the integrated intensity of the T_2 modes I_{T2}(free) of NCs with free surfaces, and the same two quantities for NCs with fixed surfaces ω_{T2}(fixed) and I_{T2}(fixed). All intensities listed are Raman intensity per atom. All frequencies are in the unit of cm^{-1}

d(nm)	N	ω_{T2}(free)	I_{T2}(free)	ω_{T2}(fixed)	I_{T2}(fixed)
0.934	29	289.0	0.9507	290.9	0.2286
1.952	167	296.6	0.6387	297.1	0.2286
2.914	633	299.1	0.5077	299.2	0.2286
3.985	1503	299.9	0.4361	300.0	0.2286
4.977	2917	300.3	0.3995	300.3	0.2286
5.983	5011	300.5	0.3707	300.5	0.2286
6.993	8105	300.6	0.3524	300.6	0.2286

20.3.3 Size Effects on the Highest Phonon Frequencies of Si

The calculated Raman spectra of Si NCs are shown in Figs. 20.6~20.8. The intensities of the A_2 and T_1 modes are very small, which is consistent with the group theory prediction. All Raman intensities for NCs with three different symmetries, A_1, E, and T_2 and with free surfaces and different sizes are calculated and investigated. In general, the major peaks in the high-frequency range always exhibit T_2 symmetry. The highest peak corresponds to the T_2 phonon modes with the highest frequencies. As the NC size increases, this highest frequency approaches the optical phonon frequency of bulk Si. Theoretically speaking, as the NC size approaches infinity, the total Raman spectrum of the NCs approaches the Raman spectrum of bulk Si; and, in that limit, this will be the only remaining peak.

In our previous calculations (Ren et al., 2000, 2001; Qin and Ren, 2001, 2002a, 2002b), we have discussed size dependence of phonon modes as a function of symmetry. We have observed that phonon modes with different symmetry have different size dependence, and A_1 modes usually have the greatest size effect. For a zinc-blend semiconductor NC, such as GaAs, when the size of the NC is relatively large, the mode with the highest frequency has the A_1 symmetry. However, as the size decreases, there change in symmetries; and the mode with the highest frequency has T_2 symmetry. For the Si NCs studied in the size range up to 7.6 nm, the highest frequency corresponds to the A_1 symmetry. However, the Raman intensity of the A_1 modes decreases as the NC size increases, so the high-frequency mode with the largest Raman intensity has the T_2 symmetry.

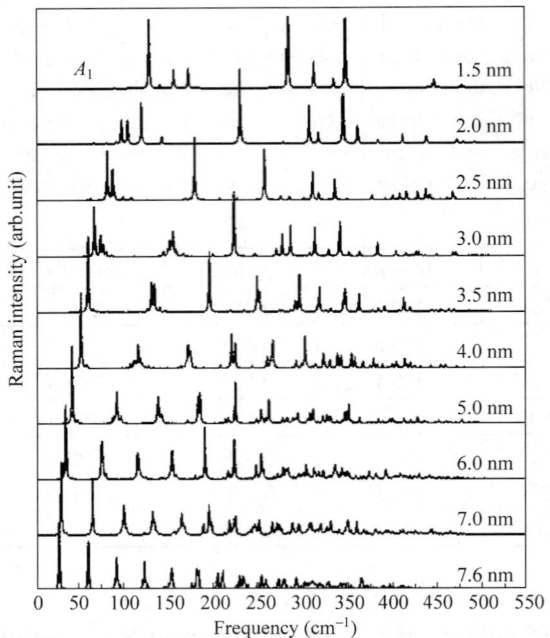

Figure 20.6 The reduced Raman intensities of the A_1 modes for Si NCs of varying diameter (1.5 – 7.6 nm) are shown

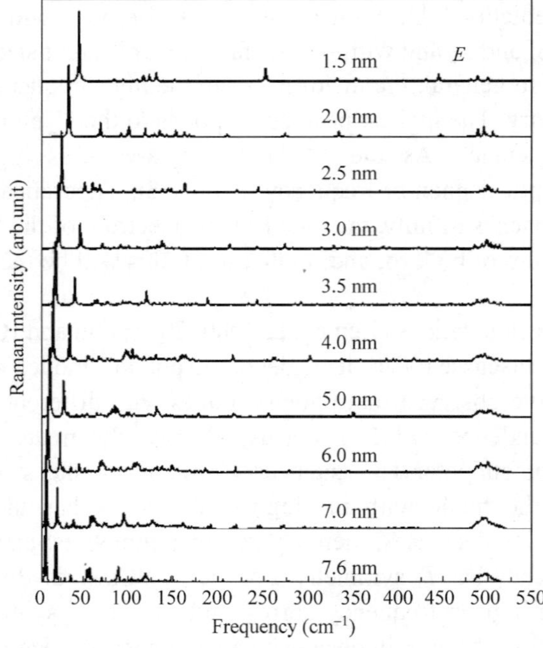

Figure 20.7 The reduced Raman intensities of the E modes for Si NCs with varying diameter are shown

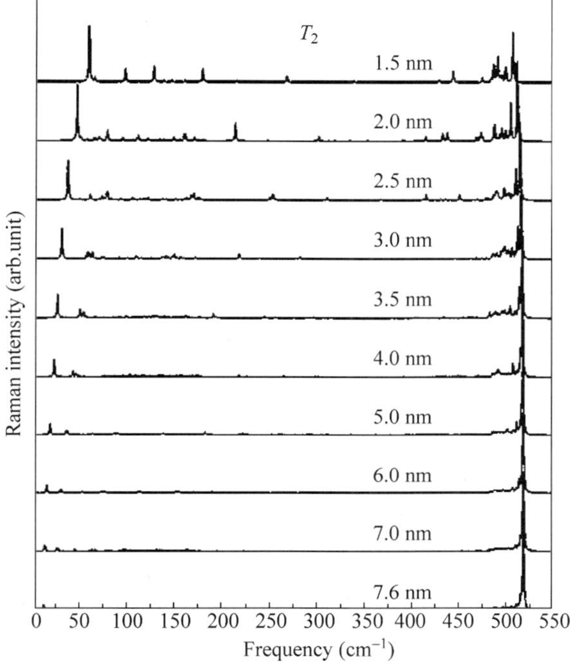

Figure 20.8 The reduced Raman intensities of the T_2 modes for Si NCs with varying diameter are shown

As the NC size decreases, the frequency of the T_2 peak decreases. To show this more clearly, the high-frequency portion of Fig. 20.8 is shown in Fig. 20.9. From the data listed in Table 20.3, we know that when the diameter of Si NCs decreases from 0.76 nm to 1.41 nm, the frequency of the highest Raman peak shifts from 518.3 cm^{-1} to 506.4 cm^{-1} (the Raman peak of bulk Si is at 518.9 cm^{-1} in our model). The systematic redshift of the longitudinal (LO) phonon peaks due to spatially confined phonon modes in nanocrystals in the size range of a few nanometers has been observed (Freire et al., 1997; Hwang et al., 1996; Blandin et al., 2000); and it has also been observed using resonant Raman scattering in three Ge nanocrystals in the size range of 4 – 10 nm (Teo et al., 2000). An additional observation is that weaker peaks appear at the same time as the highest intensity peak redshifts occur as NC size decreases.

It may be difficult, experimentally, to resolve all of the weaker peaks due to broadening resulting from a fluctuation in dot sizes. As a result, one may observe an asymmetric broadening of the Raman peak corresponding to the optical phonon as the dot size is reduced. This has indeed been exhibited in the measured Raman intensities of Ge NCs (Yu). One could interpret this as an indication that the quality of the dots may be poor, leading to larger inhomogeneous broadening as the NC size gets smaller. However, from our calculations on Raman intensities of NCs, the redshift of the strongest T_2 Raman peak is smaller than the frequency spread of the weaker peaks which appear. In other words, the broadening as the dot size decreases of the Raman peak is larger than the redshift. This indicates that the observed broadening in Raman measurements is not only due to the redshift of the peak alone, but there is also a contribution to this broadening from quantum size effects.

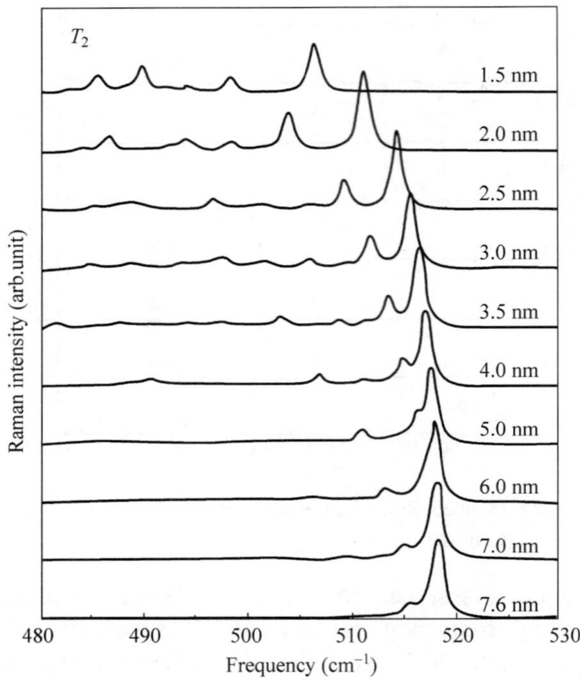

Figure 20.9 The high frequency portion of the reduced Raman spectrum for the T_2 modes of Si NCs with varying diameters is shown

20.3.4 Size Effects on the Lowest Frequencies Phonon for Si

In Figs. 20.6 through 20.8, we observe that the frequency of the first peak in the low-frequency range for the three different symmetries (A_1, E, and T_2) increases as the size of the NCs decreases. When the size of Si NCs decreases from 7.6 nm to 1.4 nm, the frequency of the first Raman peak of the A_1 modes shifts from 28.6 cm^{-1} to 129.8 cm^{-1}; the first Raman peak of the E modes shifts from 8.6 cm^{-1} to 46.7 cm^{-1}; and the first Raman peak with T_2 symmetry shifts from 12.4 cm^{-1} to 58.8 cm^{-1}. Size effects on the lowest phonon mode frequencies in NCs have been discussed in detail in our previous studies (Ren et al., 2000, 2001); and is again shown in the calculated Raman spectra. Furthermore, we notice that even though the frequencies of the lowest-frequency peak increase in all these three figures, the rate of increase is different for each. The lowest frequency of the A_1 peak increases much faster than the other two. The A_1 peak increases much faster than that of the other two because the A_1 modes have the strongest quantum confinement effects (Ren et al., 2000,2001). To show this more clearly, the lowest frequency peak versus NC size is plotted in Fig. 20.10.

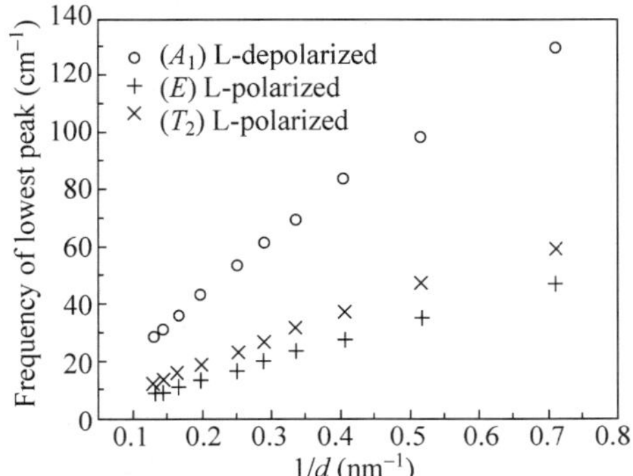

Figure 20.10 The frequency of the lowest Raman peak of A_1, E, and T_2 modes versus diameter of Si NCs is plotted

Another feature of Fig. 20.10 is that the lowest frequencies of the Raman peaks in the acoustic range are roughly proportional to the inverse of the NC diameters, which was observed (Duval, 1992). This was also observed in Si nanocrystals (Fujii et al., 1996), for which the depolarized Raman spectra were observed at much lower frequencies than the polarized spectra. Not only do our results agree with the experimental observations, but we also learned that this is actually due to the symmetry dependence of confinement of the phonon modes, i.e. the A_1 modes have the strongest confinement effects.

20.3.5 Folding of Acoustic Phonons

In Fig. 20.6, we observe that for A_1 modes in low-frequency range that the Raman spectra are dominated by a series of nearly evenly spaced peaks in the acoustical phonon range. As the NC size decreases, the spacing of these peaks increases, which can be attributed to the folding of acoustic phonons. Since the A_1 modes vibrate in the radial direction, when the radius of the NC increases by approximately one lattice constant, there will be one more folding due to confinement of the NC along the radial direction. Further study on Ge NCs shows that in the low frequency range, the Raman intensities of Ge NCs with free surfaces are similar to those of Si NCs. However, the Raman intensities for Ge NCs with fixed surfaces are too small to discuss. This indicates that the folding of A_1 acoustic phonons in NCs with free surfaces is due to the free surfaces. As shown in the next section, the peaks correspond to $l = 0$ spheroidal Lamb modes.

20.3.6 Size Effects on Si Raman Peaks

Since Raman intensities plotted in Figs. 20.6 through 20.8 are in arbitrary units, the size effects on the strength of Raman peaks are not shown clearly in these figures. To show them more clearly, we have plotted the Raman intensity per atom versus diameters of NCs for the low-frequency A_1 peaks, the low-frequency E peaks, the low-frequency T_2 peaks, and the high-frequency T_2 peaks in Fig. 20.11. For A_1 Raman spectra there are several high peaks, and we choose the strength of the highest peak (when the size is less than 3.0 nm, this peak is not the peak with the lowest frequency). In Fig. 20.11, we see that the strength of low-frequency peaks (A_1, E, and T_2) decreases quickly as the size of NCs increases, and the intensity of high-frequency peaks (T_2) remains a constant in NCs of all sizes. This indicates that even though only one major peak for bulk material can be measured, when the size of the NCs decreases, other peaks in the low-frequency range will appear. Of these low-frequency Raman peaks, the most noticeable ones are probably the evenly spaced A_1 peaks in the polarized spectra as have been observed (Kuok et al., 2003).

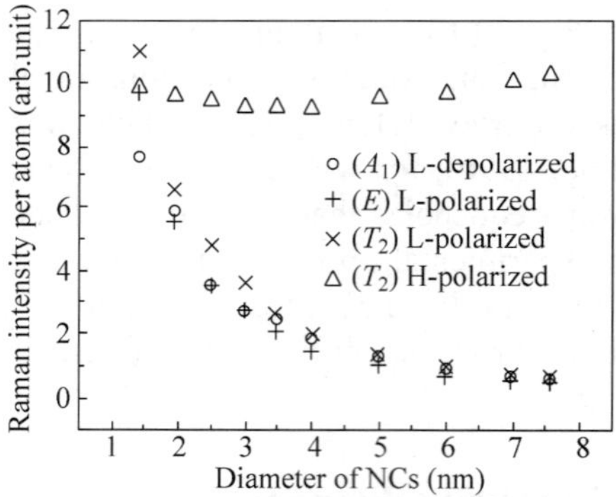

Figure 20.11 The Raman intensity per atom of the highest, low-frequency peaks for the A_1, E, and T_2 modes and the highest, high-frequency peaks of the T_2 modes versus diameter for Si NCs is plotted

We want to emphasize that in Fig. 20.11, the Raman intensity shown is from one calculated highest Raman peak, either in the low-frequency range or in the high-frequency range. The presence of multiple Raman peaks as shown in Figs. 20.6 through 20.8 may not be resolvable experimentally due to size fluctuations. However, a broadened peak can be observed. Typically, in such a situation, the Raman intensities should be integrated to obtain the total strength of the Raman peak. To compare with the experimental results, we summed the calculated Raman intensities (without broadening) for all A_1, E, and T_2 modes, respectively, and show them for NCs as a function of size in Fig. 20.12. We can see that all the Raman intensities increase when the NC size decreases. As the size of the NCs increases, the Raman intensity of the T_2 modes will approach that of the bulk crystal and other intensities go to zero. This is in qualitative agreement with what has been observed in Ge NCs (Yu).

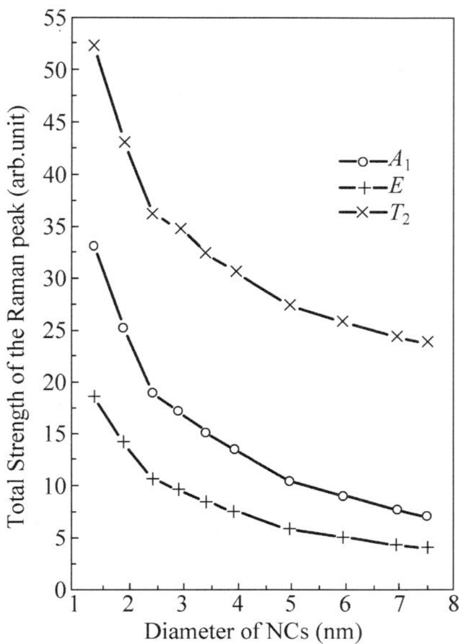

Figure 20.12 The integrated Raman intensity per atom for A_1, E, and T_2 modes versus of Si NC diameter are shown

20.3.7 Size Effects on Mode Mixing

One more point with regard to Figs. 20.6 through 20.8 and Fig. 20.9 is that, for large NCs, the major peak of the Raman spectra is derived from the T_2 high-frequency mode. This peak approaches the optical-phonon peak in the bulk Raman spectra when the NC size is large. As the NC size decreases, a number of peaks in the lower frequency range appear, which are derived from the A_1 modes in the polarized Raman spectra and the E and T_2 modes from the depolarized Raman spectra. As can be seen from Figs. 20.6 through 20.8 and Fig. 20.9, the intensities of the A_1, E, and T_2 modes are of nearly the same magnitude for small dots, which indicates mode mixing due to the quantum confinement of phonon modes in small NCs.

20.3.8 Size Effects on the Intensities of Ge Raman Peaks

All Raman intensities of Ge NCs for symmetries A_1, E, and T_2 taking into account two different surfaces and varying size have been calculated and studied.

It is found that size effects on the total strengths of Raman peaks for Ge NCs with free surfaces are similar to those of Si NCs discussed above, but different for NCs with fixed surfaces. It is found that, in general, the Raman strengths of the A_1 and E modes in NCs with fixed surfaces are much smaller (a ratio on the order of 10^{-11}) than those with free surfaces. This indicates that the A_1 and E Raman intensities in NCs with fixed surfaces can be ignored in the computational accuracy considered and are similar to the Raman intensities of bulk materials. This is the reason that the results for the A_1 and E symmetries are not listed in Table 20.4. They are too small to be considered. Not only this is true for A_1 and E modes, but it is also true for T_2 modes in the low frequency range. Because of this, there are no observable Raman peaks for the A_1 and E modes for NCs with fixed surfaces or in the low frequency range for the T_2 modes. In Fig. 20.13 and 20.14, the Raman intensities of the T_2 states for NCs with two different surfaces and different sizes are shown. From these two figures and the PDOS discussed above, we have found that Raman peaks in the lower frequency range in Fig. 20.13 are due to the free surfaces of NCs. On the other hand, for NCs with fixed surfaces, the low frequency values are more similar to that of bulk material, i.e. the low frequency Raman peaks can be ignored in NCs with fixed surfaces.

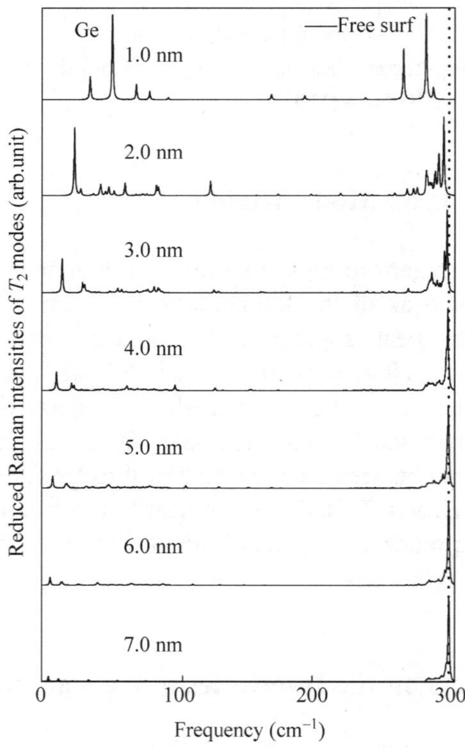

Figure 20.13 The reduced Raman intensities of the T_2 modes are shown for Ge NCs with free surfaces. The approximate diameters are indicated

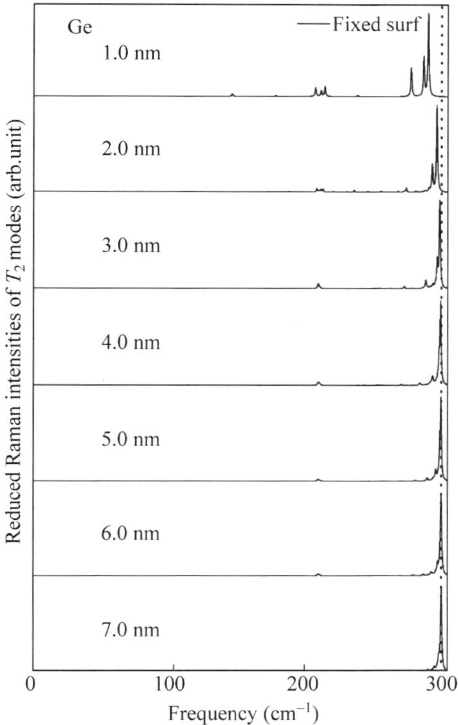

Figure 20.14 The reduced Raman intensities of the T_2 modes for Ge NCs with fixed surfaces are shown. The approximate diameters of the NCs are indicated

Since, experimentally, the presence of multiple Raman peaks, as shown in Fig. 20.13 and 20.14, may not be resolvable due to size fluctuations and only a broadened peak is observed, we have integrated the Raman intensities for each NC to obtain the total strength for the Raman peaks. To do this, we summed the calculated Raman intensities (without broadening) for all A_1, E, and T_2 modes for NCs with varying size. Our results show that for NCs with fixed surfaces, the total Raman intensities of the A_1 and E modes are very small (10^{-12}) when compared to the total strengths of T_2 modes (10^{-1}); and the integrated Raman intensities of T_2 modes remain nearly constant (see Table 7.2). This result is different than the total Raman intensities for NCs with free surfaces (Cheng and Ren, 2002), but, once again, agrees with those of the bulk material. So, we conclude that the increase of total Raman intensities in small NCs with free surfaces is mainly attributed to the free surfaces of NCs.

20.3.9 Size Effects on the Highest Raman Frequencies for Ge with Fixed or Free Surfaces

From our results, the major peaks in the high frequency range of Ge NCs with both types of surfaces always correspond to phonon modes with T_2 symmetry. The quantum confinement effects for Ge NCs with both types of surfaces are very similar to those of Si NCs. When the size of the Ge NCs decreases, the frequency of the T_2 peak decreases, which is due to confinement of the optical phonons. To show this more clearly, the high frequency portion of Figs. 20.13 and 20.14 is replotted in Fig. 20.15. The solid lines represent the data for NCs with free surfaces and the dashed lines represent NCs with fixed surfaces. The frequency of optical phonons at the center of the Brillouin Zone in our model for bulk Ge is 300.9 cm^{-1}, which is shown as a vertical dashed line in Fig. 20.15. The frequencies of the highest Raman peak for different NCs are listed in Table 3.4. The calculated values indicate that for a given NC size, the frequency of the highest Raman peak for NCs with different surfaces is quite similar. For diameters of Ge NCs that are less than 4 nm, the frequency of the highest Raman peak for those with free surfaces are slightly lower than those with fixed surfaces. This systematic red-shift of phonon peaks due to spatially confined phonon modes in nanocrystals in the size range of a few nm has been observed in several experiments (Freire et al., 1997; Hwang et al., 1996; Balandin et al., 2000; Teo et

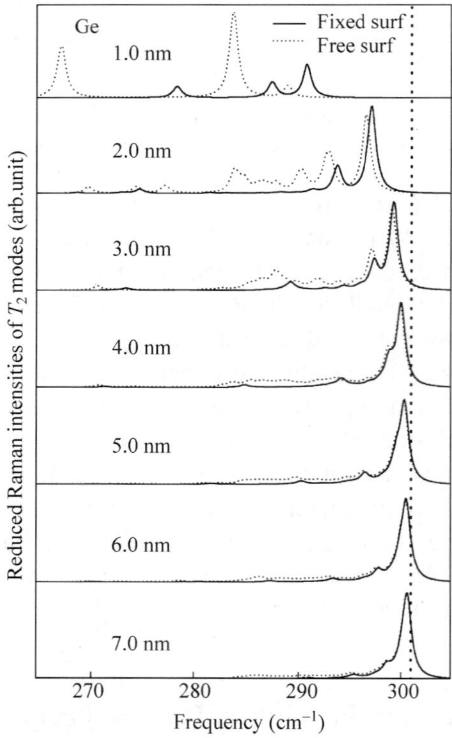

Figure 20.15 The reduced Raman intensities are shown for the T_2 modes for the higher frequencies for Ge NCs. The solid lines are for NCs with fixed surfaces, and the dashed lines are for NCs with free surfaces. The approximate NC diameters are indicated

al., 2000). Our calculations for NCs with two different types of surfaces indicate that this is a quantum confinement effect. From Figs. 20.13 through 20.15, we have also seen that Raman intensities for NCs with free surfaces have a broader tail of peaks. The corresponding plots for NCs that have fixed surfaces have fewer peaks. This shows that some of these peaks are caused by vibrations of atoms near the free surfaces.

Another thing we notice from Fig. 20.15 is that for the high frequency peaks of the T_2 modes, that the highest intensity peak that has a red shift as the size decreases and, at the same time, weak peaks appear. This is true for NCs with both types of surfaces. Experimentally, it is difficult to resolve the weaker peaks because of broadening resulting from fluctuation in NC size. Therefore, one may observe an asymmetric broadening of the Raman peak corresponding to the optical phonon as the size is reduced. This is indeed found in Raman intensities of Ge NCs (Yu). As we pointed out in our previous work, one may attempt to interpret the asymmetries broadening of Raman peaks in experimental observations as an indication that the quality of the dots may be poor, so it leads to larger inhomogeneous broadening in lower frequencies. However, from our calculations on Raman intensities of NCs, we notice that the red shift of the strongest T_2 Raman peak is smaller than the frequency spread of the weaker peaks which appear. In other words, the broadening of the Raman peak is larger than the red shift as the NC size decreases. This is true for NCs with both types of surfaces. This indicates that the observed broadening in Raman measurements is not only due to the red shift of the major peak alone, but there is probably a major contribution to the broadening from the quantum size effects.

20.3.10 Existence of Interface Modes for Nanocrystals with Fixed Surfaces

One unique feature that is observed regarding the Raman strength of NCs with fixed surfaces is that there is a Raman peak at approximately 211 cm^{-1} in NCs of all different sizes. We have also noticed that there is a major peak in the same frequency range for the PDOS of all NCs with fixed surfaces, as shown in Fig. 20.5; and we have previously discussed the interface feature of these modes.

To study the interfacial modes more carefully, we have employed the concept of average vibrational amplitude (Ren et al., 2001) to investigate it. The average vibrational amplitude A_l^i is defined as

$$A_l^i = \frac{1}{n}\sum_{k=1}^{n}\left|a_{lk}^i\right|^2 \qquad (20.33)$$

where a_{lk}^i is the vibration amplitude of atom k in the lth shell in the ith phonon mode, and n is the total number of atoms in the lth shell. In Fig. 20.16, the average vibrational amplitudes of the T_2 mode with a frequency of 210.5 cm^{-1} is shown for a 6.0-nm (diameter) NC with a fixed surface. From above figures, we believe that this is an interfacial mode. From Fig. 20.16, it is apparent that the vibrational amplitudes of this mode are small for the internal region of the NC, but very large near the interface. This indicates that this is indeed an interface mode. For comparison, we have also plotted the average amplitudes of the T_2 mode with the highest frequency of 300.5 cm^{-1} for the same NC. This is a confined optical mode, as discussed in our previous work (Ren and Cheng, 2002).

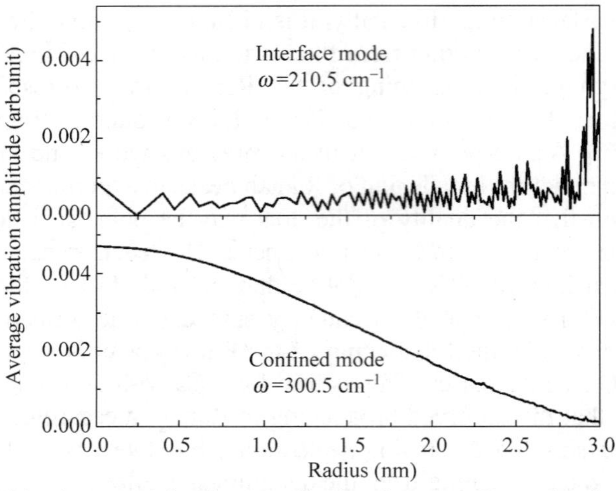

Figure 20.16 Average vibration amplitudes for two T_2 modes in a 6.0-nm (diameter) Ge NC with a fixed surface. The above amplitude has a frequency of 210.5 cm^{-1} which is an interface mode, and the second one has a frequency of 300.5 cm^{-1} which is a confined optical mode

20.4 Correspondence between the Microscopic and Macroscopic Active Raman Modes

The Raman active modes were discussed in the previous section. The macroscopic modes can be determined using Lamb theory using the Ge parameters ($C_0 =$ 47.7 eV, $C_1 = 2.8$ eV) (Harrison, 1980) and the microscopic modes can be found using the VFFM using $v_l = 5.25 \times 10^3$ m/s and $v_t = 3.25 \times 10^3$ m/s. In this section we discuss these two types of modes and their correspondence in detail.

20.4.1 Projection of the Lamb Modes

The displacements of Lamb modes for a continuous sphere of radius R can be determined using the formulas given in Section 20.2.4. The displacements of each atom in the NC modes in the microscopic model can be obtained directly from the dynamic matrices. We can compare these two calculations by projecting the atomic displacements of the NC modes obtained by VFFM along the direction of the Lamb mode displacements. The projection of each atom is then summed to obtain a quantity, which is designated the mode projection quantity (MPQ). The MPQ represents the degree of similarity between a NC mode and a Lambs mode. MPQ = 0, if we project a tangent NC mode on a spheroidal Lambs mode; and MPQ = 1, if all NC atoms have exactly the same displacement as the Lamb displacement. Modes that have MPQ values near 1 are described as NC Lamb modes; and their frequencies are NC Lamb frequencies.

For a spheroidal $l = 0$ mode, the eigenvector for atom a is $\boldsymbol{V}(a)$; and the Lamb mode displacement at the same site is $\boldsymbol{D}_{01}^{(S)}(a)$. The amplitudes of both vectors are normalized for the calculation,

$$\begin{aligned} 1 &= \sum_a \boldsymbol{V}(a) \cdot \boldsymbol{V}(a) \\ 1 &= \sum_a \boldsymbol{D}_{01}^{(S)}(a) \cdot \boldsymbol{D}_{01}^{(S)}(a) \end{aligned} \tag{20.34}$$

The dot product of the two vectors is $s(a) = \boldsymbol{V}(a) \cdot \boldsymbol{D}_{01}^{(S)}(a)$, which is summed over all atoms in the NC to obtain the mode projection quantity,

$$\mathrm{MPQ} = \left[\sum_a s(a) \right]^2 \tag{20.35}$$

Similarly, for torsional $l = 1$ modes, the projections of the NC modes on the three Lamb vectors at the atom a are

$$\begin{aligned} p_x(a) &= \boldsymbol{V}(a) \cdot \boldsymbol{D}_{11}^{(T)}(a) \\ p_y(a) &= \boldsymbol{V}(a) \cdot \boldsymbol{D}_{12}^{(T)}(a) \\ p_z(a) &= \boldsymbol{V}(a) \cdot \boldsymbol{D}_{13}^{(T)}(a) \end{aligned} \tag{20.36}$$

Summing over all projections for all atoms gives

$$\begin{aligned} q_x &= \sum_a p_x(a) \\ q_y &= \sum_a p_y(a) \\ q_z &= \sum_a p_z(a) \end{aligned} \tag{20.37}$$

Then,

$$MPQ = q_x^{\,2} + q_y^{\,2} + q_z^{\,2} \tag{20.38}$$

20.4.2 Group Theory Prediction of the Raman Intensities of the Lamb Modes

As discussed in (Duval, 1992), spheroidal modes transform as the $D_g^{(0)}$, $D_u^{(1)}$, $D_g^{(2)}, \cdots$, representations of $O(3)$; torsional modes transform as the $D_g^{(1)}$, $D_u^{(1)}$, $D_g^{(3)}, \cdots$, representations of $O(3)$. From the theory, we conclude only spheroidal Lamb modes with $l=0$ and 2 are strongly Raman active. For large NC, only these modes are observed in Brillouin scattering experiments (Kuok et al., 2003). In VFFM theory, the NC has T_{d} symmetry; and some torsional modes are also Raman active, but their strengths are much smaller than those of the spheroidal modes. This is the reason that weak torsional modes were also observed when small NCs were studied (Ovsyuk et al., 1988). In fact, these modes are $l=2$ spheroidal Lamb modes with frequencies close to the torsional Lamb modes. The structure of Ge is that of the diamond; and its lattice has octahedral (O_h) local symmetry, where only *g* modes are strongly active, so only the torsional Lamb modes with odd l values are Raman active. In the T_{d} group, $D_g^{(1)} \Rightarrow T_1$ and $D_g^{(3)} \Rightarrow A_2+T_1+T_2$. Among the A_2, T_1, and T_2 symmetries in the T_{d} group, only the T_2 modes are Raman active, so we know that the T_2 modes (with $n=0$ and $l=3$) are the strongest Raman active torsional modes. However, as we show in our Raman spectra calculations, even the intensity of these torsional modes is much smaller than the $n=0$ and $n=1$, $l=2$ spheroidal Lamb modes.

20.4.3 Identifying Lamb Modes within the VFFM-Determined Modes

To identify the Lamb modes within the calculated VFFM NC modes, the projection approach discussed in Section 20.2.4 is used. The results for six Ge NCs with the number of atoms ranging from 885 to 7289 are shown in Figs. 20.17~20.19.

In Fig. 20.17, the NC modes are projected on the spheroidal active Raman Lamb modes ($n=0$, $l=0$). From Eq. (2.20), the different n values correspond to different η values, as shown in Fig. 20.3. The projected value of the major peak of the $n=0$ Lamb mode is largest. Then, for the same ω_{NC}, but differing η, the transverse speed of sound $v_t=\omega_{\mathrm{NC}}R/\eta$ can be calculated. If $n=0$, the value is much closer to the experimental averaged transverse speed of sound. We concluded the peaks shown in Fig. 20.17 belong to $n=0$ in our earlier paper (Cheng et al., 2003). From this figure, we see that when the number of atoms is

> 2869, the NC modes with the maximum Lamb mode component contain a single major peak that is >80% of the Lamb modes. When the number of atoms is <1147, the NC modes exhibit two major peaks with the maximum Lamb mode component that is < 65% Lamb modes.

In Lamb's model, the frequency of the spheroidal $l = 0$ Lamb mode depends on both longitudinal and transverse speeds of sound. In the VFFM, the longitudinal and transverse sound speeds are directionally dependent. Therefore, the MPQ is always less than 1. In Fig. 20.17, we see that there is a critical diameter of approximately 4.0 nm, below which the ($n = 0$, $l = 0$) spheroidal Lamb modes will breakdown and that several peaks appear ($N = 1147$, $\omega = 34.2, 35.6\ \text{cm}^{-1}$). Although the VFFM calculated frequencies still approximately satisfy the linear rule (Cheng et al., 2005a, 2005b, 2005c), we can see that the NC modes with significant Lamb components are no longer of single mode character.

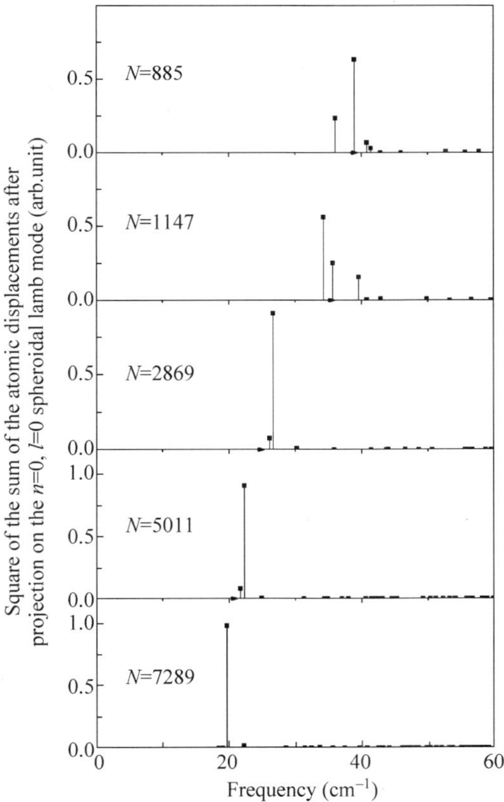

Figure 20.17 MPQ values for ($n = 0$, $l = 0$) spheroidal Lamb modes are plotted. When the number of atoms is less than 2869 (NC diameter <4.9 nm), the Lamb modes decompose into more than one NC mode, but the Lamb frequency of the major peak still follows the $1/d$ rule

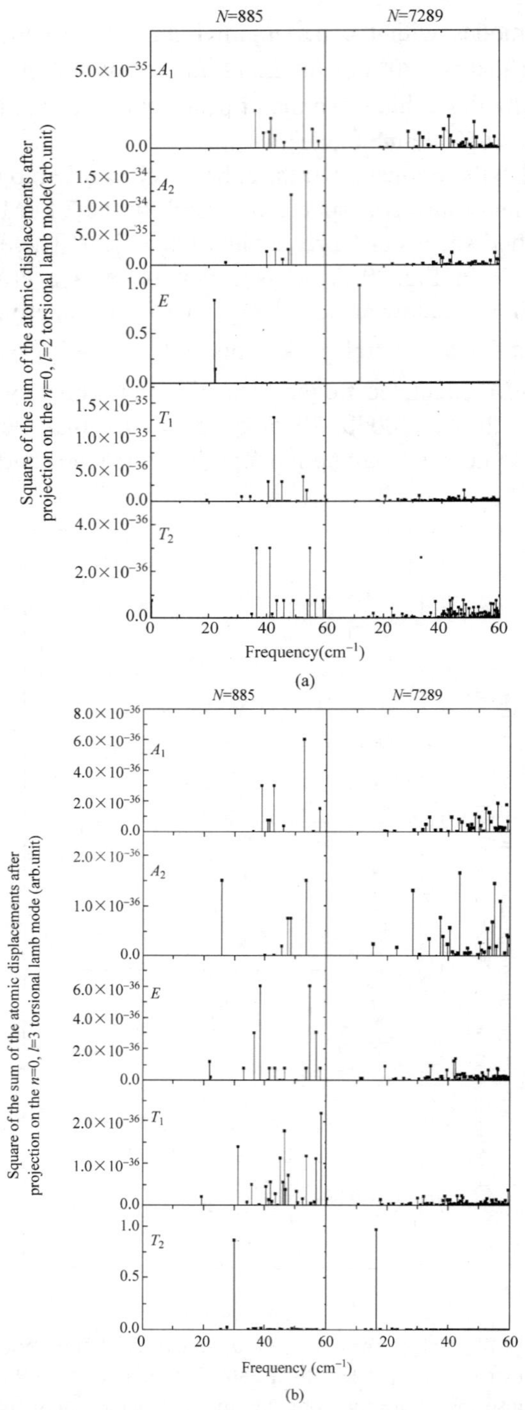

Figure 20.18 MPQ values for ($n = 0$, $l = 2$) (a); ($n = 0$, $l = 3$) (b); and ($n = 0$, $l = 4$) (c) torsional Lamb modes are plotted

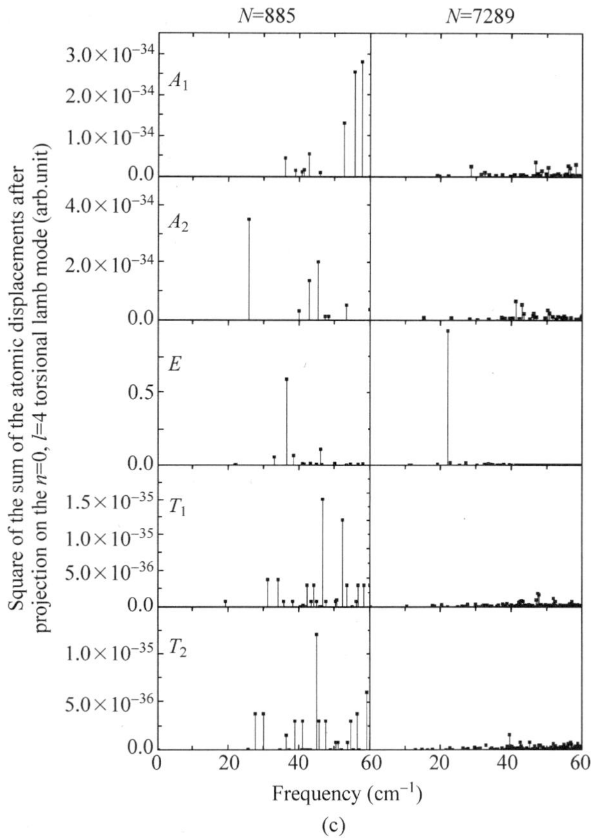

(c)

Figure 20.18 (Continued)

In Fig. 20.18, the NC modes are projected onto the three possible torsional active Raman Lamb modes with $n = 0$ and (a) $l = 2$, (b) $l = 3$, and (c) $l = 4$. In all these cases, only one of the five symmetries has a major Lamb component: when $l = 2$, it is E; when $l = 3$, it is T_2; and when $l = 4$, it is again E. The Lamb components for the other symmetries are too small to be considered. The calculation for one Lamb mode with displacements is detailed in the Appendix. This is in agreement with the symmetry properties of Lamb modes. It is also shown that for NCs of the same size, the NC modes generally contain less Lamb components with larger l values. For example, for NCs with 885 atoms, the maximum Lamb component for E symmetry ($l = 2$) is 0.84; for T_2 ($l = 3$), it is about 0.86; and for E ($l = 4$), it is about 0.6. Again, we notice that there exists a critical diameter of about 4.0 nm, below which the torsional Lamb modes tend to breakdown with more than one Lamb component. Furthermore, as the NC size increases, the maximum Lamb component value in all cases increases, which indicates the VFFM results are approaching those of the continuum model. The

MPQ for $n=0$, $l=2$ torsional modes is close to 1 for NCs with sizes > 3.3 nm, and continues to approach 1 as the NC size increases.

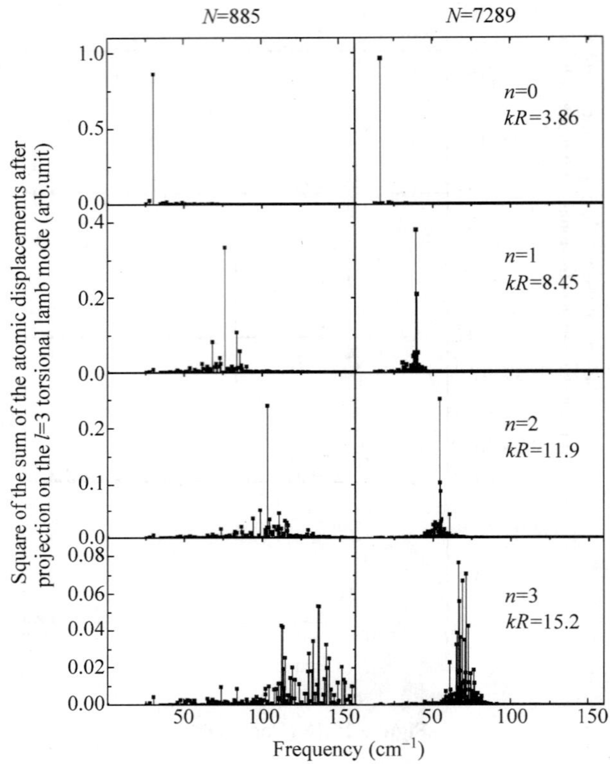

Figure 20.19 MPQ values for ($n=0$, $l=2$), ($n=1$, $l=2$), ($n=2$, $l=2$), and ($n=3$, $l=3$) torsional Lamb modes are compared with theoretical displacements. k is related to the transverse sound velocity; and the $2R$ is the diameter of the NC

In Fig. 20.19, the NC modes of two sizes are projected onto the torsional Lamb modes with different values of n, but the same l ($n=0$, 1, 2, 3 and $l=3$). We can see that the $l=3$ NC mode contains a smaller Lamb mode components as n is increased. Also, as the size of the NC increases, the frequency range with significant Lamb components decreases. This is expected since the larger n is, the larger the Lamb frequency is. In Ge NCs, there is a cutoff for torsional and longitudinal acoustic modes.

The NC modes with the maximum Lamb mode component are chosen as the NC Lamb modes; and their frequencies obey an inverse diameter rule as shown previously (Cheng et al., 2003b).

Because of the stress free boundary condition, the η values of both spheroidal and transverse Lamb modes are quantized as shown in Table 20.2 and Fig. 20.3. In reality the NC are in a matrix that the surfaces are not stress free. Therefore, the η values vary with external stress; and they may change, as shown in Fig. 20.3, and the frequency of the corresponding Lamb modes will also change.

As may be observed in Figs. 20.17 – 20.19, large NCs with low values of n and l exhibit single mode characteristics. One of the reasons for this is that, in Lamb theory, the frequency can have infinite value at large n, but in reality the bulk Ge transverse acoustic phonon cannot have a frequency greater than 100 cm^{-1}. When the NC frequency is greater than the highest transverse phonon frequency of 100 cm^{-1}, it is impossible for the NC torsional Lamb mode to retain the single mode characteristic.

20.4.4 The Radial Distribution Function of Ge Nanocrystals

In order to further understand the correspondence of an NC mode and a Lamb mode, a Radial Distribution Function (RDF) is defined for an NC mode. For a spherical NCs with T_d symmetry, there are a few equivalent N_{shl} atoms for a given radius r. The RDF for an NC mode is determined by summing the squares of the vibration amplitudes over all of the atoms with the same radius and dividing by N_{shl}. The RDF is a quantity that describes the distribution of radial amplitudes; and it is not the same as the conventional definition of the pair correlation function. The RDF for the $n=0$ torsional Lamb mode is $j_l^2(k_l r)$, where $k_1 = 5.75/R$, $k_2 = 2.51/R$, $k_3 = 3.86/R$, where R is the radius of the NC. The calculated RDFs for NCs with 7289 atoms are plotted using black dots in Fig. 20.20 and compared with the analytical results of the Lamb theory (curve). We can see that the general shapes of these two approaches produce similar results and that the RDFs of the VFFM near the surface are higher than the Lamb model values. This occurs because in the VFFM model, atoms near the surface are less restricted than the surface of the continuum model. Some differences of these two approaches are caused by the fact that the summation over discrete lattice points at radius r is not the same as integration over a continuous shell.

20.4.5 Raman Intensities for Ge NC and Lamb modes

Using the bond-polarizability approximation discussed in Section 20.2.3, we have obtained Raman intensities of Ge NCs with between 885 and 7289 atoms. The modes are separated into the A_1, E, and T_2 irreducible representations; and their Raman intensities are shown in Fig. 20.21. The parameters used in these calculations are only valid for the low frequency range; and therefore, our discussion will be limited to this range. After analyzing these results, we have found the selection rules for Raman intensities in NCs, as follows: the $l=0$ spheroidal modes belong to the A_1 representations; and they are allowed for parallel polarizations; the $l=2$ spheroidal modes belong to E and T_2 representations; and they are allowed for perpendicular polarizations.

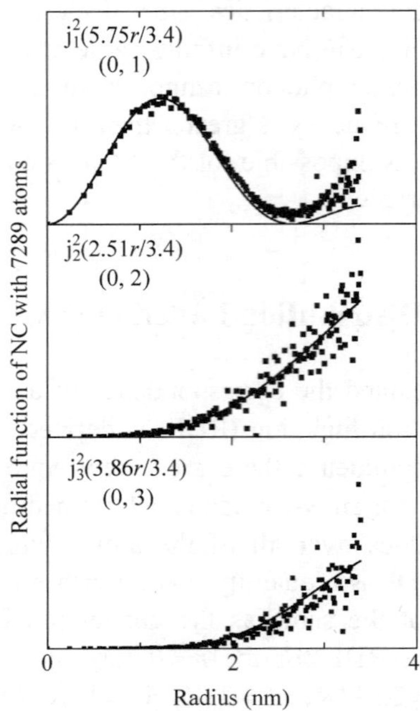

Figure 20.20 The radial amplitude distribution function of three torsional Lamb modes with (n,l) indicated in the plots are shown. These results have been computed for a Ge NC containing 7289 atoms ($R \sim 3.4$ nm). Dots represent the NC data and the curves represent the data from Lamb theory

We notice that in Fig. 20.21(a), the Raman peaks are nearly equally-spaced. As discussed in Section 20.3, this is a result of mode folding. Using the projection technique, we learned that the Raman peaks are from the $n=0$, $n=1,\cdots$ and $l=0$ spheroidal Lamb modes. They are nearly evenly spaced, as indicated by the circles at the left ($l=0$) of Fig. 20.3. In our calculations, all of the low frequency $l=0$ spheroidal Lamb modes can be found in NC modes. In Fig. 20.21(b), the first two Raman peaks of the NC with 7289 atoms are at 11.2 cm^{-1} and 19.1 cm^{-1} ($n=0$ and $n=1$, $l=2$ spheroidal Lamb modes), while the $n=0$ and $l=2$ torsional Lamb mode is at 11.7 cm^{-1}. As shown in Fig. 20.3, the η values of the two modes are nearly the same; and, as a result, the corresponding ω values are nearly the same. From the calculated intensities given in Table 20.5, we find that the $l=2$ torsional Lamb modes are Raman inactive, but the $n=0$, $l=2$ spheroidal Lamb modes that have nearly the same frequencies as the $n=0$, $l=2$ torsional Lamb modes are Raman active in the low frequency range. The results also show that the $l=3$ torsional modes are Raman active, but they are very weak when compared with the spheroidal modes.

Table 20.5 Calculated Raman intensities of some low-frequency modes that were determined using the bond-polarizability model are given

Irreducible representation	Lamb Mode	Frequency (cm^{-1})	Raman Intensity (arb. units)
A_1	$n = 0, l = 0$, spheroidal	19.6	0.904
A_1	$n = 1, l = 0$, spheroidal	47.3	0.237
A_1	$n = 1, l = 0$, spheroidal	48.1	0.316
E	$n = 0, l = 2$, torsional	11.7	0.00136
E	$n = 0, l = 2$, spheroidal	11.2	0.430
T_2	$n = 0, l = 3$, torsional	16.3	0.0197
T_2	$n = 0, l = 2$, spheroidal	12.9	0.686

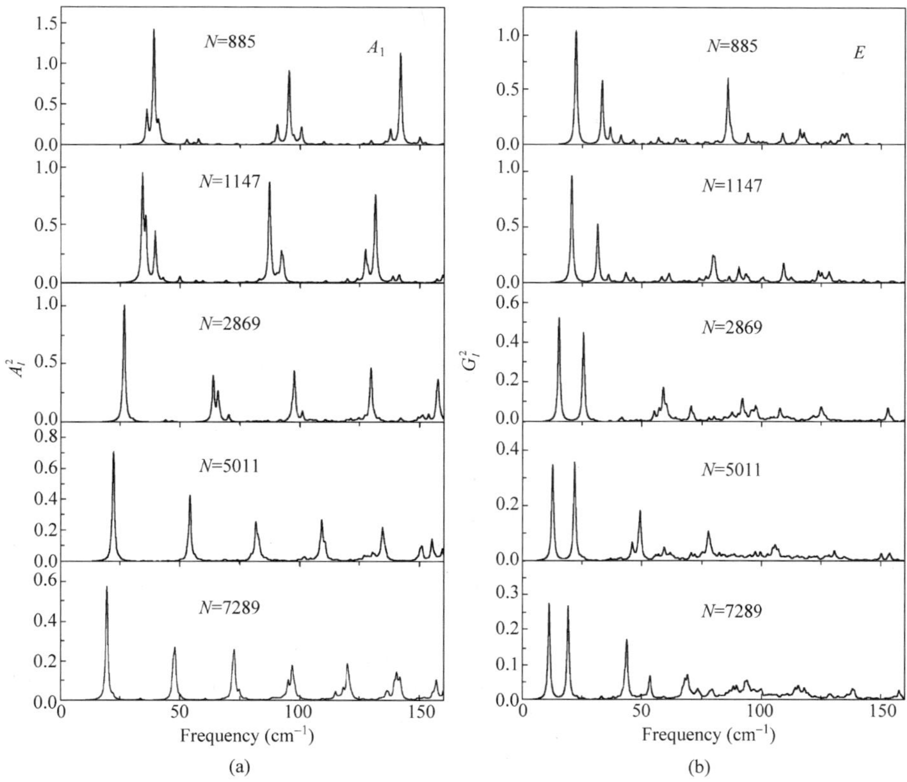

Figure 20.21 Raman intensities (the quantities A_l^2 and G_l^2 are defined in Section 20.2.3 of modes belonging to the (a) A_1, (b) E, and (c) T_2 irreducible representations of the T_d group are plotted

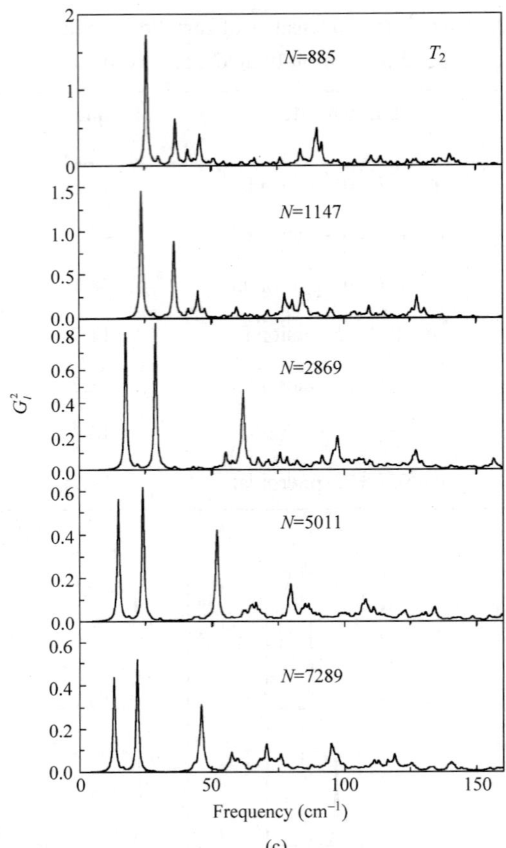

(c)

Figure 20.21 (Continued)

Also, from Table 20.5, we notice the Raman peaks for different polarizations are of the same order. Secondly, there are two NC modes with similar frequencies that have large projections on the $n = 1$, $l = 0$ spheroidal Lamb mode suggesting that this Lamb mode splits into two NC modes for the nanocrystal with $N = 7289$ atoms. Also, the intensity of the torsional $l = 2$ mode is less than that of $l = 3$ mode and the intensity of spheroidal modes are much stronger than torsional modes. The $l = 2$ Lamb modes split into E and T_2 modes with close frequencies in NC, as mentioned above.

Considering Fig. 20.21, we first notice that, in general, the E and T_2 Raman spectra are quite similar, but the frequencies of their Raman peaks are slightly different. This is because they both are derived from spheroidal and torsional $l = 2$ modes. The first two Raman peaks for an NC with 7289 atoms are at 12.9 cm^{-1} and 21.7 cm^{-1} ($n = 0$ and 1 and $l = 2$ spheroidal Lamb modes). The ($n = 0$, $l = 3$) torsional Lamb modes are at 16.3 cm^{-1}. Again this shows that the experimentally observed Raman scattering peak (Ovsyuk et al., 1988) is not from the $l = 3$ torsional modes, but are from the $l = 2$ spheroidal modes.

Returning to Fig. 20.17, we select the modes with largest Raman intensity and project them onto different n and l Lamb modes. There are only a few projections that are close to 1. Considering their transverse speeds of sound, only unique n and l values are obtained from the values represented as squares in Fig. 20.3, if all of the $l = 0$ and 2 spheroidal modes are Raman active. This conclusion does not depend on the microscopic theory. The lowest frequency peaks for the $l = 0$ and $l = 2$ spheroidal modes should be very close because the two numbers ($\eta = 2.46$ for $l = 0$ and $\eta = 2.64$ for $l = 2$) are very close as shown in Fig. 20.17. In the middle of the two peaks, lies the $n = 0$ and $l = 3$ torsional modes, which is close to the measured peak position in the experiments.

This analysis cannot explain a lower peak that was observed using perpendicular polarization (Ovsyuk et al., 1988). One possible explanation is this is a result of torsional modes, which is based on different sound speeds for transverse and longitudinal motions. This is not the result of our calculations, but results from the fact that there are a large number of lattice modes which contribute to the PDOS that are not Raman active. This is especially true for larger NCs. Lattice anharmonicity, which has been neglected in our model, allows the Raman active modes to decay into inactive modes.

From the above discussion, we conclude that the experimental Raman peak in the parallel polarization geometry is due to scattering from the $n = 0$, $l = 0$ spheroidal Lamb mode. The experimental Raman peak in the perpendicular polarization geometry arises from the $n = 0$ and $l = 2$ spheroidal Lamb mode. In principle, this lower-frequency mode may be contaminated by an E symmetry mode, which is allowed for parallel polarization, especially since the experimental spectral resolution in the low-frequency region is often 1 cm^{-1} or larger. As a result, the low-frequency E and T_2 symmetry lattice modes are not resolved. One possible explanation for the polarized nature of the experimental low-frequency mode as compared with our results is that we have neglected the lattice anharmonicity, which may cause the Raman-active $n = 0$ and $l = 2$ spheroidal Lamb mode to decay into the almost degenerate Raman-inactive torsional mode. In our earlier paper (Cheng et al., 2003), we interpreted the Raman peak observed with the crossed polarization as due to the $n = 0$ and $l = 3$ torsional Lamb mode. We now find that the $n = 0$ and $l = 3$ mode may lie close to the measured peak in position, but its strength is too weak to account for the strong experimentally observed Raman peak.

20.5 Conclusions

In this chapter, we have discussed the microscopic theory of phonon modes in semiconducting nanocrystals and shown how to obtain the vibrational dynamical matrix from VFFM theory and how to use projection matrix method to simplify the lattice dynamics matrix. We then discussed bond-charge model and Lamb theory.

Using these theories, we have investigated the vibrational properties of Si and Ge NCs, studied the phonon density of states of both Si and Ge and the Raman intensities of various NCs. The results show that asymmetrical broadening of Raman peaks is due to additional Raman active modes. In the examination of Ge NCs with both fixed and free surfaces, the results show the low-frequency peaks in the Raman spectra are from the free surface.

We have also compared NC modes and Lamb modes. By using the projection method, we demonstrated connections between the two types of phonon modes. For large Ge NCs, each Lamb mode corresponds to a dominant NC mode. For Ge NCs that are less than 4 nm, one Lamb mode degenerates into several NC modes. Finally, we have shown that the experimentally measured, so called transverse low-frequency Raman modes are in fact longitudinal phonon modes with similar frequencies.

Acknowledgements

WC is supported by the National Natural Science Foundation of China under grant Nos. 10575012, 10475009, and 10435020, and he is grateful to Illinois State University for hosting his visit. SFR is supported by the Research Enhancement Award of the College of Arts and Sciences at Illinois State University and the Cottrell College Science Award of the Research Corporation (CC6274).

Appendices

A.1 The Irreducible Matrices of the T_d Group Used in Our Calculations are as Follows

(1) Irreducible matrices for A_1:

$$\Gamma^{(A_1)}(\hat{C}_3)=1,\ \Gamma^{(A_1)}(\hat{C}_2)=1,\ \Gamma^{(A_1)}(\hat{\sigma}_d)=1$$

(2) Irreducible matrices for E:

$$\Gamma^{(E)}(\hat{C}_3)=\begin{pmatrix}\cos\left(\frac{2\pi}{3}\right) & \sin\left(\frac{2\pi}{3}\right)\\ -\sin\left(\frac{2\pi}{3}\right) & \cos\left(\frac{2\pi}{3}\right)\end{pmatrix},\ \Gamma^{(E)}(\hat{C}_2)=\begin{pmatrix}1 & 0\\ 0 & 1\end{pmatrix},\ \Gamma^{(E)}(\hat{\sigma}_d)=\begin{pmatrix}1 & 0\\ 0 & -1\end{pmatrix}$$

(3) Irreducible matrices for T_2:

$$\Gamma^{(T_2)}(\hat{C}_3)=\begin{pmatrix}\cos\left(\frac{2\pi}{3}\right) & -\sin\left(\frac{2\pi}{3}\right) & 0\\ \sin\left(\frac{2\pi}{3}\right) & \cos\left(\frac{2\pi}{3}\right) & 0\\ 0 & 0 & 1\end{pmatrix},\ \Gamma^{(T_2)}(\hat{C}_2)=\begin{pmatrix}\frac{1}{3} & 0 & \frac{2\sqrt{2}}{3}\\ 0 & -1 & 0\\ \frac{2\sqrt{2}}{3} & 0 & -\frac{1}{3}\end{pmatrix}$$

$$\Gamma^{(T_2)}(\hat{\sigma}_d)=\begin{pmatrix}1 & 0 & 0\\ 0 & -1 & 0\\ 0 & 0 & 1\end{pmatrix}$$

(4) Irreducible matrices for A_2:

$$\Gamma^{(A_2)}(\hat{\sigma}_d)=-1$$

The other two matrices are the same as A_1.

(5) Irreducible matrices for T_1:

$$\Gamma^{(T_1)}(\hat{\sigma}_d)=\begin{pmatrix}-1 & 0 & 0\\ 0 & 1 & 0\\ 0 & 0 & -1\end{pmatrix}$$

The other two matrices are the same as T_2.

A.2 Displacements for the $l = 1$ Spheroidal Lamb Modes

(1) $$\boldsymbol{A}_{11}^{(S)}=(x,y,z)xf_1(r),\quad \phi_{11}^{(S)}=g_1(r)x$$

$$\nabla\times\nabla\times\boldsymbol{A}_{11}^{(S)}=\left\{2f_1(r)+r\frac{\mathrm{d}f_1(r)}{\mathrm{d}r}\right\}\boldsymbol{i}-x\frac{\mathrm{d}f_1(r)}{\mathrm{d}r}\left(\frac{x}{r}\boldsymbol{i}+\frac{y}{r}\boldsymbol{j}+\frac{z}{r}\boldsymbol{k}\right)$$

$$\nabla\phi_{11}^{(S)}=g_1(r)\boldsymbol{i}+x\frac{\mathrm{d}g_1(r)}{\mathrm{d}r}\left(\frac{x}{r}\boldsymbol{i}+\frac{y}{r}\boldsymbol{j}+\frac{z}{r}\boldsymbol{k}\right)$$

$$\boldsymbol{D}_{11}^{(S)}=\nabla\phi_{11}^{(S)}+\alpha_1\nabla\times\nabla\times\boldsymbol{A}_{11}^{(S)}$$

(2) $$\boldsymbol{A}_{12}^{(S)}=(x,y,z)yf_1(r),\quad \phi_{12}^{(S)}=g_1(r)y$$

$$\nabla\times\nabla\times\boldsymbol{A}_{12}^{(S)}=\left\{2f_1(r)+r\frac{\mathrm{d}f_1(r)}{\mathrm{d}r}\right\}\boldsymbol{j}-y\frac{\mathrm{d}f_1(r)}{\mathrm{d}r}\left(\frac{x}{r}\boldsymbol{i}+\frac{y}{r}\boldsymbol{j}+\frac{z}{r}\boldsymbol{k}\right)$$

$$\nabla\phi_{12}^{(S)}=g_1(r)\boldsymbol{j}+y\frac{\mathrm{d}g_1(r)}{\mathrm{d}r}\left(\frac{x}{r}\boldsymbol{i}+\frac{y}{r}\boldsymbol{j}+\frac{z}{r}\boldsymbol{k}\right)$$

$$\boldsymbol{D}_{12}^{(S)}=\nabla\phi_{12}^{(S)}+\alpha_1\nabla\times\nabla\times\boldsymbol{A}_{12}^{(S)}$$

(3) $$\boldsymbol{A}_{13}^{(S)}=(x,y,z)zf_1(r),\ \phi_{13}^{(S)}=g_1(r)z$$

$$\nabla\times\nabla\times\boldsymbol{A}_{13}^{(S)}=\left[2f_1(r)+r\frac{\mathrm{d}f_1(r)}{\mathrm{d}r}\right]\boldsymbol{k}-z\frac{\mathrm{d}f_1(r)}{\mathrm{d}r}\left(\frac{x}{r}\boldsymbol{i}+\frac{y}{r}\boldsymbol{j}+\frac{z}{r}\boldsymbol{k}\right)$$

$$\nabla\phi_{13}^{(S)}=g_1(r)\boldsymbol{k}+z\frac{\mathrm{d}g_1(r)}{\mathrm{d}r}\left(\frac{x}{r}\boldsymbol{i}+\frac{y}{r}\boldsymbol{j}+\frac{z}{r}\boldsymbol{k}\right)$$

$$\boldsymbol{D}_{13}^{(S)}=\nabla\phi_{13}^{(S)}+\alpha_1\nabla\times\nabla\times\boldsymbol{A}_{13}^{(S)}$$

$\boldsymbol{D}_{11}^{(S)}$, $\boldsymbol{D}_{12}^{(S)}$, $\boldsymbol{D}_{13}^{(S)}$ belong to the T_2 modes.

where

$$f_1(r)=k\frac{j_1(kr)}{kr},\quad g_1(r)=h\frac{j_1(hr)}{hr}$$

$$\frac{\mathrm{d}f_1(r)}{\mathrm{d}r}=-k^2\frac{j_2(kr)}{kr},\quad \frac{\mathrm{d}g_1(r)}{\mathrm{d}r}=-h^2\frac{j_2(hr)}{hr}$$

$$\alpha_1=\frac{2\xi j_2(\xi)}{[-\eta j_1(\eta)+2j_2(\eta)]\eta}$$

$$D_u^{(1)}\Rightarrow T_2$$

A.3 Displacements for $l=2$ Spheroidal Lamb Modes

(1) $$\phi_{21}^{(S)}=g_2(r)xy,\quad \boldsymbol{A}_{21}^{(S)}=(x,y,z)xyf_2(r)$$

$$\nabla\phi_{21}^{(S)}=g_2(r)y\boldsymbol{i}+g_2(r)x\boldsymbol{j}+xy\frac{\boldsymbol{r}}{r}\frac{\mathrm{d}g_2(r)}{\mathrm{d}r}$$

$$\nabla\times\nabla\times\boldsymbol{A}_{21}^{(S)}=y\left[3f_2(r)+\frac{(r^2-2x^2)}{r}\frac{\mathrm{d}f_2(r)}{\mathrm{d}r}\right]\boldsymbol{i}+$$

$$x\left[3f_2(r)+\frac{(r^2-2y^2)}{r}\frac{\mathrm{d}f_2(r)}{\mathrm{d}r}\right]\boldsymbol{j}-2\frac{xyz}{r}\frac{\mathrm{d}f_2(r)}{\mathrm{d}r}\boldsymbol{k}$$

$$\boldsymbol{D}_{21}^{(S)}=\nabla\phi_{21}^{(S)}+\alpha_2\nabla\times\nabla\times\boldsymbol{A}_{21}^{(S)}$$

(2) $$\phi_{22}^{(S)}=g_2(r)yz\,,\quad \boldsymbol{A}_{22}^{(S)}=(x,y,z)yzf_2(r)$$

$$\nabla\phi_{22}^{(S)}=g_2(r)z\boldsymbol{j}+g_2(r)y\boldsymbol{k}+yz\frac{\boldsymbol{r}}{r}\frac{\mathrm{d}g_2(r)}{\mathrm{d}r}$$

$$\nabla\times\nabla\times\boldsymbol{A}_{22}^{(S)}=-2\frac{xyz}{r}\frac{\mathrm{d}f_2(r)}{\mathrm{d}r}\boldsymbol{i}+z\left[3f_2(r)+\frac{(r^2-2y^2)}{r}\frac{\mathrm{d}f_2(r)}{\mathrm{d}r}\right]\boldsymbol{j}+$$

$$y3\left[f_2(r)+\frac{(r^2-2z^2)}{r}\frac{\mathrm{d}f_2(r)}{\mathrm{d}r}\right]\boldsymbol{k}$$

$$\boldsymbol{D}_{22}^{(S)}=\nabla\phi_{22}^{(S)}+\alpha_2\nabla\times\nabla\times\boldsymbol{A}_{22}^{(S)}$$

(3) $$\phi_{23}^{(S)}=g_2(r)xz\,,\quad \boldsymbol{A}_{23}^{(S)}=(x,y,z)xzf_2(r)$$

$$\nabla\phi_{23}^{(S)}=g_2(r)z\boldsymbol{i}+g_2(r)x\boldsymbol{k}+xz\frac{\boldsymbol{r}}{r}\frac{\mathrm{d}g_2(r)}{\mathrm{d}r}$$

$$\nabla\times\nabla\times\boldsymbol{A}_{23}^{(S)}=z\left[3f_2(r)+\frac{(r^2-2x^2)}{r}\frac{\mathrm{d}f_2(r)}{\mathrm{d}r}\right]\boldsymbol{i}-2\frac{xyz}{r}\frac{\mathrm{d}f_2(r)}{\mathrm{d}r}\boldsymbol{j}+$$

$$x\left[3f_2(r)+\frac{(r^2-2z^2)}{r}\frac{\mathrm{d}f_2(r)}{\mathrm{d}r}\right]\boldsymbol{k}$$

$$\boldsymbol{D}_{23}^{(S)}=\nabla\phi_{23}^{(S)}+\alpha_2\nabla\times\nabla\times\boldsymbol{A}_{23}^{(S)}$$

(4) $$\phi_{24}^{(S)}=g_2(r)[x^2-y^2],\quad \boldsymbol{A}_{24}^{(S)}=(x,y,z)[x^2-y^2]f_2(r)$$

$$\nabla\phi_{24}^{(S)}=2g_2(r)x\boldsymbol{i}-2g_2(r)y\boldsymbol{j}+(x^2-y^2)\frac{\boldsymbol{r}}{r}\frac{\mathrm{d}g_2(r)}{\mathrm{d}r}$$

$$\nabla\times\nabla\times \boldsymbol{A}_{24}^{(S)} = x\left\{3f_2(r)+\frac{2y^2+z^2}{r}\frac{\mathrm{d}f_2(r)}{\mathrm{d}r}\right\}\boldsymbol{i} - y\left\{3f_2(r)+\frac{2x^2+z^2}{r}\frac{\mathrm{d}f_2(r)}{\mathrm{d}r}\right\}\boldsymbol{j} - z\left\{\frac{x^2-y^2}{r}\frac{\mathrm{d}f_2(r)}{\mathrm{d}r}\right\}\boldsymbol{k}$$

$$\boldsymbol{D}_{24}^{(S)} = \nabla\phi_{24}^{(S)} + 2\alpha_2\,\nabla\times\nabla\times \boldsymbol{A}_{24}^{(S)}$$

(5) $\phi_{25}^{(S)} = g_2(r)[2z^2-x^2-y^2],\ \boldsymbol{A}_{25}^{(S)} = (x,y,z)[2z^2-x^2-y^2]f_2(r)$

$$\nabla\phi_{25}^{(S)} = -2g_2(r)x\boldsymbol{i} - 2g_2(r)y\boldsymbol{j} + 4g_2(r)z\boldsymbol{k} + (2z^2-x^2-y^2)\frac{\boldsymbol{r}}{r}\frac{\mathrm{d}g_2(r)}{\mathrm{d}r}$$

$$\nabla\times\nabla\times \boldsymbol{A}_{25}^{(S)} = -\left\{f_2(r)+\frac{z^2}{r}\frac{\mathrm{d}f_2(r)}{\mathrm{d}r}\right\}\boldsymbol{r} + \left\{3zf_2(r)+zr\frac{\mathrm{d}f_2(r)}{\mathrm{d}r}\right\}\boldsymbol{k}$$

$$\boldsymbol{D}_{25}^{(S)} = \nabla\phi_{25}^{(S)} + 6\alpha_2\,\nabla\times\nabla\times \boldsymbol{A}_{25}^{(S)}$$

$\boldsymbol{D}_{21}^{(S)}$, $\boldsymbol{D}_{22}^{(S)}$, and $\boldsymbol{D}_{23}^{(S)}$ belong to the T_2 modes.

$\boldsymbol{D}_{24}^{(S)}$ and $\boldsymbol{D}_{25}^{(S)}$ belong to the E modes.

where

$$f_2(r) = k^2\frac{j_2(kr)}{(kr)^2},\quad g_2(r) = h^2\frac{j_2(hr)}{(hr)^2}$$

$$\frac{\mathrm{d}f_2(r)}{\mathrm{d}r} = -k^3\frac{j_3(kr)}{(kr)^2},\quad \frac{\mathrm{d}g_2(r)}{\mathrm{d}r} = -h^3\frac{j_2(hr)}{(hr)^2}$$

$$\alpha_2 = -\frac{2[j_2(\xi)-\xi j_3(\xi)]}{[6j_2(\eta)+2\eta j_3(\eta)-\eta^2 j_2(\eta)]}$$

$$D_g^{(2)} \Rightarrow E + T_2$$

A.4 Displacements for the $l = 2$ Torsional Lamb Modes

$\boldsymbol{A}_{21} = (x,y,z)j_2(kr)xy/r^2$ $\boldsymbol{D}_{21}^{(T)} = (xz,-yz,(y^2-x^2))j_2(kr)/r^2$

$A_{22} = (x,y,z)j_2(kr)yz/r^2$ $\boldsymbol{D}_{22}^{(T)} = ((z^2-y^2),xy,-xz)j_2(kr)/r^2$

$A_{23} = (x,y,z)j_2(kr)xz/r^2$ $\boldsymbol{D}_{23}^{(T)} = (-xy,(x^2-z^2),yz)j_2(kr)/r^2$

$A_{24} = (x,y,z)j_2(kr)(x^2-y^2)/r^2$ $\boldsymbol{D}_{24}^{(T)} = (-2yz,-2xz,4xy)j_2(kr)/r^2$

$A_{25} = (x,y,z)j_2(kr)(2z^2-x^2-y^2)/r^2$ $\boldsymbol{D}_{25}^{(T)} = (-6yz,6xz,0)j_2(kr)/r^2$

$\boldsymbol{D}_{21}^{(T)}$, $\boldsymbol{D}_{22}^{(T)}$, $\boldsymbol{D}_{23}^{(T)}$ belong to the T_1 modes.

$\boldsymbol{D}_{24}^{(T)}$, $\boldsymbol{D}_{25}^{(T)}$ belong to the E modes.

$D_u^{(2)} \Rightarrow E + T_1$

A.5 Displacements for the $l = 3$ Torsional Lamb Modes

$A_{31} = (x,y,z)j_3(kr)(x^2-y^2)z/r^3$

$\boldsymbol{D}_{31}^{(T)} = ((y^2-x^2-2z^2)y,(x^2-y^2-2z^2)x,4xyz)j_3(kr)/r^3$

$A_{32} = (x,y,z)j_3(kr)(5z^2-3r^2)z/r^3$

$\boldsymbol{D}_{32}^{(T)} = (-3(5z^2-r^2)y,3(5z^2-r^2)x,0)j_3(kr)/r^3$

$A_{33} = (x,y,z)j_3(kr)(5z^2-r^2)x/r^3$

$\boldsymbol{D}_{33}^{(T)} = (-10xyz,(10x^2-5z^2+r^2)z,(5z^2-r^2)y)j_3(kr)/r^3$

$A_{34} = (x,y,z)j_3(kr)(5z^2-r^2)y/r^3$

$\boldsymbol{D}_{34}^{(T)} = ((5z^2-10y^2-r^2)z,10xyz,-(5z^2-r^2)x)j_3(kr)/r^3$

$A_{35} = (x,y,z)j_3(kr)(3xy^2-x^3)/r^3$

$\boldsymbol{D}_{35}^{(T)} = (6xyz,3(x^2-y^2)z,3(y^2-3x^2)y)j_3(kr)/r^3$

$$A_{36} = (x, y, z) j_3(kr)(3x^2 y - y^3) / r^3$$

$$\boldsymbol{D}_{36}^{(T)} = (3(x^2 - y^2)z, -6xyz, 3(3y^2 - x^2)x) j_3(kr) / r^3$$

$$A_{37} = (x, y, z) j_3(kr) xyz / r^3$$

$$\boldsymbol{D}_{37}^{(T)} = (x(z^2 - y^2), y(x^2 - z^2), z(y^2 - x^2)) j_3(kr) / r^3$$

$\boldsymbol{D}_{31}^{(T)}$, $\boldsymbol{D}_{32}^{(T)}$, $\boldsymbol{D}_{33}^{(T)}$, $\boldsymbol{D}_{34}^{(T)}$, $\boldsymbol{D}_{35}^{(T)}$, $\boldsymbol{D}_{36}^{(T)}$ belong to the $T_1 + T_2$ modes.

$\boldsymbol{D}_{37}^{(T)}$ belongs to an A_2 mode.

$$D_g^{(3)} \Rightarrow A_2 + T_1 + T_2$$

A.6 Displacements for the $l = 4$ Torsional Lamb Modes

$$A_{41} = (x, y, z) j_4(kr)(7z^4 - 6z^2 r^2) / r^4$$

$$\boldsymbol{D}_{41}^{(T)} = (8(-7z^2 + 3r^2)yz, -8(-7z^2 + 3r^2)xz, 0) j_4(kr) / r^4$$

Rotate $\boldsymbol{D}_{41}^{(T)}$ along (1,1,1) axis two times we obtain

$$\boldsymbol{D}_{42}^{(T)} = (0, 8(-7x^2 + 3r^2)zx, -8(-7x^2 + 3r^2)yx) j_4(kr) / r^4$$

$$\boldsymbol{D}_{43}^{(T)} = (-8(-7y^2 + 3r^2)zy, 0, 8(-7y^2 + 3r^2)xy) j_4(kr) / r^4$$

$\boldsymbol{D}_{41}^{(T)}$, $\boldsymbol{D}_{42}^{(T)}$, $\boldsymbol{D}_{43}^{(T)}$ belong to A_2+E modes.

$$A_{44} = (x, y, z) j_4(kr)(7z^3 - 3zr^2)x / r^4$$

$$\boldsymbol{D}_{44}^{(T)} = ((3r^2 - 21z^2)xy, (21x^2 z^2 - 7z^4 - 3r^2 x^2 + 3r^2 z^2), (7z^2 - 3r^2)yz) j_4(kr) / r^4$$

Rotating $\boldsymbol{D}_{44}^{(T)}$ along (1,1,1) axis two times we obtain

$$\boldsymbol{D}_{45}^{(T)} = ((7x^2 - 3r^2)zx, (3r^2 - 21x^2)yz, (21y^2 x^2 - 7x^4 - 3r^2 y^2 + 3r^2 x^2)) j_4(kr) / r^4$$

$$\boldsymbol{D}_{46}^{(T)} = ((21z^2 y^2 - 7y^4 - 3r^2 z^2 + 3r^2 y^2), (7y^2 - 3r^2)xy, (3r^2 - 21y^2)zx) j_4(kr) / r^4$$

$$A_{47} = (x, y, z) j_4(kr)(7z^3 - 3zr^2) y / r^4$$

$$\boldsymbol{D}_{47}^{(T)} = ((-21y^2z^2 + 7z^4 + 3r^2y^2 - 3r^2z^2), (-3r^2 + 21z^2)xy, (-7z^2 + 3r^2)xz) j_4(kr) / r^4$$

Rotating $\boldsymbol{D}_{47}^{(T)}$ along (1,1,1) axis two times we obtain

$$\boldsymbol{D}_{48}^{(T)} = ((-7x^2 + 3r^2)yx, (-21z^2x^2 + 7x^4 + 3r^2z^2 - 3r^2x^2), (-3r^2 + 21x^2)yz) j_4(kr) / r^4$$

$$\boldsymbol{D}_{49}^{(T)} = ((-3r^2 + 21y^2)zx, (-7y^2 + 3r^2)zy, (-21x^2y^2 + 7y^4 + 3r^2x^2 - 3r^2y^2)) j_4(kr) / r^4$$

$\boldsymbol{D}_{44}^{(T)}$, $\boldsymbol{D}_{45}^{(T)}$, $\boldsymbol{D}_{46}^{(T)}$, $\boldsymbol{D}_{47}^{(T)}$, $\boldsymbol{D}_{48}^{(T)}$, $\boldsymbol{D}_{49}^{(T)}$ belong to the $T_1 + T_2$ modes.

$$D_u^{(4)} \Rightarrow A_2 + E + T_1 + T_2$$

References

Balandin, A., K. L. Wang, N. Kouklin and S. Bandyopadhyay. *Appl. Phys. Lett.* **76**: 137 (2000).

Bell, R.J. In B. Alder, S. Fernbach, and M. Rotenberg, eds. *Methods in Computational Physics*. New York: Academic p.260 (1976).

Chamberlain, M. P., C. Trallero-Giner and M. Cardona. *Phys. Rev. B* **51**: 1680 (1995).

Champagnon, B., B. Andrianasolo and E. Duval. *Mater. Sci. Eng. B* **9**, 417 (1991).

Cheng, W., S.F. Ren. *Phys. Rev. B* **65**: 205,305 (2002).

Cheng, W., S.F. Ren. *Intern. J. Nanoscience*. **2**: 37 (2003).

Cheng, W, S.F. Ren and P.Y. Yu. *Phys. Rev. B* **68**: 193,309 (2003).

Cheng, W., S.F. Ren and P.Y. Yu. *Phys. Rev. B* **71**: 174,305 (2005a).

Cheng, W., S.F. Ren and P.Y. Yu. *Phys. Rev. B* **72**: 59,901 (2005b).

Cheng, W., S.F. Ren and P.Y. Yu. AIP Conference Proceedings, 772 (2005c).

Cotton, F. A. *Chemical Applications of Group Theory*. New York: Wiley (1971).

Duval, E. Phys. Rev. *B* **46**: 5795 (1992).

Freire, P. T. C., M. A. Araujo Silva, V. C. S. Reynoso, A. R. Vaz and V. L. Lemos. *Phys. Rev. B* **55**: 6743 (1997).

Frohlich, H. *Theory of Dielectrics*. Oxford: Oxford University Press (1949).

Fu, H., V. Ozolins and A. Zunger. *Phys. Rev. B* **59**: 2881 (1999).

Fuchs, R. and K. L. Kliewer *Phys. Rev.* **140**: A 2076 (1965).

Fujii, M., Y. Kanzawa, S. Hayashi and K. Yamamoto. *Phys. Rev. B* **54**: R8373 (1996).

Harrison, W.A. *Electronic Structure and the Properties of Solids*. San Francisico: Freeman (1980).

Klein, M. C., F. Hache, D. Ricard and C. Flytzanis. *Phys. Rev. B* **42**: 11,123 (1990).

Kuok, M. H., H. S. Lim, S. C. Ng, N. N. Liu and Z. K. Wang. *Phys Rev. Lett.* **90**: 255,502 (2003).

Hwang, Y. N., S. Shin, H. L. Park, S. H. Park, U. Kim, H. S. Jeong, E. J. Shin and D. Kim. *Phys. Rev. B* **54**: 15,120 (1996).
Lamb, H. *Proc. London Math. Soc.* **13**: 189 (1882).
Li, W. S. and C. Y. Chen. *Physica B* **229**: 375 (1997).
Ovsyuk, N. N., E. B. Gorokhov, V. V. Grishchenko and A. P. Shebanin. *JETP Lett.* **47**: 298 (1988).
Qin, G. and S.F. Ren. *J. Appl. Phys.* **89**: 6037 (2001).
Qin, G. and S.F. Ren. *Solid State Commun.* **121**: 171 (2002a).
Qin, G., S.F. Ren. *J. Phys.: Condens. Matter* **14**: 8771 (2002b).
Qin, G.Y., S.F. Ren and Z.Y. Zhang. *Commun. Theo. Phys.* **38**: 91 (2002).
Ren, S.F., Z.Q. Gu and D. Lu. *Solid State Commun.* **113**: 273 (2000).
Ren, S.F., D.Y. Lu and G. Qin. *Phys. Rev. B* **63**: 195,315 (2001).
Ren, S.F., G. Qin. *Solid State Commun.* **121**: 171 (2002).
Ren, S.F., W. Cheng. *Phys. Rev. B* **66**: 205,328 (2002).
Ren, S. F., W. Cheng and P. Y. Yu. *Phys. Rev. B* **69**: 235,327 (2004).
Roca, E., C. Trallero-Giner and M. Cardona. *Phys. Rev. B* **49**: 13,704 (1994).
Ruppin, R. and R. Englman. *Rep. Prog. Phys.* **33**: 144 (1970).
Saviot, L., D. B. Murray. *Phys. Rev. B* **72**: 205,433 (2005).
Tanaka, A., S. Onari and T. Arai. *Phys. Rev. B* **47**: 1237 (1993).
Tang, A.C., F.Q. Huang. *Chem. Phys. Lett.* **243**: 387 (1995).
Tang, A.C., F.Q. Huang. *Chem. Phys. Lett.* **263**: 733 (1996a).
Tang, A.C., F.Q. Huang. *Chem. Phys. Lett.* **258**: 562 (1996b).
Tang, A.C., F.Q. Huang. *Intern. J. Quantum Chem.* **63**: 367 (1997).
Teo, K. L., S. H. Kwok, P. Y. Yu and S. Guha. *Phys. Rev. B* **62**: 1584 (2000).
Trallero-Giner, C., F. Garcia-Moliner, V. R. Velasco and M. Cardona. *Phys. Rev. B* **45**: 11,944 (1992).
Trallero-Giner, C., A. Debernardi, M. Cardona, E. Menendez-Proupin and A. I. Ekimov. *Phys. Rev. B* **57**: 4664 (1998).
Yang, Y. M., X. L. Wu, L. W. Yang, G. S. Huang, G. G. Siu and P. K. Chu. *J. Appl. Phys.* **98**: 64,303 (2005).
Yoffe, A.D. *Adv. Phys.* **42**: 173 (1993).
Yoffe, A.D. *Adv. Phys.* **50**: 1 (2001).
Yoffe, A.D. *Adv. Phys.* **51**: 799 (2002).
Yu, P. private communication.
Zi, J., H. Buscher, C. Falter, W. Ludwig, K. Zhang and X. Xie. *Appl. Phys. Lett.* **69**: 200 (1996).
Zi, J., K. Zhang, and X. Xie. *Phys. Rev. B* **58**: 6712 (1998).

21 Fracture Processes in Advanced Nanocrystalline and Nanocomposite Materials

I.A. Ovid'ko

Institute of Problems of Mechanical Engineering, Russian Academy of Sciences, St. Petersburg 199178, Russia

Abstract An overview of experimental data, computer simulations, and theoretical models of fracture processes in nanocrystalline metals and ceramic nanocomposites is presented. The key experimentally detected facts in this area are discussed. Special attention is paid to computer simulations and theoretical models of nucleation of elemental nanocracks/nanovoids in nanocrystalline metals and ceramic nanocomposites. Also, we consider mechanisms for fracture suppression and toughness enhancement in these materials.

21.1 Introduction

Nanocrystalline metals and ceramic nanocomposites often exhibit extremely high strength, superhardness and good fatigue resistance (Koch et al., 1999, Gleiter, 2000; Veprek and Argon, 2002; Kumar et al., 2003a; Milligan, 2003; Valiev, 2004; Gutkin and Ovid'ko, 2004a; Han et al., 2005, Tjong and Chen, 2004; Ovid'ko 2005a, 2005b, Wolf et al., 2005; Meyers et al., 2006; Lu et al., 2006). The outstanding mechanical properties of these materials are desirable for a range of structural, biomedical and other applications; see, e.g. (Gleiter, 2000; Veprek and Argon, 2002; Catledge et al., 2002; Tjong and Chen, 2004; Meyers et al., 2006; Thomas et al., 2006; Webster and Ahn, 2006). At the same time, in most cases, nanocrystalline metals and ceramic nanocomposites show low ductility/ machinability and low fracture toughness, which essentially limit potential of their practical utility. For instance, good machinability and high fracture toughness are of crucial importance for bone tissue engineering applications of nanocrystalline materials (Catledge et al., 2002; Thomas et al., 2006; Webster and Ahn, 2006).

Recently several examples of substantial tensile ductility and even superplasticity of nanocrystalline metallic materials have been reported (Mayo, 1997; Mishra et

(1) Corresponding e-mail: ovidko@def.ipme.ru

al., 1998, 2001; McFadden et al., 1999; Islamgaliev et al., 2001; Valiev et al., 2001, 2002; Mukherjee, 2002; Wang et al., 2002; Champion et al., 2003; Kumar et al., 2003b; He et al., 2003, 2004; Wang and Ma, 2004a; Youssef et al., 2004, 2005, 2006; Zhan et al., 2003a, 2005; Zhan and Mukherjee, 2005; Cheng et al., 2005; Zhou et al., 2005; Hu et al., 2006; Gao et al., 2006). Also, certain progress has been reached in enhancement of fracture toughness of ceramic nanocomposites at comparatively low temperatures (Zhan et al., 2003b; Zhan and Mukherjee, 2004; Xia et al., 2004; Tjong and Chen, 2004). These experimental data serve as a basis for the technologically motivated hopes to develop new superstrong nanocrystalline materials with widely ranging chemical compositions and good machinability/toughness. To do so, of crucial interest are the specific structural features and generic phenomena responsible for optimization of mechanical characteristics (high strength, good ductility, high fracture toughness) of nanocrystalline metals and ceramic nanocomposites. In particular, it is very important to understand the fundamental fracture mechanisms operating in these materials and reveal the sensitivity of fracture processes to their structural and material parameters. The main aim of this chapter is to review experimental research, computer simulations, and theoretical models of fracture of nanocrystalline metals and ceramic nanocomposites. For shorteness, hereinafter nanocrystalline metals and ceramic nanocomposites will be often called nanomaterials.

21.2 Specific Structural Features and Plastic Deformation Behavior of Nanomaterials

The fracture processes in nanomaterials strongly depend on their structural features and phase content. This section briefly describes the specific structural features of single-phase and composite nanocrystalline materials, differentiating them from conventional coarse-grained polycrystals and composites. Also, we discuss the peculiarities of plastic deformation processes affecting fracture of nanomaterials.

First, let us consider the structural features of single-phase nanocrystalline materials, compositionally homogeneous solids consisting of nanoscale grains (nanocrystallites) divided by grain boundaries (Fig. 21.1). Grains are characterized by the grain size $d < 100$ nanometers and have the crystalline structure. In most cases, nanocrystalline materials consist of approximately equiaxed grains with a narrow grain size distribution (Fig. 21.1(a)). At the same time, there are other examples of grain geometry in nanocrystalline materials. For instance, electrodeposited nanocrystalline materials commonly consist of columnar grains (Kumar et al., 2003a, 2003b), while nanocrystalline materials fabricated by the cryomilling method typically have elongated grains with high-angle grain boundaries, which contain equiaxed subgrains with low-angle boundaries (Zghal et al., 2002). Besides, in recent years, nanocrystalline materials with a bimodal structure (consisting of both nanoscopic and microscopic grains) have been fabricated (Fig. 21.1(b)) (Tellkamp et al., 2001, Wang et al., 2002; Zhang et al., 2004; Sergueeva et al., 2004; Wang and Ma, 2004a, 2004b, Han et al., 2006; Fan et al., 2006).

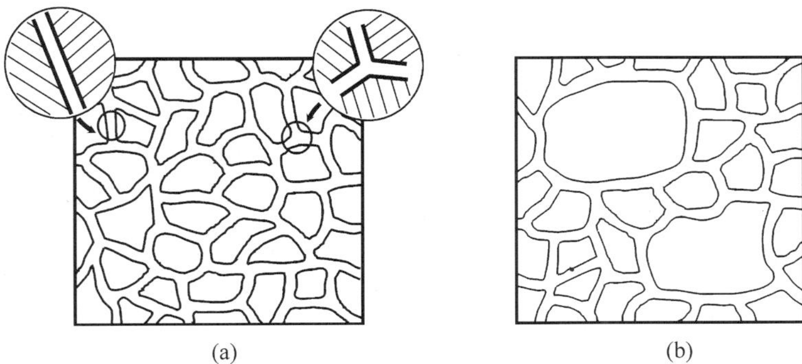

Figure 21.1 Typical single-phase nanocrystalline structures. (a) Nanocrystalline materials consisting of tentatively equiaxed grains (nanocrystallits) of the same phase. Large-scale view of typical structural elements of nanocrystalline materials—short grain boundaries and their triple junctions—are shown in circles in the upper part of figure. (d) Single-phase nanocrystalline materials with bimodal structure, a misture of equiaxed grains with nanoscopic and microscopic sizes

Crystal lattices of grains are misoriented relative each other. Neighboring grains are divided by grain boundaries, plane or faceted layers (with thickness being around 1 nm) that carry a geometric mismatch between adjacent misoriented crystalline grains (Fig. 21.1(a)). Grain boundaries have atomic structure and properties being different from those of grains. In particular, arrangement of atoms in grain boundaries is slightly or essentially disordered compared to that in grain interiors. Grain boundaries join at triple junctions that are tube-like regions with diameter being about 1 – 2 nm (Fig. 21.1(a)). Triple junctions are recognized as line defects with structure and properties commonly being different from those of grain boundaries that they adjoin; see, e.g. (Palumbo and Aust, 1989; King, 1999; Gottstein et al., 2000; Caro and Van Swygenhoven, 2001). With the nanoscale range of grain sizes, both grain boundaries and their triple junctions occupy large volume fractions in nanocrystalline materials and thereby strongly influence the mechanical proprties of these materials.

In general, one can distinguish the following specific structural features of single-phase nanocrystalline materials, differentiating them from conventional coarse-grained polycrystals:

(1) Grains have nanoscopic sizes. Grain size d does not exceed 100 nm.

(2) The volume fractions occupied by grain boundaries and their triple junctions are large in nanocrystalline materials compared to those in coarse-grained

polycrystals. In particular, the volume fraction occupied by grain boundaries is around 10% (or more) in nanocrystalline materials with grain size lower than 10 nm.

(3) Grain boundaries are very short. Grain boundary length does not exceed 100 nm.

Now let us turn to a discussion of the specific structural features of composite nanocrystalline materials, compositionally inhomogeneous solids containing nanoscale grains (nanocrystallites) of at least one component phase. Typical composite nanocrystalline bulk structures are shown in Fig. 21.2. They are a nanocrystalline composite consisting of approximately equiaxed nano-scale grains of different phases (Fig. 21.2(a)); a nanocrystalline composite consisting of grains of one phase, divided by grain boundaries with different chemical composition (second phase) (Fig. 21.2(b)); a nanocrystalline composite consisting of large grains of one phase, embedded into a nanocrystalline matrix of the second phase (Fig. 21.2(c)); a nanocrystalline composite consisting of large grains of one phase with nano-scale particles of the second phase located at grain boundaries between large grains (Fig. 21.2(d)); a nanocrystalline composite consisting of nanocrystallites of one phase, embedded into the amorphous matrix of the second phase (Fig. 21.2(e)); a nanocrystalline composite consisting of grains of two phases, divided by grain boundaries with a different chemical composition (third phase) (Fig. 21.2(f)). These and other typical classes of nanocomposite solids were discussed in detail by Niihara et al. (1993) and Kuntz et al. (2004).

Besides composite nanocrystalline bulk materials (Fig. 21.2), there are layered composite nanocrystalline structures including films and coatings deposited on substrates. In doing so, a substrate material is different from material(s) of either thin film or thick coating deposited onto the substrate. As a corollary, layered nanocrystalline structures are composite, if even a thin film or thick coating is made of single-phase material. Typical layered composite nanocrystalline structures are shown in Fig. 21.3. They are a single-phase nanocrystalline film/coating with approximately equiaxed nano-scale grains on substrate (second phase) (Fig.21. 3(a)); a composite nanocrystalline film/coating consisting of equiaxed nano-scale grains of two phases on substrate (third phase) (Fig. 21.3(b)); a composite nanocrystalline film/coating consisting of second-phase nanoparticles embedded into a film matrix on substrate (third phase) (Fig. 21.3(c)); a multilayered coating consisting of alternate nanocrystalline layers with different chemical compositions on substrate (Fig. 21.3(d)).

It is difficult to identify the generic structural features of nanocomposites, because of their variety (Figs. 21.2 and 21.3). In most cases, however, interphase and grain boundaries occupy large volume fractions in nanocomposites and thereby strongly affect the mechanical and other properties of these materials. Interphase boundaries are always characterized by geometric or, in other words, phase mismatch between different crystalline lattices of different phases matched at these boundaries. In the general situation, interphase boundaries divide misoriented crystallites of different phases. In doing so, interphase boundaries carry both misorientation and phase mismatches between crystallites matched at these boundaries.

The special case is represented by nanomaterials with amorphous intergranular boundaries. For instance, nanocrystalline ceramics typically contain amorphous

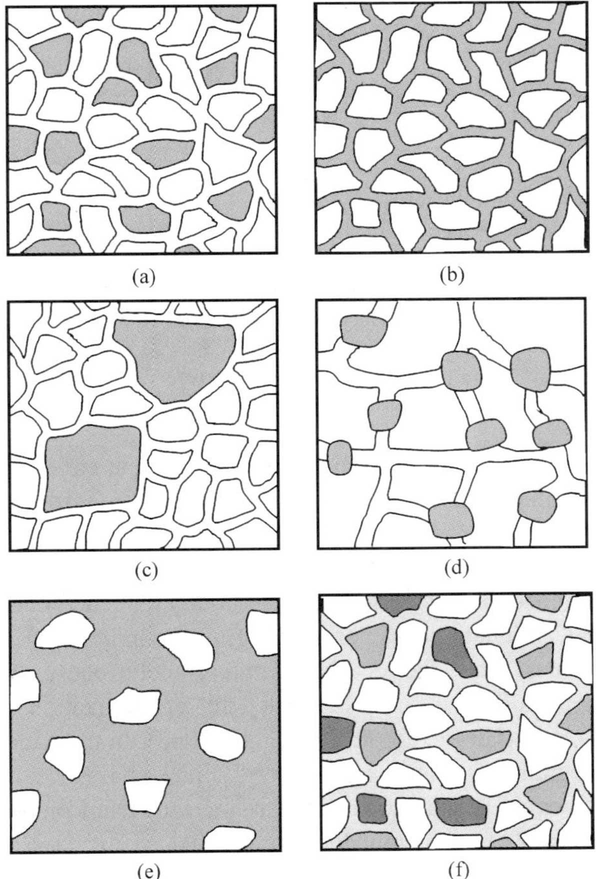

Figure 21.2 Typical composite nanocrystalline bulk structures. (a) nanocrystalline composite materials consisting of tentatively equiaxed nano-scale grains of different phases. (b) nanocrystalline materials consisting of grains of one phase, divided by grain boundaries with different chemical composition (second phase). (c) nanocrystalline composite materials consisting of large grains of one phase, embedded into a nanocrystalline matrix of the second phase. (d) nanocrystalline composite materials consisting of large grains of one phase with nano-scale particles of the second phase located at grain boundaries between large grains. (e) nanocrystalline composite materials consisting of nanocrystallites of one phase, embedded into the amorphous matrix of the second phase. (f) nanocrystalline materials consisting of grains of two phases, divided by grain boundaries with different chemical composition (third phase)

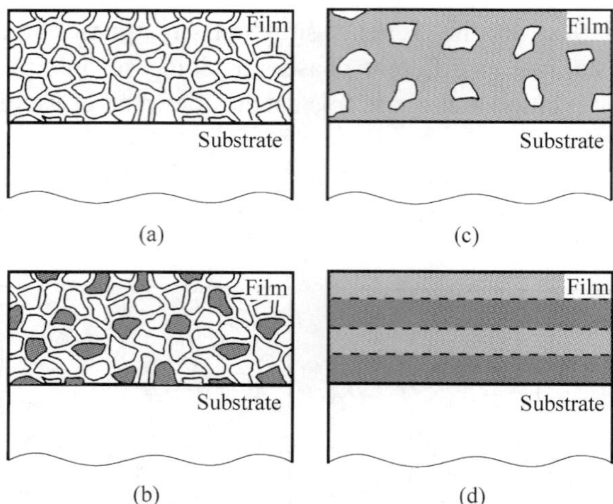

Figure 21.3 Typical nanocrystalline films and coatings: (a) single-phase nanocrystalline film (coating) with tentatively equiaxed nano-scale grains on substrate. (b) composite nanocrystalline film (coating) consisting of tentatively equiaxed nano-scale grains of two phases on substrate. (c) composite nanocrystalline film (coating) consisting of second-phase nanoparticles embedded into a film matrix on substrate. (d) multilayered coating consisting of alternate nanocrystalline layers with different chemical compositions on substrate

interganular boundaries whose chemical composition can either coincide with or be different from that of nanocrystallites. The width of amorphous intergranular boundaries ranges rather widely (from around one to several nanometers) depending on the chemical composition and fabrication conditions. Amorphous triple junctions in such nanoceramics are essentially extended compared to triple junctions of conventional (non-amorphous) grain boundaries in nanocrystalline metals and ceramics. Also, the amorphous intergranular phase often presents in nanocrystalline metallic materials fabricated by crystallization of the initially amorphous materials (Glezer, 1998; Svec et al., 2003). In the nanomaterials with amorphous intergranular boundaries, the crystalline phase occupies the largest part of volume fraction. Besides such materials, there are nanocomposites consisting of the amorphous matrix with embedded nanoparticles (Fig. 21.2(e)) (Calin et al., 2003; Inoue et al., 2005). The amorphous phase in these nanocomposites occupies the largest part of volume fraction.

The structural features and phase content cause significant effects on fracture processes in nanomaterials. In particular, these effects manifest themselves through the effects of both the structural features and phase content on plastic deformation processes that compete and interact with fracture processes in nanomaterials. Let us discuss the plastic deformation behavior of nanomaterials. With nanoscale sizes of grains and the large amount of grain boundaries, the lattice dislocation slip is hampered or even suppressed in nanocrystalline materials. In these circumstances, plastic deformation in nanocrystalline materials is characterized by very high values of the flow stress. These values are very close to those initiating crack nucleation and growth. Therefore, in most cases, nanomaterials tend to show the brittle behavior. Besides the lattice dislocation slip, deformation mechanisms mediated by grain and interphase boundaries contribute to plastic flow in nanomaterials (Koch, 1999; Gleiter, 2000; Veprek and Argon, 2002; Kumar et al., 2003a; Milligan, 2003; Valiev, 2004; Gutkin and Ovid'ko, 2004a; Han et al., 2004; Ovid'ko, 2005a, 2005b; Wolf et al., 2005; Meyers et al., 2006). For instance, the lattice dislocation slip is dominant in nanocrystalline metallic materials with intermediate grains having the size d in the range from d_c to 100 nm, where the critical grain size d_c(10 – 30 nm) depends on material and structure parameters. Basic carriers of the lattice dislocation slip in intermediate grains are perfect and partial dislocations emitted from grain boundaries; see, e.g. (Liao et al., 2003a, 2003b, 2004; Wu et al., 2006). Deformation mechanisms mediated by grain boundaries are dominant in nanocrystalline metallic materials with finest grains having the grain size $d < d_c$. These mechanisms are grain boundary sliding, grain boundary diffusional creep (Coble creep), triple junction diffusional creep, and rotational deformation mode; see, e.g. (Kumar et al., 2003a; Milligan, 2003; Valiev, 2004; Gutkin and Ovid'ko, 2004a; Han et al., 2005; Ovid'ko, 2005a, 2005b; Wolf et al., 2005; Meyers et al., 2006). Plastic deformation at its first stage in nanoceramics predominantly occurs in the interfacial phase; see, e.g. (Veprek and Argon, 2002; Szlufarska et al., 2005). With an increase in the applied stress level, both intergranular and intragranular deformation processes occur in nanoceramics (Szlufarska et al., 2005). Plastic deformation occurring in nanomaterials strongly competes and interacts with fracture processes that will be discussed in detail in next sections.

21.3 Brittle and Ductile Fracture Processes in Nanomaterials

In general, fracture processes involve nucleation, growth and coalescence of cracks/voids in a solid, resulting in its separation into two or more pieces under the action of mechanical stress. Brittle fracture occurs without apparent plastic deformation, in a dramatic way involving fast growth of a large crack or convergence of several cracks. The brittle behavior is commonly undesired for materials used in structural and other applications. Ductile fracture is preceeded by essential plastic deformation, and the ductile behavior of materials is commonly attractive for their practical applications. Ductile fracture occurs through a relatively slow nucleation, growth and coalescence of voids.

The fracture behavior of nanomaterials is not well understood because of its sensitivity to many internal and external factors. Nevertheless, with available experimental data in this area, one can distinguish several tendencies in the fracture behavior of nanomaterials. First, ceramic nanocomposites are commonly brittle (Veprek and Argon, 2002; Kuntz et al., 2004), as with their coarse-grained counterparts. Fracture of brittle nanoceramics occurs through the multiple generations of intergranular nano/micro-scale cracks and their convergence. Nanocrystaline metals can be either ductile or brittle, depending on both their structural characteristics and the conditions of mechanical loading. In particular, there are several examples of nanocrystaline metallic materials having an average grain size in the range from 20 to 100 nm and showing ductile fracture with preceeding neck formation and dimpled structures at fracture surfaces (Kumar et al., 2003a, 2003b, Li and Ebrahimi, 2004, 2005; Youssef et al., 2004, 2005, 2006; Cheng et al., 2005). The size of the dimples is commonly considerably larger than the grain size, and ductile fracture is viewed to occur through the microvoid coalescence mechanism. One of typical examples of ductile fracture behavior with the dimpled features at the fracture suface is exhibited by bulk nanocrystalline Al-5%Mg alloy specimens under tensile testing (Youssef et al., 2006). These artifact-free Al-5%Mg alloy bulk specimens are characterized by an average grain size of around 26 nm, a relatively narrow grain size distribution, ultrahigh strength (ultimate tensile strength is around 740 MPa) and good tensile ductility (8.5% elongation). The specimens with an average grain size of around 26 nm and a relatively narrow grain size distribution were synthesized by an in situ consolidation mechanical alloying technique (Youssef et al., 2006).

At the same time, there are nanocrystalline metallic materials showing the brittle behavior. For instance, nanocrystalline Ni-15%Fe specimens with an average grain size of around 9 nm (Li and Ebrahimi, 2004, 2005) and fatigued nanocrystalline Ni specimens with an average grain size of around 30 nm (Moser et al., 2006) exhibit intergranular brittle fracture. In these cases, the main brittle crack is treated to be formed through the multiple generations of intergranular nano/micro-scale cracks and their convergence.

Brittle and ductile fracture processes in nanomaterials are crucially influenced by grain boundaries whose amount is very large in these materials. Grainh boundaries serve as preferable places for nanocrack nucleation and growth, because the atomic density is low, and interatomic bonds are weak at boundaries compared to the bulk phase. In the case of ductile fracture carried by microvoid coalescence in nanocrystalline metals, grain boundaries with their high diffusivity enhance the microvoid growth, a process mediated by diffusion. Besides, the extra energy of grain boundaries contributes to the driving force for inergranular fracture with cracks propagating along boundaries and releasing the extra energy, compared to intragranular fracture with cracks propagating through grain interiors. At the same time, grain boundaries are short and curved at numerous triple junctions in nanocrystalline metallic and ceramic materials. Therefore, if cracks tend to nucleate and grow along grain boundaries, geometry of grain boundary ensembles causes restrictions on intergranular fracture processes.

With the large amount of grain boundaries in nanocrystalline metallic and ceramic materials, there is a strong competition between intergranular and intragranular fracture processes. Either one of these processes dominates or they occur in concurrent way in materials, depending on their material and structure parameters as well as on the conditions of loading. Besides, fracture processes in nanocrystalline materials compete and interact with plastic deformation processes that have the unique peculiarities due to both the nanoscale and interface effects. As it was noted in Section 21.2, plastic deformation in nanocrystalline materials occurs at very high stresses close to those initiating crack nucleation and growth processes. Nanomaterials are deformed by lattice dislocation slip and deformation mechanisms mediated by grain and interphase boundaries (Koch, 1999; Gleiter, 2000; Veprek and Argon, 2002; Kumar et al., 2003a; Milligan, 2003; Valiev, 2004; Gutkin and Ovid'ko, 2004a; Han et al., 2004; Ovid'ko, 2005a, 2005b; Wolf et al., 2005; Meyers et al., 2006; Lu et al., 2006). For instance, the lattice dislocation slip is dominant in nanocrystalline metallic materials with intermediate grains, while deformation mechanisms (e.g. grain boundary sliding, Coble creep, rotational deformation mode) mediated by grain boundaries are dominant in nanocrystalline metallic materials with finest grains (with $d < d_c$). In the context discussed, one expects that fracture processes in a nanocrystalline metallic material are sensitive to the grain size because of its dramatic effect on plastic deformation mode operating and competing with fracture in the material.

Li and Ebrahimi (2004, 2005) reported that reduction in grain size causes a shift in fracture mode, from ductile mode, for nanocrystalline Ni with mean grain size around 44 nm, to brittle fracture, for nanocrystalline Ni-15%Fe alloy with mean grain size around 9 nm. These experimental results are indicative of the unique fracture behavior of nanocrystalline fcc metals showing ductile-to-brittle transition, in contrast to coarse-grained fcc metals that always exhibit ductile fracture behavior. It should be noted, however, that the discussed experiments dealt with the materials—pure Ni and Ni-15%Fe alloy—having different chemical compositions. Therefore, the shift in fracture mode (Li and Ebrahimi, 2004, 2005) is influenced by both the grain size and chemical composition effects. In these circumstances, the grain size effect can not be unambigiously identified. Nevertheless, the grain refinement commonly leads to increase in the flow stress. (One exception is the case of inverse Hall-Petch relationship demonstrated by nanocrystalline metallic materials with the grain size lower than 10 – 15 nm (see, e.g. reviews Kumar et al., 2003a; Meyers et al., 2006; Gutkin and Ovid'ko, 2004a). In these circumstances, with reduction in grain size, values of the flow stress become closer to those needed to induce fast fracture processes, and fracture mode tends to shift from slow ductile mode to fast brittle fracture. It is just a tendency (but not a rule) that needs further investigation.

Besides grain size, other factors strongly affect fracture in nanocrystalline materials. In particular, crack nucleation and propagation can be dramatically enhanced due to fabrication-produced pores and contaminations. This effect of artifacts has been demonstrated in the experiments (Hugo et al., 2003) dealing with fracture of nanocrystalline Ni films fabricated by DC magnetron sputtering and pulsed laser deposition. Following Hugo et al. (2003), the nanocrystalline Ni film material fabricated by DC magnetron sputtering and characterized by a narrow distribution in grain size (with an average grain size of around 19 nm) contains pores and behaves in a brittle manner, with failure occurring via rapid coalescence of intergranular cracks. At the same time, the nanocrystalline Ni film material fabricated by pulsed laser deposition and characterized by a narrow distribution in grain size (with an average grain size of around 17 nm) is free from pores and behaves in a ductile manner, with failure occurring via slow ductile crack growth (Hugo et al., 2003).

Also, Ebrahimi et al. (2006) have experimentally revealed a ductile-to-brittle transition in nanocomposite layered structures. In particular, copper/siver nanolayered composites with bilayer thickness of $\lambda = 110$ nm ($\lambda_{Cu} = 90$ nm, $\lambda_{Ag} = 20$ nm) were fabricated using electrodeposition techniques. As-fabricated specimens and specimens after 6 hours annealing at 100℃ and 150℃ were mechanically tested (for details, see Ebrahimi et al., 2006). These specimens have differences in the microstructure and fracture behavior. The microstructure of as-fabricated multilayer composite consists of columnar copper nanoscale grains having with around 20 nm and length equal to layer thickness (90 nm). Annealing leads to an increase in the copper grain size. In particular, the increase was pronounced, and signs of silver layer spherodization was found in specimens annealed at 150℃ (Ebrahimi et al., 2006). In mechanical tests, as-fabricated and 100℃ annealed specimens showed the brittle behavior with layers of copper and silver detected easily at fracture surfaces (Figs. 21.4(a) and (b)). At the same time, near the edges of these specimens, where the constraint through the width of the specimen was lost, extensive necking was observed and fracture resembled a microvoid coalescence mechanism. The 150℃ annealed specimens showed the ductile fracture behavior with the dimpled structures at fracture surfaces (Fig. 21.4(c)) (Ebrahimi et al., 2006). These experimental results demonstrated a ductile-to-brittle transition in the copper/silver layered nanocomposites, with sensitivity of the fracture behavior to their microstructure (influenced by annealing) as well as a change in the stress state from plane-strain to plane-stress.

To summarize, with available experimental data, one can distinguish several tendencies in the fracture behavior of nanomaterials. First, nanocrystalline materials are deformed at very high stresses close to those initiating crack nucleation and growth. Therefore, nanocrystalline materials tend to show the brittle behavior. For instance, a ductile-to-brittle transition is experimentally detected in fcc nanocrystalline metals (Li and Ebrahimi, 2004, 2005; Ebrahimi et al., 2006), in contrast to their coarse-grained counterparts which are always ductile. In general, nanocrystaline metals with various crystal lattices (fcc, bcc, hcp) can be either ductile or brittle, depending on both their structural characteristics and the conditions of mechanical loading. Ceramic nanocomposites are commonly

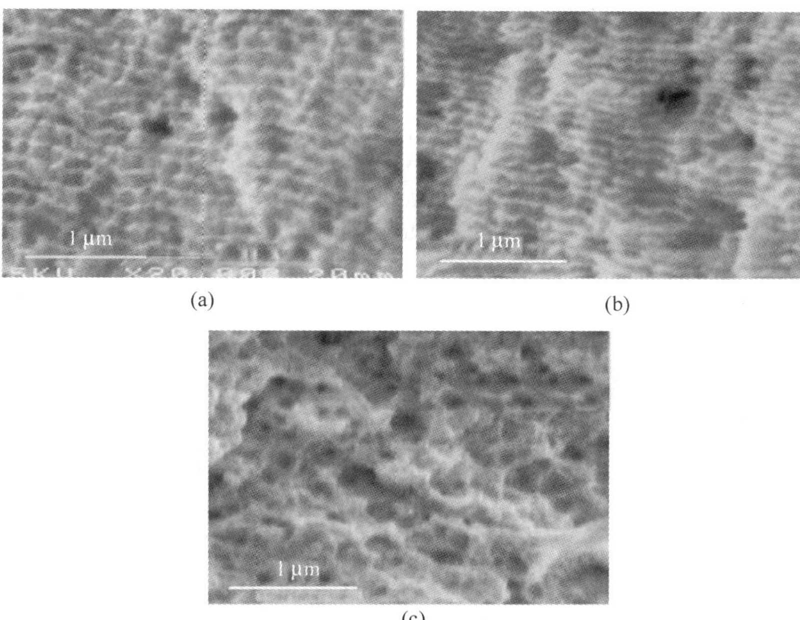

(a) (b) (c)

Figure 21.4 Scanning electron microscope micrographs showing the fracture surfaces of the Cu/Ag nanolayered specimens in (a) as-deposited, (b) annealed at 100 ℃ and (c) annealed at 150 ℃. (Reprinted from Reviews on Advanced Materials Science, Volume 13, F. Ebrahimi, A.J. Liscano, D. Kong, Q. Zhai and H.Li. Fracture of bulk face centered cubic (fcc) metallic nanostructures, Pages 33 – 40, Copyright (2006), with permission from Advanced Study Center)

brittle (Veprek and Argon, 2002; Kuntz et al., 2004; Cheng et al., 2005), as with their coarse-grained counterparts. Brittle fracture of nanomaterials occurs through the multiple generations of intergranular nano/micro-scale cracks and their convergence. Ductile fracture of nanomaterials occurs through the nucleation, growth and coalescence of microvoids whose typical size is commonly considerably larger than the grain size.

21.4 Nucleation of Nanocracks at Grain Boundaries and Their Triple Junctions

To understand the specific fracture behavior of the nanomaterials, results of microstructural experimental characterization of these materials under mechanical load are of crucial importance. Following experimental data by Kumar et al. (2003b), nanovoids in ductile nanocrystalline Ni commonly nucleate and grow at grain boundaries and their triple junctions during tensile deformation (Fig. 21.5). In these experiments, nanocrystalline Ni specimens (with an average grain size of around 30 – 40 nm and a narrow grain size distribution) fabricated by electrodeposition were subjected to tensile tests performed in situ in the transmission electron microscope (TEM). Damage evolution at the nanoscale level in these specimens is presented in Fig. 21.5 showing a sequence of in situ TEM images of the microstructure of a nanocrystalline Ni specimen during plastic deformation. As follows from the images (Fig. 21.5), grain boundaries and their triple junctions serve as preferred places for nucleation of nanoscale voids in vicinity of a large crack. The large crack grows along grain boundaries and absorbs the nanovoids (Fig. 21.5).

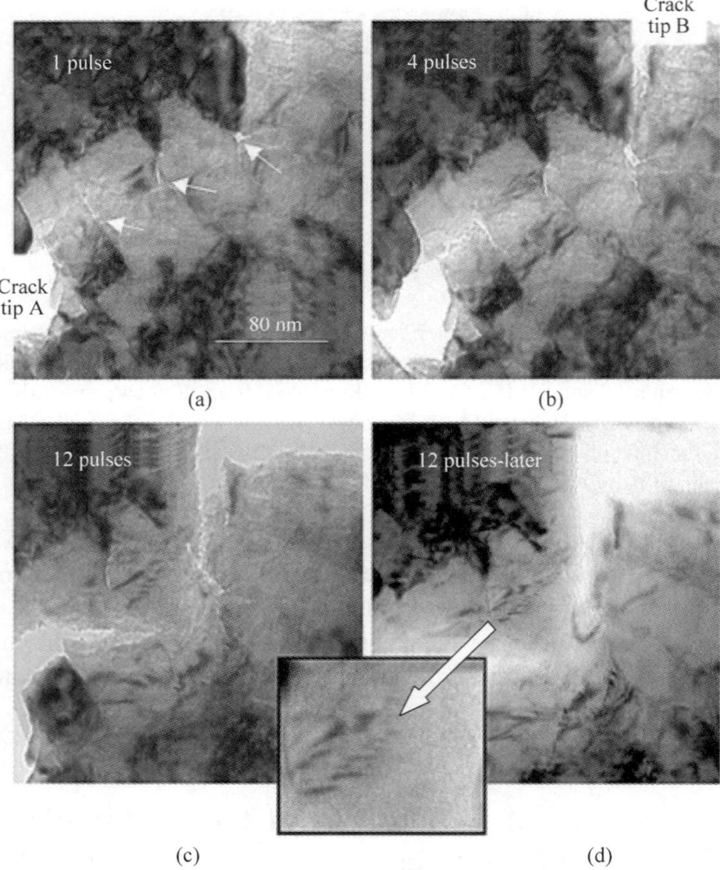

Figure 21.5 Sequence of freeze-frame images captured during an in situ deformation test in the transmission electron microscope of a nanocrystalline Ni specimen. Images (a) – (d) show the microstructural evolution and progression of damage with an increase in the plastic strain induced by applied displacement pulses. The presence of grain boundary cracks and triple-junction voids (indicated by white arrows in (a)), and their growth in (b) – (d) are shown. The magnified inset in (d) highlights the dislocation activity. (Reprinted from Acta Materialia, Volume 51, Kumar K.S., S. Suresh, M.F. Chisholm, J.A. Horton, P. Wang P. Deformation of electrodeposited nanocrystalline nickel, Pages 387 – 405, Copyright (2003), with permission from Elsevier)

A similar view on nanocale fracture processes in nanocrystaline metals is given by molecular dynamics simulations (Van Swygenhoven et al., 2003; Latapie and Farkas, 2004). These simulations show that nanocracks tend to be generated at triple junctions of grain boundaries near tips of pre-existent large cracks in nanocrystalline Ni and nanocrystalline α-Fe with grain size ranging from 5 to 12 nm and from 6 to 12 nm, respectively. In the context discussed, with a very high volume fraction of triple junctions of grain boundaries in nanomaterials, nanocracks at triple junctions can be treated as typical elemental carriers of fracture in such materials. This causes particular interest in understanding the mechanisms for nanocrack generation at triple junctions and their correlation with plastic deformation processes mediated by grain boundaries.

In paper (Ovid'ko and Sheinerman, 2004a), a theoretical model has been suggested describing nucleation and growth of nanocracks at triple junctions in nanocrystalline materials in which grain boundary sliding essentially contributes to plastic flow. Grain boundary sliding commonly occurs by either local shear events (Sutton and Balluffi, 1996; Conrad and Narayan, 2000; Bobylev et al., 2006) or movement of grain boundary dislocations (Sutton and Balluffi, 1996, Fedorov et al., 2003; Gutkin et al., 2004a, 2004b) and leads to accumulation of sessile dislocations at triple junctions (Gutkin et al., 2004b; Bobylev et al., 2006). In the case of dislocation mode of grain boundary sliding, mobile grain boundary dislocations (with the Burgers vectors parallel to grain boundary planes) move causing the sliding in a mechanically loaded specimen (Fig. 21.6(a)). They are stopped at triple junctions of grain boundaries, where boundary planes are curved and thereby dislocation movement is hampered (Fig. 21.6(a)). Further movement of grain boundary dislocations needs an increase of the applied stress. When the applied stress increases, grain boundary dislocations reach a triple junction and come into dislocation reaction resulting in the formation of a sessile dislocations at the junction (Fig. 21.6(b)) (Gutkin et al., 2004; Bobylev et al., 2006). This process is an elementary act of (super)plastic deformation involving grain boundary sliding in nanocrystalline materials where amount of triple junctions is large. The process repeatedly occurs in a deformed nanocrystalline specimen and gives rise to an increase of the Burgers vector of the sessile dislocation (Figs. 21.6(c), (d) and (e)). (Also, accumulation of the sessile dislocations at triple junctions occurs in a similar way in the situation where grain boundary sliding is carried by local shear events (Bobylev et al., 2006)) Following Ovid'ko and Sheinerman (2004a), a nanocrack at the triple junction is generated to release the strain energy of the sessile dislocation when its Burgers vector magnitude achieves a critical value (Fig. 21.6(f) and (g)). In doing so, the nanocrack may nucleate either in the grain interior (Fig. 21.6(f)) or along a grain boundary adjacent to the triple junction (Fig. 21.6(g)).

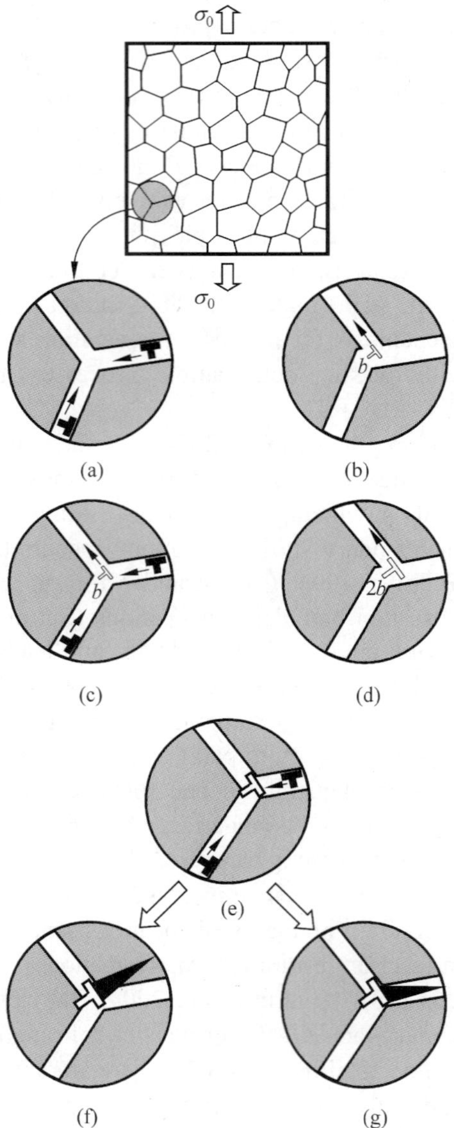

Figure 21.6 Nucleation of a triple junction nanocrack in a nanocrystalline specimen. Grain boundary sliding causes (a) – (e) formation of triple junction dislocation whose stress field induces generation of nanocrack either (f) in grain interior or (g) along a grain boundary

In general, the energetically favorable generation of a crack/nanocrack is characterized in the first approximation by its equilibrium length L_e; see, e.g. Indenbom, (1961); Gutkin and Ovid'ko (1994); Ovid'ko and Sheinerman (2004a). The equilibrium length L_e of a nanocrack is defined as the nanocrack length corresponding to the maximum or minimum energy of the system. In the first case, a nanocrack tends to rapidly grow (shrink), if its length L is larger (lower, repectively) than the equilibrium length L_e. That is, the equilibrium state of the nanocrack with the length $L = L_e$ is unstable. In the second case (the system energy has a minimum at $L = L_e$), the generation and growth of a nanocrack with the length $L < L_e$ are energetically favorable until its length L reaches L_e. That is, the equilibrium state of the nanocrack with the length $L = L_e$ is stable. This case includes, in particular, the generation and growth of a triple junction nanocrack (Figs. 21.6 (f) and (g)). These processes are energetically favorable, if the nanocrack length L is lower than the equilibrium length L_e. The equilibrium state of the triple junction nanocrack with the length $L = L_e$ is stable, because the dislocation stress field rapidly falls with increasing distance from the dislocation line, while the external stress weakly influences the nanocrack generation (Ovid'ko and Sheinerman, 2004a).

The notion of a nanocrack (or, more generally, crack) has its sense when the nanocrack length is larger than some critical minimum length L_c at which the binding between the atoms of the opposite surfaces of the nanocrack is completely broken. (L_c is around $5a = 15b$, where a is the crystal lattice parameter.) In this context, the generation of a nanocrack is treated to occur, if its equilibrium length $L_e > L_c$. In the opposite case ($L_e < L_c$), the binding between the atoms of the opposite surfaces of the nanocrack causes it to shrink and disappear.

Ovid'ko and Sheinerman (2004a) calculated the dependences of the equilibrium length L_e of a nanocrack at a dislocated triple junction on the parameter n, the number of passes of mobile grain boundary dislocations through the triple junction. These dependences are shown in Fig. 21.7, for the shear stress $\tau = 0.01G$, the Poisson ratio $\nu = 0.3$ and different values of the angle α_1 between the nanocrack plane and one of grain boundary planes. As follows from Fig. 21.7, the equilibrium length L_e rapidly increases with rising parameter n in both the cases of the nanocrack growing in the grain interior and along a grain boundary. The dashed horizontal line in Fig. 21.7 corresponds to the critical minimum length $L_c = 15b$ of a nanocrack. The points where this horizontal line intersects the curves L_e (n) correspond to the values of n at which the nanocracks are generated. These values are close to 5, indicating that a stable nanocrack is nucleated at a triple junction after just several (about 5) acts of the grain boundary dislocation transformation (Fig. 21.6) have occurred at the triple junction.

Following calculations (Ovid'ko and Sheinerman, 2004a), the equilibrium length L_e rapidly falls with increasing the free surface energy density γ_e. In general, the equilibrium length L_e^{gb} of a nanocrack nucleating along a grain boundary plane can be either larger or lower than the equilibrium length L_e^{vol} of a nanocrack nucleating in grain interior. The former case ($L_e^{gb} > L_e^{vol}$) is realized at large values of the grain boundary energy density γ_s. In doing so, the nucleation of the triple junction nanocrack growing along a grain boundary is energetically preferred compared to the nanocrack growing in the grain interior. The second case ($L_e^{gb} < L_e^{vol}$) is realized at low values of γ_s. In this case, the nucleation of the triple junction nanocrack growing in the grain interior is preferred.

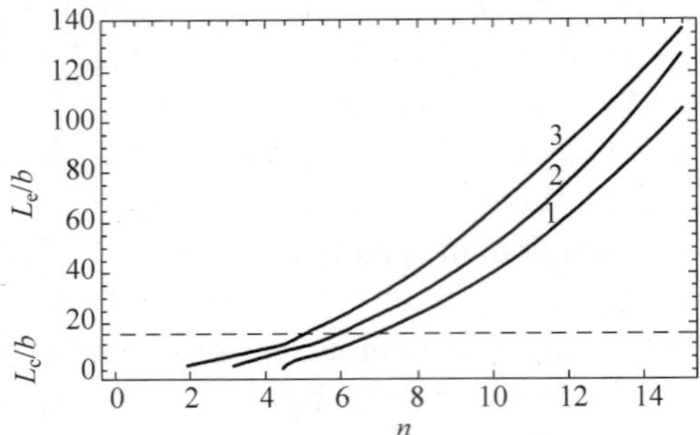

Figure 21.7 Dependencies of non-dimensional equilibrium nanocrack length L_e/b on parameter n, for the applied shear stress $\tau = 0.01G$, $\nu = 0.3$; $\alpha_1 = -\pi/3$, 0 and $2\pi/3$ (see curves 1, 2 and 3, respectively). The dashed horizontal line corresponds to the minimum critical length $L_c = 15b$ at which the nanocrack is generated. (Reprinted from *Acta Materialia*, Volume 52, I.A. Ovid'ko, A.G. Sheinerman. Triple junction nanocracks in deformed nanocrystalline materials, Pages 1201 – 1209, Copyright (2004), with permission from Elsevier)

We have considered the nucleation of nanocracks at triple junctions of grain boundaries in nanocrystalline materials in the situation where grain boundary sliding effectively operates. Recently, theoretical models (Ovid'ko and Sheinerman, 2006a, 2006b) have been suggested describing the generation and evolution of nanovoids at grain boundaries in such nanocrystalline materials. In particular, in the framework of the model (Ovid'ko and Sheinerman, 2006a), nanovoids are generated in the stress fields of dipoles of dislocations characterized by large Burgers vectors and formed at both grain boundary steps and junctions due to intensive grain boundary sliding (Fig. 21.8).

The theoretical models (Ovid'ko and Sheinerman, 2004a, 2006a) account for experimental observation (Kumar et al., 2003b) of nanocracks nucleated at grain boundaries and their triple junctions in deformed nanocrystalline Ni specimens exhibiting a substantial ductility. These specimens were fabricated by elecro-deposition methods, taking care about absence of nanocracks and nanovoids in the as-prepared state. Therefore, nanocracks observed by Kumar et al. (2003b) in in-situ experiments during plastic deformation in nanocrystalline Ni are induced by deformation processes. Notice that the models (Ovid'ko and Sheinerman, 2004a, 2006a) predict a certain stability of nanocracks generated at grain boundaries and their triple junctions in deformed nanocrystalline materials. This prediction is in agreement with experiments (Kumar et al., 2003b) in which a good ductility of nanocrystalline Ni and a non-catastrophic character of failure processes have been detected.

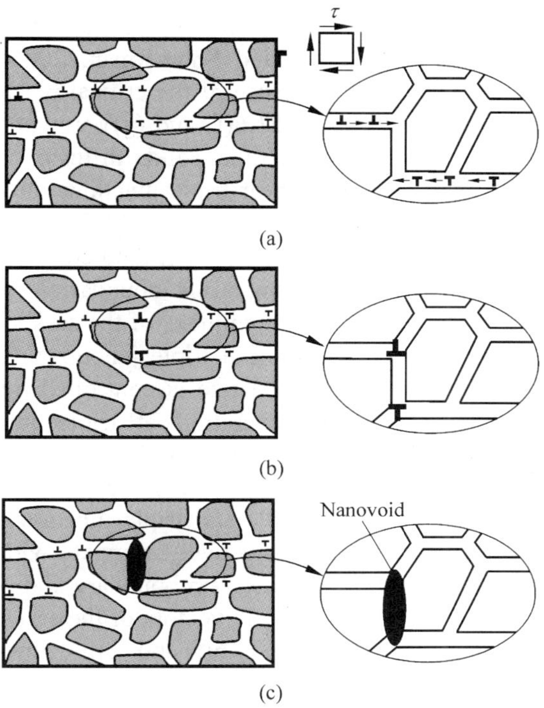

Figure 21.8 Grain boundary sliding (a) is carried by grain boundary dislocations and (b) causes the formation of dipole of dislocations with large Burgers vectors at a grain boundary step. (c) Stress fields of dislocations at grain boundary step induce the generation of nanovoid

Generally speaking, the nanocrack generation can be suppressed in nanomaterials showing good ductility or superplasticity. The suppression is naturally attributed to the effects of diffusion on the generation of triple junction nanocracks treated as typical elemental carriers of fracture in nanomaterials (Ovid'ko and Sheinerman, 2005). Diffusivity of nanocrystalline materials is highly accelerated, because of accelerated diffusivity along grain boundaries (compared to the bulk diffusivity) whose amount is large in such materials. Besides, grain boundary diffusion can be highly enhanced in deformed materials due to the action of lattice dislocation slip which 'supplies' dislocations to grain boundaries where these trapped dislocations climb, split into grain boundary dislocations and annihilate. These transformations of dislocations cause the intensive generation of excess grain boundary point defects that carry diffusion in grain boundaries; see, e.g. (Ovid'ko and Reizis, 2001; Ovid'ko and Sheinerman, 2003; Perevezentsev et al., 2005). The accelerated grain boundary diffusion gives rise to the three following effects responsible for suppression of nucleation of triple junction nanocracks: (1) The enhanced diffusion provides both intensive flow of vacancies from the local regions where high tensile stresses of the sessile triple junction dislocations exist and intensive flow of interstitial atoms in the opposite direction (Fig. 21.9).

In these circumstances, the tensile stresses, in part, are relaxed, and the nucleation of nanocracks is hampered (Ovid'ko and Sheinerman, 2005). The discussed effect of diffusion gives rise to an increase of the critical plastic strain value at which triple junction nanocracks (Fig. 21.6(f) and (g)) are generated. In certain ranges of parameters of a nanocrystalline solid, diffusion is able of even suppressing the nanocrack generation near triple junctions during the extensive stage of plastic deformation (Ovid'ko and Sheinerman, 2005). (2) Sessile dislocations formed at triple junctions due to grain boundary sliding come into reactions with dislocations that intensively climb along grain boundaries. These dislocation reactions diminish the Burgers vector magnitudes of the sessile dislocations and thereby decrease the stress concentration at triple junctions. Consequently, the grain boundary dislocation climb, whose rate is controlled by grain boundary diffusion, hampers the nanocrack generation at triple junctions of grain boundaries (Ovid'ko and Sheinerman, 2004b). (3) The enhanced grain boundary diffusion provides the effective action of Coble creep (Masumura et al., 1998; Kim et al., 2000; Yamakov et al., 2002) and triple junction diffusional creep (Fedorov et al., 2002) which thereby effectively compete with grain boundary sliding. Consequently, the contribution of grain boundary sliding to plastic flow decreases, in which case growth of Burgers vectors of the sessile dislocations—nuclei of triple junction nanocracks (Fig. 21.6(f) and (g))—slows down or stops.

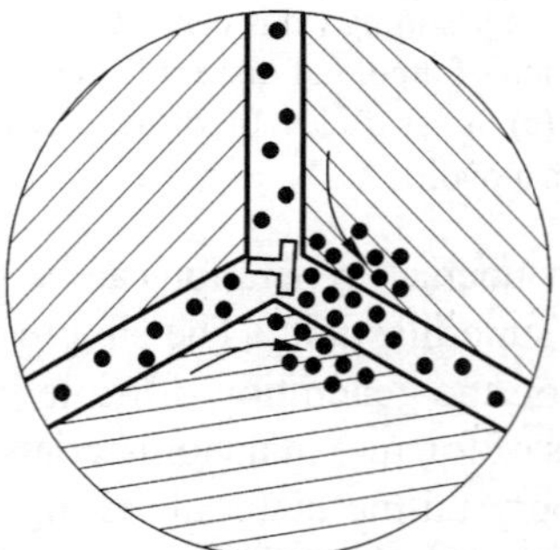

Figure 21.9 Diffusional flow of interstitial atoms causes a partial relaxation of tensile stresses created by triple junction dislocation

It is natural to think that the three effects (1) – (3) of grain boundary diffusion (enhanced owing to the action of conventional lattice dislocation slip) give rise to superplasticity exhibited by some nanocrystalline materials with intermediate grains. In doing so, the combined action of lattice dislocation slip and grain boundary sliding as dominant deformation modes is crucial. These deformation modes cause mutually consistent plastic flow of both grain interiors and grain boundaries. In addition, the lattice dislocation slip provides bombardment of grain boundaries by lattice dislocations which lead to enhancement of boundary diffusion. The enhanced diffusion suppresses nucleation of grain-boundary-sliding-induced nanocracks in nanocrystalline materials which thereby can exhibit a good ductility or even superplasticity (for details, see Ovid'ko and Sheinerman, 2005). In particular, the discussed theoretical representations about the diffusion effects on ductility/superplasticity of nanocrystalline materials are indirectly supported by the experimental data (Islamgaliev et al., 2001) showing degradation of superplastic properties of nanocrystalline materials after a short thermal treatment. More precisely, Islamgaliev et al. (2001) reported that nanocrystalline materials fabricated by severe plastic deformation method and then subjected to a short heat treatment do not show superplastic behavior, in contrast to as-fabricated materials. In the experiment (Islamgaliev et al., 2001), heat treatment is not intensive enough to cause grain growth but is sufficient to induce annihilation of the non-equilibrium grain boundary vacancies generated in nanocrystalline materials during their fabrication by severe plastic deformation. In terms of the model (Ovid'ko and Sheinerman, 2005), after heat treatment, the density of grain boundary vacancies abruptly decreases and thereby the grain boundary diffusion (occurring mostly by vacancy transport) becomes a low-intensity process which is not able to suppress the nanocrack nucleation. As a result, though a nanocrystalline specimen in its as-fabricated state shows superplasticity, heat treatment leads to its dramatic degradation.

Similar effects of diffusion can enhance ductility of materials with bimodal structure; see, e.g. (Han et al., 2006). In general, a material with bimodal structure consists of either ultrafine-grained or nanocrystalline matrix and large (micron-sized) grains embedded into the matrix (Tellkamp et al., 2001; Wang et al., 2002; Wang and Ma, 2004a; Zhang et al., 2004; Sergueeva et al., 2004; Han et al., 2006; Fan et al., 2006). Such materials are often characterized by both high strength and good ductility; for a review, see (Han et al., 2005). Recently Han et al. (2006) have experimentally revealed that a decrease of plastic strain rate in mechanical tests enhances ductility of bimodal 5083 Al alloys processed by cryomilling. Also, they found that the higher ductility at lower strain rate is caused by effective diffusion-mediated stress relaxation, which hamper microcrack nucleation and growth.

To summarize, nanocracks at triple junctions of grain boundaries serve as typical elemental carriers of fracture in nanocrystalline materials. They are generated due to grain boundary sliding which effectively operates in nanomaterials. The triple junction nanocracks are stable against their rapid growth and thereby can conduct ductile fracture. The nucleation of nanocracks can be effectively suppressed by diffusion in nanomaterials showing good ductility or superplasticity.

21.5 Intergranular Brittle Fracture Through Nucleation and Convergence of Nanocracks in Nanomaterials

The behavior of nanocracks and plastic flow processes under mechanical load are responsible for the fracture mode operating in a nanocrystalline specimen. In most cases, nanomaterials are brittle. In doing so, flat nanocracks are generated along grain boundaries in the specimen at the first stage of loading, (Fig. 21.10 (a)). Plastic flow is not intensive in brittle nanomaterials, and the flat nanocracks serve as dangerous stress concentrators inducing new flat nanocracks to be generated in their vicinities (Figs. 21.10(b) and (c)). Then nanocracks located in one specimen section fastly converge resulting in brittle intergranular fracture through the formation of a catastrophic crack (Fig. 21.10(d)).

If plastic flow and diffusion are intensive, as-generated flat nanocracks (Fig. 21.10(a)) are gradually transformed into nanovoids (Fig. 21.10(e)). Nanovoids grow and are transformed into microvoids (Fig. 21.10(f)). Then ductile fracture occurs though both plastic flow localization and coalescence of microvoids located in one section of a nanocrystalline specimen (Fig. 21.10(g)).

In the context discussed, besides the generation of individual nanocracks, their convergence is expected to strongly influence the brittle fracture behavior of nanomaterials. In a paper (Morozov et al., 2003), a theoretical model was suggested focusing on intergranular brittle fracture associated with evolution of nanocrack ensembles in mechanically loaded nanocrystalline materials. In the framework of this model, events of the nanocrack convergence in a nanocrystalline solid are described as elemental events of a percolation process resulting in the formation of catastrophic macroscale crack and separation of the solid into two pieces.

Following the model by Morozov et al. (2003), let us consider a nanocrystalline solid under tensile stress σ_0. At some critical values of the external stress, nanocracks—elemental carriers of intergranular brittle fracture—are formed in the mechanically loaded nanocrystalline solid (Fig. 21.10(a)). Following Veprek and Argon (2002), it is assumed that stable nanocracks are formed along grain boundaries and do not penetrate into grain interiors. In doing so, with nanoscopic scales of nanocracks at grain boundaries and large angles made by adjacent grain boundary planes at triple junctions, the formation of a flat nanocrack at a grain boundary is assumed to be independent of the events of the formation of a nanocrack at any other grain boundaries. Consequently, when the external stress increases, new stable flat nanocracks at grain boundaries are formed (Fig. 21.10(b) and (c)). Then the formation of a macroscopic crack—a carrier of the catastrophic failure—occurs (Fig. 21.10(d)) which results from elementary independent events of the formation of flat nanocracks at grain boundaries of a quasi-statically loaded nanocrystalline solid.

The macroscopic crack formation under consideration is a partial case of percolation described by the standard mathematical methods of the theory (Ziman, 1979; Stauffer and Aharony, 1992; Sahimi, 1994) of percolation in physical systems. Using these methods, Morozov et al. (2003) theoretically described evolution of the nanocrack ensemble in a deformed nanocrystalline solid. In doing so, according to the general representations of the percolation theory (Ziman, 1979; Stauffer and Aharony, 1992; Sahimi, 1994), the macroscopic

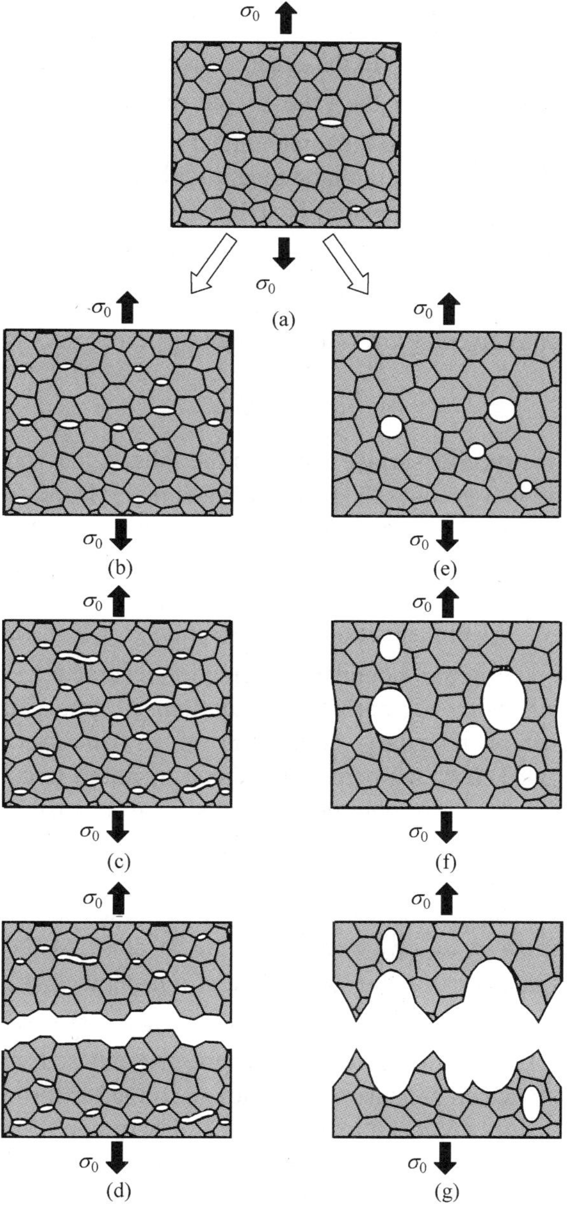

Figure 21.10 Intergranular brittle fracture and ductile fracture modes in nanocrystalline materials (schematically): (a) flat nanocracks are generated along grain boundaries in the specimen at the first stage of loading. (b) and (c) flat nanocracks serve as dangerous stress concentrators inducing new flat nanocracks to be generated in their vicinities. (d) formation of a catastrophic crack through convergence of nanocracks. (e) – (g) ductile fracture in nanocrystalline material occurs through formation of nanocracks, their transformation into pores, growth of pores and formation of local necks between large pores (microvoids)

crack is supposed to be formed when the concentration ρ of stable nanocracks reaches some critical value $\rho_{c.}$ (In the situation under consideration, the nanocrack concentration ρ is defined as the ratio of the number of grain boundaries at which nanocracks are formed to the total number of grain boundaries.)

A nanocrack of length d at a grain boundary with length d and normal n (vetor perpendicular to the boundary plane) is stable, if $\sigma_{nn} \geqslant \sigma_c(d)$. Here σ_{nn} is the stress tensor component at the boundary, and σ_c (a) is the critical normal stress characterizing the formation of a stable nanocrack. The critical stress $\sigma_c(d)$ in the first approximation is given by Griffith's formula; see, e.g. Veprek and Argon (2002):

$$\sigma_c(d) = k(\gamma E / d)^{1/2} \tag{21.1}$$

where γ denotes the specific surface energy of the solid, E the Young modulus, and k the factor taking into account the nanocrack geometry. Here, for simplicity, one considers the only normal failure mode Ⅰ, neglecting the shear fracture mode Ⅱ.

For a grain boundary (and, therefore, a nanocrack formed at this boundary) whose plane has the normal n making the angle α with axis x, we have: $\sigma_{nn} = \sigma_0$ (cos $\alpha)^2$. In this situation, the condition $\sigma_{nn} \geqslant \sigma_c(d)$ is sensitive to both grain size and grain boundary orientation characterized by a and α, respectively. With both log-normal distribution in grain size and random distribution in grain boundary orientation in a nanocrystalline specimen, Morozov et al. (2003) used the percolation theory methods to calculate the stress $\sigma_{catastrophic}$ at which a catastrophic crack results from independent events of the nucleation of stable nanocracks. The main result of these calculations is that the distributions in grain size and grain boundary orientation, inherent to nanocrystalline solids, do not essentially influence the macroscopic crack formation in the solid. Values of the stress $\sigma_{catastrophic}$ were found to be close to the critical normal stress $\sigma_c(\langle d \rangle)$ characterizing the stable state of a nanocrack at a grain boundary with the length equal to the mean grain size $\langle d \rangle$. That is, the crucial effect on the macroscopic crack formation is due to the mean grain size which causes the stress $\sigma_{catastrophic}$ at which a catastrophic crack is formed (Morozov et al., 2003). The percolation theory approach to a theoretical description of fracture processes in nanocrystalline materials is worth being developed in the future to take into account both the interaction between nanocracks and plastic flow effects.

21.6 Crack Growth in Nanomaterials. Toughening Mechanisms

There is considerable interest in developing new nanocrystalline metals and ceramic nanocomposites with outstanding mechanical properties (superior strength, fracture toughness, ductility, etc.) for various engineering and biomedical applications. Of crucial importance is their fracture toughness, the resistance of a material against growth of a pre-existent crack. In this section, we consider experimental data, computer simulations and theoretical models of crack growth processes and toughening mechanisms operating in nanomaterials.

Computer simulations (Farkas et al., 2002; Van Swygenhoven et al., 2003) of crack growth in nanocrystalline Ni with grain size ranging from 5 to 12 nm show the intergranular fracture to be dominant. Intergranular nanocracks at grain boundaries and their triple junctions are found to be generated near the tip of a pre-existent crack (a semi-infinite crack artificially formed in a nanocrystalline simulation block in its initial state) due to stress concentration at the tip. The crack grows by joining the nanocracks at grain boundaries and their triple junctions in its front. In the situation where the pre-existent crack ends at a triple junction in a nanocrystalline Ni sample with the grain size $d = 5$ nm, at the first stage of loading, the crack tip remains at the triple junction, and blunting is observed (Farkas et al., 2002). With increase of the applied mechanical stress, two new nanocracks are formed at a grain boundary located in vicinity of the crack tip. With further increase of the applied mechanical stress, the crack grows (by joining the nanocracks) along a path entirely constituted by grain boundaries. In the situation where the pre-existent crack ends in the grain interior in a nanocrystalline Ni sample with the grain size $d = 10$ nm, the crack emits several partial lattice dislocations that blunt the crack tip region. With increase of an applied load, the stress concentration in vicinity of the crack tip causes the formation of nanocracks ahead of the crack front at neighboring grain boundaries. At later stages of loading, these cracks join the main crack (Farkas et al., 2002).

Following computer simulations (Farkas et al., 2002; Van Swygenhoven et al., 2003), intergranular fracture processes occurring through growth of a pre-existent crack along grain boundaries is characterized by the energy release rate being approximately three times the expected Griffith value for brittle intergranular fracture. It is indicative of a significant role of plastic flow (realized via emission of partial lattice dislocations and structural transformations in grain boundaries) processes in the intergranular fracture observed in computer simulations (Farkas et al., 2002; Van Swygenhoven et al., 2003) of nanocrystalline metals under mechanical load.

Also, toughness of nanocrystalline materials has been theoretically examined in papers (Pozdnyakov, 2003; Pozdnyakov and Glezer, 2005) describing brittle crack growth in such materials. Focuses were placed on the competition between intergranular and intragranular fracture modes. In terms of the surface energy density γ_e and grain boundary energy density γ_s, intragranular and intergranular fracture modes (Figs. 21.11(a) and (b), respectively) in a coarse-grained polycrystal release the specific energies (per unit area of fracture surface) 2γ and $\gamma_e = \eta(2\gamma - \gamma_s)$, respectively, where η is the factor characterizing fracture surface curvature in the case of intergranular fracture. Nanocrystalline materials

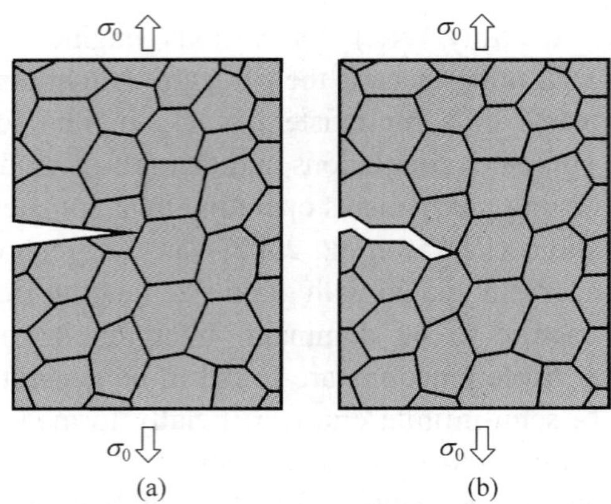

Figure 21.11 Crack growth modes in nanocrystalline materials: (a) for flat cracks and (b) for curved cracks growing along grain boundaries

with the finest grains are specified by very large volume fractions occupied by grain boundaries and their triple junctions. In these circumstances, pure intragranular fracture mode can not be realized. When a flat crack grows in such a material (Fig. 21.11(a)), it propagates through regions occupied by grain interiors, grain boundaries and triple junctions. In doing so, a crack releases the energy density:

$$\gamma_{\text{flat}} \approx f_{\text{b}}\gamma_{\text{e}} + f_{\text{gb}}\gamma_{\text{s}} + f_{\text{tj}}\gamma_{\text{tj}} \tag{21.2}$$

where $f_{\text{b}}, f_{\text{gb}}$ and f_{tj} are the volume fractions occupied by grain interiors, grain boundaries and triple junctions, respectively, and γ_{tj} is the specific energy density of triple junctions. In the context discussed, the toughness of a nanocrystalline sample with a flat crack is characterized by parameter (Pozdnyakov and Glezer, 2005):

$$G_{\text{c}} \approx G_{\text{b}}f_{\text{b}} + G_{\text{gb}}f_{\text{gb}} + G_{\text{tj}}f_{\text{tj}} \tag{21.3}$$

where $G_{\text{b}}, G_{\text{gb}}$ and G_{tj} are the critical energy release rates for the bulk, grain boundary and triple junction phases, respectively.

The models (Pozdnyakov, 2003; Pozdnyakov and Glezer, 2005) are focused on sensitivity of the fracture toughness to volume fractions occupied by grain interiors, grain boundaries and triple junctions in nanomaterials. It is a rather simplified approach taking into account the static structural characteristics $(f_{\text{b}}, f_{\text{gb}}, f_{\text{tj}})$. Also, recently, Gutkin and Ovid'ko (2004b) and Gutkin et al. (2007) have suggested theoretical models describing a change of nanocrack growth direction at triple junctions of interfaces—a critical elemental process of the brittle intergranular fracture—and its sensitivity to static structural characteristics in single-phase nanocrystalline materials and nanocomposites.

At the same time, besides the static structure, plastic deformation processes and structural transformations are known to strongly influence toughness of materials. These aspects have been considered in an excellent review (Zhan and Mukherjee, 2004) focused on toughening mechanisms in ceramic nanocomposites. Following Zhan and Mukherjee (2004), the key problem in structural applications of ceramic nanocomposites (especially for turbo engine parts and pumps, exhaust liners, ship and aerospace hardware) is related to their low fracture toughness and poor machinability. In recent years, however, several examples of enhanced fracture toughness, good machinability and even superplasticity of nanostuctured ceramic composites have been reported; see, e.g. (Zhan et al., 2003b; Xia et al., 2004; Zhan and Mukherjee, 2005a; Zhou et al., 2005; Xu et al., 2006; Gao et al., 2006; Wan et al., 2006). In this context, of particular interest are mechanisms for toughness enhancement in nanostructured ceramic composites serving as strong candidates for use in diverse high technologies. The research of such toughening mechanisms is in its infancy. Therefore, in the rest of this section, we will just briefy discuss mechanisms that potentially can enhance the fracture toughness of ceramic nanocomposites.

In general, one expects conventional and new toughening mechanisms to operate in ceramic nanocomposites. The conventional toughening mechanisms—ductile phase toughening, fiber toughening, transformation toughening, and microcrack toughening—have their analogs operating in microcrystalline ceramics (Zhan and Mukherjee, 2004). At the same time, the action of these conventional mechanisms in nanocomposites has its specific features due to the specific structural features (first of all, the presence of nanoscale crystallites and a large amount of the interfacial phase) of the nanocomposites. For instance, in contrast to ductile micron-sized grains deformed by mostly lattice dislocations that nucleate and move in grain interiors at rather low external stresses, plastic deformation in ductile nanoscale crystallites is often conducted by lattice dislocations emitted from interfaces at high external stresses (see, e.g. reviews by Kumar et al. (2003a), Gutkin and Ovid'ko (2004a), Wolf et al. (2005), Meyers et al. (2006)). Also, phase transformations in zirconia in nanostructured ceramics are highly sensitive to grain-size and interface effects (Shukla and Seal, 2003).

Besides the conventional mechanisms, special (new) toughening mechanisms are expected to effectively operate in ceramic nanocomposites due to the nanoscale and interface effects. In particular, strong candidates for such special mechanisms are the toughening by interface-mediated plastic deformation, the toughening by formation of stable nanocracks, the toughening by local lattice rotation in nanoscale crystallites, the toughening by stress-driven migration of grain boundaries, and the toughening by enhanced interfacial diffusion (Fig. 21.12). The special toughening mechanisms in ceramic nanocomposites should be controlled by processes occurring on the scales of elementary defects carrying plastic flow and fracture. These processes result in nanoscale structural inhomogeneities releasing in part the stresses near the propagating crack tip. In particular, intense interfacial sliding and Coble creep processes carried by interfacial defects as well as transformations of such defects (e.g. nucleation and climb of interfacial dislocations) create nanoscale defect configurations (Fig. 21.12(b) and (c)) whose stress fields in part accommodate the stresses near the propagating crack tip. Also, local lattice rotation in nanoscale crystallites (Fig. 21.12(a)) and stress-driven migration of grain boundaries create nanoscale configurations of disclinations (defects of the rotational type) causing a similar stress relaxation near the propagating crack. All these relaxation mechanisms enhance the toughening behavior of ceramic nanocomposites and are not typical in microcrystalline ceramics. Besides, the stresses near a pre-existent crack propagating in a ceramic nanocomposite can effectively relax through the formation of nanocracks (Fig. 21.12(d) and (e))—elementary carriers of fracture—distant from the crack tip. Such nanocracks nucleate at triple junctions containing defects generated by interfacial sliding and are stable relative either shrinking or further growth. In this case, nanocracks represent stable structural elements that do not converge with the propagating crack, and their formation can be treated as a new toughening mechanism different from the conventional microcrack toughening.

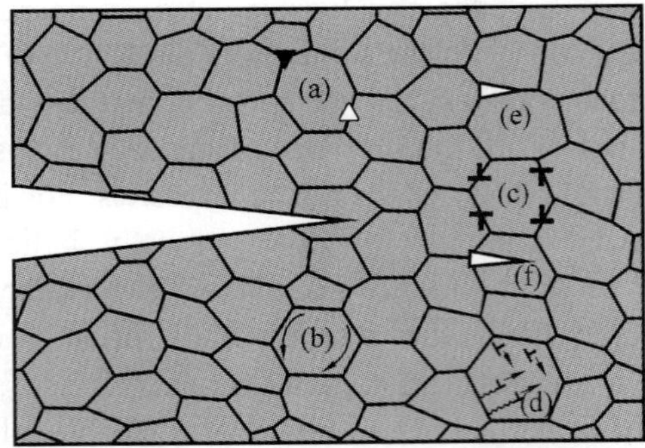

Figure 21.12 Nano-scale processes enhancing the fracture toughness of ceramic nanocomposites (schematically): (a) local lattice rotation in nanoscale crystallites creates disclinations (full and open triangles) whose stress fields in part accommodate stresses near a pre-existent crack tip. (b) enhanced diffusional mass transfer along interfaces. (c) interfacial sliding and transformations of interfacial dislocations structures. (d) nucleation of perfect and partial lattice dislocations at interfaces and their further movement in grain interiors. (e) and (f) formation of stable nanoscale cracks along interface and in grain interior, respectively

We discussed the conventional and new toughening mechanisms as potentially effective in ceramic nanocomposites. Future research efforts in this area should experimentally identify and theoretically describe those mechanisms that really enhance the fracture toughness of ceramic nanocomposites.

21.7 Concluding Remarks

Thus, intergranular brittle fracture and ductile fracture modes were experimentally observed in nanocrystalline materials. Plastic flow in such materials occurs at very high stresses close to those needed to induce fracture. Therefore, nanocracks and nanovoids are easily nucleated in nanocrystalline materials, as with brittle coarse-grained polycrystals (Ashby et al., 1979; Gandhi and Ashby, 1979). Typical elemental carriers of fracture in deformed nanocrystalline materials are nanocracks nucleated at grain boundaries and their triple junctions due to grain boundary sliding (Fig. 21.5). Besides such deformation-produced nanocracks, fabrication-produced nanocracks and pores often exist in these materials and decrease their ductility. Evolution of typical nanocracks and nanovoids in a mechanically loaded nanocrystalline specimen causes fracture mode operating in the specimen and depends on its structural characteristics (first of all, grain size), diffusivity and material parameters.

In nanocrystalline metallic materials with finest grains and nanoceramics, plastic flow (conducted by mostly grain boundary processes) is not intensive. Deformation mechanisms mediated by curved and short grain boundaries in such materials do not provide effective relaxation of stress buildup at grain boundary steps, triple junctions and elemental flat nanocracks. In these circumstances, new flat nanocracks are easily generated at triple junctions due to intergrain sliding and stress concentration at neighboring flat nanocracks (Figs. 21.10(a) – (d)). Consequently, intergranular brittle fracture tends to occur in metallic nanomaterials with finest grains and nanoceramics.

In nanocrystalline metallic materials with intermediate grains, plastic flow is often conducted by both lattice dislocation slip and grain boundary processes. If plastic flow and diffusion are intensive in these materials, they can provide effective relaxation of stress buildup at triple junctions and elemental flat nanocracks. These flat nanocracks gradually transform into ball-like and elliptic pores (Fig. 21.10(e)). Due to their shape geometry, stress concentration at ball-like and elliptic nanopores is not so dramatic compared to flat nanocracks. Consequently, such pores slowly grow (by vacancy coagulation at pores and lattice dislocation emission from pores) and cause ductile fracture (Fig. 21.10(f) and (g)). However, if plastic flow and diffusion are not intensive in nanocrystalline materials with intermediate grains and/or these materials contain pre-existent nanocracks and pores, brittle fracture tends to occur.

The research of mechanisms for toughness enhancement in nanostructured ceramic composites is in its infancy. Conventional and new toughening mechanisms are expected to operate in ceramic nanocomposites. The conventional toughening mechanisms—ductile phase toughening, fiber toughening, transformation toughening, and microcrack toughening—have their analogs operating in microcrystalline ceramics (Zhan and Mukherjee, 2004). Besides, special (new) toughening mechanisms are expected to effectively operate in ceramic nanocomposites due to the nanoscale and interface effects. In particular, strong candidates for such special mechanisms are the toughening by interface-mediated plastic deformation, the toughening by formation of stable nanocracks, the toughening by local lattice rotation in nanoscale crystallites, the toughening by stress-driven migration of grain boundaries, and the toughening by enhanced interfacial diffusion (Fig. 21.12). These mechanisms involve nanoscale processes conducted by mostly interfaces (grain and interphase boundaries) in ceramic nanocomposites and commonly are not effective in microcrystalline ceramics.

Acknowledgements

This work was supported, in part, by the Office of US Naval Research (grant N00014-07-1-0295), INTAS-AIRBUS (grant 04-80-7339), Civilian Research and Development Foundation (grant # RUE2-2684-ST-05), Russian Academy of Sciences Program Structural Mechanics of Materials and Construction Elements, and the National Science Foundation (grant CMMI #0700272).

References

Ashby, M.F., C. Gandhi and D.M.R. Taplin. *Acta Mater*. **27**: 699 (1979).

Bobylev, S.V., M.Yu. Gutkin and I.A. Ovid'ko. *Phys.Rev*. B **73**: 064,102 (2006).

Calin, M., J. Eckert, L. Schultz. *Scr. Mater*. **48:** 653 (2003).

Caro, A. and H. Van Swygenhoven. *Phys.Rev*. B **63**: 134,101 (2001).

Catledge, S.A., M.D. Fries, Y.K. Vohra, W.R. Lacefield, J.E. Lemons, S. Woodard and R. Venugopalan. *J. Nanosci. Nanotechnol*. **2**: 293(2002).

Champion, Y., C. Langlois, S. Guerin-Mailly, P. Langlois, J.-L. Bonnentien and M. Hytch. *Science* **300**: 310 (2003).

Cheng, S., E. Ma, Y.M. Wang, L.J. Kecskes, K.M. Youssef, C.C. Koch, U.P. Trociewitz and K. Han. *Acta Mater*. **53**: 1521 (2005).

Conrad, H. and J. Narayan. *Scr. Mater*. **42**: 1025 (2000).

Ebrahimi, F., A.J. Liscano, D. Kong, Q. Zhai and H.Li. *Rev. Adv. Mater. Sci*. **13**: 33 (2006).

Fan, G.J., H. Choo, P.K. Liaw and E.J. Lavernia. *Acta Mater*. **54**: 1759 (2006).

Farkas, D., H. Van Swygenhoven and P.M. Derlet. *Phys. Rev*. B **66**: 060,101 (2002).

Fedorov, A.A., M.Yu. Gutkin and I.A. Ovid'ko. *Scr. Mater*. **47**: 51 (2002).

Fedorov, A.A., M.Yu. Gutkin and I.A. Ovid'ko. *Acta Mater.* **51**: 887 (2003).

Gan, Y. and B. Zhou. *Scripta Mater*. **45**: 625 (2001).

Gandhi, C. and M.F. Ashby. *Acta Mater*. **27**: 1565 (1979).

Gao, L., X. Jin, J. Li, Y. Li and J. Sun. *Mater. Sci. Eng*. A **415**: 145 (2006).

Gleiter, H. *Acta Mater.* **48**: 1 (2000).
Glezer, A.M. In: G.M. Chow and N.I. Noskova, eds. *Nanostructured Materials: Science and Technology*. Dordrecht: Kluwer, p.163 (1998).
Gottstein, G., A.H. King and L.S. Shvindlerman. *Acta Mater.* **48**: 397 (2000).
Gutkin, M.Yu. and I.A. Ovid'ko. *Phil. Mag.* A **70**: 561 (1994); *Plastic Deformation in Nanocrystalline Materials*. Berlin-Heidelberg-New York: Springer (2004a); *Phil. Mag. Lett.* **84**: 655 (2004b).
Gutkin, M.Yu., I.A. Ovid'ko and N.V. Skiba. *Acta Mater.* **52**: 1711 (2004); *Phys. Sol. State* **49**: 261 (2007).
Han, B.Q., E. Lavernia and F.A. Mohamed. *Rev. Adv. Mater. Sci.* **9**: 1 (2005).
Han, B.Q., J.Y. Huang, Y.T. Zhu and E.J. Lavernia. *Acta Mater.* **54**: 3015 (2006).
Islamgaliev, R.K., R.Z. Valiev, R.S. Mishra and A.K. Mukherjee. *Mater. Sci. Eng.* A **304 – 306**: 206 (2001).
He, G., J. Eckert, W. Loeser and L. Schultz. *Nature Mater.* **2**: 33 (2003).
He, G., M. Hagiwaga, J. Eckert and W. Loeser. *Phil. Mag. Lett.* **84**: 365 (2004).
Hugo, R.C., H. Kung, J.R. Weertman, R. Mitra, J.A. Knapp and D.M. Follstaedt. *Acta Mater.* **51**: 1937 (2003).
Indenbom, V.I. Sov. *Phys. Sol. State* **3**: 1506 (1961).
Inoue, A., W. Zhang, T. Tsurui, A.R. Yavari and A.L. Greer. *Phil. Mag. Lett.* **85**: 221 (2005).
Kim, H.S., Y. Estrin and M.B. Bush. *Acta Mater.* **48**: 493 (2000).
King, A.H. *Interf. Sci.* **7**: 251 (1999).
Koch, C.C., D.G. Morris, K. Lu and A. Inoue. *MRS Bullet.* **24**: 54 (1999).
Kumar, K.S., S. Suresh and H. Van Swygenhoven. *Acta Mater* **51**: 5743 (2003a).
Kumar, K.S., S. Suresh, M.F. Chisholm, J.A. Norton and P. Wang. *Acta Mater.* **51**: 387 (2003b).
Kuntz, J.D., G.-D. Zhan and A.K. Mukherjee. *MRS Bullet.* **29**: 22 (2004).
Latapie, A. and D. Farkas. *Phys. Rev.* B **69**: 134,110 (2004).
Li, H. and F. Ebrahimi. *Appl. Phys. Lett.* **84**: 4307 (2004); *Adv. Mater.* **17**: 1969 (2005).
Liao, X.Z., F. Zhou, E.J. Lavernia, S.G. Srinivasan, M.I. Baskes, D.W. He and Y.T. Zhu. *Appl. Phys. Lett.* **83**: 632 (2003a).
Liao, X.Z., F. Zhou, E.J. Lavernia, D.W. He and Y.T. Zhu. *Appl. Phys. Lett.* **83**: 5062 (2003b).
Liao, X.Z., S.G. Srinivasan, Y.H. Zhao, M.I. Baskes, Y.T. Zhu, F. Zhou, E.J. Lavernia and H.F. Hu. *Appl. Phys. Lett.* **84**: 3564 (2004).
Lu, C., Y.W. Mai and Y.G. Shen. *J. Mater. Sci.* **41:** 937 (2006).
Masumura, R.A., P.M. Hazzledine and C.S. Pande. *Acta Mater.* **46**: 4527 (1998).
Mayo, M.J. *Nanostruct. Mater.* **9**: 717 (1997).
McFadden, S.X., R.S. Mishra, R.Z. Valiev, A.P. Zhilyaev and A.K. Mukherjee. Nature **398**: 684 (1999).
Meyers, M.A., A. Mishra and D.J. Benson. *Progr. Mater. Sci.* **51**: 427 (2006).
Milligan, W.W. In: I. Milne, R. O. Ritchie and B. Karihaloo, eds. *Mechanical Behavior of Bulk Nanocrystalline and Ultrafine-Grain Metals, in Comprehensive Structural Integrity* Amsterdam: Elsevier, p.529 (2003).
Mishra, R.S., R.Z. Valiev, S.X. McFadden and A.K. Mukherjee. *Mater. Sci. Eng.* A **252**: 174 (1998).

Mishra, R.S., R.Z. Valiev, S.X. McFadden, R.K. Islamgaliev and A.K. Mukherjee. *Phil. Mag.* A **81**: 37 (2001).

Morozov, N.F., I.A. Ovid'ko, Yu.V. Petrov and A.G. Sheinerman. *Rev. Adv. Mater. Sci.* **4**: 65 (2003).

Moser, B., T. Hanlon, K.S. Kumar and S. Suresh. *Scr. Mater*. **54**: 1151 (2006).

Mukai, T., S. Suresh, K. Kita, H. Sasaki, N. Kobayashi, K. Higashi and A. Inoue. *Acta Mater.* **51**: 4197 (2003).

Mukherjee, A.K. *Mater. Sci. Eng.* A **322**: 1 (2002).

Niihara, K., A. Nakahira and T. Sekino. In: S. Kormaneni, J.C. Parker and G.J. Thomas, eds. *Nanophase and Nanocomposite Materials*, MRS Symp. Proc. **286** Pittsburg: MRS, p.405 (1993).

Ovid'ko, I.A. and A.B. Reizis. *Phys. Sol. State* **43**: 35 (2001).

Ovid'ko, I.A. and A.G. Sheinerman. *Phil. Mag.* **83**: 1551 (2003); *Acta Mater.* **52**: 1201 (2004a); *Rev. Adv. Mater. Sci.* **6**: 21 (2004b); *Acta Mater.* **53**: 1347 (2005); *Phil. Mag.* **86**: 3487 (2006a); *Phil. Mag.* **86**: 1415 (2006b).

Ovid'ko, I.A. *Int. Mater. Rev.* **50**: 65 (2005a); *Rev. Adv. Mater. Sci.* **10**: 89 (2005b).

Palumbo, G. and K.T. Aust. *Mater. Sci. Eng.* A **113**: 139 (1989).

Perevezentsev, V.N., A.S. Pupynin and J.V. Svirina. *Mater. Sci. Eng.* A **410 – 411**: 273 (2005).

Pozdnyakov, V.A. *Tech. Phys. Lett.* **29**: 151 (2003).

Pozdnyakov, V.A. and A.M. Glezer. *Phys. Sol. State* **47**: 817 (2005).

Rybin, V.V. and I.M. Zhukovskii. *Sov. Phys. Sol. State* **20**: 1056 (1978).

Sahimi, M. *Applications of Percolation Theory*. London: Taylor and Francis (1994).

Sergueeva, A.V., N.A. Mara and A.K. Mukherjee. *Rev. Adv. Mater. Sci.* **7**: 67 (2004).

Shukla, S. and S. Seal. *Rev. Adv. Mater. Sci.* **5**: 117 (2003).

Szlufarska, I., A. Nakano and P. Vashishta. *Science* **309**: 911 (2005).

Stauffer, D. and A. Aharony. *Introduction to Percolation Theory*. London: Taylor and Francis (1992).

Sutton, A.P. and R.W. Balluffi. *Grain Boundaries in Crystalline Materials*. Oxford: Oxford Sci., (1996).

Svec, P., K. Kristiakova and M. Deanko. In: T. Tsakalakos, I.A. Ovid'ko and A.K. Vasudevan, eds. *Nanostructures: Synthesis, Functional Properties and Applications*. Dordrecht: Kluwer, p. 271 (2003).

Tellkamp, V.L., A. Melmed and E.J. Lavernia. *Metall. Mater. Trans.* A **32**: 2335 (2001).

Thomas, J.B., N.A. Peppas, M. Sato and T.J. Webster. In: Y. Gogotsi, ed. *Nanomaterials Handbook*. London: Taylor and Francis, p.605 (2006).

Tjong, S.C. and H. Chen. *Mater. Sci. Eng. R* **45**: 1 (2004).

Valiev, R.Z., C. Song, S.X. McFadden, A.K. Mukherjee and R.S. Mishra. *Phil. Mag. A* **81**: 25 (2001).

Valiev, R.Z., I.V. Alexandrov, Y.T. Zhu and T.C. Lowe. *J. Mater. Res.* **17**: 5 (2002).

Valiev, R.Z. *Nature Mater*. **3**: 511 (2004).

Van Swygenhoven, H., P.M. Derlet, A. Hasnaoui and M. Samaras, In: T. Tsakalakos, I.A. Ovid'ko and A.K. Vasudevan, eds. *Nanostructures: Synthesis, Functional Properties and Applications*. Dordrecht: Kluwer, p.155 (2003).

Veprek, S. and A.S. Argon. *J. Vac. Sci. Technol.* **20**: 650 (2002).

Wan J., R.-G. Duan, M.J. Gasch and A.K. Mukherjee. *J. Amer. Ceram. Soc.* **89**: 274 (2006).

Wang, Y., M. Chen, F. Zhou and E. Ma. *Nature* **419**: 912 (2002).

Wang, Y.M. and E. Ma. *Acta Mater.* **52**: 1699 (2004a); *Appl. Phys. Lett.* **85**: 2750 (2004b).

Webster, T. and E.S. Ahn. *Advances in Biochemical Engineering/Biotecyhnology* **103**: 275 (2006).

Wolf, D., V. Yamakov, S.R. Phillpot, A.K. Mukherjee and H. Gleiter. *Acta Mater* **53**: 1 (2005).

Wu, X.-L., Y.T. Zhu and E. Ma. *Appl. Phys. Lett.* **88**: 121,905 (2006).

Xia, Z., L. Riester, W.A. Curtin, H. Li, B.W. Sheldon, J. Liang, B. Chang and J.M. Xu. *Acta Mater.* **52**: 931 (2004).

Xu, X., T. Nishimura,. N. Hirosaki, R.-J. Xie, Y. Yamamoto and H. Tanaka. *Acta Mater.* **54**: 255 (2006).

Yamakov, V., D. Wolf, S.R. Phillpot and H. Gleiter. *Acta Mater.* **50**: 61 (2002).

Youssef, K.M., R.O. Scattergood, K.L. Murty and C.C. Koch. *Appl. Phys. Lett.* **85**: 929 (2004).

Youssef, K.M., R.O. Scattergood, K.L. Murty, J.A. Horton and C.C. Koch. *Appl. Phys. Lett.* **87**: 091,904 (2005).

Youssef, K.M., R.O. Scattergood, K.L. Murty and C.C. Koch. *Scr. Mater.* **54**: 251 (2006).

Zghal, S., M.J. Hytch, J.-P. Chevalier, R. Twesten, F. Wu and P. Bellon. *Acta Mater.* **50**: 4695 (2002).

Zhan, G.-D., J.D. Kuntz, J. Wan and A.K. Mukherjee. In: C.C. Berndt, T. Fisher, I.A. Ovid'ko, G. Skandan and T. Tsakalakos, eds. *Nanomaterials for Structural Applications*, MRS Symp. Proc. **740**. Warrendale: MRS, p.49 (2003a).

Zhan, G.-D., J.-D. Kuntz, J. Wan and A.K. Mukherjee. *Nature Mater.* **2**: 38 (2003b).

Zhan, G.-D. and A.K. Mukherjee. *Int. J. Appl. Ceram.Technol. Sci.* **1**: 161 (2004); *Rev. Adv. Mater.* Sci. **10**: 185 (2005).

Zhan, G.-D., J.E. Garay and A.K. Mukherjee. *Nano Lett.* **5**: 2593 (2005).

Zhang, X., H. Wang and C.C. Koch. *Rev. Adv. Mater. Sci.* **6**: 53 (2004).

Zhou, X., D.M. Hulbert, J.-D. Kuntz, R.K. Sadangi, V. Shukla, B.H. Kear and A.K. Mukherjee. *Mater.Sci.Eng.* A **394**: 353 (2005).

Ziman J. *Models of Disorder*. Cambridge: Cambridge University Press (1979).

22 Synthesis, Properties and Application of Conducting PPY Nanoparticles

Xingui Li, Meirong Huang and Yunbin Xie

Key Laboratory of Advanced Civil Engineering Materials,
College of Materials Science and Engineering, Tongji University,
Shanghai 200092, China

Abstract The successful fabrication, various structure, unique properties, and wide application potential of novel conducting polypyrrole (PPY) nanoparticles and nanocomposites with an intrinsically electrical conductivity have been systematically reviewed. Wholly new pyrrole (PY) copolymer nanoparticles were synthesized by a chemical oxidative precipitation polymerization from 20 mol% PY and 80 mol% 4-sulfonic diphenylamine (SD) in HCl aqueous solution without any external stabilizer. Their structure and morphology were characterized by laser particle-size analyzer and transmission electron microscopy. Unique effects of polymerization temperature on the polymerization yield, particle size, and bulk electrical conductivity were systematically studied. The number-average diameter of the particles in water depends on the polymerization temperature from 0 to 25℃, reaching a minimum of 78 nm with an extremely low polydispersity index of 1.033 by laser particle-size analyzer. Dry particles exhibit much smaller size of around 10 nm based on a high-resolution transmission electron microscopy observation. The PY/SD(20/80) copolymer has a gradually increased conductivity from 1×10^{-4} to 5×10^{-3} S/cm with lowering polymerization temperature from 25℃ to 0℃. The relatively low purity, poor self-stability, and high cost of the nanoscale PPYs with intrinsic electroconductivity could be overcome by effortlessly incorporating a certain amount of SD comonomer as internal emulsifier during PY polymerization in emulsifier-free HCl aqueous solution.

Keywords polypyrrole, copolypyrrole, conducting nanoparticle, nanotechnology, nanobiomaterial

(1) Corresponding e-mail: adamxgli@yahoo.com

22.1 Introduction

Polypyrrole (PPY) has been most widely studied in recent years (Benabderrahmane et al., 2005) for many potential applications such as antistatics (Bhat and shaikh, 1994), electromagnetic and microwave shieldings (Pomposo et al., 1999), sensors and actuators (Jager et al., 2000), rechargeable batteries (Susumu and Masahide, 2002), supercapacitors, corrosion protection, and anhydrous electrorheological fluids due to its reasonably high conductivity and excellent thermal and environmental stability, as well as easy synthesis. The unique electrical conductivity of PPY is attributed to the electrons hopping along and across the PPY polymer chains with conjugating bonds. As a result, more positively charged PPY, more electron holes available, longer polymer chains and better co-planarity between interchains, are favorable for a higher conductivity performance. However, a lack of processability is one of the major problems associated with practical applications of conductive and electroactive PPY. Besides, pyrrole (PY) monomer is much more expensive than aniline (AN) and its derivatives. Fortunately, their low processibility and high cost of the PY polymers could be easily overcome by simply dispersing a very small amount of their nanoparticles into some traditional polymers. Many attempts, on the one hand, have been made to obtain soluble PPY, including the use of dopants (Lee et al., 1995), the introduction of substituent groups (Kiskan et al., 2005), and the copolymerization with a second comonomer. On the other hand, various kinds of PPY nanomaterials such as nanoparticles (Jang et al., 2002; Shi et al., 2004; Hong et al., 2001), nanotubes (He et al., 2005; Wan et al., 2002), nanowires (Bocharova et al., 2005; C.Jerome, and R. Jérôme, 1998; Zhong et al., 2006; Johnson et al., 2004), nanofibers (Ikegame et al., 2003), nanorods (Maeda et al., 2004), hollow nanosphere (Cheng et al., 2004; Yang and Yu, 2005), nanofilms and nanocomposites (Yang et al., 2006; Xu et al., 2004; Jang and Oh, 2005) have been prepared, looking forward to an integration of their respective advantages of PPY and nanomaterials by a unique way of facilely and greatly improving processibility and largely lowering the cost of PPY. The synthesis of PPY nanoparticles could be traditionally performed by microemulsion and dispersion polymerizations. The PPY nanoparticles could be very useful for the preparation of transparent electrical conducting materials, modified electrode materials, and biologically conductive materials.

22.1.1 Synthesis of PPY Nanoparticles

22.1.1.1 Microemulsion Polymerization

As comparison with conventional emulsion polymerization, microemulsion polymerization could be an omnipotent method due to its fast reaction, small particle size, and narrow size distribution. It is reported that ultrafine PPY particles with the diameter of around 2 nm have been successfully fabricated by the microemulsion polymerization—a surfactant-mediated methodology (Jang et al., 2002). Low polymerization temperature of around 3℃ would be optimal. The effective oxidants are $FeCl_3$ and $(NH_4)_2S_2O_8$, and many traditional cationic surfactants including sodium dodecyl benzene sulfonate, sodium dodecyl sulfonate, octyltrimethylammonium bromide, decyl trimethyl ammonium bromide, and dodecyl trimethyl ammonium bromide would be used in the polymerization. Note that the surfactants with hydrocarbon chains of longer than C16 are not suitable for the microemulsion polymerization due to their liquid-crystalline state and high viscosity. The average size of PPY particles prepared by microemulsion polymerization varied from 149 to 119 to 67 nm with changing polymerization temperature/dodecyltrimethylammonium bromide concentration from 25℃/0.44 M to 3℃/0.44 M to 3℃/0.8 M (Wang et al., 2005). When a fixed low synthesis temperature (3℃) and a high surfactant concentration (0.8 M) were accompanied by a high-speed stirring, an average particle size of 10 – 15 nm of PPY nanoparticles was achievable. Therefore, the polymerization temperature and surfactants should be carefully chosen to efficiently control the morphology and size of nanoparticles because the micells formed by the surfactants can be served as novel nanoreactors whose stabilization can prevent the ultrasmall nanoparticles from conglomeration. The formation mechanism of the nanoparticles is that hydrophobic oligomer radicals formed in aqueous phase could penetrate organic micells and polymerize in site. Apparently, the microemulsion polymerization could be used to synthesize very small and almost monodisperse PPY nanoparticles, as shown in Fig. 22.1(a).

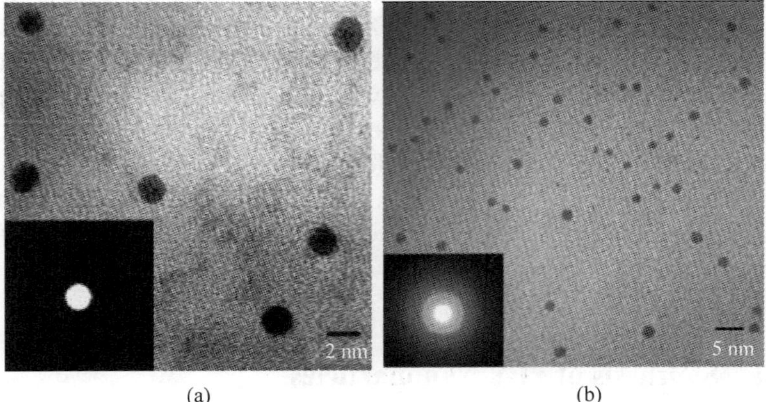

(a) (b)

Figure 22.1 TEM images and nanobeam electron diffraction patterns (inset) of initial PPY nanoparticles (a) and graphite nanoparticles (b) fabricated by the carbonization of the PPY nanoparticles prepared using decyl trimethyl ammonium bromide (0.4 M) (Jang et al., 2002)

Recently, it has been reported that the inner-structure of PPY nanoparticles can be straightly adjusted by a simple alcohol-assisted microemulsion polymerization (Liu et al., 2006). TEM and SEM images suggest that the PPY nanoparticles obtained without using alcohol during the experiment process are basically spherical particles with average particle diameter ranging from 50 to 70 nm. The PPY nanoparticles obtained in the presence of *n*-amyl alcohol are uniform monodisperse particles with average diameter of about 30 nm. The conjugation and order of PPY chains were improved directly in the presence of alcohols and adjusted by the alkyl unit of alcohols. These changes in the molecular structure lead to the improvement in the electrical conductivity of as-prepared PPY nanoparticles obviously. The conductivities of PPY nanoparticles synthesized in the presence of *n*-amyl alcohol, iso-amyl alcohol, *n*-butyl alcohol, iso-butyl alcohol, tert-butyl alcohol, and without alcohol are 9.60, 5.77, 8.72, 5.83, 1.81, and 0.067 S/cm, respectively. However, a large amount of surfactants must be added into the polymerization system, possibly leading to a complicated post treatment procedure, impure nanoparticles, imperfect performance, and also poor redispersancy.

22.1.1.2 Dispersion Polymerization

The main advantage of dispersion polymerization for the preparation of intrinsically electrical conducting PPY nanoparticles is simple preparing technology, controllable particle diameter, and narrow size distribution. Although the oxidants used in the dispersion polymerization are exactly the same as those in the microemulsion polymerization, the dispersion media are generally water or ethanol aqueous solution. The most important additives are disperser or stabilizer such as polyvinyl alcohol and ethyl hydroxyethyl cellulose. During the dispersion polymerization, PY concentration, oxidant and stabilizer species, and polymerization temperature strongly influence the polymerization rate, diameter, and size distribution of the PPY particles formed. The influence of the dispersion polymerization of PY in aqueous PVA solutions on the size of the forming PPY nanoparticles is illustrated in Table 22.1 and Fig. 22.2 (Men'shikova et al., 2003). It is seen that the capability of PVA to stabilize aqueous PPY dispersion largely depends on the molecular weight and acetate group content of the PVA. It seems that the PVA with low molecular weight and low acetate-group content could not successfully stabilize the dispersion of PPY nanoparticles because the nanoparticles may coagulate in the course of the synthesis. Fortunately, high molecular-weight PVA having high acetate-group content at the same concentration efficiently stabilize the dispersion of PPY nanoparticles with a narrow particle-size distribution or even monodispersivity because the more acetate groups may surface-activate the high molecular-weight PVA and then result in a unique amphiphilicity. Therefore, as the PY concentration decreased from 2.7 to 1.0 wt%, PVA content increased from 0.3 to 1.6 wt%, or polymerization temperature rose from 4 to 23℃, the forming PPY particles all become smaller (Table 22.1). Furthermore, a seed dispersion polymerization of PY on Fe_3O_4 nanoparticles in argon allows fabrication of uniform PPY particles with the diameter as small as 20 nm.

Table 22.1 Influence of the reaction mixture composition and temperature in dispersion polymerization of pyrrole in aqueous PVA solution with $FeCl_3$ as oxidant in the air on the diameter of the forming PPY nanoparticles (Liu et al., 2006)

PY(wt%)	Molecular mass	Acetate content of PVA	PVA (wt%)	Reaction temperature (℃)	Diameter of PPY particles (nm)
2.0	17,000	11%	0.6	23	Much bigger
2.0	50,000	10%	0.6	23	80
1.0	50,000	10%	0.9	23	60 – 100
2.7	50,000	10%	0.8	4	60 – 100
1.0	50,000	10%	0.3	4	90
1.0	50,000	10%	0.5	4	90
1.0	50,000	10%	0.8	4	70
1.0	50,000	10%	1.6	4	70
1.0	50,000	10%	0.8	23	60
1.0	50,000	10%	1.6	23	50 – 70
1.4(1)	50,000	10%	0.7	23	30 – 50
1.4(2)	50,000	10%	0.7	23	20 – 40

(1) Seed polymerization of pyrrole on 0.7 wt% Fe_3O_4 nanoparticles in 0.28 M HCl solutions in the air;

(2) Seed polymerization of pyrrole on 0.7 wt% Fe_3O_4 nanoparticles in 0.28 M HCl solutions in the argon before adding pyrrole monomer.

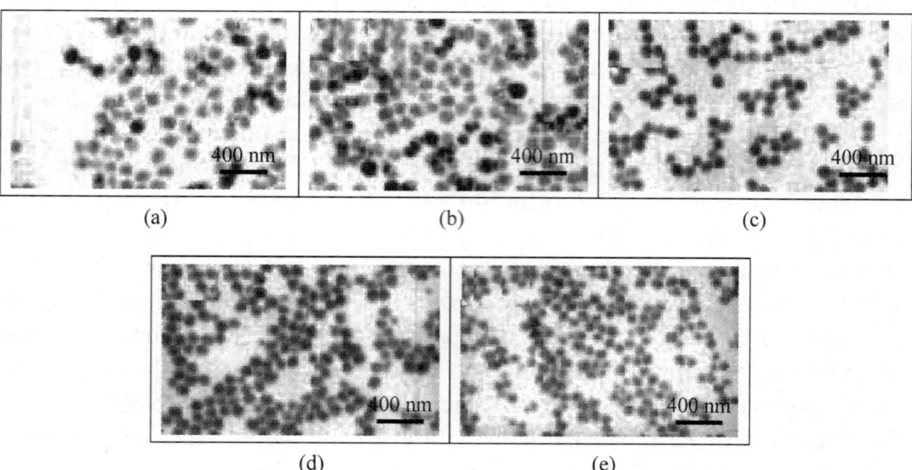

Figure 22.2 Transmission electron micrographs of PPY particles prepared at PVA(50,000) concentration of (a) 0.3, (b) 0.5, (c) 0.8, and (d) 1.6 wt% at Polymerization temperature of 4℃ and pyrrole concentration 1.0 wt%, and (e) at PVA(50,000) concentration of 0.7 wt % at polymerization temperature of 23℃ and pyrrole concentration 1.4 wt% (Merishikova et al., 2003)

It can be concluded that the dispersion polymerization will give much bigger PPY particles than microemulsion polymerization. In fact, there are only a few reports on the study on the dispersion and microemulsion polymerizations for the synthesis of PPY nanoparticles worldwide. Very recently, integrating anisotropically aligned PPY nanoparticles have been fabricated by a templated chemical polymerization strategy (Chen et al., 2006). Not only parallel arranged but also crosswise-aligned PPY nanobelts composed of anisotropically arranged PPY nanoparticles could be integrated easily over a large silicon surface. More importantly, the width of the parallel aligned PPY nanobelts and the interspace between them can be dexterously regulated by using distinct silicon substrates with different hydrophobicities or by altering the polymerization process.

22.1.2 Properties and Application of PPY Nanoparticles

Intrinsically electrical conducting PPY nanoparticles and nanocomposites have drawn much attention of scientists over last few years due to their facile preparation and unique properties involving high char yield, good redispersibility in many media, electrochemical and photoelectrochemical reversibilities, biocompatibility and biostability, reactive functionality, magnetism, thermostability, high specific capacitance, reversible charging/discharging effect, dye adsorption, and mediation of Li-ion transport. All of these strongly suggest that the nano-sized PPYs could exhibit a widely potential application in electronic materials and devices(modified electrode, supercapacitor, semiconductor, rechargeable battery, electrostatic dissipation, and mediating Li-ion transport), biomaterials and devices(artificial nerves, artificial blood vessels, artificial muscle, biomedicine, bioconductor, bioelectronics, biosensor, and immunodiagnosis), tissue engineering, controllable ion-exchanger for water purification, and conducting textiles.

The spherical PPY nanoparticles exhibit novel combination of intrinsically electrical conductivity with nano effect. It is reported that the PPY nanotubes and nanoribbons coated surfaces showed both superhydrophobic and superoleophilic properties (Yang et al., 2005). The PPY nanoparticles as very efficient conducting additives have been successfully applied in functional composites and blends. On the other hand, the ultrasmall amorphous PPY nanoparticles mentioned above as the carbon precursor can be transformed into novel graphite nanoparticles with dimensions less than 2 nm in the presence of an iron complex dopant (Jang et al., 2002), which promotes the graphitization of amorphous PPY during carbonization. The graphite PPY nanoparticles prepared thus are shown in Fig. 22.1(b). It is interesting that the graphite nanoparticles as a replacement for carbon nanofibers could be directly applied as an anodic material in Li-ion battery because of their high conductivity and large specific surface area. The graphite nanoparticles (1 – 10 wt%)/polycarbonate blend film has also demonstrated higher transparence and conductivity than carbon nanofibers(1 – 10 wt%)/ polycarbonate film although the latter displays higher conductivity but also weaker transparency than the amorphous PPY nanoparticles(1 – 10 wt%)/ polycarbonate film. The reason is that the amorphous and graphite PPY nanoparticles are much smaller (around 2 nm) than half (approximately 200 nm) of the shortest wavelength of visible light, while the carbon nanofibers with large diameter and high aspect ratio easily form bulky aggregates, causing blackening of the as-prepared films. Therefore, the highly transparent and conducting blend films of the polycarbonate/graphite PPY nanoparticles could be used as a substitute for indium-tin oxide that has been widely served as a transparent electrical conducting coating of glass electrode.

In fact, PPY nanoparticles could be used in a novel electrode that is fabricated by electrochemically cycling scanning the glass carbon electrode covered with a macroporous alumina membrane in a solution containing PY and $PMo_{12}O_{40}^{3-}$ (Wang et al., 2004). It is revealed that the PPY nanoparticles-modified electrode possesses many characteristics such as improved reversibility of the cyclic voltammogram, high sensitivity, favorable electrocatalysis toward NO_2^-, very low detection limit (1 nmol/L) of NO_2^-, good reproducibility, performance stability, and wide linearity range from 800 nmol/L to 10 mmol/L. As a comparison, the similar electrode without PPY nanoparticles exhibits higher detection limit (100 nmol/L).

The chemical polymerization of PY in the presence of chitosan has been used to form applicable PPY/chitosan hybrid materials (Khor and Whey, 1995). The hybrid materials derived from the interaction of biopolymers with conducting PPY nanomaterials may generate interesting biomaterials that can find applications where charge or electrical conductivity is desirable such as artificial nerves or blood vessels.

A PPY nanoparticle/poly(D,L-lactide) (PLA) composite membrane prepared by emulsion polymerization of PY in a PLA solution has been reported to fabricate a novel biodegradable electrical bioconductor (Wang et al., 2003; shi et al., 2004). The PPY nanoparticles formed aggregations that in turn organized into constituted microdomains and conductive networks embedded in the PLA. With the 1% – 17% increase in the PPY content, the conductivity of the composite increased by six orders of magnitude. The electrical stability of the PPY/PLA(5/95) composite was studied in vitro. It is found that the PPY/PLA composite in Ringer's solution sustained a relatively stable conductivity up to 8 weeks after an initial period of 'conditioning'. The non-nanosized PPY-coated polyester fabrics as a reference experienced a rapid loss of conductivity when subjected to electrical circulation and regained part of it when disconnected. The volume conductivity of the nonincubated PPY/PLA membrane behaved as a typical conductor in the low-frequency range. The electrical stability was significantly better in the PPY nanoparticle/PLA composite than in the non-nanosized PPY-coated fabrics. For the composite with 5% PPY, the test membrane retained 80% and 42% of the initial conductivity in 100 and 400 h, respectively, compared to 5% and 0.1% for the non-nanosized PPY-coated fabrics. Under 100 mV, a composite membrane 3.0cm × 2.5cm × 0.03 cm in size and containing 5% PPY sustained a biologically meaningful electrical conductivity in a typical cell culture environment for 1000 h. Therefore the PPY nanoparticle/PLA composite membrane may be considered as a first-generation synthetic biodegradable bioconductor. The growth of fibroblasts on such composite membranes was up regulated by the direct electron current applied through the membranes. This type of material may be potentially useful in tissue engineering and bioelectronics.

Indeed, electrically conductive PPY is very attractive for tissue engineering because of its potential to modulate cellular activities through electrical stimulation. In vivo biocompatibility and biostability of PPY nanoparticles-coated polyester fabrics prepared using phosphonylation, plasma activation, and plasma activation plus heparin treatment, have been investigated (Jiang et al., 2002). The level of acid and alkaline phosphatase showed a less intensive cellular reaction by a thin, uniform PPY nanoparticles-coated fabrics, when compared to the controls. Histology supported the enzymatic results and showed a fast collagen infiltration at 28 days for the PPY-phosphonylation fabric and an overall decrease of inflammation over time, with a thin, uniform PPY-coated fabrics showing mild inflammation in contrast to the non-PPY coated fabrics.

Redox enzyme-glucose oxidase-initiated polymerization was applied for the synthesis of PPY nanoparticles (Almira et al., 2006). The shape, flexibility and size of the formed PPY nanoparticles on the SiO_2 and Pt surfaces were also monitored by means of contact mode AFM. The highest increase in the diameter of the PPY nanoparticles was detected during 15-day period. It seems that after drying at 50℃ the PPY particles are more flexibly deposited on the Pt electrode than those on the SiO_2 substrate. The application of well-shaped PPY nanoparticles in biomedicine and bioanalysis may be predicted.

Carboxylated PPY colloids with the diameters between 100 and 200 nm have been synthesized by post-modification of PPY latex in organic media (Tarcha et al., 2001a, 2001b). PPY latex is synthesized by an oxidative polymerization of PY by $FeCl_3$ in aqueous media containing a steric stabilizer such as polyvinyl alcohol (MW = 125,000 – 186,000 and 99% hydrolyzed). The attractive thing is that conjugated PPY imparts intense and intrinsic black coloration to the colloid and the surface carboxylic groups allow the covalent attachment or immobilization of biological ligands of interest such as antibodies in active form on the particle surface. Apparently, these functional black PPY nanoparticles can be acted as colored 'markers' for immunodiagnostic assays or linked bioligands for imaging of immunochemical reactions instead of colloidal gold particles. In addition, conjugates of PPY particles with biospecific ligands can be used for development of biosensors with an electric response on variation of the concentrations of biologically active substances (C.Jérôme and R. Jérôme, 1998).

PPY-poly(*N*-vinylcarbazole) core-shell particle nanocomposites with excellent electrical and optical properties have been fabricated through PPY nanoparticle-seeded dispersion polymerization (Jang et al., 2005). The monodisperse PPY nanoparticles as the nanoseed were prepared by micelle templating in an oil/water emulsion. The poly(*N*-vinylcarbazole) shell thickness of the core-shell nanocomposites can be tuned within the range of a few nanometers. The important thing is that the core-shell nanocomposites showed superior conductivity as PPY and similar fluorescence as poly(*N*-vinylcarbazole).

PY monomer can oxidatively polymerize on the poly(methyl methacrylate)-block-poly(acrylic acid) latex, forming unique nanoparticles with PPY shell (Sonmez et al., 2003). The amazing thing is that the presence of the carboxylate groups on the latex provides stable and uniform PPY dispersions.

Electrically magnetic and conducting Fe_3O_4-PPY nanoparticles with core-shell structure have been prepared in the presence of Fe_3O_4 magnetic fluid in PY aqueous solution containing sodium dodecylbenzene-sulfonate as surfactant and dopant (Deng et al., 2003). The Fe_3O_4-PPY nanoparticles fabricated thus are spherical particles with diameters 30 to 40 nm with PPY shell thickness of around 10 nm. The properties of the composite nanoparticles depend strongly on the Fe_3O_4 content and the doping degree. With increasing Fe_3O_4 content in the composites, the conductivity decreases, but the saturated magnetization, coercive force, and thermal stability all increase.

Fe_2O_3-PPY core-shell composite nanoparticles were successfully prepared by a simple chemical oxidative polymerization of PY with $FeCl_3$ as oxidant in colloidal Fe_2O_3 particles with the diameter of 25 – 50 nm (Gangopadhyay and De, 1999). It is found that a series of subtle modification has revealed itself in the improvement in different physical properties of PPY such as its compactness, morphology, mechanical, electrical and thermal properties because of the presence of Fe_2O_3 as core in the nanoparticles. For example, the Fe_2O_3-PPY core-shell nanoparticles with the lowest PPY content of 61.1 wt% exhibit the highest conductivity of 85.3 S/cm at room temperature, while pure PPY exhibits the lowest conductivity of 23.6 S/cm. The special mechanism of electrical transport in these materials and thermoelectric power data have been investigated. However, the improvements of different physical properties of the nanocomposites are expected to enhance the application potential of the polymer without hampering its chemical properties.

The high specific capacitance and high electrical conductivity of the PPYs in the oxidized form allow applications as high-performance electrochemical supercapacitor in the field of energy storage and conversion system (Mallouki et al., 2005). Unlike carbon supercapacitor in which the energy storage is electrostatic in origin, PPYs are pseudo-capacitor materials with faradic processes by a reversible electrochemical doping-dedoping reaction and good electrochemical stability, exhibiting greater capacitance than carbon with high specific surface. It is reported that Fe_2O_3-PPY hybrid nanocomposite materials synthesized by a simple chemical method in the presence of colloidal Fe_2O_3 nanoparticles using paratoluenesulfonate as a dopant and $FeCl_3$ as an oxidant possess greater specific capacitance than pure PPY. Hybrid nanocomposite materials are obtained as a black powder. The Fe_2O_3 content and morphology of the materials are correlated to the storage charge capacity. A capacitance higher than 420F/g and an electrochemical stability of 97% after 1000 cycles have been revealed.

An in-situ miniemulsion polymerization of PY monomer on singlewall carbon nanotubes has been used to facilely fabricate novel nanotubes partially enveloped with PPY nanoparticles and the PPY ultrathin film (Ham et al., 2005). The nanotubes covered with the PPYs doped with $LiClO_4$ and mixed with a binder, Kynar FLEX 2801, could be utilized to make composite electrode for supercapacitor. The pelletized powder of the composite with Li^+ ions but without adding other conducting material like carbon black exhibited higher electrical conductivity and lower percolation threshold than pristine PPY, and also higher specific capacitance than PPY/binder/carbon black composite. All of these could be attributed to the existence of bare surfaces of the singlewall carbon nanotubes with high electrical conductivity as well as large surface area.

Recently, noble metal nanoparticles are attracting much attention from scientific and technological viewpoints because of their interesting optical, electrochemical, photoelectrochemical and electronic properties. It is reported that PPY can be electrodeposited on Au substrates in an aqueous solution containing 0.1 mol/L PY monomer and positively charged Au nanocomplexes from the redox-cycle procedure for roughening the Au substrate. It is revealed that the PPY electrodeposited on the Au substrate exhibits particularly steric morphology with nanoparticle structures (Liu et al., 2003), which is distinct from the typically granular raspberry morphology of perchlorate-doped PPY. This special structure should be favorable for its practical applications. Similarly, the electrochemical polymerization of PY monomer on Au substrates in aqueous solutions containing additives of preparing Ag nanoparticles with a diameter less than 2 nm has also been reported for the fabrication of Au/Ag-PPY core-shell composite nanoparticles (Liu and Lee, 2005). Because the unique effect of Ag nanoparticles can provide a catalytic electro-oxidation pathway for the PY polymerization, the PPY film synthesized thus demonstrates some novel characteristics involving: (1) a finer and granular raspberry morphology with nano-scaled particles, (2) a rougher surface, (3) much higher conductivity (~8 times). These specific characteristics would result from particular mechanism of the nucleation and growth of the PPY films on the Au/Ag nanoparticles.

In situ formed composites of PPY nanoparticle/amphiphilic elastomer of poly(ethylene glycol) (Mn = 2000)/poly(tetramethylene ether glycol) (Mn = 2000) multiblock copolymer have been prepared and optimized based on the synthetic conditions of PPY nanoparticles in the presence of the multiblock copolymer and their conductivity, processability and mechanical properties of resultant composites (Lee et al., 2004). It is demonstrated that composite PPY film formed from the PPY nanoparticle suspension exhibited the highest conductivity of 3.0 S/cm and also elastomeric properties that are influenced by the amount of multiblock copolymer added during nanoparticle synthesis. The synthetic conditions of PPY nanoparticles/elastomer composites, including polymerization time and concentration of multiblock copolymer and oxidant, reaction medium composition, were optimized in terms of conductivity. The tensile strength and elongation at break of the composites increased with increasing amount of multiblock copolymer. This novel PPY composite could be applied to biosensor, semiconductor, artificial muscle, polymeric battery and electrostatic dissipation because of its processability and reasonable conductivity.

A controllable preparation of polyelectrolyte multilayer ultrathin films containing PPY nanoparticles has been reported by a layer-by-layer adsorption of PY monomer and subsequent polymerization with 12-molybdophosphoric acid (Wang et al., 2006). It is indicated that the growth of PPY nanoparticles was regular and occurred within the polyelectrolyte films. The size of prepared PPY nanoparticles was found to increase with increasing polymerization cycles. The electrochemistry of the multilayer thin films was studied in detail on ITO electrodes, suggesting that the layer-by-layer adsorption/polymerization method is an effective way to prepare PPY nanoparticles in the ultrathin polymer matrix.

The charging and discharging effect of PPY accompanied by the exchange of ions could be used to develop an electrochemically switchable ion-exchanger for water purification (Weidlich et al., 2001), especially for softening drinking water. The dependence of ion-exchange behavior and capacity of electrochemically and chemically prepared PPY nanoparticles on the incorporated large counterions of polystyrenesulfonate is characterized and an ion-exchanger electrode based on modified PPY-nanoparticles with a high specific surface area was tested in a laboratory loop. In particular, the ion concentrations in the test solutions were investigated by atomic absorption spectroscopy and ion-selective electrodes with respect to an application for softening drinking water. The application of this PPY-based ion-exchanger for water softening, i.e. removal of Ca^{2+} and Mg^{2+} ions, offers certain ecological and economic advantages compared to conventional ion-exchangers because electrochemical polarization permits an electrochemical regeneration without any chemical additives or water electrolysis. Furthermore, the regeneration of the ion-exchanger obviously succeeds at relatively low oxidation potentials, which is advantageous for the stability and lifetime of the PPY.

PPY nanoparticles-embedding conducting textiles of natural and regenerated cellulose-based fibres, such as cotton, viscose, cupro and lyocell, have been prepared by means of in situ polymerization of PY vapor and liquid phase with

$FeCl_3$ and disodium antraquinone-2,6-disulfonate as oxidant and dopant (Dall'Acqua et al., 2006) respectively at room temperature for 15 h. It is found that vapor phase prepared fabrics show more uniform PPY coating on the viscose fibre surface and better partial penetration inside the amorphous zones of the fibre bulk than liquid phase method. The conducting fabrics prepared by vapor phase preserve the crystalline structure of the cellulose matrix, while SAXS results validate the presence of dispersed PPY nanoparticles with average radius of 3 nm and average interparticle distance of 8 nm in the cellulose matrix. This PPY nanoparticles-containing conducting cellulose composite textile shows good performances to light exposure, dry rubbing and washing fastness tests.

The dye adsorption properties onto the PPY nanoparticles prepared by microemulsion polymerization have been studied (Wang et al., 2005). It is clearly seen that the PPY nanoparticles dedoped by a 10% NaOH solution, followed by a redoping process using a nuclear fast red kernechtrot dye($C_{14}H_8NNaO_7S$) having a sulfonate group exhibit 1.4 times stronger adsorption ability and 1.2 times higher conductivity than the untreated nanoparticles. This method could be utilized to functionalize the PPY nanoparticles.

The PPY nanoparticles synthesized in the presence of its substituted homologue with oxyethylene oligomers as the substitute groups in a tetrahydrofuran aqueous solution of oxidant and the monomers possess brush-like architectures in the dispersing medium, and their sizes in dry state range between 10 to 40 nm (Pang et al., 2001). When dispersed by a low content of less than or equal 0.1 wt % in an aprotic organic solvent, the nanoparticles are found to affect the conduction of Li ion possibly due to a significant reduction in the electrical resistance at the electrode/electrolyte interface according to gain-phase impedance measurement. This could be attributed to the mediating role of the graft oxyethylene oligomers chains on the colloidal particles. That is to say, the PPY nanoparticles display a novel effect on mediating Li ion transport from liquid electrolyte to cathode.

Copolymer microparticles of PY and several AN derivatives have been successfully synthesized in order to remarkably enhance solubility and lower the cost of PY polymers (Li et al., 2004a, 2004b). However, to the best of our knowledge, nano-scaled copolymer particles of PY with AN or its derivatives have not been reported so far. Interestingly, the size of the copolymer particles could be sharply reduced by the use of some sulfonic acid-containing comonomers (Kim et al., 1992; Sunkara et al., 1994). Furthermore, conducting AN copolymer nanoparticles have been really obtained when 4-sulfonic diphenylamine with a relatively free sulfonic group was employed (Li et al., 2006). Note that SD homopolymer has an excellent solubility in water and a medium conductivity of 10^{-3} S/cm. The SD may be a good comonomer for the improvement of solubility and the preparation of nanoparticles of conducting copolymers. However, no attention has been paid for the copolymerization of SD and PY comonomers.

In this article, a dispersible self-stabilized nanoparticles of the PY/SD(20/80) copolymer has been facilely obtained by a chemical oxidative copolymerization in HCl aqueous medium without any external emulsifier. Relationships between the polymerization temperature and polymerization yield, particle size, bulk electrical conductivity would be systematically studied. The size and its distribution and morphology of the copolymer nanoparticles were analyzed by laser particle-size analysis (LPA) and transmission electron microscopy (TEM). Moreover, mechanism of the formation and self-stabilization of the nanoparticles would be proposed.

22.2 Experimental

22.2.1 Materials

Pyrrole, sodium-4-diphenylamine sulfonate, oxidant(ammonium peroxydisulfate, $(NH_4)_2S_2O_8$), and HCl were purchased as analytical reagents and employed without further purification. All aqueous solutions were made with freshly deionized water.

22.2.2 Polymerization

The PY/SD(20/80) copolymers were prepared through the chemical oxidative polymerization. A typical example is as follows: Firstly, 0.14 mL (2 mmol) PY and 2.17 g (8 mmol) SD were dissolved in 75 mL 1 mol/L HCl solution at 10℃ for 30 min, accompanied with a continual stir, while the oxidant solution was prepared by dissolving 1.14 g (5 mmol) $(NH_4)_2S_2O_8$ in 25 mL 1 mol/L HCl solution in the same water bath. Then, the oxidant solution was added dropwise to the comonomer mixture. The mixture color became yellowish green soon after the first several drops of the oxidant solution, then darkening blackish-blue, and finally turned to bluish black in about 20 min. After a reaction time of 24 h, the reaction mixture was filtrated and washed with deionized water to remove the residual oxidant and oligomers. Finally, the sediment was dried under an IR lamp at 40℃ for 2 days.

22.2.3 Characterization

Polymer particle size in water was analyzed by an LS230 laser particle-size analyzer from Beckman Coulter, Inc. The morphology of the copolymer particles was observed by a Jeol JEM-2010 high-resolution transmission electron microscope by a water suspension of the initial particles dropped on a copper network. The bulk electrical conductivity of the pressed copolymer salt pellets was measured by a two-disk method with a UT 70A multimeter at room temperature.

22.3 Results and Discussion

22.3.1 The Effect of Polymerization Temperature on the Yield of the Nanoparticles

The process of PY/SD(20/80) copolymerization at an initial reaction temperature of 10℃ was in-situ tracked by measuring temperature. With a continual dropwise addition of the oxidant solution, the solution temperature kept on rising to a maximum for the first 15 min, then went down gradually to a nearly constant temperature that is the same as the water bath temperature, as shown in Fig. 22.3. This suggests that the PY/SD copolymerization is an exothermic reaction. Similar exothermic phenomena have been observed during the copolymerization of PY with other AN derivatives (Li et al., 2004a, 2004b). Therefore, the polymerization yield of PY/SD (20/80) copolymerization yield depends significantly on the polymerization temperature, as shown in Fig. 22.4. As the polymerization temperature rises from 0 to 25℃, a notable increase in polymerization yield is observed for both copolymers due to the facilitation of higher temperature to copolymerization and then production of more active

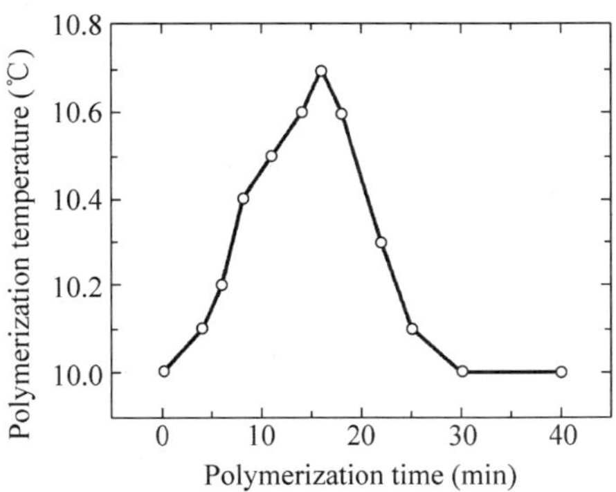

Figure 22.3 Variation of the reaction solution temperature of PY/SD(20/80) copolymerization with an oxidant/monomer ratio of 1/2 prepared by $(NH_4)_2S_2O_8$ oxidant in 1.0 mol/L HCl solution at an initial polymerization temperature of 10℃ with the polymerization time

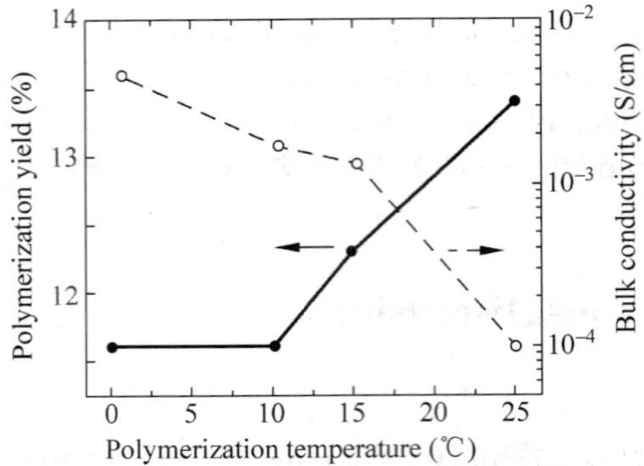

Figure 22.4 Variation of the polymerization yield and bulk electroconductivity of PY/SD(20/80) copolymers with an oxidant/monomer ratio of 1/2 prepared by $(NH_4)_2S_2O_8$ oxidant in 1.0 mol/L HCl solution for 24 h with the polymerization temperature

centers at a higher temperature. Especially, the chemical oxidative polymerizability of the SD monomers could be remarkably strengthened at an elevated temperature. This has been verified by increased water swelling effect in Section 22.3.2 but a lowered conductivity in Section 22.3.5.

22.3.2 Size and Its Distribution of the PY/SD Copolymer Nanoparticles

The influence of polymerization temperature on the size and its polydispersity index of PY/SD(20/80) copolymer particles is shown in Fig. 22.5. There exists a nonlinear variation of the particle size with the polymerization temperature between two copolymers. The decrease of the D_n with elevating temperature should be a direct result of a lower polymerization degree of the obtained copolymers due to the formation of more active centers and faster chain termination at a higher temperature. However, the higher temperature is advantageous to the polymerization of the SD monomers to some extent, leading to the formation of the slightly swelling copolymer particles with too more sulfonic groups. Consequently, the D_n increases slightly with elevating temperature from 10 to 25℃. Note that the size polydispersity index(PDI) of the copolymer particles maintain at a low value of 1.033 – 1.105. The nanoparticles could be considered monodispersible because the PDI(1.033) is smaller than 1.05. It could be concluded that 10℃ is the optimal polymerization temperature for the formation and stabilization of PY/SD copolymer nanoparticles with a monodispersity. Similar relationship between the particle size and polymerization temperature has been observed for aniline/SD (50/50) copolymer nanoparticles synthesized with a fixed $(NH_4)_2S_2O_8$/monomer molar ratio (1/4) in 1.0 mol/L HCl (Li et al., 2006).

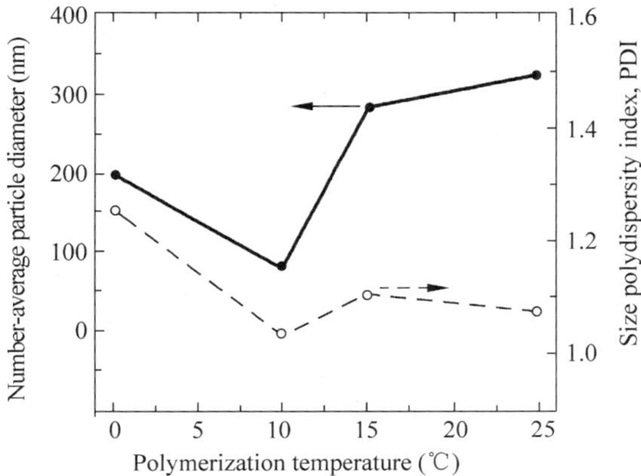

Figure 22.5 Variation of the number-average diameter and its polydispersity index of the PY/SD(20/80) copolymer particles with an oxidant/monomer ratio of 1/2 prepared by $(NH_4)_2S_2O_8$ oxidant in an aqueous 1.0 mol/L HCl solution for 24 h with the polymerization temperature by laser particle-size analyzer

22.3.3 Morphology of the PY/SD Copolymer Nanoparticles

Morphology of the dry nanoparticles of the PY/SD (20/80) copolymers was observed by means of a high-resolution TEM, as shown in Fig. 22.6. It seems that the TEM image is filled with very small particles, most of which are ellipsoidal or spherical particles with a diameter ranging from 5 to 17 nm.

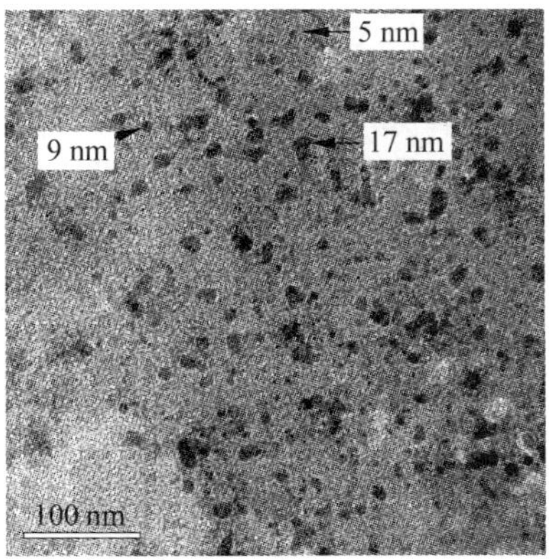

Figure 22.6 High-resolution TEM image of PY/SD (20/80) copolymer nanoparticles prepared with an oxidant($(NH_4)_2S_2O_8$)/monomer molar ratio of 1/2 in 1.0 mol/L HCl at 10℃ for 24 h

Considering a relatively high accuracy or veracity of TEM results and the easy congregating property of the nanoparticles, it can be concluded that results of LPA are actually those of aggregates consisting of several swollen nanoparticles in water. That is to say, very small nanoparticles of PY/SD copolymer could be effortlessly synthesized by this simple method without any external additives such as emulsifier or stabilizer or dispersant. Because the contamination from the external additives would be totally eliminated, the nanoparticles obtained thus must be relatively self-stabilized.

22.3.4 Mechanism of the Formation and Self-Stabilization of the Nanoparticles

As mentioned above, the formation and stabilization of PY/SD copolymer nanoparticles are mainly ascribed to the static repulsion and steric effect from the bulky negative sulfonic group in SD units (Li et al., 2004b), which hinder the further growth of the polymer nanoparticles. A more detailed process has been described in our earlier article (Li et al., 2007).

22.3.5 Bulk Electrical Conductivity

It is reported that the ordered conjugated structure of PPY is vulnerable to be destroyed as the polymerization temperature ascends (Kassin et al., 2002). Here, a loss of more than 2 orders of magnitude of the conductivity occurs when the polymerization temperature increases from 0 to 25℃ (Fig. 22.4), probably due to the decreased molecular weight (Li et al., 2004a, 2004c). Therefore, a proper temperature of (10 ± 5) ℃ should be chosen for the synthesis of the PY/SD(20/80) copolymer nanoparticles with high intrinsic conductivity and internal self-stabilizer. It can be concluded that a novel nanoscale PY copolymer conductor with relatively high purity, high self-stability, and good redispersibility has been simply synthesized because the contamination from external emulsifier, stabilizer, or dispersant that are indispensable for the preparation of nanoscale PPY conductor by a traditional complicated microemulsion polymerization has been completely eliminated.

22.4 Conclusions

Novel self-stabilized nanoparticles of PY/SD(20/80) conducting copolymers were directly and successfully fabricated by an effortless emulsifier-free technique, i.e. chemical oxidative precipitation polymerization in HCl medium without any external emulsifier or stabilizer. The polymerization temperature could be effectively optimized to synthesize small copolymer nanoparticles. PY/SD copolymer nanoparticles with small number-average diameter (10 nm), very narrow size distribution, and high self-stability have been facilely under the following conditions: a PY/SD molar ratio of 20/80, an oxidant[$(NH_4)_2S_2O_8$]/ monomer molar ratio of 1/2, and a temperature of 10℃.

Acknowledgements

The project was supported by the National Natural Science Foundation of China (20274030).

References

Benabderrahmane, S., S. Bousalem, C. Mangeney, A. Azioune, M. J. Vaulay, M. M. Chehimi. *Polymer* **46**: 1339 (2005).

Bhat, N.V., Y. B. Shaikh. *J. Appl. Polym. Sci.* **53**: 187 (1994).

Pomposo, J.A., J. Rodriguez, H. Grande. *Synth. Met.* **104**: 107 (1999).

Jager, E.W.H., E. Smela, O. Inganas. *Science* **290**: 1540 (2000).

Susumu, K., T. Masahide. *J. Electrochem. Soc.* **149**: A988 (2002).

Lee, J.Y., D. Y. Kim, C. Y. Kim. *Synth. Met.* **74**: 103 (1995).

Kiskan, B., A. Akar, N. Kizilcan, B. Ustamehmetoglu. *J. Appl. Polym. Sci.* **96**: 1830 (2005).

Jang, J., J. H. Oh, G. D. Stucky. *Angew. Chem. Int. Ed.* **41**: 4016 (2002).

Shi, G.X., R. Rouabhia, Z. X. Wang, L. H. Dao, Z. Zhang. *Biomaterials* **25**: 2477 (2004).

Hong, S.H., B. H. Kim, J. Joo, J. W. Kim, H. J. Choi. *Curr. Appl. Phys.* **1**: 447 (2001).

He, Y.H., J. Y. Yuan, G. Q. Shi. *J. Mater. Chem.* **15**: 859 (2005).

Wan, M.X., K. Huang, L. J. Zhang, Z. M. Zhang, Z. X. Wei, Y. S. Yang. *Int. J. Nonlinear Sci. Numerical Simul.* **3**: 465 (2002).

Bocharova, V., A. Kiriy, H. Vinzelberg, I. Mönch, M. Stamm. *Angew. Chem. Int. Ed.* **44**: 6391 (2005).

Jérôme, C. R. Jérôme. *Angew. Chem. Int. Ed.* **37**: 2488 (1998).

Zhong, W.B., S. M. Liu, X. H. Chen, Y. X. Wang, W. T. Yang. *Macromolecules* **39**: 3224 (2006).

Johnson, B.J.S., J. H. Wolf, A. S. Zalusky, M. A. Hillmyer. *Chem. Mater.* **16**: 2909 (2004).

Ikegame, M., K. Tajima, T. Aida. *Angew. Chem. Int. Ed.* **42**: 2154 (2003).

Maeda, Y., F. Chiba, K. Iida, K. Totani, K. Ogino, T. Ishibashi, H. S. Nalwa, T. Watanabe. *Electrochemistry* **72**: 430 (2004).

Cheng, D.N., H.B. Xia, H. S. O. Chan. *Langmuir* **20**: 9909 (2004).

Yang, X.M., Y. Lu. *Polymer* **46**: 5324 (2005).

Yang, X.M., T. Y. Dai, Y. Lu. *Polymer* **47**: 441 (2006).

Xu, X.J., L. M. Gan, K. S. Siow, M. K. Wong. *J. Appl. Polym. Sci.* **91**: 1360 (2004).

Jang, J., J. H. Oh. *Adv. Funct. Mater.* **15**: 494 (2005).

Wang, H.X., T. Lin, A. Kaynak. *Synth. Met.* **151**: 136 (2005).

Liu, Y., Y. Chu, L. K. Yang. *Mater. Chem. Phys.* **98**: 304 (2006).

Men'shikova, A.Y., B. M. Shabsel's, T. G. Evseeva. *Russian J. Appl. Chem.* **76**: 822 (2003).

Chen, P.L., P. Gao, M. H. Liu. *Polymer* **47**: 7446 (2006).

Yang, Y., M. Suzuki, H. Shirai, K. Hanabusa. *Polym. Prepri.* Japan **54** (1): 1020 (2005).

Wang, S.T., Y. H. Qin, S. Y. Zhai, L. H. Zhou, H. D. Xu, J. H. Li. *Chem. J. Chinese Universities* **25**: 841 (2004).

Khor, E., J. L. H. Whey. *Carbohydrate Polym.* **26**: 183 (1995).

Wang, Z.X., C. Roberge, Y. Wan, L. H. Dao, R. Guidoin, Z. Zhang. *J. Biomed. Mater. Res.* **66A**: 738 (2003).

Shi, G.X., M. Rouabhia, Z. X. Wang, L. H. Dao, Z. Zhang. *Biomaterials* **25**: 2477 (2004).

Jiang, X., Y. Marois, A. Traoré, D. Tessier, L. H. Dao, R. Guidoin, Z. Zhang. *Tissue Eng.* **8**: 635 (2002).

Almira, R., S. Wolfgang, R. Arunas. *Colloids Surf. B. Biointerfaces* **48**: 159 (2006).

Tarcha, P.J., L. Salvati, R. W. Johnson. *Surf. Sci. Spectra* **8**: 312 (2001a).

Tarcha, P.J., L. Salvati, R. W. Johnson. *Surf. Sci. Spectra* **8**: 323 (2001a).

Jang, J., Y. Nam, H. Yoon. *Adv. Mater.* **17**: 1382 (2005).

Sonmez, H.B., G. Sonmez, B. F. Senkal, A. S. Sarac, N. Bicak. *Synth. Met.* **135 – 136**: 807 (2003).

Deng, J.G.,Y. X. Peng, C. L. He, X. P. Long, P. Li, A. S. C. Chan. *Polym. Int.* **52**: 1182 (2003).

Gangopadhyay, R., A. De. *Eur. Polym. J.* **35**: 1985 (1999).

Mallouki, M., F. Tran-Van, C. Sarrazin, P. Simon, A. De, C. Chevrot, J. F. Fauvarque. 207th Meeting of the Electrochemical Society - Meeting Abstracts, 1677 (2005).

Ham, H.T., Y. S. Choi, N. Jeong, I. J. Chung. *Fluid Phase Equilibria* **234**: 6308 (2005).

Liu, Y.C., C. E. Tsai, W. H. Chiu. 207th Meeting of the Electrochemical Society—Meeting Abstracts 1673 (2005).

Liu, Y.C., H. T. Lee, *Polymer* **46**: 10,727 (2005).

Lee, E.S., J. H. Park, G. G. Wallace, H. B. You. *Polym. Int.* **53**: 400 (2004).

Wang, E.B., Y. Lan, Y. H. Song, Y. L. Song, Z. H. Kang, L. Xu, Z. Li. *Polymer* **47**: 1480 (2006).

Weidlich, C., K.-M. Mangold, K. Juttner. *Electrochim. Acta* **47**: 741 (2001).

Dall'Acqua, L., C. Tonin, A. Varesano, M. Canetti, W. Porzio, M. Catellani. *Synth. Met.* **156**: 379 (2006).

Pang, Y., N. Chen, L. Hong. Materials Research Society Symposium—Proceedings **635**: C691 (2001).

Li, X.G., R. F. Chen, M. R. Huang, M. F. Zhu, Q. Chen. *J. Polym. Sci. Part A. Polym. Chem.* **42**: 2073 (2004a).

Li, X.G., M. R. Huang, M. F. Zhu. *Polymer* **45**: 385 (2004b).

Kim, J.H., M. Chainey, M. S. El-Aasser, J. W. Vanderhoff. *J. Polym. Sci. Part A: Polym. Chem.* **30**: 171 (1992).

Sunkara, H.B., J. M. Jethmalani, W. T. Ford. *J. Polym. Sci. Part A: Polym. Chem.* **32**: 1431 (1994).

Li, X.G., Q. F. Lü, M. R. Huang. *Chem. Eur. J.* **12**: 1349 (2006).

Kassim, A., Z. B. Basar, H. N. M. E. Mhamud. *Proc. Indian Acad. Sci.* (Chem Sci) **114** (2): 155 (2002).

Li, X.G., H. J. Zhou, M. R. Huang, M. F. Zhu, Y. M. Chen. *J. Polym. Sci. Part A: Polym. Chem.* **42**: 3380 (2004c).

Li, X.G., F. Wei, M.R. Huang, Y.B. Xie. *J. Phys. Chem.* **B111**: 5829 (2007).

23 Field Emission of Carbon Nanotubes

Baoqing Zeng[1] and Zhifeng Ren[2]

[1] Vacuum Electronics National Laboratory, School of Physical Electronics, University of Electronic Science and Technology of China, Chengdu 610054, China

[2] Department of Physics, Boston College, Chestnut Hill, MA 02467, USA

Abstract Carbon nanotubes have attracted the interest of many scientists worldwide. The small diameter, high aspect ratios, strength and the remarkable physical properties of these structures make them a very unique material with a whole range of promising applications. Field emission from carbon nanotube is expected to be its first possible application in industry. In this chapter we present carbon nanotube growth methods, the relationship between carbon nanotube structure and field emission and review the state of the art of current research on the electron field emission properties of carbon nanotube. Finally, we discuss the future directions.

Keywords Carbon Nanotube, Field emission, Cathode, Field enhancement factor, work function

23.1 Introduction

Due to their small diameters (a few nanometers) and relatively long lengths (up to many micrometers), carbon nanotubes, with high aspect ratios can generate a large electric field enhancement at the tips to obtain electron emission at low electric fields (De Heer et al., 1995; Teo et al., 2005). This provides a great opportunity for using such a material to obtain electron emission at rather low fields. Moreover, such nanotip arrays may be grown using fairly simple deposition techniques (Ren et al., 1998) compared to another field emission cathode such as diamond films and spindt arrays cathodes (Xu and Ejaz, 2005). It is believed that CNTs are ideally suited for vacuum microelectronic devices, such as large area field emission flat panel displays (Baughman et al., 2002; Talin et al., 2001; Eden, 2006), vacuum microwave tubes (Teo et al., 2005; Kim et al., 2006), *x*-ray sources (Yue et al., 2002), etc. These structures make them very attractive for producing field emission cold cathodes.

(1) Corresponding e-mail: renzh@bc.edu

Until now, several techniques have been developed for the synthesis of CNTs. Several forms of CNTs, including powders, paste, randomly oriented, aligned nanotube films, and patterned aligned nanotube films have been prepared for field emission (Milne et al., 2004; Bonard et al., 2001). It has been confirmed that CNTs have several physical properties in favor of field emission. Firstly, the CNTs have either metallic or semiconducting conductivity. Secondly, the geometrical field enhancement factor of the currently available CNTs may be higher than 1000. However, the field emission properties can be strongly affected by the property of CNTs and the films they form. Thus, recently the issue of controlled growth has attracted increasing attention. In addition, for applications such as in field emission displays, how to prepare or grow CNTs in designed pattern on large substrate surface is a very important issue.

The organization of this chapter is as follows: in Section 23.1, we briefly introduce field emission. In Section 23.2, we describe carbon nanotube growth methods. In Section 23.3, we describe the relationship between carbon nanotube structure and field emission. In Section 23.4, we discuss how to improve field emission of carbon nanotubes. Finally, future directions are discussed.

23.2 Field Emission

Electron field emission is a quantum process where, under a sufficiently high external electrical field, electrons can escape from a solid surface to the vacuum level by tunneling. As shown schematically in Fig. 23.1, the potential barrier is square when no electric field is present. However, it becomes triangular when a negative potential is applied to the solid surface, with a slope that depends on the amplitude of the local electric field F just above the surface. The local electric field F is not simply $E = V/d$, which is the macroscopic field obtained with an applied voltage V between two planar and parallel electrodes separated by a distance d. The local field, in most cases, will be higher by a factor of β, which is termed the field enhancement factor. β is determined solely by the geometrical shape of the emitter, and the field at the emitter surface is often written as $F = \beta E = \beta V/d$, where E is the macroscopic field. Tunneling through the surface barrier becomes significant when the thickness of the barrier is comparable to the electron wavelength in the solid. Field emission will most likely peak at the Fermi level and is influenced by the work function (ϕ), as shown in Fig. 23.1. The basic physics of field emission is summarized by a simple model, normally, Fowler-Nordheim model, which describes the electron emission from metals (Fowler and Nordheim, 1928). The assumptions were: the temperature is 0 K, the free-electron approximation inside the metal surface is smooth and planar, and the potential barrier closing the surface in the vacuum region consists of an image force potential and a potential due to the applied electric field. Field emission current can then be expressed as (Spindt et al., 1976).

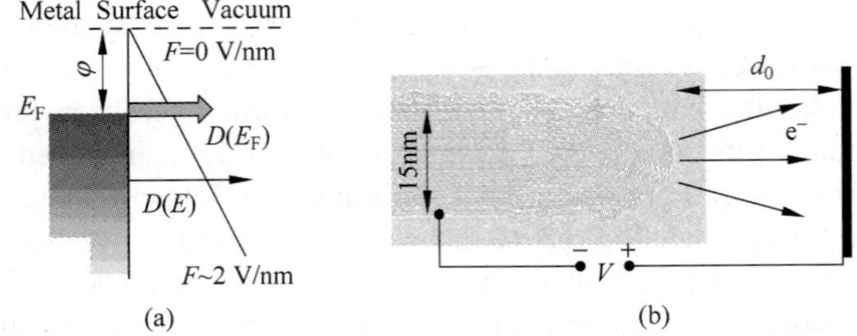

Figure 23.1 (a) Standard field emission model from a metallic emitter. (b) Schematic of a field emission experiment: A potential is applied between a nanotube (TEM micrograph) and a counter electrode located at distance d_0 (Bonard et al., 2002)

$$J = \frac{AF^2}{\phi t^2(y)} \exp\left[\frac{-B\phi^{\frac{3}{2}}}{F} v(y)\right] \tag{23.1}$$

and

$$y = \frac{3.79 \times 10^{-4} F^{\frac{1}{2}}}{\phi} \tag{23.2}$$

Where J is expressed in terms of A/cm^2, $A = 1.54 \times 10^{-6}$, $B = 6.78 \times 10^{-7}$, E is the normal components of the local electric field at the emitter surface in V/cm, ϕ is the work function of the emitter in eV. $v(y)$ and $t(y)$ are elliptic function but varying only slightly, so, in most cases, the varies of $v(y)$ and $t(y)$ can be neglected (Spindt et al., 1976).

Take $E = F/\beta$ as a macro field of the cathode, a curve of log (J/E^2) versus 1/E is called the Fowler-Nordheim plot. In general, the F-N plot of the field emission is a linear relationship given by

$$\log\left(\frac{J}{E^2}\right) = \log\left(\frac{A\beta^2}{\phi}\right) - \frac{B\phi^{\frac{3}{2}}}{\beta E} \tag{23.3}$$

For a given material, the work function of a nanotube or nanowire can be assumed equal to the same bulk material, e.g. for carbon nanotubes, work function ϕ can be taken as 5 eV, the field enhancement factors β can be evaluated from the slope of F-N plots. Note that the Fowler-Nordheim model is valid only for flat surfaces at 0 K, and in many cases is not satisfactory. The model is, however, simple and widely used. Some numerical approaches have been developed (Jensen et al., 2002).

For a metal with a flat surface, the field enhancement factor $\beta = 1$, the turn-on field, which is defined as an electric field to obtain current density of 0.01 mA/cm^2, is typically around 10^4 V/μm, which is too high to practice for a flat surface. As we know, carbon nanotubes have atomically sharp tips and large aspect ratios ($h/r \sim 10^2 - 10^4$) and, as a result, very high enhancement factor can be obtained. So, the electric field to obtain an emission current density of 1 mA/cm^2, which is the minimum emission current density required to produce the luminance of 300 cd/m^2 for video graphics array (VGA) field emission panel displays with typical high-voltage phosphor screen efficacy of 9 lm/W, are in the order of 1 – 10 V/μm that can be achieved easily.

Figure 23.2 shows the commonly used field emission tip shapes. It has been evaluated by Utsumi (1991), and has indicated that the best field emission tip should be whisker-like, followed by the sharpened pyramid, hemi-spheroidal, and pyramidal shapes. Indeed, nanotubes are whisker-like as shown in Fig. 23.1 (b). For this case the enhancement factor can be numerically amounts to h/r (h is the height of the emitter and r is the tip radius of curvature).

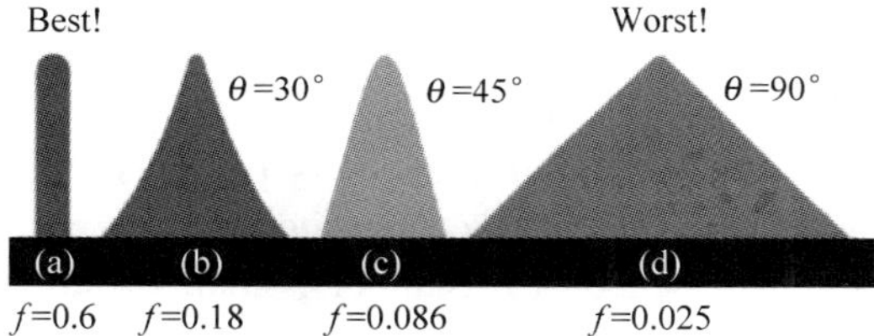

Figure 23.2 Various Shapes of field emitters and their figures of merit compared with an idealized 'floating' sphere where $f = 1$. (a) rounded whisker, (b) sharpened pyramid, (c) hemi-spheroidal, (d) pyramidal (Utsumi, 1991)

In the case of an isolated vertically aligned CNT or nanowire in the diode setup presented in Fig. 23.3, the local field of the tip depends on the height h, radius r and anode-substrate separation D. Shown in Fig. 23.3(b) are the results of electrostatic simulation for the variation of b with D for three metallic tubes of heights 2, 4 and 6 μm capped with a hemisphere by Silva et al., (2004). It is apparent that the enhancement factor in this case is only constant when D is lager than 2.5 h. As a result, care must be taken when analyzing field emission measurements on electrode geometries similar to the one described in Fig. 23.3(a) to ensure that the anode is sufficiently far away from the emitter for this effect to be ignored. The discussion above is based on a single isolated emitter. When there are a large number of emitters nearby, screening of the applied field can occur. This has been observed experimentally by Nilsson et al. who concluded that screening is an important factor when the intertube separation is less than twice the nanotube length (Nilsson et al., 2000).

Field emitters have several advantages over widely used cathodes, such as thermo electronic emitter cathodes. First, the field emitter does not have to be heated, which eliminates the need for a heat source or a heating loop. The energy spread of the emitted electrons is also far smaller. Such emitters are easy to realize in microscopic dimensions and incorporate in emitter arrays, and the emitted current can be controlled with the applied voltage. Therefore, it is apparent that researchers are aiming at replacing thermo electronic emitters with

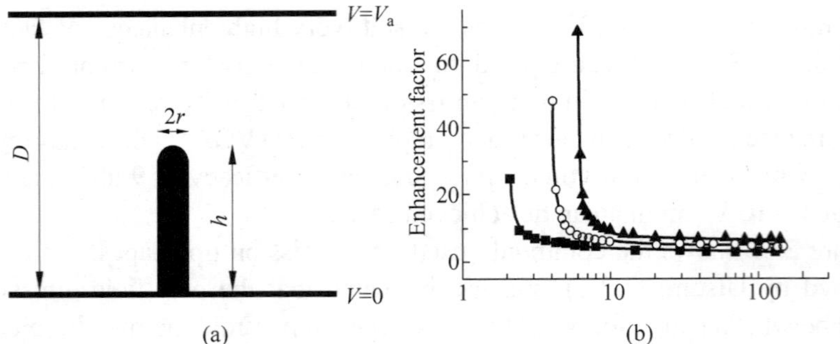

Figure 23.3 Electrode geometry and simulated field enchantment factor. (a) electrode geometry of a grounded nanotube of height h and radius r with a substrate-anode separation D. The substrate and nanotube represent a grounded equipotential surface with a potential V_a applied to the anode. Far from the nanotube the electric field E_0 is V_a / D, (b) simulated value of the ratio of the field at the tip of the nanotube to E_0 'field enhancement factor' against D for three tubes of length 2 μm (▪), 4 μm (○), and 6 μm (▲) (Silva et al., 2004)

field emitters in various applications, such as displays (with one or several electron sources for each pixel), X-ray tube and vacuum microwave tubes. On the other hand, as a consequence of F-N theory, small variations of the shape or surrounding of the emitter (which determine the geometric field enhancement β) and/or the chemical state of the solid or of its surface (which influence the work function), have a strong impact on the emitted current. The field emission current density of a single carbon nanotube can be as high as 10^7 A/cm^2 (Teo et al., 2005), but for the macroscopic situation, the current density is far less.

23.3 Carbon Nanotube Growth Technologies

There are three main techniques for growth of CNTs, namely electric arc discharge, laser ablation and chemical vapor deposition.

The electric arc discharge (Fig. 23.4a) was the first method used for the production of both multi wall nanotubes (MWNTs) (Iijima, 1991) and single wall nanotubes (SWNTs) (Iijima and Ichihashi, 1993). This method grows nanotubes through arc-vaporization of two carbon electrodes separated by approximately 1 mm, in a chamber that is usually filled with inert gas (e.g. helium, argon) at low pressure (between 50 and 700 mbar, 1bar = 10^5 Pa). A direct current of 50 to 100 A driven by approximately 20 V creates a high temperature discharge between the two electrodes. The discharge vaporizes one of the carbon electrodes and forms a small rod shaped deposit on the other rod. Producing nanotubes in high yield depends on the uniformity of the plasma arc and the temperature of the deposit formed on the carbon electrode (Ebbesen and Ajayan, 1992). Depending on the exact technique, it is possible to selectively grow SWNTs or MWNTs.

For SWNTs growth, the anode has to be doped with a metal catalyst, such as

Fe, Co, Ni, Y or Mo. A lot of elements and mixtures of elements have been tested by various authors (Journet and Bernier, 1998) and it is noted that the results vary a lot, even though they use the same elements. The quantity and quality of the nanotubes obtained depend on various parameters such as the metal concentration, inert gas pressure, kind of gas, the current and system geometry. Usually the diameter is in the range of 1.2 to 1.4 nm. The most common problems with SWNT synthesis are that the product contains a lot of metal catalysts; SWNTs have defects and purification is hard to perform.

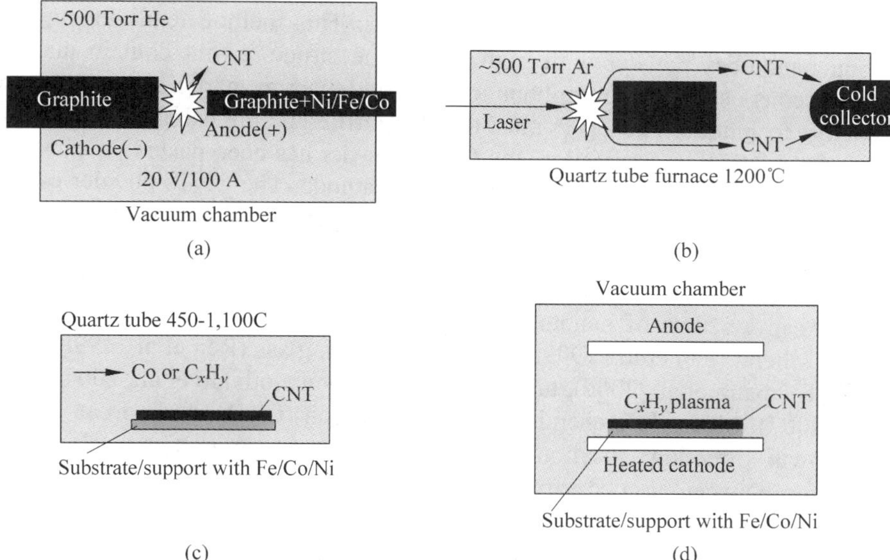

Figure 23.4 Methods of CNT production: (a) Electric arc discharge. (b) laser ablation method. (c) thermal chemical vapor deposition. (d) plasma enhanced chemical vapor deposition

If both electrodes are pure graphite, the main product will be MWNTs. Typical sizes for MWNTs are an inner diameter of 1 – 3 nm and an outer diameter of approximately 10 nm. Because no catalyst is involved in this process, there is no need for a heavy acidic purification step. This means the MWNT can be synthesized with a low amount of defects. But this method tends to synthesize MWNTs, fullerenes, amorphous carbon, and some graphite sheets. There are some modified methods that have been developed to gain pure MWNTs in a large-scale process without purification. For example, (1) magnetic field synthesis: synthesis of MWNTs in a magnetic field (Anazawa et al., 2002) gives defect-free and high purity MWNTs that can be applied as nanosized electric wires or as a field emitter for device fabrication. In this case, the arc discharge synthesis was controlled by a magnetic field around the arc plasma. (2) Plasma rotating arc discharge (Lee et al., 2002): the centrifugal force caused by the rotation generates turbulence and accelerates the carbon vapor perpendicular to the anode. In addition, the rotation distributes the micro discharges uniformly and generates stable plasma. Consequently, it increases the plasma volume and raises the plasma temperature. At a rotation speed of 5000 rpm, a yield of 60% was found at a formation temperature of 1025℃without the use of a catalyst. The yield increases up to 90% after purification if the rotation speed is increased and the temperature is increased to 1150℃.

The laser ablation technique (Thess et al., 1996) (Fig. 23.4(b)) uses a laser to evaporate a graphite target, which is usually mixed with a catalyst metal powder. The growing CNTs are carried away by the argon (Ar) flow and collected on a water cooled collector at the end of apparatus. This method tends to produce carbon nanotubes powder with high crystalline structure, but contain another carbonaceous, such as amorphous carbon and carbon particles, just as arc discharge technique. The CNTs must then be purified before using.

For field emission application, the CNTs powder has been pasted on substrate or pressed with something in solid bulk as a cathode. The CNTs powder can be made into printable inks; the inks may be screen-printed onto substrates to form arrays of emitters.

The chemical vapor deposition process (Dai et al., 1999) (Fig. 23.4(c)) is ideally suited to grow films of nanotubes on planar, nonplanar or flexible substrates, such as silicon (Fan et al., 1999; Zeng et al., 2006), glass (Ren et al., 1998), bulk metal (Talapatra et al., 2006), tungsten coil or carbon cloth (Jo et al., 2004a; Lyth et al., 2007). Meanwhile chemical vapor deposition (CVD) method can control the growth direction, location and films' structural properties such as the separation between aligned carbon nanotubes, the length and the ratio of length over diameter of the carbon nanotubes.

Thermal CVD is a simple pyrolysis, usually performed in a flow reactor inside a tubular oven. Usually, catalyst is necessary to promote growth. A variant of this method is plasma enhanced chemical vapor deposition (PECVD, Fig. 23. 4(d)) (Ren et al., 1998), the process can also be assisted by a hot filament and/or by a microwave (Kuttel et al., 1998; Chung et al., 2001) or rf plasma (Jiang et al., 2006). The method can grow aligned CNT, which is suitable to be used as a field emission cold cathode.

The first step of the CVD process involves the generation of metal catalyst nanoparticles on a substrate and these can either be prepared from metal salt solutions (Kind et al., 1999), colloidal suspensions (Cheung et al., 2002), metal organic gases (Zhang et al., 2000) or as metal thin films (Chhowalla et al., 2001). Figure 23.5 shows the schematic of a chemical vapor process, in which a thin film metal catalyst is used. At the growth temperature, the metal sinters to form nanoclusters due to the cohesive forces of the metal atoms. Two types of growth mechanism are possible based on the metal interaction with the substrate (e.g. wetting or non-wetting of the metal with the surface), leading to base growth or tip growth (Baker et al., 1989; Rodriguez, 1993) as shown in Fig. 23. 5. As the catalyst decomposes the hydrocarbon gas, the carbon dissolves in the catalyst and precipitates out from its circumference as the CNT (Baker et al., 1989). Carbon tubes tend to form when the catalyst particle is less than 100 nm, because if a filament of graphitic sheets were to form, it would contain an enormous percentage of 'edge' atoms in the structure. These edge atoms have dangling bonds, which makes the structure unstable. The closed structure of tubular graphene shells is a stable, dangling bond-free solution to this problem, and hence the CNT is the energetically favorable and stable structural form of carbon at these tiny dimensions (Tibbetts, 1984). Thus, the catalyst acts as a 'template' from which the CNT is formed, and by controlling the catalyst size, position and reaction time, one can easily control the CNT diameter, length and pattern to meet the desire (Chhowalla et al., 2001).

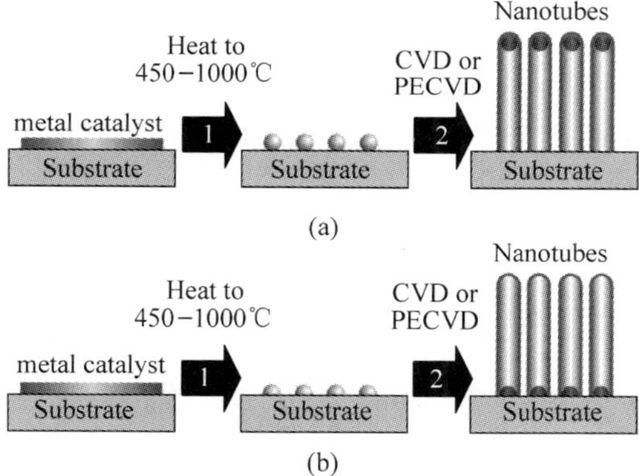

Figure 23.5 Two types of growth mechanism commonly observed in CVD: (a) Tip growth. (b) base growth

As mentioned above, in CVD, metal nanoparticles (namely iron, cobalt, and nickel) are required to catalyze the growth of CNTs, so the ability to control the size and patterning of surface bound metal nanoparticles is an essential task. One of the most common routes for creating the surface arrays of metal nanoparticles involves, as a first step, depositing a thin layer of metal on a surface using magnetron sputtering (Ren et al., 1998). Upon heating, the metal film forms metal nanoparticles, which are then capable of catalyzing the growth of CNTs. Although this method is straightforward, it offers little control over the size or spacing of the metal nanoparticles, and patterned nanoparticle arrays are not achievable. The electron beam lithography (Ren et al., 1999; Teo et al., 2005) has been used to define the catalyst location and size precisely, but it is too expensive to be used in many cases. Alternative procedures for creating metal nanoparticles have been developed recently in an attempt to gain control over the size and spacing of the metal nanoparticles. Ren and co-workers (Huang et al., 2003) have used polystyrene nanosphere masks to deposit large periodic arrays of nickel nanoparticles with diameters between 50 and 100 nm. Ren and co-workers (Tu et al., 2002) have also used electrochemical deposition to create Ni nanoparticles with controlled site density between about 10^6 and 10^8 nanoparticles per cm^2, although the nanoparticles are randomly located and have diameters ranging from less than 50 nm to up to 200 nm. Lieber and co-workers (Cheung et al., 2002) created nearly monodispersed diameter iron nanoclusters with diameters between 3 and 13 nm in organic solvents by thermal decomposition of iron pentacarbonyl, and then deposited the nanoparticles onto a silicon substrate. In another approach, Dai and co-workers (Choi et al., 2003) created iron oxide nanoparticles with diameters of 1 – 2 nm by soaking silicon oxide substrates in a solution of hydroxylamine and $FeCl_3$. Dai and co-workers (Li et al., 2001) have also used the iron-storage protein, ferritin, to create discrete iron oxide nanoparticles which are catalytically active toward single wall CNT growth. Hinderling et al. (2004) used a specially synthesized polystyrene-poly (ferrocenyldimethylsilane) diblock copolymer to produce 30-nm iron oxide nanoparticles on silicon substrates that could be subsequently used to catalyze carbon nanotube growth. Cohen and co-workers (Bennett et al., 2004) used block copolymer micelles as a template to create large area arrays of metal nanoclusters.

For field emission application, it is important to grow vertically aligned CNTs. PECVD can be used to grow aligned CNTs (Fig. 23.6) and thermal CVD may be used to grow both aligned and non-aligned CNT films (Fig. 23.7). (Xiong et al., 2006; Xiong et al., 2005).

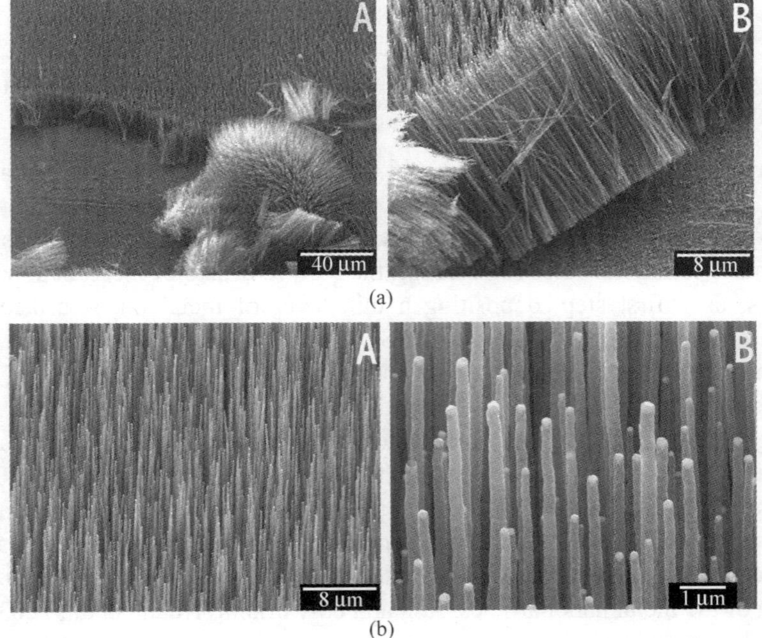

Figure 23.6 SEM micrograph of carbon nanotubes aligned perpendicular to the substrate. This is believed to be due to the electric field inherent in the plasma sheath which guides the CNTs upwards during growth (Ren et al., 1998)

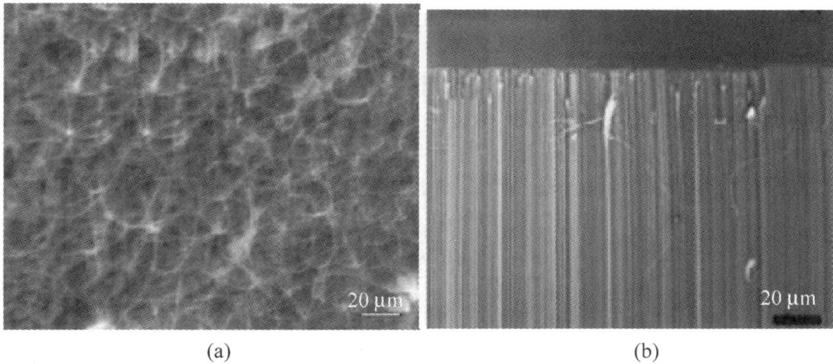

Figure 23.7 SEM images of CNTs film: (a) Random CNTs film. (b) aligned CNTs

Additionally, the high density of CNTs in the films can give rise to a field screening effect (Nilsson et al., 2000), i.e. the minimization of field enhancement resulting from the high aspect ratio of the CNTs. In order to avoid the screening effect, the separation between two neighboring CNTs should be about twice their height (Nilsson et al., 2000).

To overcome the field screening effect, several studies have been carried out to find ways to grow CNTs with designed separation. The current methods used to reduce the site density of CNTs array are to reduce the catalyst site density by electron-beam lithography (Ren et al., 1999), photolithography (Murakami et al., 2000), micro contact printing (Fan et al., 1999), shadow mask (Nilsson et al., 2000), etc. However, all these methods either require expensive equipment and intensive labor or can not control the site density in large area. Ren and Co-workers (Tu et al., 2002) developed a pulse-current electrochemical deposition technique for the preparation of Ni nanoparticles (catalyst) with a fine degree of control. Many factors may affect the result, such as the composition of the electrolytic solution, the surface morphology of the substrate, magnitude of the applied pulse current density and the time of deposition. When the solution composition and the substrates are fixed, the site density and the size of Ni nanoparticles are determined by the combined effect of applied pulse current density and the time. Thus, if the applied pulse current density is fixed, one may vary the CNT site density by controlling the time. A typical example is shown below. At different current densities, one may see different rates of increase of the site density, e.g. at 1.0 mA/cm^2, the CNT site density increased by a factor of eight when the time of deposition was increased from 1.0 to 2.0 s, while at 2.0 mA/cm^2 it increased 100 times when the time was increased from 0.8 to 1.8 s. The critical control parameter of this technique is the electrochemical deposition time—it is in the fraction of a seconds scale. The range of well-aligned CNT site density that was achieved is from 10^5 to 10^8 site/cm^2.

For some applications of field emission, such as field emission panel display, the controlled growth of CNTs in a designed pattern is a key to the fabrication of emitter arrays. In order to grow CNT emitters in a pattern, thin film deposition and photolithography techniques are employed. Several attempts have been developed (Wei et al., 2001). Fan et al., (1999) grew vertically oriented bundles of CNTs in array (Fig. 23.8) form on silicon substrates by thermal CVD and demonstrated that these bundles were good field-emitters. A process to grow aligned and patterned CNT emitters on nickel-based metal lines on glass substrates has been developed (Ren et al., 1999; Murakami et al., 2000). Since nickel is a catalyst for CNT growth, the CNTs grew locally on the metal lines and not on the glass substrate. Another development included the uniformly patterned growth of single CNTs (Fig. 23.9) on Si substrates by Teo et al., (2004). The key feature of their technique is to form one catalyst nanoparticle on a designed location. Using e-beam lithography techniques produces the Ni catalyst

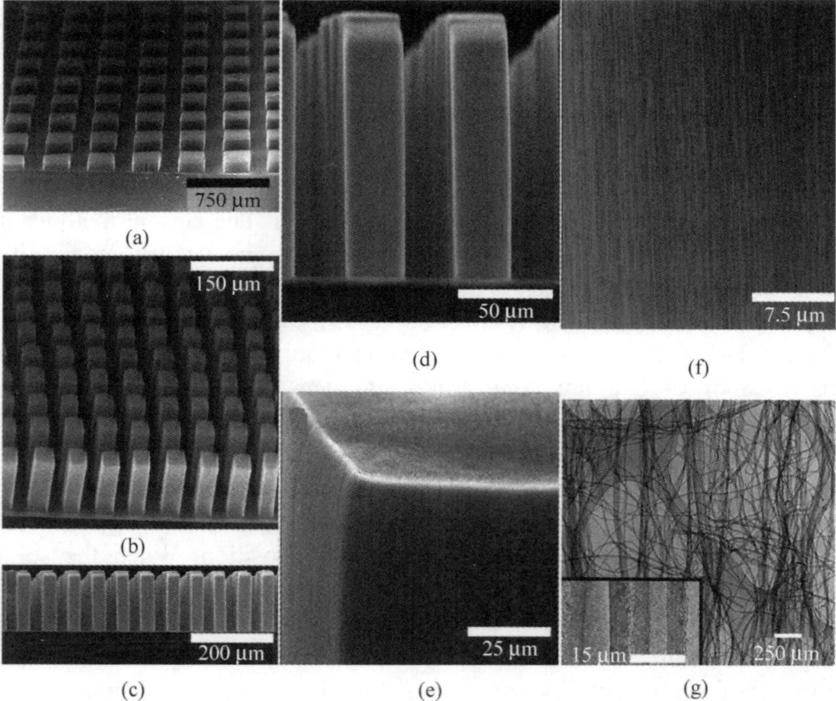

Figure 23.8 (a) SEM image of nanotube blocks synthesized on 250 μm by 250 μm catalyst patterns. The nanotubes are 80 μm long and oriented perpendicular to the substrate. (b) SEM image of nanotube towers synthesized on 38 μm by 38 μm catalyst patterns. The nanotubes are 130 μm long. (c) Side view of the nanotube towers in (b). The nanotubes self-assemble such that the edges of the towers are perfectly perpendicular to the substrate. (d) Nanotube twin towers, a zoom-in view of (c). (e) SEM image showing sharp edges and corners at the top of a nanotube tower. (f) SEM image showing that nanotubes in a block are well aligned to the direction perpendicular to the substrate surface. (g) TEM image of pure multi walled nanotubes in several nanotube blocks grown on a n-type porous silicon substrate. The inset is a high-resolution TEM image that shows two nanotubes bundling together. The well-ordered graphitic lattice fringes of both nanotubes are resolved (Fan et al., 1999)

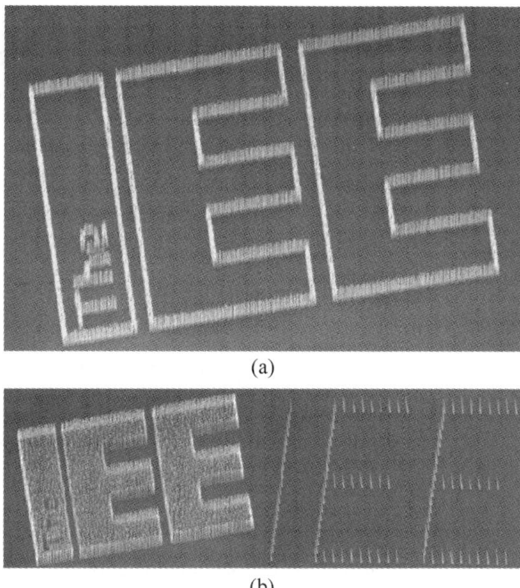

(a)

(b)

Figure 23.9 Using lithography to define the catalyst areas, the placement of the nanotubes can be accurately controlled. The IEE logo is used to illustrate this: (a) only the borders of the logo (actual size 49 – 29 μm) were patterned with Ni catalyst and hence lines or 'hedges' of nanotubes were grown. (b) the Ni catalyst was patterned into the shape of the logo (actual size 28 – 17 μm) and a dense forest of nanotubes formed in the 'shaded areas' of the logo. (c) 100 nm small catalyst dots were patterned (logo size 27 – 19 μm) and these nucleated individual nanotubes (Teo et al., 2004)

dots. The size of the Ni dot determines the diameter and number of CNTs per dot. Provided the diameter of the Ni catalyst dots are <100 nm each dot produces one MWCNT as shown by Teo et al., (2003). Such arrays have the potential of being suitable in the high current density electron sources needed in high power amplifiers (Zhu, 2001).

23.4 Characterization of Field Emission From CNTs

Most reports on field emission describe the fabrication of film emitter and present a typical I – V curve. Basically, all studies show that field emission is excellent for nearly all types of nanotubes, whether SWNTs or MWNTs. An emission current density of 1 mA/cm^2 that can be used in field emission displays has been observed at macroscopic field of several V/μm, and the turn-on field may be as low as 1 V/μm. Nanotube films are capable of emitting current densities up to a few A/cm^2 at fields below 10 V/μm (Chen et al., 2005). Two tables summarizing the results obtained can be found (Bonard et al., 2001).

Several parameters have an impact on the emission. First, the intrinsic structural and chemical properties of the individual tubes play a role, as marked differences were found depending on the diameter (Bonard et al., 1999), crystallization (Minoux et al., 2005), and surface treatment (Dimitrijevic et al., 1999; Jo et al., 2004b) as well as between closed and open tubes (Bonard et al., 1999). Second, the density and orientation of the tubes on the film (Jo et al., 2003) influence the emission. Third, the contact between the CNT and substrate also influence the emission (Minoux et al., 2005).

23.4.1 Effect of Structure on Field Emission

It is well known that carbon nanotubes appear in a variety of forms, with one or several graphitic sheets, with closed or opened tips, with well-ordered (graphitic) or disordered structure. The influence of these structural properties on the field emission should be important for applications. Bonard et al., (1999) used four types of nanotubes to study the relationship of the field emission and structure. Figure 23.10 shows the structure; first, SWNTs have a mean diameter of $\approx$ 1.4 nm, lengths up to several microns, and end in a spherical cap. Second, closed MWNTs as-produced by the arc discharge have typically 5 to 10 times larger diameters, and show tips with a polyhedral shape. Third, opened MWNTs, with their tips removed by oxidation, and consequently exposed graphitic layers and inner cavity. Finally, MWNTs produced by catalytic reactions, which show in this case large diameters and partially ordered layers containing extended structural defects.

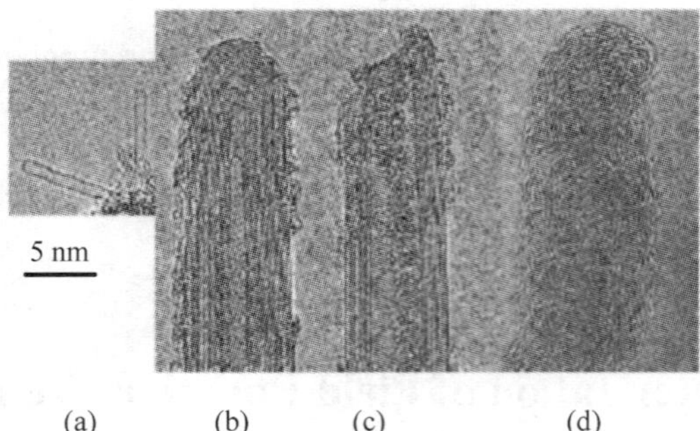

(a) (b) (c) (d)

Figure 23.10 TEM images of carbon nanotube tips for (a) a SWNT (mean diameter: $\approx$ 1.4 nm). (b) tip-closed arc discharge MWNT (14 $\pm$ 5 nm). (c) tip-opened arc-discharge MWNT (15 $\pm$ 6 nm). (d) catalytically grown MWNT (22 $\pm$ 7 nm). All images are reproduced at the same final magnification (Bonard et al., 1999)

The turn-on field, E_{to} and the threshold field E_{thr}, taken as a useful parameter to compare the field emission performance. Figure 23.11 shows the I – V characteristics around E_{to} and E_{thr}. It can be observed that closed MWNT films displayed lower emission voltages, followed by SWNTs, opened MWNTs and finally catalytic MWNTs. The results can be explained as follows: the catalytic tubes showed high macroscopic field mainly because of their larger average diameter. The small diameter of SWNT should lead to very low macroscopic field, whereas the SWNT films show 'only' comparable performances to closed MWNT films. It is supposed that this relative inefficiency arises from the fact that most SWNTs are bundled in ropes, and that these ropes mostly end in catalyst particles. Only few SWNT tips are detected by TEM, and these protrude only by a few tens of nm at most from the sample, as in Fig. 23.10(a). This in turn means that the density of free SWNT tips, and thus of potential emission centers, is far lower than for MWNTs. As for the huge difference between closed and opened MWNTs, they noted that the best film emitter with opened tubes didn't even come close in performances to the worst emitter with closed tubes. The observed difference can therefore not be assigned to the quality of the films, and it can be concluded that it is due in great part to the state of the tip.

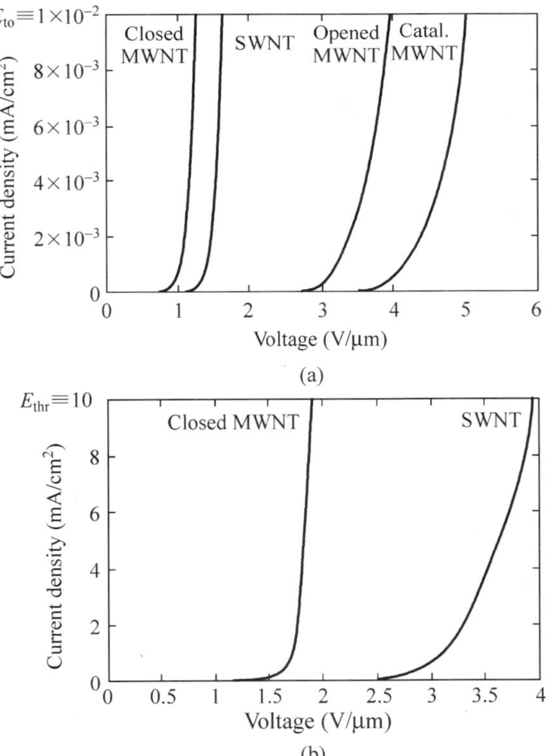

Figure 23.11 I – V characteristics around (a) the turn-on field E_{to} and (b) the threshold field E_{thr} for different nanotube films (Bonard et al., 1999)

23.4.2 Effect of Length and Space

As stated above, well aligned CNTs should make excellent field emitters.

However, as has been shown by Groening (Groening et al., 2000), Nilsson (Nilsson et al., 2000) and Bonard (Bonard et al., 2001) such closely packed arrays of CNTS are not ideal for field emission applications as the close packing of the tubes screens the applied field effectively reducing the field enhancement of the high aspect ratio tubes (Fig. 23.12(a)), which has been defined as screening effect.

In order to study the screening effect, Nilsson and co-workers (Nilsson et al., 2000) performed electrostatic calculations of the field penetration between parallel standing tubes, as shown in Fig. 23.12. They assumed tubes of 1 μm length with a tip apex of 2 nm and decreased the distance between the tubes. The equipotential lines, and thus the field enhancement factor, seem to be strongly affected as the intertube distance is decreased. The field enhancement factor β is displayed as a function of the distance in Fig. 23.12(b), along with the density of emitting sites. Inserting β and emitter density into the Fowler-Nordheim equation yields the current density as a function of the distance and applied macroscopic field, shown in Fig. 23.12(c). They calculated that it is necessary to have individual vertically aligned tubes spaced apart by twice their height to minimize screening effects and to optimize emitted current density.

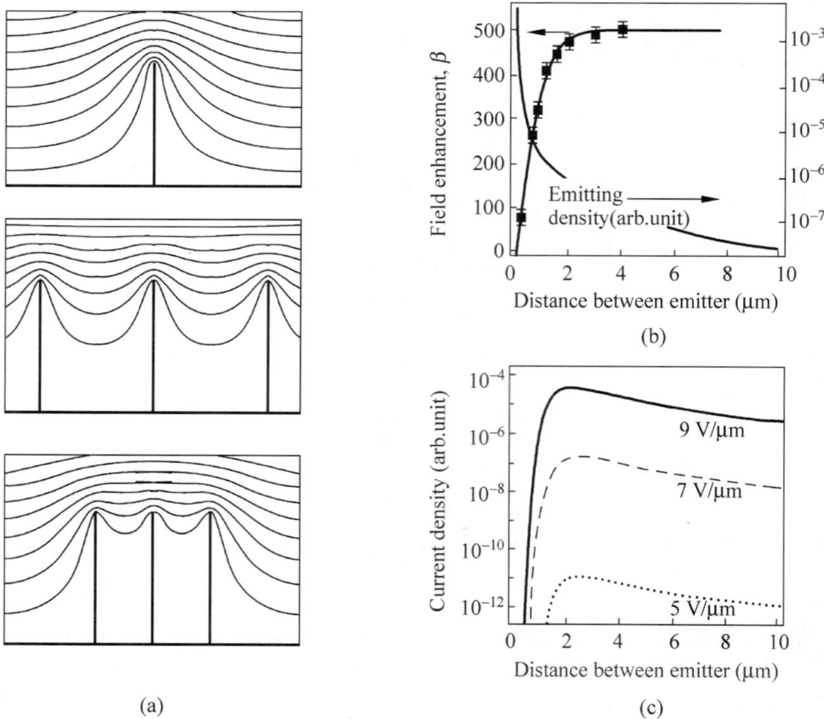

Figure 23.12 (a) Simulation of the equipotential lines of the electrostatic field for tubes of 1 μm height and 2 nm radius, for distances between tubes of 4, 1, and 0.5 μm; along with the corresponding changes of the field enhancement factor β and emitter density (b), and current density (c) as a function of the distance (Nilsson et al., 2000)

Ren and co-workers (Jo et al., 2003) varied the length and the spacing of vertically aligned CNTs independently by the electrochemical process and compare the field-emission characteristics. Vertically aligned CNT films have been grown on silicon substrate by plasma-enhanced hot filament chemical vapor deposition using the pulse-current electrochemically deposited Ni dots. Multi walled CNTs were obtained and the diameter of the nanotubes is in the range of 50 to 80 nm. In their study, eight samples have been prepared. Figure 23.13 shows some of the scanning electron microscope (SEM) micrographs of these samples. From the SEM images, we have estimated the length and site density that are listed Table 23.1. It is worth noting that the site density of sample H is much higher than any other samples, as shown in Fig. 23.13(d). The measured current densities as a function of the macroscopic electric field are shown in Fig. 23.14. The horizontal line corresponds to the current density of 1 mA/cm^2, and the values of electric field required to obtain this current density are 10.9, 9.95, 7.30, 6.05, 5.40, 6.50, and 12.8 V/μm for samples B to H, respectively. The emission current of sample A never reached 1 mA/cm^2 due to short length and high density.

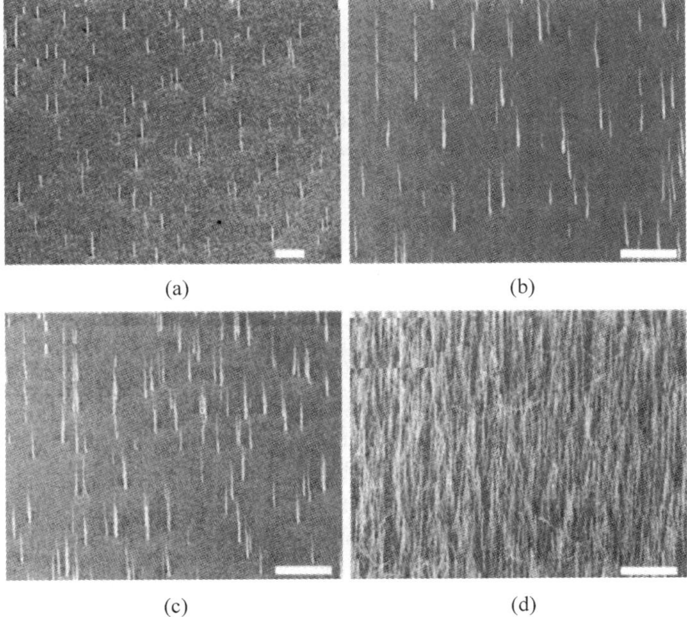

Figure 23.13 SEM micrographs at grazing incidence of 45° to the substrate of (a) sample D, (b) sample F, (c) sample G, and (d) sample H. These images show that the CNT films have different site densities and lengths. The white scale bar is corresponding to 10 μm (Jo et al., 2003)

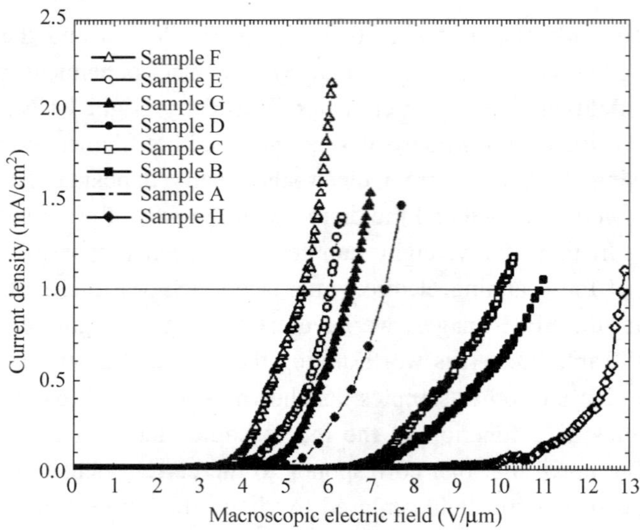

Figure 23.14 The measured current densities as a function of the macroscopic electric field for eight samples (Jo et al., 2003)

Table 23.1 Morphological characteristics of CNT films of eight samples

Sample	Length (μm)	Density (cm^{-2})
A	4.0	6×10^6
B	5.5	5×10^6
C	7.0	2×10^6
D	8.5	1×10^6
E	10.5	1×10^6
F	12.5	3×10^6
G	12.5	6×10^6
H	8.5	4×10^7

They used macroscopic field E_{mac} and local electric field E_{local} to compare the field emission from CNTs with different lengths and spacing. E_{local} is defined as the electric field at the tip of a CNT when the emission current density reaches certain value. It has been reported that E_{local} is nearly constant over samples fabricated by the same method (Bonard et al., 2001), and is related to the macroscopic electric field E_{mac} by the field enhancement factor. As a result, if we compare E_{mac} at certain current density for CNT films with different lengths and spacing, they can indirectly compare the field-enhancement factors of those CNT films. They chose the current density to be 1 mA/cm^2. The macroscopic electric field and the local electric field to obtain the current density of 1 mA/cm^2 are denoted by $E_{mac,1}$ and $E_{local,1}$, respectively.

Firstly, $E_{mac,1}$ for samples A – G are plotted in Fig. 23.15 in order to investigate the effect of the length of CNTs on emission properties. The measured data show that the same current density can be obtained at lower macroscopic electric field as the length of CNTs is increased.

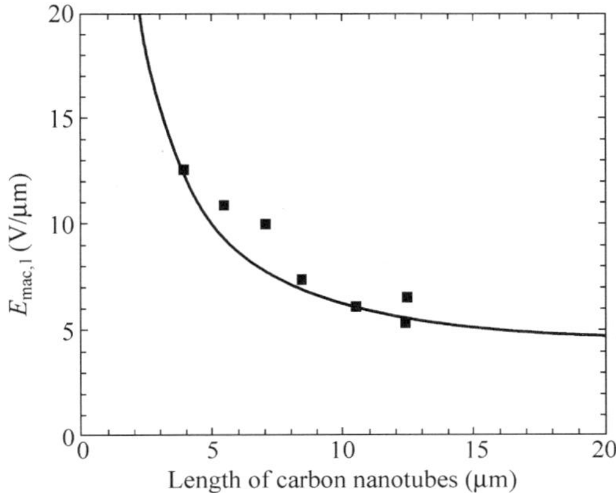

Figure 23.15 The macroscopic electric fields $E_{mac,1}$ at the average current density of 1 mA/cm^2 as a function of the length of CNTs (Jo et al., 2003)

Secondly, $E_{mac,1}$ for sample D, and F – H are plotted in Fig. 23.16 in order to investigate the effect of the spacing of CNTs on emission properties.

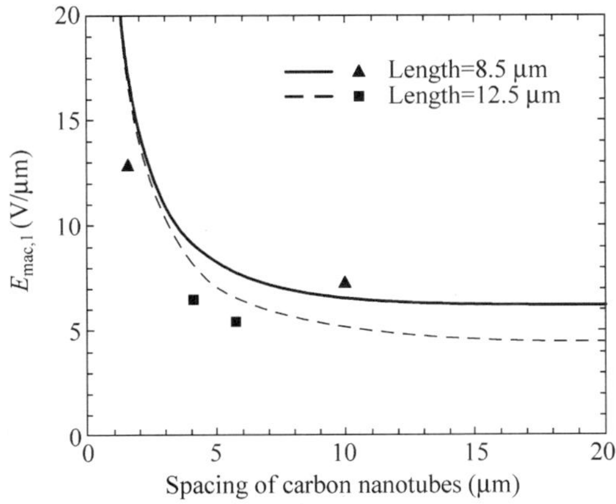

Figure 23.16 The macroscopic electric fields $E_{mac,1}$ at the average current density of 1 mA/cm^2 as a function of the spacing of CNTs. Triangles represent samples D and H, and squares represent samples F and G (Jo et al., 2003)

The measured data show that the same current density can be obtained at lower macroscopic electric field as the spacing of CNTs is increased. $E_{mac,1}$ is calculated for a wider range of lengths and spacing using r = 8 nm and $E_{local,1}$ = 3.9 V/nm. From this figure, it can be seen that the increase of spacing does not effectively reduce $E_{mac,1}$ for the short CNT film. It can also be seen that $E_{mac,1}$ is nearly saturated to be about 3 V/ μm when the density is lower than

10^6/cm^2 and the length is longer than 10 μm. This means that the increase of the length and spacing can effectively reduce $E_{mac,1}$ up to a certain level. In order to decrease $E_{mac,1}$ further, it is required to reduce the diameter of the vertically aligned CNTs.

One interesting point to be noticed from Fig. 23.17 is that $E_{mac,1}$ is increased as the length of CNTs are increased if the density is very high, for example, 10^8/cm^2 or higher. This behavior at very high density is qualitatively in agreement with the result reported by Suh et al., (2002).

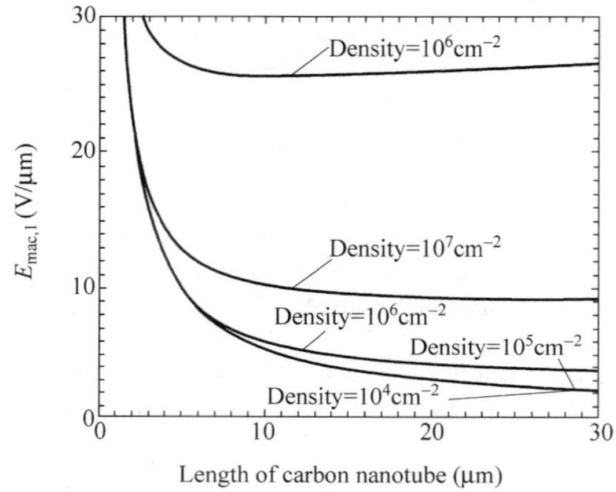

Figure 23.17 The macroscopic electric fields $E_{mac,1}$ at the average current density of 1 mA/cm^2 as a function of the length and the density of CNTs (Jo et al., 2003)

23.4.3 Method of field emission enhancement

To enhance the field emission properties of CNTs, some effective methods can be used, such as annealing in vacuum and air or oxygen (Zeng et al., 2006), plasma treatment after growth (Cheng et al., 2006; Chen et al., 2005), depositing alkali metals to reduce the work function (Wadhawan et al., 2001), laser treatment (Liu and Fan, 2004) and so on.

Ren and co-workers (Zeng et al., 2006) have demonstrated a simple annealing process in vacuum plus in air for significant improvement of field emission current density of CNTs by a factor of 4 from 19 to 79 mA/cm^2 (Fig. 23.18). Figure 23.19(a) and (b) show the top view of the morphologies of the as-grown and annealed CNTs films. From the SEM images, we determined that the nanotubes are about 60 μm long and 30 nm in diameter. Annealing seems to roughen the surface of the CNTs (Fig .23.19 (b)). The density of the CNTs seems to decrease after annealing. Moreover, from the tilted view (Fig. 23.19(c) and (d)), it looks like some intertwisted carbon nanotubes on the surface in the as-grown sample (Fig. 23.19(c)) have been separated by annealing (Fig. 23.19(d)).

It was believed that the high temperature (e.g. 850℃) annealing in vacuum could improve the bonding of CNTs with the substrate (Zhang et al., 2006) and graphitization of CNTs (Minoux et al., 2005) (Fig. 23.20), whereas the annealing in air would remove the amorphous carbon and purify CNTs (Li et al., 2004). All of this would enhance the field emission.

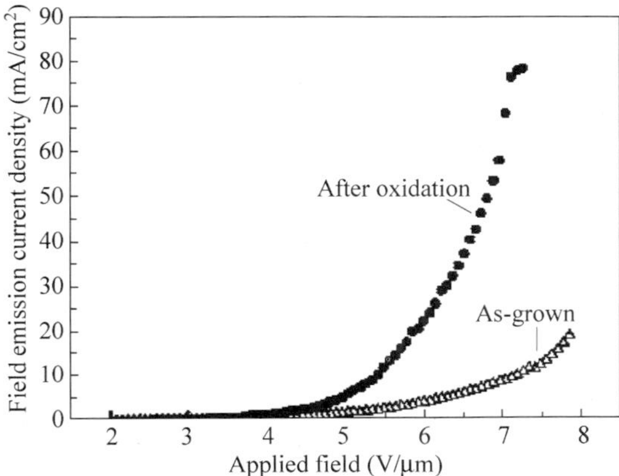

Figure 23.18 Field emission current density (up to 80 mA/cm^2) dependence of electric field (Zeng et al., 2006)

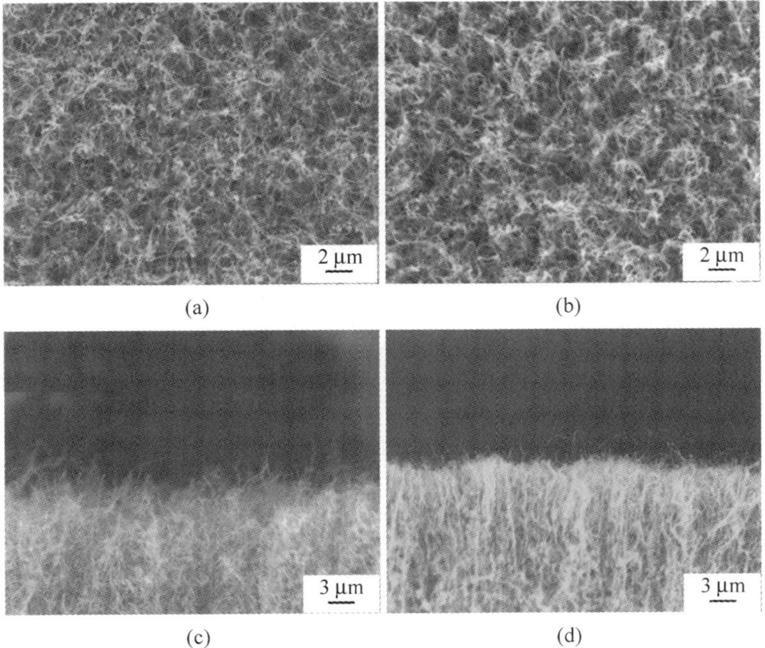

Figure 23.19 SEM micrographs of aligned carbon nanotubes: (a) Top view of the as-grown sample, (b) top view of the annealed sample, (c) side view of the as-grown sample, and (d) side view of the annealed sample (Zeng et al., 2006)

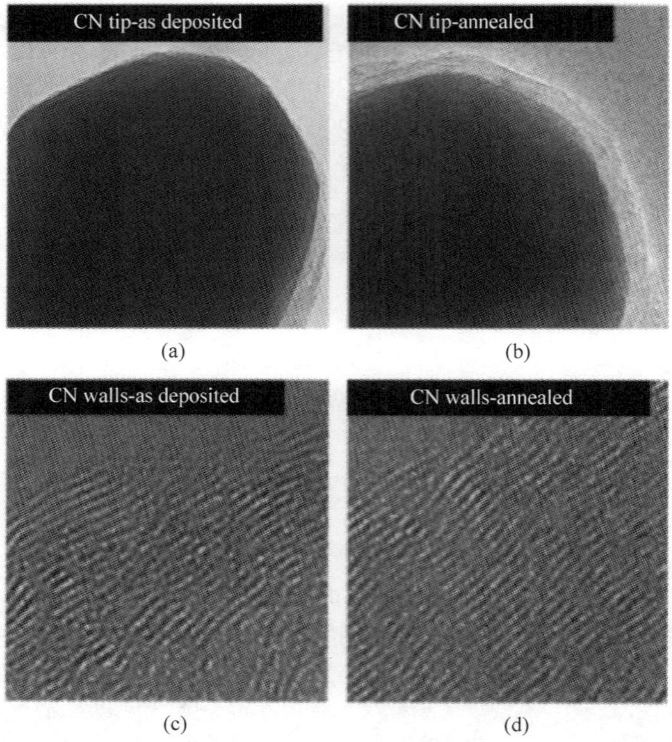

Figure 23.20 TEM images of (a) as-grown and (b) post-annealed CNT's apex, and (c) as-grown and (d) post-annealed CNT's walls (in these cases, rapid thermal annealing was performed at 850℃) (Minoux et al., 2005)

When the field emission current increases to a high level (typically at currents above 1 μA for a single CNT), a saturation of the emitted current is observed and the curves deviate significantly from FN law.

Two explanations for this observation have been proposed in the literature: (a) the presence of adsorbates (adsorbed molecules or impurities) at the CNT apex can enhance field emission at low fields, which are then removed at high fields, causing the current to saturate, (Semet et al., 2002) or (b) the presence of a resistance in series with the emitter, for example a bad CNT/substrate electrical contact, can induce a saturation at high applied fields (Bonard et al., 2003). Minoux and co-workers (Minoux et al., 2005) demonstrated both experimentally and through simulations that the emitter current saturation is due to a large voltage drop along the CNT emitter and/or at the CNT/substrate interface.

A voltage drop may appear at two places: (1) along the CNT or (2) at the CNT/substrate interface. To study the effect of both these voltage drops on the emitter field enhancement factor, the distribution of electrostatic potentials between a CNT and an anode for 3 different configurations has been simulated using CPO 3D software. First, the case where no potential drop exists in the system is presented in Fig. 23.21(a). In this case, the CNT has a field enhancement factor of β_0. Next, a potential difference, V_d, is introduced at the CNT/substrate contact. From Fig. 23.21(b), one can see that only equipotentials above V_d run around the CNT's apex. This situation is equivalent to a reduced apparent effective length of CNT, resulting in a lower field enhancement factor β_d.β_d for various V_d has been simulated, a linear dependence of β_d / V_d versus V_d shows on Fig. 23.21(c). By studying various CNT geometries, the following relationship has been deduced:

$$\frac{\beta_d}{\beta_0} = 1 - \alpha \frac{V_d}{hE_a} \tag{23.4}$$

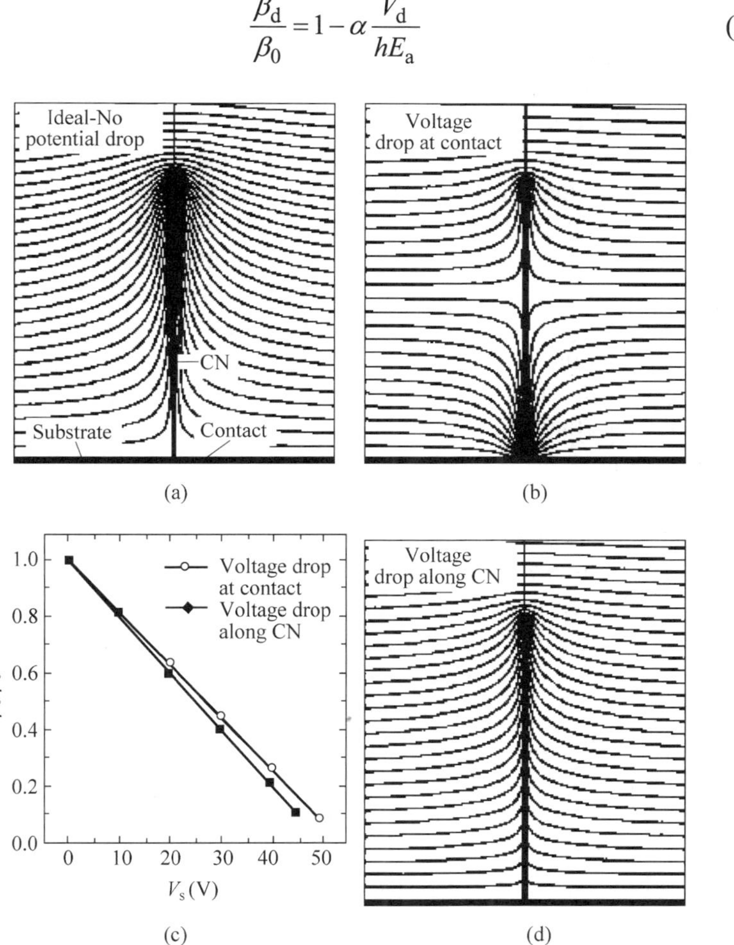

Figure 23.21 Simulations show the distribution of equipotential lines between the CNT and the anode: (a) depicts the case of a perfect emitter where there is no potential drop along it, (b) an emitter with a voltage drop at the emitter/substrate interface, and (d) an emitter with a voltage drop along its length. The graph in (c) plots the reduction of field enhancement factor as a function of the voltage drop. In this particular case, the emitter height was 5 μm, its radius was 25 nm, and the applied electric field was 10 V/μm (Minoux et al., 2005)

where h is the emitter height (m), E_a is the applied electric field (V/m), and α, which is equal to 0.92. Last, we assume that the voltage drop is generated along the CNT's length (see Fig. 23.21(d)) rather than just at the contact. The same relationship is found to apply except with α equal to 1. Hence, a voltage drop occurring at the CNT/substrate interface or along the CNT length has, in practical terms, almost the same effect on the I-E_a characteristics.

Note that this effect is prominent here because the CNT voltage drop (a few volts at μA) along the CNT length (a few microns) now generates a canceling electric field of the same order of magnitude of the applied field (a few volts/micron).

From the contact $\mathrm{I-V}$, it is deduced that the total resistance between the substrate and the CNT apex is on the order of ~100 MΩ at 1 V, and thus, the conductivity is around $0.3\ \Omega^{-1}\cdot \mathrm{cm}^{-1}$. If we assume that the as-grown CNTs were well crystallized, they should exhibit a conductivity value close to graphite ($10^4\,\Omega^{-1}\cdot \mathrm{cm}^{-1}$) and possess a resistance ~3 kΩ. This small resistance would generate insignificant voltage drops (~m V) for currents in the μA range, which implies that most of the voltage drop is occurring at the CNT/substrate interface. However, such large voltage drops (~7 V) are unlikely to exist only at the thin interface between the 8 nm TiN film and the CNT. Thus, it is believed that the voltage drop occurs along the CNT in this case. The development of a voltage drop may also lead to heating effects that determine the maximum current a CNT can support (Purcell et al., 2002).

To improve the emission behavior of the as-grown CNTs, rapid thermal annealing in high vacuum (10^{-6} mbar) at high temperature (850℃) was performed, followed by a high-resolution scanning anode field emission microscope (SAFEM) (Nilsson, 2000) measurements. Several nanotubes were measured, and the field enhancement factors were virtually the same before and after annealing in the low-current range (<0.1 μA). However, saturation was observed in high-current range (>0.1 μA) (see Fig. 23.22(a)) for as-grown sample, meanwhile no saturation was observed until a current of ~20 μA for annealed one (see Fig. 23.22(b)). The field-emitted current now follows the FN characteristic over 8 orders of magnitude (see Fig. 23.22(c)). The contact $\mathrm{I-V}$ measurements on the post-annealed CNT reveal that, at the same applied voltages, the post-annealed CNT has current approximately 3 orders of magnitude larger than that of the as-grown CNT (see Figs. 23.22(b) and 23.22(d)).

23.4.4 Gated Field-Emission Arrays with Carbon Nanotubes

For many applications including field emission flat panel display and microwave devices, it is important to fabricate arrays of addressable gated electron sources. Up to now, for the gated structure, there are mainly two types of fabrication

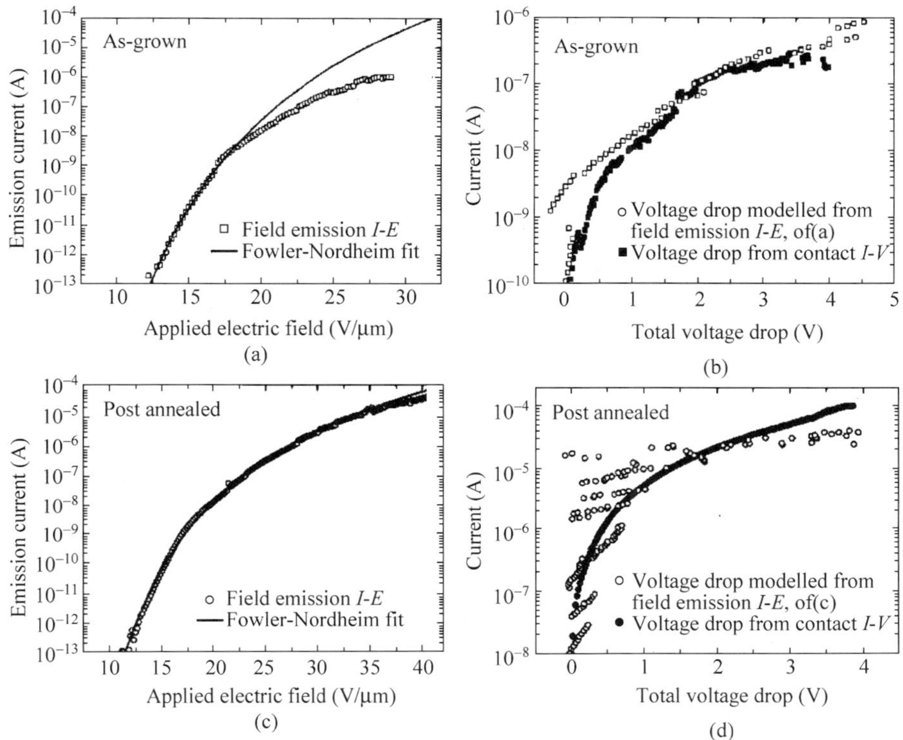

Figure 23.22 Field emission I-E_a characteristic obtained from an as-deposited CNT (a) and post-annealed CNT (c). The line corresponds to the fit to the FN model at low currents for (a) and best fit for (c). Measured (by touching the probe with the CNT) and calculated (from field emission I-E_a characteristic with $\alpha = 1$) voltage drops for the same as-deposited CNT from an as-grown CNT (b) and postannealed (d)

processes. One involves screen printing CNT cathodes with a relatively large-sized gate. The other is to directly grow vertically aligned CNTs in integrated gate apertures (Hsu and shaw, 2002). Two types of gated CNT field-emission arrays (FEAs) were fabricated, with a number of randomly oriented CNTs: one with CNTs on Si posts and the other with CNTs inside open apertures (Hsu and Shaw, 2002; Hsu, 2002). Other integrated gate structures with multiple aligned CNTs in each aperture have been demonstrated (Bower et al., 2002 and Pirio et al., 2002 and Shirator et al., 2003). In contrast to multiple CNT emitters, single CNT emitters in an integrated gate structure are desirable in a number of fields, such as, microwave amplifiers, and electron beam lithography.

Legagneux and co-works (Gangloff et al., 2004) used a self-aligned process to fabricate micro-gated nanocathodes arrays which have a single carbon nanotube per gate aperture. At first, fabricated a sandwich structure containing gate electrode (250 nm n-doped polysilicon), on insulator (1 μm silicon dioxide), on emitter electrode (100 nm TiW/Mo/TiW metal). An array of 300 nm diameter holes, with a pitch of 5 μm, is then patterned using e-beam lithography. Fig. 23.23 a showing a single resist hole on top of the sandwich structure. A reactive ion etching (RIE) is used to isotropically etch the polysilicon gate to form an 800 nm aperture. The silicon dioxide insulator is then isotropically etched in buffered hydrofluoric acid (Fig. 23.23(b)). Both gate and insulator should be over-etched to produce an undercut in order to prevent CNT from touching the gate and the silicon dioxide from being charged during field emission. A 15 nm thick conductive TiN layer is then deposited by sputtering, followed by 7 nm of Ni, which acts as a catalyst for carbon nanotube growth (Fig. 23.23(c)). The role of the TiN is to prevent Ni diffusion into the back metal electrode during carbon nanotube growth. The unwanted TiN and Ni over the gate are then removed by lifting off the e-beam resist. Carbon nanotubes are then grown by PECVD using a mixture of C_2H_2 and NH_3 (54: 200 sccm, respectively) at 5 mbar, 675℃, with – 600 V sample bias (Fig. 23.23(d)). This process typically produces straight, vertically aligned carbon nanotubes (Fig. 23.24(a), growth time 15 min). Fig. 23.24(b) and 24(c) show the carbon nanotubes selectively grown inside the self-aligned gated structure (growth time 3 min). The growth time was chosen to grow carbon nanotubes with their apex approximately equal in height to the extraction gate (i.e. 1 μm) as this is the optimal configuration for gated cathodes (Fig. 23.24(c)).

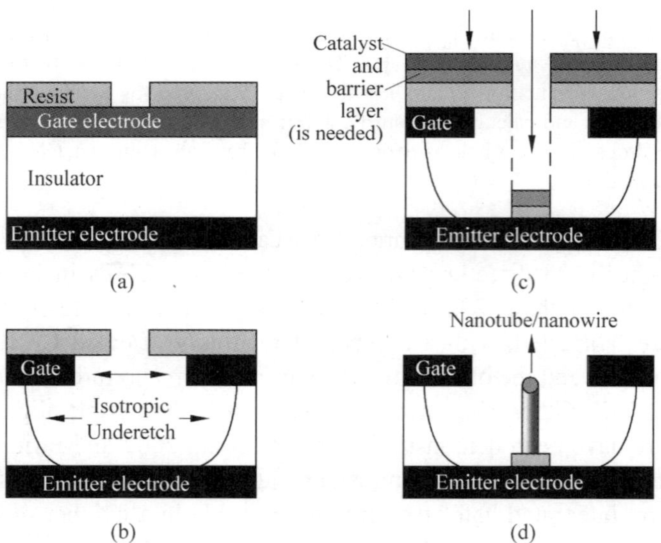

Figure 23.23 The self-aligned process for fabricating integrated gate, individual nanotube/nanowire cathodes: (a) a resist hole is first patterned on a gate electrode/ insulator/emitter electrode sandwich; (b) the gate and insulator material are then isotropically etched; (c) a thin film of catalyst, and diffusion barrier (if required), are deposited on the structure; (d) a lift-off is then performed to remove the unwanted catalyst on top of the gate followed by the nanotube/nanowire growth inside the gate cavity (Gangoff et al., 2004)

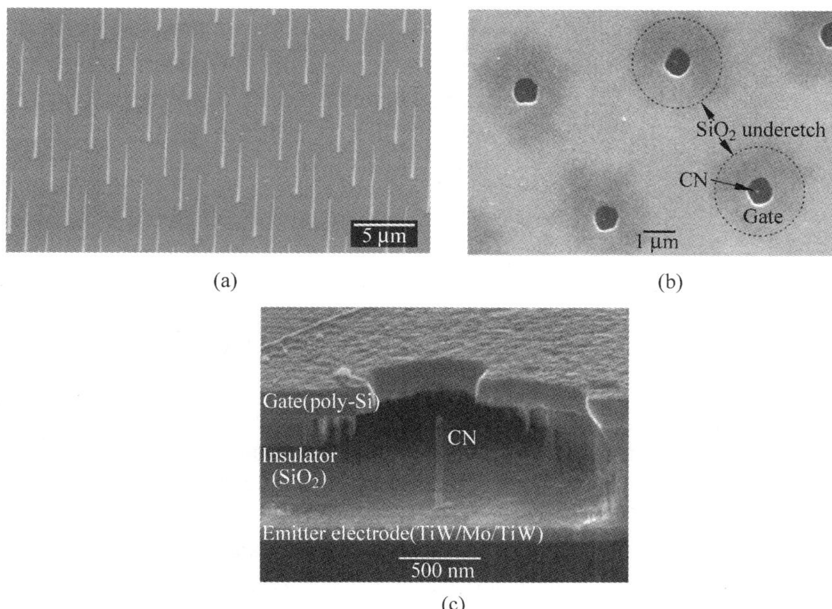

(a) (b) (c)

Figure 23.24 (a) Array of carbon nanotubes, with 5 μm pitch, deposited by PECVD of C_2H_2:NH_3 at 675℃for 15 min. (b) Top view of the integrated gate carbon nanotube cathode. The pitch of the gate apertures is 5 μm. The nanotube appears as a bright dot in each gate aperture. The dark contrast around the gate (within the dotted circle) arises from absence of the underlying SiO_2 insulator which has isotropically under-etched. (c) Cross section SEM view of the integrated gate carbon nanotube cathode, showing the gate electrode, insulator, emitter electrode, and vertically standing nanotube (CNT). The isotropic etching of the gate and the insulator prevent short circuits between the gate and emitter (Gangloff et al., 2004)

Using a scanning anode field emission microscope, field emission measurements were performed on an integrated gate carbon nanotube cathode containing 100×100 apertures with 5 μm pitch, under the base pressure of the chamber was 10^{-8} to 10^{-9} Torr, and show that a low turn-on voltage of 25 V and a peak current of 5 μA at 46 V, with a gate current of 10 nA (i.e. 99% transparency). These low operating voltage cathodes are potentially useful as electron sources for field emission displays or miniaturizing electron-based instrumentation.

Ding et al. (2005) recently developed another potentially useful technique to fabricate this structure by conventional optical lithography, and the fabrication process is very similar to that Mo-Spindt cathode arrays were made. The process started with oxidation of N-type Si wafers with 1.0 μm-thick SiO_2, followed by deposition of a 0.2 μm Mo gate layer. Then, arrays of 1 – 2 μm diameter apertures were formed using conventional optical lithographical patterning and etching processes. Next, a sacrificial layer was deposited at a glancing angle to decrease the diameter of the aperture followed by depositing Mo to form Mo tip with a height ranging from 0.3 to 1.0 μm, after that a small catalyst (Fe) dot was placed on the pre-deposited Mo tips. Before deposition of the catalyst, a 40 nm Ti thin film was evaporated as a buffer layer. Finally, vertically aligned CNTs were grown by a dc plasma-enhanced chemical vapor deposition following a lift-off process of the sacrificial layer. A turn-on voltage of 36 V and a peak current of 36 μA at 100 V have been obtained for an arrays with 25 tips.

23.5 Summary

The study of field emission from carbon nanotube and the potential applications is still a hot topic for research. Most of the current research in the field emission of carbon nanotubes focuses on fabrication techniques for the preparation of effective emitter arrays such as a well-aligned nanotubes, suitable density, structure and post-treatment to decrease the turn-on field and increased current density and total current. The other potential quasi one-dimensional nanomaterials are investigated for field emission application. These include metallic nanowires, semiconductor nanowire or nanobelt arrays such as ZnO, Si materials and so on. Compared to carbon nanotubes, they may have lower electron affinity, and their electronic property can be modified relatively easily.

Meanwhile, mechanism for low field emission electric field from CNTs is a subject of intensive research. To understand some of the fundamental issues, it will be necessary to grow single CNTs with near-perfect structure for field emission studies. It is now known that emission currents from CNTs are strongly influenced by the presence of defects in the material.

Acknowledgement

The work performed by B.Q.Z is partially supported by NSFC (Grant No. 60071043 and 60532010), the National Laboratory for Vacuum Electronics, the Sichuan Young Scientists Foundation (Grant No. 05ZQ026-047) and the Overseas Scholarship Programmer of UESTC. The work performed at Boston College is supported by DOE DE-FG02-00ER45805.

References

Anazawa, K., K. Shimotani, C. Manabe, H. Watanabe and M. Shimizu. *Appl. Phys. Lett.* **81**: 4 (2002).

Baker, R.T.K. *Carbon* **27**: 315 (1989).

Baughman, R.H., A.A. Zakhidov and W.A. de Heer. *Science* **297**: 787 (2002).

Bennett, R.D., G.Y. Xiong, Z.F. Ren and R.E. Cohen. *Chem. Mater.* **16**: 5589 (2004).

Bonard J.M., H. Kind, T. Stockli and L.O. Nilsson. *Solid State Electron* **45**: 893 (2001).
Bonard J.M., J.P.Salvetat, T. Stockli, L. Forro and A. Chatelain. *Appl. Phys.* A **69**: 245 (1999).
Bonard, J.M., C. Klinke, K.A. Dean and B.F. Coll. *Phys. Rev.* B **67**: 115,406 (2003).
Bonard, J.M., M. Croci, C. Klinke, R. Kurt, O. Noury and N. Weiss. *Carbon* **40**: 1715 (2002).
Bonard, J.M., N. Weiss, H. Kind, T. Stockli, L. Forro, K. Kern and A. Chatelain. *Adv. Mater.* **13**: 184 (2001).
Bower, C., W. Zhu, D. Shalom, D. Lopez, L.H. Chen, P.L. Gammel, Y. Chen, D.T. Shaw and L. Guo. *Appl. Phys. Lett.* **76**: 2469 (2000).
Bower, C., W. Zhu, D. Shalom, D. Lopez, L.H. Chen, P.L. Gammel and S. Jin. *Appl. Phys. Lett.* **80**: 3820 (2002).
Chen, Z., D.D. Engelsen, P. K. Bachmann, V. V. Elsbergen, I. Koehler, J.Merikhi and D. U. Wiechert. *Appl. Phys. Lett.* **87**: 243,104 (2005).
Cheng, T.C., J. Shieh, W.J. Huang, M.C. Yang, M.H. Cheng, H.M. Lin and M.N. Chang. *Appl. Phys. Lett.* **88**: 263,118 (2006).
Cheung, C. L., A. Kurtz, H. Park and C.M. Lieber. *J. Phys. Chem.* B **106**: 2429 (2002).
Chhowalla, M., K.B.K. Teo, C. Ducati, N.L.Rupesinghe, G.A.J. Amaratunga, A.C. Ferrari, D. Roy, J. Robertson and W.I. Milne. *J. Appl. Phys.* **90**: 5308 (2001).
Choi, H. C., S. Kundaria, D.W. Wang, A. Javey, Q. Wang, M. Rolandi and H.J.Dai. *Nano Lett.* **3**: 157 (2003).
Chung, S.J., S.H. Lim, C.H. Lee and J. Jang. Diam. *Relat. Mater.* **10**: 248 (2001).
Dai, H., J. Kong, C. Zhou, N. Franklin, T. Tombler, A. Cassell, S. Fan and M. Chapline. *J. Phys. Chem.* B **103**: 11,246 (1999).
De Heer, W.A., A. Chatelain and D. Ugarte. *Science* **269**: 1179 (1995).
Dimitrijevic, S., J. C. Withers, V. P. Mammana, O. R. Monteriro, J. W. Ager and I. G. Brown. *Appl. Phys. Lett.* **75**: 2680 (1999).
Ding, M.Q., W.S. Shao, X.H. Li, G.D. Bai, F.Q. Zhang, H.Y. Li and J.J. Feng. *Appl. Phys. Lett.* **87**: 233,118 (2005).
Ebbesen, T.W. and P.M. Ajayan. *Nature* **358**: 220 (1992).
Eden, J.G. *P. IEEE* **94**: 567 (2006).
Fan S, Chapline MG, N.R. Franklin, T.W. Tombler, A.M. Cassell and H. Dai. *Science*, **283**: 512 (1999).
Fowler, R.H. and L.W. Nordheim. *Proc. Roy. Soc.* A **119**: 173 (1928).
Gangloff, L., E. Minoux, K.B.K. Teo, P. Vincent, V.T. Semet, V.T. Bin, M.H. Yang, I.Y. Y. Bu, R.G. Lacerda, G. Piro, J.P. Schnell, D. Pribat, D.G. Hasko, G.A.J. Amaratunga, W.I. Mine and P. Legagneux. *Nano Lett* 4: 1575 (2004).
Groening, O., O.M. Kuettel, C. Emmenegger, P. Groening and L. Schlapbach. *J. Vac. Sci. Technol. B* **18**: 665 (2000).
Hinderling, C., Y. Keles, T. Stockli, H.F. Knapp, T. de los Arcos, P. Oelhafen, I. Korczagin, M.A. Hempenius, G.J. Vancso, R. Pugin and H. Heinzelmann. *Adv. Mater.* **16**: 876 (2004).
Hsu, D. S. Y. *Appl. Phys. Lett.* **80**: 2988 (2002).
Hsu, D.S.Y. and J. Shaw. *Appl. Phys. Lett.* **80**: 118 (2002).
Huang, Z. P., D.L., Carnahan, J. Rybczynski, M. Giersig, M. Sennett, D.Z., Wang, J.G., Wen, K., Kempa, Z.F., Ren. *App. Phys. Lett.* **82**: 460 (2003).

Iijima, S., T., Ichihashi. *Nature* **363**: 603 (1993).
Iijima, S. *Nature* **354**: 56 (1991).
Jensen, K.L., Patrick G. O'Shea and Donald W. Feldman. *Appl. Phys. Lett.* **81**: 3867 (2002).
Jiang, J., T. Feng, J.H. Zhang, X.H. Cheng, G.B. Chao, B.Y. Jiang, Y.J. Wang, X. Wang, X.H. Liu and S.C. Zou. *Appl. Surf. Sci.* **252**: 2938 (2006).
Jo, S.H., Y. Tu, Z.P. Huang, D.L. Carnahan, D.Z. Wang and Z.F. Ren. *Appl. Phys. Lett.* **82**: 3520 (2003).
Jo, S.H., D.Z. Wang, J.Y. Huang, W.Z. Li, K. Kempa and Z.F. Ren. *Appl. Phys. Lett.* **85**: 810 (2004a).
Jo, S.H., Y. Tu, Z.P. Huang, D.L. Carnahan, J.Y. Huang, D.Z. Wang and Z.F. Ren. *Appl. Phys. Lett.* **84**: 413 (2004b).
Journet, C. and P. Bernier. Applied Physics A-Materials Science & Processing **67**: 1 (1998).
Kim, H.J., J.J. Choi, J.H. Han, J.H. Park and J.B. Yoo. *IEEE Trans*. ED **53:** 2674 (2006).
Kind, H., J.M. Bonard, C. Emmenegger, L.O. Nillsson, K. Hernadi, E. Maillard-Schaller, L.L. Forro and K. Kern. *Adv. Mater.* **11**: 1285 (1999).
Kuttel, O. Goenong, C. Emmenegger and L. Schlapbach. *Appl. Phys. Lett.* **73**: 2113 (1998).
Lee, S.J., H.K. Baik, J.E. Yoo and J.H. Han. *Diam. Relat. Mater.* **11**: 3 (2002).
Li, S., D.Z. Wang, T.X. Liang, X.F. Wang, J.J. Wu, X.Q. Hu and J. Liang. *Powder Technol.* **142**: 175 (2004).
Li, Y. M., W. Kim, Y.G. Zhang, M. Rolandi, D.W. Wang and H.J. Dai. *J. Phys. Chem.* B **105**: 11,424 (2001).
Liu, Y. M. and S. S. Fan. *Nanotechnology* **15**: 1033 (2004).
Lyth, S. M., R.A. Hatton and S.R.P. Silva, *Appl. Phys. Lett.* **90**: 013,120 (2007).
Milne,W. I., K.B.K. Teo, G.A.J. Amaratunga, P.Legagneux, L. Gangloff, J.P. Schnell, V. Semet, V. Thien Binh and O. Groening. *J. Mater. Chem.* **14**: 933 (2004).
Minoux, E., O. Groening, K.B.J. Teo, S.H. Dalal, L. Gangloff, J. P.Schnell, L. Hudanski, I.Y.Y. Bu, P. Vincent, P. Legagneux, G.A.J. Amaratunga and W.I. Milne. *Nano Lett.* **5**: 2135 (2005).
Murakami, H., M. Hirakawa, C. Tanaka and H. Yamakawa. *Appl. Phys. Lett.* **76**: 1776 (2000).
Nilsson, L., O. Groening, C. Emmernegger, O. Kuettel, E. Schaller, L. Sclapbach, H. Kind, J.M. Bonard and K. Kern. *Appl. Phys. Lett.* **76**: 2071 (2000).
Nilsson, L., O. Groening, O. Kuettel, P. Groening and L. Schlapbach. *J. Vac. Sci. Technol.* B **20**: 326 (2002).
Nilsson, L., O. Groning, C. Emmenegger, O. Kuttel, E. Schaller, L. Schlapbach, H. Kind, J.M. Bonard and K. Kern. *Appl. Phys. Lett.* **76**: 2071 (2000).
Pirio, G., P. Legagneux, D. Pribat, K. B. K. Teo, M. Chhowalla, S.T. Purcell, P. Vincent, C. Journet and V.T. Binh. *Phys. Rev. Lett.* **88**: 105,502 (2002).
Purcell, S.T., P. Vincent, C. Journet, and V.T. Binh. *Phy. Rev. Lett.* **88**: 105502 (2002)
Ren, Z.F., Z.P. Huang, J.W. Xu, D.Z. Wang, J.G. Wen, J.H. Wang, L. Calvet, J. Chen, J.F. Klemic and M.A. Reed. *Appl. Phys. Lett.* **75**: 1086 (1999).
Ren, Z.F., Z.P. Huang, J.W. Xu, J.H. Wang, P. Bush, M.P. Siegal, P.N. Provencio. *Science* **282**: 1105 (1998).
Rodriguez, N.M. *J. Mater. Res.* **8**: 3233 (1993).

Shirator, Y., H. Hiraoka, Y. Takeuchi, S. Itoh and M. Yamamoto. *Appl. Phys. Lett.* **82**: 2485 (2003).
Silva, S.R.P., J.D. Carey, G.Y. Chen, D.C. Cox, R.D. Forrest, C.H.P. Poa, R.C. Smith, Y.F. Tang and J.M. Shannon. *IEE Proc.-Circuits Devices Syst.***151**: 489 (2004).
Spindt, C.A., I. Brodie, L. Humphrey and E.R. Westerberger. *J. Appl. Phys.* **47**: 5248 (1976).
Suh, J. S., K.S. Jeong, J.S. Lee and I. Han. *Appl. Phys. Lett.* **80**: 2392 (2002).
T. Utsumi. IEEE Trans. *Electron Dev.* **38:** 2276 (1991).
Talapatra, S., S. Kar, S.K. Pal, R. Vajal, L. Ci, P. Victor, M.M. Shaijumon, S. Kaur, O. Nalamasu and P.M. Ajayan. *Nature Nanotechnology* **1**: 112 (2006).
Talin, A.A., K.A. Dean and J.E. Jaskie. *Solid State Electron* **45**: 3 (2001).
Teo, K.B.K., R.G. Lacerda, M.H. Yang, A.S. Teh, L.A.W. Robinson, S.H. Dalal, N.L. Rupesinghe, M. Chhowalla, S.B. Lee, D.A. Jefferson, D.G. Hasko, G.A.J. Amaratunga, W.L. Milne, P. Legagneux, L. Gangloff, E. Minoux, J.P. Schnell and D. Pribat. *IEE Proc.-Circuits Devices Syst.* **151**: 443 (2004).
Teo, K.B.K., S.B. Lee, M. Chhowalla, V. Semet, V.T. Binh, O.Groening, M. Castignolles, A. Loiseau, G. Pirio, P. Legagneux,D. Pribat, D.G. Hasko, H. Ahmed, G.A.J. Amaratunga and W.I. Milne. *Nanotechnology* **14:** 204 (2003).
Teo, Kenneth B. K., E. Minoux, L. Hudanski and F. Peauger. *Nature* **437**: 968 (2005).
Thess, A., R. Lee, P. Nikolaev, H.J. Dai, P. Petit, J. Robert, C.H. Xu, Y.H. Lee, S.G. Kim, A.G. Rinzler, D.T. Colbert, G.E. Scuseria, D. Tomanek, J.E. Fischer and R.E. Smalley. *Science* **273**: 483 (1996).
Tibbetts, G.G. *J. Cryst. Growth* **66**: 632 (1984).
Tu, Y., Z.P. Huang, D.Z. Wang, J.G. Wen and Z.F. Ren. *Appl. Phys. Lett.* **80**: 4018 (2002).
Semet, V., V.T. Binh, P. Vincent, D. Guillot, K.B.K. Teo, M. Chhowalla, G.A.J. Amaratunga, W. I. Milne, P. Legagneux and D. Pribat. *Appl. Phys. Lett.* **81**: 343 (2002).
Wadhawan, A., R. E. Stallcup II and J. M. Perez. *Appl. Phys. Lett.* **78**: 108 (2001).
Wei,Y.Y., G. Eres, V.L. Merkulov and D.H. Lowndes. *Appl. Phys. Lett.* **78**: 1394 (2001).
Xiong, G.Y., D.Z. Wang and Z.F. Ren. *Carbon* **44**: 969 (2006).
Xiong, G.Y., Y. Suda, D.Z. Wang, J.Y. Huang, Z.F. Ren. *Nanotechnology* **16**: 532 (2005).
Xu, N. S. and S. Ejaz Huqb. *Mater. Sci. Eng.* R **48**: 47 (2005).
Yue, G.Z., Q. Qiu, B. Gao, Y. Cheng, J. Zhang, H. Shimoda, S. Chang, J. P. Lu and O. Zhou. *Appl. Phys. Lett.* **81**: 355 (2002).
Zeng, B.Q., G.Y. Xiong, S. Chen,W.Z. Wang, D.Z. D.Z. Wang and Z.F. Ren. *Appl Phys Lett.* **89**: 223,119 (2006).
Zhang, J.H., X. Wang, W.W. Yang, W.D. Yu, T. Feng, Q. Li, X.H. Liu and C. R. Yang. *Carbon* **44**: 418 (2006).
Zhang, Z.J., B.Q. Wei, G. Ramanath and P.M. Ajayan. *Appl. Phys. Lett.* **77**: 3764 (2000).
Zhu, W. *Vacuum Microelectronics.* Wiley, New York (2001).

24 Flexible Dye-Sensitized Nano-Porous Films Solar Cells

Dongshe Zhang[1], Tony Pereira[2], Torsten Oekermann[3], Katrin Wessels[3], Changyong Qin[4] and Jun Lu[5]

[1]Department of Chemical and Materials Engineering, University of Cincinnati, Cincinnati, OH 45221-0012, USA.

[2]Department of Mechanical and Aerospace Engineering, University of California Los Angeles, Los Angeles, CA 90095, USA.

[3]Leibniz University Hannover, Institute of Physical Chemistry and Electrochemistry, Hannover 30167, Germany;

[4]Department of Chemistry, Washington State University, Pullman, WA 99164, USA.

[5]Howard Hughes Medical Institute, The University of Chicago, Chicago, IL 60637, USA.

Abstract This chapter reviewed the progress in the flexible dye-sensitized nanostructured thin film solar cells (DSSCs). Flexible DSSCs show potential to be commercialized in the field of DSSCs. It attracts many efforts to study on it in recent years. So in this chapter, we reviewed the flexible DSSCs and their current status. Further reviewed on the low temperature preparation of the nanostructured thin film methods and technology, which is the key point for the flexible DSSCs. Moreover, electron transport and back reaction at the TiO_2 / electrolyte interface, interfacial electron transfer, charge separation and recombination also has been reviewed, which would help to go insight into the essential of the flexible DSSCs. The further improvement of the conversion efficiency of the flexible DSSCs has been discussed, and outlook was presented based on the review study.

24.1 Introduction

In times of decreasing fossil fuel reserves and increasing air pollution caused by the global use of energy obtained by burning fossil fuels, the interest and research in renewable and clean energies continues to grow. A very clean energy source is the direct conversion of sunlight to electrical energy with solar cells

(1) Corresponding e-mail: dongshe88@yahoo.com

The photovoltaic effect was first observed in 1839 by the French physicist Alexandre-Edmond Becquerel, with the first 1% efficient solar cell only being built almost a half century later in 1883 by Charles Fritts. The modern solar cell was first patented in 1954 by Russell Ohl, following his work at Bell Labs. The Russians took the lead once more by being the first to utilize solar cells on their Sputnik 3 satellite launched into earth orbit in 1957. Solar cells have been in continuous development since 1953 and have reached efficiencies of up to 25% (Green et al., 2007).

The overall light-to-electricity conversion efficiency η of solar cells is given by the equation:

$$\eta = \frac{I_{\mathrm{MPP}} \cdot V_{\mathrm{MPP}}}{\Phi} = \frac{I_{\mathrm{SC}} \cdot V_{\mathrm{OC}} \cdot \mathrm{FF}}{\Phi}$$

where Φ *is* the intensity of the incident light, I_{SC} the short circuit current, V_{OC} the open circuit voltage, FF the fill factor, and I_{MPP} and V_{MPP} are the current and voltage at the maximum power point (Fig. 24.1). Efficiencies of solar cells are usually given for the AM 1.5 sun spectrum (often referred to as 1 sun light intensity).

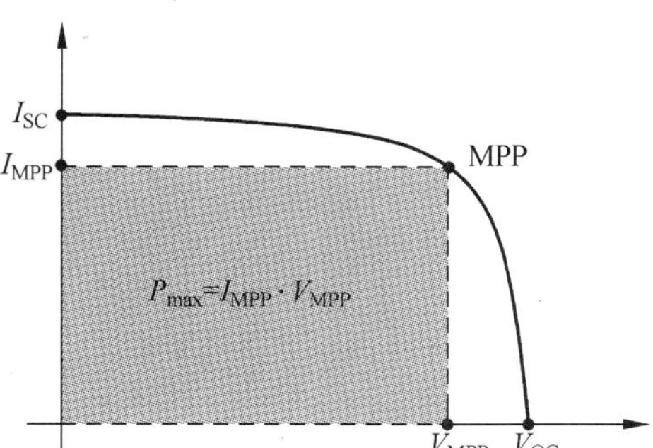

Figure 24.1 Typical I - V -curve of a solar cell

One disadvantage of the silicon solar cell is that its production costs and therefore the cost of the electricity it generates are rather high. The production of silicon pure enough to be used for solar cells from SiO_2 involves several high-temperature steps (up to 2000℃), which are very energy consuming. Dye-sensitized solar cells (DSSC) have emerged in the last two decades as a possible cost-effective alternative. Contrary to conventional p-n solar cells where the used materials need to have good light absorption as well as charge carrier transport properties, light harvesting and charge carrier transport are separated in DSSC. While an inorganic semiconductor serves as the electron transport medium, the photo excitation of the electrons occurs in dye molecules attached to the surface.

The working principle of a DSSC is shown in detail in Fig. 24.2. A porous film of a wide band gap n-type semiconductor is prepared on a transparent conducting oxide (TCO) electrode, e.g. indium tin oxide (ITO) or F-doped tin oxide (FTO) on glass. The film is sensitized by dye molecules, which are adsorbed in a monolayer on the semiconductor surface. If the lowest unoccupied molecular orbital (LUMO) of the dye is energetically higher than the conduction band edge of the semiconductor, photo excited electrons can be injected from the dye to the semiconductor and transported to the conducting back contact. The dye is regenerated by hole injection into a redox electrolyte (e.g. I^- / I_{3^-}), whose redox potential has to be energetically higher than the highest occupied molecular orbital (HOMO) of the dye. The redox electrolyte is regenerated by electron transfer from the counter electrode, in most cases a platinum (Pt) electrode or platinized TCO/glass electrode in order to catalyze the charge transfer. Since the Fermi level of the counter electrode is determined by the redox potential of the electrolyte and the maximum quasi-Fermi level of electrons in the semiconductor is close to the conduction band, the maximum reachable photovoltage of the DSSC is the difference between the conduction band edge and the redox potential of the electrolyte.

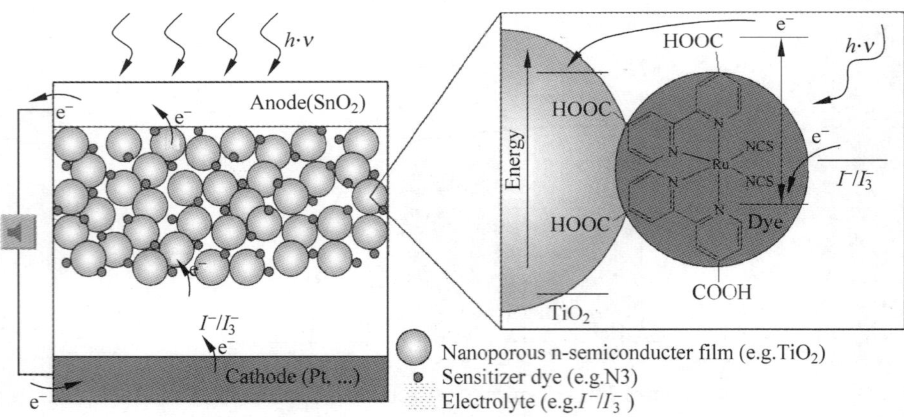

Figure 24.2 Scheme and working principle of a DSSC

Photosensitization is actually known since the discovery of the photographic process in the 19th century and was first associated with dye molecules when Vogel sensitized silver halide emulsions by adding dyes in 1883 (West, 1974). The first dye-sensitized photoelectrode device followed only four years later (Moser, 1887). However, the possibilities of dye-sensitization were not fully recognized for a long time, until it was 're-discovered' in the early 1960s. Many new findings were reported at the International Conference on Photosensitization of Solids in Chicago in 1964, e.g. dye-sensitization of ZnO with cyanine dyes (Namba and Hishiki, 1965) and the necessity of an adsorbed dye monolayer to reach maximum efficiency (Nelson, 1965). The question if sensitization taking place due to the transfer of electrons or energy was answered by Gerischer and

Tributsch (Gerischer et al., 1968), who demonstrated the electron transfer mechanism on a single crystal ZnO electrode. In 1971, Tributsch investigated the photochemical reactions of chlorophyll and suggested dye-sensitization for solar cells (Tributsch, 1971). In 1984, the sensitization of TiO_2 particles with Ru (II) complexes for water splitting started (Dung et al., 1984), and the first photoelectrode consisting of this combination was reported one year later (Desilvestro et al., 1985). However, the breakthrough only came with the preparation of a TiO_2 film with considerably higher surface area by using TiO_2 nanoparticles, leading to the famous paper published in Nature (O'Regan and Grätzel, 1991) reporting efficiencies over 7%. Since then, the efficiency has increased to about 11 % by further development of TiO_2 nanoparticles, sensitizer dyes and film preparation techniques. The efficiency record for dye-sensitized solar cells, which was held by Grätzel and co-workers for more than two decades, was recently taken over by the research group of Sharp Corp., where 11.1% was reached with a 0.22 cm^2 cell. The highest 'official' efficiency (for cells of the standard size of 1 cm^2) of 10.4% was also reached by this group (Koide et al., 2006; Green at al., 2007).

Besides the further development of the 'conventional' DSSC, two topics within the field have gained special attention in recent years, which could lead to the main breakthrough in the field of DSSC regarding their commercialization. The first topic is the replacement of the liquid redox electrolyte by solid or quasi-solid hole conducting materials, the second is the development of flexible dye-sensitized solar cells. Solid-state DSSC are sought in particular because the problems associated with the long-term sealing of the liquid electrolytes used in DSSCs are still not fully solved. A review of material development for the replacement of liquid electrolytes in DSSC can be found in (Li et al., 2006). Flexible DSSCs have become the topic of much interest due to their great advantages. Firstly, conductive plastic substrates, e.g. indium tin oxide coated on polyethylene terephthalate (PET) or polyethylene naphthalate (PEN), can be processed by a continuous process like roll-to-roll production for porous nanocrystalline film coating, therefore greatly decreasing the production cost of the solar cells. Secondly, flexible DSSCs would significantly widen the application possibilities of solar cells. Flexible DSSCs can become part of a variety of every day products and turn them into energy sources. One example is 'wearable solar cells', i.e. flexible solar cells as a part of clothing. The possibility to produce the flexible DSSCs in any colour and in transparent as well as non-transparent versions would open almost endless opportunities to the designers of such products. The 'wearable solar cells' could, for example, be used to charge the electrical batteries of cellular phones, mobile personal computers, watches, calculators, PDAs, iPods, portable stereo walkmans, etc. Even without being flexible, DSSC using (rigid) plastic substrates would have advantages compared to DSSC based on glass due to their lightweight character. As a last point to be mentioned, the flexible and lightweight solar cells may also present great advantages in military applications in the pursuit of energy sources to partly replace troublesome use of heavy batteries in the battlefield front.

Due to all these possibilities and advantages, commercialization of flexible DSSCs indeed has attracted a lot of efforts so far. However, the conventional method for the preparation of TiO_2 electrodes for DSSC using colloidal suspensions of TiO_2 nanoparticles typically includes high-temperature sintering at 450℃ or higher. This method cannot be applied to prepare films on flexible plastic substrates, which only endure temperatures of up to around 150℃. The necessary low-temperature preparation of porous nanocrystalline metal oxides semiconductor films has been a well highlighted and on-going challenge up to today. There have been a number of studies concerned with the preparation of such low-temperature films, and various kinds of flexible DSSCs have been fabricated. In this chapter, we will describe the flexible DSSCs and the current efforts of low temperature preparation of porous nanocrystalline films (Section 24.2). The specific concerns besides low-temperature preparation are electron transport and recombination of photogenerated electrons in low-temperature films as well as electron injection and recombination between the dye and the semiconductor, which will therefore be discussed in separate chapters (Section 24.3 and Section 24.2, respectively with and 4). We expect that this work will help to understand the science behind DSSCs and contribute to the further improvement of the efficiency of flexible DSSCs.

24.2 Flexible DSSCs and Low Temperature Preparation

Conventional dye-sensitized solar cells are based on a porous nanocrystalline semiconductor metal oxide film such as TiO_2, ZnO and SnO_2. Typically, these films are prepared by a sol-gel method with a high temperature > 450℃ sintering process. There are two different preparation methods that can be used generally. One is film preparation starting from commercially available nanocrystalline particles; the other is starting from oxide precursors of organic or inorganic salts. Methods starting from precursor salts have an advantage that the process parameters, like particle size, porosity, surface area, crystallinity, density and so on can be modified, and therefore the microstructure of films can be optimized for photosensitization. For instance, porous nanocrystalline TiO_2 films can be obtained starting from Ti(Ⅳ) tetraisopropoxide (TTIP) (Barbé et al., 1997): With hydrolysis of TTIP a white precipitate is formed; then after about 8 h at about 80℃, a TiO_2 gel can be obtained. Following a hydrothermal process at 180 – 220℃ overnight, particles with a perfect crystalline structure are formed. Finally, certain amounts of organic additives, typically a poly(ethylene glycol)-based surfactant, are added and mixed together, forming the paste ready for coating. The surfactant decreases the surface stress of nanoparticles resulting from their large surface area, leading to forming a homogenous film without cracks during the next step of high temperature sintering. Meanwhile, the surfactant can modify the porosity of the films. Without surfactant, the films are easy to crack during sintering. The coated raw films must be sintered at high temperature to get robust films with strong interconnection between particles and strong adhesion between films and the substrates such as conductive glass. Most importantly, the electrical connections between the particles will be improved by this high temperature sintering, which will benefit the electron transport in films.

The other method starting from commercially available nanocrystalline particles has the advantage of being a fast and convenient process. The nanocrystalline particles of oxides are mixed with water by mechanical blending with the addition of a surfactant such as Triton-100, achieving an appropriate paste for coating under ambient conditions, then sintered at a temperature of 450℃ or higher.

In summary, both processes described above require the following three items:

(1) Medium: must be employed for hydrolyzing, reacting and blending (water is used in most cases)

(2) Surfactant: must be added for appropriate paste preparation and to assure crack-free film formation

(3) High temperature sintering process: must be employed to form films with good electrical interconnections and to remove the (water) medium and surfactant.

It has been shown that the high temperature sintering process is essential for achieving a high performance nanocrystalline porous film, which in fact is responsible for the high conversion efficiency of DSSC. The sintering process not only enables the formation of good electrical connections between the particles, it also decreases the number of surface states that might act as electron traps, leading to more efficient electron transport in the film. This is mainly due to the removal of the (water) medium and the surfactants, which, if present, would represent extrinsic surface states, resulting in the significant reduction of the recombination of electrons at the interface of film and electrolyte.

However, flexible DSSCs employ plastic conductive PET/PEN substrates instead of rigid glass, therefore the vital step of high temperature sintering cannot be employed. In other words, without the high temperature sintering process, the efficient electrochemical interconnection would not be achieved, and the medium plus the surfactant in the film therefore have to be removed by some other process at low or room temperature. With the use of ITO-PET electrodes, the thermal treatment is limited to 150℃, because above this temperature the polymer undergoes thermal degradation, loosing its transparency and becoming completely distorted.

The ongoing challenge to prepare high performance efficient nanocrystalline porous films at low or room temperature has been highlighted in the literature. Effective low temperature processes that is as efficient as the above mentioned high temperature sintering have yet to be developed in order to realize high efficiency flexible DSSCs. So far the oxide films prepared with low temperature methods are not as efficient as those prepared at high temperature, therefore this vital process of high temperature sintering has been used in the preparation of one kind of flexible solar cell that is based on metal foils such as titanium foil (Ito et al., 2006), tungsten and stainless steel (Kang et al., 2005, 2006).Even though metal substrates can be sintered at high temperature, and the conventional film preparation methods can be employed without further development, they are not transparent. Therefore, light has to be directed to the front side of the films (through the counter electrode) and the counter electrodes have to use transparent PET/PEN. As anticipated, these flexible DSSCs still have lower conversion efficiency of about 2.2% – 7.2% because electrons originating from the front side illumination have to travel longer distances before they are collected, therefore the possibilities of recombination are higher than in the case of back side illumination (through the conducting substrate of the oxide film), which is usually employed for conventional DSSCs. Obviously, this kind of flexible metal substrate DSSCs cannot fulfill the advantages of real flexible DSSCs based on whole ITO/PET or PEN structures.

There is an interesting method of lift-off and transfer (Dürr et al., 2005) that has been proposed to fulfill the goal of flexible DSSCs on PET/PEN using the conventional high temperature sintering process. The high performance films were prepared by the conventional high temperature method on Au/glass as the supporting substrate, then transferred to ITO/PET substrates, resulting in the highest efficiency of 5.8% for a flexible DSSC based on whole plastic substrates under the illumination of AM 1.5 simulated sun light. However, this procedure may not be suitable for practical applications due to the complications in transferring a nanocrystalline TiO_2 layer from Au/glass to ITO/PET.

Electrodeposition has also been employed to prepare nanocrystalline porous oxides films at low temperature. A one-step electrodeposition technique (Yoshida et al., 2004). was developed for the preparation of hybrid dye/ZnO films at low temperature. Since dye aggregates were formed in the pores of the ZnO in the as-prepared films, the dyes had to be extracted to achieve a porous ZnO film, then dipped into dye solutions to re-absorb the dye. Even tough this method can prepare highly porous crystalline ZnO films with effective electron interconnections at low temperature, the efficiency of the films is still considerably lower than that of conventional TiO_2 films, since the efficient Ru-complexes usually used for TiO_2-based cells cannot be used as sensitizers for ZnO as they tend to aggregate on the ZnO surface (Keis et al., 2000). On the other hand, electrodeposition of crystalline TiO_2 does not work at low temperature or yields films with very small pores not suitable for DSSC (Wessels et al., 2006). The method does not work at all for other oxides which might be suitable for DSSC such as SnO_2 since they cannot be crystallized at low temperature.

From the above mentioned efforts, it is clear that low temperature preparation methods have to be developed to achieve high performance nanocrystalline porous oxides films to fulfill the full advantages of flexible DSSCs. The high temperature sintering process must be put aside for now, though it has been proven to be very efficient so far. In fact, a number of efforts have been made towards the development of efficient porous nanocrystalline semiconductor metal oxides such as TiO_2 and ZnO films without high temperature sintering. The easiest way is simply by reducing the annealing temperature to less than 150℃ and to employ coatings from colloidal pastes free of any organic surfactants, while compensating for the lower temperatures with longer annealing times up to overnight or more. Following this method, Pichot et al. (2000) have fabricated a flexible porous nanocrystalline TiO_2 film onto ITO-coated poly(ethylene terephthalate) substrates by spin coating from a surfactant-free nanocrystalline TiO_2 colloidal suspension, and then sintered at a low temperature of 100℃ for 24 h. Unfortunately, only very thin films with a maximum film thickness of 1 μm were achieved, which are much thinner than the optimal thickness (10 – 15 μm) obtained by the high temperature sintered film, which is necessary to achieve a sufficient dye loading for maximizing the device conversion efficiency in a typical rigid DSSC. Because of this very thin TiO_2 electrode, the overall device efficiency (1.22%) was much lower than that (11%) of the sintered rigid DSSC. Sintering at various temperatures less than 150℃ and varying sintering times were also investigated. However, a significant increase in the conversion efficiency was not achieved.

A different low-temperature method proposed by De Paoli and co-workers (Longo et al., 2002, 2003) takes advantage of the photocatalytic activity of TiO_2 which was exposed to UV irradiation in order to eliminate organic substances present in the commercial TiO_2 colloidal precursor used. The as-prepared TiO_2 thick film fabrication is completed by following heating at 140℃ during a 2 h period. A solid state flexible DSSC based on this process was able to achieve a 0.32% conversion efficiency. Without any annealing, another study showed that the films were simply dried at room temperature, and only 1.2% conversion efficiency was achieved (Kim et al., 2005).

A smart method without any sintering was proposed by Hagfeldt and co-workers for the preparation of a porous nanocrystalline semiconductor film onto ITO-PET substrates at room temperature (Lindström et al., 2001). Instead of sintering, a mechanical compression technique consisting of statically or continuously pressing powder films of metal oxides such as TiO_2 or ZnO, free from organic surfactant and previously dispersed in ethanol, has been successfully developed. The typical pressure for preparing efficient solar cells is 1000 kg/cm for a few seconds. Interestingly, the same mechanical and morphological properties and porosities like those of films prepared by the conventional high temperature annealing technique were found for films prepared with the pressing technique. This method achieved overall cell conversion efficiencies as high as 4.9% with a weak illumination of 10 mW/cm^2. This compression technique can not only be applied to a plastic substrate, but also to glass. The DSSCs on glass substrates assembled using compressed films with additional heat treatment ('annealed'), or with compressed films without further heat treatment ('non-annealed') exhibit similar performance. The great advantage is that this pressing technique can be employed to prepare porous nanocrystalline films on plastic substrates by the continuous method such as the roll-to-roll process.

Novel approaches for surface activation methods used instead of the high temperature sintering process were also developed and investigated to prepare porous nanocrystalline films or to further improve their performance. Electrophoretic deposition (Miyasaka et al., 2002; Miyasaka and Kijitori, 2004; Yum et al., 2005) was employed to prepare porous nanocrystalline metal oxide films at low temperature. The electrophoretic deposition method is a combination of electrophoresis and deposition. With this method, charged particles in a suspension including an electrolyte, particles, additives and solvent are moved toward an oppositely charged electrode and are then deposited onto a substrate under an applied DC electric field. The porous films prepared by this method have shown lower performance, and further treatment of the as-prepared films such as following a chemical treatment, thermal treatment of 150 ℃ or compression can further improve its performance. DSSCs based on the aforementioned method obtained more then 3% conversion efficiency after such post-treatment. Microwave processing offers the possibility of achieving sintering at lower temperatures and in shorter times. A multi-mode microwave heating system operating at a frequency of 28 GHz (Uchida et al., 2004; Miyasaka et al., 2002; Miyasaka and Kijitori, 2004) was employed to produce rapid synthesis of the porous nanocrystalline films on a transparent conductive PET-ITO electrode. Photoelectron energy conversion efficiency of 2.16% is achieved in an electrode prepared by 28 GHz microwave irradiation at 1.0 kW for 5 min. When electrophoretic deposition is used following the microwave post treatment, conversion efficiencies as high as 4.1% can be achieved under AM 1.5 illumination with simulated sun light (Miyasaka et al., 2002; Miyasaka and Kijitori, 2004). Low-accelerating electron beam showers (Kado et al., 2003) at room temperature were successfully utilized for the preparation and cure of the porous nanocrystalline TiO_2 films on conductive plastic. No substrate deterioration was found by the employment of this physical method. Short circuit photocurrents for dye sensitized solar cells increased from 3.50 to 7.38 mA/cm^2 after the TiO_2 films were exposed to electron beam showers. Chemical vapor deposition (CVD) of TiO_2 combined with UV light irradiation was also employed as activation method to improve the performance of the films (Takurou et al., 2003). Applying this treatment to the nanocrystalline TiO_2 particle films coated on plastic film electrodes (ITO-PET) drastically enhanced dye-sensitized photocurrent and improved photovoltage up to 750 mV, achieving an energy conversion efficiency of 3.8%. Likewise, a UV-mediated low-temperature sintering method (Lewis et al., 2006) has been shown for the fabrication of porous nanocrystalline films at low temperature. UV irradiation appears to facilitate the clean oxidation of residual organic materials in the titania precursor pastes. UV treatment has also been employed by Murakami et al. (Murakami et al. 2002; Murakami and Kijitori, 2004) in order to eliminate adsorbed organic impurities in the TiO_2 obtained using an electrophoretic method and improved the efficiency of their DSSC. A UV laser sintering technique was also used and a laser direct-write technique (Kim et al., 2006) was developed to fabricate nanocrystalline TiO_2 films. An advantage of this approach is that the same UV laser direct-write setup is used for both transferring the TiO_2 colloidal suspensions and low-temperature sintering of the TiO_2 films. The overall conversion efficiency of the cells based on the laser-sintered TiO_2 electrodes was double than that of the devices with non-laser-treated TiO_2 electrodes. The above indicates that this method can be used to remove the organic additives and to form an electrically connected network structure without damaging the substrates underneath.

In addition, wet chemical approaches are developed for the porous nanocrystalline film preparation. A wet technique (Takenaka et al., 2003) of crystals directly grown on a substrate in an aqueous solution has been applied and shown to be able to fabricate porous nanocrystalline films for dye-sensitized solar cells. An acid-base chemistry also was used to prepare a binder-free TiO_2 paste, which can be used to fabricate thick films at low temperature (Park et al., 2004). Thick porous TiO_2 films have also been prepared at low temperature from a mixture of a commercial TiO_2 powder and an easy-to-handle water-soluble titania precursor, such as titanium(Ⅳ) bis (ammonium lactato)dihydroxide. A post-treatment by ultraviolet (UV) light irradiation using a medium-pressure mercury vapor lamp leads to the decomposition of the titania precursor as a result of the photocatalytic activity of nanocrystalline TiO_2 present in the blend (Gutierrez-Tauste et al., 2005).

Another low-temperature chemical method for the fabrication of mesoporous TiO_2 films grown on ITO/PET substrates at 100℃ employs a hydrothermal reaction at the solid/gas interface (Zhang et al., 2002, 2003, 2004). Nanocrystalline TiO_2 particles mixed with Ti monomers such as $TiCl_4$, $TiOSO_4$, and TiIV tetraisopropoxide were coated on the substrate and exposed to hot steam in the gas phase of an autoclave. The added Ti monomers are hydrolyzed and converted into crystalline TiO_2, which can act as a 'glue' to chemically connect the TiO_2 particles as well as promote adherence of the film to the substrate. A flexible DSSC with a conversion efficiency of 2.3% under illumination of AM 1.5 simulated sunlight (100 mw/cm^2) can be successfully prepared by applying an ethanolic paste containing TTIP as the Ti monomer onto an ITO/PET conductive film substrate. Firm attachment of the TiO_2 particles by the newly formed crystalline TiO_2 has been thought to be the reason for the high efficiency. More details about the electron transport in these films are given in Section 24.3.

Furthermore, based on the low temperature preparation by hydrothermal crystallization, fast processing of high-performance porous TiO_2 thick-film electrodes at room temperature was achieved (Zhang et al., 2006a). In this process, a small amount of titanium salt like TTIP was mixed with nanocrystlline titanium powders in an ethanolic solution that can be coated under ambient conditions to form robust films very fast at room temperature. With the elimination of the hydrothermal treatment, 1.8% conversion efficiency was achieved for a flexible solar cell under 1 sun illumination with AM 1.5 simulated sun light. It was also found that the pre-treatment of commercial nanocrystalline powders of TiO_2 with high temperature sintering can improve the conversion efficiency to levels as high as 2.55%. The contamination found in commercial nanocrystalline powders can be removed by this high temperature pre-treatment. Further, the UV-ozone post-treatment of the films resulted in a remarkable improvement of the cell efficiency up to 3.27% for all-flexible DSSCs. The rigid version of the same DSSC using conductive glass showed a conversion efficiency as high as 4.00% without any sintering. UV-ozone post-treatment removed the residual organics originating from the hydrolysis of TTIP. Research work on the preparation of porous nanocrystalline films at room temperature is ongoing. Very recently it was found that even the addition of the titanium precursor TTIP can be eliminated. While the TTIP is thought to produce the glue for effective interconnection, it can also result in small organic molecules remaining in the film as recombination centers (Zhang et al., 2006b). With thorough mixing and dispersion, films were prepared at room temperature employing only nanocrystalline powders with ethanol solvent, and still very robust films could be obtained. Figure 24.3 presents the AFM image of the nanocrystalline TiO_2 film prepared at room temperature by this method. One can see that the film is very homogenous with individual particles of the same size connected with each other.

In summary, conversion efficiency of up to about 4% under AM 1.5 simulated sun light illumination (100 mW/cm^2) has been achieved so far for all-flexible DSSCs based at room or low temperature preparation (150℃) on conductive polymer films. The efficiencies of the flexible DSSCs on polymer films were lower than the efficiencies of DSSCs on FTO (F-doped tin oxide) glass substrates sintered at high-temperature. The low performance of the low temperature porous nanocrystalline films can be attributed to the following factors: (1) poor mechanical stability of the films, (2) weak electrical interconnections between nanocrystalline particles and adhesion with substrates, (3) contamination from ex-situ processes such as storage or transport, (4) organics resulting from the additives used for film preparation, (5) low level of crystallization, (6) weak coupling between dye molecules and semiconductor films, (7) intrinsic surface states in a much higher density compared to high temperature sintered films. All these factors have an effect on the efficiencies of injection/recombination, transport/recombination and collection of electrons. So, in the following parts we will analyze in detail the electron transport and the electron recombination at the interface of low temperature films and electrolytes (Section 24.3) as well as the electron injection and recombination pathways between the dye and film (Section 24.4).

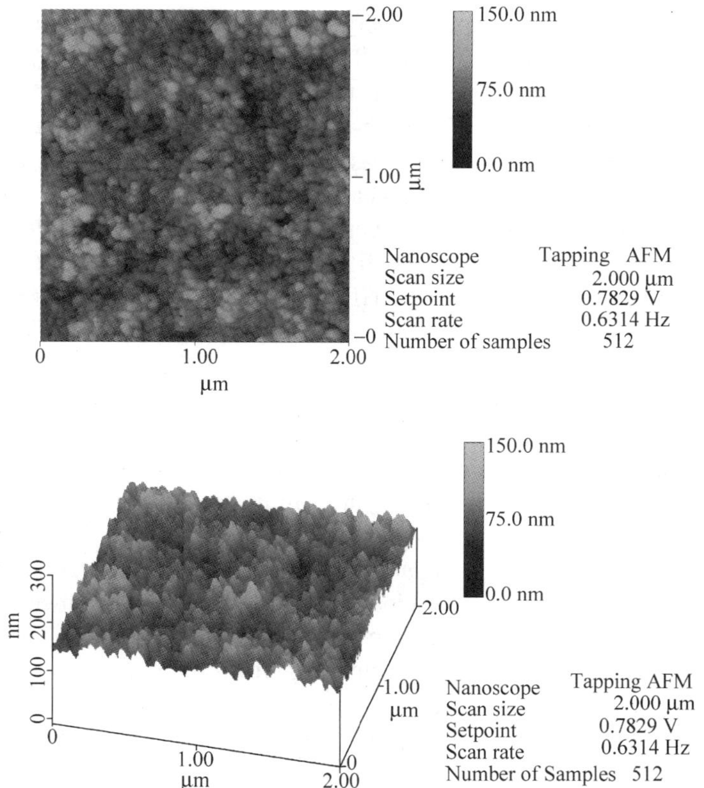

Figure 24.3 AFM image of nanocrystalline TiO_2 films with 10 μm film thickness prepared at room temperature and ambient conditions

24.3 Electron Transport and Back Reaction at the TiO_2/ Electrolyte Interface

24.3.1 Factors that Determine Efficiency

In this chapter, the factors that determine the efficiency of DSSC will be discussed in more detail. Beside the overall efficiency η, one way to measure the performance of solar cells is the incident photon to current conversion efficiency (IPCE), which can also be described by the equation

$$\mathrm{IPCE}(\lambda) = \mathrm{LHE}(\lambda) \cdot \Phi_{\mathrm{inj}} \cdot \eta_{\mathrm{c}} \tag{24.1}$$

where LHE stands for the light harvesting efficiency, Φ_{inj} is the efficiency of electron injection, and η_{c} is the collection efficiency of injected electrons. Since the LHE depends on the absorption coefficient of the dye, the LHE as well as the IPCE change with the wavelength λ of the incident light.

All three factors can depend on the preparation method of the films. Comparing low-temperature with high-temperature TiO_2 films made from the same nanoparticles, similar surface areas, dye loadings and therefore LHE values can be expected, given that both films have the same thickness. This is the reason why it is important to develop techniques for the preparation of stable thick films at low temperature, since a lower film thickness would lead to less light absorption and therefore to a lower LHE. The second factor, Φ_{inj}, was found to depend on the crystallinity of the TiO_2, since low crystallinity of the TiO_2 surface leads to a weaker adsorption of the dye molecules and therefore to a less efficient electron injection into the TiO_2 (Kim et al., 2002). This problem, however, is not important for most low-temperature preparation techniques, where highly crystalline TiO_2 nanoparticles prepared by high-temperature methods are used for the low-temperature preparation of the films, or if the nanoparticles are pre-treated by annealing.

The most important problem regarding the efficiency of low-temperature TiO_2 films is the electron collection efficiency η_c, which can be described in terms of the electron lifetime τ_n and the electron transit time τ_D. While τ_n is determined by the back reaction of photogenerated electrons from the conduction band of the TiO_2 to the redox electrolyte, τ_D is a measure for the time that photoinjected electrons need to reach the back contact. Consequently, τ_n should be higher than τ_D in order to collect all photoinjected electrons.

In general, electron transport has been found to be slow in the nanoporous TiO_2 films. Since no electric field is present in the films due to screening by the redox electrolyte in the pores, electron transport takes place solely by diffusion. The electron transport can therefore be described by an electron diffusion coefficient D_n and the continuity equation (Södergren et al., 1994; Oekermann et al., 2004)

$$\frac{\partial n}{\partial t} = \Phi_{\mathrm{inj}} \alpha I_0 \mathrm{e}^{-\alpha x} + D_n \frac{\partial^2 n}{\partial x^2} - \frac{n - n_0}{\tau_n} \qquad (24.2)$$

The three terms of this equation describe electron generation, electron diffusion and electron back reaction with α as absorption coefficient, I_0 as incident light intensity, n as electron density under illumination and n_0 as equilibrium electron concentration in the dark. D_n is often called efficient or apparent diffusion coefficient, since it is determined by trapping and detrapping events of the electrons on their way through the film. It can be defined by

$$D_n = D_{\mathrm{cb}} \frac{k_{\mathrm{d}}}{k_{\mathrm{t}}} \qquad (24.3)$$

where k_t and k_d are the first-order rate constants for the trapping and detrapping, respectively, and D_{cb} is the diffusion coefficient of electrons in the conduction band (Fisher et al., 2000). It has been estimated that the time spent in traps by photogenerated electrons on their way through a nanoporous TiO_2 film is about 100 times higher than the time spent as free electrons in the conduction band. Knowing D_n and τ_n, the diffusion lengths L_n of the electrons can be calculated according to the equation (Peter and Vanmaekelbergh, 1999)

$$L_n = \sqrt{D_n \tau_n} \tag{24.4}$$

The diffusion length is a useful value to discuss the collection efficiency of DSSC, since it has to be higher than the film thickness in order to collect all photoinjected electrons.

24.3.2 Techniques for Measuring Electron Transport and Back Reaction

Several techniques are available for the measurement of τ_n, τ_D and D_n. The first measurements of electron transit times have been performed by Solbrand, Hagfeldt and coworkers (Solbrand et al., 1997; Solbrand et al., 1999) by illuminating the dye-sensitized porous TiO_2 films with short laser pulses from the electrolyte side and monitoring the resulting photocurrent transients in the millisecond- to second-regime. Assuming that most photons are absorbed near the geometrical surface of the film and have to diffuse through the whole film, the diffusion coefficient can be simply calculated by

$$D_n = \frac{d^2}{6 \cdot t_{\text{peak}}} \tag{24.5}$$

where d is the film thickness and t_{peak} is the time delay between the laser pulse and the maximum of the photocurrent response. The disadvantage of this method is that the system is driven far from the equilibrium by the laser pulse, which makes an exact analysis of the results difficult. For example, the electron density and therefore the trap occupancy and the apparent diffusion coefficient D_n along the film thickness are expected to change during such a measurement.

This problem has been overcome by measurements under working conditions, i.e. under constant illumination, using small changes (up to $+/-$ 10%) of the illumination level. This can be a small step in the light intensity or a light modulation with small amplitude. Under these conditions, D_n can be treated as constant for a given bias light intensity (Dloczik et al., 1997). Especially, intensity modulated photocurrent spectroscopy (IMPS), which uses a mostly sinusoidal modulation of the light intensity, has often been used for the investigation of electron transport in DSSC. The modulation of the light is described by the periodic illumination function

$$I(t) = I_0\left[1 + (\delta e^{i\omega t})\right] \tag{24.6}$$

where I_0 is the bias light intensity, $\omega = 2\pi f$ is the modulation frequency and δ is $\ll 1$. The photocurrent response is measured in terms of its amplitude and phase shift with respect to the illumination function under variation of the modulation frequency, and it can be represented in the IMPS complex plane plots, which are characterized by a semicircle in the positive/negative quadrant. A typical example with flattened semicircles, which is caused by a certain distribution of electron transit times, is given in Fig. 24.4. The transit times τ_D can be calculated directly from the IMPS response since $\tau_D = 1 / \omega_{min}(\text{IMPS}) = 1 / 2\pi f_{min}(\text{IMPS})$ where f_{min}(IMPS) is the frequency of the minimum of the semicircle, i.e. the frequency of the lowest imaginary component in the IMPS plot (Peter and Vanmaekelbergh, 1999).

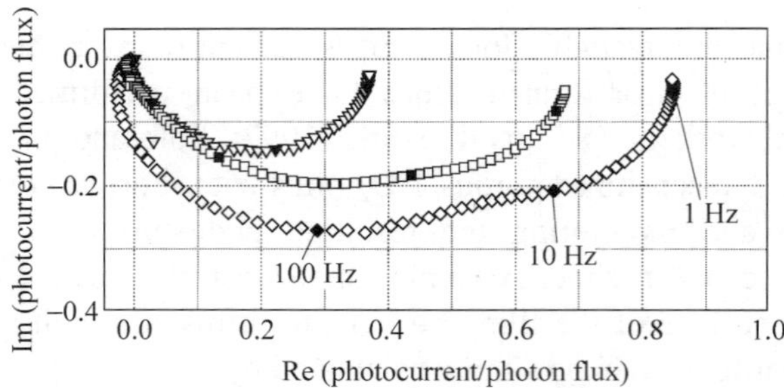

Figure 24.4 IMPS plots measured with an incident dc light intensity of 2.6 mW/cm^2 for dye sensitized TiO_2 films prepared by hydrothermal crystallization (▽ on FTO / glass; ◇ on FTO/glass, sintered at 450℃ for 1 h after preparation). For comparison the IMPS plot of a film prepared from TiO_2 nanoparticles (Degussa P25) by the conventional method including high-temperature sintering (□) is also shown (Oekermann et al., 2004)

The electron back reaction to the electrolyte can be measured by a similar method, intensity modulated photovoltage spectroscopy (IMVS), where the open-circuit photovoltage is analyzed instead of the short-circuit photocurrent. The open-circuit voltage in a DSSC is the difference between the quasi Fermi level of the electrons in the TiO_2 and the redox potential of the electrolyte. It therefore depends on the electron concentration in the TiO_2, which in turn solely depends on the electron generation rate and the rate of electron back reaction to the redox electrolyte under open-circuit conditions. Based on these considerations, it has been shown that the electron lifetime τ_n can be calculated from the f_{min} of the IMVS response by $\tau_n = 1 / \omega_{min}(\text{IMVS}) = 1 / 2\pi f_{min}(\text{IMVS})$ (Schlichthörl et al., 1997).

Based on the illumination function in Eq. (24.6), analytical solutions of the continuity equation Eq. (24.2) for short-circuit conditions (IMPS) have been published in the literature (Dloczik et al., 1997). Using τ_n from the IMVS measurements, these analytical solutions can be used to fit the IMPS response and calculate D_n. The normalized solution for the photocurrent j_{photo} and therefore the IMPS response for illumination through the back contact of the film are

$$\frac{j_{\text{photo}}}{q\delta\Phi_{\text{inj}}I_0} = \frac{\alpha}{\alpha+\gamma}\cdot\frac{e^{\gamma d} - e^{-\gamma d} + 2\alpha\dfrac{e^{-\alpha d} - e^{-\gamma d}}{\gamma - \alpha}}{e^{\gamma d} + e^{-\gamma d}} \tag{24.7}$$

with

$$\gamma = \left[\frac{1}{D_n \tau_n} + \mathrm{i}\frac{\omega}{D_n}\right]^{\frac{1}{2}} \tag{24.8}$$

where q is the elementary charge. Since dye-sensitized solar cells are usually illuminated through the back contact due to the higher resulting photocurrent, IMPS measurements under this condition are also preferable. Figure. 24.5 shows Bode plots of the fitting results for one of the IMPS plots shown in Fig. 24.4. It can be seen that the IMPS response is affected by RC attenuation at high frequencies, which can be taken into account by multiplying Eq. (24.7) with the complex attenuation function

$$A(\omega) = \frac{1}{1 + \mathrm{i}\omega RC} \tag{24.9}$$

where R is the series resistance and C is the capacitance of the electrode.[24.10]

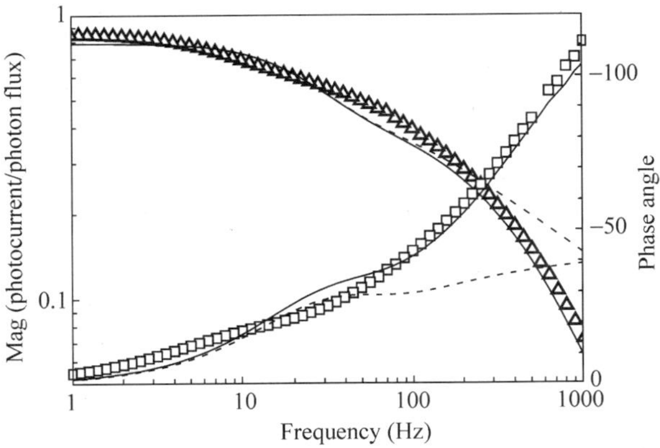

Figure 24.5 IMPS bode plots (△ magnitude; □ phase angle) of a dye-sensitized TiO_2 film prepared by hydrothermal crystallization and subsequent sintering at 450℃ for an incident dc light intensity of 2.6 mW/cm^2. The lines show fits according to Eqs. (24.17), (24.18) and (24.19). (---- RC attenuation neglected; — RC attenuation with $C = 9$ μF, $R = 37$ Ω) (Oekermann et al., 2004)

It has been found that, under short circuit conditions, R and C are mostly due to the SnO_2 / TiO_2 and SnO_2 / electrolyte interfaces with typical values of around 10 to 20 Ω and 30 μF/cm.

Due to the availability of light emitting diodes (LED) with high light intensity and fast response as light sources for illumination of the cells, the measurement of small amplitude photocurrent and photovoltage transients has become increasingly popular for the measurement of electron transport and back reaction in recent years. In these measurements, the small step in the illumination level can simply be generated by a small change in the voltage applied to the LED. Transient methods using pulsed light (O'Regan and Lenzmann, 2004; van de Lagemaat and Frank, 2001) as well as square-wave modulation (Nakade et al., 2005; Boschloo et al., 2006) have been developed. The calculation of the electron lifetimes and transit times from the transients can be done by determining the time constants of the photovoltage or photocurrent decay after the light pulses based on fitting to exponential functions. In general, the time constants derived from these calculations were found to be comparable to the τ_D and τ_n values extracted from IMPS and IMVS measurements. It has further been shown that the electron diffusion coefficient D_n can be estimated from the photocurrent transient response by

$$D_n = \frac{d^2}{2.35 \cdot \tau_c} \tag{24.10}$$

for illumination through the counter electrode, where τ_C is the time constant of the photocurrent decay.

In general, apparent electron diffusion coefficients around 10^{-4} cm^2/s have been found at high light intensities (around '1 sun' = 100 mW/cm) for nanoporous TiO_2 films prepared by standard preparation methods that include high-temperature annealing. The value is about 1 order of magnitude lower if the illumination level is in the range of a few mW/cm. Measurements at such light intensities have often been done due to limitations by the LEDs used as light sources. Although such measurements at low light intensities underestimate the diffusion coefficients under 'real' working conditions, they are still useful to compare the electron transport in films prepared from different kinds of nanoparticles, e.g. particles of different size (Nakade et al., 2003), crystal structure and shape (Kambe et al., 2002), or films prepared under otherwise different conditions like different temperatures, as will be shown in detail in the following part of this chapter.

24.3.3 Results Obtained with Low-Temperature Films

While electron transport in nanoporous TiO_2 films is slow in general, it has been found to be even slower in films prepared by low-temperature methods. This is often attributed to a low degree of neck growth at low temperature and a resulting low electric contact between the particles (Kim et al., 2002; Nakade et al., 2002; Park et al., 2000). At first glance, one could think that the collection efficiency and therefore the overall efficiency of low-temperature films could be increased if measures are taken to make electron transport faster. In fact, comparing low-temperature and high-temperature films made from the same materials, the high temperature films are generally found to exhibit increased diffusion lengths and efficiencies (Park et al., 1999). However, to discuss the reasons for this increase, it has to be considered that electron transport in the nanoporous TiO_2 films is limited by trapping and detrapping events as mentioned above. Faster electron transport does not mean that the free electrons in the conduction band move faster, but that the electrons spend less time in traps. The time that electrons need to spend as free electrons in order to diffuse to the back contact is not changed, and therefore the recombination probability of the electrons, their diffusion length and the electron collection efficiency also remain the same. In other words, if the electron transit time τ_D decreases due to less trapping of electrons, the electron lifetime τ_n, will be changed by the same factor. This has been shown quantitatively by Frank and co-workers (Kopidakis et al., 2003). It should be noted that this theory is based on the assumption that electron traps are mainly located within the TiO_2 particles. If they would be located mainly at the surface, electron recombination would essentially involve trapped electrons and not free electrons in the conduction band, so that less trapping would lead to longer, not shorter, electron lifetimes.

Due to the above considerations, a higher electron collection efficiency cannot be achieved by improving electron transport, but only by suppressing back reaction. In fact, the effect of additives, which are used in the electrolytes of dye-sensitized solar cells since long time such as pyridine, is at least partly based on a blocking of the surface, which leads to less back reaction (Neale et al., 2005; Kopidakis et al., 2006). The same effect is seen if the TiO_2 particles are covered by thin barrier coatings, e.g. thin alumina layers (Fabregat-Santiago et al., 2004). However, preparation of these barrier layers has to be done on the surface of the readily prepared porous TiO_2 films, and also requires high-temperature treatment. Coating the TiO_2 nanoparticles before low-temperature preparation of the films did not lead to satisfactory efficiencies (Kim et al., 2005) since the coatings also hinder the electron transport between the particles in this case. Concerning low-temperature films, the further development of additives in the electrolyte to suppress back reaction might therefore be a more realistic approach to further improve the performance (Kansai et al., 2006).

Based on all these considerations, the effects of the different measures taken during the preparation of low-temperature films as described earlier of this contribution can be discussed in detail. The low-temperature preparation of nanoparticulate TiO_2 films by hydrothermal crystallization and the post-treatment of low-temperature films by UV-ozone treatment are given as an example in the following. Figure 24.6 shows the electron lifetimes and transit times for low-temperature films treated by hydrothermal crystallization in comparison with those of a conventional high-temperature film. Without post treatment, the electron transit times of the low-temperature film are lower than those of the conventional high-temperature film. On the other hand, electron lifetimes are lower than electron transit times by factors between 2 and 4, which should enable the collection of almost all photogenerated electrons even if a certain distribution of transit times and lifetimes is considered. The low-temperature films prepared by hydrothermal crystallization are therefore much more efficient in dye-sensitized solar cells than low-temperature films prepared only by low-temperature sintering (150℃) without hydrothermal treatment. Similar differences between transit times and lifetimes were reported for low-temperature TiO_2 films prepared by compression of TiO_2 powder films at high pressures of up to 1900 kg/cm^2 in IMPS and IMPS measurements (Hagfeldt et al., 2004), and both hydrothermally treated and compressed TiO_2 films lead to similar overall efficiencies η of 4 to 5% (Oekermann et al., 2004; Hagfeldt et al., 2004).

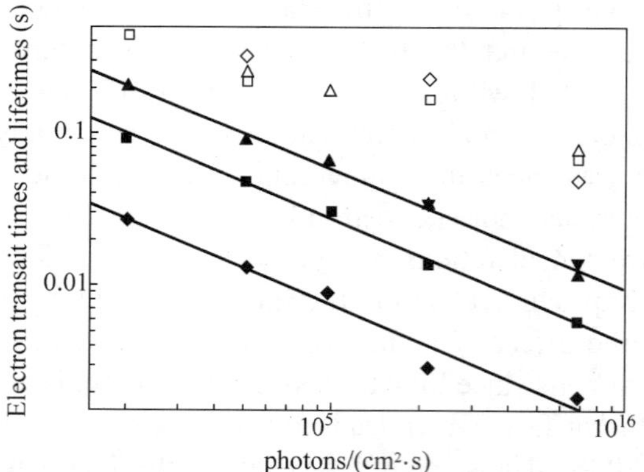

Figure 24.6 Electron transit times τ_D at different light intensities for dye sensitized TiO_2 films prepared by hydrothermal crystallization (▼ on FTO / glass; ▲ on ITO / glass ◆on FTO / glass, sintered at 450℃ for 1 h after preparation). The respective open symbols show the electron lifetimes τ_n of the films (△ on ITO/ glass; ◇ on FTO/glass, sintered at 450℃). For comparison the electron transit times (■) and lifetimes (□) of a film prepared by the conventional method including high-temperature sintering are also shown. The lines were calculated by linear regression (Oekermann et al., 2004)

Figure 24.7 shows the apparent diffusion coefficients and the electron diffusion lengths of the films for which IMPS plots, electron lifetimes and transit times were shown in Figs. 24.4 and 24.6. Films prepared by the conventional high-temperature preparation method exhibit L_n values of about 10 μm, which is the film thickness usually used in dye-sensitized solar cells, towards higher light intensities. Rather low L_n values are found for the films prepared by the low-temperature hydrothermal crystallization method. On the other hand they compare rather favorably with diffusion lengths reported in the literature for P25-based TiO_2 films prepared by the conventional method and low-temperature sintering (150℃). The highest efficiencies for such films so far have been reported for films where the addition of larger TiO_2 particles allowed the formation of thicker films up to 7 μm, and an electron diffusion length of 2.8 μm was measured at these films using high bias light intensities (close to 1 sun) (Kambe et al., 2002). It is seen in Fig. 24.7 that the films prepared by hydrothermal crystallization without heat treatment in this study already reach a comparable diffusion length at a rather low light intensity used in the IMPS measurements (2×10^{15} photons/(cm · s) ≈ 2.6 mW/cm^2). Therefore, compared to the films prepared by the conventional method and low-temperature sintering, enhanced electron transport properties are indicated for the hydrothermally prepared film. The higher overall efficiency of the hydrothermally prepared films under white light illumination (4.2% (Zhang et al., 2002)) compared to films prepared by low-temperature sintering without hydrothermal treatment (3.1% (Kambe et al., 2002)) is therefore understood.

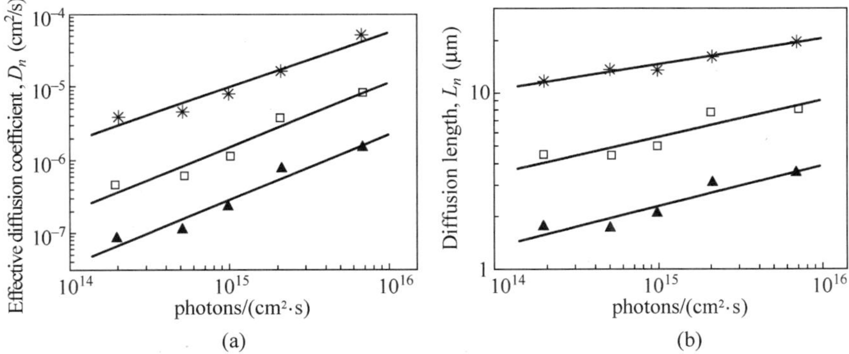

Figure 24.7 Effective diffusion coefficients D_n (a) and electron diffusion lengths L_n (b) at different light intensities for dye sensitized TiO_2 films prepared by hydrothermal crystallization (▲ on ITO / glass; * on FTO / glass, film sintered at 450℃ for 1 h after preparation). For comparison the diffusion lengths of a film prepared by the conventional method including high-temperature sintering (□) are also shown. The lines were calculated by linear regression (Oekermann et al., 2004)

Figures 24.4 to 24.7 also show the IMPS plots and electron transport and back reaction properties of the film prepared by hydrothermal treatment after its high-temperature treatment at 450℃. Interestingly, the electron transit times of this film are much lower than those of the film prepared by the conventional high-temperature method. This shows the high potential of the films prepared by hydrothermal treatment, however, a low-temperature pre-treatment method had to be found in order to improve the performance and still use these films for flexible solar cells. Figure 24.8 shows the electron lifetimes and transit times of low-temperature films prepared by hydrothermal crystallization before and after UV-ozone treatment. After the UV/ozone treatment the electron transport is only slightly improved, which can be seen in the almost unchanged electron transit times. On the other hand, a significant increase is seen for the electron lifetimes. This has been attributed to the removal of residual organics, which represent surface states that can act as recombination centers and therefore reduce the electron lifetime. XPS measurements on films prepared by hydrothermal crystallization show the existence of these residual organics, which probably originate from the titanium isopropoxide used as Ti precursor.

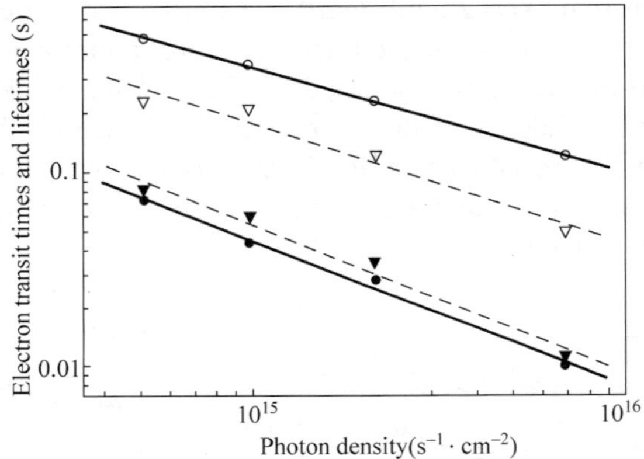

Figure 24.8 Influence of UV/ozone treatment on the electron transit times τ_D and electron lifetimes τ_n of a film prepared by hydrothermal crystallization on FTO/glass. The values were measured before ($\tau_D = \blacktriangledown; \tau_n = \triangledown$) and after ($\tau_D = \bullet$; $\tau_n = \circ$) UV/ozone treatment. The lines were calculated by linear regression (Oekermann et al., 2004)

In first view, it is astonishing that only small differences in the electron lifetimes have been found for films that show so different electron transport properties as seen in Fig. 24.6, given the fact that, in general, faster electron transport should lead to faster back reaction. Considering the effect of surface state removal as observed after UV-ozone treatment, however, can perfectly explain this observation. It can be expected that high-temperature sintering not only improves electron transport, but that it also efficiently removes surface states. The effect of faster transport, which should lead to a shorter electron lifetime, is compensated by the suppression of back reaction due to the removal of recombination centers.

24.3.4 Recent Developments and Outlook

One weakness of the studies published on charge transport and back reaction at low-temperature films so far is that electron transit times and lifetimes have been compared at the same light intensities or current densities, which were seen as a measure for the electron concentrations in the films. This is also the case for most of the studies presented in this contribution. However, in the last few years it has become common sense that it is better to compare electron transport properties at light intensities which cause the same photovoltages in different films, since the photovoltage should directly depend on the concentration of electrons in the TiO_2, while the photocurrent density depends itself on electron transport.

Another weakness of almost all measurements of electron transport and back reaction to date is that they are performed under different conditions: electron transport has been studied under short circuit conditions, while measurements of electron lifetimes have been done atopen circuit. Although there is no electric field in the porous TiO_2 layers as discussed above, there is a gradient in the quasi-Fermi level of electrons in the TiO_2 at least near to the conducting back contact, which strongly depends on the Fermi-level of the back contact, i.e. the external bias applied to it. Changing electron transport properties and therefore also changing electron lifetimes can therefore be expected along the I - V -curve of a dye-sensitized solar cell. Very recently some studies have been published which take these considerations into account. O'Regan et al. suggested the measurement of transient photovoltage rise times as a new tool to investigate electron transport at open circuit conditions (O'Regan et al., 2006). Measurements of electron transit times and lifetimes at different potentials along the I - V - curve by small square-wave light intensity modulation were performed by Boschloo and co-workers (Nissfolk et al., 2006). In both studies a considerable change of transit times and lifetimes with potential has been found. Furthermore, impedance measurements under illumination along the I - V -curve have been suggested as a new tool for the investigation of dye-sensitized solar cells (Bisquert and Vikhrenko, 2004; Wang et al., 2006).

Although these new techniques have not been applied for the detailed investigation of low-temperature films yet, they are a big step forward towards an even better understanding of dye-sensitized solar cells. It is believed that the knowledge gained by the new techniques will eventually lead to the development of a more comprehensive model of dye-sensitized solar cells, which, for example, can also fully explain the fill factor and therefore predict the maximum power achievable with a cell. Such a comprehensive understanding should also greatly benefit the further development of low-temperature TiO_2 films and flexible dye-sensitized solar cells in the future.

24.4 Interfacial Electron Transfer, Charge Separation and Recombination

For DSSCs, the electron transfer scheme is displayed in Fig .24.9. The attached dye is firstly excited by absorbing photons, then oxidized by ejecting electrons to the semiconductor conduction band, and finally regenerated by accepting electrons from the redox couples. However, the actual energy conversion efficiency is sharply reduced by electron back transfer from the semiconductor conduction band to dye cations and redox couples, making the practical efficiency (11%) much lower than the theoretical maximum (30%) (Shockley and Queisser, 1961). Therefore, to achieve high photovoltage, the electron transfer from redox anion (E^-) to dye cation (D^+) must be faster than that from the film conduction band to dye cation (RD ≫ RC1) and the electron diffusion in the semiconductor film should be fast enough to retard charge recombination at the semiconductor/redox interface (ED ≫ RC2).

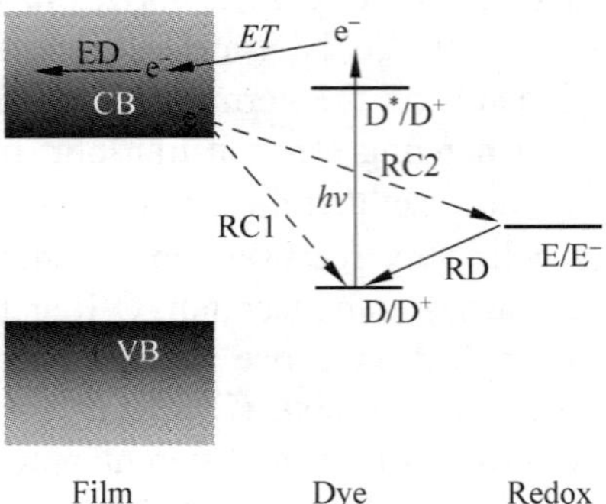

Figure 24.9 Scheme of the electron transfer in DSSCs

Theoretically (Huang et al., 1997), the observed photocurrent density J_{pd} is given by

$$J_{\mathrm{pd}} = J_{\mathrm{ei}} - J_{\mathrm{rc}} \tag{24.11}$$

where J_{ei} is the electron injection current from the excited dye to the semiconductor conduction band and J_{rc} is the interfacial charge recombination of injected electrons with the redox couple and dye cation. Since the concentration of redox anions is much higher than that of dye molecules, the charge recombination of the latter is relatively negligible (Hagfeldt et al., 1994; Hagfeldt and Grätzel., 1995). J_{ei} is related to the incident photo flux I_0 by

$$J_{\mathrm{ei}} = qAI_0 \tag{24.12}$$

where q is the electronic charge and A is the ratio of absorbed photon flux to I_0, which is proportional to the incident radiant power (mW/cm^2) P_0 ($P_0 = (kT)^{-1}\int_0^\infty h\nu I(h\nu)\mathrm{d}(h\nu)$). The recombination current is determined by the Butler-Volmer equation (Bard and Faulkner, 1980),

$$J_{\mathrm{rc}} = qK_{\mathrm{et}}C_{\mathrm{ox}}^{m}(n^{ua} - n_0^{ua}) \tag{24.13}$$

where K_{et} is the rate constant of back electron transfer, C_{ox} is the concentration of oxidized half of the redox couple, and n_0/n is the electron population in the semiconductor present in the dark/light. The order of the recombination reaction is m for C_{ox} and u for n_0/n, while α is the electron-transfer coefficient.

Assuming $J_{pd} = 0$ (open circuit, $V = V_{OC}$), we obtain

$$qAI_0 = qK_{et}C_{ox}^m(n^{ua} - n_0^{ua}) \tag{24.14}$$

The electron population n is exponentially related to the photovoltage V by the equation

$$n = n_0 \exp(qV / kT) \tag{24.15}$$

where $qV = E_f - E_{f0}, E_f / E_{f0}$ are Fermi levels of the semiconductor film in the light/dark. Combining Eqs. (24.14) & (24.15) gives

$$V_{OC} = \frac{kT}{qua}\ln\left(\frac{AI_0}{n_0^{ua}k_{et}C_{ox}^m} + 1\right) \tag{24.16}$$

and

$$V_{OC} = \frac{kT}{qua}\ln\left(\frac{AI_0}{n_0^{ua}k_{et}C_{ox}^m}\right) \quad (\text{generally, } AI_0 \gg n_0^{ua}k_{et}C_{ox}^m) \tag{24.17}$$

However, it should be kept in mind that here surface electrons and those in the conduction band are not separated, so a lower V_{OC} is expected if taking trapped electrons into account (Huang et al., 1997).

Now we understand that three factors determine the energy conversion efficiency of DSSCs in view of electron transfer dynamics. They are high efficient heterogeneous electron injection from the excited dye to film conduction band, maximum charge separation at the film/dye interface and minimum charge recombination of injected electrons with the dye sensitizer and redox couple. In the following subsections, we will discuss each one of them separately in detail.

24.4.1 Heterogeneous Electron Transfer

Heterogeneous electron transfer (HET) at the dye/film interface is the most important step in DSSCs. To make it thermodynamically favorable, the dye excited state energy must be higher than that of the film conduction band edge (Fig. 24.9). Therefore, when considering a particular dye as a DSSC sensitizer, its ground and excited state redox potentials are key parameters. Nowadays, theoretical quantum chemistry has advanced to the point where these parameters can be well estimated by density functional theory (DFT) (Labanowski and

Andzehn, 1991) calculations, giving opportunities for designing DSSC dye sensitizers at the molecular level. For instance, calculated excited state energy levels of fully deprotonated cis-[Ru(dcb)$_2$L$_2$] (dcb = 4,4'-dicarboxyl-2,2' -bipyridine, L = NCS ($N3^{4-}$), CN (complex 1) and dcb (complex 2)) are shown in Fig. 24.10 (Zhang et al., 2007). All are more negative than the TiO_2 conduction band edge. Therefore, such theoretical calculations could provide direct suggestions for selecting dye sensitizers for high efficiency DSSCs.

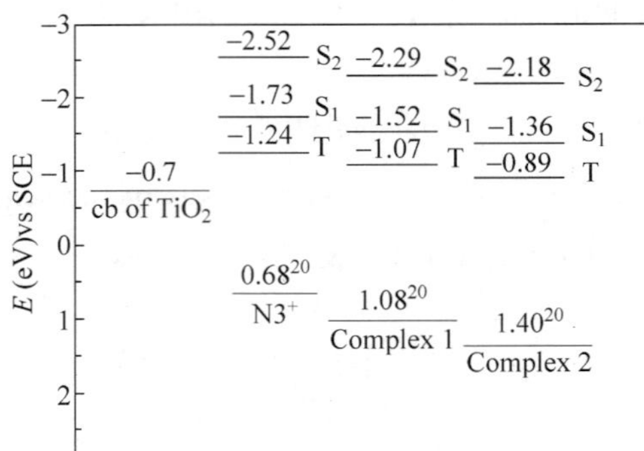

Figure 24.10 DFT excited state energy levels of N3 and its derivatives

Effects of film preparation processes on HET have been discussed in previous sections. However, selecting dye sensitizers is of equal importance. These molecules must have large absorption efficiency, high light harvesting capability, strong coupling with the semiconductor film and good charge separation at the dye/film interface. Numerous dyes have been sought as DSSC photo-sensitizers, including ruthenium organometallic complexes and organic chromophores. The efficient metal-ligand (M-L) electron transfer in the excited state Ru-based dyes and strong couplings of their ligands with semiconductor surfaces identify them as the current best photo-sensitizers with an energy conversion efficiency of 11%. However, their large scale application is limited by their high costs and resource limitations. In contrast, organic dyes have a wide absorption band, efficient light harvesting and low costs, which make them very suitable for DSSCs, but currently organic based DSSCs are less efficient than those based on Ru-dyes. However, the abundance of such organic molecules, both synthetic and natural, provides opportunities for lower cost and higher efficiency replacements for Ru-dyes in DSSCs.

To secure an efficient HET, strong interfacial coupling between the dye-sensitizer and semiconductor film is required, which can be controlled by employing different anchoring groups. Quantumly, an overlap between the dye excited state wavefunction with the semiconductor conduction band should exist. Mostly used binding groups of dye molecules to the oxide surfaces are —P(OH)$_3$, —COOH, —SH, —OH and so on. The coupling strength order is —COOH > —P(OH)$_3$ > —OH > —SH. Density functional theory calculations shows —COOH has the strongest coupling and therefore the highest electron transfer (ET) rate

(Lundqvist et al., 2006). The dye/film coupling strength also depends on the preparation conditions of the dye/film complexes.

To study dynamics and spectroscopy in the HET process, the vibrational coupling to the electronic transition should also be taken into account (Kondov et al., 2006). There is experimental evidence that the electron injection process occurs at a rate faster than the geometric relaxation. As such, the electronic-vibrational coupling constants $K_l^{(n)}$ can be computed from the gradients of the potential energy of the nth electronic state with respect to the normal mode Q_l at the optimized ground state geometry,

$$K_l^{(n)} = \left(\frac{\partial E_n}{\partial Q_1} \right)_0 \tag{24.18}$$

In practice, $K_l^{(n)}$ is calculated from the analytical Cartesian gradients of the energy $\left(\frac{\partial E_n}{\partial x_i} \right)$, Cartesian displacements (L_{il}) and frequencies (ω_l) as shown in Eq. (24.19),

$$K_l^{(n)} = \sum_{i=1}^{3N} \left(\frac{\partial E_n}{\partial x_i} \right)_0 L_{il} \omega_l^{-1/2} \tag{24.19}$$

where N is the number of atoms and x_i denotes the Cartesian nuclear coordinates. The reorganization or stabilization energy of the l th mode, $\lambda_l^{(n)}$, then can be computed by Eq. (24.20),

$$\lambda_l^{(n)} = \frac{1}{2} \frac{(K_1^{(n)})^2}{\omega_l}. \tag{24.20}$$

The contribution of a vibrational mode to an ET process is determined by the stabilization energy of this mode for a transition from the donor to the acceptor state. In DSSCs, the donor state is the excited state of the dye sensitizer and its cation is the acceptor. The organization energy of the lth vibrational mode for the ET process is given by

$$\lambda_l^{\mathrm{ET}} = \frac{1}{2\omega_l} (K_l^{D_0} - K_l^{S_1})^2, \tag{24.21}$$

which provides a quantitative measure of the role of the lth normal mode in the ET process. Since the potential energy surface at low frequency is pretty flat, artificial large displacements could be produced in frequency calculations, which could overestimate the reorganization energies of low frequency modes. For example, betanidin natural dye (Fig. 24.11) as a DSSC sensitizer and its vibrational coupling to the ET process is shown in Fig. 24.12 (Qin and Clark, 2007).

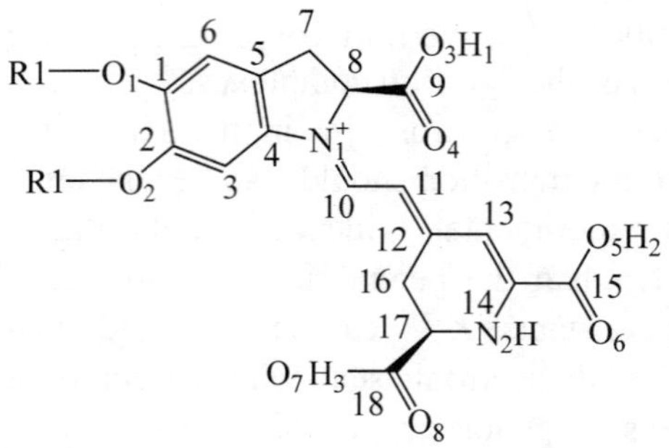

Figure 24.11 2-D structure of betanidin (R1 = R2 = H)

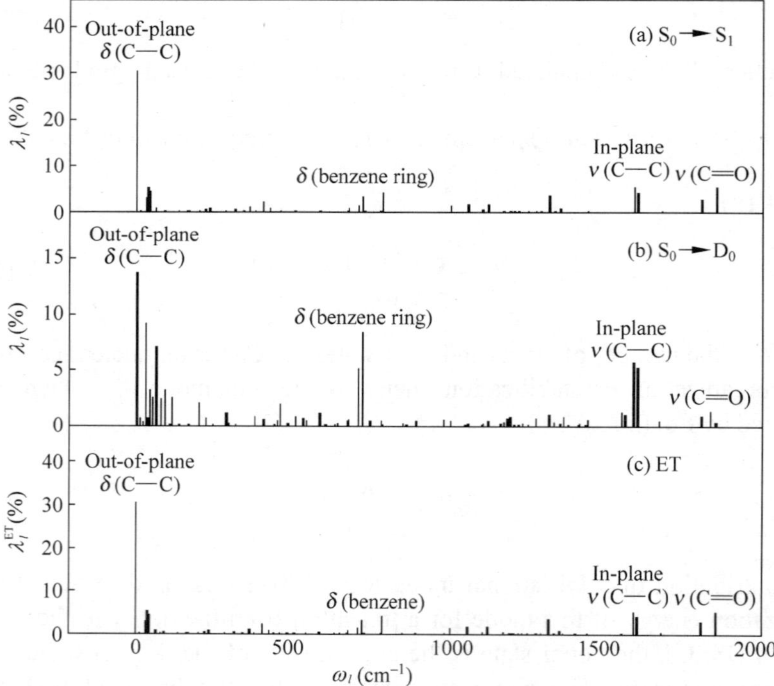

Figure 24.12 Calculated reorganization energies of deptotonated betanidin: (a) ground state→lowest singlet excited state. (b) ground state→cation. (c) electron transfer

24.4.2 Charge Separation at the Film/Dye Interface

The excited state electron injection from the dye to semiconductor conduction band is determined by the charge separation at the film/dye interface. Here, charge separation means two processes, a high efficient electron injection (ET in Fig. 24.9) and a minimum charge recombination at the film/dye interface (RC1 in Fig. 24.9). Since the second value is associated with the back electron transfer from the conduction band to the redox couple, we will discuss them together in the next section. In this section, the details about the charge separation at the film/dye interface will be discussed.

For a DSSC photo-sensitizer, it is expected that the electron density be redistributed after photon excitation. Functional groups with high electron density in the excited state can then be anchored to the semiconductor surface, and the overlap between the excited state wavefunction and the semiconductor conduction band directly leads to the electron injection. For example, time-dependent density functional theory (TDDFT) calculations show that a HOMO→LUMO transition is dominant in the excited state of natural betalain dyes (shown in Fig. 24.13) (Qin et al., 2007). The HOMO is mainly localized in the benzene ring while the LUMO has maximum density at pyridine moiety. After excitation, a partial electron transfer from the benzene to pyridine is achieved. If the pyridine ring could be connected to the semiconductor surface, an excited state electron injection from the dye to semiconductor conduction band would be anticipated. For Ru-based dyes, their lowest energy allowed excited state is delocalized to many configurations, including metal-ligand (M→L) and inter-ligand (L→L) charge transfer pairs. The Ru center is an electron donor and its ligands are electron acceptors. After photo excitation, electrons are transferred from Ru to its ligands, and finally injected to the semiconductor film conduction band. For N3, details about its photo excitation can be found in Ref. (Monat et al., 2002; Persson and Lundqvist, 2005; Persson et al., 2006).

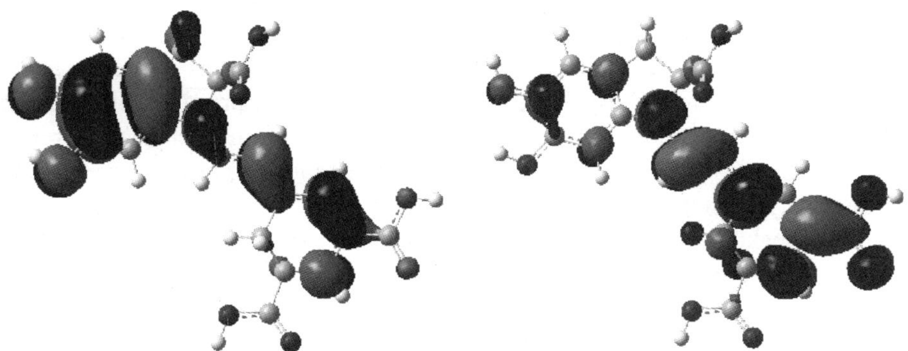

Figure 24.13 HOMO and LUMO of natural dye betanidin (color Fig. 27)

24.4.3 Charge Recombination at the Film/Redox/Dye Interface

Once electrons are injected to the semiconductor conduction band, to retard the back charge transfer (RC1 and RC2 in Fig. 24.9) becomes the most important aspect in DSSCs. Alternatively, to speed the electron diffusion in the semiconductor conduction band can also reduce the charge recombination at the film/redox/dye interface. Tai et al. (Tai et al., 2001; Tai, 2002) examined a SnO_2/TiO_2 coupled system and found higher performance than a single TiO_2 based DSSC. SnO_2 itself is a poor DSSC semiconductor film because of high charge recombination rate at the SnO_2/dye/redox interface. However, it can promote electron diffusion to the anode collector and improve the DSSC IPCE value.

To retard the charge recombination at the film/dye/redox interface, the best way is to keep them separated in space. This can be achieved by an insulator film on TiO_2, functional groups in dye molecules to push redox cations away from the TiO_2 surface and a proper redox couple (Wang et al., 2004). Although DSSCs are improved by these measurements, the actual efficiency is still low and far from the theoretical limit.

24.5 Summary

So far, conversion efficiencies of up to about 4% under AM 1.5 simulated sun light illumination (100 mW/cm^2) have been achieved for all-flexible DSSCs based on room or low temperature preparation (150℃) on conductive polymer films. Although the efficiency is lower than that of rigid and high temperature sintered versions, it nevertheless promises the possibility for commercialization in new and unique niche markets. Because of its flexibility, DSSCs can be uniquely designed for specific products, while satisfying special shape and color needs. DSSCs could be made as attachments or in combination with other emerging technologies for autonomous systems (wireless communication).

Low temperature preparations of nanocrystalline porous films are nearly at the verge of a breakthrough. At the time of this writing, the prepared films are as robust as high temperature sintered ones, and have very strong mechanical stability. Active methods should be developed to significantly decrease the ex- and intrinsic surface states which hinder electron injection, transport and collection. With the breakthrough of low/room temperature preparation, flexible DSSCs can realize all the great advantages of such as a wide spectrum of applications, light weight and colorful designs at low production costs.

References

Barbé, C. J., F. Arendse, P. Comte, M. Jirousek, F. Lenzmann, V. Shklover, M. Grätzel. J. Am. Ceram. Soc. **80**: 3157 (1997).

Bard, A. J., L. R. Faulkner, *Electrochemical Methods*. New York: John Wiley and Sons, p.103 (1980).

Bisquert, J. and V.S. Vikhrenko. *J. Phys. Chem. B* **108**: 2313(2004).

Boschloo, G., L. Häggman and A. Hagfeldt. *J. Phys. Chem. B* **110**: 13,144 (2006).
Desilvestro, J., M. Grätzel, L. Kavan and J. Moser, J. Am. Chem. Soc. **107**: 2988 (1985).
Dloczik, L., O. Ileperuma, I. Lauermann, L.M. Peter, E.A. Ponomarev, G. Redmond, N.J. Shaw and I. Uhlendorf. *J.Phys.Chem. B* **101**: 10,281 (1997).
Dung, D.H., N. Serpone and M. Grätzel. Helv. Chim. Acta **67**: 1012 (1984).
Dürr, M., A. Schmid, M. Obermaier, S. Rosselli, A. Yasuda and G. Nelles. Nat. Mater. **4**: 607 (2005).
Fabregat-Santiago, F., J. Garcia-Canadas, E. Palomares, J.N. Clifford, S.A. Haque, J. Durrant, G. Garcia-Belmonte and J. Bisquert. *J. Appl. Phys.* **96**: 6903(2004).
Fisher, A.C., L.M. Peter, E.A. Ponomarev, A.B. Walker and K.G.U. Wijayantha. *J. Phys. Chem. B* **104**: 949 (2000).
Gerischer, H. and H. Tributsch, Ber. Bunsenges. Phys. Chem. **72**: 437 (1968).
Green, M.A., K.Emery, D.L. King, Y. Hishikawa and W. Warta. Prog. Photovolt: Res. Appl. **15**: 35 (2007).
Gutierrez-Tauste, D., I. Zumeta, E. Vigil, M.A. Hernandez-Fenollosa, X. Domenech, J.A. Ayllon., J. Photochem. Photobiol. A: Chem. **175**: 165 (2005).
Hagfeldt A., M. Grätzel. *Chem. Rev.* **95**: 49 (1995).
Hagfeldt, A., G. Boschloo, H. Lindström, E. Figgemeier, A. Holmberg, V. Aranyos, E. Magnusson and L. Malmqvist. *Coord. Chem. Rev.* **248**: 1501 (2004).
Hagfeldt, A., S. E. Lindquist, M. Grätzel. *Sol. Energy Mater. Sol. Cells* **32**: 245 (1994).
Huang, S. Y., G. Schlichthörl, A. J. Nozik, M. Grätzel, A. J. Frank. *J. Phys. Chem. B* **101:** 2567 (1997).
Ito, S., N.-L.C. Ha, G. Rothenberger, P. Liska, P. Comte, S.M. Zakeeruddin, P. Pechy, M.K. Nazeeruddin and M. Grätzel. Chem. Commun. **4004** (2006).
Kado, T., Yamaguchi, M., Yamada Y., and Hayase S. Chem. Lett. **32**: 1056 (2003).
Kambe, S., S. Nakade, Y. Wada, T. Kitamura and S. Yanagida. J. Mater. Chem. **12**: 723 (2002).
Kang, M. G., N.-G. Park, K. S. Ryu, S.H. Chang and K.-J. Kim. Sol. Energy Mater. Sol. Cells. **90**: 574 (2006).
Kang, M. G., N.-G. Park, K.S. Ryu, S. H. Chang and K.-J. Kim. Chem. Lett. **6**: 34 (2005).
Kanzaki, T., S. Nakade, Y. Wada and S. Yanagida. *Photochem. Photobiol. Sci.* **5**: 389 (2006).
Keis, K., J. Lindgren, S. E. Lindquist and A. Hagfeldt. Langmuir **16**: 4688 (2000).
Kim, K.-J., K.D. Benkstein, J. van de Lagemaat and A.J. Frank. *Chem.Mater.* **14**: 1042 (2002).
Kim, R.C.Y., M. Auyeung, G.P. Ollinger, Z.H. Kushto, A. P. Kafafi. Appl. Phys. A **83**: 73 (2006).
Kim, S.-S., J.-H. Yum and Y.-E. Sung. J. Photochem. Photobiol. A Chem. **171**: 269 (2005).
Kim, S.S., J.H. Yum and Y.E. Sung. J. Photochem. *Photobiol. A: Chem.* **171**: 269 (2005).
Koide, N., A. Islam, Y. Chiba and L. Han. J. Photochem. Phobiol. A: Chem. **182**: 296 (2006).
Kondov, I., H. Wang, M. Thoss. *Inter J. of Quantum Chem.* **106**: 1291 (2006).
Kopidakis, N., K.D. Benkstein, J. van de Lagemaat and A.J. Frank. *J. Phys. Chem. B* **107**: 11,307 (2003).
Kopidakis, N., N.R. Neale and A.J. Frank. *J. Phys. Chem. B* **110**: 12,485 (2006).
Labanowski, J. K., J. W. Andzehn, Density Functional Methods in Chemistry. New York: Springer-Verlag (1991).

Lewis, L. N., J. L. Spivack, S. Gasaway, E. D. Williams, J. Y. Gui, V. Manivannan, O. P. Siclovan. Sol. Energy Mater. Sol. Cells. **90**: 1041 (2006).

Li, B., L.D. Wang, B.N. Kang, P. Wang and Y. Qiu. Sol. Energy Mater. Sol. Cells **90**: 549 (2006).

Lindström. H., A. Holmberg, E. Magnusson, S.-E. Lindquist, L. Malmqvist and A. Hagfeldt. Nano Lett. **1**: 97 (2001).

Longo, C., A. F. Nogueira, M.-A. De Paoli and H. Cachet. J. Phys. Chem. B **106**: 5925 (2002).

Longo, C., Freitas J., De Paoli M.-A., J. Photochem. Photobiol. A: Chem. **159**: 33 (2003).

Lundqvist, M. J., M. Nilsing, S. Lunell, B. Akermark, P. Persson. *J. Phys. Chem. B* **110**: 20,513 (2006).

Miyasaka, T. and Y. Kijitori. J. Electrochem. Soc. **151**: A1767 (2004).

Miyasaka, T., Y. Kijitori, T. N. Murakami, M. Kimura and S. Uegusa. Chem. Lett. **31**: 1250 (2002).

Monat, J. E., J. H. Rodriguez, J. K. McCusker. *J. Phys. Chem. A* **106**: 7399 (2002).

Moser, J. Monatsh. Chem. **8**: 373 (1887).

Nakade, S., M. Matsuda, S. Kambe, Y. Saito, T. Kitamura, T. Sakata, Y. Wada, H. Mori and S. Yanagida. *J. Phys. Chem. B* **106**: 10,004 (2002).

Nakade, S., T. Kanzaki, Y. Wada and S. Yanagida. *Langmuir* **21**: 10,803 (2005).

Nakade, S., Y. Saito, W. Kubo, T. Kitamura, Y. Wada and S. Yanagida. *J. Phys. Chem. B* **107**: 8607 (2003).

Namba, S. and Y. Hishiki. J. Phys. Chem. **69**: 774 (1965).

Neale, N.R., N. Kopidakis, J. van de Lagemaat, M. Grätzel and A.J. Frank. *J. Phys. Chem. B* **109**: 23,183 (2005).

Nelson, R.C. J. Phys. Chem. **69**: 714 (1965).

Nissfolk, J., K. Fredin, A. Hagfeldt and G. Boschloo. *J. Phys. Chem. B* **110**: 17,715 (2006).

O'Reagan, B. and M. Grätzel. Nature **353**: 737 (1991).

O'Regan, B., K. Bakker, J. Kroeze, H. Smit, P. Sommeling and J.R. Durrant. *J. Phys. Chem. B* **110**: 17,155 (2006).

O'Regan, B.C. and F. Lenzmann. *J. Phys. Chem. B* **108**: 4342 (2004).

Oekermann, T., D. Zhang, T. Yoshida and H. Minoura. *J. Phys. Chem. B* **108**: 2227 (2004).

Park, N.G., G. Schlichthörl, J. van de Lagemaat, H.M. Cheong, A. Mascarenhas and A.J. Frank. *J. Phys. Chem. B* **103**: 3308 (1999).

Park, N.G., J. van de Lagemaat and A.J. Frank. *J. Phys. Chem. B* **104**: 8989 (2000).

Park, N-G., K. M. Kim, M. G. Kang, K.S. Ryu, S. H. Chang, Y. J. Shin. Adv. Mater. **17**: 2349 (2004).

Persson, P., M. J. Lundqvist, M. Nilsing, A. C. T. van Duin, W. A. Ⅲ. Goddard *Proc. of SPIE*, 2006, 6325, 63250P-3.

Persson, P., M. J. Lundqvist. *J. Phys. Chem. B* **109**: 11,918 (2005).

Peter, L.M. and D. Vanmaekelbergh, In: R.C. Alkire and D.M. Kolb eds. *Advances in Electrochemical Science and Engineering*, Vol. 6. Weinheim: Wiley-VCH (1999).

Pichot, F., J. R. Pitts and B. A. Gregg. Langmuir **16**: 5626 (2000).

Qin, C., A. E. Clark. *Chem. Phys. Letts.* 2007, doi:10.1016/j.cplett.2007.02.063.

Schlichthörl, G., S.Y. Huang, J. Sprague and A.J. Frank. *J. Phys. Chem. B* **101**: 8141 (1997).

Shockley, W., H. Queisser. *J. Appl. Phys.* **32**: 510 (1961).

Södergren, S., A. Hagfeldt, J. Olsson and S.E. Lindquist. *J. Phys. Chem.* **95**: 5522 (1994).

Solbrand, A., A. Henningsson, S. Södergren, H. Lindström, A. Hagfeldt and S.E. Lindquist. *J. Phys. Chem. B* **103**: 1078 (1999).

Solbrand, A., H. Lindström, H. Rensmo, A. Hagfeldt, S.E. Lindquist and S.J. Södergren. *J. Phys. Chem. B* **101**: 2514 (1997).

Sommeling, P.M., M. Späth, J. Kroon, R. Kinderman and J. van Roosmalen. In: H. Scheer, ed. 16th *European Photovoltaic Solar Energy Conference Proceedings*. James & James Science Publishers Ltd., London (2000).

Tai, W.-P. *Mater. Lett.* **51**: 451 (2001).

Tai, W.-P., K. Inoue, J.-H. Oh. *Sol. Energy Mater. Sol. Cells* **71**: 553 (2002).

Takenaka, S., Y. Maehara, H. Imai, M. Yoshikawa, S. Shiratori. Thin Solid Films. **438**: 346 (2003).

Takurou, N. M., Y. Kijitori, N. Kawashima. and T. Miyasaka. Chem. Lett. **32**: 1076 (2003).

Tributsch, H. Photochem. Photobiol. **14**: 95 (1971).

Uchida, S., M. Tomiha, H. Takizawa and M. Kawaraya. J. Photochem. Photobiol. A Chem. **164**: 93 (2004).

van de Lagemaat, J. and A.J. Frank. *J. Phys. Chem. B* **105**: 11,194 (2001).

Wang, P., S. M. Zakeeruddin, J.-E. Moser, R. Humphry-Baker, M. Grätzel. *J. Am. Chem. Soc.* **126**: 7164 (2004).

Wang, Q., S. Ito, M. Grätzel, F. Fabregat-Santiago, I. Mora-Sero, J. Bisquert, T. Bessho and Imai, H.J. *J. Phys. Chem. B* **110**: 25,210 (2006).

Wessels, K., A. Feldhoff, M. Wark, J. Rathousky and T. Oekermann. *Electrochem. Solid-State Lett.* **9**: C93 (2006).

West, W. Proc. Vogel Centennial Symp. Photogr. Sci. Eng. **18**: 35 (1974).

Yamaguchi, K. M., Y. Yamada and S. Hayase. Chem. Lett. **32**: 1056 (2003).

Yoshida, T., M. Iwaya, H. Ando, T. Oekermann, K. Nonomura, D. Schlettwein, D. Wöhrle and H. Minoura. Chem. Commun. 400(2004).

Yum, J.-H., S.-S. Kim, D.-Y. Kim and Y.-E. Sung J. Photochem. Photobiol. A Chem. **173**: 1 (2005).

Zhang, D., J. A. Downing, F. Knorr, J. L. McHale. J. Phys. Chem. B **110**: 21,890 (2006b).

Zhang, D., T. Yoshida and H. Minoura. *Chem.Lett.* 874 (2002).

Zhang, D., T. Yoshida, H. Minoura. Adv. Mater. **15**: 814 (2003).

Zhang, D., T. Yoshida, H. Minoura. Chem. Lett. 874 (2002).

Zhang, D., T. Yoshida, K. Furuta, H. Minoura. J. Photochem. Photobiol.A Chem. **164**: 159 (2004).

Zhang, D., T. Yoshida, T. Oekermann, K. Furuta and H. Minoura. Adv. Funct. Mater. **16**: 1228 (2006a).

Zhang, X., J. Zhang, Y. Xia. *J. Photochem. & Photobiol. A*: *Chem.* **185**: 283 (2007).

25 Magnetic Nanofluids: Synthesis and Structure

L. Vékás[1,2], M.V. Avdeev[3], Doina Bica[1]

[1]Laboratory of Magnetic Fluids, Center for Fundamental and Advanced Technical Research, Romanian Academy, Timisoara Division, Timisoara, Romania

[2]National Center for Engineering of Systems with Complex Fluids, University Politehnica Timisoara, Timisoara, Romania

[3]Frank Laboratory of Neutron Physics, Joint Institute for Nuclear Research, Dubna, Russia

Abstract Recent results are reviewed concerning the synthesis of magnetic nanoparticles (MNP) and various types of magnetic nanofluids (MNF) or ferrofluids, their structural properties and behavior in an external magnetic field, specially tailored to meet the requirements of some specific engineering and biomedical applications. There are described the chemical co-precipitation procedure and the liquid- and gas-phase thermal decomposition methods to obtain magnetic nanoparticles (Fe_3O_4, γ-Fe_2O_3, $CoFe_2O_4$, Co, Fe and Fe-C) of adequate size distribution to prepare magnetic nanofluids. Sterical stabilization of MNPs in organic and water carrier liquids is discussed in details, related to the diagrams of magnetic nanofluid synthesis procedures. The macroscopic behavior, especially the magnetic and flow properties of magnetic fluids and their compatibility with various media and exploitation conditions in magnetofluidic devices are described related to composition and structural characteristics, such as nature and size of magnetic nanoparticles, nature and chain length of surfactants used for ultrastable dispersion of magnetic nanoparticles in various non-polar and polar carrier liquids, hydrodynamic size of particles, as well as the formation and characteristics of agglomerates induced by an applied magnetic field.

Manifold results of structural investigations of MNFs by small angle neutron scattering (SANS), including specific techniques (contrast variation, scattering of polarized neutrons) are presented concerning particle structure (size, surfactant shell thickness, composition of core and shell, solvent rate penetration in surfactant layer, micelles), magnetic structure (magnetic size and composition), particle interaction (interparticle potential, magnetic moment correlation, phase separation) and cluster formation (aggregation and chain formation). Long-term colloidal stability of magnetic nanofluids and their properties are discussed in terms of the above structural characteristics.

---

(1) Corresponding e-mail: vekas@acad-tim.tm.edu.ro

25.1 Introduction

25.1.1 Ferrofluids—Magnetically Controllable Nanofluids

Ferrofluids or magnetic (nano)fluids (M(N)F)—a category of smart fluids, in particular magnetically controllable nanofluids (Shliomis, 1974; Rosensweig, 1979; Charles and Popplewell, 1980; Rosensweig, 1985, 1988; Berkovski and Bashtovoy, 1996; Blums et al., 1997; Odenbach, 2002, 2006)—are rather attractive for a large variety of applications, which require simultaneously fluid and magnetic properties.

Such a material, i.e. a liquid medium easily controllable by a magnetic field, was not found in nature but synthesized in laboratory conditions in the early 1960s. The magnetic control of a liquid medium may be considered (Odenbach, 2006) as the employment of Kelvin forces to change the flow and the properties of a liquid. The experimental investigations led finally to ferrofluids—ultrastable suspensions of nanosized magnetic dipolar particles in appropriate carrier liquids—actually an achievement of colloid science (Davalos-Orozco and Castillo, 2002). Macroscopically, these fluids manifest themselves as magnetizable liquid media due to the 'integration' in the structure of the carrier of nanosized permanent magnetic dipolar particles.

25.1.2 Early History of Magnetic Fluids (A Short Review)

A number of colloidal magnetic fluids having stability against settling and agglomeration in or out of a magnetic field were independently invented at around the same time in the United States in the 1960s. The best known patent is that of S. S. Papell of NASA who used long term ball milling of a mixture of large particles of magnetite (Fe_3O_4), carrier liquid, and a surfactant (Papell, 1965). His objective was to provide a positive feed of liquid rocket fuel to the intake of pumps in the reduced gravity conditions of outer space. Magnetic fluids use a surface-sorbed layer of a long-chain surfactant, polymer, or protein molecule to provide a short-range repulsion preventing particles from sticking to each other. These magnetic fluids incorporate a particle size on the order of 10 nm.

Starting in 1963 E. L. Resler, Jr., a Cornell University professor on sabbatical and R. E. Rosensweig at Avco Corporation in Wilmington, Massachusetts proposed a magnetocaloric thermodynamic cycle to efficiently convert heat to electricity with no moving mechanical parts to be used on spacecraft (Resler and Rosensweig, 1964, 1967). The regenerative heat transfer steps required to implement the cycle were envisioned to be done using a dispersion of ferromagnetic particles in a liquid metal carrier.

R.E. Rosensweig and J.L. Neuringer developed a mathematical theory broadening the Navier-Stokes equation to include force on a magnetic fluid regarded as a continuum and published the first paper on this idea terming the word 'Ferrohydrodynamics' (Neuringer and Rosensweig, 1964). In addition to finding as a corollary a generalization of the celebrated equation of Bernoulli published in his Hydrodynamica of 1737, the paper compared a prediction of the ferrohydrodynamic theory with an experiment in which a pool of magnetic fluid climbed a current-carrying wire creating a meniscus having a predicted shape. The pair coined the term 'ferrofluid' as a descriptor of the colloidal magnetic fluid.

Starting from the generalized Bernoulli equation, the phenomena of magnetic levitation where introduced by R. E. Rosensweig (1966a, 1966b), broadening concepts of buoyancy introduced in antiquity by Archimedes. In one form a magnet repels a nonmagnetic object immersed in a ferrofluid in circumvention of Earnshaw's theorem (Earnshaw, 1842). In another manifestation, a magnet more dense than the ferrofluid it is immersed in levitates itself to a stable equilibrium at the center of the fluid space in the containing vessel. The effects find practical application in mineral separation, inclinometers, and other instrumentation.

Concomitantly, R. E. Rosensweig, J. W. Nestor and R. S. Timmins elucidated the physical make-up and magneto-physical properties of the ferrofluids characterizing the particle size, energetics of the colloidal stability, diffusive properties, magnetization curve, and viscosity in an archival paper presented in London in 1965 (Rosensweig et al., 1965). Under a grant from NASA Rosensweig together with R. Kaiser broadened the range of ferrofluid compositions to include other ferrites, other surfactants, and other carrier liquids including water (Rosensweig and Kaiser, 1967).

An early historical account of progress on the fronts of magnetic fluid mechanics, physical chemistry, new phenomena, and novel applications can be found in the 1966 review articles (Rosensweig, 1966c—the last paragraph of this review reads '*The number of workers in the field of ferrohydrodynamics is very few, and for the most part their efforts are intermittent. However, when the peculiarities of magnetic fluids are better known we may expect an increase of interest and participation, hopefully with benefits on a wide front.*'; Rosensweig 1966d), including the discovery of the normal field instability, perhaps the best known and most characteristic response of a ferrofluid (Cowley and Rosensweig, 1967). The instability can onset only in a ferrofluid whose magnetization exceeds a characteristic threshold. A themed session at Dynamics Days Europe 2007, Loughborough, England was held on this phenomenon in honor of the 40th anniversary publication of the paper. The phenomenon furnishes a singular example of fluid patterning in the absence of a dissipative process.

World interest in ferrofluids was further stimulated by the first commercial application of ferrofluids, the leakage-free rotating seals, an excellent component today of many high-tech devices (Rosensweig, 1971). The invention discloses a means for constructing compact rotary shaft seals in which a single magnet supplies magnetic field to a multiplicity of discrete stages, each retaining a liquid O-ring of magnetic fluid, such that the device is capable of sustaining large pressure differences. The seals are hermetic and utterly free of mechanical wear.

Described as 'a modern machine element' the seals furnished the most important product line of the Ferrofluidics Corporation (today Ferrotec Co.) and have been widely copied around the world.

The described early activity and others created the framework of a new science and technology and stimulated a world effort in the study of magnetic fluids, though news of those efforts was slow to diffuse until B. M. Berkovsky of Minsk and UNESCO organized what has been later termed the first International Conference on Magnetic Fluids in Udine, Italy in 1977 (Berkovsky and Rosensweig, 1978). The first book on ferrofluids and their applications appeared in 1978 in Romania (Luca et al., 1978), where systematic application orientated researches began already in 1970s (Anton et al., 1980). A second conference was held in the U.S. in Orlando, Florida in 1980 and subsequent meetings at three year intervals have been held in the UK (1983), Japan (1986), Latvia (1989), France (1992), India (1995), Romania (1998), Germany (2001), Brazil (2004) and Slovakia (2007).

In the following beside the well known names 'ferrofluid' or 'magnetic fluid', we will use also the term 'magnetic nanofluid', starting from the concept of 'nanofluid' introduced much later by U.S. Choi of Argonne NL (U.S.) (Choi, 1995), for non-magnetic nanoparticle suspensions developed for advanced cooling systems.

25.1.3 Composition, Structure and Macroscopic Behavior

The macroscopic behavior of magnetic fluids and their compatibility with various media and exploitation conditions of devices with magnetic fluids are determined by composition and structural characteristics. Sometimes, e.g. for rotating seals, biomedical applications or nanocomposite synthesis, the tailoring of the nanoscale characteristics and macroscopic (magnetic and flow) behavior of MNFs to the requirements of envisaged applications becomes essential. The basic aspects of the fundamental relation between structural characteristics and macroscopic behavior of MNFs are systematically presented in a recent comprehensive work (Odenbach, 2006) and are illustrated with a lot of experimental data, referring mainly to commercial ferrofluids.

This chapter will review some recent results concerning the synthesis of magnetic nanoparticles (MNP) and various types of magnetic nanofluids (MNF), their structural properties and behavior in an external magnetic field, specially tailored to meet the requirements of some specific engineering and biomedical applications. These types of nanofluids are colloids of magnetic nanoparticles, such as Fe_3O_4, γ-Fe_2O_3, $CoFe_2O_4$, Co, Fe or Fe-C, stably dispersed in a carrier liquid (Charles, 2002) (Fig. 25.1). At nanoscale, a specific difficulty associated with the preparation of magnetic fluids is that the nanoparticles have large surface area-to-volume ratios and thus tend to aggregate to reduce their surface energy. In particular, magnetic metal oxide surfaces have extremely high surface energies (>100 dyn/cm, 1 dyn = 10^{-5} N) that make the production of nanoparticles very challenging. In addition, magnetic dipole-dipole attractions between particles enhance the difficulties experienced in the production of ferrofluids in comparison to suspensions of nonmagnetic nanoparticles (usual nanofluids). Macroscopically, the introduction of magnetic forces into the fundamental hydrodynamic equations for the quasi-homogeneous magnetizable liquid medium gives rise to the magnetohydrodynamics of magnetic nanofluids, known as ferrohydrodynamics and opens up an entire field of new phenomena (Rosensweig, 1985) and a lot of promising applications (Raj and Moskowitz, 1990; Anton et al., 1990; Rosensweig, 1996; Raj, 1996). From a microscopic point of view, long-range, attractive van der Waals and magnetic forces are ubiquitous and therefore must be balanced by Coulombic, steric or other interactions to control the colloidal stability of dispersed nanoparticle system, even in intense and strongly non-uniform magnetic field.

Many of the applications (Raj and Moskowitz, 1990; Raj et al., 1995; Piso, 1999; Popa et al., 1999) e.g. rotating seals, bearings, dampers or sensors, require magnetic fluids with high magnetization and at the same time, with long-term colloidal stability. In case of MNF cooled and damped HIFI loudspeakers, colloidal stability of MNFs have to be ensured up to relatively high temperatures (150 – 180℃). These requirements are difficult to fulfill simultaneously and implies severe conditions on the MNP synthesis/stabilization/dispersion procedures applied during the preparation of magnetic nanofluids. The size of nanoparticles can be controlled by systematically adjusting the reaction parameters, such as time, temperature and the concentrations of reagents and stabilizing surfactants. In general, particle size increases with increasing reaction time, because more monomeric species are generated, and with increasing reaction temperature because

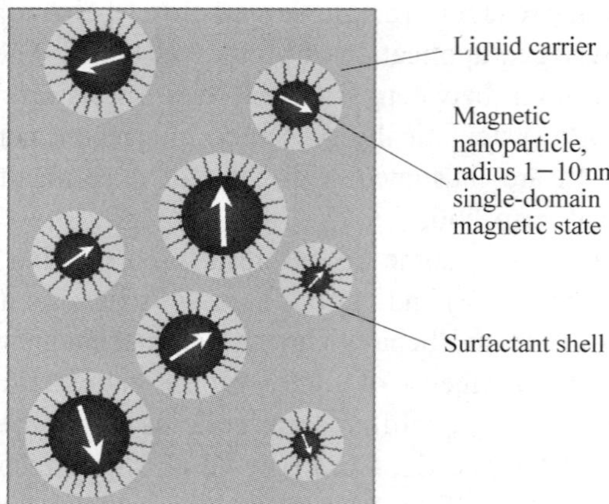

Figure 25.1 Main components of a magnetic fluid (schematic view): magnetic nanoparticles, surfactant and carrier liquid

the rate of reaction is increased (Hyeon, 2003). Surface coating with surface active molecules play important roles in dictating nanoparticle size, shape, and interparticle spacing, and also in determining the properties of both the interface between the stabilizing layer and the nanoparticle surface and the interface between the nanoparticle and carrier liquid. While the atomic composition of nanoparticles is most important in determining their physical properties, it is the chemical nature of the coating layer(s) that dictates how nanoparticles will be stably dispersed in various non-polar and polar carriers (Grubbs, 2007).

The agglomeration processes, in particular irreversible chain formation by alignment of dipolar nanoparticles under the action of an applied magnetic field (Fig. 25.2), are not desired in the case of magnetic fluids (Chantrell et al., 1981) used in most of the applications; therefore the characterization methods are mainly focused on these processes and on their consequences on the macroscopic behavior of the fluids (Cabuil et al., 1996). When the dipolar interactions are much stronger than the thermal energy, the fluid develops clusters, like dimers, trimers, and longer chains (Fig. 25.2). Indeed, dipolar structure formation is expected when the dipolar potential energy exceeds thermal energy, i.e. when the dimensionless magnetic interaction energy, $\lambda_{\text{int}} = \mu_0 m^2 /(2\pi k_{\text{B}} T d_m^3)$ becomes greater than unity, $\lambda_{\text{int}} > 1$. Here, $\mu_0 = 4\pi \times 10^{-7}$H/m-permeability of the vacuum, m is magnetic dipole moment of one particle, T is absolute temperature, k_{B} is Boltzmann constant, d is physical diameter fo a particle, d_{m} is magnetic diameter of a particle. The microstructural processes in a particular fluid are hardly to be observed experimentally, although some techniques can probe the small scale structure of the fluid, such as the thickness of the surfactant layer that is responsible for the steric stabilization of the magnetic colloid. One of the most efficient methods of nanostructural investigation is based on small-angle neutron scattering (SANS) (Holm and Weiss, 2005). This advanced method is applied to

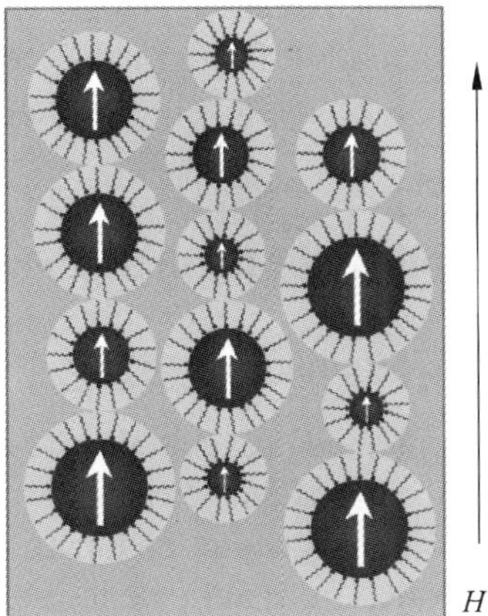

Figure 25.2 Magnetic fluid in applied magnetic field: alignment of magnetic moments and chain formation

reveal structural features at the scale of 1 – 100 nm regarding both atomic and magnetic organization of magnetic fluids. The sizes of magnetic particles in magnetic fluids (3 – 15 nm), as well as the characteristic correlation length between particles are mostly in this dimensional range, consequently SANS investigations are conducted to obtain valuable data on the particle structure and agglomerate formation processes in magnetic nanofluids.

In what follows, the composition, synthesis procedures, structure and properties of various types of magnetic fluids are reviewed.

25.2 Synthesis of Magnetic Nanofluids

25.2.1 Generalities

MNFs are colloidal systems composed of isolated particles with nanometer-sized dimensions that are stabilized by surfactant molecules and dispersed in solvent media. In the ideal case, these non-interacting systems derive their unique magnetic properties mostly from the reduced size of the isolated nanoparticles, and contributions from interparticle interactions are negligible.

The synthesis of magnetic fluids has two main steps (Charles, 2002): (1) the preparation of nano-sized magnetic particles and (2) the subsequent stabilization/dispersion of the nanoparticles in various non-polar and polar carrier liquids. In what concerns the ferrite nanoparticles, such as magnetite, maghemite or cobalt ferrite, the most efficient route is the chemical co-precipitation process (Khalafalla and Reimers, 1973, 1980), while for Fe or Co nanoparticles physical-chemical methods, such as thermal decomposition of Fe or Co carbonyls (Griffiths et al., 1979; Papirer et al., 1983) proved to be advantageous, with special care on particle surface passivation against oxidation. Fe or Co nanoparticles are envisaged for very high magnetization nanofluids. Thermal decomposition procedures are applied also for the synthesis of iron or cobalt oxid nanoparticles.

25.2.2 Synthesis of Nanosized Magnetic Particles

25.2.2.1 Chemical Co-Precipitation

The chemical coprecipitation method proved to be versatile for the preparation of magnetite, maghemite and substituted ferrites nanoparticles suitable for magnetic fluid preparation. In the case of magnetite, nanoparticles can be prepared from the coprecipitation of hydroxides from an aqueous solution of Fe^{3+} and Fe^{2+} in the mole ratio of approximatively 2:1 using a base (Khalafalla and Reimers, 1973). The reaction is complex and involves the conversion of the hydroxide particles to magnetite. Particles produced may be in fact a mixture of magnetite and maghemite. Studies were performed concerning the effect of precipitation temperature on the nature and size of particles, the effect of heating the precipitate in the alkaline medium and the effect of addition of surfactant to the reaction medium (Davies et al., 1993; Charles, 1995; Bica, 1995). An essential feature related to the synthesis of magnetite ferrofluids is to ensure the optimum temperature of 80 – 82℃ (Bica, 1995; Bica, 1985; Moeser et al., 2002) for co-precipitation and stabilization (usually with oleic acid) in order to obtain only magnetite nanoparticles with adequate chemisorbed stabilizing layer. To produce substituted ferrite nanoparticles to be used in magnetic fluid preparation, the Fe^{2+} ion is simply replaced by another divalent metal ion, M^{2+}, such as Co^{2+} or also Mn^{2+}, Ni^{2+}, Zn^{2+}. Cobalt ferrite and γ-Fe_2O_3 nanoparticles may be prepared, but applying a similar procedure and using NaOH in excess, instead of NH_4OH. A different procedure was developed by Pileni and coworkers (Pileni, 1989; Moumen and Pileni, 1996a, 1996b; Pileni et al., 1997) for the synthesis of cobalt ferrite, maghemite and magnetite nanoparticles using a microemulsion technique, e.g., for cobalt ferrite aqueous methylamine (CH_3NH_3OH) was added to sodium dodecylsulfate solution containing cobalt(Ⅱ) dodecyl-sulfate ($Co(DS)_2$) and iron(Ⅱ) dodecyl-sulfate ($Fe(DS)_2$) to generate a precipitate. The size of the nanoparticles was controlled from 2 to 5 nm by changing the sodium dodecyl sulfate concentration and by maintaining constant concentrations of $Co(DS)_2$, $Fe(DS)_2$, and methylamine. In case of maghemite and magnetite instead of using mixed micelles, the synthesis was performed using iron dodecyl sulfate micelles, $Fe(DS)_2$ and the average size of particles varied between 3.7 and 11.6 nm (Pileni et al., 1997).

25.2.2.2 Thermal Decomposition. Size Selection Procedures

Thermal decomposition of organo-metallic compounds (e.g. iron or cobalt carbonyl) in organic solvents is an important strategy of making monodisperse iron/cobalt-containing nanoparticles and finally, high magnetization magnetic fluids. The composition, size and size distribution can be finely controlled by varying the reaction mixtures and synthetic conditions. Several groups have focused their researches on the size and composition control of iron, cobalt, iron and cobalt oxide nanoparticles obtained by this method (Jeong et al., 2007). Iron carbonyl, acetate, acetylacetonate, carboxylate, and chloride are some of the commonly used precursors for making monodisperse nanoparticles of iron and/or iron oxides, with diameters ranging from 3 to 50 nm. Among all these precursors, $Fe(CO)_5$ is particularly versatile. In (Hyeon, 2003; Hyeon et al., 2001) a thermal decomposition based procedure is described for the synthesis of monodisperse iron nanoparticles. The procedure started from the high temperature (300℃) aging of an iron-oleic acid metal complex, which was prepared by the thermal decomposition of iron pentacarbonyl in the presence of oleic acid at 100℃.

Monodisperse nanoparticles resulted with sizes ranging from 4 to 20 nm without using any size selection process. Using a similar procedure, based on the thermal decomposition of a metal-surfactant complex followed by mild oxidation, highly crystalline and monodisperse maghemite and cobalt ferrite nanocrystals were also obtained.

Spherical γ-Fe_2O_3 nanoparticles can also be directly generated with size ranging from 4 to 16 nm by introducing an oxidation agent, trimethylamine *N*-oxide or $(CH_3)_3NO$, into the reaction solution. Both XRD and X-ray photoelectron spectroscopy (XPS) spectra were used to confirm that the as-made iron oxide particles were γ-Fe_2O_3.

It was shown (Teng and Yang, 2004) that γ-Fe_2O_3 nanoparticles with diameter around 3 nm may be synthesized by substituting the oleic acid with stearic acid in octyl ether solution at 200℃ through a similar thermal decomposition approach. Also, highly monodisperse maghemite nanoparticles were obtained through the decomposition of iron pentacarbonyl in dioctyl ether (Taboada et al., 2007), in the presence of oleic acid. The mean diameter obtained was 4.9 ± 0.7 nm, with a standard deviation of 14%, where 94% of the particles display sizes between 3.5 and 5.75 nm, and none of them was larger than 8 nm. To stabilize the particles in an aqueous solution at physiological pH, the organic nonpolar surfactant was displaced by an electrolyte, tetramethyl-ammonium-hydroxide (TMA)OH.

For magnetic fluids to be used in future highly sensitive magnetic nanodevices and biomedical applications, various size-selective synthesis procedures were developed (Sun et al., 2004; Sun and Zeng, 2002; Neveu et al., 2002) to obtain mono-disperse MFe_2O_4 nanoparticles with diameters smaller than 20 nm and a tight size distribution (sometimes less than 10% standard deviation). High-temperature solution phase reaction of iron (Ⅲ) acetylacetonate, $Fe(acac)_3$, with 1,2-hexadecanediol in the presence of oleic acid and oleylamine leads to monodisperse magnetite (Fe_3O_4) nanoparticles (Sun et al., 2004). Similarly, reaction of $Fe(acac)_3$ and $Co(acac)_2$ or $Mn(acac)_2$ with the same diol results in monodisperse $CoFe_2O_4$ or $MnFe_2O_4$ nanoparticles. Particle diameter can be tuned from 3 to 20 nm by varying reaction conditions or by seed-mediated growth. The process does not require a low-yield fractionation procedure to achieve the desired size distribution. The hydrophobic nanoparticles can be transformed into hydrophilic ones by mixing with bipolar surfactants, allowing preparation of aqueous nanoparticle dispersions. Their long-term colloidal stability in non-uniform magnetic field and in physiological conditions is still not proved.

Referring to biomedical applications of magnetic nanoparticles (Neuberger et al., 2005), using metallic nanoparticles, only small amounts of nanoparticles would be required for effective drug targeting due to the excellent magnetic characteristics, minimizing potential side effects. Clearly, in vitro applications such as magnetic cell separation will be the first field of application for metallic magnetic fluids while therapeutic and diagnostic in vivo treatments will appear in the far future. One of the main challenges besides the synthesis of monodisperse metal nanoparticles is their transfer into aqueous phase and stabilization under physiological conditions.

25.2.2.3 Iron and Cobalt Nanoparticles

Co nanoparticles for technical grade high magnetization magnetic fluids, e.g., for ferrohydrostatic bearings, were prepared by thermolysis of $Co_2(CO)_8$ in the presence of $Al(C_8H_{17})_3$ (Bönnemann et al., 2003). For a typical synthesis, 171 g $Co_2(CO)_8$ were added to 88 mL $Al(C_8H_{17})_3$ in 3000 mL toluene at 80 – 90℃ and heated at 110℃ for 18 h under stirring. After cooling the reaction mixture to room temperature, the particles were smoothly oxidized by synthetic air introduced through a small capillary. The resulting black precipitate was washed two times with 1500 mL toluene. The precipitate was allowed to settle, the supernatant was decanted, and the Co particles were isolated as a suspension in 100 mL toluene. Bimetallic Fe/Co nanoparticles were synthesized according to the following procedure (Bönnemann et al., 2005). 50 g $Fe(CO)_5$ (255.2 mmol/L) and 21.81 g $Co_2(CO)_8$ (63.8 mmol/L) were stirred in 500 mL tetrahydronaphthalene at room temperature for 3 days. After adding 20.3 mL $Al(C_8H_{17})_3$ (38.4 mmol/L), the reaction mixture was heated slowly to 90°C, followed by stepwise heating at 10℃/h to 120℃ releasing CO. The temperature was carefully raised to 150℃ to finalize the gas evolution. 'Smooth oxidation' of the nanoparticles was performed by applying oxygen (3.5 vol% O_2 in argon) through a thin capillary. The precipitate was washed two times with 500 mL toluene and isolated as a suspension in 100 mL toluene.

Various gas-phase synthesis methods were also applied to obtain iron/iron oxide nanoparticles. The IR laser pyrolysis is recommended as a versatile technique for producing iron-based nanoparticles (Bi et al., 1993; Leconte et al., 2007). In case of preparation of iron/iron oxide core-shell nanostructures by a two-steps procedure (Fig. 25.3(a)) the laser pyrolysis was first acting on the iron pentacarbonyl (vapors) gas mixture (Dumitrache et al., 2005). The freshly formed iron nanoparticles are entrained downstream and retained by a microporous filter. A careful in situ passivation process was performed in a second step on the primary collected nanoparticles.

By introducing a liquid toluene bubbler downstream and in front of the collection filter, selective particle collection was achieved mainly by the trapping of large particle aggregates (Popovici et al., 2007).

Due to the exposure of the liquid surface to air, toluene immersion creates conditions for nanoparticle mild surface oxidation. Structural investigations carried on by electron microscopy (TEM, HRTEM), Fig. 25.3(b), revealed small aggregates of the dispersed iron-based particles, most of them presenting the core-shell morphology. X-ray diffraction patterns showed that the samples have a spinel structure, similar to magnetite or maghemite.

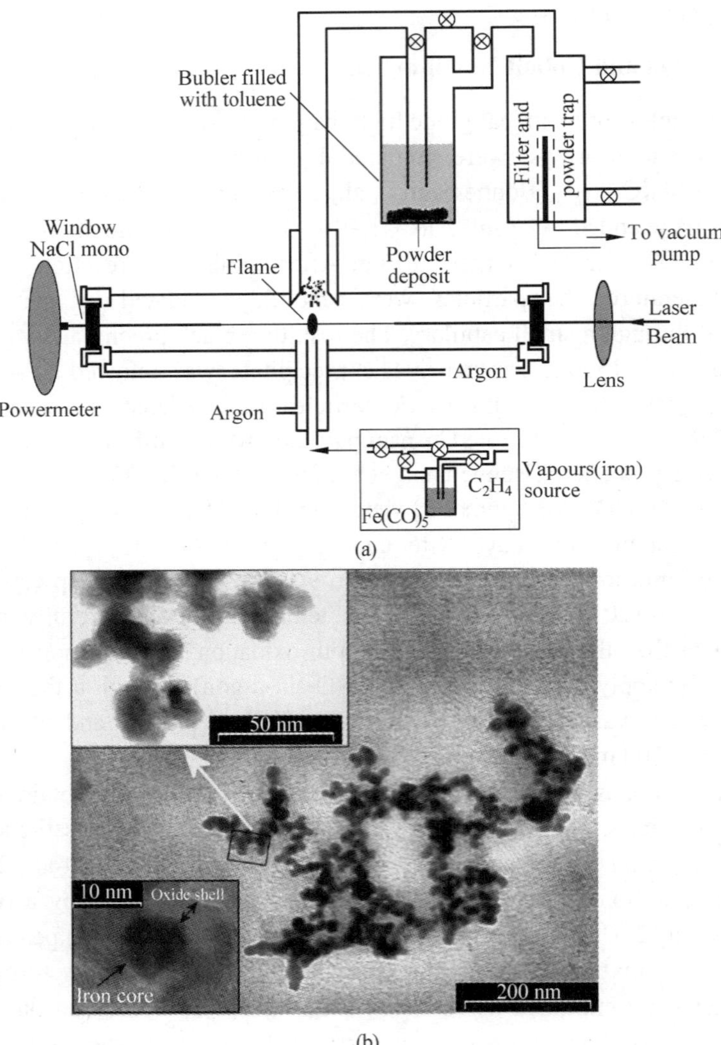

Figure 25.3 (a) Experimental setup for the laser pyrolysis synthesis procedure of iron/iron oxide nanoparticles and the system for powder collection in the toluene bubbler (after Popovici et al., 2007). (b) TEM images revealing an individual assembly of iron/iron oxide core-shell nanoparticles obtained; enhanced magnification TEM image, revealing the encapsulated feature of the nano-Fe powder-higher inset; HRTEM image for a single nanoparticle showing a dark core with a lighter shell-lower inset; TEM image after agglomerates removal (after Popovici et al., 2007)

25.2.3 Magnetic Nanofluids with Organic Carriers

25.2.3.1 Colloidal Stability, Sterical Stabilization

The surfactant coating on magnetic nanoparticles prevents clustering due to steric repulsion. Stabilization-dispersion of nanoparticles in organic liquids using various chain length organic surface-active molecules (e.g. fatty acids, polymers)—steric stabilization—is dependent on the liquid carrier properties and it should ensure long-term colloidal stability of magnetic nanofluids, even in an intense and strongly non-uniform magnetic field. This is a key feature of magnetic nanofluid synthesis and it has to take into account the specific conditions of the envisaged application.

Long-term colloidal stability of magnetic nanofluids, especially at high volume fraction of magnetic nanoparticles, is a complex issue connected to the synthesis procedure followed, including the nature of surfactant(s) and carrier liquid used. The dimensionless magnetic interaction energy, λ_{int}, which is half the ratio of the dipolar energy of two aligned magnetic dipoles at close contact to the thermal energy, should be kept below 1 to ensure highly stable magnetic fluids. During preparation repulsive forces due to coating of magnetic cores are introduced to prevent irreversible aggregation of particles produced by attractive van der Waals and dipolar interactions. When the dipolar interactions are much stronger than the thermal energies, $\lambda_{int}>2$ (Chantrell et al., 1980), particle chains start growing and forming more complex structures, including also flux-closure rings (Klokkenburg and Ernè, 2006), depending on the particle volume fraction, size distribution, temperature and magnetic field applied. Consequently, the colloidal stability of magnetic nanofluids is dependent on this interplay between isotropic van der Waals and anisotropic dipolar forces. An interesting feature of magnetic nanofluid synthesis is that the relative strengths and ranges of various interaction potentials can be controlled by the diameter of magnetic cores and the thickness of the stabilizing layer. The effects of the size of magnetic particles on aggregation phenomena were investigated using cryo-TEM and complex magnetic susceptibility measurements (Klokkenburg and Ernè, 2006) on two kind of magnetic colloids. In oxidized iron colloid systems in zero field irreversible aggregation was evidenced, while in magnetite dispersions the dipolar chains break up upon dilution.

In the case of weakly stabilized magnetic colloids at relatively high volume fraction when the contact distance between nanoparticles is short enough, due to the van der Waals interactions clusters are formed. These clusters exhibit large dipole moments compared to individual particles and favour development of larger structures and formation of chain-like agglomerates, especially under the influence of an applied field. Tailoring of magnetic nanofluids for various applications has to take into account all these structural features.

E.g., magnetic fluids for sealing applications have to be prepared in such a way to ensure high magnetization, low viscosity, low or very low vapour pressure and long-term colloidal stability in intense (magnetic induction 1 – 1.5 T) and strongly non-uniform magnetic field (field gradient $10^8 - 10^9$ A/m^2). These requirements are sometimes difficult to fulfil simultaneously and impose special conditions on the stabilization procedure applied in MNF preparation, to avoid irreversible magnetic field induced structural processes.

25.2.3.2 Synthesis Procedures

The synthesis of magnetic fluids with organic carriers (Bica, 1995; Bica and Vékás, 1994; Bica et al., 2002, 2004) has the following main steps (Diagrams 1 (Fig. 25.4) and 2 (Fig.25.5)):

- Synthesis of surface coated magnetite nanoparticles: co-precipitation (at $t \approx 80$℃) of magnetite from aqueous solutions of Fe^{3+} and Fe^{2+} ions in the presence of concentrated NH_4OH solution (25%)→ subdomain magnetite particles → sterical stabilization (chemisorbtion of oleic acid; 80 – 82℃) → phase separation → magnetic decantation and repeated washing → monolayer covered magnetite nanoparticles + free oleic acid → extraction of monolayer covered magnetite nanoparticles (acetone added; extraction) → stabilized magnetite nanoparticles.
- Dispersion of magnetic nanoparticles in non-polar carriers (hydrocarbons) (Diagram 1, Fig. 25.4): dispersion of oleic acid monolayer coated magnetite nanoparticles in various hydrocarbon (kerosen, toluen, cyclohexan, transformer oil etc.) carriers at $t \approx 120 - 130$℃→ magnetic decantation/ filtration → repeated flocculation and re-dispersion of magnetic nanoparticles (elimination of free oleic acid; advanced purification process) → non-polar magnetic nanofluid.
- Dispersion of magnetic nanoparticles in polar carriers (such as diesters, alcohols, ketones, amins, mixtures of various mineral and synthetic oils (e.g. high vacuum oils) (Diagram 2, Fig. 25.5): primary purified magnetic fluid on light hydrocarbon carrier obtained through repeated flocculation and redispersion of magnetic nanoparticles (elimination of free oleic acid; advanced purification) → monolayer stabilized magnetic nanoparticles → dispersion in polar solvent (stabilization with secondary surfactant, e.g. dodecylbenzensulphonic acid (DBSA) for alcohols and ketones, poly-isobutilene-succinanhydride (PIBSA) or poly-isobutilene-succinimide (PIBSI) for diesters and high vacuum oil, physically adsorbed to the first layer) → polar magnetic nanofluid.

The dispersion of chemisorbed oleic acid coated magnetic nanoparticles in organic polar carriers (e.g. diesters, C3 – C10 alcohols) was ensured by the proper choice of a secondary surfactant layer (Bica, 1995; Bica and Vékás, 1994; Bica et al., 2002) in order to screen the combined action of van der Waals and lyophobic attractions, which become increasingly significant in polar carriers

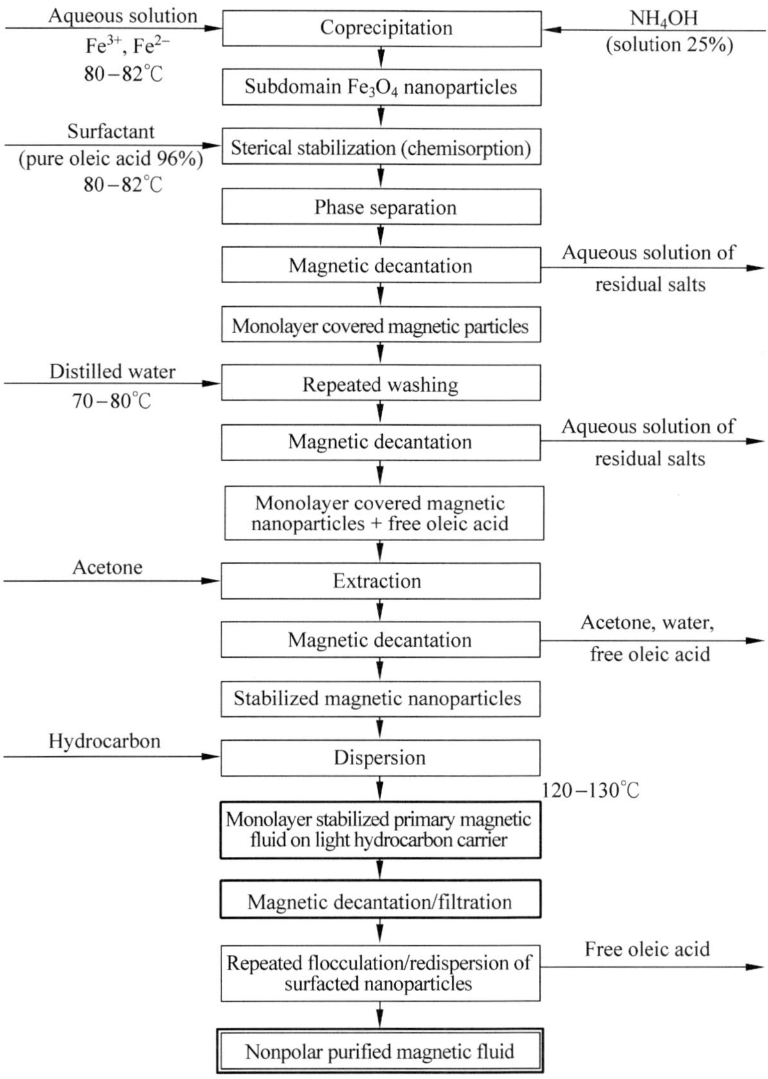

Figure 25.4 Diagram 1: main steps of the synthesis procedure of magnetic nanofluids with non-polar organic carriers (Bica, 1995; Vékás et al., 2007)

(with relative dielectric constant $\varepsilon_r > 9$) (Lopez-Lopez et al., 2005) and become dominant for very polar solvents. Combinations of chemisorbed oleic acid first layer with DBSA, PIBSA or PIBSI ensured the long-term colloidal stability of magnetic nanofluids with polar carriers, including very polar ones such as methyl-ethyl-ketone (Vékás et al., 2005). Also, a combination of oleic acid (OA) covered magnetite nanoparticles with beeswax ensured their stable dispersion in lanoline, giving a biocompatible magnetic nanocompund experimented as UV protective ointment for skin (Sincai et al., 2007).

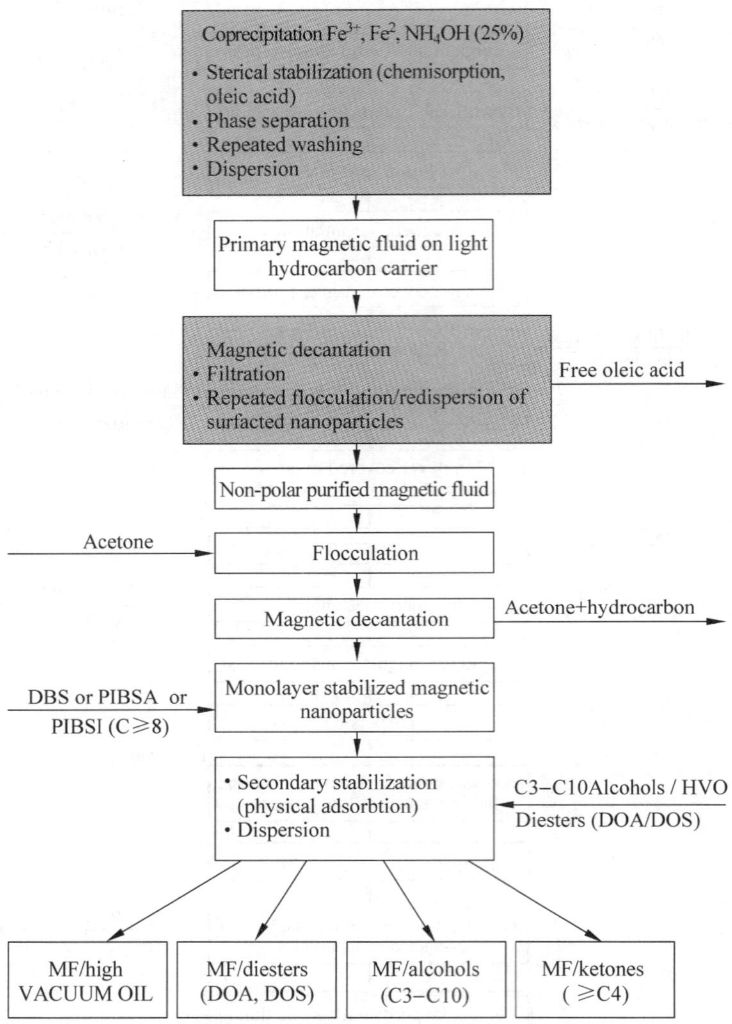

Figure 25.5 Diagram 2: main steps of the synthesis procedure of magnetic nanofluids with polar organic carriers (Bica, 1995; Bica and Vékás, 1994; Bica et al., 2002)

According to the synthesis procedures described above, transformer oil (TR30), diesters (DOA = dioctyl adipate (bis(2-ethylhexyl)adipate), $C_{22}H_{42}O_4$; DOF = dioctyl phtalate (bis(ethylhexyl)phtalate), $C_{24}H_{38}O_4$ and DOS = dioctyl sebacate (bis(2-ethylhexyl)sebacate), $C_{26}H_{50}O_4$) and high vacuum oil (HVO (KW, Merck)) based magnetic fluids were prepared for various type of magnetic fluid seals (MFSs) (Borbáth et al., 2006; Vékás et al., 2007). The high boiling point (over 200℃) carriers, especially DOS, DOF and HVO, were selected for high vacuum and/or for very long duty seals, while TR30 for pressure seals. Mono- and double layer sterical stabilization procedures were applied taking into account the non-polar (Fig. 25.4) or polar (Fig. 25.5) character of the carriers: TR30- non-polar; DOA, DOF and DOS—weakly polar; HVO—non-polar with some polar additives. The stabilization/dispersion of magnetite nanoparticles in TR30 required monolayer sterical stabilization with chemisorbed oleic acid, while in the case of polar diester carriers double layer sterical stabilization with oleic acid (chemisorbed primary surfactant) + dodecylbenzene-sulphonic acid (DBSA; physically adsorbed secondary surfactant) proved to be efficient. In the case of HVO carrier a polymeric secondary surfactant was used to achieve long-term colloidal stability of the resulted magnetic fluid. This type of magnetic fluid with very low vapour pressure, below 10^{-7} mbar at 20℃, was developed specially for vacuum MFSs. The saturation magnetization of these specially tailored MNFs, with long-term colloidal stability, was set between 20 and 60 kA/m, depending on the sealing device application. Several years long leakage-free operating period of rotating seals for high vacuum in crystal growth equipments and for moderate pressure differences (~ 10 bars) in high power electric switches with SF_6 gas (Borbáth et al., 2006) proved the efficiency of magnetic fluids preparation/stabilization procedures given in diagrams 1 and 2 (Figs. 25.4, 25.5).

The preparation of MNFs from magnetite, maghemite and Fe-C nanoparticles obtained by laser pyrolisis conducted to promising results. TEM analysis of MNFs obtained, starting from Fe-based nano aggregates in toluene (Fig. 25.6(a),(b)), by stabilization with oleic acid in hydrocarbon carrier. Fig. 25.6(c) reveals a satisfactory dispersion of the iron based nanoparticles, containing single particles or aggregates with a few numbers of particles, observed on the microscopic grid. Mean cluster diameters of 7 nm may be estimated. This two-step procedure of MNF synthesis based on gas-phase laser pyrolisis has direct control on size of magnetic nanoparticles, however implies more difficulties in their stabilization-dispersion in various carriers.

Co, FeCo, and Fe nanoparticles synthesized by thermolysis (Behrens et al., 2006a, 2006b) of the carbonyl precursors in the presence of aluminium organics can be peptized after 'smooth oxidation' yielding magnetic fluids which were remarkably stable and which showed a high saturation magnetization and high volume concentrations (e.g. 10 vol% Co) (Bönemann et al., 2005). Several surfactants such as KorantinSH (N-oleyl sarcosine, BASF AG), or AOT (sodium dioctyl sulfosuccinate, SERVA2), LP4 (fatty acid condensation polymer, ICI Ltd.) were applied to prepare magnetic fluids in various organic media, e.g. kerosene, vacuum and mineral oil. Referring to magnetic fluids based on metallic Co, Fe/Co, and Fe nanoparticles in various organic media (Behrens et al., 2006a), their saturation magnetization attains 190 kA/m, the highest value reported up to now.

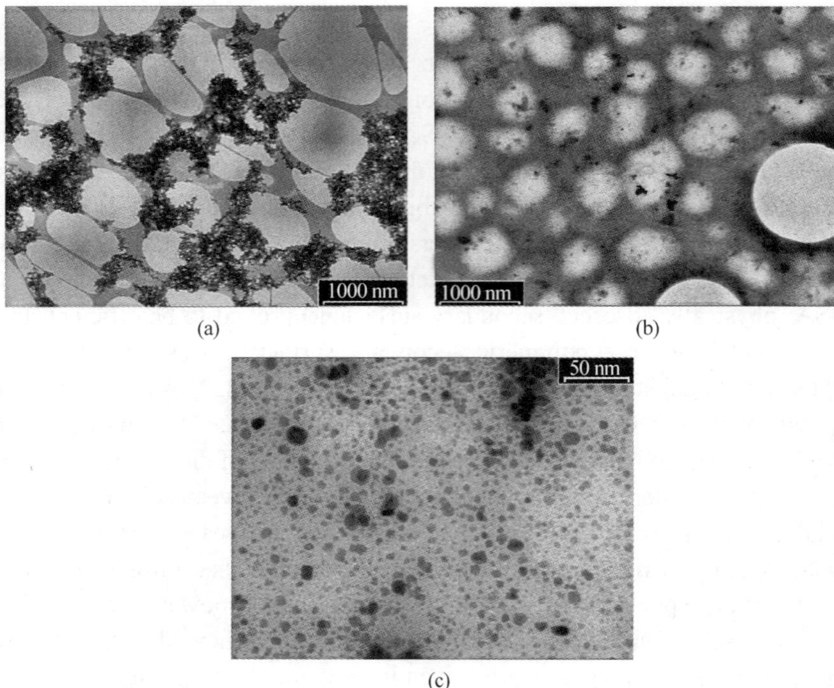

(a) (b) (c)

Figure 25.6 TEM images: Fe-based nano aggregates, collected from the bubbler (a) and clear solution (b) and (c) of the hydrocarbon-based magnetic nanofluid prepared from laser-pyrolisis magnetic nanoparticles, revealing almost single particles or assemblies of a few nanoparticles (after Popovici et al., 2007)

25.2.4 Water Based Magnetic Nanofluids

25.2.4.1 Stabilization Mechanisms

Electrostatic and steric stabilization procedures are both applicable for water based magnetic nanofluids.

Formation of similarly charged electric double layer and/or of adsorption layers on the particle surface enhances the stability of magnetic colloids in aqueous medium. Massart (1981, 1996), Shimoiizaka and coworkers (Shimoiizaka et al., 1980), Khalafalla and Reimers (1980), Bica (1995, 1985), Wooding and coworkers (Wooding et al., 1991, 1992) and Hatton and coworkers (Shen et al., 1999b; Moeser et al., 2002) used various kind of stabilizing bilayers to produce stable water based magnetic fluids.

Preparation procedures of stable aqueous alkaline and acidic magnetic liquids by free precipitation, with electric bilayer stabilized magnetic nanoparticles were presented in (Massart, 1981; Massart et al., 1995). The nature of the counterions and the pH of the suspensions played a vital role in stabilizing the charged magnetic particles through interactions between their electrical double layers. The applications of magnetic fluids stabilized solely by electrostatic repulsion are somewhat restricted since this stabilizing mechanism is overly sensitive to conditions such as pH and ionic strength and offers little flexibility for tuning the surface properties of the particles.

Double layer steric and electrostatic (combined) stabilization of magnetic nanoparticles in water carrier proved to be efficient when colloidal stability had to be ensured up to relatively large values (over 0.10) of the particle volume fraction (Bica et al., 2002). Improved colloidal stability in a wide range of pH and enhanced salt tolerance is expected for these nanofluids based on a manifold analysis of the mechanism of combined stabilization of magnetite particles in aqueous systems (Illés and Tombácz, 2006). For most of biomedical uses the magnetic nanoparticles (Pankhurst et al., 2003) should be below 15 nm in size and stably dispersed in water (Neuberger et al., 2005). The attractive interactions between magnetic particles, when preponderant, may lead to various types of agglomerates, usually in the shape of linear chains quasi-parallel to the applied magnetic field or drop-like aggregates (Cabuil et al., 1996; Socoliuc and Bica, 2001). The ferrofluid becomes a biphasic system i.e. condensed-phase droplets form in equilibrium with the uncondensed phase matrix. The density of the condensed phase droplets increases with decreasing temperature and increasing magnetic field intensity. The kinetics of phase condensation was found to be influenced mainly by the temperature. The growth process of condensed-phase drops evolves in two stages: small primary agglomerates grow and stick together into large secondary drop-wise agglomerates, as it was evidenced also by SANS investigations (Avdeev et al., 2006). Particle condensation have to be impeded by advanced stabilization of water based magnetic fluids for biomedical applications, because the agglomeration processes are much intensified under physiological conditions (Jurgons et al., 2006).

25.2.4.2 Synthesis Procedures, Technical Grade and Biocompatible Water Based MNFs

Synthesis of sterically stabilized aqueous magnetic fluids applying a two-step procedure (Shen et al., 1999b, 2000; Moeser et al., 2002) is resumed in what follows. First, Fe_3O_4 nanoparticles coated with a primary surfactant were produced by chemical coprecipitation from an aqueous solution of Fe (II) and Fe (III) chloride in the presence of the molecularly dispersed surfactant. Then, following removal of the excess primary surfactant, the particles were coated with a secondary surfactant to form self-organized bilayers of the two surfactants on the iron oxide nanoparticle surfaces. It was found that the reliability of the synthesis improved significantly with the initial presence of primary surfactant during the precipitation process. Fatty acids and polymers were used as stabilizants.

Fatty acids are sparingly soluble in water and their solubility is enhanced by the presence of acetone, which is an excellent solvent for fatty acids and is completely miscible with water. The solubility enhancement increases the possibility of direct interactions between individual molecules of the acid and the iron oxide crystal, which is especially important for preventing agglomeration during the early stages of crystal growth. Under vigorous stirring at 80℃, rapid evaporation of acetone ensures a large contact area between the freshly precipitated particles and surfactant. Meanwhile, the extremely high affinity between iron oxide and the carboxylic acid group of the surfactant makes not only the orientation of the surfactant at the particle/surfactant interface favorable but also the chemisorption reaction between them. Once the surfactant is adsorbed on the iron oxide particles, the number of accessible sites for further crystal growth is reduced, leading to termination of crystal growth. Owing to the rapid kinetics of the precipitation process and the strong tendency of naked magnetic nanoparticles to agglomerate, the initial presence of molecularly dispersed fatty acids provides an effective means to keep the particles apart during the crystal growth process.

The synthesis conditions, such as the precipitation temperature of 80℃ (Bica 1995, Bica, 1985) and the excess amount of NH_4OH ensure the formation of Fe_3O_4 over Fe_2O_3, which has a smaller magnetic susceptibility.

For example, precipitation at temperatures below 60℃ typically produces an amorphous hydrated oxyhydroxide that can be easily converted to Fe_2O_3, while higher reaction temperatures (>80℃) favor the formation of Fe_3O_4 (Ziolo et al., 1992; Zhang et al., 1997). The necessary pH value for the rapid formation of Fe_3O_4 is attained by addition of excess NH_4OH. A straightforward procedure for the synthesis of technical grade water based MNF's, using DBSA + DBSA coating of magnetite nanoparticles, is given in Fig. 25.7(a) Diagram 3(a) (Bica, 1995; Bica, 1985).

Biocompatible MNFs were synthesized using lauric acid (LA), myristic acid (MA) or oleic acid (OA) as double layer surfactant (Bica et al., 2007; Tombácz et al., 2008). The oleate coating on magnetite is favored because of the surface complex formation between the Fe-OH sites (Tombácz et al., 2004) and carboxylate groups, especially if the aim is to further functionalize the magnetic nanoparticles (Moeser et al., 2004; Lattuada and Hatton, 2007).

Less attention was paid until now to the adsorption of fatty acids, the charge neutralization and overcharging due to the first and second layer formation. The effect of dilution, pH and salt concentration has also remained in the background, although these are the most important factors in biomedical application. The procedures and specific conditions of stabilization/dispersion of magnetite nanoparticles in water carrier to obtain stable magnetic fluids, such as nature and quantity of surfactant(s) added for unit mass of nanoparticles, pH value, temperature and elimination of excess surfactant, depend on the surfactant combination. Synthesis and characterization of nanosized magnetite in water based systems (Illés and Tombácz, 2006; Tombácz et al., 2007a) and preparation of biocompatible water based MNFs present several particularities (Bica et al., 2007; Tombácz et al., 2007b). The preparation procedure for magnetic fluids with magnetite (or cobalt ferrite) nanoparticles having LA + LA, MA + MA or OA + OA biocompatible stabilizing double layer is different from that with DBSA + DBSA double layer used for technical grade fluids (diagram 3(a), Fig. 25.7(a)). The main difference is the formation of a magnetic organosol, similar to that encountered in the preparation process of oleic acid stabilized magnetic fluid with hydrocarbon carrier (preparation diagram 1; Fig. 25.4 (Bica, 1995)).

The main steps of the preparation route (diagram 3(b); Fig. 25.7(b)) for the biocompatible MF/W/MA+MA (also for (LA + LA) or (OA + OA)) samples with magnetite nanoparticles are exemplified below: 215 mL solution of 1 M $FeSO_4$ and 130 mL solution of 2.8 M $FeCl_3$ were used under atmospheric conditions, with $Fe^{3+}/Fe^{2+} = 1.7$; heating up to 80 – 82℃ under continuous stirring; addition

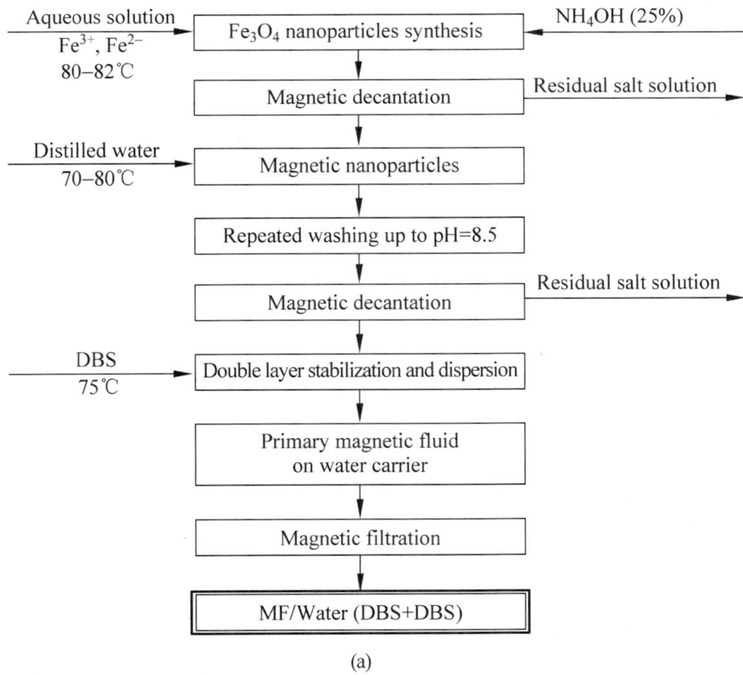

(a)

Figure 25.7 Diagram 3: main steps of the synthesis procedure of water based magnetic nanofluids with magnetic nanoparticles coated by double layer of surfactants: (a) DBSA (Bica, 1995; Vékás et al., 2005); (b) carboxylic acids (C12, C14, C16, C18) and mixed carboxylic acid + DBSA double layers (Vékás et al., 2006, 2007; Bica et al., 2007)

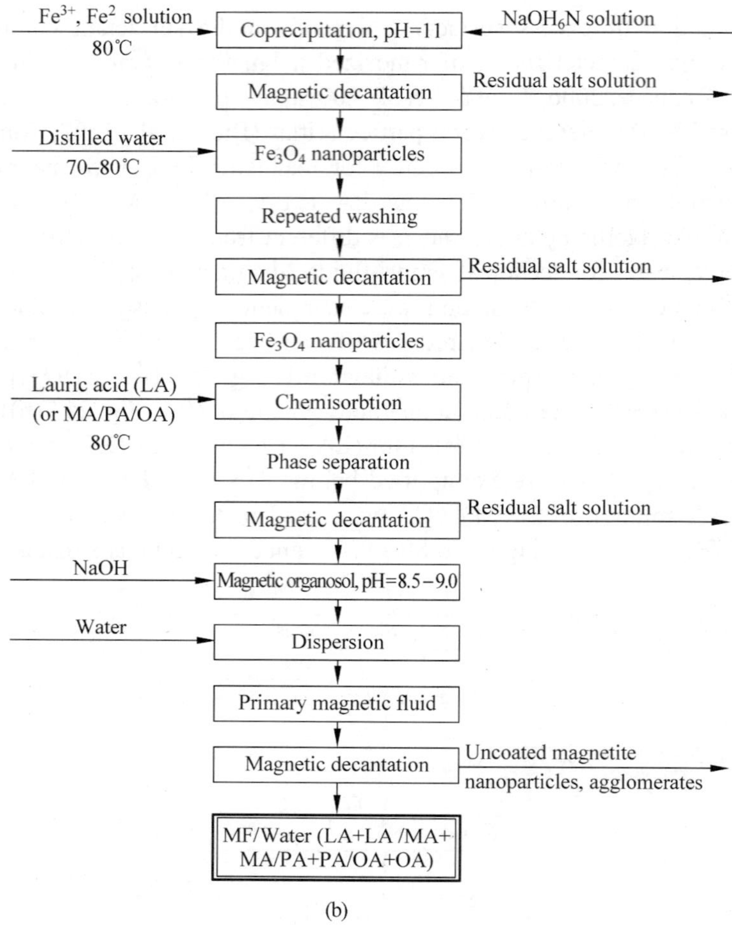

(b)

Figure 25.7(Continued)

of 300 mL NaOH(6N)(or 160 mL solution of NH_4OH 25% in excess up to 50%); surfactant coating of magnetite nanoparticles by addition, shortly after the co-precipitation reaction, of 24 g MA (or LA, OA) at 80℃; separation of phases (after about 20 min); decantation; washing of the resulting magnetic organosol (distilled water); elimination of residual salts; dispersion of double layer coated magnetite (or cobalt ferrite) particles in a weak solution of NaOH or NH_4OH (correction of pH); purification of the resulting magnetic fluid by magnetic decantation/filtration. The result of this laboratory scale procedure was 100 mL water based magnetic fluid with appoximate. 12 kA/m saturation magnetization.

25.2.4.3 Surfactant Layers and Colloidal Stability

Four samples of water based magnetic nanofluids, prepared according to the procedure given in diagram 3b, consisting of cobalt ferrite and magnetite nanoparticles coated with MA + MA, OA + OA and MA + DBS, LA + LA double layers of surfactants, respectively, were subsequently characterized by X-ray diffraction (XRD) and Mössbauer spectroscopy (Kuncser et al., 2007). The XRD data provide proof of the crystalline state and yield, by Scherer formula, average physical diameters of about 11 nm for all nanoparticle systems, somewhat overestimated compared to transmission electron microscopy (TEM) and magneto-granulometric analyses.

Mössbauer spectroscopy results obtained at 4.2 K in zero external field support a correct site occupation in the inverse spinel structure of the both ferrites. The temperature dependent Mössbauer data reveal the most pronounced magnetic relaxation behaviour for the sample prepared with magnetite nanoparticles double coated with lauric acid surfactant. The blocking temperature in this system was estimated to be about 195 K, by employing two alternative procedures which are based on the temperature evolution of the magnetic hyperfine field distribution. The time constant τ_0 in the Néel formula for superparamagnetic relaxation, $\tau = \tau_0 \exp (KV/k_B T)$, was estimated purely from Mössbauer spectroscopy data in zero external field. Here, τ is superparamagnetic (Néel) relaxation time, K is effective anisotropy constant of the magnetic material, V is volume of magnetic particle. Information on both the relative size dispersion of the particles and their magnetic anisotropy energy were obtained from the Mössbauer spectra in the temperature regime of collective excitations. The results support the formation of a magnetic dead layer at the surface of the nanoparticles and suggest that the thickness is dependent on the ferrite type and on the surfactant type. Hence, the much higher crystalline magnetic anisotropy constant of the cobalt ferrite (as compared with the anisotropy constant of magnetite) cannot improve substantially the magnetic performances of the cobalt ferrite based magnetic fluids at ambient temperature. The use of an inappropriate surfactant for magnetite particles could enhance substantially the superparamagnetic relaxation behaviour, leading to a low saturation magnetization of such magnetic nanofluids at ambient temperature.

Colloidal stability of dilute water based magnetic fluids prepared applying the procedures given in diagrams 3(a), (b) (Fig. 25.7), in particular pH dependence and salt tolerance were examined using dynamical light scattering (DLS) technique (Tombácz et al., 2008). DBS acid stabilized MNF samples are not biocompatible and were considered for comparative investigations. Besides an attempt for the direct sizing of dense MNFs with NanoZS apparatus (Malvern Co.) working in backscattering mode, the samples were characterized concerning the pH-dependent stability and salt tolerance of these MNFs in dilute aqueous systems.

The double DBSA layer stabilized MNF was found to be strongly aggregated, the average size of hydrodynamic units varied between 160 and 270 nm depending on the pH from 3.4 to 7 and the salt concentration up to 0.15 M NaCl. The combined layers of DBSA with LA and MA resulted also in relatively large aggregates (~64 nm at pH ~6.2) and (~33 nm at pH ~6.3) respectively, in accordance with SANS result (Avdeev et al., 2006). The best stabilization was reached with the MA and OA double layers.

It can be stated that the hydrophobic interactions are favored in the case of OA + OA and MA + MA double layer stabilized magnetic fluids, the magnetite nanoparticles with their coating are dispersed well, significant aggregation cannot be observed even in fairly dilute systems up to the physiological salt concentration in the favored pH region.

The salt tolerance of the oleic acid double layer stabilized magnetic nanofluids was investigated in dilute systems at pH~6 to test particle aggregation in time, whether the surfactant double layers provide suitable colloidal stability under physiological condition. It should be noted that the salt tolerance of naked magnetite particles is very low (~0.001 M NaCl) under this condition. Coagulation kinetics measurements were performed to determine quantitatively the stabilization effect of surfactant double stabilization on magnetite particles as explained before (Illés and Tombácz, 2006). The surfactant double layer can hinder effectively the aggregation of magnetite particles due to the combined steric and electrostatic stabilization, and the resistance against electrolytes is enhanced above the critical salt tolerance (>0.150 M) expected under physiological conditions. Such oleic acid covered magnetite nanoparticles in stable water based colloidal systems are rather favored for further functionalization (Lattuada and Hatton, 2007), due to the outward carboxyl group in the second physically adsorbed stabilizing layer.

Different procedures for transferring the metallic nanoparticles obtained by thermal decomposition and 'pre-stabilized' by 'smooth oxidation' into the aqueous phase were worked out recently (Behrens et al., 2006b). One approach is the formation of bi- or polylayers around the air-stable Co- and FeCo nanoparticles by using ionic, non-ionic, or double layer of surfactants. Firstly, surfactants such as oleic acid or KorantinSH were applied forming a first lipophilic layer around the particles, followed by addition of sodium oleate, sodium dodecylsulfonate, or dodecylamine resulting in a hydrophilic second or polylayers. Dispersions of 'pre-stabilized' Co (0) nanoparticles in water which were obtained by this procedure were stable for over one year.

Alternatively, water-based Co- and FeCo magnetic fluids have been obtained *via* phase transfer, using e.g TMAOH (tetramethylammonium hydroxide). TMAOH has been a popular stabilizer for the preparation of ferrofluids, mainly for those based on iron oxide nanoparticles (Tourinho et al., 1990), but it has been also applied successfully for phase transfer of FePt nanoparticles from organic into aqueous phase (Salgueirino-Marceira et al., 2004). It has been suggested that the mechanism of colloidal stabilization changed when TMAOH was applied. Upon addition of TMAOH, the hydrophobic surfactant layer consisting of KorantinSH, or oleic acid and oleylamine is replaced by negative hydroxide ions which in turn are surrounded by positively charged tetramethylammonium counterions, resulting in a stabilization of the particles by formation of a double layer. Possibly, the formation of the double layer is favoured by the presence of the thin oxide shell surrounding the metallic core of the particles.

Furthermore, the Co, Fe, and Fe/Co particles could be peptized directly with L-cysteine ethyl ester yielding a water-based magnetic fluid. The concentration in the aqueous phase, however, remained quite low up to now. The particles were peptized by thiol groups of cysteine with the amino groups remaining free which was confirmed by infrared spectra.

25.2.5 Long-Term Colloidal Stability of Magnetic Nanofluids

25.2.5.1 Effects of Surface Coating and Size of Magnetic Nanoparticles

The quality of surface coating of magnetic nanoparticles is of utmost significance for colloidal stability and aging of magnetic nanofluids. The most used surfactant for stabilization of magnetic nanoparticles in non-polar organic carriers is the oleic acid, while in case of polar carriers (alcohols, diesters) OA is the first chemisorbed surfactant combined with a secondary physically adsorbed one, as it was shown in Section 25.2.1. Transformer oil based samples were prepared according to the procedure given in preparation diagram 1(Fig. 25.4), using technical grade (TOA) and chemically pure oleic acid (POA). TOA contains only about 70% oleic acid, while the remaining 30% consists mostly of saturated shorter chain length carboxylic acids. The weak solvation of saturated acids, in comparison with OA reduces the steric repulsion or even changes the sign of interaction to an attractive one between surface coated particles, favoring agglomerate formation and slow structure formation in TOA stabilized samples.

The effects of these microstructural processes, as well as the differences between POA and TOA stabilized MNF samples, were evaluated by detailed magnetic, rheological, magnetorheological and magnetooptical investigations (Vékás et al., 1999, 2000; Socoliuc and Bica, 2002, 2005, Rasa et al., 2002; Socoliuc et al., 2003). E.g. in case of POA stabilized transformer oil based samples the effect of interactions on the magnetization curve is negligible and the magnetogranulometry and TEM data are in good agreement, while in TOA stabilized samples accelerated aging and drop-like agglomerates were evidenced (Vékás et al., 2000). Rheological and magnetorheological measurements on these samples (Vékás et al., 1999, 2000) evidenced non-Newtonian behavior and large magnetorheological effect in the case of TOA stabilized samples. Moreover, static magnetization (Rasa et al., 2002; Socoliuc et al., 2003) and magnetic induced linear dichroism experiments (Socoliuc and Bica, 2002, 2005) show that

TOA, having also shorter chain length saturated carboxylic acids in composition beside OA, has lower efficiency in steric repulsion mechanism, compared to OA. Detailed analysis of magnetization data, starting from a MNF model with chain-like aggregates of monodispersed magnetic nanoparticles (Zubarev and Iskakova, 1995), conducted to quantitative evaluation of the effective surfactant layer thickness (Socoliuc et al., 2003), which show that POA layer is almost two times larger than TOA. This result explains the qualitatively different colloidal stability, as well as magnetic and flow behavior of the two kind of samples, due to the difference evidenced in particle surface coating efficiency of POA and TOA surfactants.

The role and stabilizing efficiency of shorter chain length saturated carboxylic acids was further investigated, both in case of polar and non-polar carriers, as it will be shown below.

According to TEM analyses of different water based MNFs (Fig. 25.8), having magnetite nanoparticles stabilized with MA + MA, LA + LA, MA + DBSA, LA + DBSA and DBSA + DBSA surfactant double layers, and the log-normal size distributions show that the mean size and standard deviation depend mainly on the nature of the first (chemisorbed) stabilizing layer. By varying the first chemisorbed surfactant, the mean size of magnetic nanoparticles may be reduced from approximate 8 nm (with DBS first layer) close to 4 nm (with MA or LA first layer) (Bica et al., 2007; Turcu et al., 2007b).

Various chain length mono-carboxylic acids (e.g. lauric (LA; C12), myristic (MA; C14), palmitic (PA; C16) or stearic (SA; C18) saturated acids) may be applied also for stabilizing magnetic fluids with organic carriers, evidencing an efficient particle size-regulating procedure. As a first step, these surfactants were probed to coat magnetite nanoparticles in non-polar organic liquids by the usual procedure of MNF synthesis described in this work (preparation diagram 1, Fig. 25.4). The most effective stabilizing agent in such type of magnetic fluids is OA, $C_{18}H_{34}O_2$, having C18 (oleic) tail with a cis-double-bound in the middle, forming a kink. The kink plays a crucial role in the organization of the surfactant on the surface of magnetic particles, which results in proper steric repulsion (Tadmor et al., 2000). This is confirmed by the fact that the saturated stearic acid (SA) of the same tail length, $C_{18}H_{34}O_2$, but without this kink, is a weak stabilizer. It can be seen during the procedure (Avdeev et al., 2007a) that the preparation of magnetic fluids with short chain saturated surfactants is characterized by a larger amount of non-dispersed material in comparison with the case of OA and requires more cycles to achieve the same concentration. Nevertheless, in principle no difficulties to concentrate samples up to magnetic volume fraction 20% were found. The fluids show excellent stability in time (at least 2 years), as well as under effect of magnetic field (up to 2.5 T). However, the same procedure for SA resulted in significantly less stable fluid.

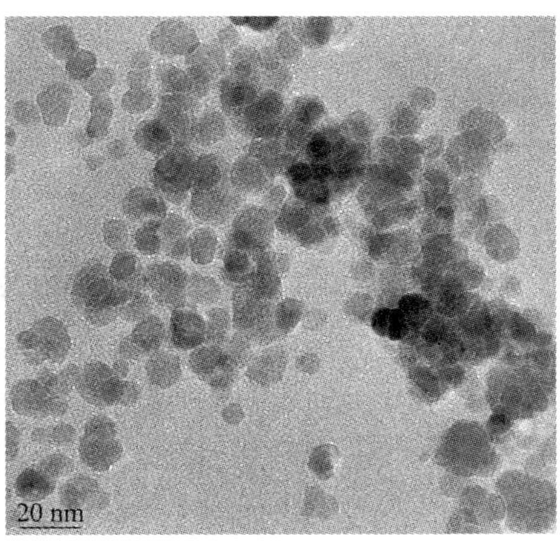

(a)

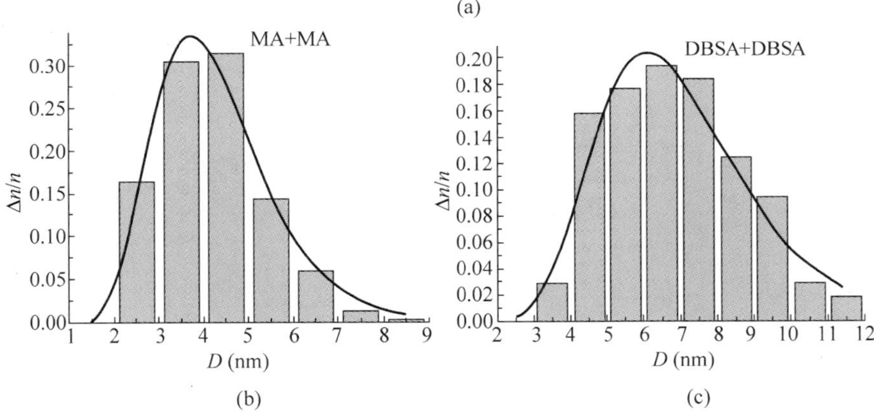

Figure 25.8 (a) TEM image of MNF/W (DBSA + DBSA) and the size distributions of (b) MA + MA and (c) DBSA+DBSA stabilized magnetite nanoparticles dispersed in water (Craciun et al., 2007)

The results show that short chain length saturated mono-carboxylic acids (LA and MA) can be used for the synthesis of highly stable magnetic fluids in organic non-polar media. The surfactant length is an important parameter that determines the molecules organization on the surface of magnetic particles. In comparison with the classical surfactant OA the shorter surfactants stabilize the magnetite particles of smaller size and reduce poly-dispersivity in organic media. This feature is well illustrated by the qualitative difference concerning the influence of applied magnetic field on the viscosity curves of MA and OA stabilized transformer oil MNFs (Vékás et al., 2006), Fig. 25.9.

The magnetoviscous effect (Fig. 25.10), i.e. the relative increase of viscosity in magnetic field, is much reduced in the case of MA stabilized sample compared to that with OA, due to lower mean size and standard deviation of dispersed magnetite nanoparticles in the MA stabilized sample.

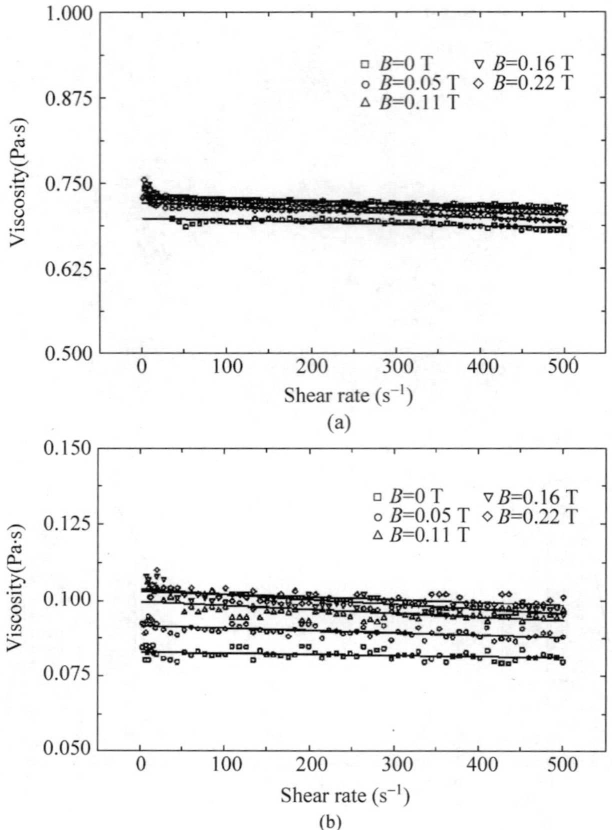

Figure 25.9 Influence of applied magnetic field (plate-plate MR cell, MCR300 PHYSICA rheometer) on the viscosity curves of MA and OA stabilized transformer oil based MNFs (Vékás et al., 2006): (a) MA. (b) OA

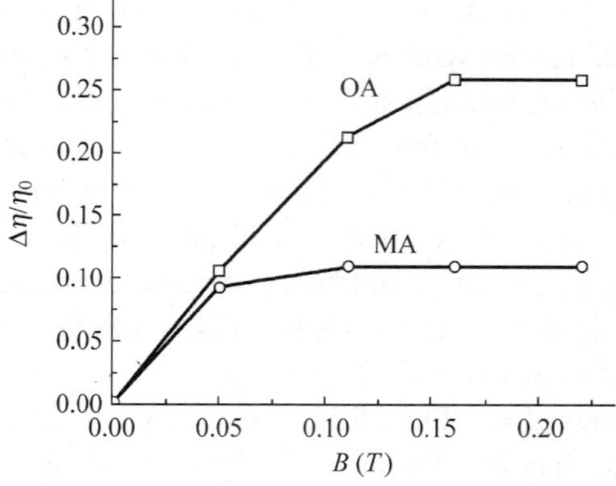

Figure 25.10 Influence of the nature of surfactant (MA or OA) on the magnitude of the magnetoviscous effect

A more detailed analysis, referring to the influence of the series of surfactants LA, MA, PA, SA and OA implied also magnetogranulometry and SANS investigations (Avdeev et al., 2008). The main structural difference revealed for the fluids with saturated acids as compared to the OA case concerns the size distribution function of stabilized magnetite. This function was estimated by the magnetization analysis and the data of small-angle neutron scattering (SANS) at room temperature from magnetic fluids based on decahydronaftalene (DHN) and diluted down to volume fraction of magnetite $\varphi_p \sim 1.5\%$. Such fraction allowed us to neglect interaction effects during the data interpretation for both methods. The data show that while OA is highly efficient surfactant for stabilizing nanomagnetite over a wide size range of 1 – 20 nm, saturated acids partially stabilize this interval dispersing in the carrier only a fraction of smaller particles, i.e. a size regulation effect of the surfactant was observed. The effect was proved also by using mixed surfactants (e.g. OA and MA, in various molar ratios) in mono-layer coating the dispersed particles. Depending on the relative fraction of shorter chain length surfactant (MA), the mean size of magnetite nanoparticles can be moved from about 8 nm (100% OA) to approx. 4 nm (100% MA) (Avdeev et al., 2008).This procedure proved to be an efficient one to tailor the properties of surface coated magnetic nanoparticles, as well as of magnetic nanofluids to the requirements of various applications.

25.2.5.2 Functionalized Coatings

Magnetic-electroconducting core-shell nanostructures were synthesized starting from well stabilized water based magnetic nanofluids.

The conducting polymer-inorganic hybrid materials have attracted increasing interest due to their synergistic properties difficult to get from individual components. The combination of conducting polymers and magnetic nanoparticles represents a new strategy to obtain composites possessing both conducting properties and magnetic response, which are suitable for a wide range of applications like: electromagnetic interference shielding and microwave absorbing, actuators, magnetic separation, biotechnology (Turcu et al., 2007b). Furthermore, the development of magnetic core-shell nanoparticles with a magnetic core and a polymeric shell offers the advantage of tailoring the magnetic properties, functionalizing and protecting the magnetic particles. Among conducting polymers, polypyrrole (PPY) was intensively used in association with magnetic nanoparticles like Fe_2O_3, Fe_3O_4 to get new nanocomposites by using different synthesis methods (Goiti et al., 2006). Different surfactants and oxidants could be used for the magnetic nanoparticles stabilization and pyrrole polymerization process and as a consequence, the properties of the composites differ with the synthesis conditions. Sterically stabilized water based magnetic fluids were used as primary nanoparticle system for synthesis of core-shell type nanostructured composites (Turcu et al., 2007a; Goiti et al., 2006). Water based magnetic fluids with magnetite nanoparticles carrying DBSA + DBSA, LA + DBSA, MA + DBSA or OA + DBSA stabilizing double layer were prepared for further nanocomposite synthesis, applying the procedure given in diagram 3 (Fig. 25.7).

Polypyrrole coated magnetic nanoparticles, which constitute in magnetic core-electroconducting core-shell type nanostructures, were prepared (Turcu et al., 2006, 2007b) by the oxidative polymerization of pyrrole (PY) and functionalized pyrrole (monomer pyrrole with attached COOH group) in aqueous solution containing an oxidant, ammonium peroxodisulfate (APS) and water based magnetic nanofluid. The ratio of MNF/PY was varied in the range 2 – 20 (v/v). The reaction proceeded at room temperature under magnetic stirring for different time intervals between 6 to 20 h. The reaction was terminated by adding excess methanol to the reaction flask. The resulting black precipitate was separated by centrifugation, washed with water and dried at 60℃ for 24 h. The HRTEM images (Fig. 25.11) of functionalized magnetic copolymer nanostructures show a

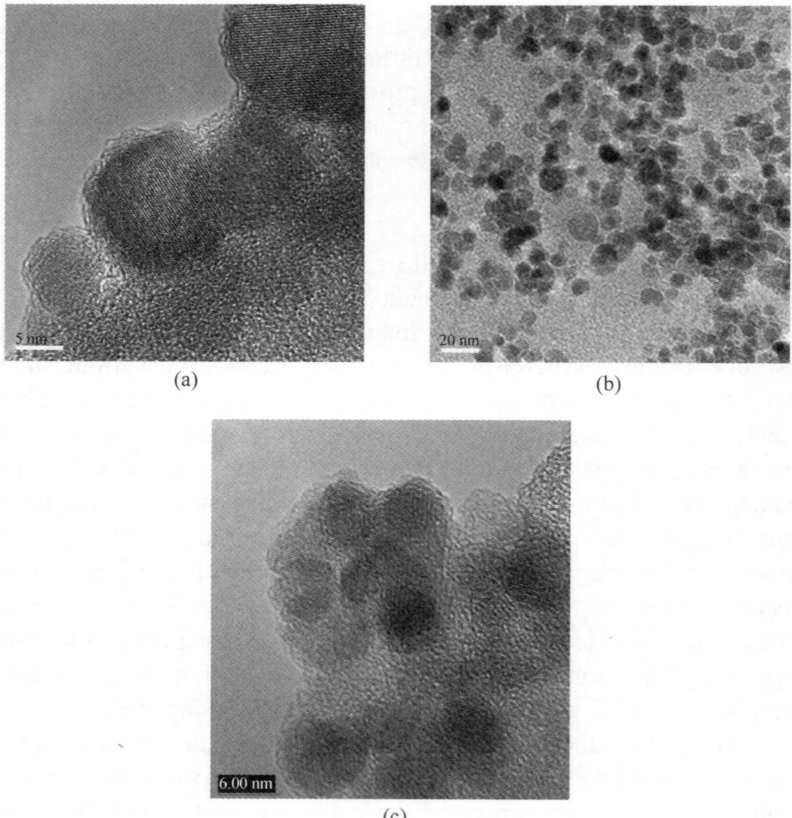

Figure 25.11 (a) HRTEM of MNF/W(DBS+DBS) showing the crystalline magnetite core covered by the surfactant double layer 1 – 2 nm thick (b) HRTEM images of the magnetic core-pyrrole copolymer shell hybrid nanostructures (Chauvet et al., 2007)

core-shell structure with Fe_3O_4 crystalline magnetic core covered by a thin (1.5 – 3 nm) copolymer shell. The thickness of the copolymer is mainly influenced by the polymerization time. E.g. the FPco1 sample (Turcu et al., 2007b) was obtained from MNF with MA + DBS coated Fe_3O_4 nanoparticles, applying APS/PY(v/v) = 0.5, PY/substituted PY ratio 1 : 5 and 10 h polymerization time.

The magnetite-conducting polypyrrole core-shell nanostructure proved to be a biocompatible one (Khan et al., 2007). Recently it was shown that superparamagnetic magnetite nanoparticles encapsulated inside conducting polypyrrole are cyto-compatible (Wuang et al., 2007) and present enhanced specific power absorption rates (SAR) by the combination of magnetic losses and inductive heating, offering great promise for use in the hyperthermia treatment of cancer tumors. FTIR spectra of magnetic-copolymer samples contain the characteristic absorption bands of both component materials, namely functionalized pyrrole copolymer and Fe_3O_4. The conjugation length of the copolymer chains is influenced by the unsubstituted pyrrole/substituted pyrrole ratio. The missing hysteresis loop in the magnetization vs applied magnetic field shows the superparamagnetic behavior for the functionalized magnetic nanostructures based on pyrrole copolymers. The superparamagnetic behavior is also evidenced from FC and ZFC dependences of the magnetization vs temperature.

Magnetite nanoparticles of ~7 nm synthesized by chemical coprecipitation were coated with a bifunctional graft copolymer composed of a poly(acrylic acid) (PAA) backbone and grafted poly(ethylene oxide) (PEO) and poly(propylene oxide) (PPO) side chains (Moeser et al., 2004). The outer hydrophilic PEO layer is for colloidal stability, while the inner hydrophobic PPO region is for solubilization of organic compounds, to be removed by magnetic separation from water.

A different procedure was used for the encapsulation of poorly water soluble drugs in magnetic biodegradable polymer, e.g. poly(D,L-lactide) polymer (PLA) (Zavisova et al., 2007) or poly(D,L-lactide-co-glycolide) polymer (PLGA) (Koneracka et al., 2007). The main issue is the proper ratio between the encapsulated drug and magnetite nanoparticles content of polymer nanospheres, to satisfy the requirements of magnetic carrier technology.

Surface modification or encapsulation procedures of magnetite or maghemite nanoparticles using biocompatible/biodegradable polymers is a promising strategy for biomedical applications.

25.2.6 Dilution Stability

The colloidal stability of various magnetic fluids with organic non-polar (hydrocarbons) and polar (diesters, alcohols), prepared according to Figs. 25.4 and 25.5 (Bica, 1995; Bica et al., 2002) was thoroughly investigated by magnetic, magneto-optical and rheo/magnetorheological measurements (Vékás et al., 1999, 2000, 2001; Rasa, 1999, 2000; Susan-Resiga Daniela, 2001; Raşa et al., 2002;

Socoliuc and Bica, 2002; Socoliuc et al., 2003; Bica et al., 2004). A qualitative study of magnetization and flow curves was performed to establish the influence of interactions or the presence of agglomerates in a large variety of MNF samples. The physical particle volume fraction was varied between large limits (0.01% to 20%) in order to investigate the dilution stability of mono- and double-layer sterically stabilized magnetic nanofluid samples. A quantitative study using several models for ideal and interacting particles was performed to select the best method and dimensional distribution function for magneto-granulometric analysis as well as for accurately determining macroscopic quantities of samples (initial susceptibility, saturation magnetization, particle number density or magnetic volume fraction) and properties of nanoparticles (mean magnetic diameter, thickness of the nonmagnetic layer, effective thickness of stabilizing layer and particle distribution).

Magnetization curves can be extensively used for the study of both particle interactions and agglomerate formation, processes which strongly influence the rheological and magnetoheological behaviour of magnetic fluids. Saturation magnetization (M_s), initial magnetic susceptivity (χ_i), full magnetization curves ($M = M(H)$ or $M/M_s(H)$, (H—intensity of applied magnetic field, M—magnetization of magnetic fluid) and magneto-granulometric analysis (mean magnetic diameter $\langle d_m \rangle$ and standard deviation of size distribution of particles σ), at various values of the volumic concentration of magnetic nanoparticles, give an insight on microstructural characteristics of various samples to be compared. For example, the initial susceptivity is influenced by particle diameter and size distribution, particle interactions, existence of preformed aggregates during the preparation process and aggregate formation at zero field or induced by the applied magnetic field. The comparison of the dependence of the initial susceptivity, χ_i, on the physical volume fraction, φ_ρ, of magnetic nanoparticles for samples of different types of magnetic fluids, reveals interesting microstructural aspects. The initial susceptivity in the framework of the thermodynamic perturbation theory (TPT) (Ivanov, 1992; Ivanov and Kuznetsova, 2001; Rasa et al., 2002) is given by

$$\chi_i = \chi_{iL}\left(1 + \frac{1}{3}\chi_{iL}\right) \tag{25.1}$$

where

$$\chi_{iL} = \frac{\mu_0 \pi M_d^2 d_m^3 \varphi_m}{18 k_B T} \tag{25.2}$$

Here M_d is spontaneous magnetization, φ_m is magnetic volume fraction, $M = M_s L(\xi)$ where $L(\xi)$ is the Langevin function. Equations (25.1) and (25.2) show the strong influence of the mean 'magnetic' volume/diameter of particles, as well as of the size distribution on the low field part of the magnetization curve.

In particular, particle agglomerates, which behave as large particles will determine this part of the magnetization curve.

Composition details, in particular the quality of the surfactant used, as well as its particular adsorbtion properties to the nanoparticle surface, influence particle agglomeration processes. E.g., double layer sterically stabilized pentanol magnetic fluids have smaller initial susceptivity, compared to other, less well stabilized samples of the same concentration and quasilinear $\chi_i = \chi_i(\varphi_m)$ dependence, at least for small φ_m values, i. e. agglomerates are practically absent in this case. In this context, it is worthwile to examine the volume fraction (dilution) dependence of magnetization curves, which indicate, if any, the presence of agglomerates as a function of mean interparticle distance (particle volume fraction).

In Fig. 25.12 the superposition of non-dimensional magnetization curves for a series of transformer oil based MNFs stabilized with OA, in a large domain of particle volume fraction, indicates that agglomerate formation is practically negligible in this case, i.e. the MNF remains highly stable under dilution (Rasa, 1999; Rasa et al., 2002).

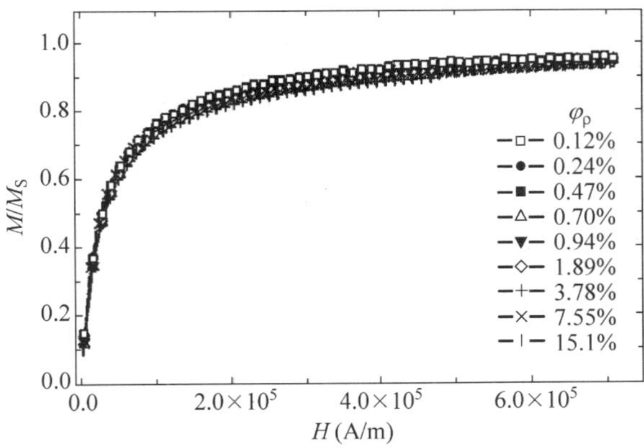

Figure 25.12 Reduced magnetization curves of transformer oil based MNF/TR30 (OA) series having the physical volume fraction φ_ρ as a parameter (after Rasa, 1999; Rasa et al., 2002)

The dependence of non-dimensional viscosity, η / η_0, where η is dynamic viscosity of the magnetic fluid and η_0 is the dynamic viscosity of the carrier liquid, on the solid particle volume fraction, φ_ρ, may be determined using the Vand formula (Vékás et al., 2001). In order to determine the hydrodynamic volume fraction, φ_h i.e. the effective volume fraction of the surface coated Fe_3O_4 nanoparticles, the experimental data were fitted to the Vand formula (Vand, 1948; Barnes et al., 1989) using the fit parameter $p = \varphi_h / \varphi_\rho$:

$$\eta / \eta_0 = \exp\left[(2.5 p\varphi_\rho + 2.7 p^2 \varphi_\rho^2)\right] / (1 - 0.609 p\varphi_\rho) \tag{25.3}$$

The fitted $\eta/\eta_0 = f(\varphi_\rho)$ curves at various temperatures, together with the detailed results of the fits with the formulae of Vand, Krieger-Dougherty, Quemada, Chong, Rosensweig and Chow, were used to evaluate various magnetic fluid samples (Vékás et al., 1999, 2000, 2001; Rasa et al., 2002). Using the fitted p values, the effective mean surfactant layer thickness may be obtained, $h = (p^{1/3} - 1)d/2$.

The values of the maximum hydrodynamic volume fraction, φ_{hm}, were determined by fitting the data to the well-known two-parameter formula of Krieger and Dougherty (Krieger and Dougherty, 1959; Barnes et al., 1989),

$$\eta/\eta_0 = \left(1 - \varphi_{\text{h}}/\varphi_{\text{hm}}\right)^{-[\eta]\varphi_{\text{hm}}} \tag{25.4}$$

or to the even simpler formula of Quemada (Barnes et al., 1989)

$$\eta/\eta_0 = \left(1 - \varphi_{\text{h}}/\varphi_{\text{hm}}\right)^{-2} \tag{25.5}$$

where $[h]$ is intrinsic viscosity.

Theoretical analysis in the framework of a liquid lattice model of concentrated suspensions (Chow, 1993, 1994), taking into account the contribution of many-body particle interactions on the effective viscosity, conducted to the following expression of the low-shear limiting viscosity

$$\frac{\eta}{\eta_0} = \exp\left(\frac{2.5\varphi_{\text{h}}}{1-\varphi_{\text{h}}}\right) + \frac{A\varphi_{\text{h}}^2}{1 - A\varphi_{\text{h}}^2\varphi_{\text{hm}}} \tag{25.6}$$

where A is the coupling coefficient. Without considering magnetic dipole-dipole type interactions between particles, the theoretical value of A was found to be 4.67.

The theoretical formula (Eq. (25.6)) obtained by Chow proved to be well fitted by viscosity data for various magnetic fluids, as it follows from detailed investigations on various type of magnetic fluids (Susan-Resiga, 2001). The fitted values of A are close to the theoretical one for $\varphi_{\text{h}} \leqslant 0.45$. At higher values of the hydrodynamic volume fraction, the resulting A value is lower, evidencing the role of dipolar interactions at close packing. The volume fraction (mean interparticle distance) dependence of the viscosity for a highly stable pentanol based MNFs series is given in Fig. 25.13. The very good fit to the theoretical formula Eq. (25.6) indicates the absence of agglomerates of OA + DBS double layer coated magnetite nanoparticles in the polar carrier liquid (pentanol). The fitted value of the interaction parameter $A = 3.63$ is somewhat lower than the theoretical value ($A_{\text{theor}} = 4.67$) due to the effect of dipolar interactions between suspended particles. The analysis was extended to other highly stable non-polar and polar magnetic nanofluids. It can be seen from Fig. 25.14 (Susan-Resiga,

2001) that the solid particle volume fraction dependence of dynamic viscosity values determined at different temperatures fit well the formula Eq. (25.6), illustrating the dilution stability of the investigated concentrated MNF samples. As in the previous case, the fitted value of the interaction parameter $A = 3.52$ is somewhat lower than the theoretical value ($A_{theor} = 4.67$) due to the effect of dipolar interactions between suspended particles.

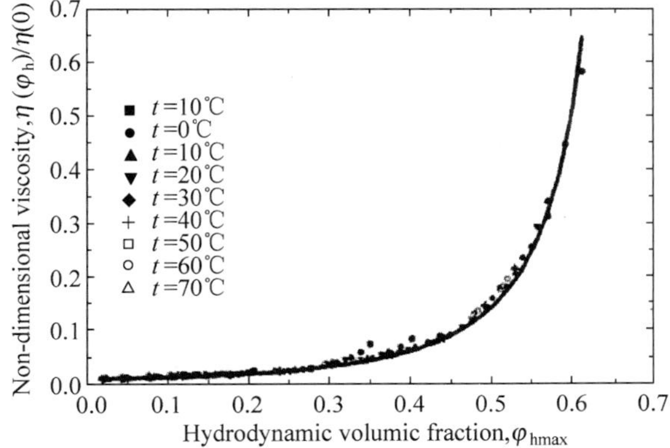

Figure 25.13 Dilution stability: non-dimensional viscosity vs hydrodynamic volume fraction of OA + DBS double layer surfactant covered magnetite nanoparticles in pentanol carrier. Fit to Chow formula Eq. (25.6) (Susan-Resiga, 2001) using the maximum hydrodynamic volume fraction $\varphi_{hm}^{K} = 0.66$ fitted from Krieger-Dougherty formula Eq. (25.4) supposing the nanoparticles are spherical

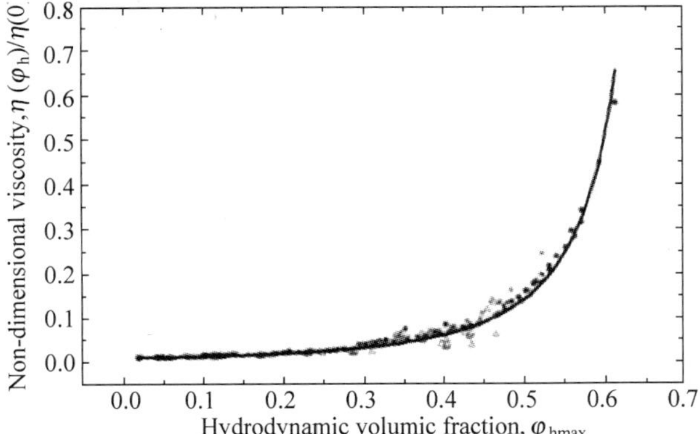

Figure 25.14 Dilution stability: non-dimensional viscosity vs hydrodynamic volume fraction of mono- or double layer covered magnetic nanoparticles in non-polar (transformer oil) and polar (pentanol, heptanol and dioctyl-sebacate) carrier liquids. Fit to Chow formula Eq. (25.6) (Susan-Resiga, 2001) using the maximum hydrodynamic volume fraction $\varphi_{hm}^{Q} = 0.69$ fitted from Quemada's formula Eq. (25.5)

25.3 Structure Investigations

Small angle neutron scattering is one of the most efficient methods of nanostructural investigation of magnetic fluids. During the SANS experiment a widening of the neutron beam passed through the sample is studied in terms of the differential scattering cross-section. The latter is a function of vector $\boldsymbol{q}$ with the module $q = (4\pi/\lambda)\sin(\theta/2)$, where λ is the incident neutron wavelength and θ is the scattering angle. Usually, in practice one uses the differential scattering cross-section per sample volume which is conventionally called scattering intensity $I(\boldsymbol{q})$. This dependence is quite sensitive to structural features of the studied system at the scale of 1 – 100 nm. Indeed, the sizes of magnetic particles in magnetic fluids (3 – 15 nm), as well as the characteristic correlation length between particles are mostly in this dimensional range. SANS investigations including specific techniques (contrast variation, scattering of polarized neutrons) give information about particle structure (size, surfactant shell thickness, composition of core and shell, solvent rate penetration in surfactant layer, micelles), magnetic structure (magnetic size and composition), particle interaction (interparticle potential, magnetic moment correlation, phase separation) and cluster formation (aggregation and chain formation). Major advantages of SANS in comparison with other structural methods are connected with possibilities of the contrast variation in the studied systems by substitution hydrogen/deuterium, as well as with magnetic scattering of neutrons. The other important feature of this method is a high penetration depth of neutrons into the sample, which makes it possible to investigate non-modified bulk magnetic fluids in a wide range of magnetic volume fraction of 1% – 20%.

Early applications of SANS were focused on different aspects of the MNFs structure including interaction and aggregation effects (Hayter and Pynn, 1982; Cebula et al., 1983; Pynn et al., 1983; Potton et al., 1983; Akselrod et al., 1986; Rosman et al., 1990). The present review covers recent achievements in the structural investigations by SANS and other complementary methods.

25.3.1 Particle Structure

25.3.1.1 Non-Polarized Neutrons

In the small-angle neutron scattering from magnetic nanoparticles there are two components corresponding to the interaction of neutrons with atomic nuclei (nuclear scattering) and interaction of magnetic moments of neutrons and atoms (magnetic scattering). As a first step in the analysis of the particle structure in magnetic fluids, the interference effects connected with the particle interaction are neglected at small particle concentration (volume fraction of magnetic material $\varphi_m < 3\%$), so MNFs are considered as systems consisted of non-interacting spherical particles. In the absence of external magnetic field the particle magnetic moments are disoriented, thus both scattering components are isotropic with respect to the orientation of the **q**-vector, which is schematically shown in Fig. 25.15. In this case the differential cross-section of the scattering per one particle depends only on the module of the momentum transfer, q:

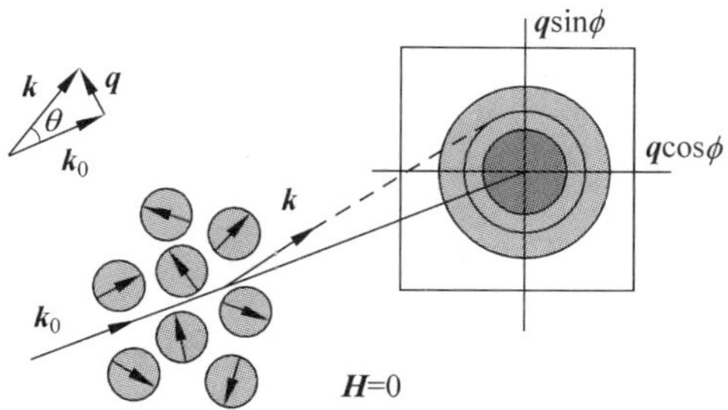

Figure 25.15 Schematic view of SANS experiment on system of magnetic nanoparticles. In case of unmagnetized system scattering pattern is isotropic over radial angle φ on detector plane

$$\frac{\mathrm{d}\sigma}{\mathrm{d}\Omega}(q) \approx F_N^2(q) + (2/3)F_M^2(q) \tag{25.7}$$

where F_N and F_M are amplitudes of nuclear and magnetic scattering, the corresponding Fourier transforms of the scattering length distributions (nuclear and magnetic, respectively) within the particle. Since the magnetic scattering length is dependent on the angle between the momentum transfer and the magnetic moment of the particle, the chaotic orientation of the moment results in coefficient 2/3 in formula Eq. (25.7).

The model representation of the particle from the scattering viewpoint is shown in Fig. 25.16. For the nuclear form-factor of the particle the core-shell model gives

$$F_N^2(q) = [(\rho_0 - \rho_1)V\Phi(qR) + (\rho_1 - \rho_s)V_1\Phi(qR_1)]^2 \tag{25.8a}$$

$$\Phi(x) = 3\,(\sin(x) - x\cos(x))/x^3 \tag{25.8b}$$

Here ρ_0, ρ_1, ρ_s are densities of the nuclear scattering lengths for 'the core' (magnetic nanoparticles), surfactant shell and the solvent (liquid carrier), respectively; V, V_1 are the volumes restricted by the corresponding radii R, R_1. The difference $h = R_1 - R$ determines the effective thickness of the surfactant shell.

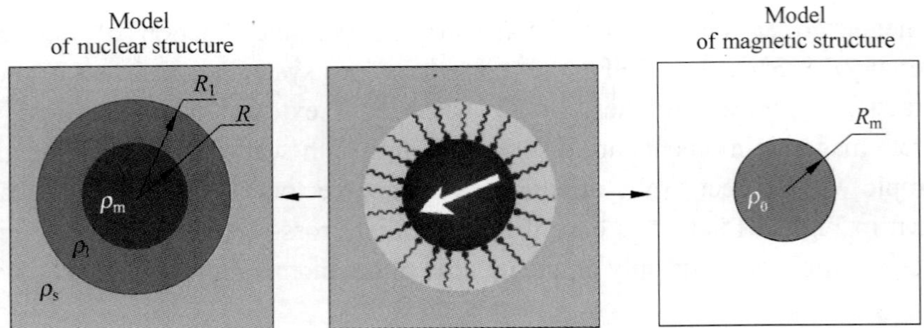

Figure 25.16 Model representation of nuclear and magnetic particle structures in MFs

Since the surfactant shell and the carrier are non-magnetic, the magnetic form-factor is described by simpler spherical model:

$$F_{\mathrm{M}}^2(q) = \rho_{\mathrm{m}}^2 V_{\mathrm{m}}^2 \Phi^2(qR_{\mathrm{m}}) \tag{25.9}$$

Here, ρ_{m} is the density of the magnetic scattering length in the magnetic nanoparticles distributed within volume V_{m} with the corresponding radius R_{m}. It is usually assumed that R_{m} differs from R because of the non-magnetic layer at the particle surface, which is a result of the spin canting from the orientation of domain magnetization at the interface. Such hypothesis explains naturally results of various experiments including magnetization analysis (Kaiser and Miskolczy, 1970; Berkowitz et al., 1975; Mollard et al., 1977; Han et al., 1994), Mössbauer spectroscopy (Haneda and Morrish, 1988; Tronc and Jolivet, 1998), diffraction of polarized neutrons (Lin et al., 1995) and others. Indirect confirmation of such layer comes from theoretical calculations (Kodama et al., 1996). However, one should note that still the direct experimental evidence of the magnetically dead layer is not demonstrated.

The difficulty in SANS for MNFs is a strong polydispersity of magnetic nanoparticles dispersed in liquids, so the additional averaging of Eq. (25.7) over the particle size distribution function, $D_N(R)$, is required. Usually the log-normal distribution is used:

$$D_N(R) = (1/\sqrt{2\pi}SR)\exp[-\ln^2(R/R_0)/2S^2] \tag{25.10}$$

where parameters R_0 and S characterize the most probable radius and dispersion of the distribution, respectively. Sometimes the Schultz distribution is probed as well. Thus, the model formula for the whole scattering intensity (nuclear plus magnetic) for low concentrated and non-magnetized MNF has the form:

$$I(q) \approx (4/3)^2 \pi^2 N \int [(\rho_0 - \rho_1)R^3 \Phi(qR) + (\rho_1 - \rho_s)(R+h)^3 \Phi(q(R+h))]^2 D_N(R)\mathrm{d}R + (4/3)^2 \pi^2 N \rho_{\mathrm{m}}^2 \int (R-\delta)^6 \Phi^2(q(R-\delta)) D_N(R)\mathrm{d}R \tag{25.11}$$

where N is the mean particle number density (ratio of the particle volume fraction to their mean volume), and δ is the thickness of non-magnetic surface layer. The ρ_s value can be easily changed for the MNF samples in SANS. This is done by a substitution of hydrogen (H) with deuterium (D) in the carrier. The two isotopes have very different scattering lengths, which makes it possible to vary ρ_s in a wide interval. The typical ratios between nuclear scattering length densities of different components in MNFs in the cases of H- and D-carriers are given in Fig. 25.17. One can see that for the analysis of the surfactant shell structure experiments should be done in D-carriers; in usual H-carriers the contrast between the carrier and the shell $(\rho_1 - \rho_s)$ is small, so no effect on the scattering curve from the shell can be seen.

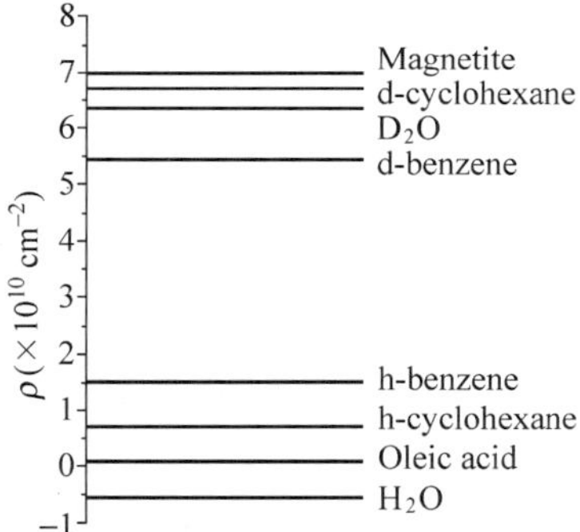

Figure 25.17 Map of scattering length densities for typical components in MFs

In the general case formula Eq. (25.11) for the direct modeling of the particle structure has quite a number of free parameters. For reliable fits to experimental data one has to fix some of them taking into account the complementary information obtained by other methods. Thus, for MNF based on D-benzene (magnetite covered by a single layer of oleic acid) (Avdeev et al., 2002) parameters of the $D_N(R)$ function were taken from the data of electron microscopy, and δ was supposed to be zero. Such simplifications lead to stable fits (Fig. 25.18), from which h and ρ_1 are derived. The obtained values for 1% MNF ($h = 1.85 \pm 0.05$ nm and $\rho_1 = (0.26 \pm 0.15) \times 10^{10}\,\text{cm}^{-2}$) are close to those expected. The deviation of the obtained ρ_1 from that for pure surfactant ($\rho_1 = 0.077 \times 10^{10}\,\text{cm}^{-2}$) was interpreted as a result of the penetration of the solvent into the surfactant shell. Despite this difference one can conclude that such penetration does not exceed 5% of the shell volume. The interesting feature was revealed, when SANS was applied for MNF in usual H-carriers (Avdeev et al., 2006; Gazeau et al., 2003). Besides the fact that the scattering from the shell can be neglected, the fits are not sensitive to the magnetic scattering term. The

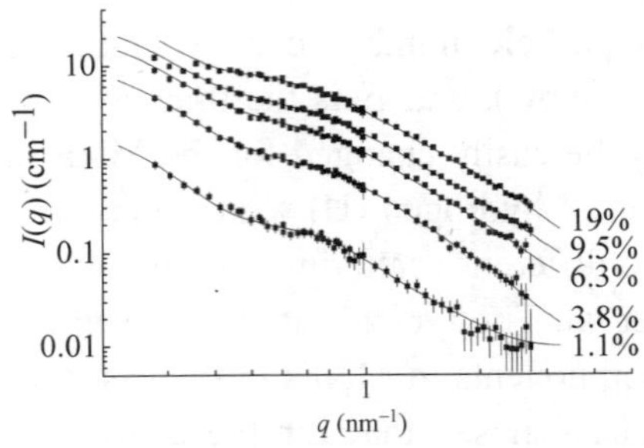

Figure 25.18 Experimental (points) and model (lines) scattering curves for MF magnetite/oleic acid/D-benzene. Different volume fractions of magnetite are given to the right of the curves. Model 'core-shell' was used. Structure-factor effect was not taken into account

best agreement with the experimental data is achieved, when the last term is not taken into account, i.e. formula Eq. (25.11) has the simple form:

$$I(q) \approx (4/3)^2 \pi^2 N(\rho_0 - \rho_s)^2 \int R^6 \Phi^2(qR) D_N(R) \mathrm{d}R \qquad (25.12)$$

The conclusion is that the magnetic scattering is negligibly small as compared to nuclear scattering in the case of the H-carrier. This conclusion is confirmed in experiments on the scattering of polarized neutrons (see below). The reason, as it will be shown further, is connected with significant magnetic correlations in MNF even for low-concentrated samples. In a whole, this results in a decrease in the magnetic scattering. Thus, the magnetic term in Eq. (25.11) is not correct, and one should consider the fit by Eq. (25.11) as a first approximation for revealing characteristic values of the particle parameters. Equation (25.12) makes it possible to determine well the parameters of the $D_N(R)$ function for magnetic nanoparticles by the SANS curves from MNFs in H-carriers. Examples of the corresponding fits are given in Fig. 25.19 for the same type of MNF based on H-benzene (Török et al., 2006), as well as for MNF based on polar organic solvent pentanol (magnetite covered by double shell of OA and DBS) (Avdeev et al., 2006; Török et al., 2006). In comparison with the data of transmission electron microscopy SANS gives lower sizes of magnetic nanoparticles (Avdeev et al., 2005; Shen et al., 2001; Moeser et al., 2004). The reason, on our opinion, can be connected with different size resolution limits of the techniques. The sensitivity of SANS is limited by 1 nm, while for TEM it can be larger, which results in an effective increase in the observed size in the last case. Also, a possible influence of the sample preparation procedure in TEM, namely the aggregate formation should be taken into account. In (Shen et al., 2001) it is supposed that the discussed reason is a result of the deviation in the particle shape from spherical. The other well-known method for determining $D_N(R)$, which also deals with bulk samples, is the magnetization analysis. It gives information about the magnetic size of the particles, and, as a rule, results in

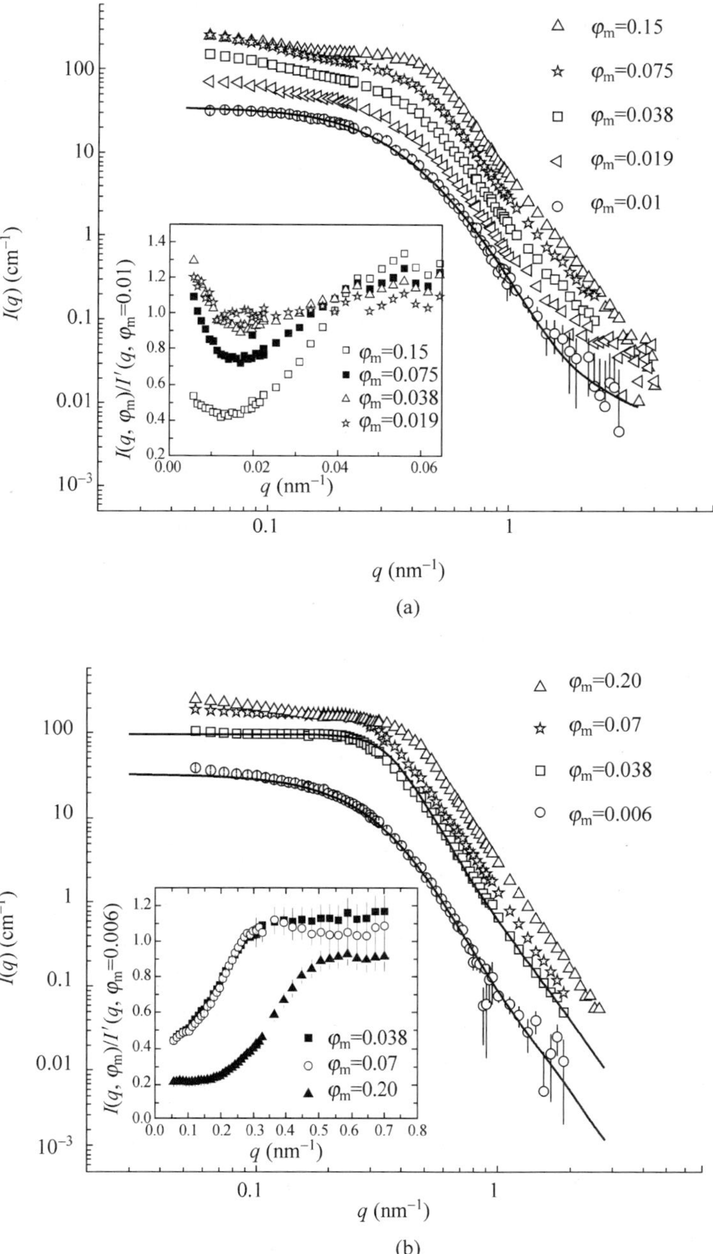

Figure 25.19 SANS curves from MF based on non-polar and polar organic H-solvents. Insets show ratios of intensities I' referred to one concentration. (a) magnetite/OA/H-benzene; line at $\varphi_m = 0.01$ shows the fit of the model of independent spheres, $R_0 = 4.0$ nm; $S = 0.31$; ($\langle R \rangle = 4.2$ nm; $\sigma = 1.3$ nm); (b) magnetite/OA+DBS/H-pentanol; line at $\varphi_m = 0.006$ shows the fit of the model of independent spheres, $R_0 = 3.4$ nm; $S = 0.38$; ($\langle R \rangle = 3.7$ nm; $\sigma = 1.4$ nm); line at $\varphi_m = 0.038$ shows the fit of the model of interacting spheres (hard spheres potential)

smaller sizes than SANS (Shen et al., 2001; Avdeev et al., 2004). This fact can be related to the existence of the non-magnetic layer in magnetic nanoparticles. Thus, from the comparison of the $D_N(R)$ from SANS and magnetization analysis one can estimate the thickness of the non-magnetic layer.

So, one should be careful when applying Eq. (25.11) in the SANS data treatment. It concerns the use of the data of other complementary methods for the $D_N(R)$ function, as well as the form of the magnetic scattering. In this connection, quite good results are obtained (Avdeev et al., 2002; Balasoiu et al., 2004; Avdeev et al., 2008) for the scattering from organic non-polar MNF based in D-solvents, when the magnetic term is neglected, and parameters of the $D_N(R)$ function are varied. They are consistent well with the data for MNFs based on H-solvents and the data of the scattering of polarized neutrons. Significant deviations of the model curves from the experimental data are observed only at small q-values, where the effect of magnetic scattering contribution is still large.

The direct modeling of the SANS curves for non-magnetized MNFs was used for ferrites with single and double layers in water (Mehta et al., 1995; Upadhyay et al., 1997), for magnetite dispersed in deuterated organic carrier covered with double layer OA + OA (Aswal et al., 2004) and for barium hexaferrite MF with oleic acid as surfactant (Müller et al., 2002).

Other methods complementary to SANS are used for reliable conclusions about the particle nanostructure. Besides the magnetization analysis and electron microscopy mentioned above, among them is the X-ray diffraction from crystalline structure of magnetic particles. The analysis of widening of the diffraction peaks gives additional information about the mean particle size (Bläsing et al., 1994; Amaral and Tourinho, 1995; Upadhyay et al., 1997; Itri et al., 2001; Wagner et al., 2002; Aswal et al., 2004). At last, the combined use of SANS and small-angle X-ray scattering (SAXS) is the most reliable combination. In SAXS there is no magnetic scattering component. Also, because of the small contrast between electron density of the surfactant shell and the solvent the main scattering is from the magnetic nanoparticles. So, the SAXS experiment is identical to the SANS experiment for H-carriers and can be used for determining parameters of $D_N(R)$ (Bläsing et al., 1994; Eberbeck and Bläsing, 1999; Itri et al., 2001; Butter et al., 2002, 2004; Wagner et al., 2002; Kruse et al., 2003; Bonini et al., 2004). In comparison with the laboratory SAXS instruments, the modern SANS set-ups cover smaller q-values, which is quite important for exact estimates of the $D_N(R)$ function. Also, in contrast to SAXS the SANS method provides easy and quite precise calibrations for obtaining absolute scattering cross-section. On the other hand, the covered q-range is the same as in SANS, if SAXS experiments are performed at a synchrotron source, but the experimental time is significantly less.

If in MNF, which is initially the dispersion of separate particles, aggregates are formed under some conditions, the main changes in the scattering curves take place at small q-values. It is known as a structure-factor effect, which is discussed below. At the same time, for sufficiently large q-values, where such effect is small or negligible, the model fitting described above can be made. This was done (Neto et al., 2005) for maghemite dispersed in cyclohexane and covered with a single layer of oleic acid, as well as for MNF based on MEK with magnetite covered by double layer OA+DBS (Avdeev et al., 2006).

25.3.1.2 Polarized Neutrons

When a magnetic field is applied to MNF during the SANS experiment, the magnetic scattering contribution becomes partially anisotropic over the radial angle φ on the detector plane (approximately $\boldsymbol{q}$-direction), as shown by details of the SANS description for this case (Wiedenmann, 2000). After the sample is fully magnetized the scattering intensity can be written as

$$I(q,\varphi) \sim \langle F_{\mathrm{N}}^2(q)\rangle + \langle F_{\mathrm{M}}^2(q)\rangle \sin^2 \varphi \tag{25.13}$$

where brackets $\langle\cdots\rangle$ denote the averaging over the polydispersity function, and φ is the radial angle on the scattering plain. From the analysis of the $\sin^2$-type of the φ-anisotropy of the 2D scattering patterns one can separate the nuclear and magnetic scattering contributions. The important notice is that some structural changes under the magnetic field influence can take place in MNF, so $\langle F_{\mathrm{N}}^2(q)\rangle$ and $\langle F_{\mathrm{M}}^2(q)\rangle$ terms are not the same as in the non-magnetized sample. For purely superparamagnetic systems where no aggregates are formed under the magnetic field the sum of the both contributions $\langle F_{\mathrm{N}}^2(q)\rangle + 2/3\,\langle F_{\mathrm{M}}^2(q)\rangle$ should give the scattering curve obtained in the absence of the magnetic field. The described procedure for separating nuclear and magnetic scattering contributions was applied for classical MNF (magnetite/OA/D-benzene) (Aksenov et al., 2002; Avdeev et al., 2004).

The additional equations for anisotropic scattering in the magnetic field can be obtained, when polarized neutrons are used (see scheme of experiment in Fig. 25.20). The corresponding technique is known as SANSPOL (Wiedenmann, 2000). In

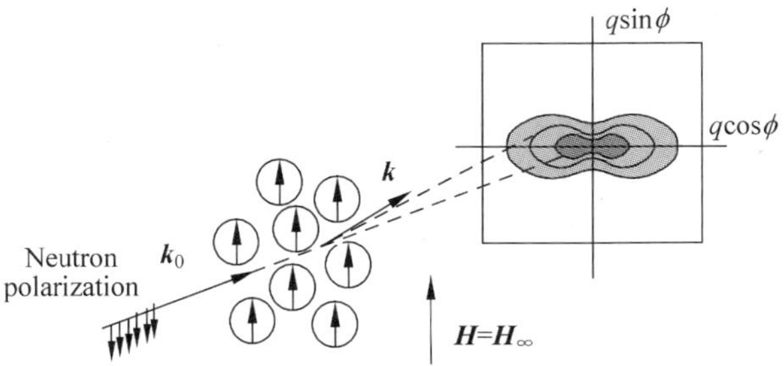

Figure 25.20 Schematic view of SANSPOL experiment on system of magnetic nanoparticles. Anisotropy in the scattering pattern over radial angle φ is caused by magnetization of the system

this case the neutron magnetic moments in the incident beam are oriented in one direction, which is collinear to the magnetic field, ***H***, at the sample. This is done by a special device (neutron polarizer). The other device, spin-flipper, regulates whether the magnetic moment has the same or opposite orientation as ***H***. These two polarization states of the neutron beam produce two kinds of the scattering intensity:

$$I^+(q,\varphi) \sim \langle F_{\mathrm{N}}^2(q)\rangle + \{\langle F_{\mathrm{M}}^2(q)\rangle - 2P\langle F_{\mathrm{N}}(q)F_{\mathrm{M}}(q)\rangle\}\sin^2\varphi \qquad (25.14a)$$

$$I^-(q,\varphi) \sim \langle F_{\mathrm{N}}^2(q)\rangle + \{\langle F_{\mathrm{M}}^2(q)\rangle + 2P\varepsilon\langle F_{\mathrm{N}}(q)F_{\mathrm{M}}(q)\rangle\}\sin^2\varphi \qquad (25.14b)$$

where P is the polarization rate of the beam, and ε is the efficiency of the spin-flipper with respect to change of the neutron polarization. As compared to Eq. (25.13), Eq. (25.14) contain the cross-term $\langle F_{\mathrm{N}}(q)F_{\mathrm{M}}(q)\rangle$ with the nuclear and magnetic scattering amplitudes. Unfortunately, because of the polydispersity smearing this term cannot be used so efficiently as for the monodisperse case, where the important parameter $F_{\mathrm{N}}(q)/F_{\mathrm{M}}(q)$ is obtained from equations of type Eq. (25.14).

The simplest way to determine experimentally the isotropic and anisotropic parts in Eq. (25.14) is the radial averaging in the vicinity of $\varphi = 0$ and $\pi/2$ directions on the detector plane, which are parallel and perpendicular to the field direction, respectively. It gives a system of four equations:

$$I^+(q,0) = I_{\parallel}^+(q) = \langle F_{\mathrm{N}}^2(q)\rangle \qquad (25.15a)$$

$$I^+(q,\pi/2) = I_{\perp}^+(q) = \langle F_{\mathrm{N}}^2(q)\rangle + \langle F_{\mathrm{M}}^2(q)\rangle - 2P\langle F_{\mathrm{N}}(q)F_{\mathrm{M}}(q)\rangle \qquad (25.15b)$$

$$I^-(q,0) = I_{\parallel}(q) = \langle F_{\mathrm{N}}^2(q)\rangle \qquad (25.15c)$$

$$I^-(q,\pi/2) = I_{\perp}^-(q) = \langle F_{\mathrm{N}}^2(q)\rangle + \langle F_{\mathrm{M}}^2(q)\rangle + 2P\varepsilon\langle F_{\mathrm{N}}(q)F_{\mathrm{M}}(q)\rangle \qquad (25.15d)$$

which makes it possible to find out and analyze three functions $\langle F_{\mathrm{N}}^2(q)\rangle$, $\langle F_{\mathrm{M}}^2(q)\rangle$ and $\langle F_{\mathrm{N}}(q)F_{\mathrm{M}}(q)\rangle$. Here, $I^+(\boldsymbol{q}), I^-(\boldsymbol{q})$ are scattering intensities corresponding to two neutron polarizations, along $(-)$ and opposite $(+)$ to magnetic field direction on the sample, P is beam polarization rate. For checking out the $\sin^2$-type of the φ-anisotropy the averaging of Eq. (25.14) over the whole φ-angle can be made. In this case, one substitutes $\sin^2\varphi$ with its mean value of 1/2:

$$\langle I^+(q,\varphi)\rangle_{\varphi} = I^+(q) = \langle F_{\mathrm{N}}^2(q)\rangle + (1/2)\langle F_{\mathrm{M}}^2(q)\rangle - P\langle F_{\mathrm{N}}(q)F_{\mathrm{M}}(q)\rangle \qquad (25.16a)$$

$$\langle I^-(q,\varphi)\rangle_{\varphi} = I^-(q) = \langle F_{\mathrm{N}}^2(q)\rangle + (1/2)\langle F_{\mathrm{M}}^2(q)\rangle + P\varepsilon\langle F_{\mathrm{N}}(q)F_{\mathrm{M}}(q)\rangle \qquad (25.16b)$$

One can see that function $\langle F_{\mathrm{N}}(q)F_{\mathrm{M}}(q)\rangle$ can be obtained from Eqs. (25.16) and 25.14. It requires that no additional anisotropy beside $\sin^2\varphi$ (corresponding to the magnetic scattering) takes place. If $\langle F_{\mathrm{N}}(q)F_{\mathrm{M}}(q)\rangle$ obtained from the two Equation systems is different, this means that linear aggregates form and oriented under the effect of the external magnetic field.

The data interpretation is the most transparent for non-aggregated MNFs such as magnetite covered by OA and MA in d-cyclohexane (Avdeev et al., 2007a; Balasoiu et al., 2006b). 2D scattering patterns from these fluids ($\varphi_{\mathrm{m}} \sim 1\%$) for different polarization states of the neutron beam are given in Fig. 25.21. After the procedure according to Eq. (25.15) one obtains form-factors of the nuclear and magnetic scattering (Fig. 25.22). The nuclear scattering curves in both fluids are fitted well with the previously described core-shell model. The model gives parameters of the $D_N(R)$ function for magnetic particles (Table 25.1) and the thickness of the surfactant shell $h \sim 1.4$ nm, the same for the two fluids. The magnetic scattering component reflects complex correlations between magnetic moments in the fluids. As one can see in Fig. 25.22, their length exceeds the characteristic size of magnetic nanoparticles. This is demonstrated for both components in Fig. 25.22 in terms of the radius gyration, the parameter obtained from the Guinier approximation to the initial parts of the curves:

$$I(q) = I(0)\exp(-(R_{\mathrm{g}}q)^2/3) \tag{25.17}$$

Parameter $I(0)$ is the forward scattering intensity and R_{g} is the radius of gyration regarding to the scattering length density distribution. The reason for the observed effect is, probably, connected with the influence of the dipole-dipole interaction on the mutual orientations of the magnetic moments even at comparatively small

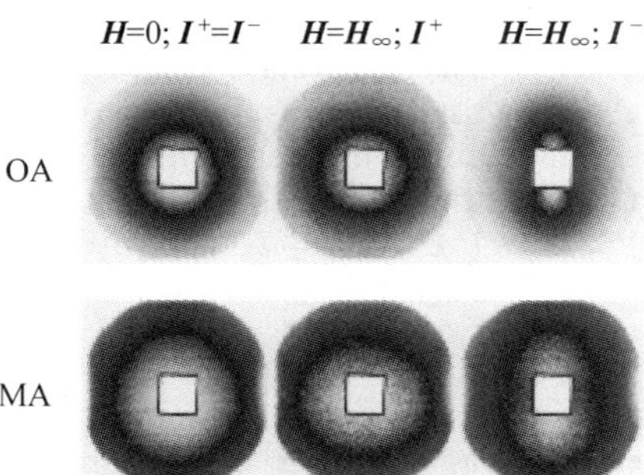

Figure 25.21 2D experimental SANS patterns for two neutron polarization states in the case of magnetic fluids ($\varphi_{\mathrm{m}} = 2.8\%$) based on D-cyclohexane and stabilized by oleic and myristic acids. Detector area is 55 cm × 55 cm. Sample-detector distance is 4.5 m. Wavelength of incident neutrons is 0.81 nm. White rectangle spot in the center of images is a shadow of the beam stop, which prevents the harmful effect of the direct neutron beam passing through the sample on the detector. Small side spots along the left and right edges are the shadows from the units of the magnetic system at the instrument

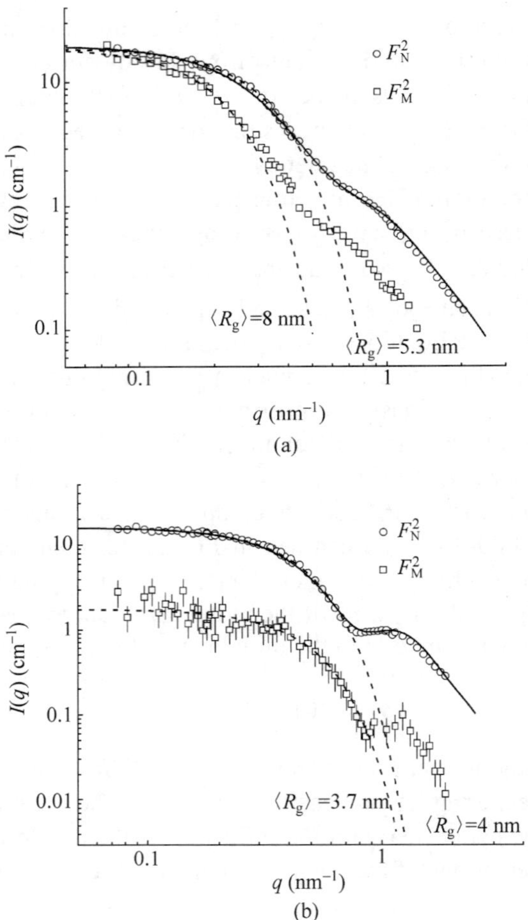

Figure 25.22 Separated nuclear and magnetic scattering components from SANSPOL for magnetic fluids ($\varphi_m = 2.8\%$) based on D-cyclohexane and stabilized by oleic (a) and myristic (b) acids. Solid lines show fits of 'core-shell' model, which takes into account the particle size distribution function of log-normal type; results of the fits are (OA) $R_0 = 3.4$ nm; $S = 0.38$; ($\langle R \rangle = 3.7$ nm; $\sigma = 1.4$ nm) $h = 1.38$ nm; (MA) $R_0 = 2.3$ nm; $S = 0.28$; ($\langle R \rangle = 2.4$ nm; $\sigma = 0.7$ nm), $h = 1.35$ nm. Dashed lines show Guinier approximations; obtained radii of gyration are given

Table 25.1 Parameters of log-normal size distribution obtained by SANS and magnetization analyses for organic non-polar MFs (cyclohexane) stabilized by two different surfactants (OA, MA)

Sample	R_0		δ	S	
	Scattering	Magnetization		Scattering	Magnetization
OA	3.4 nm	2.7 nm	0.7 nm	0.38	0.37
MA	2.4 nm	2.3 nm	0.1 nm	0.28	0.28

concentration ($\varphi_m \sim 1\%$) in the magnetic field. The particle polydispersity seems to be a significant factor, which determines the unexpectedly complicate picture of the magnetic correlations in MNF (Avdeev et al., 2004). At the same time, locations of the particles at the discussed concentrations can be considered as weakly correlated. The further decrease in the particle concentration for reducing magnetic correlations requires a special consideration, since the scattering decreases significantly, which results in low statistics and poor precision. The interesting feature is that the observed correlation in the magnetic structure is the same when the field is turned off. It is followed from the fact that the sum $\langle F_N^2(q)\rangle + 2/3\langle F_M^2(q)\rangle$ repeats well the curves obtained in the absence of the magnetic field. The only correlations in MNF, which can hold out in the magnetic field, are those determined by the interaction along the magnetic moment orientations. This means that the chain like orientation formations (short ordering) in the magnetic structure of MNF take place even without particle contact. This conclusion is testified also by the analysis of the structure-factor, which is presented below.

From the viewpoint of the particle structure the dipole-dipole interaction in MNF complicates the possibility for estimating directly the characteristic magnetic size of the particles and comparing it with the analogous nuclear size. Nevertheless, the nuclear size found in the given experiments with the high precision can be compared well with the results of the magnetization analysis. Such a comparison is presented in Table 25.1. The difference in the mean sizes obtained by the two methods gives estimation for the thickness of the non-magnetic layer at the particle surface. From Table 25.1 one can conclude that δ depends on the particle size, the greater is the particle size, the greater is δ. However, one should take into account that existence of small aggregates in MNF (number of particles does not exceed ten), which comprise some part of particles (~10%), can result also in the difference between nuclear and magnetic sizes observed in SANS. The reason is that the magnetic correlation length within the clusters of magnetic nanoparticles is in most cases less than the cluster size. The influence of the indicated small aggregates does not change the character of the scattering curves, but still it effectively increases the experimental nuclear size.

The same approach for the separation of the nuclear and magnetic scattering components was used (Perzinsky et al., 2006) for water-based MNF with charged stabilization. In this fluid the relation between the nuclear and magnetic scattering is quite different in comparison with the previous case.

At present, SANSPOL is intensively used for characterization magnetic fluids regarding their nuclear and magnetic microstructures. The method is usually applied together with the change in the contrast between different components of the particles and the carrier. It is achieved by the substitution hydrogen/deuterium in the carrier. Examples are the SANSPOL analysis for the silica coated cobalt ferrite nanoparticles in water (Bonini et al., 2004), oleic-acid-coated iron particles in decalin (Butter et al., 2004), cobalt ferrofluids in various carriers (Wiedenmann et al., 2002; Kammel et al., 2006, 2002; Heinemann and Wiedenmann, 2003), barium hexaferrite in dodecane stabilized by oleic acid (Hoell et al., 2002), water-based ferrofluids with magnetite covered by double layer dodecanoic acid plus C_{12} ethoxylated alcohol and covered by single layer of dextrane (Kammel et al., 2001). It should be pointed out that in all last examples together with single particles large aggregates are found in solutions. In comparison with the previous cases this complicates significantly the model and requires additional number of free parameters. To conclude about the reliability of the results a special treatment of the SANSPOL data is suggested (Heinemann and Wiedenmann, 2003).

The interesting idea (Heinemann et al., 2004) is the use of the dependence of the scattering on the magnetization rate of the MNF to obtain additional equations connecting the nuclear and magnetic scattering components. The technique was called the magnetic contrast variation.

At last, polarized neutrons can be used in the full polarization analysis. In SANSPOL the neutron polarization is fixed before the sample. After the scattering the depolarization takes place, which is not taken into account in SANSPOL. It is possible to analyze the change in the polarization after the scattering by the polarization analyzer, so four kinds of intensities corresponding to different combinations of the magnetic moment of neutrons before and after the scattering $(I^{++}, I^{+-}, I^{+}, I^{-})$ should be considered. The corresponding system of equations (Gazeau et al., 2003) allows one to separate the nuclear and magnetic scattering contributions without magnetization of the sample, but a strong influence of the background and large exposition times make this technique quite complicated. Examples, which cover also the interaction effects in magnetic fluids, can be found in several works (Hayter and Pynn, 1982; Pynn et al., 1983; Akslerod et al., 1986; Gazeau et al., 2003).

25.3.1.3 Contrast Variation

The contrast variation in SANS experiments can be made in terms of the basic functions approach. The latter implies the analysis of changes in scattering curves when varying the contrast, $\Delta\rho = \overline{\rho} - \rho_s$, the difference between the mean scattering length densities of the studied particles, $\overline{\rho}$, and homogeneous medium ('solvent'), ρ_s, where the particles are located. For monodisperse particles in the general case the scattering intensity is represented as a function of the contrast (Stuhrmann, 1995):

$$I(q) = I_s(q) + \Delta\rho I_{cs}(q) + (\Delta\rho)^2 I_c(q) \qquad (25.18)$$

where $I_c(q), I_s(q), I_{cs}(q)$ are basic functions. The $I_c(q)$ function corresponds to the scattering from the particle shape; the $I_s(q)$ corresponds to the scattering from fluctuations of the scattering length density from its mean value inside the particle; the $I_{cs}(q)$ function is the cross-term. Basic functions can be found experimentally by measuring $I(q)$ at least at three contrast values. The contrast is varied by changing ρ_s with the isotopic hydrogen/deuterium substitution. Basic functions approach makes it possible to write in convenient form the contrast dependence of integral parameters of the scattering curves including the radius of gyration. First applications of the SANS contrast variation for magnetic fluids were made in terms of the classical approach neglecting the particle polydispersity (Cebula et al., 1983; Grabcev et al., 1994). Then, dependence of the scattering parameters on the contrast in the system was estimated for the defined particle size distribution function of the lognormal type (Grabcev et al., 1999). In the general case for magnetic fluids the polydispersity in magnetic core of particles results in the fact that the mean scattering length density of one particle depends on the size of its core, and the scattering cross-section from such systems is the average of expression Eq. (25.18) over the corresponding polydispersity function. Thus, the contrast is size dependent, which makes it impossible to apply directly the classical approach based on expression Eq. (25.18) for polydisperse systems. Additionally, the magnetic scattering contribution independent of the nuclear contrast, affects Eq. (25.18). Recently, the basic functions approach was developed for the case of polydisperse and superparamagnetic systems (Avdeev, 2007). It was shown that the scattering cross-section from such systems can be transformed into the expression of type Eq. (25.18) with the use of modified contrast, $\Delta\tilde{\rho} = \bar{\rho}_e - \rho_s$, where $\bar{\rho}_e$ is the effective mean scattering length density corresponding to the minimum in the scattering intensity as a function of the solvent density. Basic functions are modified. Their interpretation is not so transparent like in the case of monodisperse non-magnetic systems; still the function $\tilde{I}_c(q) = \langle I_c(q) \rangle$ can be used well to judge about the particle form averaged over the polydispersity function. The analysis of the contrast dependence of integral parameters differs qualitatively from the monodisperse case. Thus, for the forward scattering intensity and radius of gyration one has

$$I(0) = N\langle V_c^2 \rangle (\Delta\tilde{\rho})^2 + N\langle V_c^2 \rangle D \tag{25.19a}$$

$$R_g^2 = \left(\frac{\langle V_c^2 R_c^2 \rangle}{\langle V_c^2 \rangle} + \frac{A}{\Delta\tilde{\rho}} - \frac{B}{(\Delta\tilde{\rho})^2} \right) \Bigg/ \left(1 + \frac{D}{(\Delta\tilde{\rho})^2} \right) \tag{25.19b}$$

where $\Delta\tilde{\rho}$ is the modified scatting contrast, and $\langle V_c^2 \rangle$ is the averaged squared particle volume, and $\langle V_c^2 R_c^2 \rangle / \langle V_c^2 \rangle$ is the weighted average value of the squared radius of gyration of the particle shape; *A*, *B*, *D* are the parameters connected with different averages over the polydispersity function. Unlike the monodisperse case, dependence Eq. (25.19b) has a limit, $-B / D$, at $\Delta\tilde{\rho} \to 0$. This is demonstrated in Fig. 25.23, where changes in the experimental SANS data and radius of gyration with the contrast are followed for magnetic fluid magnetite/MA/benzene (Avdeev et al., 2007b). The experimentally found values of $\langle V_c^2 R_c^2 \rangle / \langle V_c^2 \rangle$ and other parameters (see legend to Fig. 25.23) confirm the results of the direct modeling. Thus, the contrast variation technique makes it possible to check out in terms of several averages the model used for the particles in magnetic fluids. The new approach was recently applied also to water-based magnetic fluids with double layer sterical stabilization (Balasoiu et al., 2004) and with charged stabilization (Perzinsky et al., 2006).

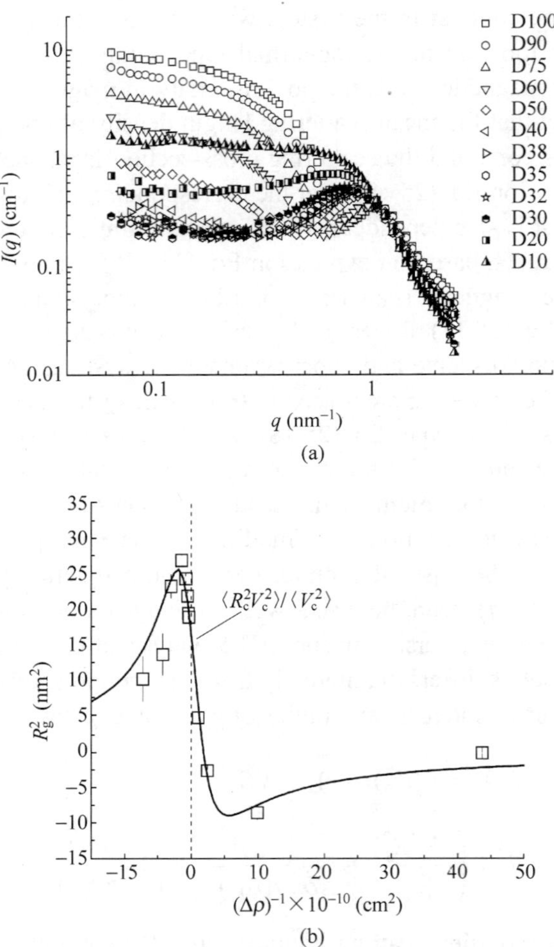

Figure 25.23 (a) Scattering curves obtained during the SANS contrast variation for 0.8% MF magnetite/myristic acid/benzene. In the sample names the content of deuterated benzene is indicated. (b) Squared visible radius of gyration as a function of the inversed modified contrast. Line is a result of fitting with Eq. (25.19b). Arrow shows characteristic radius of gyration for the particle shape, $(\langle R_c^2 V_c^2 \rangle / \langle V_c^2 \rangle)^{1/2} =$ 4.1 nm. Other parameters are $A = 900 \times 10^{-6}$, $B = 0$, $D = 0.09 \times 10^{20}$ cm^{-4}

25.3.2 Interaction

25.3.2.1 Interaction Potential

The interaction character between particles in magnetic fluids can be judged by the correlation between particle locations, as well as between orientations of particle magnetic moments. Both correlation types influence the scattering intensity. In SANS the interaction effects start to be significant at $\varphi_m > 5\%$. They are a result of the competition between attraction (atomic Van der Waals interaction and magnetic dipole-dipole interaction) and stabilizing repulsion (temperature and shell interaction). It is well known that for isotropic interaction between monodipserse particles an additional so called structure-factor, $S(q)$, appears in the scattering intensity. In the case of magnetic fluids two principle difficulties restrict the analysis of the interaction effects. First, particles in magnetic fluids are polydisperse. Second, magnetic interaction, which depends on the relative orientation of particles, is not isotropic. The exact description of the interaction effects in magnetic fluids is extremely complicated. In practice qualitative estimates of the structure-factor are done under some simplifying assumptions. Thus, if one neglects the polydispersity and takes into account that the magnetic scattering is isotropic in unmagnetized magnetic fluids, the equation, which is an analog of the monodisperse case, can be written as

$$I(q) \approx NF_N^2(q)S_N(q) + (2/3)NF_M^2(q)S_M(q) \qquad (25.20)$$

where $S_N(q)$ and $S_M(q)$ are effective structure-factors corresponding to the nuclear and magnetic scattering contributions, respectively. As it was noticed above, in magnetic fluids based on H-solvents the magnetic scattering is comparatively small, so, according to Eq. (25.20) the $S_N(q)$ function can be analyzed in this case separately. For this purpose the scattering from concentrated samples is divided by the curve obtained at a small volume fraction of particles when $S_N(q) \approx 1$ (non-interacting particles). In Fig. 25.19 this is shown for two types of magnetic fluids based on non-polar and polar organic carriers. The effective structure-factors are smeared in comparison with monodisperse systems. As one can see, the fluids reveal different types of interaction. For non-polar fluid (single layer sterical stabilization) the character of the structure-factor points out a significant attractive component in the interaction potential, which is followed from the increase in $S_N(q)$ at smallest q-values. In another case the double layer sterical stabilization screens fully this attraction, so there is no increase in the initial parts of the curves, moreover, a significant decrease in $S_N(q)$ with the concentration growth is observed. The discussed difference in the interaction character of the two types of MNF explains the difference in their magnetorheological properties (Bica et al., 2004; Vékás et al., 2007). In the same way changes in the effective structure factor with the concentration were observed in ionic water-based magnetic fluids (Bacri et al., 1993; Boue et al., 1993; Dubois et al., 1999, 2000; Cousin et al., 2001a, 2001b; Meriguet et al., 2005) and oil-based MNF (Dubois et al., 1999). Data on the effective $S_N(q)$ in these works were used for studying gas-liquid transition in electrostatically stabilized MNFs.

Possibilities of exact description of the effective structure-factor were considered for non-magnetized MNF based on H-pentanol (Avdeev et al., 2006). It was shown that the simplest model of the hard-sphere interaction in terms of the Vrij formalism (Vrij, 1979; Frenkel et al., 1986) for polydisperse systems could be applied only for samples with $\varphi_m < 6\%$. Despite some cumbersome calculations, still there are no principle difficulties in calculation of the structure-factor in this case. During the fitting procedure the hard sphere radius $R + h$, where R is the magnetic particle radius and h is the effective thickness of the surfactant shell, was varied by changing h. The found value $h \approx 2.3$ nm is significantly less than the sum of surfactant lengths constituting the double layer (2×1.8 nm $= 3.6$ nm), which indicates a strong interpenetration of the sublayers. For higher concentration, as it was mentioned, the softening of the structure factor takes place, which was related to the interpenetration of surfactant layers of particles at their contacts. For the moment, no quantitative model exists for such type of interaction, which would take into account the particle polydispersity. The same situation takes place for other kinds of MNF even for intermediate concentrations.

In D-solutions of MNF, according to Eq. (25.20), one deals with the mixed effect of the nuclear and magnetic structure-factors. In the treatment of SANS from magnetic fluids containing magnetite stabilized by alkanoic acid (Shen et al., 2001), by copolymers (Moeser et al., 2001) and by the double layer of oleic acid and oleylamine (Klokkenburg et al., 2007) it was suggested that $S_N(q) = S_M(q)$. However, there are indications that the two structure-factors are significantly different. As it was shown above, a significant correlation between magnetic moments in magnetic fluids takes place even for low concentrated samples, while, at the same time, $S_N(q) \sim 1$. It seems that, if the $S_N(q)$ factor is known from measurements with the H-solutions, then it can be used to treat the scattering from D-solutions and extract the exact behavior of the $S_M(q)$ factor in Eq. (25.20). However, because of the polydispersity, Eq. (25.20) is quite conventional, and cannot be applied for quantitative estimates.

In a magnetic field both nuclear and magnetic effective structure-factors become anisotropic. It should be noted that at sufficiently high particle concentration the formation of chain like aggregates takes place. They are oriented along the field, which should cause a significant anisotropy in the scattering intensity. But it is interesting that in H-solutions of MNF an anisotropy appears (Meriguet et al., 2006a, 2006b; Gazeau et al., 2002), even when no chains are formed. This means that the effect is related to anisotropy in the short-range ordering in the system. In D-solutions, when the magnetic scattering contributes much, the additional anisotropy comes from the orientation of particle magnetic moments (magnetic form-factor), so the picture becomes extremely difficult to describe. One should mention that the problem of the full 2-dimensional structure-factor comprising nuclear and magnetic correlations is not solved until now even for monodisperse magnetic particles. Several theoretical and modeling works in this direction can be mentioned (Davies et al., 1986; Camp and Patey, 2000; Huang et al., 2005).

25.3.2.2 Cluster Formation

As was mentioned in the previous sections, the colloidal nature of magnetic fluids suggests under some conditions the cluster formation in these systems. Scattering methods reflect well this process and give new insight into the inner structure of the clusters, as well to their growth dynamics. For monodisperse systems, the particle aggregation leads to appearance of the structure-factor in the scattering intensity, like in the case of interacting particles. This factor reflects a correlation between monomers in the cluster. Again, for neutron scattering its magnetic scattering contribution corresponds now to a correlation of magnetic moments in the cluster. In the case of magnetic fluids the polydispersity affects the indicated factorization. One should use the structure-factor conventionally, as in the case of interaction between particles in liquid (Section 25.3.2.1). While the analysis of nuclear SANS contribution from clusters in magnetic fluids is quite clear, the full understanding of the magnetic correlation is again a problem. Typical SANS curves for aqueous magnetic fluids (Avdeev et al., 2006) with a small volume fraction of magnetite, based on conventional light water, are shown in Fig. 25.24(a). Since the contrast between the liquid carrier and surfactant molecules is negligible in comparison with the contrast between the carrier and magnetite particles; the curves correspond to the scattering from magnetite. Again, the contribution of the magnetic scattering can be neglected. The linear behavior of the scattering in the double logarithm scale at small q-values in Fig. 25.24(a) corresponds to the power law $S_N(q) \sim q^{-\alpha}$, where exponent α determines the type of clusters. The case $\alpha = -1$ can be related to the elongated aggregates, while the case $1 < \alpha < 3$ corresponds to the branched fractal clusters of the mass fractal dimension $D = \alpha$. Also, $\alpha = 2$ can corresponds to flat lamellar-like particles. Such kind of analyses can be found in recent works (Neto et al., 2005; Lecommandoux et al., 2006).

More detailed analysis of the clusters is possible by the direct modeling of the SANS data obtained both in the non-polarized (Shen et al., 1999a; Moeser et al., 2004) or polarized (Butter et al., 2004; Wiedenmann et al., 2002; Heinemann and Wiedenmann, 2003; Kammel et al., 2002, 2006, 2001; Hoell et al., 2002) modes with changing the contrast in the system. But in this case the magnetic correlations in the clusters are simplified. The magnetic moments of particles in the clusters are considered either independent or strongly correlated. Recently, the approach where the alternating magnetic field is used for studying the response

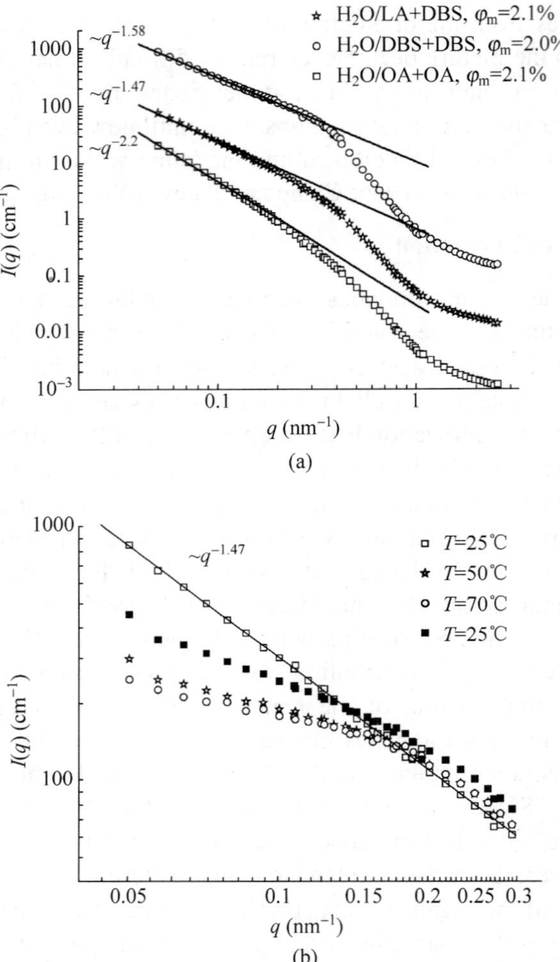

Figure 25.24 (a) Experimental (points) SANS curves for water-based MFs with different stabilization. For convenient view data for H_2O/DBS + DBS and H_2O/OA + OA are divided by factors of 10 and 100, respectively. Solid lines show power law dependences. (b) Changes of the scattering for water-based MF H_2O/DBS + DBS with temperature. Temperature was increased sequentially from 25 to 70℃ and, then, returned to initial value. Straight solid line shows the power-law fit in initial sample

in the SANSPOL from particle assemblies in MNFs was proposed and was applied to concentrated Co-magnetic fluids (Wiedenmann et al., 2006). Such stroboscopic SANSPOL technique allowed the observation of the magnetic ordering of nanosized objects during magnetic relaxation processes on a time scale of few hundred ms.

The SANS applications with other complementary methods show that there is a variety in the cluster organization for different types of MNFs. Sometimes such organization is more complicated than the simple aggregation of separate magnetic particles initially dispersed in liquids. Thus, for water-based MNFs mentioned above it seems that a specific first aggregation of several particles takes place (Avdeev et al., 2006; Balasoiu et al., 2006a). These initial aggregates can form secondary large clusters which are observed in the scattering in Fig. 25.24(a). It was shown, that while initial aggregates are stable with respect to temperature, the secondary clusters are destroyed when increasing the temperature. It is demonstrated in Fig. 25.24(b). When temperature is returned back to the room value the growth of secondary clusters starts again. These clusters can develop, when magnetic field is applied to magnetic fluids. Unfortunately, the power of modern neutron sources does not allow us to follow this process in detail. Thus, in water-based MNF with double layer sterical stabilization of magnetite the characteristic time scale of changes initiated by the magnetic field is of order of minutes, which is not enough to obtain statistically good scattering curve over wide q-interval. Nevertheless, the integrated scattering intensity can be analyzed (Aksenov et al., 2003) for such times, which reflects basic dynamic features of the cluster growth. More complex assemblies like spokes and spirals (Neto et al., 2006), agglomerates (Kammel et al., 2001, 2002, 2006; Wiedenmann et al., 2002; Hoell et al., 2002; Heinemann and Wiedenmann, 2003; Butter et al., 2004) and ordered pseudo-crystalline structures initiated by the external magnetic field (Wiedenmann et al., 2003, 2004; Wiedenmann and Heinemann, 2005; Heinemann and Wiedenmann, 2005; Klokkenburg et al., 2007) are reported.

For the moment it is difficult to classify and relate the cluster formation in MNFs to their structure type or the kind of preparation procedure. In most cases it is a specific problem of the given system. The thorough study of the clustering process is to be done for model and well-defined MNFs.

As one can see, the observation and analysis of the chain-like aggregation under magnetic field by means of scattering methods is a non-trivial problem. The main difficulty comes from the fact that the interaction potential anisotropy in MNF under magnetic field coincides with the anisotropy of the formed elongated aggregates. Attempts on separation of the corresponding scattering components are connected with the shearing experiments (Odenbach et al., 1999; Pop et al., 2004, 2005; Pop and Odenbach, 2006). The dependence of the scattering on the angle between directions of the flow and applied magnetic field makes it possible to conclude about the appearance of the elongated particles in the system. However, the quantitative analysis of such particles is still under development.

Acknowledgements

We are indebted to Prof. R. E. Rosensweig (MIT, USA), Prof. K. Stierstadt (LMU Münich, Germany) and Prof. S. Odenbach (TU Dresden, Germany) for many fruitful and illuminating discussions on the properties and applications, as well as on the development of science and technology of magnetic fluids.

Grateful thanks are due to Prof. I. Anton (CFATR Timisoara and Politehnica Univ. Timisoara, Romania) for the initiation and continuous support of magnetic fluids researches in Timisoara and for the foundation and development of the Laboratory of Magnetic Fluids from Timisoara.

The authors are thankful to Prof. V. L. Aksenov (FLNP JINR) and Dr. L. Rosta (Research Institute for Solid State Physics and Optics, Hungarian Academy of Sciences, RISP HAS) for the support of the work and fruitful discussions on the structure research of magnetic fluids.

References

Akselrod, L.A., G.P. Gordeyev, G.M. Drabkin, I.M. Lazebnik, V.T. Lebedev. *JETP* **91**: 531 (1986).

Aksenov, V., M. Avdeev, M. Balasoiu, L. Rosta, G. Torok, L. Vekas, D. Bica, V. Garamus, J. Kohlbrecher. *Applied Physics* A **74**: 943 (2002).

Aksenov, V.L., M.V. Avdeev, M. Balasoiu, D. Bica, L. Rosta, Gy. Török, L. Vékás. *J. Mag. Mag. Mater*. **258**: 452 (2003).

Amaral, L.Q., F.A. Tourinho. *Brazilian J. Phys*. **25**: 142 (1995).

Anton, I., Vékás L., Potencz I., Suciu E.. *IEEE Trans. on Magnetics*, **MAG-16** : 283 (1980).

Anton, I., I. De Sabata, L. Vékás. *J. Magn. Magn. Mater*. **85**: 219 (1990).

Aswal, V.K., J.V. Joshi, P.S. Goyal, R. Patel, R.V. Upadhyay, R.V. Mehta. *Pramana-J. Phys*. **63** (2): 285 (2004).

Avdeev, M., M. Balasoiu, Gy. Torok, D. Bica, L. Rosta, V. Aksenov, L. Vékás. *J. Mag. Mag. Mater*. **252**: 86 (2002).

Avdeev, M.V., M. Balasoiu, V.L. Aksenov, V.M. Garamus, J. Kohlbrecher, D. Bica, L. Vékás. *J. Magn. Magn. Mater*. **270**: 371 (2004).

Avdeev, M.V., V.L. Aksenov, M. Balasoiu, V. Garamus, A. Schreyer, Gy. Torok, D. Hasegan, A. Schreyer, L. Rosta, D. Bica, L. Vékás. *J. Coll. Interface Sci*. **295**: 100 (2006).

Avdeev, M.V., D. Bica, L. Vékás, O. Marinica, M. Balasoiu, V.L. Aksenov, L. Rosta, V.M. Garamus, A. Schreyer. *J. Magn. Magn. Mater*. **311**: 6 (2007a).

Avdeev, M.V., A.V. Feoktystov, V. Garamus. In: GeNF Annual Report 2006, GKSS (2007b).

Avdeev, M.V. *J. Appl. Cryst*. **40**: 56 (2007).

Avdeev, M.V., D.Bica, L. Vekas, V.L.Aksenov, A.V. Feoktystov, L.Rosta, V.M.Garamus, R. Willumeit, submitted to *J. Magn. Magn. Mater.* (2008).

Bacri, J.-C., F. Boue, V. Cabuil, R. Perzynski. *Colloids Surf. A* **80**: 11 (1993).

Balasoiu, M., M.V. Avdeev, A.I. Kuklin, V.L. Aksenov, D. Bica, L. Vekas, D. Hasegan, Gy. Torok, L. Rosta, V. Garamus, J. Kohlbrecher. Magnetohydrodynamics **40**: 359 (2004).

Balasoiu, M., M.V. Avdeev, V.L. Aksenov, D. Hasegan, V.M., Garamus A. Schreyer, D. Bica, L. Vékás. *J. Magn. Magn. Mater.* **300**: e225 (2006a).

Balasoiu, M., M.V. Avdeev, A.I. Kuklin, V.L. Aksenov, D. Hasegan, V. Garamus, A. Schreyer, D. Bica, L. Vékás, V. Almasan. *Romanian Reports in Physics* **58**: 305 (2006b).

Barnes, H. A., J. F. Hutton, K. Walters. *An Introduction to Rheology*. Amsterdam: Elsevier (1989).

Behrens, S., H. Bönemann, N. Matoussevitch, E. Dinjus, H. Modrow, N. Palina, M. Frerichs, V. Kempter, W. Maus-Friedrichs, A. Heinemann, M. Kammel, A. Wiedenmann, L. Pop, S. Odenbach, E. Uhlmann, N. Bayat, J. Hesselbach, J. M. Guldbakke. *Z. Phys. Chem.* **220**: 3 (2006a).

Behrens, S., H. Bönemann, N. Matoussevitch, A. Gorschinski, E. Dinjus, W. Habicht, J. Bolle, S. Zinoveva, N. Palina, J. Hormes, H. Modrow, S. Bahr, V. Kempter. *J. Phys: Condens. Matter* **18**: S2543 (2006b).

Berkovski, B., V. Bashtovoy (Eds). *Magnetic Fluids and Applications Handbook*. Washington: Begell House (1996).

Berkovsky, B. M., R. E. Rosensweig. *J. Fluid Mech.* **87** (3): 521 (1978).

Berkowitz, A.E., J.A. Lahut, I.S. Jacobs, L.M. Levinson, D.W. Forester. *Phys. Rev. Lett.* **34**: 594 (1975).

Bi, X.- X., B. Granguly, G.P. Huffman, F.E. Huggins, M. Endo, P.C.Ecklund. *J. Mater. Res.* **8**: 1666 (1993).

Bica, D. RO Patent 90078 (1985).

Bica, D. *Romanian Reports in Physics* **47**: 265 (1995).

Bica, D.,L. Vékás. *Magnitnaia Ghidrodinamika* (Magnetohydrodynamics) **30** (3): 194 (1994).

Bica, D., L. Vékás, M. Rasa. *J. Magn. Magn. Mater.* **252**: 10 (2002).

Bica D., L. Vékás, M.V. Avdeev, M. Balasoiu, O. Marinica, F.D. Stoian, D. Susan-Resiga, G. Török, L. Rosta. *Prog. Coll. Polym. Sci.* **125**: 1 (2004).

Bica, D, L.Vékás, M. V. Avdeev, O. Marinica, M. Balasoiu, V. M. Garamus. *J. Magn. Magn. Mater.* **311**: 17 (2007).

Bläsing, J., G. Strassburger, D. Eberbeck. *Phys. Status Solidi* **146**: 595 (1994).

Blums, E., A. Cebers, M.M. Mayorov. *Magnetic fluids*, Walter de Gruyters, Berlin (1997).

Bonini M., A. Wiedenmann, P. Baglioni. *Journal of Physical Chemistry* B **108**: 14,901 (2004).

Bonini M., A. Wiedenmann, P. Baglioni. Physica A **339**: 86 (2004).

Bönnemann, H., W. Brijoux, R. Brinkmann, N. Matoussevitch, N.Waldöfner, N. Palina, H. Modrow. *Inorg. Chim. Acta* **350**: 617 (2003).

Bönnemann, H., R. A. Brand, W. Brijoux, H. W. Hofstadt, M. Frerichs, V. Kempter, W. Maus-Friedrichs, N. Matoussevitch, K. S. Nagabhushana, F. Voigts V. Caps. *Appl. Organomet. Chem.* **19**: 790 (2005).

Borbáth, I., Z. Kacsó, L. Dávid, I. Potencz, D. Bica, O. Marinica, L.Vékás. In: *Convergence of micro-nano-biotechnologies, Series Micro- and Nanoengineering*, Bucharest: Romanian Academy Publ. House (2006). p.200.

Boue, F., V. Cabuil, J.-C. Bacri, R. Perzynski. J. Magn. Magn. Mater. **122**: 78 (1993).

Butter, K., A. Hoell, A. Wiedenmann, A.V. Petukhov, G.-J. Vroege. *J. Appl. Cryst.* **37**: 847 (2004).

Butter, K., A.P. Philipse, G.J. Vroege. *J. Mag. Mag. Mater.* **252**: 1 (2002).

Cabuil, V., J.C. Bacri, R. Perzynsky, Yu. Raikher. In: B. Berkovski, V. Bashtovoy (Eds.). *Magnetic Fluids and Applications Handbook,* Begell House, Washington (1996) p.33.

Camp, P.J., G.N. Patey, *Phys. Rev. E.* **62**: 5403 (2000).

Cebula, D.J., S.W. Charles, J. Popplewell. *J. Magn. Magn. Mater*. **39**: 67 (1983).

Chantrell, R. W., A. Bradbury, J. Popplewell, S.W. Charles. *J. Phys. D* **13**: L119 (1980).

Chantrell, R. W., A. Bradbury, J. Popplewell, S. W. Charles. *J. Appl. Phys*. **53**: 2742 (1981).

Charles, S. W. *Romanian Reports in Physics* **47**: 249 (1995).

Charles, S. W. In: S. Odenbach (Ed). *Ferrofluids. Magnetically controllable fluids and their applications.* Springer-Verlag (2002) p.3.

Charles, S. W., J. Popplewell. Ferromagnetic liquids. In: E.P. Wohlfarth (Ed). *Ferromagnetic materials*, vol.**2**. Amsterdam: North-Holland (1980) pp.509 – 559.

Chauvet, O., E. Gautron, R. Turcu. (National RD Institute for Isotopic and Molecular Technologies Cluj-Napoca, Romania) personal communication. 2007.

Choi, U. S. Enhancing Thermal Conductivity of Fluids with Nanoparticles. In: D. A. Siginer, H. P. Wang (eds). *Developments and Applications of Non-Newtonian Flows*. New York: The American Society of Mechanical Engineers. FED-VO1. 23 VM.D-VO1.66 (1995) p.99.

Chow, T.S. *Phys. Rev*. E **48**: 997 (1993).

Chow, T. S. *Phys. Rev*. E **50**: 1274 (1994) .

Cousin F., E. Dubois, V. Cabuil. *J. Chem. Phys*. **115**: 6051 (2001a).

Cousin F, E. Dubois, V. Cabuil, F. Boué, R. Perzynski. *Braz. J. Phys* **31**: 350 (2001b).

Cowley, M. D., R. E. Rosensweig. *J. Fluid Mechanics* **30** (4): 671 (1967).

Craciun, C., L. Barbu, R. Turcu personal communication (2007).

Davalos-Orozco, L. A., L. F. del Castillo. In: *Enciclopedia of Surface and Colloid Science*. New York: Marcel Dekker Inc. (2002) p.2375.

Davies P., J. Popplewell, A. Bradbury, R.W. Chantrell, *J. Phys. D: Appl. Phys*. **19**: 469 (1986).

Davies, K. J., S. Wells, S.W. Charles. *J.Magn.Magn.Mater*. **122**: 24 (1993).

Dubois, E., V. Cabuil, F. Boue, R. Perzynski. *J. Chem. Phys*. **111**: 7147 (1999).

Dubois, E., R. Perzynski, F. Boue, V. Cabuil. *Langmuir* **16** : 5617 (2000).

Dumitrache, F., I. Morjan, R. Alexandrescu, V. Ciupina, G. Prodan, I.Voicu, C. Fleaca, I. Albu, M. Savoiu, I. Sandu, E. Popovici, I. Soare. *Appl.Surf. Sci*. **247**: 25 (2005).

Earnshaw, S. *Trans. Camb. Phil. Soc*. **7**: 97 (1842).

Eberbeck, D., J. Bläsing. *J. Appl. Cryst*. **32**: 273 (1999).

Frenkel, D., R.J. Vos, C.G. de Kruif, A. Vrij *J. Chem. Phys*. **84**: 4625 (1986).

Gazeau, F., E. Dubois, J.C. Bacri, F. Boue, A. Cebers, R. Perzynski. *Phys. Rev.* E **65**: 031,403 (2002).

Gazeau, F., F. Boue, E. Dubois, R. Perzynski. *J. Phys.*: *Cond. Matter* **15**: S1305 (2003).

Goiti, E., R. Hernández, R. Sanz, D. López, M. Vázquez, C. Mijangos, R. Turcu, A.Nan, D. Bica, L.Vékás. *Journal of Nanostructured Polymers and Nanocomposites* **2**: 5 (2006).

Grabcev, B, M. Balasoiu, A. Tirziu, A.I. Kuklin, D. Bica *J. Magn. Magn. Mater*. **201**: 140 (1999).

Grabcev, B., M. Balasoiu, D. Bica, A. I. Kuklin. *Magnetohydrodynamics*. **30**: 156 (1994).

Griffiths, C. H. M.P. O'Horo, T.W. Smith. *J. Appl. Phys*. **50**: 7108 (1979).

Grubbs, R. B. *Polymer Reviews* **47**: 197 (2007).

Han, D.H., J.P. Wang, Y.B. Feng, H.L. Luo. *J. Appl. Phys.* **76**: 6591 (1994).

Haneda, K., A.H. Morrish. *J. Appl. Phys.* **63**: 4258 (1988).

Hayter, J., R. Pynn. *Phys. Rev. Lett.* **49**: 1103 (1982).

Heinemann, A., A. Wiedenmann. *J. Appl. Cryst.* **36**: 845 (2003).

Heinemann, A., A. Wiedenmann. *J. Magn. Magn. Mater.* **289**: 149 (2005).

Heinemann, A., A. Wiedenmann, M. Kammel. *Physica* B **350**: e207 (2004).

Hoell, A., R. Muller, A. Wiedenmann, W. Gawalek. *J. Magn. Magn. Mater.* **252**: 92 (2002).

Holm, C., J.-J. Weiss. Current Opinion in Colloid & Interface Science **10**: 133 (2005).

Huang, J.P., Z. Wang, C. Holm. *Phys. Rev. E* **71**: 061,203 (2005).

Hyeon, T. *Chem. Commun.* 927 (2003).

Hyeon, T., S. S. Lee, J. Park, Y. Chung, H. B. Na. *J. Am. Chem. Soc.***123**: 12,798 (2001),

Illés, E., E. Tombácz. *J. Colloid Interface Sci.* **295**: 115 (2006).

Itri, R., J. Depeyrot, F.A. Tourinho, M.H. Sousa. *Eur. Phys. J.* E **4**: 201 (2001).

Ivanov, O. A. *Magn. Gidr.* **4**: 39 (1992).

Ivanov, O. A., O. B. Kuznetsova. *Colloid J.* **63**: 60 (2001).

Jeong, U., X. Teng, Y. Wang, H. Yang, Y. Xia. *Adv. Mater.***19**: 33 (2007).

Jurgons, R., C. Seliger, A. Hilpert, L. Trahms, S. Odenbach,C. Alexiou. *J. Phys.: Condens. Matter* **18**: S2893 (2006).

Kaiser, R., G. Miskolczy. *J. Appl. Phys.* **41**: 1064 (1970).

Kammel, M., A. Hoell, A. Wiedenmann. *Script. Mater.* **44:** 2341 (2001).

Kammel, M., A. Wiedenmann, A. Heinemann, H. Bönneman, N. Matoussevitch. *Physica B: Condensed Matter* **385**: 457 (2006).

Kammel, M., A. Wiedenmann, A. Hoell. *J. Mag. Mag. Mater.* **252**: 89 (2002).

Khalafalla, S. E., G.W. Reimers. US Patent 3,764,540 (1973).

Khalafalla, S. E., G.W. Reimers. *IEEE Trans. Magn.* **MAG-16**: 178 (1980).

Khan, W., M. Kapoor, N. Kumar. *Acta Biomaterialia* 3: 541 (2007).

Klokkenburg, M., B.H. Ernè. *J. Magn. Magn. Mater.* **306**: 85 (2006).

Klokkenburg, M., B.H. Erné, A. Wiedenmann, A.V. Petukhov, A.P. Philipse. *Phys. Rev.* E **75**: 051,408 (2007).

Kodama, R.H., A.E. Berkowitz, E.J. McNiff Jr, S. Foner. *Phys. Rev. Lett.* **77**: 394 (1996).

Koneracka, M., M. Muckova, V. Zavisova, N. Tomasovicova, P. Kopcansky, M. Timko, A. Jurikova, K. Csach, V. Kavecansky. Submitted (2007).

Krieger, I. M., T. I. Dougherty. *J. Rheology* **3**: 137 (1959).

Kruse, T., H. G. Krauthauser, A. Spanoudaki, R. Pelster. *Phys. Rev.* B **67**: 094,206 (2003).

Kuncser, V., G. Schinteie, B. Sahoo, W. Keune, D. Bica, L. Vekas, G. Filoti. *J. Phys.: Condens. Matter* **19**: 016,205 (2007).

Lattuada, M, T A. Hatton. *Langmuir* **23**: 2158 (2007).

Lecommandoux, S., O. Sandre, F. Checot, J. Rodriguez-Hernandez, R. Perzynski *J. Magn. Magn. Mater.* **300** (1) : 71 (2006).

Leconte, Y., S. Veintemillas-Verdaguer, M. P. Morales, R. Costo, I. Rodríguez, P. Bonville, B. Bouchet-Fabre, N. Herlin-Boime. *J. Coll.Int.Sci.* **313**: 511 (2007).

Lin D., A.C. Nunes, C.F. Majkrzak, A.E. Berkowitz. *J. Mag. Mag. Mater.* **145**: 343 (1995).

Lopez-Lopez, M. T., J.D. G. Duran, A.V. Delgado, F. Gonzalez-Caballero. *J. Coll. & Int.* Sci. **291**: 144 (2005).

Luca, E., Gh. Calugaru, Gh. Badescu, C. Cotae, V. Badescu. *Ferrofluids and their industrial applications* (in Romanian). Bucuresti: Ed. Tehnica (1978).

Massart, R. IEEE Trans. Magn. **MAG-17**: 1247 (1981).

Massart, R. In: B. Berkovski, V. Bashtovoy,eds. *Magnetic Fluids and Applications Handbook* Begell House Inc., New York: Wallingford, (UK) (1996) 24.

Massart, R. E. Dubois, V. Cabuil, E. Hasmonay. *J.Magn.Magn.Mater*. **149**: 1 (1995).

Mehta, R.V., R.V. Upadhyay, G.M. Sutariya, P.S. Goyal, B.A. Dasannacharya, V.K. Aswal. *J. Magn. Magn. Mater.* **149** (1): 47 (1995).

Meriguet, G., E. Dubois, A. Bourdon, G. Demouchy, V. Dupuis, R. Perzynski. *J. Magn. Magn. Mat*. **289**: 39 (2005).

Meriguet, G., F. Cousin, E. Dubois, F. Boue, A. Cebers, B. Farago, R. Perzynski. *J. Phys. Chem. B* **110 :** 4378 (2006a).

Meriguet, G., E. Dubois, M. Jardat, A. Bourdon, G.. Demouchy, V. Dupuis, B. Farago, R. Perzynski, P. Turq. *J. Phys. Cond. Matter* **18**: S2685 (2006b).

Moeser, G.D., K. A. Roach, W. H. Green, P. E. Laibinis, T.A. Hatton. *Ind. Eng. Chem. Res*. **41**: 4739 (2002).

Moeser, G.D., W.H. Green, P.E. Laibinis, P. Linse, T.A. Hatton, *Langmuir*. **20**: 5223 (2004).

Mollard, P, P. Germi, A. Rousset, Physica B **86 – 88**: 1393 (1977).

Morales, M. P., S. Veintemillas-Verdaguer, M.I. Montero, C.J. Serna, A.Roig, L. Casas, B. Martinez, F. Sandiumenge. *Chem. Mater*. **11**: 3058 (1999).

Moumen, N., M. P. Pileni. *Chem. Mater*. **8**: 1128 (1996a).

Moumen, N., M. P. Pileni. *J. Phys. Chem*., **100**: 1867 (1996b).

Müller R., R. Hiergeist, W. Gawalek, A. Hoell, A. Wiedenmann. *J. Mag. Mag. Mater.*, **252**: 43 (2002).

Neto, C., M. Bonini, P. Baglioni. *Coll. Surf. A* **269**: 96 (2005).

Neuberger, T., B. Schöp, H. Hofmann, M. Hofmann, B. von Rechenberg. *J. Magn. Magn. Mater*. **293**: 483 (2005).

Neuringer, J. L., R. E. Rosensweig. Ferrohydrodynamics. *Phys. Fluids* **7** (12): 1927 (1964).

Neveu, S., A. Bee, M. Robineau, D. Talbot. *J.Coll.Int.Sci*. **255**: 293 (2002).

Odenbach, S., H. Gilly, P. Lindner. *J Magn. Magn. Mater*. **201**: 353 (1999).

Odenbach, S. *Ferrofluids. Magnetically controllable fluids and their applications*. Springer-Verlag (2002) p.252.

Odenbach, S., Ferrofluids, In: K.H.J. Buschow, Ed. *Handbook of Magnetic Materials*, vol.16, Chap.3 (2006) pp.127 – 208.

Pankhurst, Q. A., J. Connolly, S.K. Jones, J. Dobson. *J. Phys. D. Appl. Phys*. **36**: R167 (2003).

Papell, S. S. US. Patent 3,215,572 (1965).

Papirer, E., P. Horny, H. Balard, R. Anthore, R. Petipas, A. Martinet. *J. Coll. Int. Sci*. **94**: 207 (1983).

Perzinsky, R., E. Dubois, V. Garamus, G. Mériguet, E. Wandersman, M.V. Avdeev, In: GeNF Annual Report 2005, GKSS (2006).

Pileni, M.-P. *Langmuir* **13**: 639 (1997).

Pileni, M.-P., N. Feltin, N. Moumen, In: U. Häfeli, W. Schütt, M. Zborowski, eds. *Scientific and Clinical Applications of Magnetic Carriers* New York, London: Plenum Press pp.117 – 133 (1997).

Pileni, M.-P. *Structure and Reactivity of Reverse Micelles*. Elsevier, Amsterdam (1989).

Piso, M.-I. *J.Magn.Magn.Mater*. **201**: 380 (1999).

Pop, L.M., J. Hilljegerdes, S. Odenbach, A. Wiedenmann. *Appl. Organomet. Chem.* **18** (10): 523 (2004).

Pop, L.M., S. Odenbach. *J. Phys.*: *Condens. Matter*. **18**: S2785 (2006).

Pop, L.M., S. Odenbach, A. Wiedenmann, N. Matoussevitch, H. Bönnemann. *J. Magn. Magn. Mater*. **289**: 303 (2005).

Popa, N. C., I. De Sabata, I. Anton, I. Potencz, L. Vékás. *J.Magn.Magn.Mater.* **201**: 385 (1999).

Popovici, E., F. Dumitrache, I. Morjan, R. Alexandrescu,V. Ciupina, G. Prodan, L. Vékás, D. Bica, O. Marinica, E. Vasile. *Appl. Surf. Sci.* (2007), doi:10.1016/j.apsusc.2007.09.022

Potton, J.A., G.J. Daniell, A.A. Eastop, M. Kitching, D. Melville, B. Rainford, H. Stanley. *J. Magn. Magn. Mat*. **39**: 95 (1983).

Pynn, R., J. Hayter, S.W. Charles. *Phy. Rev. Lett*. **51**: 710 (1983).

Raj, K., R. Moskowitz. *J.Magn.Magn.Mater*. **85**: 233 (1990).

Raj, K., B. Moskowitz, R. Casciari. *J. Magn. Magn. Mater.* **149**: 174 (1995).

Raj, K. In: B. Berkovski, V.Bashtovoy, eds. *Magnetic Fluids and Applications Handbook,* New York, Wallingford: Begell House, Inc. (1996) pp.657 – 751.

Rasa, M. PhD Thesis. West University Timisoara (1999).

Rasa, M. *Eur. Phys. J. E* **2**: 265 (2000).

Raşa, M., D. Bica, A. Philipse, L. Vékás. *Eur. Phys. J.* E **7**: 209 (2002).

Resler, E. L., Jr., R. E. Rosensweig. *J. Eng. Power* **89**: 399 (1967).

Resler, E. L., Jr. R. E. Rosensweig. *AIAA Journal* **2** (8): 1418 (1964).

Rosensweig, R. E. *AIAA Journal* **4** (10): 1751 (1966a).

Rosensweig, R.E. *Nature* (London) 210 (5036): 613 (1966b).

Rosensweig, R. E. *New Scientist*, **20** (7): 146 (1966c).

Rosensweig, R. E. *Int. Sci. Tech*. **48** (7): (1966d).

Rosensweig, R. E. US Patent 3,260,584(1971).

Rosensweig, R. E. In: M. Martin, ed. *Advances of Electronics and Electron Physics*, vol.**48**. Martin New York: Academic Press. 103 – 199 (1979).

Rosensweig, R. E. *Ferrohydrodynamics* Cambridge Univ. Press, Cambridge (1985) p.344. reprinted with slight corrections by Dover, Mineola, New York (1997).

Rosensweig, R. E., *Chem. Eng. Comm*. **67**: 1 (1988).

Rosensweig, R. E. In: B. Berkovski, V. Bashtovoy, Eds. *Magnetic Fluids and Applications Handbook.* New York, Wallingford: Begell House, Inc. 591 – 656 (1996).

Rosensweig, R. E., J. W. Nestor, R. S. Timmins. In: Mater. Assoc. Direct Energy Convers. Proc. AIChE—IChemE Symposium Series No. 5. London, 104 – 118; discussion 133 – 137 (1965).

Rosensweig, R. E., R. Kaiser. Study of ferromagnetic liquid, Phase I. NTIS Rep. No. NASW-1219, NASA Rep. NASA-CR-91684. NASA Office of Advanced Research and Technology, Washington, D.C. (1967).

Rosman R., J.J.M. Janssen, M.T. Rekveldt. *J. Appl. Phys.* **67**: 3072 (1990).

Salgueirino-Marceira, V., L. M. Marźan, M. Farle. *Langmuir* **20**: 6946 (2004).

Shen L., P.E. Laibinis, T.A. Hatton. *J. Magn. Magn. Mater.* **194**: 37 (1999a).

Shen, L., P. E. Laibinis, T. A. Hatton. *Langmuir* **15**: 447 (1999b).

Shen L., A. Stachowiak, S.-E.K. Fateen, P.E. Laibinis, T.A. Hatton. *Langmuir* **17**: 288 (2001).

Shen, L.,A. Stachowiak, T. A. Hatton, P. E. Laibinis. *Langmuir* **16**: 9907 (2000).

Shimoiizaka, J., K. Nakatsuka, T. Fujita, A. Kounosu. *IEEE Trans. Magn.* **MAG-16**: 368 (1980).

Shliomis M. I. *Soviet Phys. Uspekhi* (*Engl. Transl*) **17**: 34 (1974).

Sincai, M., D. Argherie, D. Ganga, D. Bica, L. Vékás. *J. Magn. Magn. Mater.* **311**: 363 (2007).

Socoliuc, V., D. Bica. *Progr. Colloid Polym.Sci.***117**: 131 (2001).

Socoliuc, V., D. Bica. *J. Magn. Magn. Mater.* **252**: 26 (2002).

Socoliuc, V., D. Bica. *J. Magn. Magn. Mater.* **289**: 177 (2005).

Socoliuc, V., D. Bica, L. Vékás. *J. Coll.Int. Sci.* **264**: 141 (2003).

Stuhrmann, H.B. In: H. Brumberger, ed. *Modern Aspects of Small-angle Scattering*. Kluwer Acad. Publishers, Dordrecht, 221 (1995).

Sun, S., H. Zeng. *J. Am. Chem. Soc.***124**: 8204 (2002).

Sun, S., H. Zeng, D. B. Robinson, S. Raoux, P. M. Rice, S. X. Wang, G. Li. *J. Am. Chem. Soc.***126**: 273 (2004).

Susan-Resiga, Daniela. PhD Thesis. West University, Timisoara (2001).

Taboada, E., E. Rodríguez, A. Roig, J. Oró, A. Roch, R. N. Muller. *Langmuir* **23**: 4583 (2007).

Tadmor, R., R.E. Rosensweig, J. Frey, J. Klein. *Langmuir* **16**: 9117 (2000).

Teng, X. W., H. Yang. *J. Mater.Chem.* **14**: 774 (2004).

Tombácz, E., Zs. Libor, E. Illés, A. Majzik, E. Klumpp. *Organic Geochemistry* **25**: 257 (2004).

Tombácz, E., E. Illés, A. Majzik, A. Hajdú, N. Rideg, M. Szekeres. *Croatica Chemica Acta CCA*, 1249 (2007a).

Tombácz, E., D. Bica, A. Hajdú, E. Illés, A. Majzik, L. Vékás. *J. Phys.: Condens. Matter* (2007b, accepted).

Török, Gy., A. Len, L. Rosta, M. Balasoiu, M.V. Avdeev, V.L. Aksenov, I. Ghenescu, D. Hasegan, D. Bica, L. Vékás. *Romanian Reports in Physics* **58**: 293 (2006).

Tourinho, F. A., R. Franck, R. Massart. *J. Mater. Sci.* **25**: 3249 (1990).

Tronc, E., J.P. Jolivet. *Hyperfine Interactions* **112**: 97 (1998).

Turcu, R., D. Bica, L. Vékás, N. Aldea, D. Macovei, A. Nan, O. Pana, O. Marinica, R. Grecu, C.V.L. Pop. *Romanian Reports in Physics* **58**: 359 (2006).

Turcu R., O. Pana, A. Nan, L. M. Giurgiu, In: H.S. Nalwa, ed. *Polymeric Nanostructures and Their Applications,* vol. 1. American Scientific Publishers, p.337 (2007a).

Turcu, R., A. Nan, I. Craciunescu, S. Karsten, O. Pana, I. Bratu, D. Bica, L. Vékás, O. Chauvet, D. Eberbeck, H. Ahlers. *Journal of Nanostructured Polymers and* Nanocomposites **3** (2): 55 (2007b).

Upadhyay, T., R.V. Upadhyay, R.V. Mehta, V.K. Aswal, P.S. Goyal. *Phys. Rev. B* **55**: 5585 (1997).

Vand, V. J. Phys.*Colloid Chem.* **52**: 277 (1948).

Vékás, L., Doina Bica, Daniela Gheorghe, I. Potencz, M. Raşa. *J. Magn. Magn. Mater.* **201**: 159 (1999).

Vékás, L., M.Raşa, D. Bica. *J. Coll.Int. Sci.* **231**: 247 (2000).

Vékás, L., D. Bica, I.Potencz, D. Gheorghe, O. Bălău, M. Raşa. *Progr. Colloid Polym. Sci.* **117**: 104 (2001).

Vékás, L., Doina Bica, Oana Marinica, M. Rasa, V. Socoliuc, Floriana D. Stoian. *J. Magn. Magn. Mater.* **289**: 50 (2005).

Vekas, L., D. Bica, O. Marinica. *Romanian Reports in Physics* **58**: 257 (2006).

Vékás, L., D. Bica, M.V. Avdeev. *China Particuology* **5**: 43 (2007).

Vrij, A. *J. Chem. Phys.* **71**: 3267 (1979).

Wagner, J., T. Autenrieth, R. Hempelmann. *J. Mag. Mag. Mater.* **252**: 4 (2002).

Wiedenmann, A. *J. Appl. Cryst.* **33**: 428 (2000).

Wiedenmann, A., A. Heinemann. *J. Magn. Magn. Mater.* **289**: 58 (2005).

Wiedenmann, A., A. Hoell, M. Kammel. *J. Mag. Mag. Mater.* **252**: 83 (2002).

Wiedenmann, A., A. Hoell, M. Kammel, P. Boesecke. *Phys Rev.* E **68**: 031,203, 1 (2003).

Wiedenmann, A., M. Kammel, A. Hoell. *J. Magn. Magn. Mat.* **272** – **274**: 1487 (2004).

Wiedenmann, A., U. Keiderling, R.P. May, C. Dewhurst. *Physica B: Condensed Matter* **385**: 453 (2006).

Wooding, A, M. Kilner, D. B. Lambrick. *J. Coll. Int. Sci.* **144**: 236 (1991).

Wooding, A, M. Kilner, D.B. Lambrick. *J. Coll. Int. Sci.* **149**: 98 (1992).

Wuang, S. C., K. G. Neoh, E.T. Kang, D.W. Pack, D.E. Leckband. *J. Mater. Chem.* 17: 3354 (2007).

Zavisova, V., M. Koneracka, O. Strbak, N. Tomasovicova, P. Kopcansky, M. Timko, I. Vavra. *J. Magn. Magn. Mater.* **311**: 379 (2007).

Zhang, L, G. C. Papaefthymiou, J. Y. Ying. *J. Appl. Phys.* **81**: 6892 (1997).

Ziolo, R. F., E. P. Giannelis, B. A. Weinstein, M. P. O'Horo, B. N. Ganguly, V. Mehrotra, M. W. Russell, D. R. Huffman. *Science* **257**: 219 (1992).

Zubarev A. Yu and Iskakova L. Yu., J. Exp. Theor. Phys. **80**: 857 (1995).

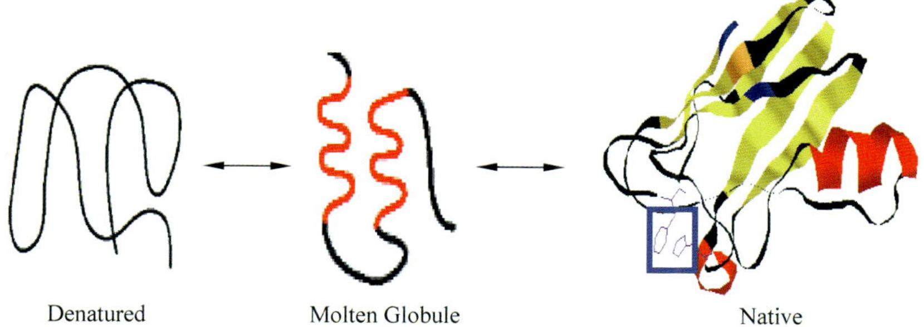

Color figure 1 Schematic representation of the interactions that direct protein (plastocyanin) assembly during initial folding. The structure is color- coded by the types of noncovalent interactions. Hydrogen bonding is represented by red (α-helix) or yellow (β-sheet), salt bridges are shown between lysine (blue) and glutamate (orange) residues, and π-π interaction is shown in purple (included in the blue box) between the side chains of histidine and phenylalanine residues. The protein crystal structure is from the Protein Data Bank (PDB ID: 1KDI)

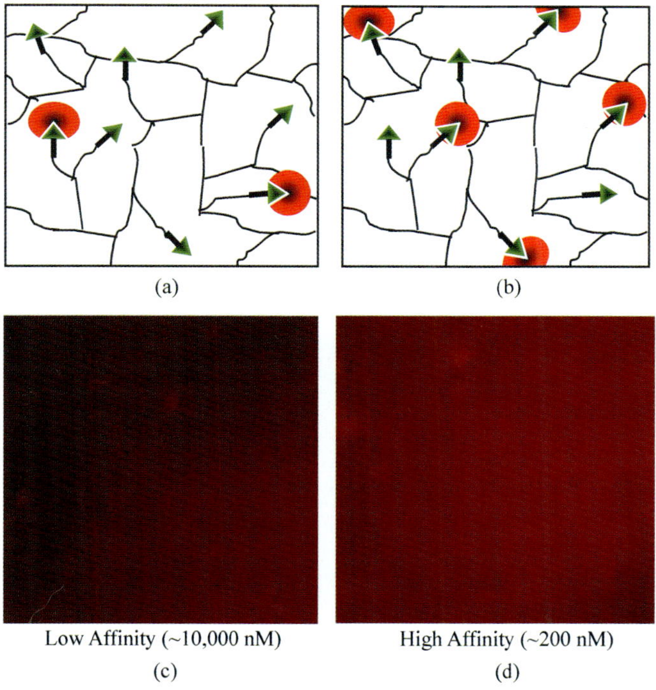

Color figure 2 Schematic representation of sequestering Rhodamine-labeled VEGF (●) in PEG hydrogels containing (a) a low affinity peptide ligand (K_d ~10,000 nM); and (b) a high affinity ligand (K_d ~200 nM) (▲). Also shown are the fluorescence images of hydrogels containing low affinity (c) and high affinity (d) peptide ligands after incubation in 10 nM VEGF and rinsing with PBS. Results suggest that the amount of VEGF sequestered in a hydrogel is dependent on the affinity of the ligand-VEGF interaction

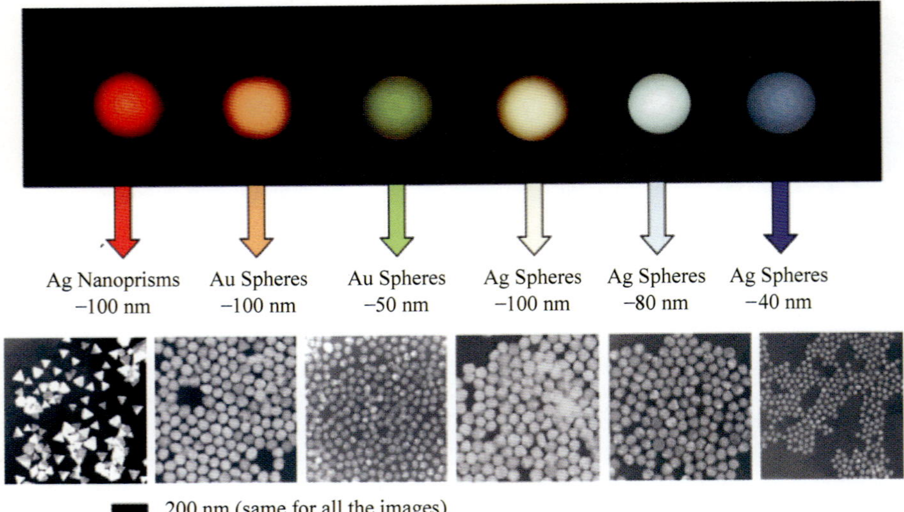

Color figure 3 The sizes, shapes, and compositions of metal nanoparticles can be systematically varied to produce materials with distinct light-scattering properties (Rosi and Mirkin, 2005)

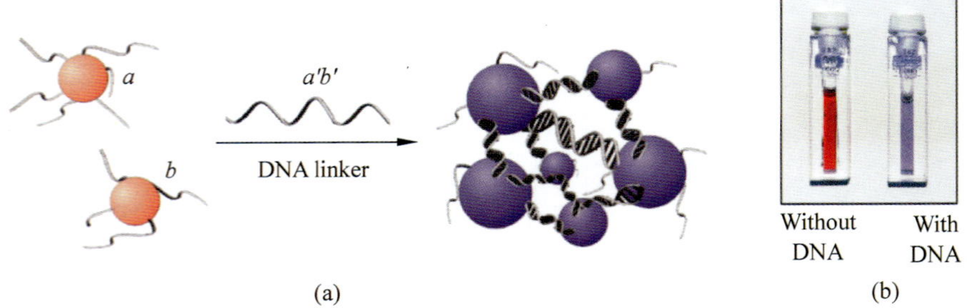

Color figure 4 Scheme for (a) DNA-directed nanoparticle assembly (Elghanian et al., 1997) and (b) colorimetric detection. When target DNA (*a*'*b*') is added to a solution of gold nanoparticles modified with DNA '*a*' and DNA '*b*,' the particles aggregate results in a change of color from red to blue that can be monitored visually (Rosi and Mirkin, 2005)

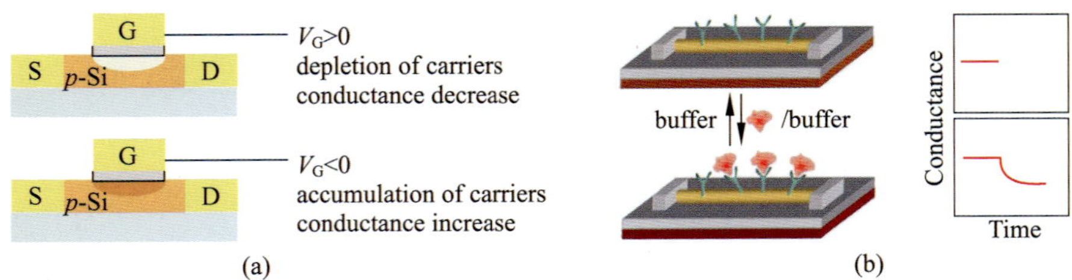

Color figure 5 Principle of the FET NWs sensor. (a) schematic of a regular planar FET. (b) schematic of an NWs FET sensor (Patolsky and Lieber, 2005)

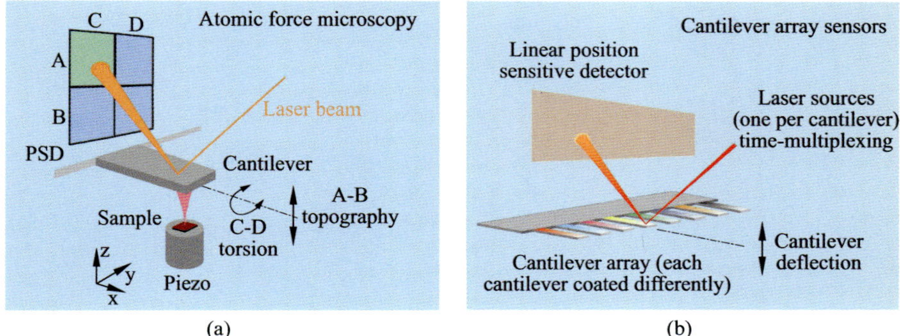

(a) (b)

Color figure 6 Schematic of the AFM technique (a) and the cantilever-array sensor readout (b). Different sensing layers are shown in different colors (Lang et al., 2005)

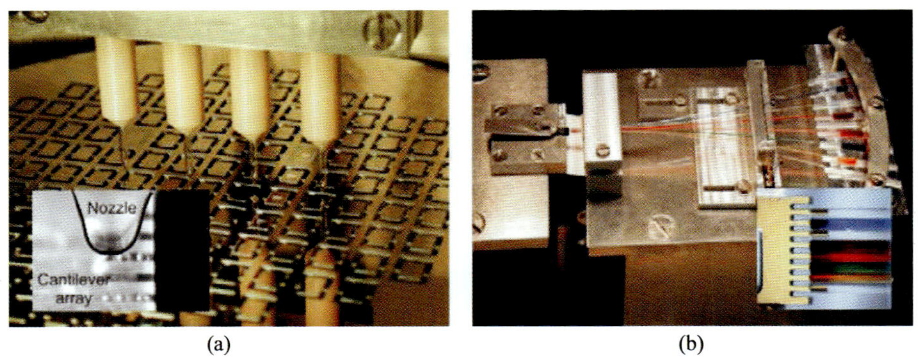

(a) (b)

Color figure 7 Cantilever array functionalization using (a) a four-nozzle ink-jet device (the inset shows spotted liquid droplets at the upper surface of the cantilever) and (b) an array of eight microcapillaries (the inset shows how the individual cantilevers of the array are inserted into the array of microcapillaries; the colored liquids are for visualization purposes only) (Lang et al., 2005)

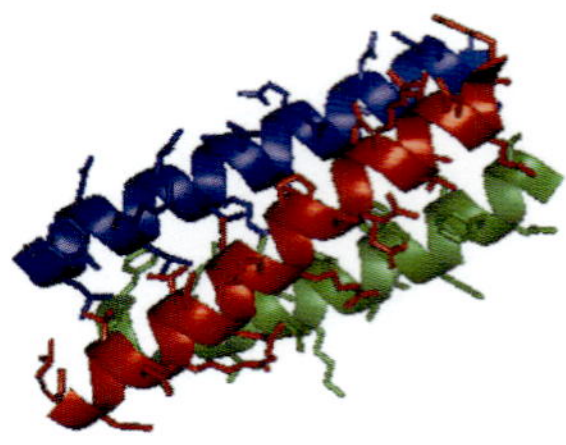

Color figure 8 Ribbon diagram of a short parallel triple helical coiled coil from the central region of bovine fibrinogen. The N-termini of each chain is to the right. Side chains are displayed

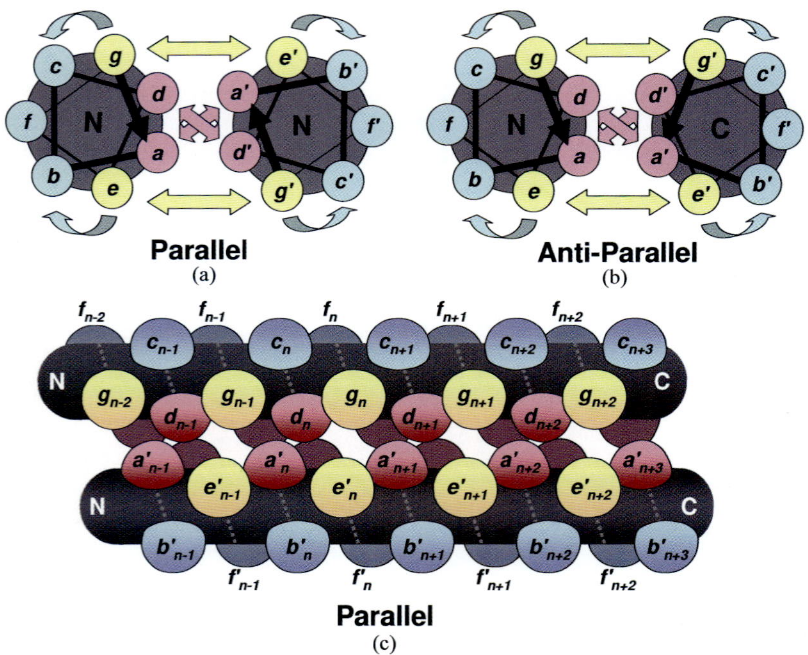

Color figure 9 Intermolecular and intramolecular interactions in parallel and anti-parallel coiled coils. (a-b) helical wheel projections. (c) 3-D representation. Coiled coil folding is primarily driven by hydrophobic interactions (pink arrows) between ***a*** and ***d*** residues (pink residues). Hydrophobic interactions are stabilized by additional electrostatic interactions between ***e*** and ***g*** residues (yellow arrows and residues) and by tertiary interactions between ***g-c*** and ***e-b*** pairs (blue arrows and residues)

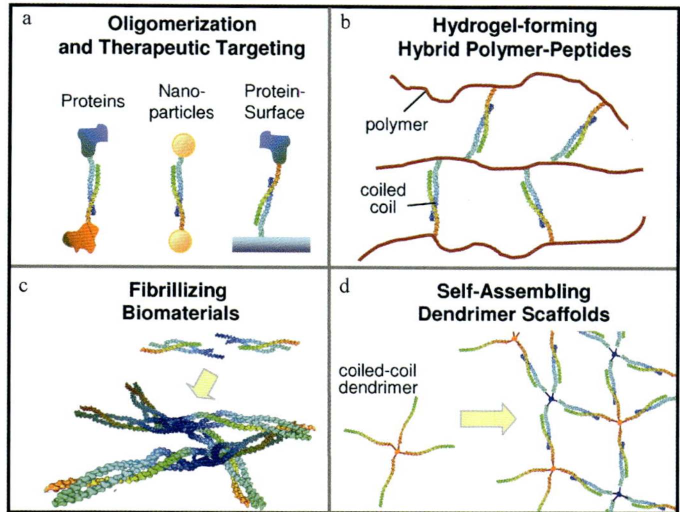

Color figure 10 Applications of coiled-coils in Biomaterials. Coiled-coils are useful folding motifs for tethering proteins, nanoparticles, or surfaces together (a) and for nanostructured scaffold construction (b-d). For scaffolds, coiled-coils can be utilized to cross-link biocompatible polymers into stimulus-responsive hydrogels (b), to form fibrillar networks through sticky-ended assemby (c), or to form networks by the oligomerization of multi-arm molecules (d). See text for corresponding references

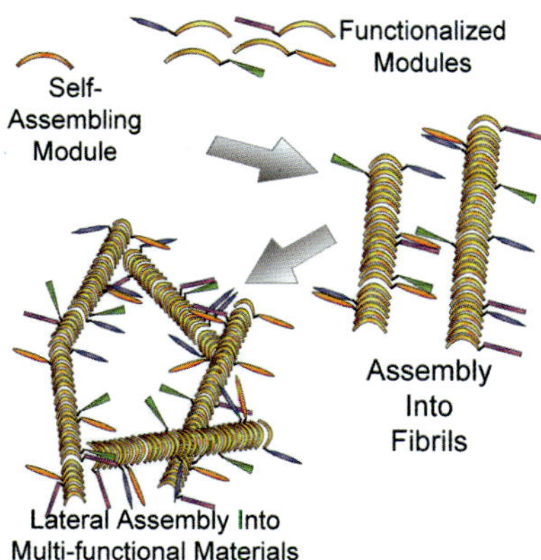

Color figure 11 Modularity in β-sheet peptide systems. Functionalized co-assembling peptides form mixed fibrils, which laterally associate into gel materials. Adapted with permission from Jung, JP et al., (submitted, 2007)

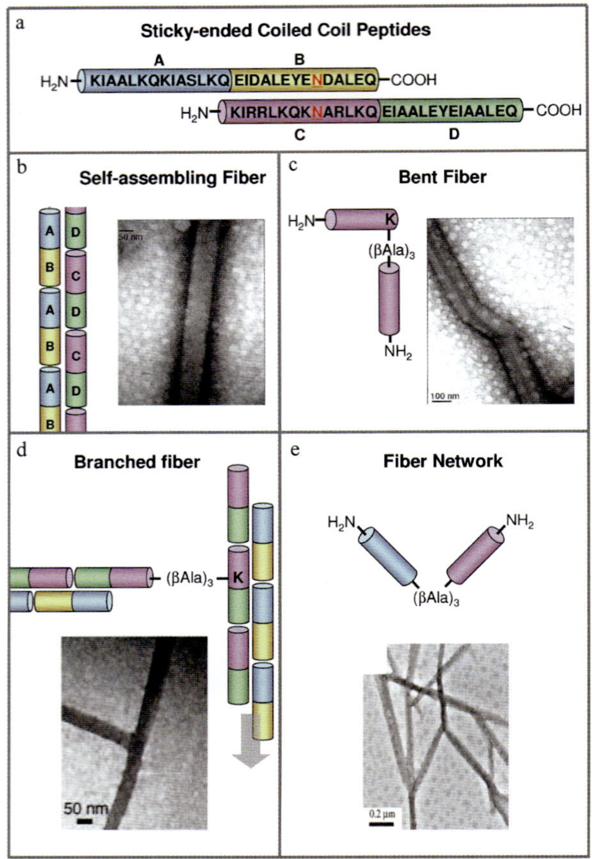

Color figure 12 Modularity in coiled coil fibrils described by Woolfson and coworkers. Sticky ended coiled coil dimers (a) form straight fibers (b), the morophology and interconnectedness of which can be varied through the addition of one or more modifying peptide modules (c-e). See text for details. TEM images in (b-c) reprinted by permission from Macmillan Publishers Ltd: Ryadnov et al., *Nature Materials* **2**, 329-332 (2003). TEM image in (d) reprinted by permission from Wiley-VCH: Ryadnov et al., *Angewandte Chemie, Int'l Ed.* **42**, 3021-3023 (2003). TEM image in (e) reprinted with permission from Ryadnov et al., *J. Am. Chem. Soc.* **127** (35), 12407-12415 (2005). Copyright 2005 American Chemical Society

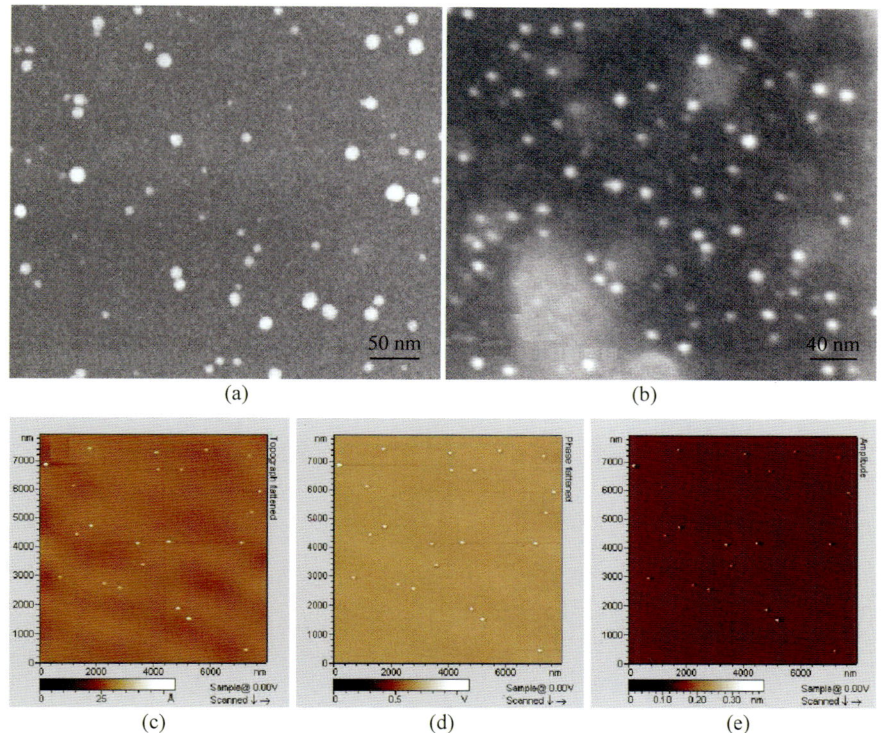

Color figure 13 Representative S-TEM images of carbon dots surface-passivated with (a) PEG_{1500N} and (b) PPEI-EI, and AFM images of carbon dots surface-passivated with PPEI-EI (c) topography, (d) phase, and (e) amplitude. (Reproduced from (Sun et al., 2006) with permission. Copyright ©2006 American Chemical Society)

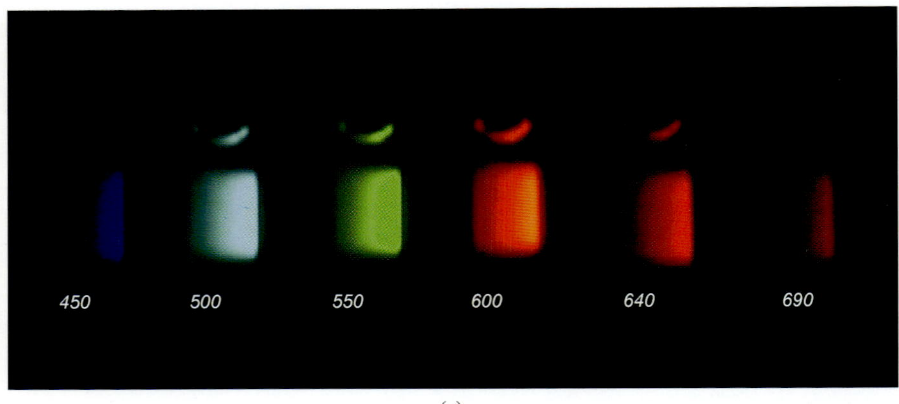

(a)

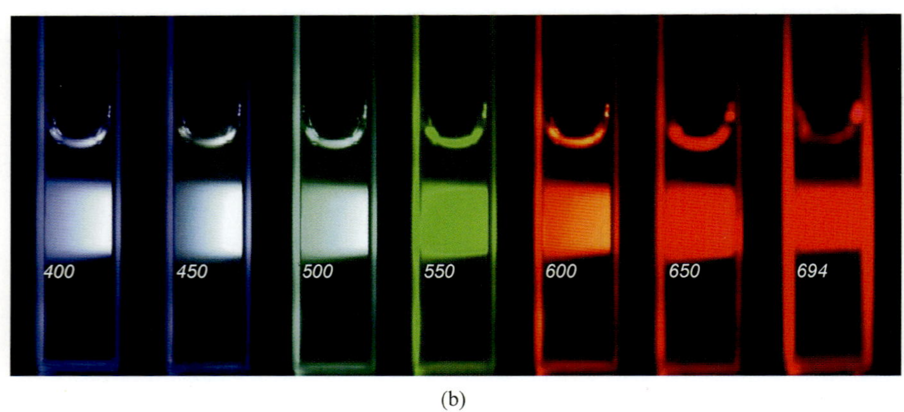

(b)

Color figure 14 Aqueous solutions of the PEG_{1500N}-attached carbon dots, (a) excited at 400 nm and photographed through band-pass filters of different wavelengths as indicated, and (b) excited at the indicated wavelengths and photographed directly (Reproduced from (Sun et al., 2006) with permission. Copyright ©2006 American Chemical Society)

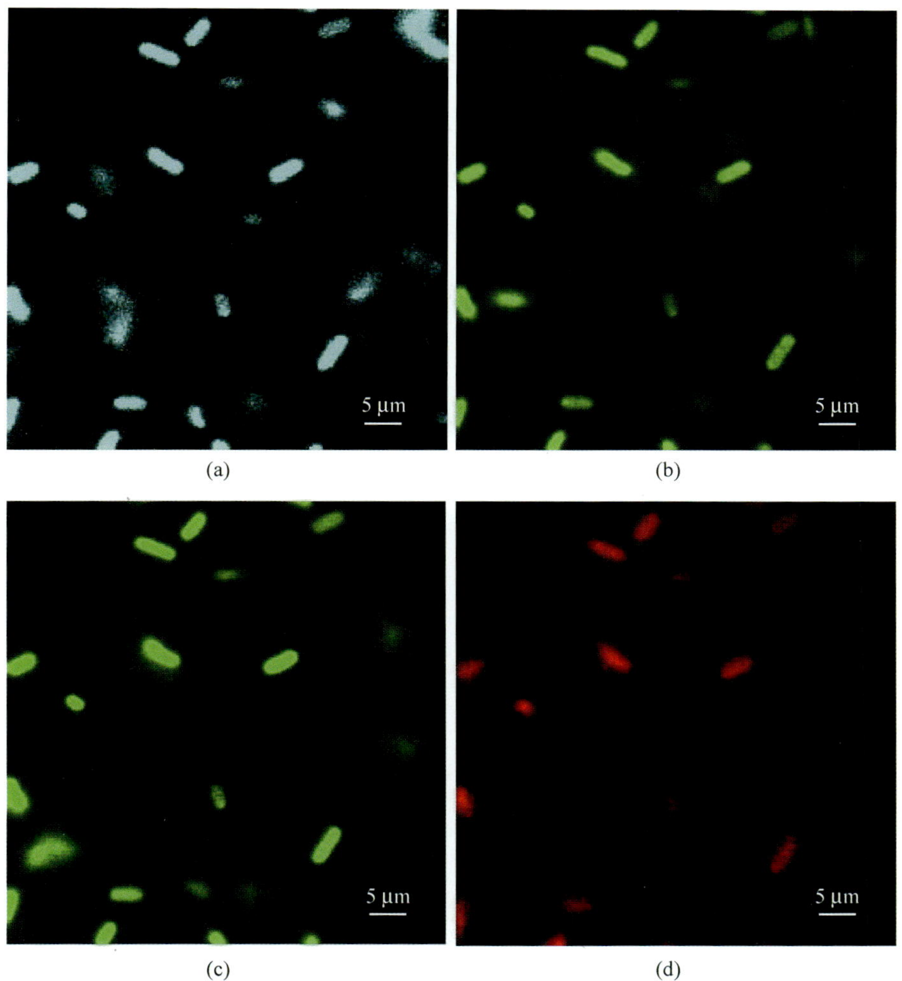

(a) (b) (c) (d)

Color figure 15 Confocal microscopy images of E. coli ATCC 25922 cells labeled with luminescent carbon dots (Color Fig.10): (a) $\lambda_{EX} = 458$ nm, detected with 475 nm long pass filter. (b) $\lambda_{EX} = 477$ nm, detected with 505 nm long pass filter. (c) $\lambda_{EX} = 488$ nm, detected with 530 long pass filter (d) $\lambda_{EX} = 514$ nm, detected with 560 nm long pass filter (Reproduced from (Sun et al., 2006) with permission. Copyright © 2006 American Chemical Society)

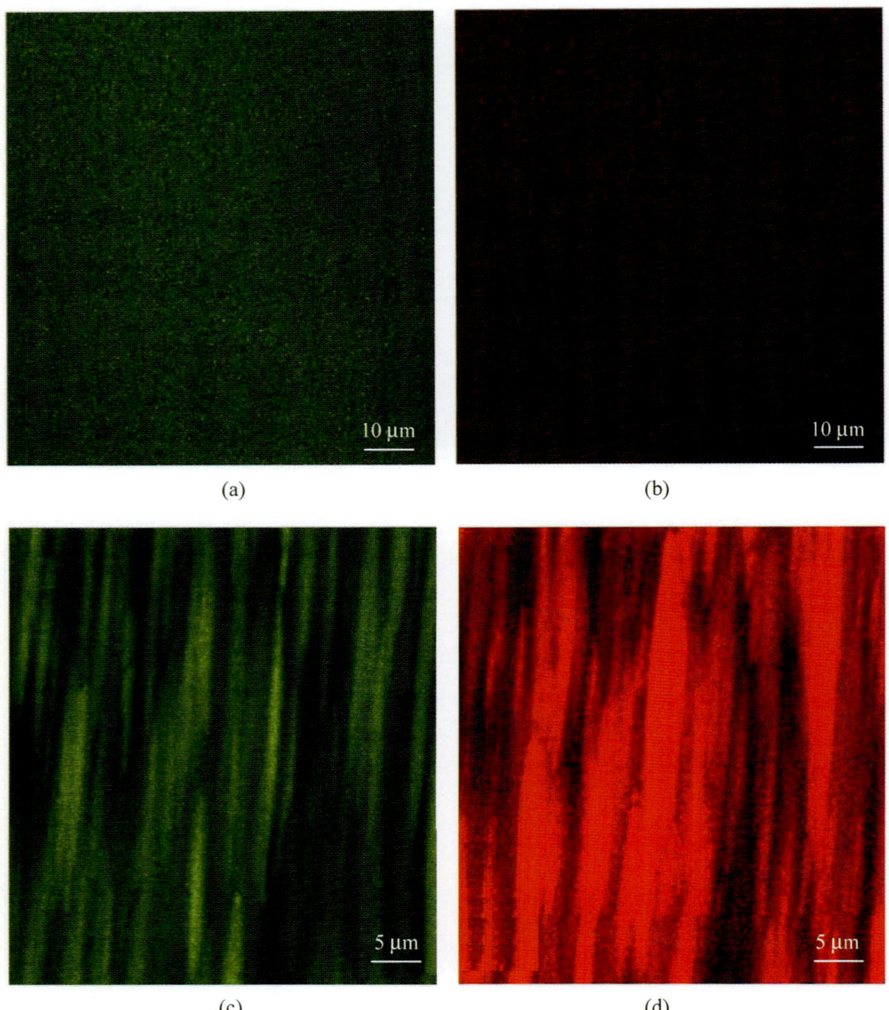

(a) (b)

(c) (d)

Color figure 16 Confocal microscopy images of PPEI-EI-SWNT in PVA film (a), (b) before and (c), (d) after mechanical stretching to a draw ratio of about 5. (a), (b): 514 nm excitation, >530 nm detection. (b), (d): 633 nm excitation, >650 nm detection (Reproduced from (Zhou et al., 2006) with permission. Copyright © 2006 American Chemical Society)

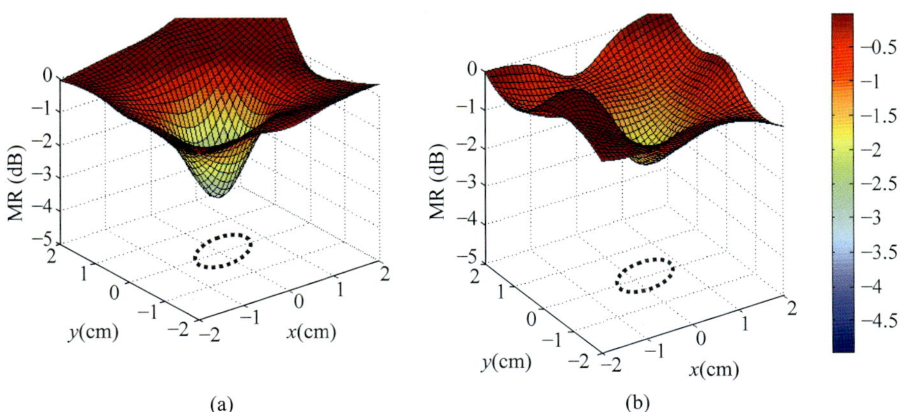

Color figure 17 Optical contrasts created by an empty Vitamin K capsules (oval shape with a dimension of 1.0 cm × 1.0 cm × 1.5 cm) filled with (a) 0.1wt% of 150 nm NGP and (b) 0.1wt% of Fe_3O_4, placed 1 cm deep in an experimental breast model whose optical property was adjusted to those of human breast tissue. NIR-TRS spectra, at the wavelength of 788 nm were obtained in transmittance and the spectra were transferred to frequency domain. The modulation frequency analyzed here is at 100 MHz. The black dashed ellipsoids indicate the tumor model size and position

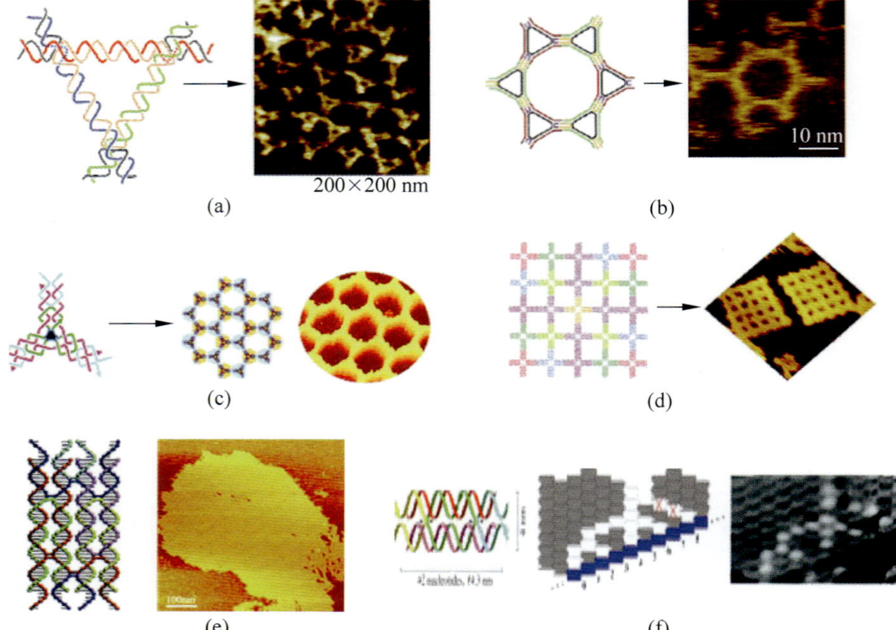

Color figure 18 Schematic drawings of DNA tiles and atomic force micrographs of two-dimensional periodic arrays that were fabricated using these tiles. (a) A DNA triangle tile that is composed of three four-arm junctions is shown on the left, and a two-dimensional array that was formed by self-assembly of these DNA triangles is shown on the right. (b) Schematic drawing and atomic force micrograph of a single hexagonal structure composed of six equilateral triangle complexes that are attached to one another. (c) A three-pointed star DNA motif is shown on the left, and hexagonal two-dimensional DNA lattices that were formed by self-assembly of three-point-star motifs with sticky ends are shown on the right. (d) Schematic drawing and atomic force micrograph of a 5×5 fixed-size array that was assembled from a cross-shaped tile structure with *C*4 symmetry. (e) A diagram of DNA double-double crossover tiles, which consist of eight strands that form four double helices, is shown on the left. These helices are connected by six reciprocal exchanges. Planar structures fabricated using the DNA double-double crossover structures are shown on the right. (f) A diagram of a binary pattern formed from rule tiles on a linear scaffold is shown in blue. Red crosses indicate tiles that exhibit mismatch with their neighbors. A corresponding atomic force micrograph is shown on the right. Figure (a) reprinted with permission from Liu, D., M.S. Wang, Z.X. Deng, R. Walulu and C.D. Mao. *J. Am. Chem. Soc.* 126: 2324 (2004). Copyright 2004 American Chemical Society. Figure (b) reprinted with permission from Chelyapov, N., Y. Brun, M. Gopalkrishnan, D. Reishus, B. Shaw and L. Adleman. *J. Am. Chem. Soc.* 126: 13,924 (2005). Copyright 2005 American Chemical Society. Figure (c) reprinted with permission from He, Y., Y. Chen, H. Liu, A. E. Ribbe and C. Mao. *J. Am. Chem. Soc.* 127: 12,202 (2005). Copyright 2005 American Chemical Society. Figure (d) reprinted with permission from Liu, Y., Y.G. Ke and H. Yan. *J. Am. Chem. Soc.* 127: 17,140 (2005). Copyright 2005 American Chemical Society. Figure (e) reprinted with permission from Reishus, D., B. Shaw, Y. Brun, N. Chelyapov and L. Adleman. *J. Am. Chem. Soc.* 127: 17,590 (2005). Copyright 2005 American Chemical Society. Figure (f) reprinted with permission from Barish, R.D., P.W.K. Rothemund and E. Winfree. *Nano Lett.* 5: 2586 (2005). Copyright 2005 American Chemical Society

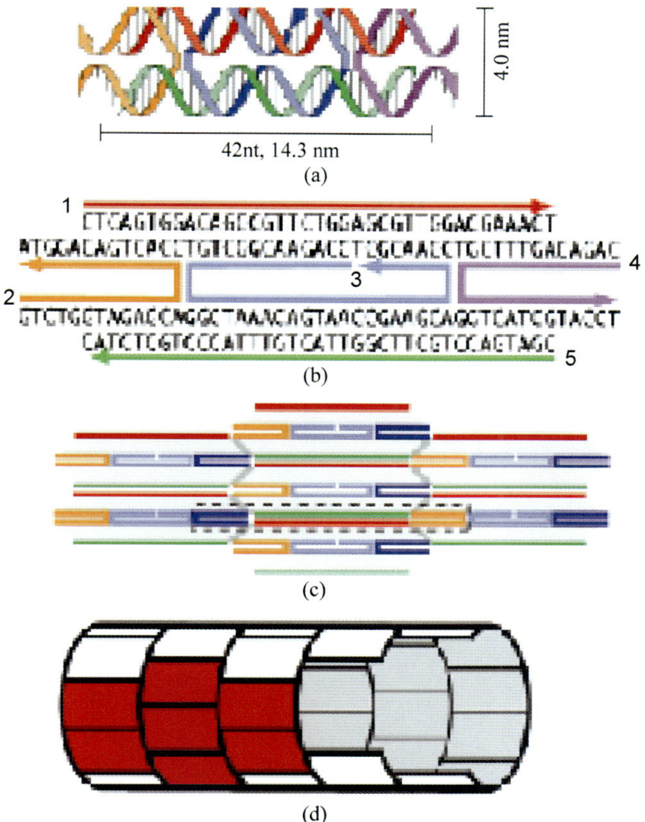

Color figure 19 Schematic of DNA nanotube structure. Reprinted with permission from Rothemund, P.W. K., A. Ekani-Nkodo, N. Papadakis, A. Kumar, D. K. Fygenson and E. Winfree. *J. Am. Chem. Soc.* 126: 16,344(2004). Copyright 2004 American Chemical Society

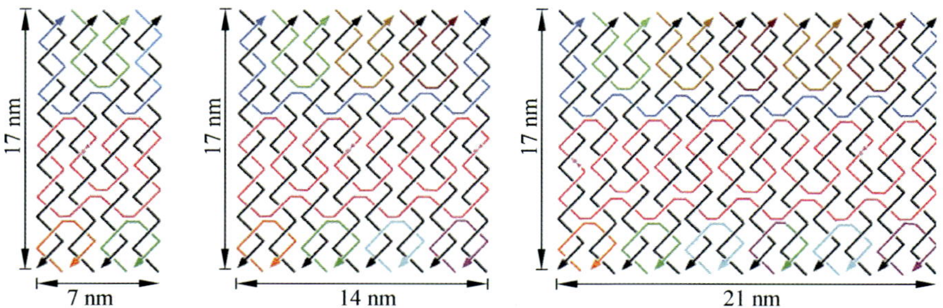

Color figure 20 Schematics of (a) 4-helix tile, (b) 8-helix tile, and (c) 12-helix tile (Color Fig. 15). Reprinted with permission from Ke, Y.G., Y. Liu, J.P. Zhang, H. Yan. *J. Am. Chem. Soc.* 128: 4414 (2006). Copyright 2006 American Chemical Society

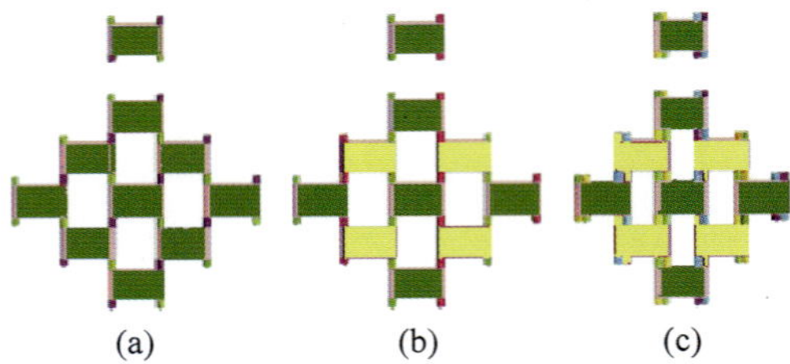

Color figure 21 Schematics of three sticky end connections for each tile. (a) 1SE. (b) 1SE-C. (c) 2SE-C. Sticky ends with identical colors are complementary to one another. Sticky ends with different colors contain tiles with opposite planes. Reprinted with permission from Ke, Y.G., Y. Liu, J.P. Zhang, and H. Yan. *J. Am. Chem. Soc.* 128: 4414 (2006). Copyright 2006 American Chemical Society

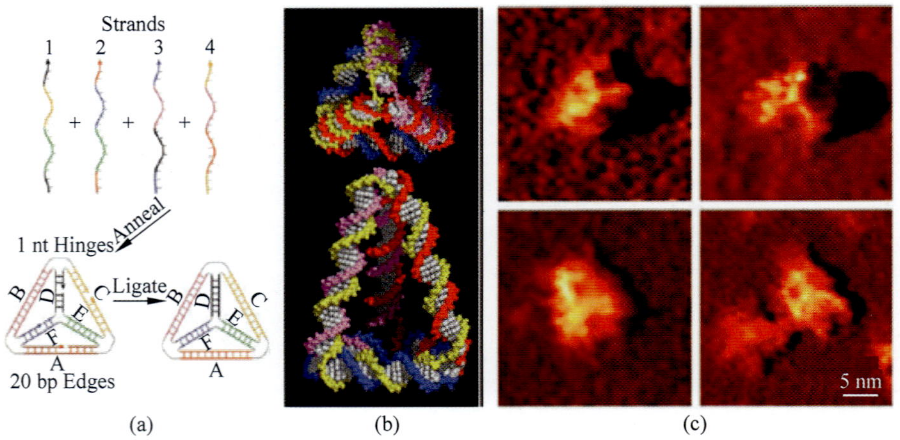

Color figure 22 (a) Schematic depicting formation of DNA tetrahedron from four oligonucleotides. The colored complementary subsequences underwent hybridization to form the edges of the tetrahedron structure. (b) Schematics of the DNA tetrahedron. (c) Atomic force microscopy images of four tetrahedra. In these images, three upper edges of the tetrahedra are visible. From Goodman, R.P., I.A.T. Schaap, C.F. Tardin, C.M. Erben, R.M. Berry, C.F. Schmidt, A.J. Turberfield. *Science* 310: 1661 (2005). Reprinted with permission from AAAS

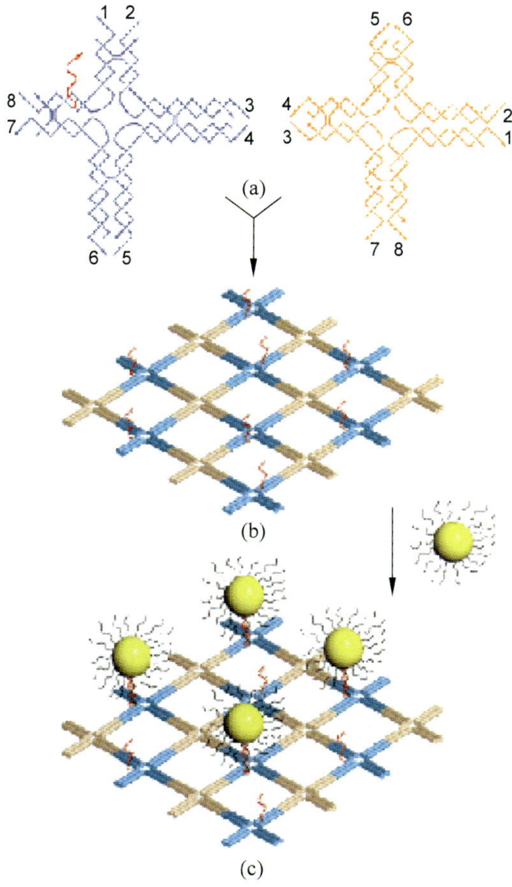

Color figure 23 Mechanism for arraying gold nanoparticles on DNA nanogrids. (a) In this figure, tile A is blue, and tile B is orange. The short strand A15 on tile A serves as a hybridization site for gold nanoparticles. (b) A DNA nanogrid formed from cross-shaped tiles. (c) Assembly of 5 nm gold particles on DNA nanogrids. Reprinted with permission from Zhang, J.P., Y. Liu, Y.G. Ke, H. Yan. *Nano. Lett.* 6: 248 (2006). Copyright 2006 American Chemical Society

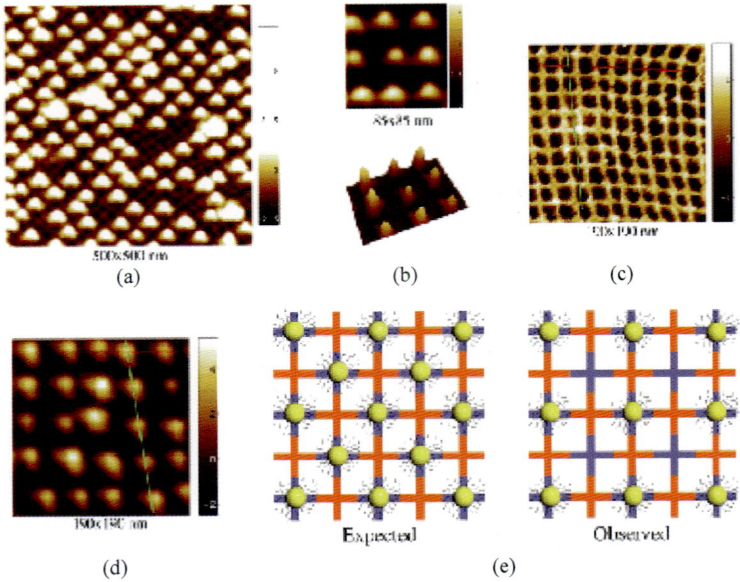

Color figure 24 Atomic force micrographs showing gold nanoparticles assembled on two-dimensional DNA grids. Reprinted with permission from Zhang, J.P., Y. Liu, Y.G. Ke, H. Yan. *Nano. Lett.* 6: 248 (2006). Copyright 2006 American Chemical Society

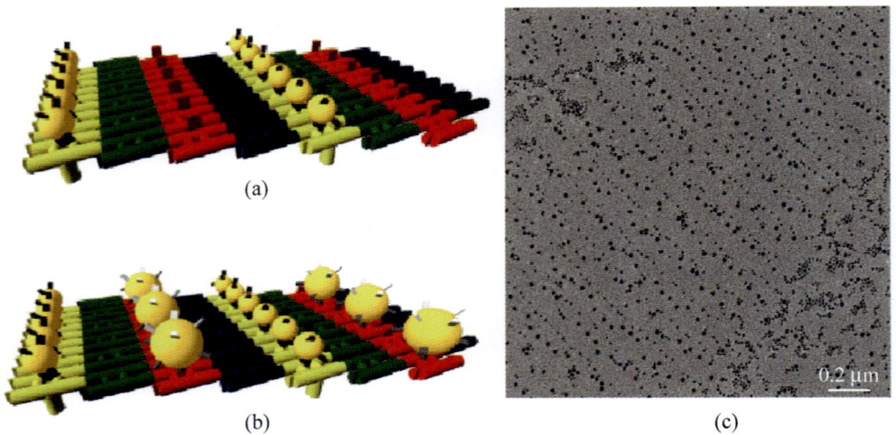

Color figure 25 (a) A diagram of a two-dimensional lattice fabricated from four different double-crossover tiles, in which 5 nm gold particles are occupying the D tiling rows. (b) A diagram of a two-dimensional lattice fabricated from four different double-crossover tiles, in which 5 nm gold particles are occupying the D tiling rows and 10 nm gold particles are occupying the B tiling rows. (c) Transmission electron micrograph of array containing 5 nm gold particles and 10 nm gold particles. (Color Fig. 20) Reprinted with permission from Pinto, Y.Y., J.D. Le, N.C. Seeman, K. Musier-Forsyth, T.A. Taton, R.A. Kiehl. *Nano Lett.* 5: 2399 (2005). Copyright 2005 American Chemical Society

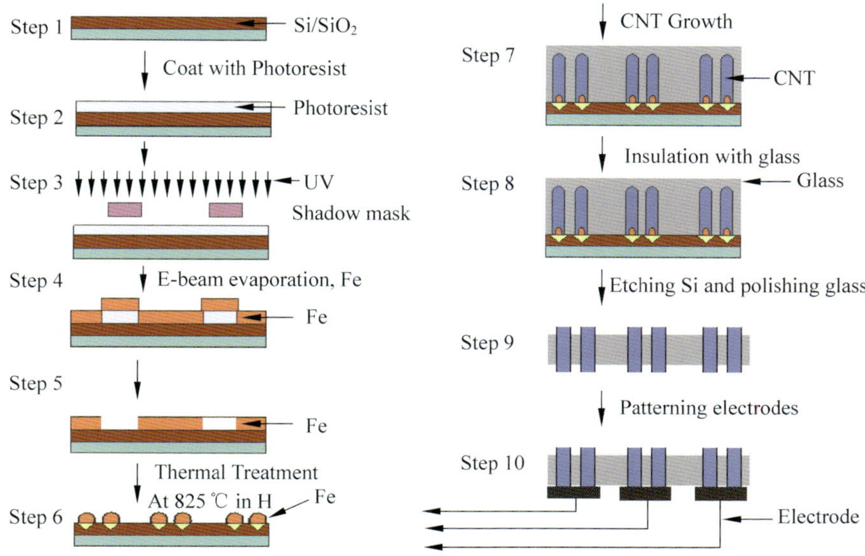

Color figure 26 Fabrication steps for the vertically grown nanotube array

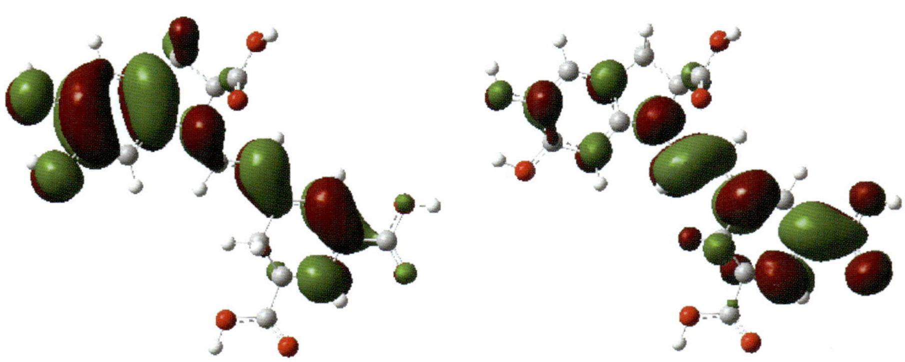

Color figure 27 Homo and lumo of natural dye betanidin